RADIOLOGY
of the
KIDNEY
and
URINARY
TRACT

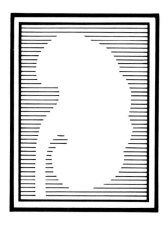

RADIOLOGY
of the
KIDNEY
and
URINARY
TRACT

SECOND EDITION

ALAN J. DAVIDSON, MD
Senior Scientist
Department of Radiologic Pathology
American Registry of Pathology
Armed Forces Institute of Pathology
Washington, DC

DAVID S. HARTMAN, MD
Professor of Radiology
Department of Radiology
Penn State College of Medicine
The Milton S. Hershey Medical Center
Hershey, PA

W.B. SAUNDERS COMPANY
A Division of Harcourt Brace & Company
Philadelphia ■ London ■ Toronto ■ Montreal ■ Sydney ■ Tokyo

W.B. SAUNDERS COMPANY
A Division of Harcourt Brace & Company

The Curtis Center
Independence Square West
Philadelphia, Pennsylvania 19106

Library of Congress Cataloging-in-Publication Data

Davidson, Alan J.
Radiology of the kidney and urinary tract/Alan J. Davidson,
David S. Hartman.—2nd ed.

p.   cm.

Includes bibliographical references.

ISBN 0–7216–3552–0

1. Kidneys—Radionuclide imaging.   2. Kidneys—
  Radiography.   I. Hartman, David S.   II. Title. [DNLM: 1.
  Kidney Diseases—radiography.   2. Kidney Diseases—
  radionuclide imaging.   3. Kidney—radiography.
  4. Kidney—radionuclide imaging.   WJ 302 D252r   1994]
RC904.5.R32D38 1994   616.6'10757—dc20

DNLM/DLC   93-28371

Radiology of the Kidney and Urinary Tract, Second Edition   ISBN 0–7216–3552–0

Printed in the United States of America.

Last digit is the print number: 9   8   7   6   5   4   3   2   1

To
our families

CONTRIBUTORS

PETER L. CHOYKE, MD
Professor of Radiology
Uniformed Services University of the Health Sciences
Deputy Director, Clinical Radiology
National Institutes of Health
Bethesda; Maryland

MICHAEL P. FEDERLE, MD
Professor of Radiology
University of Pittsburgh Medical Center
Pittsburgh, Pennsylvania

WENDELIN S. HAYES, DO
Visiting Professor
Department of Radiologic Pathology
Armed Forces Institute of Pathology
Washington, D.C.

R. BROOKE JEFFREY, Jr., MD
Professor of Radiology
Stanford University School of Medicine
Chief of Abdominal Imaging
Stanford University Medical Center
Stanford, California

MIKE McBILES, MD
Chief, Nuclear Medicine Service
Fitzsimons Army Medical Center
Aurora, Colorado

EUGENE T. MORITA, MD
Associate Clinical Professor of Radiology and Nuclear Medicine
School of Medicine, University of California, San Francisco
Director, Nuclear Medicine Laboratory
Mount Zion Hospital and Medical Center
San Francisco, California

PREFACE

This book has been written to provide the kind of information that is necessary for an informed, organized, and efficient approach to the radiologic diagnosis of diseases of the kidney and urinary tract, the retroperitoneum, and the adrenal glands. At the time of its original publication as *Radiologic Diagnosis of Renal Parenchymal Disease* in 1977, the text focused on the application of the excretory urogram, then the mainstay of uroradiologic diagnostic techniques, to abnormalities of the renal parenchyma in the adult. Revised in 1985, *Radiology of the Kidney* reflected the striking impact of the new and then still evolving applications of computed tomography and ultrasonography on the diagnosis of diseases of the renal parenchyma and added new sections on the pelvocalyceal system and retroperitoneum and some essays on a variety of uroradiologic topics. This edition, with the title *Radiology of the Kidney and Urinary Tract*, further expands the previous contents with chapters on the bladder, the urethra, and the adrenal gland; revises the entire text to include diseases of infancy and childhood; and incorporates all of the now mature technologic advances of the previous two decades.

Two concepts have been fundamental to all these editions. First, the organizational approach taken is that of the radiologist's point of view—how the greatest amount of information can be derived from a given set of careful observations and applied to the resolution of a well-formed clinical question. Second, we adhere to the concept that an informed radiologic interpretation is more dependent on a thorough understanding of the underlying pathologic process and less on a particular imaging modality—acknowledging pathology as the "mother church" of radiology.

Part I, Techniques and Anatomy, discusses the excretion of the contrast material used in uroradiology, the hazards that attend its use, and the precautions needed to minimize adverse reactions. The first part also covers the proper performance and application of excretory urography, ultrasonography, computed tomography, magnetic resonance imaging, angiography, and radionuclide imaging. The final chapter in Part I presents the normal radiologic anatomy of the kidney and ureter. Here, the embryogenesis and anatomy of a single, prototypic renal lobe is used as a model for understanding the radiologic appearance of the entire kidney and its ureter and their anomalous development. A thorough familiarity with the material in Part I is fundamental to the radiologic evaluation of the upper urinary tract and the retroperitoneum.

Part II, Renal Parenchymal Disease, is organized according to a scheme for the diagnosis of renal parenchymal disease that is derived from an analysis of the manner in which pathologic processes alter renal size and contour, and according to the *inherent* distribution of a given disease or abnormality. This approach results in a group of categories called "diagnostic sets," each of which contains a limited number of abnormal states that have common features of renal size, contour, and lesion distribution. Other radiologic observations, such as the appearance of the pelvocalyceal system, the papillae, and the nephrogram, are used to differentiate entities within each diagnostic set.

Although a list of abnormal conditions constitutes each diagnostic set, the reader is urged not to treat these as "gamuts" to be memorized. While gamuts may have rhyme, they do not necessarily have reason. Assignment of entities to each diagnostic set has been rationally derived by consideration of specific pathologic and clinical features; these must be understood thoroughly for the system to work. Nevertheless, it is difficult to fit all diseases neatly into any given system of classification. The approach used in Part II is no exception. Some assignments to diagnostic sets are based on arbitrary considerations, such as the most common form of presentation of each entity, the stage at which the radiologist is most likely to encounter the abnormality in the usual clinical setting, and the *elemental distribution* of the specific lesion. For example, angiomyolipoma is discussed as a cause of unifocal, unilateral enlargement of the kidney rather than as multifocal and/or bilateral lesions, since the former is the common presentation, and the latter is the uncommon. Acute cortical necrosis is placed in the diagnostic set of bilaterally enlarged, smooth kidneys because the radiologist is most likely to see this condition here rather than at a later time when chronic renal failure and small kidneys develop. Similarly, listing reflux nephropathy under the diagnostic set of small kidney with unifocal scar recognizes the fact that a single scar is the elemental lesion; multifocal and/or bilateral lesions may occur as chance events that are randomly distributed.

The five chapters of Part III, The Pelvocalyceal System and Ureter, describe abnormalities of these structures as they appear to the radiologist, using the same approach as that for Part II, Renal Parenchymal Disease. The first three chapters discuss abnormalities by their site of origin in the upper tract: intraluminal, mural, or renal sinus–periureteral space. The concluding two chapters analyze the meaning of the pelvocalyceal system and ureter that are abnormally dilated or effaced.

Part IV, The Lower Urinary Tract, presents in two chapters the normal anatomy and anomalies and diseases of the bladder and the urethra, including trauma. Here, the emphasis is on the limited number of radiologic abnormalities that develop in response to a wide variety of pathologic processes. This gives rise to broad differential diagnoses rather than the more precisely defined diagnostic groupings found in other parts of the book.

Part V, The Retroperitoneum and Adrenal, discusses the relevant normal anatomy and diseases in these two areas that have been so strikingly elucidated by the development of computed tomography, magnetic resonance imaging, ultrasonography, and, in the case of the adrenal gland, radionuclide imaging. Each of these two subjects lends itself well to diagnostic approaches based on categories derived from radiologic observations.

Part VI contains five essays on topics that either are not included in other parts or require integration of material from diverse chapters. These subjects include nephrographic analysis, imaging approaches to the patient in renal failure, diagnostic strategies in evaluating renal masses, the use of angiography in renal parenchymal disease, and the radiologic evaluation of the traumatized patient.

For readers so inclined, the Appendix contains a historical review of the development of contrast material and data on the chemistry of compounds previously and currently used to opacify the urinary tract, including low-osmolality agents.

The bibliographies for each chapter have been structured to provide the reader with both detailed references that support the text and a starting point for independent search of the literature. In most chapters, references that provide a historical perspective are included as well.

It is our hope that these chapters, taken together, will help physicians develop a solid understanding and enjoyment of the contemporary radiologic evaluation of the kidney and urinary tract—and that, in turn, their patients will be served efficiently and well.

ALAN J. DAVIDSON
DAVID S. HARTMAN

SPECIAL ACKNOWLEDGMENT

More than any other book, Davidson's *Radiologic Diagnosis of Renal Parenchymal Disease* profoundly influenced my professional development and sparked my interest in uroradiology. In 1977 most uroradiology textbooks were organized either by disease or by category of disease. Few other textbooks were designed specifically to assist the radiologist in the evaluation of an unknown abnormal image. Davidson's "user-friendly" diagnostic sets were revolutionary and proved invaluable to me when I was confronted with a perplexing case. Since then, I have freely adapted this pragmatic approach and now utilize diagnostic sets in lectures and teaching seminars and in publications.

Over the next several years, Dr. Davidson and I frequently exchanged cases and collaborated on research projects. In 1986 Dr. Davidson joined the faculty of the Department of Radiologic Pathology at the Armed Forces Institute of Pathology, where, at the time, I was Chairman. We have worked closely together since then. His healthy skepticism of uroradiologic "dogma," his academic integrity, and his clarity of thought as well as his scholarly presentations have been vital to my own professional maturation. I am deeply honored to join him as coauthor of this most recent update of his original landmark book.

In addition, I offer special thanks to my wife, Anne Marie, and my children, Matt and Kate; to my parents, Amabelle and Herbert Hartman; and to my stepmother, Irene. Each has been a loyal and dedicated supporter whose tolerance, guidance, encouragement, and love have made my contributions to *Radiology of the Kidney and Urinary Tract* possible.

DAVID S. HARTMAN

ACKNOWLEDGMENTS

A task that began more than two decades ago, and produced *Radiologic Diagnosis of Renal Parenchymal Disease* in 1977 and *Radiology of the Kidney* in 1985, is now complete with the publication of this book. A large number of people are owed a debt of gratitude for their support of this effort.

Much of the text of the earlier editions, now revised and expanded, has been retained in *Radiology of the Kidney and Urinary Tract*. The quality and the enduring nature of this material reflect the contributions of those experts who were invited to review the prior manuscripts. Helen C. Redman, Hugh Saxton, Thomas Sherwood, and Lee B. Talner gave generously while holding true to their reputations for unrestrained criticism and excellence.

Both of us have had the good fortune and honor to serve as faculty in the Department of Radiologic Pathology at the Armed Forces Institute of Pathology in Washington, D.C. Our professional lives have been singularly enriched in this unique environment. Fathollah K. Mostofi, Charles J. Davis, Jr., and Isabelle A. Sesterhann, three of the world's most eminent uropathologists, have been patient, accessible teachers as well as research collaborators. Our students, residents in radiology from nearly all educational institutions in the United States and Canada as well as many in Europe, the Middle East, and Latin America, have been at the core of our intellectual growth and pleasure. And by no means least, we hold an enduring gratitude and affection for John E. Madewell, Joel E. Lichtenstein, William D. Wehunt, Richard P. Moser, Jr., James C. Smirniotopoulos, Michael J. McCarthy, Pablo R. Ros, Melissa L. Rosado de Christenson, James L. Buck, Mark J. Kransdorf, Paula J. Kessler, and Peter C. Buetow. These colleagues in the Department of Radiologic Pathology have shared with us their collegiality, integrity, and selfless support as well as their academic excellence.

Many individuals have provided important assistance in particular areas. Peter L. Choyke contributed his expertise in modern imaging techniques in uroradiology to the section on magnetic resonance imaging in Chapter 1 and also reviewed other related portions of the text. Our ideas regarding the impact of recent technical advances on contemporary uroradiologic diagnosis have been honed by the give-and-take that we enjoy with Dr. Choyke in our regular review of material as it is accessioned in the archives of the Department of Radiologic Pathology at the Armed Forces Institute of Pathology. Wendelin S. Hayes has also been an important participant in these conferences. She has enhanced this book with her valuable chapters on the bladder and urethra. The chapters on radionuclide imaging and renal trauma contain fine contributions in areas in which our personal experience is limited. Our appreciation for these noteworthy efforts is extended to Mike McBiles and Eugene T. Morita and to Michael P. Federle and R. Brooke Jeffrey, Jr. Valuable information on uroradiologic procedures in pediatric practice was graciously provided by Robert Lebowitz.

Hundreds of educational institutions enroll their residents as students in the Armed Forces Institute of Pathology Course in Radiologic-Pathologic Correlation. As a result of the support of the Chairpeople and the Program Directors of these departments of radiology and the earnestness of our resident-students, nearly 400 new cases are accessioned each year in the uroradiologic archives of the Department of Radiologic Pathology. This is the material—with complete radiologic, clinical, and pathologic documentation—on which our research and teaching are based. We have borrowed freely from this valuable and unique collection in illustrating this book. We are grateful to all who have directly or indirectly made contributions over the nearly 50 years that the archives have been in existence. In addition, many colleagues have generously allowed us the use of fine illustrations from their personal experience to supplement the text. Each is acknowledged individually in the legend to the illustration.

The research and publications of our fellow members of the Society of Uroradiology also underlie much of the information contained in this book. We are particularly indebted to these colleagues for their extensive contribution to the literature and for the rich professional relationship that we share with so many.

Our efforts have been greatly enhanced by the dedicated support and high standards of four individuals. We are most grateful to Earlene Turner, Administrative Assistant, and Adahlia Glover, Research Assistant, both of the Department of Radiologic Pathology at the Armed Forces Institute of Pathology; to Henri C. Hessel, photographer in the Department of Radiology and Radiologic Sciences, The Johns Hopkins University; and to Karen Rank, secretary in the Department of Radiology at Hershey Medical Center, Penn State University.

Finally, Lisette Bralow, Vice President and Editor in Chief; Carolyn Naylor, Assistant Director of Production; Gina Scala, Senior Copy Editor; Peg Shaw, Illustration Specialist; Paul Fry, Designer; Robert Keller, Marketing Manager; and Roger Wall, Indexer, are W. B. Saunders Company staff who have lent welcome support and expert guidance at each stage of the writing and production of this book. We are most pleased by the long association that *Radiology of the Kidney and Urinary Tract* and its predecessors have enjoyed with this leading medical publishing house.

CONTENTS

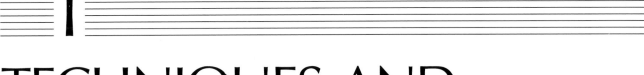

I

TECHNIQUES AND ANATOMY

DIAGNOSTIC URORADIOLOGIC TECHNIQUES

CONTRAST MATERIAL	ULTRASONOGRAPHY
Physiology of Excretion	COMPUTED TOMOGRAPHY
Practical Considerations	MAGNETIC RESONANCE IMAGING
Adverse Reactions	
EXCRETORY UROGRAPHY	ANGIOGRAPHY

This chapter describes the principal diagnostic methods for studying the kidneys and surrounding structures. Presented first are the events that follow the intravenous administration of contrast material and their influence on the quality of the excretory urogram and computed tomogram of the kidney. Following that is a discussion of the hazards associated with the use of contrast material and the means by which these may be minimized or treated. The remaining sections review the technique, applications, and limitations of excretory urography, ultrasonography, computed tomography, magnetic resonance imaging, and angiography. Nuclear medicine techniques are discussed in Chapter 2. The application of Doppler and duplex ultrasound examination of the kidney and its blood vessels has not been sufficiently clarified to warrant inclusion in this text, although some references to these techniques are included in several chapters.

The discussion on contrast material covers both the ionic, monomeric high osmolality compounds as well as the various nonionic and ionic forms of low osmolality agents. The chemical characteristics of these compounds are described in the Appendix.

CONTRAST MATERIAL

Physiology of Excretion

Until 1967, a thorough understanding of the physiology of excretory urography was hampered by the absence of a simple, reproducible, and accurate method for the measurement of contrast material in plasma and urine. In that year, Purkiss and colleagues devised a spectrographic technique that met these re-

quirements. This method was applied by Purkiss's colleagues, Cattell and Fry, to the study of contrast material excretion in a group of patients with normal renal function. The conclusions drawn from their data have been confirmed and expanded upon by others. The spaces of distribution of intravenously injected contrast material, the relationship of dose to plasma level, the rate of plasma disappearance, the mode of renal excretion, and the impact of contrast material on urine formation are clearly defined for both high and low osmolality compounds. These insights provide the basis for the rational conduct and knowledgeable interpretation of contrast material–enhanced examinations of the kidney.

Following the rapid intravenous injection of a bolus of contrast material, a peak plasma level is reached almost immediately. This is followed by a rapid decline (Fig. 1–1). Plasma level decline is multifactorial. An immediate drop is due to initial rapid mixing in the vascular compartment. Concomitantly there is loss of plasma contrast material by diffusion into the extravascular, extracellular fluid space. That distribution in this space occurs has been deduced from the experimental observation that the distribution volume of contrast material is equal to 20 per cent of body weight, a figure identical to the extravascular and extracellular fluid compartment. The time for equalization with this space has not been conclusively established. Estimates based on experimental observations have ranged from near instantaneous to 120 minutes. Finally, decrease in plasma contrast material levels obviously occurs from renal excretion, the third factor contributing to the plasma decay curve illustrated in Figure 1–1. Injection of iodine equivalent doses of high and low osmolality contrast material may yield

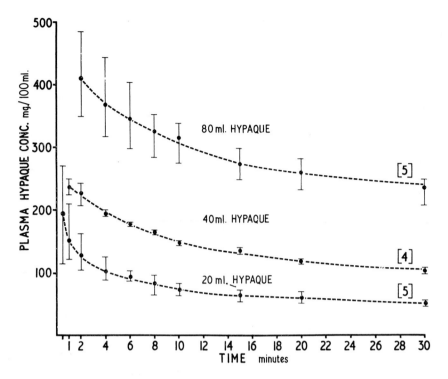

Figure 1–1. Mean plasma sodium diatrizoate (Hypaque) concentrations and range of values following intravenous injection of varying volumes. Figures in brackets represent the number of subjects studied. The decline in plasma level represents vascular mixing, extravascular diffusion, and renal excretion. (From Cattell, W. R., Fry, I. K., Spencer, A. G., and Purkiss, P.: Br. J. Radiol. 40:561, 1967. Reproduced with kind permission of the authors and the *British Journal of Radiology.*)

a slightly higher peak plasma level for the low osmolality agents. The apparent difference between these two classes of contrast material suggests that low osmolality compounds may have a volume of extravascular distribution that is smaller than that of high osmolality contrast material. This has not been fully elucidated, however, and does not represent a practical issue in terms of clinical applications.

One of the most important determinants of the diagnostic quality of an excretory urogram is the level of contrast material present in the plasma and available to the kidney for excretion. This concept actually was derived empirically through clinical experience before the clarification of the physiologic principles involved and has been popularized as the "high dose" or "drip infusion" urographic technique. The advantage of this technique is based on the phenomenon demonstrated in Figure 1–2. In that illustration, the 10-minute plasma concentration of sodium diatrizoate is shown to have a positive linear correlation (r = .85) with the amount of contrast material (adjusted for body surface area) injected in patients with normal renal function. These data clearly indicate that a dose can be calculated precisely to achieve any given plasma level and illustrate the basis for the value of "high dose" urography.

One of the major accomplishments of Cattell, Fry, and their colleagues was to demonstrate conclusively that for all practical purposes contrast material is excreted by glomerular filtration alone. This has subsequently been shown to also be true for low osmolality compounds. Previously this fact had been a subject of speculation and was not universally accepted. Rearrangement of the mathematical equation expressing the glomerular filtration rate brings out the importance of the relationship between the plasma level of contrast material and the glomerular filtrate:

$$GFR = \frac{UV}{P}$$

where GFR = glomerular filtration rate (ml/min)
    U = concentration of contrast material in urine (mg/ml)
    V = flow rate of urine (ml/min)
    P = plasma concentration of contrast material (mg/ml)

rearranges into:

$$UV = GFR \times P$$

Clearly, the diagnostic quality of an excretory urogram is a function of UV, the amount of iodine-containing contrast material excreted by the kidney in a volume of urine that distends the pelvocalyceal system and ureters. It is important to note that of the determinants of UV, contrast material plasma concentration (P) is the only variable that the radiologist can manipulate by adjustment of dose. Glomerular filtration rate is a given value in any individual, although it varies with each patient.

Another important determinant of the diagnostic quality of an excretory urogram is the volume of urine formed to distend the pelvocalyceal system and ureters. A collapsed collecting system does not reflect surrounding anatomic structures and may obscure abnormalities within its lumen. Adequate distention is basic to optimal urographic technique and can be achieved by a mechanical device such as a ureteral compression balloon, by taking advantage of the diuretic effect of the urographic contrast material, or by

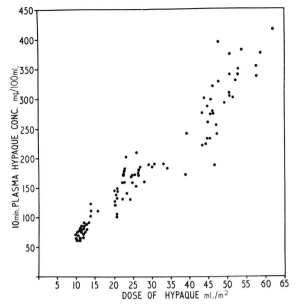

Figure 1–2. Plasma sodium diatrizoate (Hypaque) concentration related to dose expressed as ml/m² body surface. A positive correlation between dose and 10-minute plasma levels is shown. (From Cattell, W. R., Fry, I. K., Spencer, A. G., and Purkiss, P.: Br. J. Radiol. *40*:561, 1967. Reproduced with kind permission of the authors and the *British Journal of Radiology*.)

both. High osmolality contrast material is a potent osmotic diuretic because it freely dissociates into two particles when in solution. The iodine-bearing anion is an osmotically active, nonreabsorbable solute that produces a diuresis of salt and water. The degree of diuresis produced varies directly with the dose administered. However, considerably less diuretic effect occurs following the use of sodium salts than after the use of meglumine salts. The cation meglumine is not reabsorbed by the renal tubules to any significant degree and thus provides added osmotic force within the tubule lumen to potentiate the diuretic effect of the nonreabsorbable anion. The cation sodium, on the other hand, is freely reabsorbable by the renal tubules. The additional available sodium in the proximal tubule following the use of a sodium salt enhances water reabsorption. For this reason, a smaller urine volume and higher urine concentration of contrast material follows the use of the sodium salt when compared with a meglumine salt of contrast material. One important difference between low and high osmolality agents is the markedly reduced osmotic diuretic effect of the former compared with the latter. This is true for nonionic monomers and dimers as well as for the ionic dimers. Decreased urine volume translates into enhanced radiodensity of the pelvocalyceal system and ureter because there is less dilution of the iodine-bearing molecule by urine. Decreased urine volume also means less distention of the pelvocalyceal system with low osmolality agents compared with ionic, high osmolality compounds. As a result, when using low osmolality contrast material, ureteral compression to distend the pelvocalyceal system is particularly important to compensate for the relatively small volume of urine being formed by the kidneys.

The foregoing considerations represent events that occur in the proximal renal tubule where the volume of glomerular filtrate is reduced by approximately 85 per cent. The final concentration of contrast material is influenced further by additional water reabsorption, which takes place in the distal tubules and collecting ducts. Here, the major influence on water reabsorption is the level of activity of antidiuretic hormone. This, in turn, reflects the state of hydration. The well-dehydrated, volume-depleted individual will experience less of a diuresis following contrast material injection and will excrete a higher concentration of this material than the volume-expanded individual. Dehydration, on the other hand, potentiates the risk for contrast material–induced nephrotoxicity.

Practical Considerations

With this knowledge of the physiology of contrast material excretion, what can the radiologist do to maximize the diagnostic information derived from the excretory urogram or contrast material–enhanced computed tomogram of the kidneys?

Regarding the choice of high osmolality ionic contrast material, it is clear that sodium salts, rather than meglumine salts, provide a higher concentration of radiopaque material in the urine. Additionally, there is some evidence that fewer adverse reactions occur with sodium salts than with meglumine salts. A number of reports claim that pelvocalyceal density, but not nephrographic density, is superior with sodium rather than meglumine salts. This is disputed by others, who assert that although this superiority may be true at low and medium dosage schedules, the difference is obliterated when maximum doses are used. Yet another point of view is that even if concentration differences do exist, they are insignificant because opacity is a function of the number of radiopaque atoms, regardless of the volume in which they are distributed; small differences in the number of atoms of iodine are hard to detect with the eye. From a practical point of view, these opposing opinions are of no importance, and the use of sodium salts is favored in most situations if high osmolality contrast material is to be used. Two differences of practical importance are apparent when the physiology of excretion of low osmolality contrast material is compared with that of high osmolality compounds. First, radiopacity of urine is greater with low osmolality agents because a smaller urine volume yields higher iodine concentration. Although this is generally considered advantageous, a high level of radiodensity carries the undesirable potential of obscuring small filling defects in the pelvocalyceal system. Second, reduced osmotic diuresis results in less distention of the pelvocalyceal system than occurs with high osmolality contrast material. Effective ureteral compression and, in some cases, a slight delay in filming sequences to allow time for more urine to form can compensate for this effect. For the same reason—high iodine concentration related to low urine flow rates—maximum density of the nephrogram produced by low osmolality contrast material may be greater and its appearance slower when compared with that of high osmolality agents.

Traditionally, dehydration was advocated as a means of maximizing the radiodensity of urine during excretory urography. This was an important adjunct at a time when convention held that the maximum total dose of contrast material should not exceed 7.5 gm (25 ml of sodium diatrizoate 50%). Thus, a 12-hour period of water deprivation and vigorous bowel preparation were necessary routines. As the conventional dosage of contrast material increased, the need for the radiodensity-enhancing value of dehydration diminished. In fact, dehydration is now considered a risk-potentiating factor for contrast material–induced nephrotoxicity, particularly in patients with pre-existing renal disease, hyperuricemia, or dysproteinemia. This is discussed further in a following section.

Another practical fluid problem is encountered in individuals with heart failure or other conditions associated with salt and water retention. These patients may require higher doses of contrast material to compensate for diffusion of greater than normal amounts of radiopaque material into the expanded extracellular fluid space that is present in these disorders.

How does one determine an appropriate dose of contrast material? First, it is best to think of dose in terms of grams of iodine administered, rather than volume of injectate, since iodine content is the basic determinant of radiopacity and the various products available vary considerably in their iodine concentration. Second, as emphasized previously, it is useful to relate the dosage to body size.

In adults, the question of optimal dosage has received the attention of many investigators. It is generally agreed that in the presence of normal renal function, a total dose of 15 to 25 gm of iodine will provide satisfactory opacification. This represents approximately 300 mg of iodine per kilogram of body weight. In the most commonly used forms of contrast material of both high and low osmolality, a dose of 1.0 ml/kg of body weight will result in this dosage range, as noted in Table 1–1. In patients who are obese, or who have a great deal of gas and feces, the dose can be increased, either initially or by reinjection of an additional amount of contrast material after the examination has been started and the initial films found inadequate. Historically, it has been demonstrated that a single dose of 4 ml/kg of 50% or 60% diatrizoate resulted in distinct discomfort, including tremors, irritability, and tachycardia. Thus, the convention of limiting total dose for excretory urography to 2 ml/kg evolved; in addition, many workers in this field arbitrarily limit the total volume of injectate to 170 to 200 ml. Some evidence exists, in fact, that at very large doses of high osmolality contrast material, urinary concentration of iodine levels off and may even diminish as a result of the osmotic force of the radiopaque solute's interfering with osmotic gradients in the cortex and medulla. This phenomenon is, presumably, of less importance with low osmolality contrast material. Renal failure presents a special problem in dosage determination and will be discussed subsequently.

In the pediatric patient, dosage must be based on both weight and age. The latter factor is particularly important in the premature or normal newborn in whom there is normally a reduction in glomerular filtration rate that necessitates an upward adjustment in dose. The following schedule, based on that used at Children's Hospital, Boston (R. Lebowitz, personal communication, 1991), takes these factors into account.

Weight	Dose
Up to 5.5 kg	4.0 ml/kg
5.5 to 11.5 kg	25 ml
11.5 to 23 kg	2.0 ml/kg
23 to 46 kg	50 ml
Over 46 kg	1.0 ml/kg

Table 1–1. COMMONLY USED CONTRAST MATERIAL FOR EXCRETORY UROGRAPHY AND COMPUTED TOMOGRAPHY

Generic Name	Trade Name	Sodium Content (mEq/ml)	Iodine Content (mg/ml)	Osmolality (mOsm/kg H$_2$O)
Ionic Monomers (Ratio 1.5):				
Sodium diatrizoate	Hypaque 50	0.8	300	1515
Meglumine and sodium diatrizoate	Renografin 60	0.16	292	1420
Sodium iothalamate	Conray 400	1.05	400	2300
Meglumine iothalamate	Conray		282	1400
Nonionic Monomers (Ratio 3):				
Iopamidol	Isovue 300		300	616
Iohexol	Omnipaque		300	709
Ioversol	Optiray		320	702
Iopromide	Ultravist		300	620
Ionic Dimer (Ratio 3):				
Meglumine and sodium ioxaglate	Hexabrix	0.15	320	600
Nonionic Dimers (Ratio 6):				
Iotrolan (under development)				
Iodixanol (under development)				

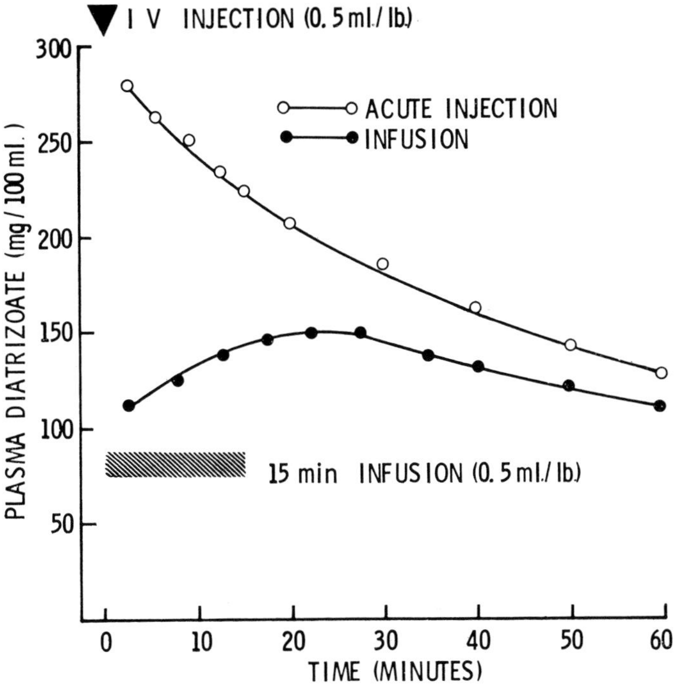

Figure 1–3. Plasma concentration of diatrizoate following rapid bolus injection and slow drip infusion. Drip infusion does not produce the same maximal level of contrast material as is achieved by direct injection. (From Cattell, W. R.: Invest. Radiol. 5:473, 1970. Reproduced with kind permission of the author and *Investigative Radiology*.)

Low osmolality agents are of value in infants to minimize the cardiovascular complications from excessive volume expansion, as discussed subsequently.

The plasma concentration of contrast material is affected materially by the speed of injection. Figure 1–3 illustrates the significant difference in peak and sustained plasma concentration following a rapid single injection compared with a 15-minute infusion of contrast material. For equivalent total doses, it is apparent that the slow, 15-minute administration never produces as high a plasma level as a rapid, 30- to 90-second injection. In addition, the slow infusion technique has no impact on either urine flow rate or urine sodium diatrizoate concentration when compared with the rapid bolus injection technique. The use of drip infusion technique is therefore unjustified except, perhaps, for its convenience. Patients at risk for contrast material–induced cardiotoxicity are an exception to this generalization. Here, risk is related directly to the speed of injection. It is important to avoid having contrast material reach the myocardium as a bolus. In this group, then, the total dose of contrast material should be delivered over a 2- to 3-minute period. This subject is discussed in greater detail in the following section on contrast material hazards.

Adverse Reactions

Untoward reactions to contrast material can be separated into two major categories: adverse systemic reactions and organ toxicity. The first group can be further subdivided into nonidiosyncratic and idiosyncratic. In the organ toxic reactions, the kidney, heart, and lungs are the organs susceptible to clinically manifested damage by urographic contrast material.

Adverse Systemic Reactions. Systemic reactions to contrast material vary from mild and inconsequen-

tial (heat and nausea) to life-threatening and fatal (bronchospasm, hypovolemic hypotension, laryngeal edema, or cardiac arrest). Collection of comprehensive epidemiologic data on serious reactions is hindered by their infrequency, methodologic weaknesses inherent in collaborative multi-institutional studies, nonuniform systems of classification, risk factors that vary with different study populations, and the availability and effectiveness of therapeutic measures that may prevent a life-threatening reaction from becoming a fatal one. Despite these limitations, it is generally held that the overall prevalence of adverse systemic reactions of *all* types may be as high as 13 per cent of patients exposed to high osmolality intravenous contrast material and approximately 3 per cent of those exposed to low osmolality intravenous contrast material. This reflects the common occurrence of minor reactions, which account for approximately 98 per cent of all reactions. Intermediate and severe reactions are much less common.

From an epidemiologic perspective, the convention is to classify reactions according to their clinical severity: minor, intermediate, severe, and fatal. These are outlined in Table 1–2. Minor reactions are of limited duration and consequence and usually require no treatment. Nausea, vomiting, a sensation of warmth, and very mild rash are examples. These occur in up to 10 per cent of individuals exposed to high osmolality contrast material, with the highest prevalence in young adults. The use of low osmolality contrast material reduces the overall prevalence of adverse systemic reactions substantially. Most of this is accomplished by up to a sevenfold decrease in minor reactions. The magnitude of reduction varies considerably among specific minor symptoms. Intermediate reactions are those that cause concern for the well-being of the patient and require some form of therapy,

Table 1–2. CLINICAL CLASSIFICATION OF ADVERSE REACTIONS TO UROGRAPHIC CONTRAST MATERIAL

Adverse Reaction	Minor	Intermediate	Severe
Systemic			
Idiosyncratic	Mild urticaria	Extensive urticaria Angioneurotic edema Bronchospasm Laryngospasm Hypovolemic hypotension	Cardiopulmonary collapse Pulmonary edema Bronchospasm Laryngospasm Hypovolemic hypotension
Nonidiosyncratic	Nausea Vomiting Heat Injection site pain Tachy/bradycardia	(?) Hypotension secondary to vasodilation	
Organ Toxic	Tachy/bradycardia	Oliguria/anuria Azotemia Myocardial ischemia Cardiac arrhythmia Bronchospasm	Ventricular tachycardia/ fibrillation Myocardial infarction

which is rapidly effective. Extensive urticaria, angioneurotic edema, bronchospasm, laryngospasm, and hypotension are included in the category. No precise data are available for the frequency of intermediate reactions, but their pattern of age distribution appears to be similar to that of minor reactions. Severe reactions are defined as those that threaten life and require intensive treatment. Cardiopulmonary collapse, pulmonary edema, severe forms of bronchospasm, laryngeal edema, and severe hypotension fall into this category. Earlier reports of the prevalence of severe reactions to high osmolality contrast material varied from 1:3000 to 1:4500 (Ansell et al., 1980; Hartman et al., 1982). More recent studies indicate that severe reactions with high osmolality agents are as frequent as from 1:200 to 1:1000 (Lasser et al., 1987; Palmer, 1988; Katayama et al., 1990; Caro et al., 1991). The use of either low osmolality contrast material or a corticosteroid pretreatment regimen, discussed subsequently, has been variably reported to reduce the prevalence of severe adverse reactions to a range of from 1:640 to 1:2500 (Lasser et al., 1987; Katayama et al., 1990; Caro et al., 1991). Unlike minor and intermediate reactions, severe reactions appear to occur uniformly in all age groups, with perhaps a slightly greater frequency among young adults. The literature, however, is not without conflict on this issue. The reported frequency of fatal reactions to high osmolality contrast material has varied between 1:14,000 and 1:110,000. The former figure is most likely inaccurate. The most generally accepted range has been between 1:40,000 and 1:100,000. However, the large study of Katayama and colleagues (1990) failed to document any fatalities unequivocally due to contrast material in nearly 170,000 patents exposed to high osmolality contrast material and an approximately equal number of patients exposed to low osmolality contrast material. The changing data on mortality rates likely reflect the inherent safety of both high and low osmolality agents as well as improved availability and effectiveness of therapy

for severe adverse reactions to both categories of contrast material.

The preceding discussion addresses only the frequency and clinical manifestations of adverse systemic reactions to intravenous contrast material, not the pathogenesis of reactions. To this end, systemic reactions are divided into two groups: nonidiosyncratic and idiosyncratic, or anaphylactoid.

Nonidiosyncratic Reactions. Nonidiosyncratic reactions are the consequence of physical and chemical characteristics of the contrast material, such as hyperosmolality, single-valence cations, and the intrinsic chemotoxicity of an iodinated benzoic acid derivative. Low osmolality contrast material is particularly effective in reducing the prevalence of nonidiosyncratic reactions, reflecting the paramount role of osmolality as a cause of this type of reaction. Examples of physicochemical systemic reactions include vasodilation, tachycardia, bradycardia, hypotension, and flushing. Specific organs or tissues may be the site of nonidiosyncratic reactions to contrast material. Examples include venous endothelium damage at the site of injection, nausea and vomiting, transient alterations in heart rate or rhythm, change in renal blood flow and glomerular filtration rate, and deformity of circulating red blood cells. In general, nonidiosyncratic reactions to contrast material are limited in nature and of minor clinical importance.

Idiosyncratic Reactions. The clinically important adverse systemic reactions to contrast material are idiosyncratic, or anaphylactoid. These comprise those intermediate, severe, and fatal reactions with clinical features usually seen with allergic reactions. They include urticaria, angioneurotic edema, bronchospasm, laryngospasm, cardiopulmonary collapse, pulmonary edema, and hypotension. Although these reactions resemble allergies in their clinical manifestations, they are neither antigen-antibody mediated nor the result of initial exposure and subsequent sensitization. Thus, it is proper to characterize this phenomenon as idiosyncratic or anaphylactoid rather than allergic or anaphylactic. Reactions in this category are the same whether provoked by either high or low osmolality contrast material.

The mechanisms that cause idiosyncratic response to contrast material have not been completely elucidated. Four broad categories of pathogenesis have been postulated: (1) nonimmunologically mediated release of a vasoactive substance such as histamine or serotonin; (2) antibody-antigen reactions; (3) disturbance of activation systems involving complement, kinins, coagulation, and fibrinolysis; and (4) psychological reactions. Of these, the overwhelming body of investigational evidence points to complement activation, release of vascular mediators, and a coagulation disturbance as the biochemical basis for idiosyncratic systemic responses to contrast material. The reader is referred to sources listed in the bibliography at the end of the chapter for a more detailed explanation of this subject.

Prophylaxis. What can be done to minimize the risk and consequences of adverse systemic reactions to contrast material? The nonidiosyncratic effects are of little consequence. The greatest impact of low osmolality contrast material is to reduce the frequency of adverse reactions in this category. When using high osmolality contrast material, some measures can be taken to mitigate nonidiosyncratic reactions. For example, venous endothelial irritation leading to arm pain can be avoided by selecting a large vein for injection, by flushing the vessel with saline after injection, or, if important, by using a meglumine salt rather than the more irritating sodium salt. Similarly, the likelihood of nausea and vomiting can be lessened by a prolonged injection time.

Idiosyncratic adverse systemic effects, on the other hand, are a major concern. Every effort must be undertaken by the radiologist to minimize the likelihood of their occurrence or, once they develop, their consequence. Because a precise understanding of the mechanism involved does not exist, only limited means are available to accomplish this. These include screening patients for epidemiologically determined risk factors; using empirically derived prophylactic measures; and having available and being familiar with all necessary measures needed to treat a reaction.

Data derived from patients exposed to high osmolality contrast material have identified certain risk factors that indicate an increased likelihood of an idiosyncratic adverse systemic reaction occurring with greater frequency than in a population free of these factors (Ansell et al., 1980; Katayama et al., 1990). A patient with a history of allergy is four to five times more likely to develop a severe, adverse idiosyncratic systemic reaction to contrast material than one without such a history. Included in this risk group are patients with a history of hay fever, hives, eczema, and various other allergies to substances such as seafood and penicillin. Current or remote asthma increases the risk of a severe reaction by as much as 8-fold, and a history of prior reaction to urographic contrast material is associated with an 11-fold increase in the risk of a severe reaction, when compared with a population without this history. These risk factors remain valid for patients exposed to low osmolality contrast material although the frequency of reactions is less than that provoked by high osmolality contrast material. These data strongly militate for taking a careful history of all patients before administration of either high or low osmolality contrast material and instituting prophylactic measures when appropriate, as discussed below. However, since most adverse reactions to contrast material occur in individuals without any history of allergy or a prior reaction to contrast material, it is important to remember that a negative screen is no assurance that a reaction will not occur.

Intravenous injection of a test dose of contrast material has not been validated as an effective screen for potential reactors, although this approach does have its advocates (Yocum et al., 1978). An *in vitro* assay of prekallikrein to kallikrein conversion rate as a predictor of contrast material reactors has been developed but has not become available for general use (Lasser et al., 1981).

In patients who are judged to be at increased risk because of a significant history of allergy or a prior contrast material reaction, the need for a diagnostic test that requires contrast material should be reassessed. If the need for the test remains justified, low osmolality contrast material should be used.

Before the development of low osmolality contrast material, pretreatment with adrenal corticosteroids was used empirically in high-risk patients to provide protection against an idiosyncratic adverse systemic reaction. Neither the validity of this approach nor its physiologic basis has ever been established. However, adrenal corticosteroids have now been shown to reduce the frequency of severe idiosyncratic adverse systemic reactions in a general population without identified risk factors to a level similar to that achieved by low osmolality contrast material (Lasser et al., 1987; Lasser, 1988). These observations apply to the high-risk population only by implication. A typical protocol is hydrocortisone, 100 mg (or its equivalent dose in other forms of corticosteroids such as methylprednisolone) administered orally or parenterally at least 12 hours before injection of contrast material. Some radiologists advocate two doses, one at 24 hours and another at 12 hours before contrast material administration. An initial dose of corticosteroid given less than 12 hours before contrast material administration is thought to be ineffective. This is the same protocol that can be used in the general low-risk population in lieu of low osmolality contrast material.

In any high-risk patient, it is advisable to maintain an open intravenous line during the contrast material examination as an access route for further medication if an adverse reaction develops. Although low osmolality contrast material and, presumably, a pretreatment protocol of adrenal corticosteroids provide a measure of protection, a major reaction may still develop and vigilance should not be relaxed. If there is extreme concern for a life-threatening reaction, the presence of a resuscitation team at the time of injection should be considered.

Antihistamines have not been generally accepted as an effective preventative measure in high-risk patients, although theoretically both H_1- and H_2-receptor antagonists may have a role in the prevention of contrast material reactions. Likewise, the possibility exists that epsilon-aminocaproic acid may reduce the risk of reaction. Rapid injection of contrast material is no more likely to precipitate an adverse systemic reaction than is a slow injection.

Treatment. The treatment of idiosyncratic adverse systemic reactions is determined by their nature and their severity. Minor reactions, by definition, are not treated. Antihistamines (H_1-receptor antagonists such as diphenhydramine) are often advocated for intermediate cutaneous reactions. However, this category of drugs has its own inherent risks, such as drowsiness developing in the ambulatory patient responsible for driving an automobile. These considerations lead some authorities not to recommend antihistamines as a treatment for minor or intermediate adverse contrast material reactions. Clearly, antihistamines have no role in the active treatment of major reactions.

Adrenal corticosteroids, as discussed previously, are used principally for prophylaxis in high-risk individuals, if at all. This category of drugs is not a first line of therapy in the treatment of adverse systemic reactions of any severity that have already developed.

The treatment of intermediate and severe adverse systemic reactions is determined by the nature of the reaction. These fall into four categories: (1) severe urticaria, (2) isolated hypovolemic hypotension, (3) isolated airway compromise due to bronchospasm, and (4) anaphylactoid reactions characterized by severe and progressive combinations of both hypotension and airway compromise (Bush and Swanson, 1991).

Severe urticaria is best treated with an H_1 antihistamine such as diphenhydramine in an intravenous or intramuscular injection of 25 to 50 mg. H_2 antihistamines (cimetidine or ranitidine) have also been advocated, although their efficacy is less well established.

Hypovolemic hypotension is associated with tachycardia and is the result of fluid loss through increased capillary permeability, which is part of the pathophysiology of adverse idiosyncratic reactions. The same mechanism accounts for the occasional appearance of pulmonary edema. Treatment of this reaction requires placing the patient in a Trendelenburg position and administering nasal oxygen and normal saline or Ringer's lactate for large volume fluid replacement. Central venous pressure should be monitored as an index of the volume of fluid required to restore blood pressure to normal and to avoid the complications of fluid overload, especially in patients with pre-existing compromised cardiac function. In most cases, fluid replacement is the only measure required to correct hypotension. If pharmacologic intervention is required because of the ineffectiveness of fluid replace-

ment, a beta-adrenergic vasopressor in the form of dopamine is ideal. However, the complicated nature of this therapy requires expertise that is usually beyond that of a radiologist. Instead, subcutaneous epinephrine (0.2 to 0.3 ml of 1:1000 solution) may be used.

Hypotension associated with bradycardia is usually vasovagal in origin and not an idiosyncratic adverse systemic reaction to contrast material per se *except in a patient treated with a beta-blocker that prevents a normal tachycardic response to hypovolemia.* Vasovagal-mediated bradycardic hypotension is a common form of hypotension seen in a radiology department under a variety of circumstances unrelated to contrast material exposure. Atropine (0.5 to 2.0 mg intravenously), not epinephrine, is the appropriate pharmacologic intervention for this phenomenon if simple measures of Trendelenburg positioning, oxygen, and volume expansion are not effective.

Mild to intermediate forms of isolated airway compromise due to bronchospasm can be treated either by epinephrine administered subcutaneously in incremental doses of 0.2 to 0.3 ml of 1:1000 solution or by one or two inhalations of a beta-agonist bronchodilator such as albuterol, metaproterenol, or terbutaline. Signs and symptoms must be carefully assessed to determine the need for additional increments. Severe and/or accelerating airway compromise due to bronchospasm or angioneurotic edema often requires a slow intravenous injection of 1 to 2 ml of 1:10,000 epinephrine.

For anaphylactoid reactions, intravenous epinephrine should be administered slowly to maximize its beta-adrenergic effect and to reduce the alpha-adrenergic effect. An initial dose of 1.0 ml of 1:10,000 epinephrine may be followed by additional doses as needed. Oxygen should be administered and blood volume restored with the rapid intravenous infusion of normal saline or Ringer's lactate.

In any of the above treatment regimens in which epinephrine is administered, particular caution should be exercised with patients who are elderly or hypoxic, which are two risk factors in which epinephrine may induce severe cardiac arrhythmia. Epinephrine should be avoided in patients who are medicated with noncardioselective beta-blocking agents such as propranolol (Inderal). The desired beta-adrenergic effect of epinephrine may be blocked in such patients with deleterious complications resulting from unopposed alpha-agonist effects.

Idiosyncratic reactions manifested as cardiopulmonary collapse require that the radiologist be expert in basic cardiopulmonary resuscitation. Diagnostic tests requiring exposure to contrast material should take place only in an environment that provides both the expertise and the facilities for the effective treatment of this most serious complication. The radiologist's role in this setting can then be limited to first-line measures, such as administering epinephrine, instituting fluid replacement, and performing basic cardiopulmonary resuscitation.

Organ Toxicity. The kidney, heart, and lung are

susceptible to damage by contrast material. In the absence of a basic understanding of the mechanisms involved, these organ toxic responses are best defined by the clinical disorders that result.

Nephrotoxicity. Oliguria or anuria with or without azotemia is the clinical manifestation of contrast material damage to the kidneys. Two very different pathogenetic mechanisms lead to this disorder: one is acute tubular necrosis; the other is acute obstruction of tubule lumina by precipitated solutes or proteins.

Nephrotoxicity in the form of acute tubular necrosis occurs mainly in patients with low flow states (congestive heart failure, hypotension), generalized vascular disease (arteriosclerosis, nephrosclerosis), or pre-existing renal failure (such as chronic glomerulonephritis, diabetic nephropathy). Dehydration potentiates the risk for nephrotoxicity and should always be avoided in patients receiving contrast material, particularly those with risk factors for nephrotoxicity. On the contrary, hydration reduces, but does not eliminate, the risk of contrast material–induced nephrotoxicity. Theory and some clinical evidence support the concept that nephrotoxicity is also influenced by time and dosage factors, with a large amount of contrast material (50 gm or greater) given as a single dose imparting the highest risk.

Speculation about the pathogenesis of contrast material–induced acute tubular necrosis has centered on two possibilities. Evidence for a direct toxic effect on proximal tubule cells by contrast material includes induction of enzymuria, reduction in sodium transport by the toad bladder, decreased extraction of para-aminohippuric acid, and vacuolization of tubule cells by these agents. A second body of data suggests that the renal damage that follows exposure to contrast material is a result of ischemia from either vasoconstriction or sludging of red blood cells in the microcirculation.

Diabetic nephropathy is a particularly important risk factor for contrast material–induced acute tubular necrosis. However, the level of risk associated with diabetic nephropathy apparently is not as high as has been previously thought. Earlier clinical investigations (Harkinen and Kjellstrand, 1977) indicated that as many as 90 per cent of patients with juvenile-onset diabetes with baseline serum creatinine levels greater than 5 mg/dl develop nephrotoxicity and that there was a positive correlation among the severity of diabetic nephropathy, the prevalence of contrast material–induced nephrotoxicity, and impaired recovery to baseline levels of renal function. Later studies (Parfrey et al., 1989; Schwab et al., 1989) have demonstrated a prevalence of only 9 per cent for contrast material–induced nephrotoxicity in patients with diabetic nephropathy with baseline serum creatinine levels of greater than 1.7 mg/dl. It is necessary to emphasize, however, that the unique risk of nephrotoxicity in the diabetic patient is limited to those with pre-existing diabetic nephropathy. The nonazotemic diabetic patient and, possibly, the nondiabetic patient with pre-existing renal insufficiency are not at increased risk for contrast material–induced nephrotoxicity when the examination is performed using standard precautions regarding dose and hydration (Shieh et al., 1982; Parfrey et al., 1989).

The other form of contrast material–induced nephrotoxicity is due to an acute obstruction of tubule lumina by precipitation of abnormal urinary proteins in patients with multiple myeloma, by Tamm-Horsfall proteins in dehydrated newborns or infants, or by uric acid precipitation in individuals with very high serum uric acid levels. Contrast material has a uricosuric effect, presumably as a result of inhibition of uric acid reabsorption by the renal tubules. Consequently, its use in patients with marked hyperuricemia potentiates the risk for acute urate nephropathy. A large fluid intake, alkaline diuresis, and reduction of serum uric acid by allopurinol are specific measures that reduce the risk of this complication. The risk of acute myeloma nephropathy and Tamm-Horsfall nephropathy can be minimized by ensuring that dehydration does not occur when at-risk patients are exposed to contrast material.

Precautions. How should a patient be approached when any of the above risk factors are identified? First, the need for a radiologic study requiring contrast material must be reassessed. Often other studies can provide the necessary information. This is particularly true in the diagnostic evaluation of the azotemic patient in which ultrasonography usually provides all of the information needed to make important management decisions. (See discussion in Chapter 24.)

If, however, the indication for a diagnostic study using contrast material remains, hydration appropriate to the patient's general physical condition should be maintained. Bowel purges should be avoided, and only the meal immediately preceding the examination should be withheld. The dose of contrast material should be held to the minimum necessary to obtain the desired information. The specific amount will vary with conditions unique to each patient and cannot be strictly prescribed. Claims that low osmolality compounds reduce the prevalence of contrast material–induced nephropathy have not been unequivocally established (Schwab et al., 1989; Barrett et al., 1993.)

Although nephrotoxicity has been reported in patients exposed to a total dose of only 30 gm of iodine, most reported cases have been associated with at least twice that amount. Furthermore, diagnostic studies should be conducted and scheduled to avoid repeated exposure to contrast material without adequate intervals for observation and recovery. Two protocols for protection against contrast material–induced nephrotoxicity have been proposed. Both merit attention.

The first one consists of a prescribed amount of intravenous hydration for 12 hours before and during the examination, a moderate dose of contrast material, and mannitol infusion 60 minutes after exposure to the contrast material (Anto et al., 1981). The other protocol uses infusions of normal saline at a rate of 550 ml/hr during angiographic procedures (Eisenberg et al., 1981). Obviously, patients with medical conditions requiring a controlled fluid intake (congestive heart failure or cerebral edema) should not be subjected to these approaches without special consideration.

The removal of contrast material by natural excretory routes is slow in the patient with renal failure. Rapid removal may be desirable for patients with a serious adverse systemic reaction or nephrotoxicity. This can be done by either hemodialysis or peritoneal dialysis. After 12 hours of dialysis perfusion through a Kiil coil, 80 to 90 per cent of the contrast material is removed.

Clinical or laboratory evidence of contrast material nephrotoxicity may not become apparent in the first 24 hours after exposure. The serum creatinine level in some patients who develop this complication does not peak until 6 days after exposure. Detection requires careful surveillance of serum creatinine and urinary output during this period.

Cardiotoxicity. Contrast material can induce cardiac arrhythmias, conduction abnormalities, and myocardial ischemia. Patients at risk include those with pre-existing myocardial, atherosclerotic, or valvular disease and those with existing conduction disturbances. Major cardiac arrhythmias and ischemia have been noted in 18 per cent of patients with cardiac disease and in 5 per cent of healthy individuals with no history of heart disease who were exposed to contrast material during excretory urography (Pfister and Hutter, 1980). Arrhythmias occur more frequently than ischemia. Premature ventricular contraction is the most common cardiac arrhythmia induced by contrast material; ventricular tachycardia and fibrillation are the most severe. Atrioventricular block has also been observed. An increase in cardiac rate leading to an increased oxygen requirement is the likely basis for ST segment depression and symptoms of ischemia.

Many symptoms, such as chest pain, loss of consciousness, and cardiac arrest, traditionally have been classified as adverse systemic reactions to contrast material. In fact, these symptoms are likely manifestations of cardiotoxicity. Similarly, the mortality rate for contrast material usage, historically thought of as the result of idiosyncratic systemic reactions, is undoubtedly composed of a significant cardiotoxic element.

The pathogenesis of contrast material–induced cardiotoxicity has not been established. The sudden introduction of a hypertonic volume load, direct toxicity to the myocardium, and stimulation of neural reflex pathways have been suggested as causative factors.

Precautions. When contrast material is administered to a patient at risk for cardiotoxicity, a low osmolality compound should be used and a bolus injection avoided. This precaution reflects the likelihood that cardiac toxicity is related to hyperosmolality, time, and dosage factors. Injection rates of 1 ml/sec can reduce the incidence of cardiotoxicity, as will even slower infusions over a 10- to 15-minute period. Electrocardiographic monitoring during the examination may also be considered an adjunctive precaution in high-risk patients.

Excessive volume expansion in the newborn or infant is a risk when high osmolality contrast material is used. This cardiovascular complication can be essentially avoided by the use of low osmolality agents in an appropriate weight-adjusted dose, as previously discussed.

Pulmonary Toxicity. Subclinical bronchospasm, manifested by decreased forced expiratory flow rates, occurs frequently with exposure to contrast material in both normal and allergic patients. As yet it is unclear whether this reaction is caused by direct pulmonary toxicity or by the mechanisms that mediate idiosyncratic adverse systemic reactions. This phenomenon occurs more often with slow infusion of the meglumine salt than with bolus injection of the sodium salt. Neither an important clinical implication for this pulmonary reaction nor the effect of low osmolality contrast material has been established.

EXCRETORY UROGRAPHY

The goal of excretory urography, to obtain clinically useful information about the urinary tract and its related structures, requires that each examination be designed to meet unique needs. The elements that contribute to a successful study include an adequate dose of contrast material; a film to record the nephrogram; a sequence of films to assess the dynamics of urine formation and propulsion; adequate distention of the opacified pelvocalyceal system; use of oblique, prone, and upright positions; use of tomography; reinjection of contrast material, if needed; and minimization of risks to the patient. Some of these have already been discussed in the earlier sections on use of contrast material.

Film Sequence

A preliminary film is a fundamental part of an examination using contrast material. This film should be exposed after the patient voids. It is then evaluated by the radiologist for proper radiographic technique and patient positioning; the presence of radiodense structures in areas of the urinary tract that may subsequently be obscured by the excreted contrast material; and assessment of organ systems other than the urinary tract.

The exact number and type of preliminary films are determined by the patient's individual circumstances. A single film of the abdomen that includes the pubis bone (the "KUB") may suffice in some patients, whereas in others an additional film coned to the kidney is needed. A full set of tomograms may be of value in a patient suspected of having small kidney stones. When tomograms are anticipated, a single preliminary cut one-third of the anteroposterior diameter from the table top is useful to determine technique. Finally, an oblique preliminary film is essential for localization of radiodense structures that overlie the kidney (see discussion in Chapter 14). All exposures should be made after the patient fully exhales, to minimize the geometric distortion of the renal image that occurs when deep inspiration causes descent and ventral rotation of the lower poles of the kidneys.

It is of great practical advantage during excretory urography to obtain a film of the kidneys as soon as possible after the administration of contrast material, preferably at 1 minute when using a high osmolality compound and somewhat later when low osmolality contrast material has been injected. It is at this time that a relatively large amount of contrast material in the proximal tubules renders radiodense the entire renal parenchyma, causing the urographic nephrogram. This is the most opportune time for the evaluation of renal size, position, contour, and parenchymal integrity (Fig. 1–4). A tomogram at this time is often useful, too.

The number and sequence of films used in excretory urography, following injection of contrast material, must be individualized to each patient. A 5-minute film without compression provides useful information about the rate of urine formation. Oblique films, including those obtained with tomographic technique, may provide important evidence of contour abnormalities, deformities of the papillae or calyces, or abnormalities of the collecting system. Prone or upright films are of value in assessing obstruction. As described in Chapter 23, a sequence of films is needed for time–density analysis of the nephrogram and the dynamics of collecting system opacification. This is a useful exercise in elucidating certain renal abnormalities and a fundamental process in the diagnosis of obstructive uropathy. In some circumstances, such as preoperative screening of patients undergoing prostatic or gynecologic surgery, a single film exposed 8 to 10 minutes after injection of contrast material will suffice; the most useful information is derived from films obtained within the first 15 minutes after injection of contrast material. After this point, reinjection may be of value if a particular suspicion must be tested.

A complete routine for an excretory urographic examination would include the following:

- 1–3 minute anteroposterior (11 × 14-inch [28 × 35-cm] film)
- 5-minute anteroposterior (11 × 14-inch film)
- Apply ureteral compression
- 10-minute anteroposterior, right and left posterior oblique (11 × 14-inch film)
- Release compression
- Post-compression anteroposterior, right and left posterior oblique (14 × 17-inch [35 × 43-cm] film)
- Upright postvoid anteroposterior (14 × 17-inch film)

Adequate distention of the pelvocalyceal system is an essential component of the well-performed excretory urogram (Fig. 1–5). This is effected, in part, by the diuresis that is induced by contrast material, especially high osmolality compounds. Additionally, external compression of the ureter by two small inflatable rubber balloons is a simple and effective way of producing distention. The balloons are held in place by a plastic foam block and a band that passes around

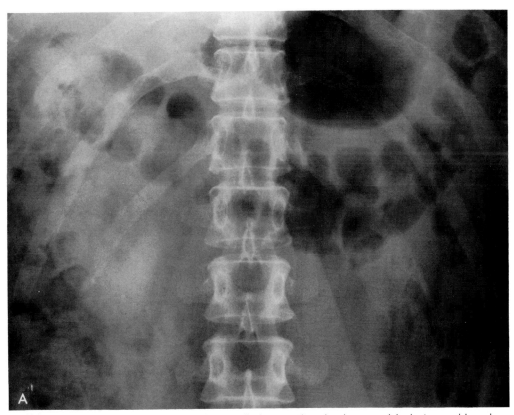

Figure 1–4. Emergency excretory urogram in a patient with acute flank pain. There has been no dehydration, and bowel preparation is poor. Sodium diatrizoate 50%, 1.0 ml/kg body weight.

A, Preliminary film.

Illustration continued on following page

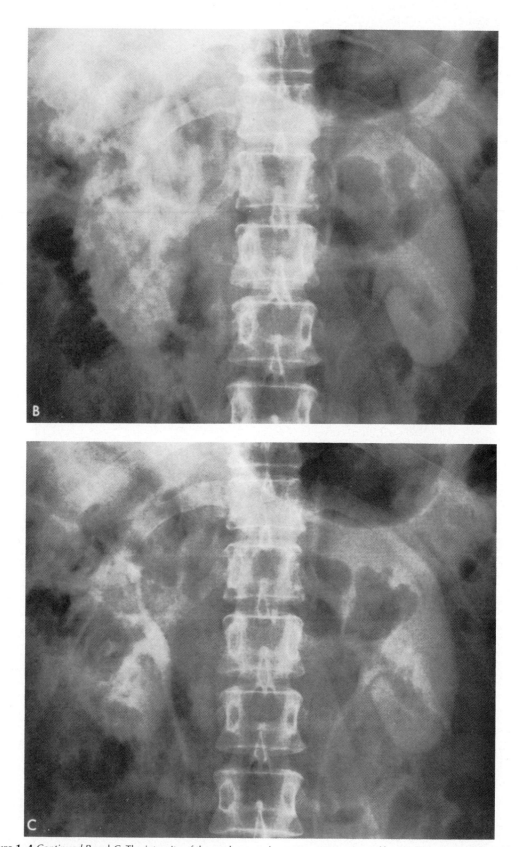

Figure 1–4 *Continued B* and *C,* The intensity of the nephrogram is greater on a 1-minute film *(B)* than on a 5-minute film *(C).*

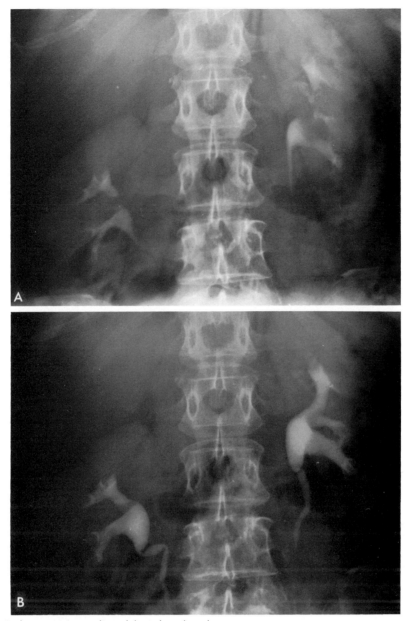

Figure 1–5. Value of abdominal compression to distend the pelvocalyceal systems.
  A, Five-minute film before application of compression device.
  B, Ten-minute film after 5 minutes of abdominal compression. Portions of the collecting systems that were collapsed on film shown in A are now distended.

the patient. The ureters are compressed at the point at which they pass over the sacral prominence. The most effective commercial devices are those that have two separate balloons that permit mobility, allowing the patient to be placed in an oblique position. External compression should be avoided in patients with recent abdominal or urinary tract surgery, ostomies, abdominal tumor, ureteral stone, or abdominal aortic aneurysm. A less effective method for producing distention is to tilt the head of the radiographic table down 10 to 15 degrees. Ureteral compression is of particular importance in patients given low osmolality contrast material to compensate for the low diuretic effect of these agents.

Value of Tomography. Tomography has been widely recognized as a valuable adjunct to excretory urographic diagnosis. Historically, a great body of literature has tended to categorize nephrotomography as something distinct from excretory urography. However, there is no need to view nephrotomography as a mysterious procedure, separate from routine excretory urography. Tomography during excretory urography should be applied whenever anatomic information is obscured, whether because of overlying bowel content (Fig. 1–6) or faint visualization in impaired renal function (Fig. 1–7) or simply to acquire better anatomic definition (Fig. 1–8). Tomography should be used the moment the need is determined.

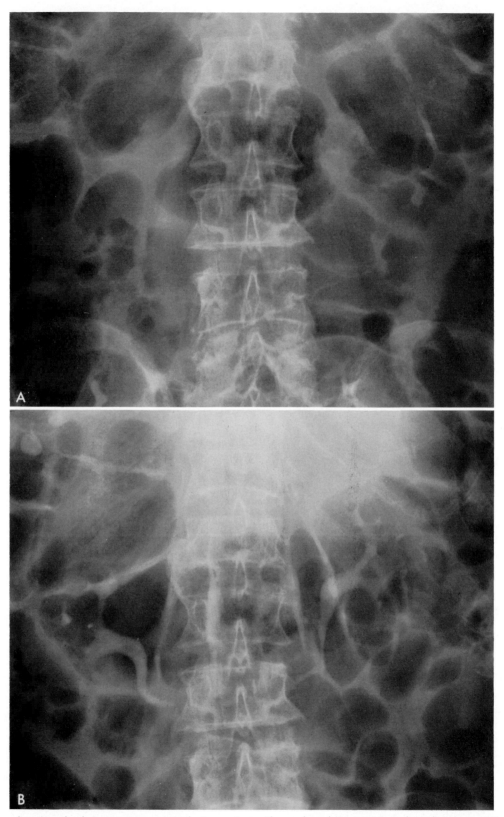

Figure 1–6. Value of tomography during excretory urography in a patient with poor bowel preparation. Sodium diatrizoate 50%, 1.0 ml/kg body weight.
  A, Preliminary film.
  B, Details of the kidneys on a 5-minute film are obscured by bowel gas.

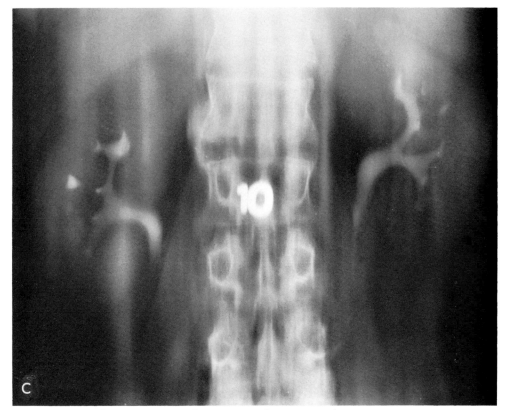

Figure 1–6 *Continued C,* Tomogram eliminates impediments seen in *B.*

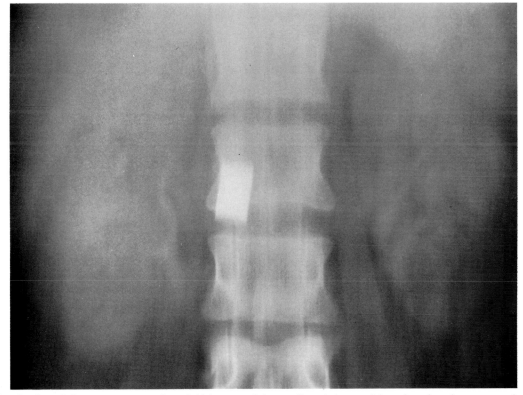

Figure 1–7. Details of renal size, contour, parenchymal thickness, and the nondistended state of the pelvocalyceal system are clearly defined by tomography in a patient with severe renal failure (serum creatinine = 11.5 mg/dl).

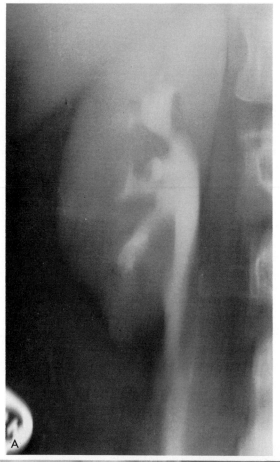

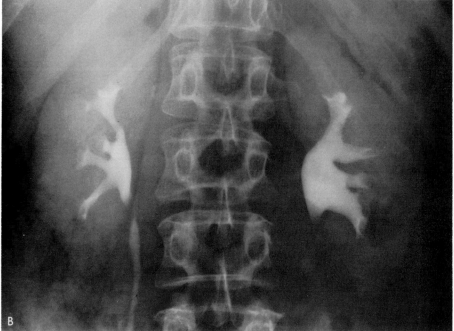

Figure 1–8. The use of tomography for improved detail is illustrated in a patient with a depression in renal contour of the right lower pole due to an old infarct.
A, Tomogram.
B, Standard film in which the deformity is not well defined.

To perform this study, exposure factors that allow discrimination of small differences in density must be chosen. Kilovoltage in the 60- to 75-kV range with a variable mAs is considered ideal. Arc may be varied from 10 to 50 degrees, depending on the desired thickness of the cut. Often it is valuable to inject additional contrast material immediately before the tomogram. Oblique projections are frequently helpful, and thick-section tomography (zonography) is often sufficient. Computed tomography–derived guidelines based on abdominal thickness are available for accurate determination of tomographic levels (Rhodes et al., 1987).

Diagnostic Value

Ultrasonography has supplanted excretory urography as the best diagnostic modality for the diagnosis of subacute or chronic obstruction; for assessing kidney size as an index of the acuity or chronicity in patients with renal failure (see discussion in Chapter 24); for evaluating patients with acute renal infections suspected to be associated with obstruction; and for preoperative assessment.

If ultrasonography or computed tomography is unavailable for the evaluation of the azotemic patient, excretory urography may be employed to assess renal size and the possibility of urinary tract obstruction. The efficacy of excretory urography for the evaluation of the azotemic patient was first suggested in 1963 by Schwartz and colleagues in a study of patients with renal failure in whom administration of a "double dose" (60 ml of 50% sodium diatrizoate) yielded useful diagnostic information without detectable deterioration in renal function. Since then, an extensive, carefully documented record has accumulated that verifies the diagnostic value of excretory urography in renal failure; but it also establishes significant associated risks, as described in the preceding section on nephrotoxicity of contrast material.

There is no level of renal function at which urography might not be useful. In fact, information of diagnostic and prognostic importance can be obtained in 90 per cent of patients with glomerular filtration rates below 15 ml/min as well as in anuric patients without measurable glomerular filtration (Van Waes, 1972). It is clear that the only prerequisite for successful excretion urography in the failing kidney is the presence of a blood supply to deliver contrast material to the remaining intact nephrons, an adequate dose of contrast material, impeccable radiographic technique, and strict precautions against dehydration. Significant diagnostic information under these circumstances may simply be limited to enough parenchymal opacification to visualize the kidney faintly or to identify one or more calyces. Often, knowing kidney size is enough to determine whether renal failure is chronic or acute; visualizing calyceal distention is often enough to determine whether renal failure is primary and nonobstructive or postrenal and obstructive.

To detect the very small amount of iodine filtered in profound nephron loss, technically superb radio-graphs must be exposed at an optimal time. The half-life of plasma iodine in the normal kidney is 30 to 60 minutes; in renal failure this value is prolonged to 20 to 40 hours or longer. The slow plasma loss of contrast material reflects whatever glomerular filtration remains and extrarenal excretion through the liver and the intestinal mucosa. Taking all these factors into consideration, the optimal time for obtaining films in patients with severe nonobstructive renal failure is generally within the first 20 minutes following injection. Some radiologists, however, have found the time of maximal opacification of the renal parenchyma in renal failure to be quite variable. In a study of 15 patients with terminal renal failure, maximal opacification occurred from 3 minutes to 32 hours after injection (Van Waes, 1972).

It has been suggested that in patients with renal failure, performing urography following dialysis gives greater diagnostic results. It was presumed that by diminishing the osmotic load of urea, the concentration of contrast material in the urine is increased. The practical usefulness of this approach has not been substantiated, however.

Whereas an adequate total dose in normal renal function is in the range of 15 to 25 gm of iodine, in renal failure urographic success requires roughly twice this dose. This can be reached by administering a dose schedule of 600 mg of iodine per kilogram of body weight. Most studies have employed between 35 and 45 gm of total iodine to opacify the failing kidney, although a few have used up to 70 gm of iodine. A dose schedule of 2 ml/kg of the commonly used urographic agents listed in Table 1–1 will produce these levels.

ULTRASONOGRAPHY

Real-time ultrasonographic imaging systems are used for examination of the kidneys and surrounding structures. Mechanical-sector or phased-array scanners have the particular advantage of being able to image through small acoustic windows such as the intercostal spaces.

A 3.5-MHz transducer is used most commonly for renal ultrasound examination. A 2.25-MHz transducer may be needed to examine very large patients, to avoid hypoechoic patterns in deeper portions of the kidney. Similarly, a higher-frequency transducer (5.0 MHz) is most valuable in studying very small patients, including infants and children.

One fundamental aspect in the assessment of the kidneys by ultrasonography is comparing the echogenicity of renal parenchyma with that of the liver and spleen. To make this analysis valid requires compensation for the exponential attenuation of sound as it penetrates the tissue. This is the function of the time–gain–control curve, which must be set to produce a uniform intensity of echoes throughout the entire thickness of the homogeneous reference tissue. For renal ultrasonography, the reference tissue is the liver. When the time–gain–control curve is properly set, the echogenicity of normal renal parenchyma should be equal to or less than that of the liver at equal depths from the transducer. This criterion maximizes the specificity of ultrasonography in the evaluation of patients for renal parenchymal disease though the sensitivity remains low. As a generality, then, renal parenchymal echogenicity greater than that of the liver reliably indicates renal disease, whereas that which is equal to or less than that of the liver does not. Comparison of relative renal-hepatic echo intensities may be distorted by the interposition of fluid (ascites or a cystic lesion) between the liver and kidney or by intrinsic alterations of hepatic echogenicity by diffuse liver disease.

Ultrasound examination of the kidney should be performed on hydrated patients with empty bladders. Some ultrasonographers claim that hydration enhances differentiation of the cortex from the medulla and will increase the likelihood of visualizing the pelvocalyceal system through diuresis. Additionally, a low-grade obstruction is more likely to be detected in a diuretic rather than antidiuretic state induced by dehydration. On the contrary, a full bladder may impede the flow of urine across the vesicoureteral junction and produce a false impression of obstruction.

The right kidney is best examined using the liver as an acoustic window. The patient is usually placed in a left posterior oblique or supine position. Longitudinal images are obtained along the anterior axillary line and transverse images are obtained along intercostal and subcostal spaces. Deep inspiration, to position the kidney below the ribs, is often a useful technique in examining the right kidney. Both longitudinal and transverse images are sequentially recorded in 1- to 2-cm steps until the entire kidney is included.

The left kidney is more difficult to examine than the right because the overlying contents of the gastrointestinal tract often block sound transmission. The most feasible acoustic approach to the left kidney is through the spleen. This requires putting the patient in a right side down decubitus position or a right anterior oblique prone position so the transducer can be placed over an intercostal space along the posterior axillary line. Deep inspiration is particularly valuable during imaging of the lower pole of the left kidney. The posterolateral approach to the left kidney results in coronal images.

Accurate measurement of renal length depends on obtaining an image that includes the extreme limits of both the upper and lower poles of the kidney on a single image. The complete examination of the kidney also includes examination in two projections at right angles to each other; evaluation of the vascular pedicle and inferior vena cava; and assessment of the contralateral kidney, the retroperitoneum, and the pelvic organs.

Some ultrasonographic evaluations require assessment of renal vessels with Doppler ultrasound. Duplex ultrasonography is especially useful in confirming flow within the renal veins or inferior vena cava. The Doppler cursor is placed within the vessel image,

and venous tracings are sought. Renal artery tracings are generally quite difficult to obtain. The cursor can be placed within the image of the renal parenchyma or renal masses for the purpose of determining vascularity. Color flow imaging greatly speeds evaluation by aiding in the detection of vessels.

COMPUTED TOMOGRAPHY

The kidney is composed of broad anterior and posterior halves, which because of their orientation in a coronal plane, cannot be completely visualized by standard radiographic techniques. The ability of computed tomography to reconstruct the anatomy of the kidney in the transverse plane overcomes this major limitation in uroradiologic diagnosis. This technique is also ideal for the study of the renal sinus and the retroperitoneum.

In addition, the superior density discrimination of computed tomography over standard radiography is particularly advantageous in assessing urolithiasis and nephrocalcinosis; in determining the nature of renal masses; and in diagnosing renal, subcapsular, and retroperitoneal hemorrhage. The enhanced density discrimination also makes computed tomography desirable for studying patients who should not be exposed to contrast material because of a high risk of adverse systemic reaction or those who can only tolerate a minimal dose of contrast material because of risk of nephrotoxicity.

The ability to derive information about renal perfusion and function from dynamic computed tomographic scanning is another distinct advantage of computed tomography over other diagnostic uroradiologic techniques. This technique can also be applied to study the vascular nature of a renal tumor.

The specific technique for performing computed tomography of the kidneys is determined in part by the characteristics of the available equipment. A standard examination should include contiguous sections of approximately 10-mm thickness and cover both poles of the kidneys. Most patients are examined with contrast material–enhanced tomography only. Pre–contrast material tomograms are essential only in assessing urolithiasis, nephrocalcinosis, calcified masses, hemorrhage, or in assessing enhancement of problematic renal masses.

Contrast material can be administered as a rapidly injected bolus or by slow infusion. The former is useful in distinguishing blood vessels from other soft tissue structures and in dynamic studies (Figs. 1–9 and 1–10). An average dose for bolus injection is 15 gm of iodine. This represents 50 ml of a contrast material solution containing 300 mg/ml of iodine. A standard infusion would deliver up to 30 gm of iodine over a 10-minute period. This amounts to 200 ml of a solution containing 150 mg/ml of iodine given at 20 ml/min. Administering contrast material orally is a useful technique when the bowel must be eliminated as a cause of confusing soft tissue structures. Ideally, oral contrast material should be given for a period

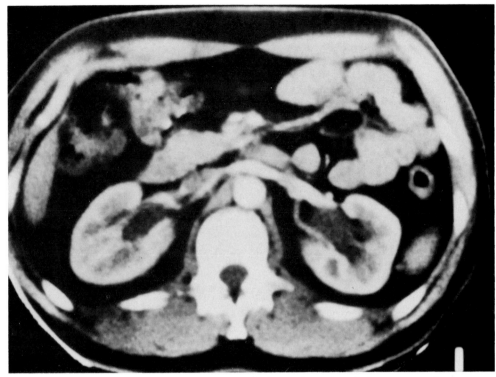

Figure 1–9. Computed tomogram with bolus injection of contrast material. The rapid injection of a large amount of contrast material renders major blood vessels opaque. The left renal veins are particularly well defined. (Courtesy of Robert Stanley, M.D., University of Alabama in Birmingham, Birmingham, Alabama.)

beginning several hours before the examination to ensure opacification of all portions of the intestine.

Two specialized computed tomographic techniques are dynamic scanning and multiformat reconstruction. Dynamic scanning is a rapid sequence of scans at a predetermined level (see Fig. 1–10). When the scanning sequence begins with a bolus injection of contrast material, sequential changes in attenuation values of the examined area permit identification of blood vessels, help characterize the vascular nature of tumors, and aid in assessment of corticomedullary perfusion and function. Multiformat reconstruction is a computational technique that reformats the image into coronal or sagittal planes.

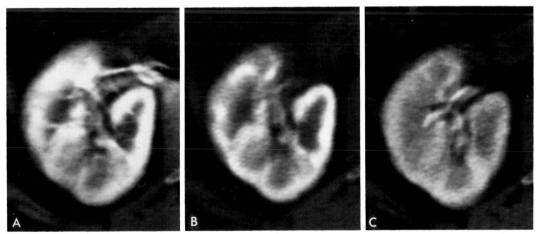

Figure 1–10. Computed tomogram with dynamic scanning. Contrast material has been injected through a catheter in the renal artery.
   A, Scan during arterial injection.
   B, Scan 4.8 seconds after *A.*
   C, Scan 9.6 seconds after *A.*
   The density of the cortex diminishes as the density of the medulla increases, reflecting transit of contrast material from the cortical microcirculation to the lumina of the proximal tubules.

MAGNETIC RESONANCE IMAGING

Peter L. Choyke

Magnetic resonance imaging of the kidney and retroperitoneum is a useful alternative to computed tomography in patients in whom the use of iodinated contrast material is contraindicated because of an increased risk of adverse reaction or nephrotoxicity and in patients in whom sagittal and coronal images might provide useful diagnostic information. Although each examination should be tailored to the patient's unique clinical problem, a renal magnetic resonance imaging study should include a T1- and T2-weighted spin-echo image in at least one plane and a T1-weighted image in at least one plane after contrast material enhancement.

Field strength is not a significant factor in obtaining good renal images, although larger fields do enable more flexibility in scan techniques. Image quality is very dependent on the motion compensation or suppression program of a particular magnetic resonance unit. T1-weighted (TR 300–500 msec; TE 5–20 msec) spin-echo images generally provide the highest quality images. Before contrast material enhancement the cortex is usually higher in signal intensity than the medulla (corticomedullary ratio = 1.2 to 1.5), depending on age and hydration status (Fig. 1–11*A*). Fat suppression, when available, should be employed since this improves the ability to detect renal lesions (see Fig. 1–11*B*). A T2-weighted (TR 1500–3000 msec; TE 60–120 msec) spin-echo image is usually obtained in the axial plane (see Fig. 1–11*C*). The medulla is slightly higher in signal intensity than the cortex, owing to its higher water content. This sequence permits evaluation of cystic and solid masses, although it alone cannot discriminate between these two. Magnetic resonance is limited in the urinary tract by an inability to detect calcifications and the nonspecificity of signal intensity. Fast spin-echo imaging may enable shorter scan times with equal or greater contrast compared with conventional T2-weighted images.

Gadolinium chelates are used as contrast material to evaluate masses considered indeterminate by other modalities or in place of iodinated contrast material when it is contraindicated. Gadopentate dimeglumine, gadoteridol, or gadodiamide (0.1 mmol/kg) can be either infused slowly and followed by conventional T1-weighted spin-echo images or delivered as a bolus with dynamic image acquisition (see Fig. 1–11*D*). The latter approach permits evaluation of the enhancement properties of a focal renal lesion or estimation of the degree of functional impairment associated with hydronephrosis or other parenchymal abnormalities. There are two types of dynamic images, the rapid spin echo and the rapid gradient echo. In the former, imaging time is decreased by shortening repetition times and halving the Fourier transformation. Even shorter repetition times are possible with dynamic gradient-echo images. In either case the images obtained after a bolus of contrast material are similar to those obtained with dynamic computed tomography (see Fig. 1–11*E*). Images are obtained during breath-holding. From one to five images can be obtained per breath depending on the length of each scan. Region of interest measurements from normal and abnormal segments are plotted as a function of time. With T2-weighted sequences, such as gradient-echo images with narrow flip angles (less than 30 degrees) and a long TE in relation to TR, renal parenchyma decreases in signal intensity with progressive renal concentration of contrast material. This enhancement pattern is more complex and susceptible to changes in relation to the patient's hydration status.

To evaluate the inferior vena cava for thrombus, thin, multiplanar T1-weighted images before and after contrast material administration are required. Orthogonal views are critical since the veins traverse several planes. If available, presaturation pulses should be utilized upstream to the area of interest to eliminate flow artifacts. Gradient-echo scans or "white blood" pulses are an alternative method of visualizing the veins.

Magnetic resonance imaging techniques continue to evolve. Faster imaging techniques such as echo planar imaging may be of particular importance in the abdomen where motion artifact can be "frozen" by images of 50 to 100 msec in duration. Magnetic resonance angiography has potential application for the noninvasive assessment of renal artery stenosis, for presurgical "road mapping," and for assessment of vascular malformations.

ANGIOGRAPHY

Angiography of the kidney is performed by the Seldinger technique. The reader may refer to standard sources for the basic principles and methodology of angiography. The discussion in this section is limited to aspects unique to renal arteriography and venography and applies to either film radiography or digital image recording.

Arteriography

A complete examination of the arterial supply to the kidney includes an aortogram and selective renal arteriograms of all renal arteries.

Aortography. For aortography, the distal curve and side hole placement of the catheter should be designed to promote mixture of contrast material with blood and to minimize the amount of contrast material flowing into the celiac and superior mesenteric arteries. A J-shaped or pigtail catheter with three or four side holes closely grouped 2 to 3 cm from the end of the straight limb meets this requirement (Fig. 1–12*C*). Many commercially available, preshaped catheters of different materials meet these specifications. The senior author's preference is for a thin-walled, opaque, polyethylene catheter (red Kifa) that has a 6.6 French outer diameter and is individually tapered, shaped, and perforated. This catheter accommodates guide wires up to 0.038 inch (0.97 mm) in diameter, depending on the taper. In straightening the

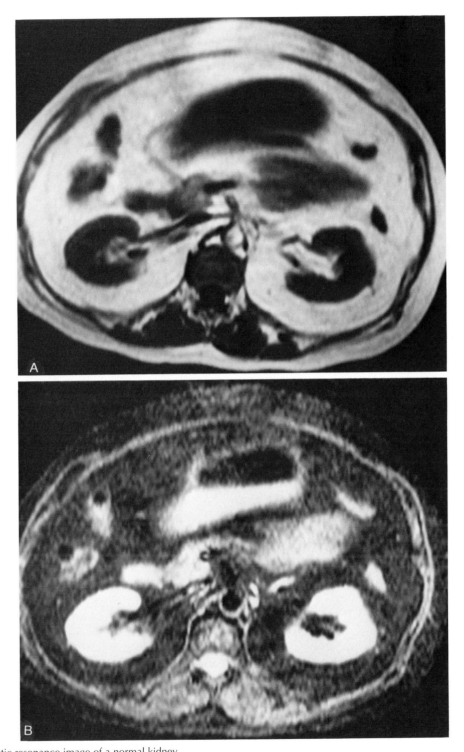

Figure 1–11. Magnetic resonance image of a normal kidney.
A, T1-weighted (TR 500 msec; TE 12 msec) image demonstrates low signal intensity medulla with slightly higher intensity cortex.
B, Fat-suppressed inversion recovery image (TR 1500 msec; T1 100 msec; TE 20 msec) demonstrates high signal intensity kidneys and absent signal from the retroperitoneal fat.

Illustration continued on following page

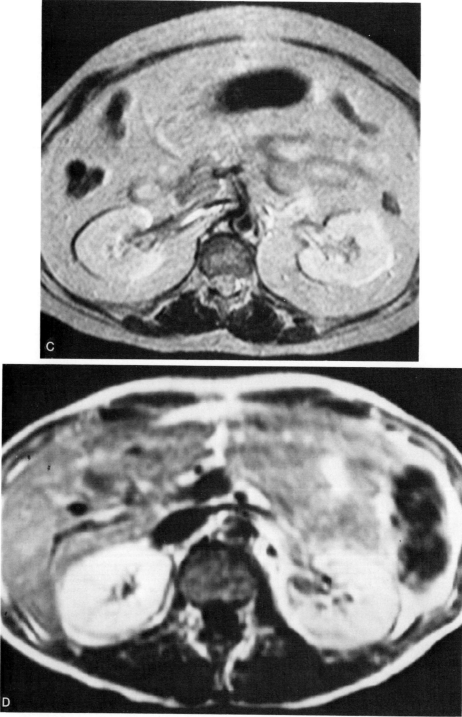

Figure 1–11 *Continued C,* T2-weighted (TR 2000 msec; TE 80 msec) image demonstrates high signal intensity within the kidneys and retroperitoneal fat.

D, Contrast-enhanced (gadopentate dimeglumine) T1-weighted image shows increased signal within the renal parenchyma and excretion of contrast material into the collecting system.

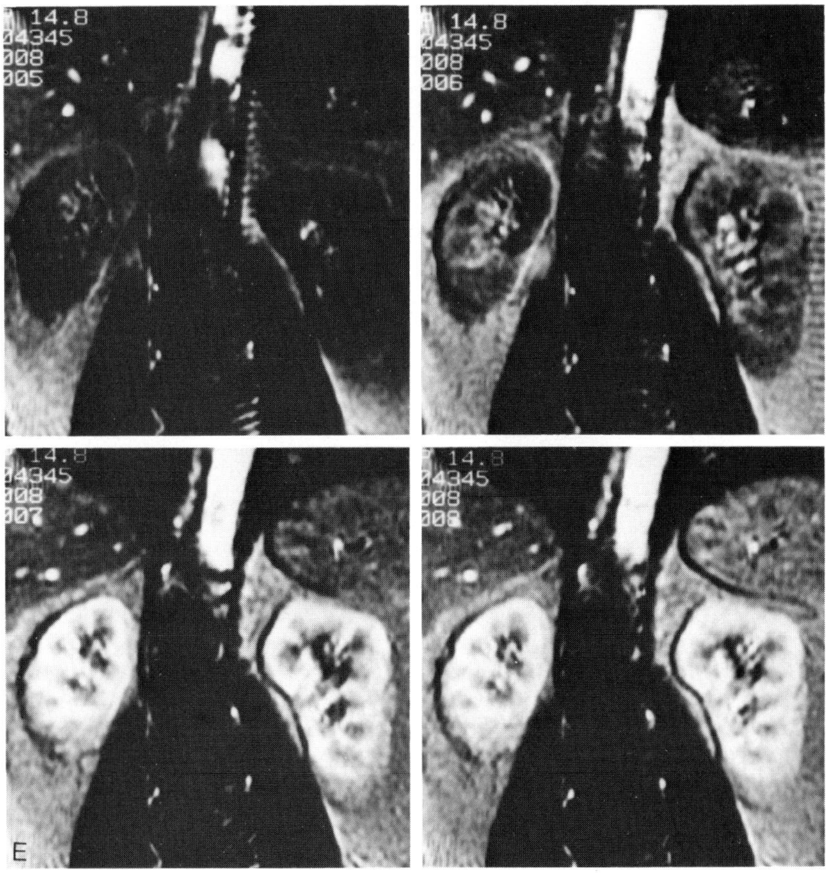

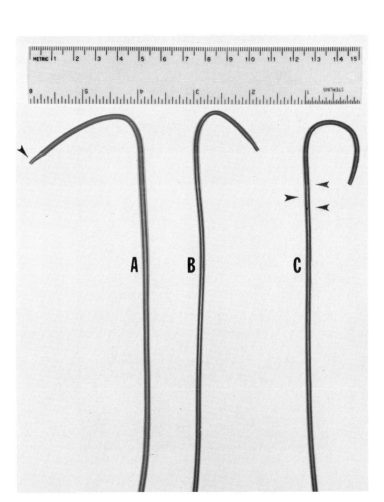

Figure 1–11 *Continued E,* Dynamic enhanced (GRASS TR 18 msec; TE 9 msec flip 60 degree) images with bolus of gadopentate dimeglumine. Images have been obtained every 2 seconds during breath-holding. Note progressive enhancement of the renal cortex on serial images.

(Kindly supplied by Peter Choyke, M.D., Department of Diagnostic Radiology, National Institutes of Health, Bethesda, Maryland.)

Figure 1–12. Catheters for renal angiography. (Arrows denote location of side holes.)
  A, Selective renal vein catheter.
  B, Selective renal artery catheter.
  C, Aortogram catheter.

catheter for introduction into the abdominal aorta, the primary curve may not re-form spontaneously when the guide wire is removed. This occurs particularly in individuals with a small-diameter aorta. In this circumstance, the curve can be reshaped by hooking its tip into any of the aortic branches, including the intercostal arteries in the distal thoracic aorta, while simultaneously advancing the catheter in a cephalic direction. Once the J shape is regained, the catheter is positioned so that the end and side holes are at the level of the most cephalic of the renal artery orifices (Fig. 1–13). This position is verified by a test injection of 5 to 10 ml of contrast material.

To perform an aortogram, contrast material is injected at 20 ml/sec for 2 seconds. A typical image sequence would be three images per second over a 3-second period and 1 image per second over a 4-second period. The initial study is usually done using the anteroposterior projection, but 20- to 30-degree posterior oblique sequences are often used, particularly when searching for stenotic lesions of the proximal renal arteries. It is often best to determine optimal oblique positioning by turning the patient under direct fluoroscopic observation. Careful coning of the recorded image to the margins of the kidneys greatly enhances diagnostic quality.

Selective Renal Arteriography. Selective arteriography is performed with a catheter shaped to conform to the renal artery. The senior author uses a catheter with only an end hole and made with the same polyethylene material and dimensions as the red Kifa aortogram catheter (see Fig. 1–12B). The orifice of the desired renal artery is searched for at the level of origin identified in an initial aortogram. If an aortogram is not done, most arteries can be located by moving the catheter up and down a segment of the aorta from the upper margin of L-1 to the lower margin of L-2. Often, continuous clockwise or counterclockwise torque must be applied to the catheter to keep the catheter tip pointing in a lateral direction. Insertion of the catheter into the renal artery is signaled by a sudden lateral movement of the catheter tip (Fig. 1–14). Injection of 2 to 3 ml of contrast material under fluoroscopic control verifies accurate positioning and ensures that the tip is not pointed into the arterial wall. This procedure may have to be repeated in kidneys with more than one renal artery.

The amount of contrast material used in selective renal arteriography depends on the size of the kidney and the renal blood flow. An average total dose is 10 ml administered over 1.5 seconds. This should be decreased in patients with low-flow states, as in chronic renal failure, and increased in those with high-flow states, as in vascular renal carcinoma or conditions with arteriovenous shunting. The rate of image recording varies with the state of renal blood flow. A sequence for average flow is four images per second over a 2-second period, two images per second over a 2-second period and one image per second over a 6-second period. Usually, an anteroposterior and posterior oblique projection are obtained for each kidney, but the actual approach is determined by individual

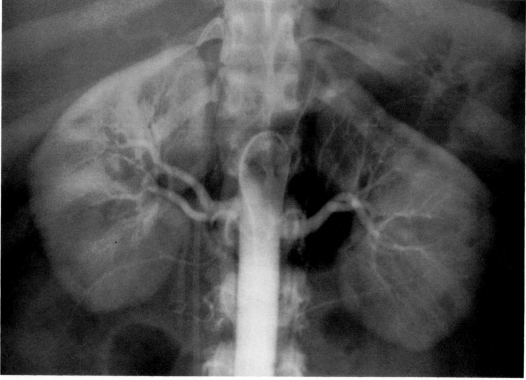

Figure 1–13. Aortogram for renal blood vessels. The J-shaped catheter illustrated in Figure 1–12C has been placed to direct the contrast material into the renal arteries and the distal aorta, thus avoiding opacification of the celiac and mesenteric arteries. The J-shape of the catheter has been distorted by the pressure of injection.

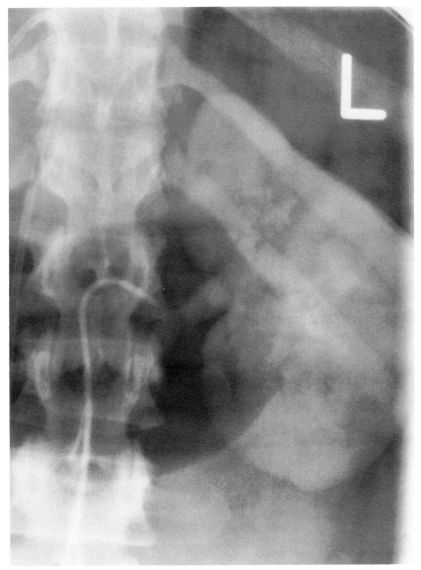

Figure 1–14. Catheter position for selective left renal arteriogram. The tip of the catheter projects lateral to the aorta. Note larger catheter in inferior vena cava.

circumstances. Again, the value of careful collimation for achieving superior quality images cannot be over-emphasized. Magnification and subtraction techniques may be employed to search for very small or obscured lesions (Fig. 1–15).

Venography

Inferior vena cavography should be performed before selective catheterization of the renal veins when venous thrombosis is suspected. Selective catheterization of the renal veins is best done with a catheter having good torque control, that is, one that is both larger and stiffer than those used for arterial studies. The senior author's preference is for a thin-walled, opaque, polyethylene catheter (green Kifa) with a 7.2 French outer diameter individually tapered over a 0.038-inch (0.97-mm) guide wire and shaped to conform to the length of the main renal vein (see Fig. 1–

12A). A single shape usually suffices for both veins. However, the left renal vein is much longer than the right, and a long-limbed catheter may be required in special circumstances. Two side holes may be placed just proximal to the tip of the catheter. A selective renal venogram is performed with contrast material injected at a rate of 10 ml/sec over a 3-second period. An image recording sequence of two images per second over a 5-second period is suitable for most circumstances. The examination is usually performed in the anteroposterior projection.

One impediment to satisfactory visualization of the renal veins is that blood flow from the kidney washes out the injected contrast material. Techniques to reduce this effect include reduction of renal blood flow by either performing the Valsalva maneuver or injecting epinephrine into the renal artery immediately before injecting contrast material into the renal vein, or by using balloon occluding selective catheters. Epi-

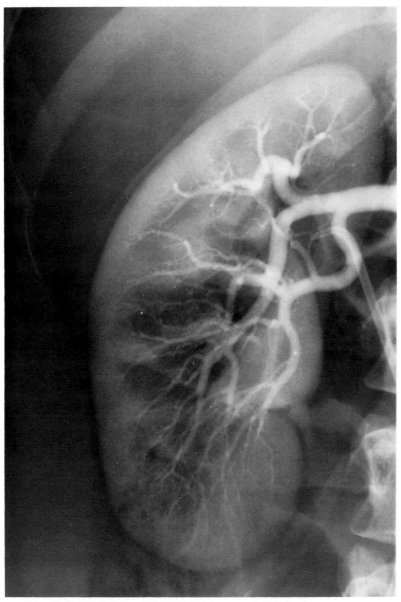

Figure 1–15. Selective right renal arteriogram magnified 1.5 times.

nephrine is given in a dose of 5 to 10 μg,* injected into the ipsilateral renal artery and followed in 10 to 20 seconds by a selective renal venogram.

Pharmacoangiography

Vasoconstrictive renal pharmacoangiography is rarely used in contemporary uroradiology. Historically, epinephrine-induced vasoconstrictive angiography was used to assess the nature of suspected neovascularity or as an adjunct to renal venography. Epinephrine is injected through a selective renal artery catheter in a dose of 5 to 10 μg.* The catheter is flushed with saline immediately after instilling the epinephrine, which is then followed by an injection of 5 to 10 ml of contrast material. A standard sequence is two images per second over 5 seconds. The normal renal arterial system constricts so that only the main renal artery and its major branches become opacified. Vasodilatory renal pharmacoangiography has not evolved into a useful diagnostic technique.

If during selective renal arteriography an excessive amount of contrast material is injected, the following protocol may be efficacious:

1. Immediately start an intravenous infusion of 5% dextrose in water and maintain it at 100 ml/hr over a 12-hour period.
2. Directly inject mannitol 10% in distilled water into the selective renal artery catheter at a rate of 10 ml/min over 5 minutes. Repeat one time if the nephrogram does not begin to diminish.
3. If the renal artery catheter is out, give 50 ml mannitol 10% intravenously at a rate of 10 ml/min. Repeat one time if nephrogram does not fade.
4. Maintain a strict intake–output record for 12 hours.

If the patient has cardiac failure or a history of cardiac failure, this protocol should be initiated but modified according to individual circumstances.

---

*Add 1.0 mg epinephrine to 500 ml normal saline. Each milliliter contains 2 μg epinephrine.

Bibliography

Contrast Material

Alexander, R. D., Berkes, S. L., and Abuelo, J. G.: Contrast media–induced oliguric renal failure. Arch. Intern. Med. 138:381, 1978.

Almén, T.: Development of nonionic contrast media. Invest. Radiol. 20(Suppl.):S2, 1985.

Andrews, E. J., Jr.: The vagus reaction as a possible cause of severe complications of radiological procedures. Radiology 121:1, 1976.

Ansari, Z., and Baldwin, D. S.: Acute renal failure due to radiocontrast agents. Nephron 17:28, 1976.

Ansell, G.: Adverse reactions to contrast agents: Scope of problems. Invest. Radiol. 5:374, 1970.

Ansell, G., Tweedie, M. C. K., West, C. R., Evans, P., and Couch, L.: The current status of reactions to intravenous contrast media. Invest. Radiol. 15(Suppl.):S32, 1980.

Anto, H. R., Shyan-Yih, C., Porush, J. G., and Shapiro, W. B.: Infusion intravenous pyelography and renal function: Effects of hypertonic mannitol in patients with chronic renal insufficiency. Arch. Intern. Med. 141:1652, 1981.

Assen, E. S. K., and Bray, K.: The release of histamine from human basophils by radiological contrast agents. Br. J. Radiol. 56:647, 1983.

Bahlmann, J., and Krüskemper, H. L.: The excretion of iodine-containing x-ray contrast material in patients on intermittent haemodialyses. In Proceedings, IV International Congress of Nephrology, Stockholm, 1969. Basel (Switzerland), Karger, 1970.

Baltzer, G., Kuni, H., Dombrowski, H., Köthe, E., Dölle, W., and Graul, E. H.: Investigations on renal function during and after intravenous administration of contrast media. Urol. Nephrol. 1:127, 1969.

Barrett, B. J., Parfrey, P. S., McDonald, J. R., Hefferton, D. M., Reddy, E. R., and McManamon, P. J.: Nonionic low-osmolality versus ionic high-osmolality contrast material for intravenous use in patients perceived to be at high risk: Randomized trial. Radiology 183:105, 1992.

Barrett, B. J., and Carlisle, E. J.: Metaanalysis of the relative nephrotoxicity of high- and low-osmolality iodinated contrast media. Radiology 188:171, 1993.

Bartley, O., Bengtsson, U., and Cederbom, G.: Renal function before and after urography and angiography with large doses of contrast media. Acta Radiol. (Diagn.) 8:9, 1969.

Becker, J. A., and Berdon, W. E.: Blood clearance of contrast material in patients with impaired renal function. Radiology 93:1301, 1969.

Becker, J. A.: Before and after dialysis urography. Radiology 109:271, 1973.

Bennett, W. M., Luft, F., and Porter, G. A.: Pathogenesis of renal failure due to aminoglycosides and contrast media used in roentgenography. Am. J. Med. 69:767, 1980.

Benness, G. T.: Urographic contrast agents: A comparison of sodium and methylglucamine salts. Clin. Radiol. 21:150, 1970.

Berdon, W. E., Baker, D. H., and Becker, J. A.: Danger of dehydration in pyelography. N. Engl. J. Med. 281:167, 1969.

Berg, G. R., Hutter, A. M., and Pfister, R. C.: Electrocardiographic abnormalities associated with intravenous urography. N. Engl. J. Med. 289:87, 1973.

Bettmann, M. A.: Clinical summary with conclusions: Ionic versus nonionic contrast agents and their effects on blood components. Invest. Radiol. 23(Suppl. 2):S378, 1988.

Bettmann, M. A.: Guidelines for use of low-osmolality contrast agents. Radiology 172:901, 1989.

Bettmann, M. A.: Ionic versus nonionic contrast agents for intravenous use: Are all the answers in? Radiology 175:616, 1990.

Brasch, R. C.: Allergic reactions to contrast media: Accumulated evidence. AJR 134:797, 1980.

Brennan, R. E., Rapoport, S., Weinberg, I., Pollack, H. M., and Curtis, J. A.: CT-determined canine kidney and urine iodine concentrations following intravenous administration of sodium diatrizoate, metrizamide, iopamidol and sodium ioxaglute. Invest. Radiol. 17:95, 1982.

Brezis, M., and Epstein, F. H.: A closer look at radiocontrast-induced nephropathy. N. Engl. J. Med. 320:179, 1989.

Brismar, J., Jacobsson, B. F., and Jorulf, H.: Miscellaneous adverse effects of low- versus high-osmolality contrast media: A study revised. Radiology 179:19, 1991.

Bush, W. H., and Swanson, D. P.: Acute reactions to intravascular contrast media: Types, risk factors, recognition, and specific treatment. AJR 157:1153, 1991.

Byrd, L., and Sherman, R. L.: Radiocontrast-induced acute renal failure: A clinical and pathophysiologic review. Medicine 58:270, 1979.

Caro, J. J., Trinade, E., and McGregor, M.: The risks of death and of severe nonfatal reactions with high- vs low-osmolality contrast media: A meta-analysis. AJR 156:825, 1991.

Carr, D. H.: Contrast media reactions: Experimental evidence against the allergy theory. Br. J. Radiol. 57:469, 1984.

Carr, D. H., Walker, A. C., and White, R. G.: Effects of radiographic contrast media on leukocyte locomotion. Invest. Radiol. 16:133, 1981.

Cattell, W. R., Fry, I. K., Spencer, A. G., and Purkiss, P.: Excretion urography: I. Factors determining the excretion of Hypaque. Br. J. Radiol. 40:561, 1967.

Cattell, W. R.: Excretory pathways for contrast media. Invest. Radiol. 5:473, 1970.

Cochran, S. T., Khodadoust, A., and Norman, A.: Cytogenetic effects of contrast material in patients undergoing excretory urography. Radiology 136:43, 1980.

Cochran, S. T., Wong, W. S., and Roe, D. J.: Predicting angiography-induced acute renal functional impairment: Clinical risk model. AJR 141:1027, 1983.

Cochran, S. T., Ballard, J. W., Katzberg, R. W., Barbaric, Z. L., Spataro, R., Iwamoto, K., and Lee, J. J.: Evaluation of iopamidol and diatrizoate in excretory urography: A double-blind study. AJR 151:523, 1988.

Cohan, R. H., and Dunnick, N. R.: Intravascular contrast media: Adverse reactions. AJR 149:665, 1987.

Cohen, M., Meyers, A. M., Milne, F. J., Disler, P. B., and Van Blerk, P. J. P.: Acute renal failure after use of radiographic contrast media. S. Afr. Med. J. 54:662, 1978.

Curry, N. S., Schabel, S. I., Reinheld, C. T., Henry, W. D., and Savoca, W. J.: Fatal reaction to intravenous nonionic contrast material. Radiology 178:361, 1991.

Cwynarski, M. T., and Saxton, H. M.: Urography in myelomatosis. Br. Med. J. 1:486, 1969.

Dacie, J. E., and Fry, I. K.: A comparison of sodium and methylglucamine diatrizoate in clinical urography. Br. J. Radiol. 44:51, 1971.

Dacie, J. E., and Fry, I. K.: Comparison of sodium and methylglucamine diatrizoate in high dose urography. Br. J. Radiol. 45:385, 1972.

Dahl, S. G., Linaker, O., Mellbye, Å., and Sveen, K.: Influence of the cation on the side effects of urographic contrast media. Acta Radiol. (Diagn.) 17:461, 1976.

Davidson, A. J., Becker, J., Rothfield, N., Unger, G., and Ploch, D.: An evaluation of the effects of high-dose urography on previously impaired renal and hepatic function in man. Radiology 97:249, 1970.

Davies, P., Roberts, M. B., and Roylance, J.: Acute reactions to urographic contrast media. Br. Med. J. 2:434, 1975.

Dawson, P.: Contrast media and enzyme inhibition: I. Cholinesterase. Br. J. Radiol. 56:653, 1983.

Dawson, P., Pitfield, J., and Britton, J.: Contrast media and bronchospasm: A study with iopamidol. Clin. Radiol. 34:227, 1983.

Dawson, P., Turner, M. W., Bradshaw, A., and Westaby, S.: Complement activation and generation of C3a anaphylatoxin by radiological contrast agents. Br. J. Radiol. 56:447, 1983.

Dawson, P.: Chemotoxicity of contrast media and clinical adverse effects: A review. Invest. Radiol. 20(Suppl.):S84, 1985.

Dean, P. B., and Kormano, M.: Intravenous bolus of 125I labelled meglumine diatrizoate: Early extravascular distribution. Acta Radiol. (Diagn.) 18:293, 1977.

Diaz-Buxo, J., Wagoner, R. D., Hattery, R. R., and Palumbo, P. J.: Acute renal failure after excretory urography in diabetic patients. Ann. Intern. Med. 83:155, 1975.

Eisenberg, R. I., Bank, W. O., and Hedgcock, M. W.: Renal failure after major angiography can be avoided with hydration. AJR 136:859, 1981.

Feldman, H. A., and McCurdy, D. K.: Recurrent radiographic dye induced acute renal failure. JAMA 229:72, 1974.

Fry, I. K., Cattell, W. R., Spencer, A. G., and Purkiss, P.: The relation between Hypaque excretion and the intravenous urogram. Br. J. Radiol. 40:572, 1967.

Gafter, V., Creter, D., Zevin, D., Catz, R., and Djaldetti, M.: Inhibition of platelet aggregation by contrast media. Radiology 132:341, 1979.

Gerstman, B. B.: Epidemiologic critique of the report on adverse reaction to ionic and nonionic media by the Japanese committee on the safety of contrast media. Radiology 178:787, 1991.

Goldstein, E. J., Feinfeld, D. A., Fleischner, G. M., and Elkin, M.: Enzymatic evidence of renal tubular damage following renal angiography. Radiology 121:617, 1976.

Golman, K., and Almén, T.: Contrast media–induced nephrotoxicity: Survey and present-state. Invest. Radiol. 20:592, 1985.

Gomes, A. S., Lois, J. F., Baker, J. D., McGlade, C. T., Bunnell, D. H., and Hartzman, S.: Acute renal dysfunction in high-risk patients after angiography: Comparison of ionic and nonionic contrast media. Radiology 170:65, 1985.

Greganti, M. A., and Flowers, W. M., Jr.: Acute pulmonary edema

after the intravenous administration of contrast media. Radiology 132:583, 1979.

Hansson, R., and Lindholm, T.: Elimination of Hypaque (sodium 3,5-diacetamido, 2,4,6-triiodobenzoate) and the effect of hemodialysis in anuria: A clinical study and an experimental investigation on rabbits. Acta Med. Scand. 174:611, 1963.

Harkonen, S., and Kjellstrand, C. M.: Exacerbation of diabetic renal failure following intravenous pyelography. Am. J. Med. 63:939, 1977.

Harkonen, S., and Kjellstrand, C. M.: Intravenous pyelography in nonuremic diabetic patients. Nephron 24:268, 1979.

Harkonen, S., and Kjellstrand, C. M.: Contrast nephropathy. Am. J. Nephrol. 1:69, 1981.

Hartman, G. W., Hattery, R. R., Witten, D. M., and Williamson, B., Jr.: Mortality during excretory urography: Mayo Clinic experience. AJR 139:919, 1982.

Heneghan, M.: Contrast-induced acute renal failure. AJR 131:1113, 1978.

Jensen, N., and Dorph, S.: Adverse reactions to urographic contrast medium: Rapid versus slow injection rate. Br. J. Radiol. 53:659, 1980.

Kappelman, N. B., Rosenfield, A. T., Putman, C. E., and Ulreich, S.: Electrocardiographic changes with intravenous pyelography in healthy individuals. Urology 9:88, 1977.

Katayama, H., Yamaguchi, K., Kozuka, T., Takashima, T., Seez, P., and Matsuura, K.: Adverse reactions to ionic and nonionic contrast media: A report from the Japanese committee on the safety of contrast media. Radiology 175:621, 1990.

Kaye, B., Howard, J., Foord, K. D., and Cumberland, D. C.: Comparison of the image quality of intravenous urograms using low-osmolar contrast media. Br. J. Radiol. 61:589, 1988.

Kelley, W. M.: Uricosuria and x-ray contrast agents. N. Engl. J. Med. 284:975, 1971.

Kelly, M., and Golman, K.: Metabolism of urographic contrast media. Invest. Radiol. 16:159, 1981.

Kennison, M. C., Powe, N. R., and Steinberg, E. P.: Results of randomized controlled trials of low- versus high-osmolality contrast media. Radiology 170:381, 1989.

Khoury, G. A., Hopper, J. C., Varghese, Z., Farrington, K., Dick, R., Irving, J. P., Sweny, P., Fernando, O. N., and Moorhead, J. F.: Nephrotoxicity of ionic and non-ionic contrast material in digital vascular imaging and selective renal arteriography. Br. J. Radiol. 56:631, 1983.

Knapp, M. S.: Renal failure after contrast radiography. Br. Med. J. 287:3, 1983.

Kormano, M.: Volume of distribution of contrast media in blood. Acta Radiol. (Diagn.) 20:33, 1979.

Kumar, S., Hull, J. D., Lathi, S., Cohen, A. J., and Pletka, P. G.: Low incidence of renal failure after angiography. Arch. Intern. Med. 141:1268, 1981.

Lang, E. K., Foreman, J., Schlegel, J. U., Leslie, C., List, A., and McCormick, P.: The incidence of contrast medium induced acute tubular necrosis following arteriography: A preliminary report. Radiology 138:203, 1981.

Lasser, E. C., Lang, J. H., and Zawadzki, Z. A.: Contrast media: Myeloma protein precipitates in urography. JAMA 198:945, 1966.

Lasser, E. C., Lang, J., Sovak, M., Kolb, W., Lyon, S., and Hamblin, A. E.: Steroids: Theoretical and experimental basis for utilization in prevention of contrast media reactions. Radiology 125:1, 1977.

Lasser, E. C., Slivka, J., Lang, J. H., Kolb, W. P., Lyon, S. G., Hamblin, A. E., and Nazareno, G.: Complement and coagulation: Causative considerations in contrast catastrophies. AJR 132:171, 1979.

Lasser, E. C., Lang, J. H., Hamblin, A. E., Lyon, S. G., and Howard, M.: Activation systems in contrast idiosyncracy. Invest. Radiol. 15(Suppl.):S2, 1980.

Lasser, E. C., Lang, J. H., Lyon, S. G., and Hamblin, A. E.: Changes in complement and coagulation factors in a patient suffering a severe anaphylactoid reaction to injected contrast material: Some considerations of pathogenesis. Invest. Radiol. 15(Suppl.): S6, 1980.

Lasser, E. C., Lang, J. H., Lyon, S. G., Hamblin, A. E., and Howard, M.: Glucocorticoid-induced elevations of CT-esterase inhibitor:

A mechanism for protection against lethal dose range contrast challenge in rabbits. Invest. Radiol. 16:20, 1981.

Lasser, E. C., Lang, J. H., Lyon, S. G., Hamblin, A. E., and Howard, M.: Prekallikrein-kallikrein conversion rate as predictor of contrast material catastrophes. Radiology 140:11, 1981.

Lasser, E. C., and Berry, C. C.: Pretreatment with corticosteroids to alleviate reactions to intravenous contrast material. N. Engl. J. Med. 317:845, 1987.

Lasser, E. C.: Pretreatment with corticosteroids to prevent reactions to IV contrast material: Overview and implications. AJR 150:257, 1988.

Lasser, E. C., and Berry, C. C.: Nonionic versus ionic contrast media: What do the data tell us? AJR 152:945, 1989.

Lawrence, V., Matthai, W., and Hartmaier, S.: Comparative safety of high-osmolality and low-osmolality radiographic contrast agents. Invest. Radiol. 27:1, 1992.

Lawton, G., Phillips, T., and Davies, R.: Alterations in heart rate and rhythm at urography with sodium diatrizoate. Acta Radiol. (Diagn.) 23:107, 1982.

Littner, M. R., Rosenfield, A. T., Ulreich, S., and Putman, C. E.: Evaluation of bronchospasm during excretory urography. Radiology 124:17, 1977.

Littner, M. R., Ulreich, S., Putman, C. E., Rosenfield, A. T., and Meadows, G.: Bronchospasm during excretory urography: Lack of specificity for the methylglucamine cation. AJR 137:477, 1981.

Longhran, C. F.: Clinical intravenous urography: Comparative trial of ioxoglate and iopamidol. Radiology 161:455, 1986.

Madowitz, J. S., and Schweiger, M. J.: Severe anaphylactoid reaction to radiographic contrast media. Recurrence despite premedication with diphenhydramine and prednisone. JAMA 241:2813, 1979.

Magill, H. L., Clarke, E. A., Fitch, S. J., Boulden, J. F., Ramirez, R., Siegle, R. L., and Somes, G. W.: Excretory urography with iohexal: Evaluation in children. Radiology 161:625, 1986.

McClennan, B. L.: Ionic versus nonionic contrast media: Safety, tolerance and rationale for use. Urol. Radiol. 11:200, 1989.

McClennan, B. L.: Low-osmolality contrast media: Premises and promises. Radiology 162:1, 1989.

Miller, D. L., Chang, R., Wells, W. T., Dowjat, B. A., Malinovsky, R. M., and Doppman, J. L.: Intravascular contrast media: Effect of dose on renal function. Radiology 167:607, 1988.

Milman, N., and Stage, P.: High dose urography in advanced renal failure: II. Influence on renal and hepatic function. Acta Radiol. (Diagn.) 15:104, 1974.

Milman, N., and Gottlieb, P.: Renal function after high-dose urography in patients with chronic renal insufficiency. Clin. Nephrol. 7:250, 1977.

Mindell, H. J., and Gibson, T. C.: ECG abnormalities during excretory urography: The effect of stress. AJR 150:1327, 1988.

Moore, R. D., Steinberg, E. P., Powe, N. R., Brinker, J. A., Fishman, E. K., Graziano, S., and Goplan, R.: Nephrotoxicity of high-osmolality versus low-osmolality contrast media: Randomized clinical trial. Radiology 182:649, 1992.

Moreau, J.-F., Droz, D., Sabto, J., Jungers, P., Kleinknecht, D., Hinglais, N., and Michel, J.-R.: Osmotic nephrosis induced by water-soluble triiodinated contrast media in man. Radiology 115:329, 1975.

Moreau, J.-F., Droz, D., Noel, L.-H., Leibowitch, J., Jungers, P., and Michel, J.-R.: Tubular nephrotoxicity of water-soluble iodinated contrast media. Invest. Radiol. 15(Suppl.):S54, 1980.

Mudge, G. H.: Nephrotoxicity of urographic radiocontrast drugs. Kidney Int. 18:540, 1980.

Mudge, G. H.: The maximal urinary concentration of diatrizoate. Invest. Radiol. 15(Suppl.):S67, 1980.

Myers, G. H., Jr., and Witten, D. M.: Acute renal failure after excretory urography in multiple myeloma. AJR 113:583, 1971.

Neoh, S. H., Sage, M. R., Willis, R. B., Roberts-Thomson, P., and Bradley, J.: The in vitro activation of complement by radiologic contrast materials and its inhibition with ε-aminocaproic acid. Invest. Radiol. 16:152, 1981.

O'Reilly, P. H., Jones, D. A., and Farah, N. B.: Measurement of the plasma clearance of urographic contrast media for the determination of glomerular filtration rate. J. Urol. 139:9, 1988.

Owens, A., and Ennis, M.: Arrhythmias occurring during intravenous urography. Clin. Radiol. 31:291, 1980.

Palmer, F. J.: The RACR survey of intravenous contrast media reactions final report. Australas. Radiol. 32:426, 1988.

Parfrey, P. S., Griffiths, S. M., Barrett, B. J., Paul, M. D., Genge, M., Withers, J., Farid, N., and McManamon, P. J.: Contrast material–induced renal failure in patients with diabetes mellitus, renal insufficiency or both: A prospective controlled study. N. Engl. J. Med. 320:143, 1989.

Pfister, R. C., and Hutter, A., M.: Cardiac alterations during intravenous urography. Invest. Radiol. 15(Suppl.):S239, 1980.

Pillay, V. K. G., Robbins, P. C., Schwartz, F. D., and Kark, R. M.: Acute renal failure following intravenous urography in patients with long-standing diabetes mellitus and azotemia. Radiology 95:633, 1970.

Postlethwaite, A. E., and Kelley, W. N.: Uricosuric effect of radiocontrast agents. A study in man of four commonly used preparations. Ann. Intern. Med. 74:845, 1971.

Powe, N. R.: Low- versus high-osmolality contrast media for intravenous use: A health care luxury or necessity? Radiology 183:21, 1992.

Purkiss, P., Lane, R. O., Cattell, W. R., Fry, I. K., and Spencer, A. G.: Estimation of sodium diatrizoate by absorption spectrophotometry. Invest. Radiol. 3:271, 1968.

Rahimi, A., Edmondson, R. P. S., and Jones, N. F.: Effect of radiocontrast media on kidneys of patients with renal disease. Br. Med. J. 282:1194, 1981.

Ramsay, A. W., Spector, M., Rodgers, A. L., Miller, R. L., and Knapp, D. R.: Crystalluria following excretory urography. Br. J. Urol. 54:341, 1982.

Rao, S. R., Mieza, M. A., and Leiter, E.: Renal failure in diabetes after intravenous urography. Urology 15:577, 1980.

Rapoport, S., Bookstein, J. J., Higgins, C. B., Carey, P. H., Sovak, M., and Lasser, E. C.: Experience with metrizamide in patients with previous severe anaphylactoid reactions to ionic contrast agents. Radiology 143:321, 1982.

Reich, N. E., Seidelmann, F. E., Lalli, A. P., Castle, L. W., and Alfidi, R. J.: Electrocardiographic changes during urography. Cleve. Clin. Q. 41:61, 1974.

Robinson, T., Waterhouse, K., and Becker, J. A.: Renal failure induced by contrast material. Urology 18:92, 1981.

Rosenfield, A. T., Littner, M. R., Ulreich, S., Farmer, W. C., and Putman, C. E.: Respiratory effects of excretory urography: A preliminary report. Invest. Radiol. 12:295, 1977.

Schrott, K. M., Behrends, B., Clauss, W., Kaufman, J., and Lehnert, J.: Iohexal in der Auscheidungsurographic: Ergelbnisse des Drug-monitoring. Fortschr. Med. 104:153, 1986.

Schwab, S. J., Hlatky, M. A., Pieper, K. S., Davidson, C. J., Morris, K. G., Skelton, T. N., and Bashore, T. M.: Contrast nephrotoxicity: A radiological controlled trial of a nonionic and an ionic radiographic contrast agent. N. Engl. J. Med. 320:149, 1989.

Shehadi, W. H., and Toniolo, G.: Adverse reactions to contrast media. Radiology 137:299, 1980.

Shehadi, W. H.: Contrast media adverse reactions: Occurrence, recurrence and distribution patterns. Radiology 143:11, 1982.

Sherwood, T., Breckenridge, A., Dollery, C. T., and Doyle, F. H.: Intravenous urography and renal function. Clin. Radiol. 19:296, 1968.

Shieh, S. D., Hirsch, S. R., Boghell, B. R., Pino, J. A., Alexander, L. J., Witten, D. M., and Friedman, E. A.: Low risk of contrast media-induced acute renal failure in nonazotemic type 2 diabetes mellitus. Kidney Int. 21:739, 1982.

Siegle, R. L., and Lieberman, P.: A review of untoward reactions to iodinated contrast material. J. Urol. 119:581, 1978.

Siegle, R. L., Lieberman, P., Jennings, B. R., and Rice, M. C.: Iodinated contrast material: Studies relating to complement activation, atopy, cellular association and antigenicity. Invest. Radiol. 15(Suppl.):S13, 1980.

Spataro, R. F.: Newer contrast agents for urography. Radiol. Clin. North Am. 22:365, 1984.

Spataro, R. F., Fischer, H. W., and Baylan, L.: Urography with low osmolality contrast media: Comparative urinary excretion of iopamidol, Hexabrix and diatrizoate. Invest. Radiol. 17:494, 1982.

Spataro, R. F., Katzberg, R. W., Fischer, H. W., and McMannis, M. J.: High-dose clinical urography with low-osmolality contrast agent Hexabrix: Comparison with conventional agent. Radiology 162:9, 1987.

Stadalnik, R., Davies, R., Vera, Z., Hilliard, G., and Da Silva, O.: Ventricular tachycardia during intravenous urography. JAMA 229:686, 1974.

Stadalnik, R., Vera, Z., Da Silva, O., Davies, R., Kraus, J. F., and Mason, D. T.: Electrocardiographic response to intravenous urography: Prospective evaluation of 275 patients. AJR 129:825, 1977.

Stanley, R. J., and Pfister, R. C.: Bradycardia and hypotension following use of intravenous contrast media. Radiology 121:5, 1976.

Swartz, R. D., Rubin, J. E., Leeming, B. W., and Silva, P.: Renal failure following major angiography. Am. J. Med. 65:31, 1978.

Talner, L. B.: Does hydration prevent contrast material renal injury? AJR 136:1021, 1981.

Tereul, J. L., Marcén, R., Onaíndía, J. M., Serrano, A., Quered, C., and Ortuño, J.: Renal function impairment caused by intravenous urography. Arch. Intern. Med. 141:1271, 1981.

Van Arsdel, P. P., Jr.: The complex world of adverse reactions. AJR 132:309, 1979.

Van Zee, B. E., Hoy, W. E., Talley, T. E., and Jaenike, J. R.: Renal injury associated with intravenous pyelography in nondiabetic and diabetic patients. Ann. Intern. Med. 88:51, 1978.

Vix, V. A.: Intravenous pyelography in multiple myeloma. Radiology 87:896, 1966.

Wagoner, R. D.: Acute renal failure associated with contrast agents. Arch. Intern. Med. 138:353, 1978.

Webb, J. A. W., Reznek, R. H., Cattell, W. R., and Fry, I. K.: Renal function after high dose urography in patients with renal failure. Br. J. Radiol. 54:479, 1981.

Weinrauch, L. A., Robertson, W. S., and D'Elia, J. A.: Contrast media–induced acute renal failure: Use of creatinine clearance to determine risk in elderly diabetic patients. JAMA 239:2018, 1978.

Wideröe, T.-E., Tetsche, K., Damgaard-Mörch, P., Jörstad, S., and Kemp, E.: Cellular and renal toxicity of a urographic contrast medium used in high concentration in uremic patients. Scand. J. Urol. Nephrol. 14:101, 1980.

Wilcox, J., Evill, C. A., Sage, M. R., and Benness, G. T.: Urographic excretion studies with nonionic contrast agents: Iopamidol vs iothalamate. Invest. Radiol. 18:207, 1983.

Wolf, G. L., Arenson, R. L., and Cross, A. P.: A prospective trial of ionic vs nonionic contrast agents in routine clinical practice: Comparison of adverse effects. AJR 152:939, 1989.

Yamaguchi, K., Katayama, H., Takashima, T., Kozuka, T., Seez, P., and Matsuura, K.: Prediction of severe adverse reactions to ionic and nonionic contrast media in Japan: Evaluation of pretesting. Radiology 178:363, 1991.

Zeman, R. K.: Disseminated intravascular coagulation following intravenous pyelography. Invest. Radiol. 12:203, 1977.

Techniques

Aronberg, D. J.: Techniques. In Lee, J. K., Sagel, S. S., and Stanley, R. J. (eds.): Computed Body Tomography. New York, Raven Press, 1983, pp. 9–36.

Becker, J. A.: The non-visualized kidney: The value of nephrotomography. Radiology 93:1301, 1969.

Benness, G. T., and Evill, C. A.: Urographic physiology and contrast materials. In Friedland, G. W., et al. (eds.): Uroradiology: An Integrated Approach. London, Churchill Livingstone, 1983, pp. 155–166.

Berdon, W. E.: Contemporary imaging approach to pediatric urologic problems. Radiol. Clin. North Am. 29:605, 1991.

Bernardino, M. E., and McClennan, B. L.: High dose urography: Incidence and relationship to spontaneous peripelvic extravasation. AJR 127:373, 1976.

Dixon, A. K., Webb, J. A. W., Cattell, W. R., and Fry, I. K.: The effect of DDAVP on intravenous urography. Br. J. Radiol. 54:484, 1981.

Doyle, F. H., Sherwood, T., Steiner, R. E., Breckenridge, A., and Dollery, C. T.: Large dose urography. Is there an optimum dose? Lancet 2:964, 1968.

Dunnick, N. R., and Korobkin, M.: Computed tomography of the kidney. Radiol. Clin. North Am. 22:297, 1984.

Engelstad, B. L., McClennan, B. L., Levitt, R. G., Stanley, R. J., and Sagel, S. S.: The role of pre-contrast images in computed tomography of the kidney. Radiology 136:153, 1980.

Ettinger, A., and Fainsinger, M. H.: Zonography in daily radiological practice. Radiology 87:82, 1966.

Evans, J. A., Dubilier, W., Jr., and Monteith, J. C.: Nephrotomography: A preliminary report. AJR 71:213, 1954.

Friedland, G. W., Gross, D., and Goris, M. L.: Intravenous urography (excretory urography) and excretion scintigraphy. In Friedland, G. W., et al. (eds.): Uroradiology: An Integrated Approach. London, Churchill Livingstone, 1983, pp. 201–232.

Fry, I. K., and Cattell, W. R.: Radiology in the diagnosis of renal failure. Br. Med. Bull. 27:148, 1971.

Fulton, R. E., Witten, D. M., and Wagoner, R. D.: Intravenous urography in renal insufficiency. AJR 106:623, 1969.

Hattery, R. R., Williamson, B., Jr., Hartman, G. W., LeRoy, A. J., and Witten, D. M.: Intravenous urographic technique. Radiology 167:593, 1988.

Lewis-Jones, H. G., Lamb, G. H. R., and Hughes, P. L.: Can ultrasound replace the intravenous urogram in preliminary investigation of renal tract disease: A prospective study. Br. J. Radiol. 62:977, 1989.

Mahalfy, R. G., Matheson, N. A., and Caridis, D. T.: Infusion pyelography in acute renal failure. Clin. Radiol. 20:320, 1969.

Matalon, R., and Eisinger, R. P.: Successful intravenous pyelography in advanced uremia: Visualization in the post-dialytic state. N. Engl. J. Med. 282:835, 1970.

Platt, J. F., Rubin, J. M., Bowerman, R. A., and Marn, C. S.: The inability to detect kidney disease on the basis of echogenicity. AJR 151:317, 1988.

Resnick, M. I., and Rifkin, M. D. (eds.): Ultrasonography of the Urinary Tract. 3rd ed., Baltimore, Williams & Wilkins, 1991.

Rhodes, R. A., Fried, A. M., Lorman, J. G., and Kryscio, R. J.: Tomographic levels for intravenous urography: CT-determined guidelines. Radiology 163:673, 1987.

Roberg-Wade, A. P., Hosking, D. H., MacEwan, D. W., and Ramsey, E. W.: The excretory urogram bowel preparation—Is it necessary? J. Urol. 140:1473, 1988.

Rosenfield, A. T., Rigsby, C. M., Burns, P. N., and Romero, R.: Ultrasonography of the urinary tract. In Pollack, H. M. (ed.): Clinical Urography. Philadelphia, W. B. Saunders Company, 1990, pp. 319–386.

Saxton, H. M.: Review article: Urography. Br. J. Radiol. 42:321, 1969.

Schenker, B.: Drip infusion pyelography: Indications and applications in urologic diagnosis. Radiology 83:12, 1964.

Schey, W. L., Shkolnik, A., White, H., and Finder, C.: Eight-minute excretory urography film: Once is enough. Urology 18:515, 1981.

Schwartz, W. B., Hurwit, A., and Ettinger, A.: Intravenous urography in the patient with renal insufficiency. N. Engl. J. Med. 269:277, 1963.

Stage, P., Milman, N., and Brix, F.: High-dose urography in advanced renal failure: I. Evaluation of diagnostic value. Acta Radiol. (Diagn.) 14:689, 1973.

Talner, L. B.: Urographic contrast media in uremia: Physiology and pharmacology. Radiol. Clin. North Am. 10:421, 1972.

Van Waes, P. F. G. M.: High Dose Urography in Oliguric and Anuric Patients. Amsterdam, Excerpta Medica, 1972.

Wells, P. N. T.: Doppler ultrasound in medical diagnosis. Br. J. Radiol. 62:399, 1989.

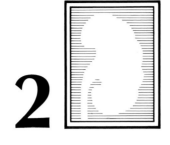

MIKE McBILES
EUGENE T. MORITA

2

RADIONUCLIDE IMAGING OF THE KIDNEY, URINARY TRACT, AND ADRENALS

When used to examine the kidneys, nuclear medicine techniques provide anatomic information as well as data on blood flow, nephron function, and urine drainage. These techniques are simple, safe, and rapid and expose the patient to minimal discomfort and levels of radiation. The discussion in this chapter focuses on the equipment and radiopharmaceuticals used in the various applications of nuclear medicine technology for the diagnosis of diseases of the urinary tract.

EQUIPMENT

Gamma camera and computer technology, especially the routine use of large field-of-view cameras (circular, rectangular, or square) and the growing use of single photon emission computerized tomography, allow the acquisition of high quality images and the rapid processing of dynamic functional data in renal scintigraphy.

The selection of the collimator used with a particular gamma camera is important and should be varied according to the isotope used and the nature of the information desired. Most collimator designs make some compromise between sensitivity and resolution. The energy of technetium (^{99m}Tc) at the usual dose allows relatively high sensitivity and resolution with an all-purpose collimator. Heavier and thicker collimators with reduced sensitivity and resolution are required for the high energy photons emitted from iodine 131 (^{131}I), gallium 67 citrate (^{67}Ga), and indium 111 (^{111}In). Parenchymal detail is best resolved in static

imaging by using pinhole collimation. However, this entails a marked loss of sensitivity. Converging collimators, on the other hand, offer an acceptable compromise by giving both improved resolution and sensitivity over parallel hole collimators and substantially better sensitivity than pinhole collimators.

Current single photon emission computed tomography systems also allow rapid acquisition and processing of three-dimensional images. These can be useful in specific situations when accurate spatial localization is important, such as in dual radiopharmaceutical studies using dimercaptosuccinic acid and ^{111}In-labeled white blood cells.

Computers interfaced with a gamma camera permit analysis of blood flow and kidney function data. Quantification of static images through selection of background correction and region-of-interest manipulation, permanent storage of digital data for quantitative analysis of serial studies, and the ability to rapidly analyze time–activity curves are essential properties of modern digital computer systems.

RADIOPHARMACEUTICALS AND STANDARD PROCEDURES

Radiopharmaceuticals labeled with ^{99m}Tc or iodine (^{131}I or ^{123}I) are most often used to evaluate the kidneys. Sodium hippurate (Hippuran) labeled with ^{123}I, although it has excellent physical characteristics, is expensive and not commonly available. Two additional radiopharmaceuticals, gallium (^{67}Ga) and indium (^{111}In), have applications in the examination of the urinary tract. Gallium 67 is used to evaluate possible infection, inflammation, and neoplasia. Indium 111–labeled white blood cells are useful in the investigation of acute infection.

Technetium-Labeled Compounds

Radiopharmaceuticals labeled with ^{99m}Tc are used to study both renal function and anatomy. This radionuclide's primary gamma photon energy of 140 keV provides an ideal combination of sensitivity and resolution when used with modern gamma camera systems. In most studies, the relatively short physical half-life of 6 hours and the lack of significant amounts of particulate energies, such as beta particles, permit a dose that allows rapid acquisition of high count density and good diagnostic images.

The selection of a particular agent labeled with ^{99m}Tc is determined by the diagnostic information that is required. Some agents best evaluate glomerular or tubular clearance rates, others that are cleared relatively quickly allow data collection about blood flow and parenchymal or collecting system clearance rates, while still others are best for anatomic detail because of their ability to bind to renal tubules. ^{99m}Tc-labeled radiopharmaceuticals that are used for nonrenal studies (pertechnetate and diphosphonates) provide incidental information about the urinary tract because of their vascular flow to and excretion by the kidneys.

Technetium 99m–labeled diethylenetriaminepentacetic acid (^{99m}Tc-DTPA) is excreted by the kidneys through glomerular filtration. Up to 95 per cent is cleared from the blood within 6 hours in patients with normal renal function. There is a close positive correlation between the clearance rate of ^{99m}Tc-DTPA and other measures of glomerular filtration, such as creatinine or inulin. Rapid kidney clearance allows for favorable dosimetry when 370 to 740 megabecquerels (MBq) (10 to 20 millicuries [mCi]) of ^{99m}Tc are given. This dose permits the collection of count rates sufficient to assess blood flow to each kidney during the first minute after injection (Fig. 2–1).

Clearance data for each kidney can be derived by computer processing of multiple sequential images obtained over 20 to 30 minutes after injection. With the use of time–activity curves derived from regions of interest drawn around each kidney, differential glomerular function can be determined by the per cent relative accumulation of ^{99m}Tc-DTPA in each kidney during the 1- through 3-minute period after injection when the radiopharmaceutical transits through the renal cortex. The normal differential function value is 50 ± 5 per cent. Differential function is valuable in the determination of kidney salvagability in chronic conditions and in the evaluation of an acutely damaged kidney for improvement or deterioration over time.

The time of radiopharmaceutical arrival to maximal kidney activity, which corresponds roughly to cortical transit time, can be used as a measure of absolute kidney function. Similar information can be derived from measurement of the slope of the rising activity curve. Measurement of the speed of renal clearance can be helpful in evaluating both kidney function and possible obstruction. A commonly used parameter is half-time, defined as the time in which one-half maximum activity remains in the kidney.

Technetium 99m–labeled glucoheptonate (^{99m}Tc-GHA) is cleared from the circulation more rapidly than ^{99m}Tc-DTPA. Approximately 20 per cent of this compound becomes fixed to the proximal tubules, a fact that precludes its use in estimating glomerular filtration rate. However, the usual dose of 370 to 740 MBq (10 to 20 mCi) permits adequate determination of blood flow as well as the functional parameters described previously for ^{99m}Tc-DTPA. Additionally, the delay in excretion of this agent permits recording of static images of the renal parenchyma for 2 to 4 hours after injection. Differential function can be measured either during the 1- to 3-minute period after injection or by analysis of delayed images acquired several hours later. When using delayed images, however, the collecting system should be free of activity to avoid error from its inclusion in the region of interest. In patients with impaired renal function, static images can be obtained for up to 24 hours after injection. Normally, enough ^{99m}Tc-GHA is excreted by the kidney to provide useful information on drainage of the collecting systems and ureters. However, with reduced renal function, ^{99m}Tc-GHA is cleared by the liver through biliary excretion as an alternative pathway. This may cause activity in the gallbladder and bowel loops to obscure kidney patterns (Fig. 2–2). Despite these drawbacks, ^{99m}Tc-GHA yields comprehensive information about blood flow, nephron function, anatomy, and urine drainage. It is often used as an excellent all-purpose agent for renal surveys.

Technetium 99m–labeled dimercaptosuccinic acid (^{99m}Tc-DMSA) is used as a parenchymal imaging agent. Approximately 50 per cent of the intravenous dose of 185 MBq (5 mCi) becomes firmly bound to the proximal tubules within 2 to 3 hours after injection. The net accumulated activity in each kidney is an estimate of vascular flow and tubule mass. ^{99m}Tc-DMSA differs from ^{99m}Tc-GHA in that only 5 to 7 per cent is excreted into the urine by glomerular filtration. This alleviates the problem of radioactivity in the collecting system erroneously affecting measurement of differential function. Because of the small dose required with ^{99m}Tc-DMSA, adequate blood flow measurements cannot be obtained. Despite additional drawbacks of *in vitro* instability, which requires injection within 30 minutes of compounding, and relatively high cost, ^{99m}Tc-DMSA is the preferred agent for parenchymal imaging. This is especially true for infants and newborns, whose immature kidneys may not accumulate sufficient amounts of ^{99m}Tc-GHA for adequate imaging.

Technetium 99m–labeled mercaptoacetylglycineglycineglycine (^{99m}Tc-MAG$_3$) is rapidly cleared by both glomerular filtration and tubule secretion. Rapid clearance allows injection doses of 370 MBq (10 mCi). The simi-

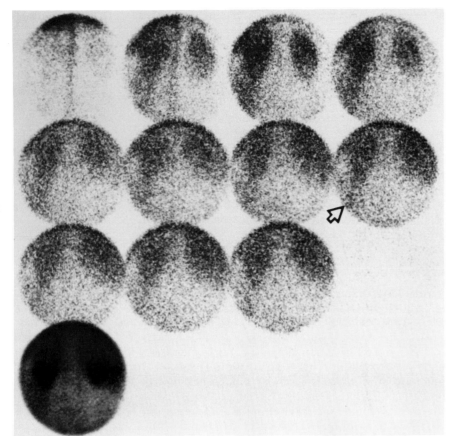

Figure 2–1. Vascular flow study showing good renal concentration immediately after aortic flow. Note the added vascular blush pattern from abdominal contents below the left kidney *(arrow).*

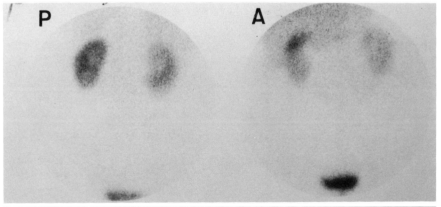

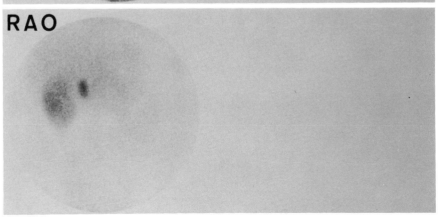

Figure 2–2. ^{99m}Tc-GHA images 40 minutes after injection in a patient with renal failure. Liver excretion and gallbladder concentration may confuse data from the right kidney. Posterior (P), anterior (A), and right anterior oblique (RAO) projections.

larity of the clearance kinetics of ^{99m}Tc-MAG$_3$ to ^{131}I-Hippuran combined with the superior imaging properties of ^{99m}Tc make it a very useful agent for the study of both blood flow and function (Fig. 2–3). Measurement of effective renal plasma flow with ^{99m}Tc-MAG$_3$ is closely correlated with that derived with ^{131}I-Hippuran. Although the values are not identical, they are proportional at all levels of renal function. The difference in the values is in part related to the higher degree of protein binding with ^{99m}Tc-MAG$_3$ and their different volumes of distribution.

Pertechnetate and ^{99m}Tc sulfur colloid are both routinely used for bladder studies, including voiding studies for reflux. Neither is absorbed by bladder epithelium. The usual dose is 37 MBq (1 mCi) instilled intravesically.

Iodine-Labeled Compounds

Iodine 131 is the most readily available radionuclide to label sodium hippurate (Hippuran) and the adrenal radiopharmaceuticals. However, ^{131}I has limitations in allowable dosage because of its long physical half-life of 8.1 days and its combination of gamma and particulate beta radiation. This is especially relevant when retention in the kidney is prolonged, as in acute tubular necrosis. Further, its primary gamma energy (364 keV) is above the level of optimal counting efficiency for most gamma cameras. ^{131}I also requires high

energy collimation, which markedly diminishes spatial resolution. Even small amounts of noncomplexed free iodine can subject the thyroid to large radiation doses, and pretreatment with Lugol's solution or supersaturated potassium iodide is mandatory. Iodine 123 is more desirable than ^{131}I because of its short physical half-life (13 hours) and primary gamma energy (159 keV), but it is very expensive and not readily available.

^{131}I-Hippuran is a low-cost, widely available radiopharmaceutical that is particularly useful in the evaluation of urinary tract outflow obstruction, renal failure, and unilateral renal artery occlusion, and in assessing the functional integrity of transplanted kidneys. ^{131}I-Hippuran, which is administered in a dose of 3.7 to 11.3 MBq (100 to 300 mCi), is particularly useful for measuring total and individual renal function because it is efficiently cleared by both glomerular filtration (20 per cent) and tubule secretion (80 per cent). Additionally, the rapid clearance of ^{131}I-Hippuran provides an excellent ratio of target to background activity. Measurement of the clearance of this radiopharmaceutical permits derivation of values for effective renal plasma flow in a manner similar to that used for ^{99m}Tc-DTPA and ^{99m}Tc-MAG$_3$.

Iodine 123– and Iodine 131–labeled metaiodobenzylguanidine (MIBG) and *iodine 131–labeled 6-beta-iodomethylnorcholesterol (NP-59)* are functional adrenal imaging agents. The protocol for these agents is dependent on

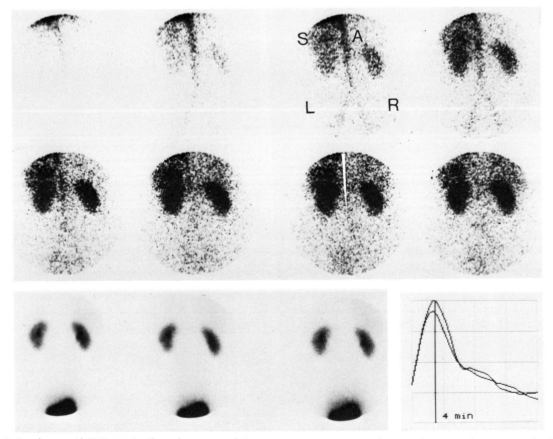

Figure 2–3. Renal scan with ^{99m}Tc-MAG$_3$. Flow, clearance, and time–activity curves are normal. Note spleen (S) and aorta (A) in the flow study.

the adrenal abnormality under investigation and often requires imaging over multiple days for the ^{131}I compounds. The usual dose is 37 to 74 MBq (1 to 2 mCi) for both ^{131}I radiopharmaceuticals. For ^{123}I-MIBG, 185 to 370 MBq (5 to 10 mCi) is used. High count anterior and posterior static adrenal images at 24 hours after injection are usually the only studies obtained. Quantification of relative adrenal activity can be performed.

Gallium- and Indium-Labeled Compounds

Gallium 67 citrate is useful in evaluating infectious and neoplastic processes in the kidneys and perinephric spaces. This radiopharmaceutical has three principal gamma emission energies (93, 184, and 296 keV) and a physical half-life of 78 hours. These physical characteristics both limit the acceptable injected dose to a range of 165 to 370 MBq (5 to 10 mCi) and impair resolution with most detecting systems because of the need for medium to high energy collimation. These disadvantages, as well as the frequent requirement for multiple-day imaging because of obscuring activity excreted into the bowel, are offset by the low radiopharmaceutical cost and an extensive experience of clinical utility.

Indium-111–labeled white blood cells are a highly sensitive and specific combination for the detection of focal inflammatory processes (Fig. 2–4). The half-life of [111]In (68 hours) and its emission energies (171 and 245 keV) are similar to those of [67]Ga. Images are obtained 18 to 24 hours after injection of 11.3 to 16.5 MBq (300 to 500 uCi). The problem of bowel activity seen with ^{67}Ga is not apparent, and the kidneys can readily be separated from expected normal white blood cell accumulations in the liver, spleen, and bone marrow. Disadvantages in the use of ^{111}In-labeled white blood cells include the tediousness and expense of the process of labeling indium to autologous white blood cells and the exposure of the technologist to the risks of blood products.

CLINICAL APPLICATIONS

Acute Renal Failure

Radionuclide imaging is often a useful adjunct to clinical evaluation and laboratory testing in the assessment of the acutely anuric and/or azotemic patient. As described in Chapter 24, prerenal and postrenal etiologies must be excluded. Here, radionuclide imaging can be applied for the documentation of both arterial inflow and urine outflow disorders. These are discussed in sections that follow. This section describes the use of radionuclide imaging in the detection of renal parenchymal causes of acute renal failure.

As stressed throughout this text, kidney size is often a valuable indicator of renal disease. Although ultrasonography is the most efficacious modality for determination of kidney size, a reasonable estimate can be obtained during a radionuclide examination by comparing the size of the kidney image with cali-

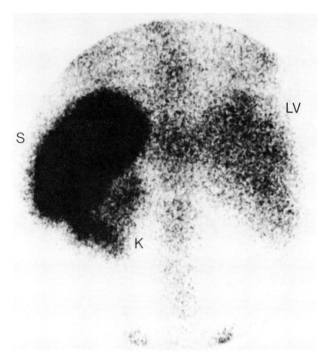

Figure 2–4. Acute left pyelonephritis studied with ^{111}In-labeled white blood cells. There is intense and diffuse uptake of radionuclide by the left kidney (K) on this posterior view of the abdomen. Note the normal activity in the spleen (S) and liver (LV).

brated markers placed on the camera. Several views may be required. Single photon emission computed tomography imaging using parenchymal agents also permits measurement of renal size. In severe renal failure, glomerular filtration of ^{99m}Tc-DTPA may be so deficient that adequate studies are not achievable. In this circumstance, delayed images using ^{99m}Tc-labeled parenchymal agents or dynamic images that take advantage of the efficient extraction of agents secreted by the tubules may better delineate the kidneys.

In patients with acute tubular necrosis there is rapid parenchymal accumulation without evidence of significant excretion of ^{99m}Tc-MAG$_3$ or ^{131}I-Hippuran (Fig. 2–5). Normal arterial blood flow but deficient accumulation and excretion is demonstrated with ^{99m}Tc-DTPA. This discordance is quite specific for acute tubular necrosis. If renal function progressively deteriorates, flow may remain close to normal while parenchymal accumulation of tubule binding agents progressively diminishes. Restoration of uptake constitutes a favorable prognostic sign of functional recovery.

Urinary Tract Obstruction

Because radiopharmaceuticals such as ^{99m}Tc-DTPA, ^{99m}Tc-MAG$_3$ and ^{131}I-Hippuran are cleared rapidly through the kidneys, they are useful for the detection of both acute and chronic urinary tract obstruction. Additionally, these agents also measure differential function, which is an important factor in both determining stability over time of a partially obstructed

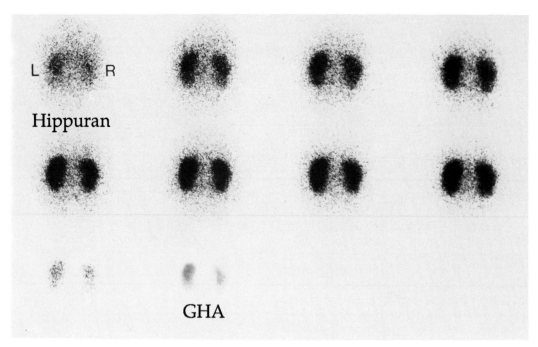

Figure 2–5. Acute tubular necrosis. The ^{131}I-Hippuran scan, represented by images in the upper two rows, demonstrates rapid parenchymal accumulation and no excretion of the radionuclide. The lower row depicts images from a study done with ^{99m}Tc-GHA in the same patient. There is minimal uptake and no excretion. (Courtesy of Mailine Chew, M.D., Ralph K. Davies Medical Center, San Francisco, California.)

kidney or predicting salvageability of a severely obstructed kidney. Patients undergoing radionuclide evaluation for obstruction must be adequately hydrated to avoid a false-positive result that can accompany dehydration.

^{99m}Tc-DTPA images interpreted in conjunction with the finding of an opaque calculus in the region of the urinary tract on a standard radiograph of the abdomen can be used to determine both the presence and the site of an acute obstruction. The absence of activity in the renal pelvis on the symptomatic side at a time when the contralateral side is detected is known as the "empty pelvis" sign. Although this is an indicator of acute obstruction, other etiologies can cause the same finding, as discussed in the section on acute urinary tract obstruction in Chapter 9. Rising time–activity curves with furosemide renography, as described later in the discussion on chronic obstruction, can also be found in acute obstruction (Fig. 2–6).

Renal imaging with ^{99m}Tc-DTPA, ^{99m}Tc-MAG₃, and ^{131}I-Hippuran reliably detects unilateral or bilateral chronic urinary tract obstruction by virtue of the findings of a dilated pelvocalyceal system and/or ureter with delayed drainage. When these findings are equivocal, the routine renal study can be augmented by the use of furosemide (Fig. 2–7). This procedure, known as diuresis renography, is based on the same principle underlying diuresis urography, which is discussed in Chapter 15. Furosemide (0.5 mg/kg) is injected intravenously, usually at the point of maximum activity in the collecting system. Alternatively, furosemide can be injected at the same time as the radionuclide agent so that the maximal diuretic effect coincides with the peak radionuclide concentration. In

the absence of renal failure, the rate of disappearance of radioactivity from the collecting system correlates with the presence or absence of obstruction. A half-time of 15 minutes or less is normal, while a half-time of 20 minutes or more confirms the diagnosis of obstruction. A half-time between 15 and 20 minutes is considered indeterminate. In addition to the radiopharmaceuticals already mentioned, ^{99m}Tc-DMSA and ^{99m}Tc-GHA can be used for the serial assessment of differential renal function in patients with chronic urinary tract obstruction. Information about the stability or progressivity of damage to renal function caused by obstruction provides a basis for decisions on the need for surgical correction.

The serial evaluation of differential renal function is particularly valuable in the management of apparently obstructed urinary tracts detected in the fetus or newborn. In addition, the maturation of function in the neonatal kidney can be estimated by the serial measurement of the half-time for ^{99m}Tc-DTPA. A value of 9 minutes is considered to represent normal maturation.

Vascular Pathology

Renal Artery Aneurysm, Embolus, and Renal Infarct. An arterial flow study using ^{99m}Tc-GHA, ^{99m}Tc-DTPA, or ^{99m}Tc-MAG₃ permits both visualization of the renal arteries and an estimate of the relative flow to each kidney. A moderate- to large-sized aneurysm or a complete interruption of blood flow can be detected by this method (Fig. 2–8). Segmental or lobar infarction of the kidney produces deficient uptake on parenchymal imaging studies in a pattern that corre-

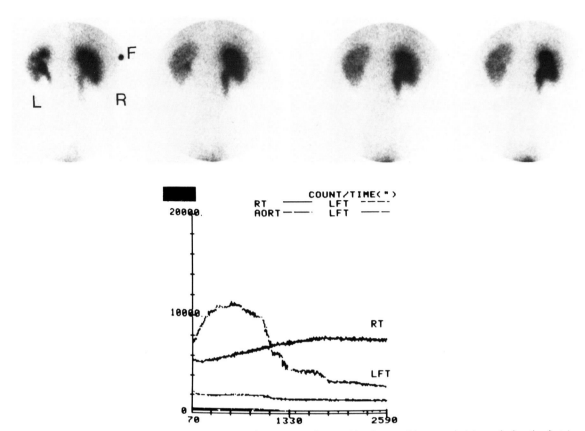

Figure 2–6. Right ureteral obstruction. Diuresis renogram and scan using furosemide. Furosemide was administered after the first image in the upper row was obtained (F). The left pelvocalyceal system loses activity thereafter, while the right does not. The time–activity curves reflect these dynamics.

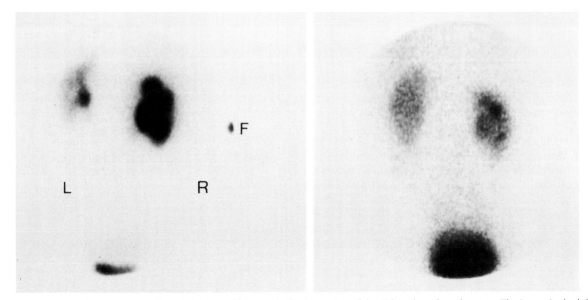

Figure 2–7. ⁹⁹ᵐTc-DTPA diuresis renography using furosemide to exclude obstruction of the right pelvocalyceal system. The image in the left panel, obtained before furosemide (F) administration, demonstrates retention of radionuclide in a dilated right pelvocalyceal system. The panel on the right shows normal drainage of both kidneys, thus eliminating obstruction as the cause of right-sided dilatation.

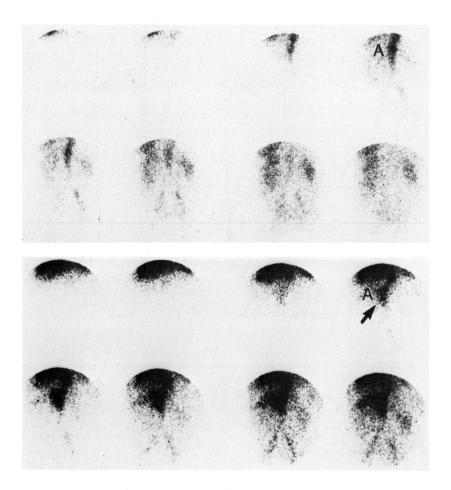

Figure 2–8. Progressive dilatation of an aortic aneurysm. Posterior flow study using ^{99m}Tc-DTPA. The upper two panels demonstrate aortic widening (A) proximal to the origin of the renal arteries. The lower two panels obtained 2 years later demonstrate progression of the aneurysm (A, *arrow*). Involvement of the left renal artery is also evident.

sponds to the zone of infarction (Fig. 2–9). A large area of infarction may be seen on perfusion studies with any ^{99m}Tc-labeled renal agent. The detection of a small infarct, however, requires the use of parenchymal agents, such as ^{99m}Tc-DMSA or ^{99m}Tc-GHA, and pinhole collimation.

Renal Vein Thrombosis. Thrombosis of the renal vein causes diminished perfusion and prolonged parenchymal retention of those radionuclide agents that are cleared by either glomeruli or tubules. These findings are not, however, specific for renal vein thrombosis, the diagnosis of which requires correlation with other morphologic findings, such as kidney enlargement, as well as clinical features.

Renovascular Hypertension. Standard renal scintigraphy is neither sensitive nor specific in investigating hypertensive patients for a renal artery stenosis etiology. Similarly, standard renal radionuclide studies cannot reliably evaluate the functional significance of a known lesion. However, the predictive accuracy of renal scintigraphy in screening patients for unilateral ischemia due to renal artery stenosis and in predicting improvement or cure with correction of the stenosis is markedly enhanced when an angiotensin converting enzyme inhibitor, either captopril or enalapril, is incorporated into the examination. In the patient with unilateral renovascular ischemia producing hypertension, glomerular filtration in the affected kidney would be diminished as a result of decreased

afferent arterial pressure if it were not for the intense vasoconstriction of the efferent arterioles in the glomeruli mediated by increased levels of angiotensin II. Angiotensin I, the precursor of angiotensin II, is made by the conversion of angiotensinogen by renin. Angio-

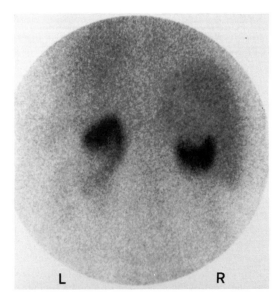

L   R

Figure 2–9. Multiple emboli. Three-hour ^{99m}Tc-GHA image showing focal areas of no uptake.

tensin converting enzyme mediates the conversion of angiotensin I to angiotensin II. An angiotensin converting enzyme inhibitor blocks efferent arteriolar vasoconstriction by reduction of angiotensin II and, thus, causes a marked decrease in the glomerular filtration rate in the affected kidney. This, in turn, accentuates differences in the uptake and washout of radionuclide by the normal and the ischemic kidney. Non–angiotensin converting enzyme inhibitor renography is compared with angiotensin converting enzyme renography. Enhanced sensitivity is realized when an initial normal renogram in a patient with renovascular hypertension is followed by an abnormal angiotensin converting enzyme–inhibited renogram (Fig. 2–10). Specificity is improved when abnormal renograms in patients with kidney dysfunction unrelated to renal artery stenosis do not change with angiotensin converting enzyme inhibitor renography. A variety of radiopharmaceuticals, including [123]I- and ^{131}I-Hippuran, ^{99m}Tc-DTPA, ^{99m}Tc-DMSA, and ^{99m}Tc-MAG$_3$ have been used for this study.

The conduct of an angiotensin converting enzyme inhibitor–enhanced renogram is similar to a routine renogram except that adequate hydration before the study must be ensured and the angiotensin converting enzyme inhibitor must be given before radiopharmaceutical injection. Captopril is given orally 1 hour before injection of the radiopharmaceutical, while enalapril is injected intravenously 15 minutes before injection of the radiopharmaceutical. Furosemide is sometimes used to enhance radionuclide washout and thereby eliminate interference with quantitative analysis by calyceal accumulation. It is important to monitor blood pressure, keep an intravenous line open, and maintain the patient in a supine position in the event that significant hypotension occurs as a possible complication of the angiotensin converting enzyme inhibitor. If the angiotensin converting enzyme inhibitor–enhanced renal study is abnormal, routine renography is repeated without angiotensin converting enzyme inhibitor enhancement on a different day. Alternatively, if a non–angiotensin converting enzyme inhibitor study is performed first with a low dose, then the angiotensin converting enzyme inhibitor study is performed immediately with a high dose.

Despite a lack of standardized criteria for interpretation, variations in study conduct (including angiotensin converting enzyme inhibitor dosage, hydration protocols, and use of diuretics) and decreased sensitivity for bilateral lesions, angiotensin converting enzyme inhibitor scintigraphy has shown potential as an efficacious screening test and prognostic indicator for therapy.

Parenchymal Function

There are numerous radionuclide-based methods for the measurement of glomerular filtration rate using ^{99m}Tc-DTPA or ^{125}I-iothalamate and for determining effective renal plasma flow using the tubule-secreted agents ^{123}I or ^{131}I-Hippuran or ^{99m}Tc-MAG$_3$. Most methods are based on a measurement of each parameter in the equation for clearance,

$$C = \frac{UV}{P},$$

where U is the radionuclide activity in a given volume of urine, V is the volume of urine output per unit of time, and P is the average plasma concentration of the

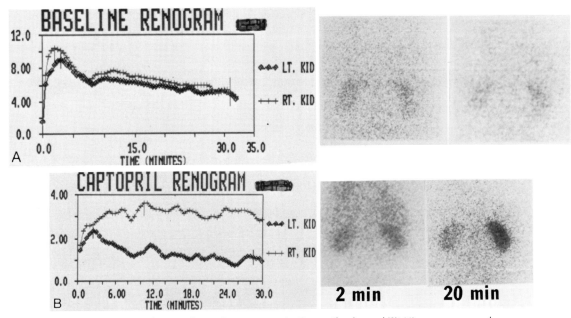

Figure 2–10. Renovascular hypertension due to right renal artery stenosis. Captopril-enhanced ^{131}I-Hippuran scans and renograms.
A, A baseline study demonstrates normal 2- and 20-minute scans and normal time–activity curves for both kidneys.
B, Repeat scans and renogram after administration of captopril demonstrate marked parenchymal retention of radionuclide by the right kidney and persistently normal findings in the left kidney.

radionuclide measured. Radionuclide techniques for measurement of renal function vary from simple counting of the radioactivity of urine and plasma samples to pure imaging methods. Imaging-only methods measure glomerular filtration rate and effective renal plasma flow by estimating the absolute parenchymal accumulation of the radionuclide agent before excretion. Sometimes, a combination of imaging and serum or urine sample counting techniques are used. The choice of method depends on the clinical situation, the need for a quick estimate of renal function during times of rapid change in critically ill patients, and the need for information that can be determined only by imaging, such as differential function.

Renal Infection

In acute pyelonephritis, decreased parenchymal uptake of ^{99m}Tc-DMSA or ^{99m}Tc-GHA is seen in those regions of the kidney in which there is an acute tubulointerstitial nephritis. The pathophysiology of these events is discussed in Chapter 9. These abnormalities may be present as a single focus or as multiple foci, often in the upper or lower poles. In some patients the diminished uptake is generalized. Radionuclide images can be useful for both initial diagnosis and follow-up (Fig. 2–11). Since infection-related changes can be minimal, pinhole, converging collimator, or single-photon emission computed tomography images are usually necessary. In addition to the parenchymal component, ^{99m}Tc-GHA also demonstrates flow abnormalities to the infected kidney, as well as incidental drainage problems. ^{99m}Tc-DMSA, on the other hand, can best evaluate parenchymal lesions when severe urinary drainage problems compromise the ^{99m}Tc-GHA parenchymal scans.

Reflux nephropathy, or chronic pyelonephritis, is characterized by focal areas of both diminished uptake and parenchymal loss associated with contour abnormalities. Overall renal mass may be diminished. Abnormal differential function may be noted in those patients in whom the process is unilateral and multifocal.

Renal or perinephric abscess may be detected by imaging with either ^{67}Ga- or ^{111}In-labeled white blood cells. Any accumulation of ^{111}In-labeled white blood cells is considered compatible with severe infection or inflammation. In addition to abscess, these agents have been utilized in the diagnosis of infection in either a simple renal cyst or in the cyst of a polycystic kidney. White blood cells labeled with ^{99m}Tc-labeled hexamethylpropyleneamine oxine (^{99m}Tc-HMPAO) have also been used for detecting renal and perirenal abscess. The advantage of this agent lies in the high photon flux of the short-lived ^{99m}Tc-labeled cell, which allows imaging as early as 2 hours and as late as 24 hours after injection. However, tracer activity in the bowel may impair later images.

Renal Mass

Radionuclide studies using ^{99m}Tc-DTPA, ^{99m}Tc-GHA, or ^{99m}Tc-DMSA provide useful information in determining the cystic or solid nature of a renal mass, in investigating the possibility of hydronephrosis as a cause of a mass, and in establishing whether there is functioning renal tissue associated with a mass. These clinical applications are often most valuable in neonatal or pediatric patients but can be applied to the adult as well (Fig. 2–12).

In the newborn, multicystic dysplastic kidney and hydronephrosis are the most common causes of a fluid-filled abdominal mass (Fig. 2–13). Both usually, but not always, involve the entire kidney. In the pelvoinfundibular atretic form of multicystic dysplastic kidney there is no radionuclide uptake at any time,

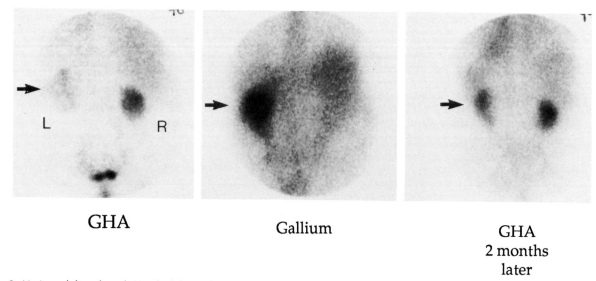

GHA   Gallium   GHA
                                                  2 months
                                                  later

Figure 2–11. Acute left pyelonephritis. The left panel represents a ^{99m}Tc-GHA scan that demonstrates poor function of the left kidney *(arrow)*. The middle panel demonstrates intense uptake by the left kidney of ^{67}Ga *(arrow)*. The right panel demonstrates return of normal uptake of ^{99m}Tc-GHA by the left kidney *(arrow)* 2 months after successful treatment. (Courtesy of Mailine Chew, M.D., Ralph K. Davies Medical Center, San Francisco, California.)

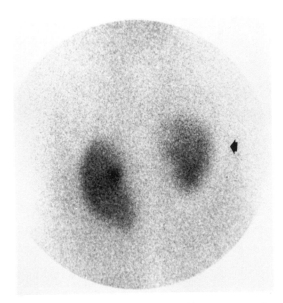

Figure 2–12. Angiomyolipoma with perirenal hematoma causing photopenic "halo" *(arrow)* surrounding the right kidney. ^{99m}Tc-DTPA image.

whereas in the hydronephrotic form faint uptake appears over time. The basis for these findings in multicystic dysplastic kidney is discussed in Chapter 11. Hydronephrosis, on the other hand, has a distinctly different appearance on radionuclide studies, as discussed earlier in this chapter.

Solid neoplasms of the kidney, both benign and malignant and in all age groups, usually demonstrate increased flow during the arterial phase of the kidney study. Since neoplasms do not have normal, functioning nephrons there is diminished to absent accumulation of the radiopharmaceutical during later phases. Uncommon exceptions have been reported in meso-

blastic nephroma with ^{131}I-Hippuran and in adenoma with a variety of agents. Burkitt's lymphoma of the kidney may show intense uptake of ^{67}Ga citrate. Lobar dysmorphism, discussed in Chapter 3, or any other cause of pseudotumor, can be distinguished from a neoplasm or a cyst by demonstrating uptake with either ^{99m}Tc-GHA or ^{99m}Tc-DMSA (Fig. 2–14). Simple renal cyst or a multiloculated cystic tumor, lacking both arterial blood supply or nephrons, does not demonstrate uptake during any phase of a radionuclide study (Fig. 2–15).

There is considerable overlap in the information derived from radionuclide evaluation of a kidney mass and that provided by other imaging modalities, most notably computed tomography and ultrasonography. In general, the latter two techniques are used preferentially and radionuclide methods are used only for supplemental information in difficult diagnostic problems (Figs. 2–16 and 2–17).

Renal Trauma

Although largely supplanted by computed tomography and ultrasonography, radionuclide procedures do provide functional and anatomic information in the acute trauma patient. ^{99m}Tc-DTPA and ^{99m}Tc-GHA permit assessment of aortic and renal arterial blood flow and the functional integrity of the renal parenchyma. Delayed images allow detection of urine leakage, which might follow disruption of the kidney, ureter, or bladder (Fig. 2–18). Contusion of the kidney causes focal defects in the uptake of parenchymal agents. Acute lobar or regional infarction can be similarly demonstrated.

A post-traumatic renal arteriovenous fistula is characterized by a prominent arterial blush, rapid fading of the venous phase, and early activity in the inferior

Figure 2–13. Multicystic dysplastic kidney. ^{99m}Tc-DMSA renal scans. The image in the left panel was obtained immediately after injection of the radionuclide and demonstrates multiple photopenic areas that correspond to cysts *(arrow)*. The right panel demonstrates images obtained after a delay of several hours in which there is no renal function on the left side and normal renal function on the right side.

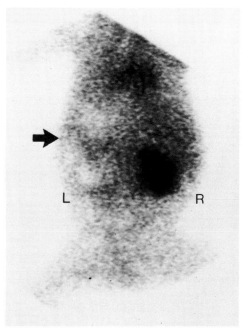

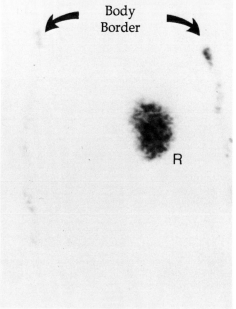

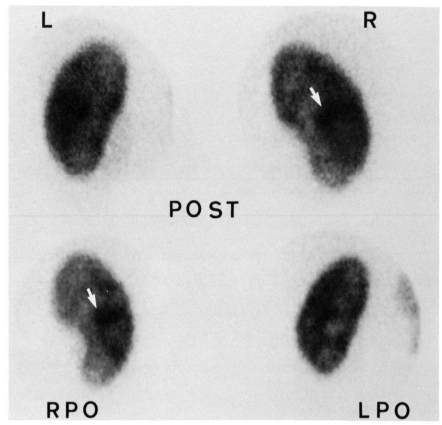

Figure 2–14. Pseudotumor. Posterior and posterior oblique pinhole images 3 hours after ⁹⁹ᵐTc-GHA injection showing kidney parenchyma *(arrows)* extending into the pelvis of the right kidney in the area of suspected tumor.

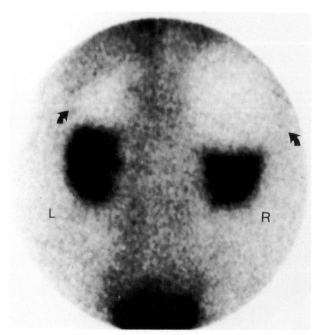

Figure 2–15. Bilateral renal cysts. ⁹⁹ᵐTc-GHA scan demonstrates large photopenic defects in the upper poles of each kidney *(arrows)*.

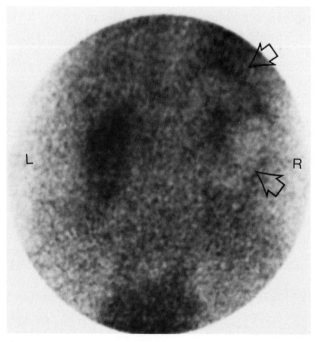

Figure 2–16. Hematoma occurring after needle biopsy in a patient with renal failure. ⁹⁹ᵐTc-GHA scan. There are multiple photopenic areas in the right kidney *(arrows)*.

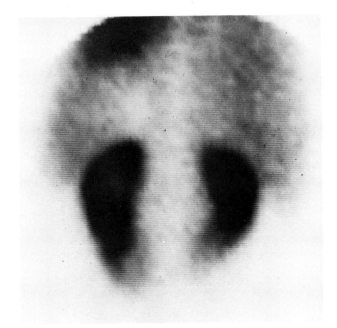

Figure 2–17. Horseshoe kidney. ^{99m}Tc-DTPA scan, posterior projection. There is medial orientation of the lower poles of both kidneys.

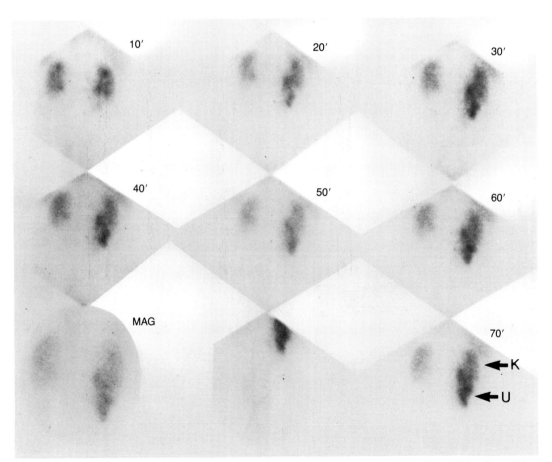

Figure 2–18. Right ureteral leak due to trauma. Scans obtained sequentially from 10 to 70 minutes after ^{99m}Tc-GHA radionuclide injection. Note collection of activity at the site of ureteral tear (U) inferomedial to the kidney (K). (Courtesy of Mailine Chew, M.D., Ralph K. Davies Medical Center, San Francisco, California.)

vena cava. This complication of penetrating wounds is usually delayed in its appearance.

Other aspects of trauma of the kidney and urinary tract are discussed in Chapter 27.

Ureteral Reflux

Direct radionuclide cystography is the most sensitive imaging method for detecting ureteral reflux, and, at the same time, involves less radiation exposure than conventional radiographic techniques. Pertechnetate or ^{99m}Tc-sulfur colloid is instilled into the bladder through a urethral catheter along with increasing volumes of normal saline. Both filling and voiding are continuously imaged. The high sensitivity of radionuclide voiding cystography for detecting transient vesicoureteral reflux is due to a high target-to-background ratio as well as the accuracy inherent in the continuous imaging that is feasible with radionuclide techniques (Fig. 2–19). The low dosimetry of radionuclide cystography compared with radiographic cystography is especially attractive in pediatric screening or when the diagnosis is already established and multiple imaging studies may be needed to evaluate for treatment efficacy or disease progression.

Indirect or antegrade cystography, which is performed in conjunction with ^{99m}Tc-DTPA or ^{99m}Tc-MAG$_3$ kidney studies can also detect ureteral reflux. This is accomplished by monitoring the time–activity curve over the ureters while the patient voids. Evidence of increased activity during voiding supports a diagnosis of vesicoureteral reflux. Although this technique avoids catheterization, it is less sensitive than direct retrograde voiding cystography because slight reflux cannot be detected against the background activity of the continuous flow of radiopharmaceutical from above. Also, this technique requires the cooperation of the patient in voiding on command.

Noninvasive estimates of bladder volume, usually within 10 per cent of true volumes, can be made by comparing the difference in counts within a region drawn surrounding a computer-acquired image of the bladder before and after voiding. The volume voided is measured and then the prevoid and postvoid volumes are calculated by comparing the counts per volume of voided urine with the counts in the prevoid and postvoid images.

Adrenal Imaging

Radiopharmaceuticals used for adrenal imaging, all of which are investigational, provide data that reflect anatomy as well as metabolic function. Both NP-59, an ^{131}I-labeled agent used for imaging the adrenal cortex, and ^{131}I- and ^{123}I-MIBG, used for imaging the adrenal medulla, become incorporated in the adrenal glands at specific metabolic sites (Fig. 2–20). It is therefore important that a patient's biochemical abnormality be well characterized so that the appropriate radiopharmaceutical and imaging protocol can be chosen.

Adrenal cortical imaging is performed to evaluate the etiology of Cushing's syndrome, primary aldosteronism, or hyperandrogenism. In Cushing's syn-

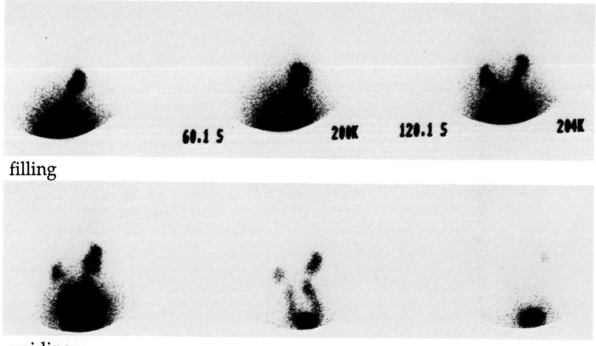

Figure 2–19. Ureteral reflux. Radionuclide cystogram using ^{99m}Tc-pertechnetate. Upper row demonstrates images obtained during passive filling with reflux into both ureters. This is accentuated on voiding, as illustrated in the lower row of images.

drome, abnormally high NP-59 uptake 5 days after administration has a 95 per cent diagnostic accuracy in distinguishing adrenal hyperplasia from adenoma or carcinoma. Bilateral, sometimes asymmetric, visualization is characteristic of adrenocorticotropic hormone–independent hyperplasia; unilateral visualization is seen in cortical adenoma; and nonvisualization often, but not always, occurs in adrenal cortical carcinoma. After surgery for any of these lesions, scintigraphy using NP-59 has been shown to be superior to venography, arteriography, and venous sampling in the localization of adrenal remnants. In primary aldosteronism and renal hyperandrogenism, prolonged suppression with dexamethasone is necessary before and during scanning. A positive diagnosis for these conditions is based on the pattern of scintigraphic "break through" of the adrenals during suppression. Normal adrenals "break through" at 5 or more days after NP-59 injection. Unilateral visualization at less

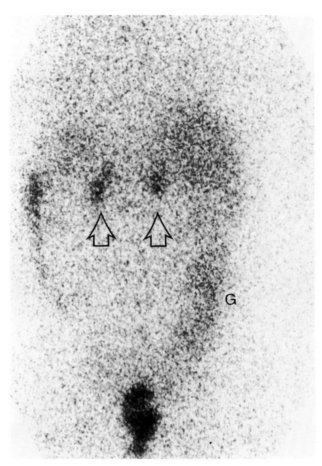

Figure 2–20. Normal NP-59 study (^{131}I). There is uptake by both adrenal glands *(arrows)* and residual activity from unbound ^{131}I in gut (G).

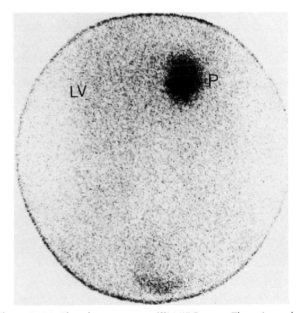

Figure 2–21. Pheochromocytoma. ^{123}I-MIBG scan. There is marked uptake of radionuclide by the tumor (P) in the left adrenal gland. Note diminished liver activity (LV). (Courtesy of Dayan Sandler, M.D., and Robert Hattner, M.D., University of California, San Francisco.)

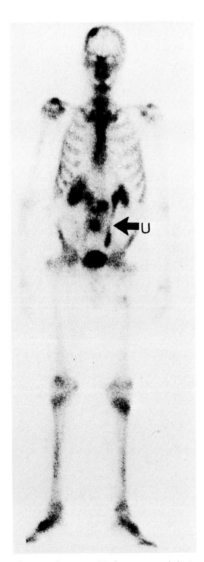

Figure 2–22. Obstructed ureters (U) demonstrated during a bone scan in a patient with carcinoma of the prostate metastatic to bone and retroperitoneum.

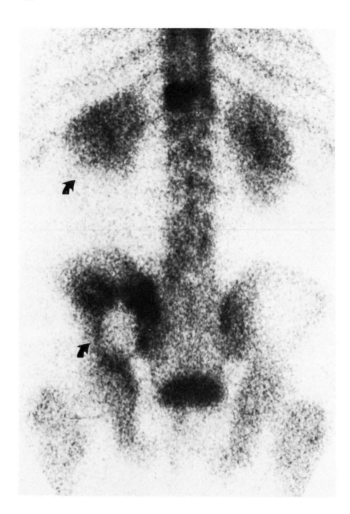

Figure 2–23. Adenocarcinoma of the kidney metastatic to bone. ^{99m}Tc-MDP bone scan, posterior view, demonstrates focal defect in the lower pole of the left kidney *(upper arrow)* and associated metastases to spine and pelvis *(lower arrow)*.

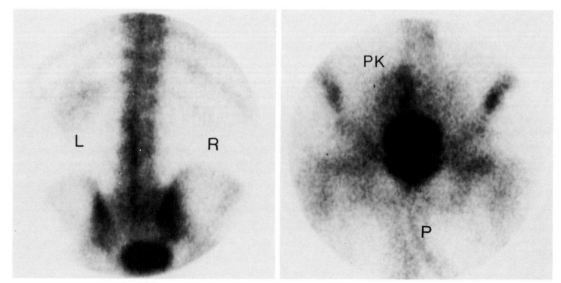

Figure 2–24. Pelvic kidney incidentally detected during a bone scan with ^{99m}Tc-MDP. The left panel, a posterior view, reveals uptake in the left kidney (L) but none in the region of the normal right kidney (R). The right panel demonstrates an anterior view of the pelvis with a pelvic right kidney (PK) and penile prosthesis with a photopenic linear defect (P).

than 5 days is indicative of adenoma, while bilateral visualization before this time is seen in hyperplasia. Diagnostic accuracy for these criteria is over 90 per cent.

Adrenal medullary imaging performed with [131]I- or ^{123}I-MIBG is used to localize neural crest tumors, particularly pheochromocytoma (Fig. 2–21). An abnormal scan is characterized by focal activity in the adrenal or a focus or foci of activity in areas that do not normally accumulate MIBG on 48-hour images. These include the heart, salivary glands, liver, spleen, bladder, and kidney. MIBG scintigraphy is very sensitive in detecting small lesions in the adrenals. It is also of value in detecting bilateral pheochromocytomas, extra-adrenal paragangliomas, and metastatic or recurrent pheochromocytomas. MIBG scintigraphy requires proper patient preparation based on careful history before injection as well as knowledge of the many drugs and conditions that affect its distribution.

Other aspects of the radiologic diagnosis of adrenal disease are discussed in Chapter 22.

Incidental Information from Other Radiopharmaceutical Studies

Radionuclide agents excreted by the kidneys may reveal unanticipated urinary tract abnormalities, including ureteral obstruction, ureteral perforation (see Fig. 2–18), a kidney mass, abnormal kidney morphology or position, or abnormal excretory function (Figs. 2–22 through 2–24). These findings may be encountered in imaging studies of the skeleton (using ^{99m}Tc-methylene diphosphonate [MDP]) and thyroid (using ^{99m}Tc-pertechnetate) as well as blood pool studies of the heart and for gastrointestinal bleeding (using ^{99m}Tc-labeled red blood cells). Thallium 201 (^{201}Tl), whose main route of excretion is through the kidneys, can demonstrate a stenosis of the renal artery.

Bibliography

General References

Blaufox, M. D., Hollenberg, N. K., and Raynaud, C. (eds.): Radionuclides in Nephrourology. Basel, Karger, 1990.

Blaufox, M. D.: Procedures of choice in renal nuclear medicine. J. Nucl. Med. 32:1301, 1991.

Kim, E. E., Pjura, G. A., and Lowry, P. A.: Principles of radionuclide studies of the G.U. system, In Gottschalk, A., Hoffer, P., and Potchen, E. (eds.): Golden's Diagnostic Radiology. Baltimore, Williams & Wilkins, 1988, p. 927.

Sfakianakis, G. N., Vonorta, K., Zilleruelo, G., Jaffe, D., and Georgiou, M.: Scintigraphy in acquired renal disorders. In Freeman, L. M. (ed.): Nuclear Medicine Annual. New York, Raven Press, 1992, pp. 157–224.

Tauxe, W. N., and Dubovsky, E. V. (eds.): Current Practice in Nuclear Medicine. Nuclear Medicine in Clinical Urology and Nephrology. East Norwalk, Connecticut, Appleton-Century-Crofts, 1985.

Williams, E. D.: Renal single photon emission computed tomography: Should we do it? Semin. Nucl. Med. 22:112, 1992.

Radiopharmaceuticals

Anghileri, L. J., Crone-Escanye, M. C., Thouvenot, P., Brunotte, F., and Robert, J.: Mechanisms of gallium-67 accumulation by tumors: Role of cell membrane permeability. J. Nucl. Med. 29:663, 1988.

Chervu, L. R., and Blaufox, M. D.: Renal radiopharmaceuticals—an update. Semin. Nucl. Med. 12:224, 1982.

de Lange, M. J., Piers, D. A., Kosterink, J. G. W., van Luijk, W. H. J., Meijer, S., de Zeeuw, D., and van der Hem, G. K.: Renal handling of technetium-DMSA: Evidence for glomerular filtration and peritubular uptake. J. Nucl. Med. 30:1219, 1989.

Dubovsky, E. V., and Russell, C. D.: [99m]Tc MAG₃: Multipurpose renal radiopharmaceutical. In Freeman L. M. (ed.): Nuclear Medicine Annual. New York, Raven Press, 1991.

Eshima, D., and Taylor, A., Jr.: Technetium-99 (^{99m}Tc) mercaptoacetyltriglycine: Update on the new ^{99m}Tc renal tubular function agent. Semin. Nucl. Med. 22:61, 1992.

Russell, C. D., Thorstad, B., Yester, M. V., Stutzman, M., Baker, T., and Dubovsky, E. V.: Comparison of technetium-99m MAG₃ with iodine-131 Hippuran by a simultaneous dual channel technique. J. Nucl. Med. 29:1189, 1988.

Tsan, M. F., and Scheffel, U.: Mechanism of gallium-67 accumulation in tumors. J. Nucl. Med. 27:1215, 1986.

Acute Renal Failure

Brezis, M., Rosen, S., and Epstein, F. H.: Acute renal failure. In Brenner, B. M., and Rector, F. C., Jr. (eds.): The Kidney. Philadelphia, W. B. Saunders, vol. 1, 1991, p. 993.

Fine, E. J.: Assessment of acute and chronic renal failure, evaluation of renal function and disease with radionuclides. In Blaufox, M. D. (ed.): The Upper Urinary Tract. 2nd rev. ed. Basel, Karger, 1989, p. 316.

Piepsz, A., Ham, H. R., and DuPont, A. G.: Renal blood flow in renal disease and hypertension: Evaluation of renal function and disease with radionuclides. In Blaufox, M. D. (ed.): The Upper Urinary Tract. 2nd rev. ed. Basel, Karger, 1989, p. 163.

Sherman, R. A.: Acute and chronic renal failure. In Tauxe, W. N., and Dubovsky, E. V. (eds.): Current Practice in Nuclear Medicine. Nuclear Medicine in Clinical Urology and Nephrology. East Norwalk, Connecticut, Appleton-Century-Crofts, 1985, p. 221.

Urinary Tract Obstruction

Brown, R. K., Bahn, D. K., Walters, B. L., Karazim, J. J., Reidinger, A. A., Shei, K. Y., Morgan, A. W., Hurd, D. B., Gontina, H., and Kling, G. A.: Nuclear scintigraphy in the evaluation of renal colic. Clin. Nucl. Med. 15:11, 1990.

Conway, J. J.: "Well-tempered" diuresis renography: Its historical development, physiologic and technical pitfalls and standardized technique protocol. Semin. Nucl. Med. 22:74, 1992.

Fine, E. J.: Interventions in renal scintirenography. Semin. Nucl. Med. 21:116, 1991.

Gordon, I., Ransley, P. G., and Hubbard, C. S.: [99m]Tc DTPA scintigraphy compared with intravenous urography in the follow-up of posterior urethral valves. Br. J. Urol. 60:447, 1987.

Homsy, Y. L., Saad, F., Laberge, I., Williot, P., and Pison, C.: Transitional hydronephrosis of the newborn and infant. J. Urol. 144:579, 1990.

Kass, E. J., Majd, M., and Belman, B.: Comparison of the diuretic renogram and the pressure perfusion study in children. J. Urol. 134:92, 1985.

Kullendorff, C. M., and Evander, E.: Renal parenchymal damage on DMSA scintigraphy in pelviureteric obstruction. Scand. J. Urol. Nephrol. 23:127, 1989.

O'Reilly, P. H.: Diuresis renography 8 years later: An update, a review article. J. Urol. 136:993, 1986.

Parkhouse, H. F., and Barratt, T. M.: Practical pediatric nephrology: Investigation of the dilated urinary tract. Pediatr. Nephrol. 2:43, 1988.

Thomsen, H. S., Hvid-Jacobsen, K., Meyhoff, H. H., and Nielsen, S. L.: Combination of DMSA-scintigraphy and Hippuran renography in unilateral obstructive nephropathy. Acta Radiol. 28:(5):653, 1987.

Vascular Abnormalities

Chen, C. C., Hoffer, P. B., Vahjen, G., Gottschalk, A., Koster, K., Zubal, I. G., Setaro, J. F., Roer, D. A., and Black, H. R.: Patients at high risk for renal artery stenosis: A simple method of renal scintigraphic analysis with Tc-99m DTPA and captopril. Radiology 176:365, 1990.

Dondi, M., Monetti, N., Fanti, S., Marchetta, F., Corbelli, C., Zagni, P., De Fabritis, A., Losinno, F., Levorato, M., and Zuccalá, A.: Use of technetium-99m-MAG₃ for renal scintigraphy after angiotensin-converting enzyme inhibition. J. Nucl. Med. 32:424, 1991.

Dondi, M., Fanti, S., De Fabritis, A., Zuccalá, A., Gaggi, R., Mirelli, M., Stella, A., Marengo, M., Losinno, F., and Monetti, N.: Prognostic value of captopril renal scintigraphy in renovascular hypertension. J. Nucl. Med. 33:11, 1992.

Erbsloh-Moller, B., Dumas, A., and Roth, D.: Furosemide ¹³¹I Hippuran renography after angiotensin converting enzyme inhibition for the diagnosis of renovascular hypertension. Am. J. Med. 90:23, 1991.

Fine, E. J.: Interventions in renal scintirenography. Semin. Nucl. Med. 21:116, 1991.

Geyskes, G. G., Oei, H. Y., Puylaert, C. B., and Mees, E. J.: Renovascular hypertension identified by captopril-induced changes in the renogram. Hypertension 9:451, 1987.

Mann, S. J., and Pickering, T. G.: Detection of renovascular hypertension—state of art—1992. Ann. Intern. Med. 117:10, 1992.

Meier, G., and Sumpio, B.: Captopril renal scintigraphy: An advance in the detection and treatment of renovascular hypertension. J. Vasc. Surg. 11:770, 1990.

Nally, J. V., and Black, H. R.: State-of-the-art review: Captopril renography: Pathophysiology considerations and clinical observations. Semin. Nucl. Med. 22:85, 1992.

Nielander, A. J., Bode, W. A., and Heidendal, G. A.: Renography in diagnosis and follow-up of renal vein thrombosis. Clin. Nucl. Med. 6:56, 1983.

Prigent, A.: The diagnosis of renovascular hypertension—the role of captopril renal scintigraphy and related issues. Eur. J. Nucl. Med. 20:625, 1993.

Saddler, M. C., and Black, H. R.: Captopril renal scintigraphy: A clinician's perspective (an editorial). In Hoffer, P. (ed.): Yearbook of Nuclear Medicine. Chicago, Mosby–Year Book, 1990, p. xiii.

Sfakianakis, G. N., Sfakianaki, E., and Bourgoignie, J.: Renal scintigraphy following angiotensin-converting enzyme inhibition in the diagnosis of renovascular hypertension (captopril scintigraphy). In Freeman, L. M., and Weissmann, H. S. (eds.): Nuclear Medicine Annual. New York, Raven Press, 1988, p. 125.

Wells, G. A., Smith, H. S., Trepashko, D. W., and MacCarthy, E. P.: Abnormal captopril renal scintigraphy in a case of renal artery branch stenosis. Clin. Nucl. Med. 15:191, 1990.

Parenchymal Function

Dubovsky, E., and Russell, C.: Quantitation of renal function with glomerular and tubular agents. Semin. Nucl. Med. 12:308, 1982.

Gates, G.: Glomerular filtration rate: Estimation from fractional renal accumulation of ⁹⁹ᵐTc DTPA (Stannous). AJR 138:569, 1982.

Jackson, J., Blue, P., and Ghaed, N.: Glomerular filtration rate determined in conjunction with routine renal scanning. Radiology 154:203, 1985.

LaFrance, N., Drew, H., and Walker, M.: Radioisotopic measurement of glomerular filtration rate in severe chronic renal failure. J. Nucl. Med. 176:1927, 1988.

Mulligan, J. S., Blue, P. W., and Hasbargen, J. A.: Methods for measuring GFR with technetium 99m DTPA: An analysis of several common methods. J. Nucl. Med. 31:1211, 1990.

Perrone, R., Steinman, T., and Beck, G.: Utility of radioisotopic filtration markers in chronic renal insufficiency: Simultaneous comparison of ¹²⁵I-iothalamate, ¹⁶⁹Yb-DTPA, ⁹⁹ᵐDTPA, and inulin. Am. J. Kidney Dis. 16:224, 1990.

Russell, C. D., Taylor, A., and Eshima, D.: Estimation of technetium-99m MAG₃ plasma clearance in adults from one or two blood samples. J. Nucl. Med. 30:1955, 1989.

Infection

Amesur, P., Castronuovo, J. J., and Chandramouly, B.: Infected cyst localization with gallium SPECT imaging in polycystic kidney disease. Clin. Nucl. Med. 13:35, 1988.

Bakir, A. A., Lopez-Majano, V., Levy, P. S., Rhee, H. L., and Dunea, G.: Gallium 67 scintigraphy in glomerular disease. Am. J. Kidney Dis. 12:481, 1988.

Conway, J. J.: The role of scintigraphy in urinary tract infection. Semin. Nucl. Med. 18:308, 1988.

Froelich, J. W.: Nuclear medicine in inflammatory diseases. In Freeman, L. M., and Weissmann, H. S. (eds.): Nuclear Medicine Annual. New York, Raven Press, 1985, p. 23.

Handa, S. P.: Drug-induced acute interstitial nephritis: Report of 10 cases. Can. Med. Assoc. J. 135:1278, 1986.

Lantto, E. H., Lantto, T. J., and Vorne, M.: Fast diagnosis of abdominal infections and inflammation with technetium-99-m-HMPAO labeled leukocytes. J. Nucl. Med. 32:2029, 1991.

Linton, A. L., Richmond, J. M., Clark, W. F., Lindsay, R. M., Driedger, A. A., and Lamki, L. M.: Gallium 67 scintigraphy in the diagnosis of acute renal disease. Clin. Nephrol. 24:84, 1985.

Majd, M., Rushton, H. G., Jantausch, B., and Wiedermann, B. L.: Relationship among vesicoureteral reflux, P-fimbriated Escherichia coli, and acute pyelonephritis in children with febrile urinary tract infection. J. Pediatr. 119:578, 1991.

Majd, M., and Rushton, H. G.: Renal cortical scintigraphy in the diagnosis of acute pyelonephritis. Semin. Nucl. Med. 22:98, 1992.

Pike, M. C.: Editorial: Imaging of inflammatory sites in the 1990s: New horizons. J. Nucl. Med. 32:2034, 1991.

Rubin, R. H., Fischman, A. J., Callahan, R. J., Khaw, B. A., Keech, F., Ahmad, M., Wilkinson, R., and Strauss, H. W.: ¹¹¹In-labeled nonspecific immunoglobulin scanning in the detection of focal infection. N. Engl. J. Med. 321:935, 1989.

Smellie, J. M., Shaw, P. J., Prescod, N. P., and Bantock, H. M.: ⁹⁹ᵐTc dimercaptosuccinic acid (DMSA) scan in patients with established radiological renal scarring. Arch. Dis. Child. 63:1315, 1988.

Tsang, V., Lui, S., Hilson, A., Moorhead, J., Fernando, O., and Sweny, P.: Gallium-67 scintigraphy in the detection of infected polycystic kidneys in renal transplant recipients. Nucl. Med. Comm. 10:167, 1989.

Verber, I. G., and Meller, S. T.: Serial ⁹⁹ᵐTc dimercaptosuccinic acid (DMSA) scans after urinary infections presenting before the age of 5 years. Arch. Dis. Child. 64:1533, 1989.

Verboven, M., Ingels, M., Delree, M., and Piepsz, A.: ⁹⁹ᵐTc DMSA scintigraphy in acute urinary tract infection in children. Pediatr. Radiol. 20:540, 1990.

Renal Mass

Felson, B., and Moskowitz, M.: Renal pseudotumors: The regenerated nodule and other lumps, bumps, and dromedary humps. AJR 107:720, 1969.

Lee, V. W., Allard, J., Foster, J., Sheahan, K., and Franklin, P.: Functional oncocytoma of the kidney: Evaluation by dual tracer scintigraphy. J. Nucl. Med. 28:1911, 1987.

Leonard, J. C., Allen, E. C., Goin, J., and Smith, C. W.: Renal cortical imaging and the detection of renal mass lesions. J. Nucl. Med. 20:1018, 1979.

Pollack, H. M., Ewdell, S., and Morales, J. O.: Radionuclide imaging in renal pseudotumors. Radiology 111:639, 1974.

Trauma

Berg, B., Jr.: Nuclear medicine and complementary modalities in renal trauma. Semin. Nucl. Med. 12:280, 1982.

Lisbona, R., Palayew, M. J., Satin, R., and Hyams, B. B.: Radionuclide detection of iatrogenic arteriovenous fistulas of the genitourinary system. Radiology 134:201, 1980.

Rosenthall, L., and Ammann, W.: Renal trauma. Semin. Nucl. Med. 13:238, 1983.

Sty, J. R., Starshak, R. J., and Hubbard, A. M.: Radionuclide evaluation in childhood injuries. Semin. Nucl. Med. 13:258, 1983.

Vesicoureteral Reflux

Goldraich, N. P., Ramos, O. L., and Goldraich, I. H.: Urography versus DMSA scan in children with vesicoureteric reflux. Pediatr. Nephrol. 3:1, 1989.

Monsour, M., Azmy, A. F., and MacKenzie, J. R.: Renal scarring secondary to vesicoureteric reflux: Critical assessment and new grading. Br. J. Urol. *60*:320, 1987.

Strife, J. L., Bisset, G. S., III, Kirks, D. R., Schlueter, F. J., Gelfand, M. J., Babcock, D. S., and Han, B. K.: Nuclear cystography and renal sonography: Findings in girls with urinary tract infection. AJR *153*:115, 1989.

Van den Abbeele, A. D., Treves, S. T., Lebowitz, R. E., Bauer, S., Davis, R. T., Retik, A., and Colodny, A.: Vesicoureteral reflux in asymptomatic siblings of patients with known reflux: Radionuclide cystography. Pediatrics *79*:147, 1987.

Adrenal Imaging

Bretan, P. N., Jr., and Lorig, R.: Adrenal imaging, computed tomographic scanning and magnetic resonance imaging. Urol. Clin. North Am. *16*:505, 1989.

Edeling, C. J., Frederiksen, P. B., Kamper, J., and Jeppesen, P.: Diagnosis and treatment of neuroblastoma using metaiodobenzylguanidine. Clin. Nucl. Med. *12*:632, 1987.

Geatti, O., Fig, L., and Shapiro, B.: Adrenal cortical adenoma causing Cushing's syndrome: Correct localization by functional scintigraphy despite nonlocalizing morphological imaging studies. Clin. Nucl. Med. *15*:168, 1990.

Gross, M. D., Shapiro, B., Bouffard, J. A., Glazer, G. M., Francis, I. R., Wilton, G. P., Khafagi, F., and Sonda, L. P.: Distinguishing benign from malignant adrenal masses. Ann. Intern. Med. *109*:613, 1988.

Gross, M. D., and Shapiro, B.: Scintigraphic studies in adrenal hypertension. Semin. Nucl. Med. *19*:122, 1989.

Ikeda, D. M., Francis, I. R., Glazer, G. M., Amendola, M. A., Gross, M. D., and Aisen, A. M.: The detection of adrenal tumors and hyperplasia in patients with primary aldosteronism: Comparison of scintigraphy, CT, and MR imaging. AJR *153*:301, 1989.

Jonckheer, M. H., Mertens, J., Ham, H. R., and Piepsz, A.: Consolidating the role of I-MIBG-scintigraphy in childhood neuroblastoma: Five years of clinical experience. Pediatr. Radiol. *20*:157, 1990.

Kazerooni, E. A., Sisson, J. C., Shapiro, B., Gross, M. D., Driedger, A., Hurwitz, G. A., Mattar, A. G., and Petry, N. A.: Diagnostic accuracy and pitfalls of [iodine-131]6-beta-iodomethyl-19-norcholesterol (NP-59) imaging. J. Nucl. Med. *31*:526, 1990.

Korobkin, M.: Overview of adrenal imaging. Urol. Radiol. *11*:221, 1989.

Kumar, R., David, R., Sayle, B. A., and Lamki, L. M.: Adrenal scintigraphy. Semin. Roentgenol. *23*:243, 1988.

Shapiro, B., Fig, L. M., Gross, M. D., and Khafagi, F.: Radiochemical diagnosis of adrenal disease. CRC Lab. Sci. *27*:265, 1989.

Velchik, M. G., Alavi, A., Kressel, H. Y., and Engelman, K.: Localization of pheochromocytoma: MIBG, CT and MRI correlation. J. Nucl. Med. *30*:328, 1989.

Incidental Findings

Bihl, H., Sautter-Bihl, M. L., and Riedasch, G.: Extrarenal abnormalities in ^{99m}Tc DTPA renal perfusion studies due to hypervascularized tumors. Clin. Nucl. Med. *13*:590, 1988.

Bocchini, T., Williams, W., and Patton, D.: Radioscintigraphic demonstration of unsuspected urine extravasation. Clin. Nucl. Med. *14*:421, 1989.

Datz, F. L. (ed.): Gamuts in Nuclear Medicine. East Norwalk, CT, Appleton & Lange, 1987, p 26.

Hurwitz, G. A., Mattar, A. G., Bhargava, R., Driedger, A. A., Hogendoorn, P., and Wesolowski, C. A.: Renal uptake of ^{201}Tl in hypertensive patients undergoing myocardial perfusion imaging. Clin. Nucl. Med. *15*:88, 1990.

Lin, D. S.: "Missing" one kidney. Semin. Nucl. Med. *21*:167, 1991.

Macpherson, R. J., and Leithiser, R. E.: Serendipitous diagnosis of childhood xanthogranulomatous pyelonephritis in a child with osteomyelitis. Pediatr. Radiol. *17*:159, 1987.

Shih, W. J., DeLand, F. H., and Biersack, H. J.: Serial bone scintigrams demonstrating obstructive uropathy and nephropathy due to transitional cell carcinoma of the urinary bladder. Radiol. Med. *7*:203, 1989.

Williamson, S. L., Seibert, J. J., Tryka, A. F., Glasier, C. M., and Williamson, M. R.: Renal imaging on liver-spleen scans. Clin. Nucl. Med. *12*:831, 1987.

Pediatric

Conway, J. J.: The role of scintigraphy in urinary tract infection. Semin. Nucl. Med. *18*:308, 1988.

Copely, D. J., Smith, R., and Murakami, M. E.: Renal scintigraphy with technetium ^{99m}Tc succimer: Clinical utility in newborns with cystic renal dysplasia. South Med. J. *81*:99, 1988.

Gordon, I.: Pediatric article: Indications for ^{99m}technetium dimercapto-succinic acid scans in children. J. Urol. *137*:464, 1987.

Heyman, S.: An update of radionuclide renal studies in pediatrics. *In* Freeman, L. M., and Weissmann, H. S. (eds.): Nuclear Medicine Annual. New York, Raven Press, 1989, p. 179.

Majd, M., and Rushton, G. H.: Renal cortical scintigraphy in the diagnosis of acute pyelonephritis. Semin. Nucl. Med. *22*:112, 1992.

Preston, A., and Lebowitz, R. L.: What's new in pediatric uroradiology. Urol. Radiol. *11*:217, 1989.

Sfakianakis, G. N.: Nuclear medicine in congenital urinary tract anomalies. *In* Freeman, L. M. (ed.): Nuclear Medicine Annual. New York, Raven Press, 1991, p. 129.

Sfakianakis, G. N., and Sfakianaki, E. D.: Nuclear medicine in pediatric urology and nephrology. J. Nucl. Med. *29*:1287, 1988.

Sty, J. R., Wells, R. G., Starshak, R. J., and Schroeder, B. A.: Imaging in acute renal infection in children. AJR *148*:471, 1987.

3

RADIOLOGIC ANATOMY OF THE KIDNEY AND URETER

The adult kidney and ureter, perhaps more than any other mammalian organ, retain evidence of the series of temporal and structural events that occur during their fetal development. A review of the embryogenesis of the kidney and ureter in this book, therefore, is no routine attempt at completeness. The reader is urged to acquire a knowledge of the process, described in the first section of this chapter, to achieve a better understanding of the architecture of the renal lobe as the basic unit for studying the gross morphology of the kidney. The section on the anatomy of the single lobe is followed by a discussion of the kidney as a union and partial fusion of many lobes. Next, variations in the anatomy of the papillae, which are of fundamental importance in the genesis of acute renal infection and scarring, are presented in detail. This material is then related to uroradiologic landmarks and measurements. The final section describes anomalous development of the kidney and ureter. The anatomy of the lower urinary tract is discussed in Chapters 19 and 20, while that of the retroperitoneum, including the renal sinus, and that of the adrenal gland are presented, respectively, in Chapters 21 and 22.

EARLY EMBRYOGENESIS OF THE KIDNEY AND URETER

Pronephros

The human excretory system has its origin in the plate of embryonic mesenchyme known as the *intermediate*

mesoderm. The first evidence of urinary tract development is a cellular condensation visible between the second and sixth somites of the 10-somite embryo. This occurs at the end of the third week of gestation. Because of the cervicodorsal position of these early excretory structures, they have been termed the *pronephroi*, meaning forward, or head, kidney (Fig. 3–1*A*). No excretory function occurs at this stage, and the pronephros involutes after a very short time. The only potential importance of the pronephroi is the occasional mediastinal cyst, which may develop as a vestige of this developmental phase of the excretory system.

Mesonephros

The second of the three phases of excretory system development begins with the differentiation of tissue, known as the *mesonephros*, immediately caudal to the involuting pronephros. In this stage, the intermediate mesoderm on each side of the midline is asymmetrically divided by a longitudinal cleft into a narrow medial structure, the *mesonephric (wolffian) duct*, and a broad lateral portion, the *nephrogenic cord*. This process occurs at slightly more than 3 weeks of gestation, between the 9th and 13th somites of the 20-somite embryo, and progresses caudally. Communication with the cloaca is established within the next few days (29 somites).

The *mesonephroi* are supplied by a series of paired vessels, the rete arteriosum urogenitale, which originate from the aorta and iliac arteries.

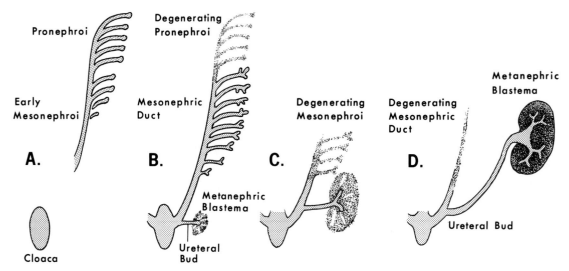

Figure 3–1. Schema of successive stages of the embryogenesis of the kidney and ureter from pronephros *(A)*, mesonephros and appearance of the ureteral bud *(B)*, to division of the ureteral bud and development of the metanephric blastema into the mature kidney *(C and D)*.

In the laterally situated nephrogenic cord, vesicles form and differentiate into functioning glomeruli and tubules, which drain directly into the mesonephric (wolffian) duct. All in all, some 40 to 42 pairs of glomeruli form in the mesonephros. However, only 30 to 32 are present at any one time, since those formed earliest, in the cranial aspect, degenerate at the same time as new glomeruli are formed caudally. These events are illustrated in Figure 3–1B and C.

With time, all the mesonephric glomeruli degenerate. Remnants of the tubules and mesonephric duct, on the other hand, persist in both sexes as structures, listed in Table 3–1.

Ureteral Bud and Metanephros

All the events described to this point occur at a site somewhat remote from where the kidney will eventually develop. Even though the pronephric and mesonephric stages do not directly influence the anatomic form of the definitive excretory organ, they are essential to the development of a small diverticulum at the caudal end of the mesonephric duct, first noted in the 5-week-old embryo. This structure is the *ureteral bud*, and its appearance signals the start of the development of the definitive ureter and kidney, the latter also known as the *metanephros*.

The ureteral bud has two components of growth:

elongation and division. As the ureteral bud elongates, the interaction between the specialized cells at its distal tip, known as the ampulla, and the surrounding *metanephric blastema*, moves progressively anterior and cephalad from its initial sacral location, eventually placing the developing kidney in the upper lumbar region (see Fig. 3–1C and D). The elongated portion of the ureteral bud eventually becomes the ureter, the thin-walled muscular tube that propels urine from the developing metanephros to the bladder as it evolves from the cloaca.

The metanephros is derived from two cell types. The first is the ureteral bud itself; the second is the metanephric blastema. The metanephric blastema differentiates into nephrons and renal connective tissue under the inductive influence of the advancing point, the ampulla, of the ureteral bud. The ureteral bud is the "prime mover" in this process, inasmuch as the metanephric blastema alone will not develop nephrons unless contacted by the ampulla. Potter (1972) has ascribed the following four activities to the ampulla of the ureteral bud: anterior extension, division, induction of nephrons from the metanephric blastema, and establishment of communications between the nephrons from the metanephric blastema and the collecting tubules derived from the ureteral bud.

The process of ureteral bud division is the focus of the remainder of this section. Division is always dichotomous and occurs from the first appearance of

Table 3–1. FATE OF MESONEPHRIC STRUCTURES IN THE ADULT

Male		Female	
Mesonephric Tubules	*Mesonephric Ducts*	*Mesonephric Tubules*	*Mesonephric Ducts*
Efferent ductules of testes (connecting seminiferous tubules to epididymis)	Vas deferens Seminal vesicle Ejaculatory duct	Epoöphoron* Paroöphoron*	Complete involution
Epididymis Paradidymis			

*Inconstant, functionless structures in the mesosalpinx.

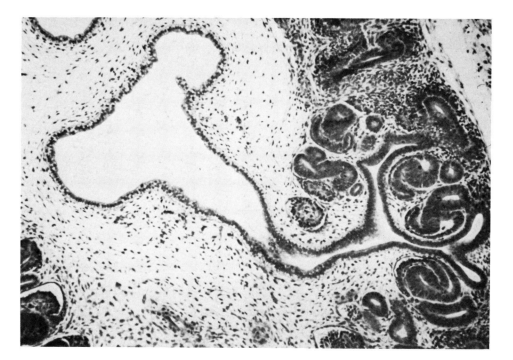

Figure 3–2. Photomicrograph of the early development of a human kidney. The ureteral bud is the bifurcating tubular structure that is dilated centrally. The ureteral bud divides peripherally and induces the formation of nephrons from metanephric blastema, seen as dark-staining tissue on the right.

the ureteral bud, at approximately 5 weeks of gestation, to the last division in the periphery of the renal medulla, at 5 months of gestation. The first three to five generations of tubes produced by this process dilate to form the renal pelvis; the next three to five generations expand to form the calyces, papillae, and cribriform plates; and the last six to nine generations become the collecting tubules. Understanding this process provides an important foundation for understanding the radiologic anatomy of the kidney.

Development of the Renal Pelvis and Infundibula

Renal function begins when the metanephric blastema, under the inductive influence of the ureteral bud ampullae, starts differentiating into nephrons. This occurs at approximately 7 weeks of gestation. The existing ureteral bud branches at this time begin to dilate, presumably as a result of the accumulation of urine. These dilating branches become the renal pelvis (Fig. 3–2).

The pattern of early ureteral bud branching has an important bearing on the features of the adult kidney.

As illustrated in Figure 3–3, more divisions of the ureteral bud occur in the polar than in the interpolar regions of the kidney. Quantitatively, four to five generations of ureteral bud branches contribute to the formation of each polar region of the renal pelvis, whereas only two to three generations are present in the interpolar region when the pelvis starts forming. The tip of each branch, it should be remembered, is the active portion of the dividing ureteral bud. With substantially more ureteral bud branches inducing nephron formation in the polar regions, it is easy to see why the renal parenchyma normally is thicker in the poles than in the central (interpolar) region of the kidney.

The infundibula that connect the pelvic elements to the calyces are derived from the next generation of ureteral bud branches after those that form the pelvis. These tubular structures do not dilate. It should be pointed out that infundibula have traditionally been called "major calyces," while in fact they are not calyces at all. *Calyx* is the Latin term for cup or chalice. Sherwood and Williams (1973) have noted that properly this word should be reserved for the structure surrounding the papilla, commonly called the "minor

Figure 3–3. Schema of early divisions of the ureteral bud. Four to five divisions form the polar regions and two to three generations form the interpolar area. Dilatation and subsequent assimilation of individual branches occur as urine formation begins. (Modified from Potter, E. L.: Normal and Abnormal Development of the Kidney, 1972, with kind permission of the author and Year Book Medical Publishers.)

DEVELOPMENT OF RENAL PELVIS

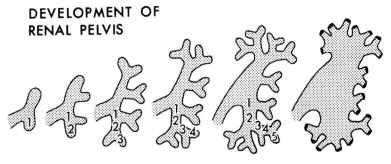

calyx." The "major calyx" is, in fact, a simple tubular conduit, embryologically a part of the renal pelvis, that links the calyx to the common chamber of the renal pelvis.

Development of the Calyces and Papillae

Following the generations of ureteral bud branches that dilate to form the renal pelvis and the infundibula, another series of three to five generations appears. According to Potter (1972), these branches differ from their predecessors in that they are formed one from the other in rapid succession. The rapidity of the dichotomous branching in this series results in little time for growth and elongation of the individual tubes. As a result, three to five generations of very short tubules are produced; these expand to form the cavity of the calyx.

The early calyx has the configuration of multiple, dilated, short fingers. With progressive distention, the calyx undergoes transformation into a saclike cavity. Dilatation is believed to progress as a result of urine filling many short tubules that open into a space having the infundibulum as a single outlet to the pelvis. As nephrons grow, there is both an increase in the bulk of tissue adjacent to the calyx and in the volume of urine formed. The dilating calyx thus becomes interposed between developing nephrons on one side and the enlarging renal pelvis on the other. The net effect is to flatten the calyceal sac and to force the margins of the space to pouch outward and partially encompass the lower ends of the collecting ducts. Thus, a cuplike structure, or calyx, is formed.

Subsequent branching is slower, allowing time for the ducts to elongate considerably. These tubules become the *papillary ducts of Bellini*, which enter the calyx through the *cribriform plate* covering the surface of the papilla. (The cribriform plate is discussed further in the section Anatomy of the Papillae.)

The progression of events in the formation of a calyx and papilla is illustrated in Figure 3–4.

Development of the Collecting Tubules and Nephrons

The papillary duct is formed from the ureteral bud branch that is immediately distal to those that have formed the calyx and cribriform plate. A single papilla bears 10 to 20 of these ducts opening into the calyx. Potter has estimated that the papillary ducts belong to the 11th generation of divisions from the original ureteral bud. Each of these 10 to 20 ducts at the papillary tip gives rise to another seven to eight generations of structures known as *collecting tubules*. One can easily visualize, then, the beginning formation of the conical renal lobe extending outward from the papillary tip. All that is lacking at this point is the investiture of this bundle of collecting tubules with a cloak of nephrons.

As the ampullae of the collecting tubules elongate and divide, they do so in close contact with the solid mass of the metanephric blastema, the anlage of the glomerulus, the proximal convoluted tubule, the loop of Henle, and the distal convoluted tubule. Collectively, these structures constitute the *nephron*. The distal convoluted tubule communicates with the last generation of collecting tubules to establish the final union of the two tissue groups, which combine to form the definitive kidney. Each of the collecting tubule branches eventually has eight to nine nephrons

DEVELOPMENT OF CALYX

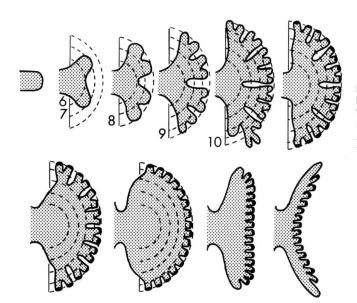

Figure 3–4. Schema of the sixth to tenth generations of ureteral bud branches, which form by rapid division. These develop into the calyx. With time, the ducts dilate, and the resultant cavity becomes invaginated by the expanding lobe. (Modified from Potter, E. L.: Normal and Abnormal Development of the Kidney, 1972, with kind permission of the author and Year Book Medical Publishers.)

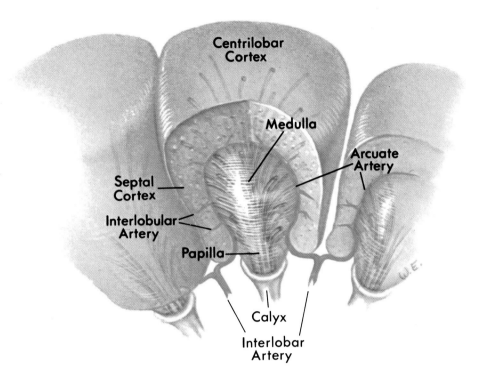

Figure 3–5. Diagram of the archetypical renal lobe. Designation of interlobar and arcuate artery based on observations of C. J. Hodson, M.D. (1976).

attached to it. There is controversy over the details of how the nephron differentiates into its several components and the various patterns of attachment to the collecting tubule. These differences of opinion, however, are beyond the scope of this book.

Development of the Renal Lobe

There are two consequences of the continued elongation and division of the collecting tubules. First, the mass of formed renal tissue expands centrifugally, in the shape of a cone, from each papilla. Second, the major portion of the nephrons induced by the advancing collecting tubules are arranged peripherally to the collecting tubules, rather than intermingled with them. As a result, a central zone of collecting tubules, the *medulla*, is formed. It becomes completely surrounded by a dense zone of nephrons, the *cortex*, which invests the medulla completely, except at the papillary tip.

The sharp demarcation between the ureteral bud derivatives (papillary ducts and collecting tubules) in the medulla and metanephric blastema derivatives (nephrons and connective tissue) in the cortex is striking. Some intermixing does occur, however; loops of Henle and connective tissue extend into the medulla. Actually, those loops of Henle derived from the earliest collecting tubule branches extend deep into the papilla. The vascular supply of the nephrons is also found in the medulla. Intermixing occurs in the cortex when the terminal branches of the collecting tubules extend outward in a radial pattern known as *cortical rays*.

It is of fundamental importance for the reader to recognize that this process of lobe formation occurs simultaneously at each site where a calyx has been formed. Basically, the number of lobes that form is determined by the number of calyces; the size of each lobe is determined by the number of papillary ducts draining into each calyx. In the adult, however, there is not a one-to-one relationship between calyces and papillae. It is common to have an arrangement in which a calyx drains two, three, or occasionally more papillae. In the fetus, on the other hand, the definitive number of primary lobes, averaging 14 per kidney, is established by the end of the fourth month of gestation. At this point, before continuing with the final events that transform these independent units into the adult kidney, it is useful to consider the architecture of the individual renal lobe.

ARCHITECTURE OF THE RENAL LOBE

The archetypical renal lobe consists of medulla, cortex, draining calyx, and vascular system, as illustrated in Figures 3–5 and 3–6.

As has already been described, the conical medulla is composed of collecting tubules derived from ureteral bud divisions and proximal and distal convoluted tubules, loops of Henle, and connective tissue arising from the metanephric blastema. The arterial blood supply to the medulla comes chiefly from the vasa recta, a system of postglomerular vessels derived from the efferent arterioles of the juxtamedullary cortex (Figs. 3–6 and 3–7). These vessels follow the descending limb of Henle's loops through the medulla and into the papilla and return with the ascending loop, where drainage into an interlobular or arcuate vein occurs. Under normal circumstances, the medulla receives less than 20 per cent of the total renal

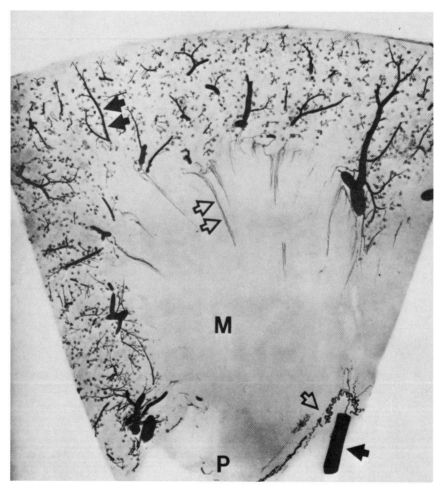

Figure 3–6. Microradiograph of a renal lobe from a human kidney injected post mortem with barium. The vasa recta of the medulla are sparsely opacified, whereas the cortical vasculature is well defined. M, medulla; P, papilla; single solid arrow, arcuate artery; double solid arrows, interlobular artery; single open arrow, spiral artery to papilla; double open arrows, vasa recta.

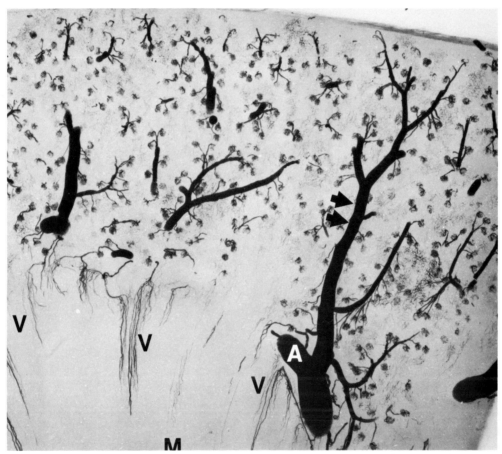

Figure 3–7. Enlargement of Figure 3–6 demonstrating details of cortical vascular anatomy. Afferent arterioles branch from the large interlobular arteries and supply glomerular tufts. Vasa recta can be seen in the corticomedullary region. V, vasa recta; A, arcuate artery; arrows, interlobular artery; M, medulla.

blood flow through this system. The remaining blood flow perfuses the cortex. This difference in regional perfusion is the basis for the radiologic appearance of the medulla as a relatively radiolucent structure surrounded by the opacified lobar cortex during the early nephrographic phase of a renal arteriogram or dynamic contrast material–enhanced computed tomogram (Fig. 3–8). The papilla also receives blood directly from the arterial branches of the interlobar artery, the *spiral arteries*, in addition to the vasa recta (see Fig. 3–6).

The cortex of the renal lobe is the cloak of dense tissue which in the pristine lobe completely surrounds the medulla except at its papillary tip. Composed largely of nephrons derived from the metanephric blastema, the cortex is interrupted at regular intervals by linear bands, *cortical rays*, representing straight terminal branches of collecting tubules extending into cortical tissue from the medulla. The portion of the cortex that forms the base of the lobe has been called the *centrilobar cortex* by Hodson (1972); that which

surrounds the sides of the medulla is called the *septal cortex*. The distinction between these two is of considerable importance: The centrilobar cortex is invariably present in the adult and is an important border-forming urographic landmark, whereas the septal cortex in the adult kidney is variably present and not always discernible during radiologic studies enhanced by contrast material. The reader will undoubtedly recognize that the septal cortex is, in fact, what is popularly called the *column of Bertin* or *Bertini*. It is both useful and correct to speak of this structure as either the "septal cortex" or the "septum of Bertin."* In its most internal extension, the septal cortex reaches the level of the papilla. Here, it may have a slight bulbous enlargement, as shown in Figure 3–5, which, if accentuated to some degree, is one explanation for the so-

---

*Hodson (1972) has provided an engaging, brief reconstruction of how Bertin's original description of this structure, using the French word for "internal partition" *(cloison),* has been transformed into the current imprecise term *"column."*

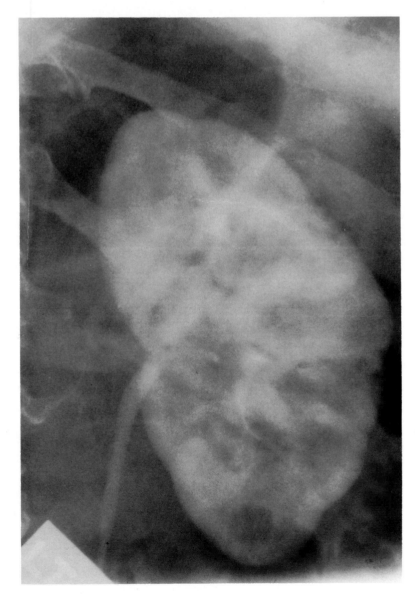

Figure 3–8. Angiographic nephrogram. The centrilobar and septal cortices are opacified, whereas the medulla of each lobe remains radiolucent. This reflects predominant blood flow to the cortex. The angiographic nephrogram is seen in the first few seconds following injection of contrast material into the renal artery and is essentially a vascular phenomenon.

called renal pseudotumor, discussed later in this chapter. As mentioned earlier, the cortex receives approximately 80 per cent of the total renal blood flow through the interlobular arteries, which give rise to the afferent arterioles (see Fig. 3–7).

In the archetypical renal lobe there is a single calyx into which a single papilla is invaginated. These two structures form the innermost landmarks of the renal lobe. In addition, they serve as a reference point for the central axis of the renal lobe, an imaginary line that extends from the tip of the papilla to the midpoint of the centrilobar cortex. The concept of a central axis will be of importance in subsequent chapters in which the impact of various pathologic processes on the renal lobe is discussed.

Each lobe receives its blood supply from *interlobar*, or *segmental*, *arteries* that branch into *arcuate arteries* while still passing through the fat of the renal sinus. The arcuate artery enters the renal substance adjacent to the papilla of the lobe and runs along the corticomedullary junction, periodically giving off branches, the *interlobular arteries*, which extend into the cortex at right angles to the arcuate artery. Several arcuate arteries serve each lobe in a pattern that allows perfusion of the lobe's full circumference. The interlobular arteries, in turn, give rise to the *afferent arterioles*, which supply the glomeruli and, in the juxtamedullary cortex, the vasa recta as well. Although the preceding description applies to a single lobe, in reality each interlobar artery supplies arcuate vessels to two adjacent lobes, and these have a roughly mirror image distribution, as shown in Figure 3–5.

LATE DEVELOPMENT OF THE KIDNEY: THE KIDNEY AS A WHOLE

The development of the renal lobes continues beyond the cessation of ureteral bud branching at approximately 20 weeks. By the 28th week of gestation the individuality of each lobe is most pronounced. At this time, most fetal kidneys have 14 lobes, also known as *renunculi*. Some have as few as 8 lobes; very few have more than 14. Inspection of the kidney at this stage reveals deep surface clefts that delineate the margins of the lobes (Fig. 3–9). In fact, the lobes can be manually separated with ease. At this stage, characteristically, there are 7 anterior and 7 posterior lobes. A longitudinal groove composed of fibrous tissue, which is well developed by the 28th week of gestation, separates the anterior from the posterior groups.

Calyceal development at this stage corresponds to the pattern of lobar clefts. In most fetal kidneys that have been studied at this stage of development, there were seven anterior and seven posterior calyces, each with a single draining papilla. That is to say, each calyx corresponded exactly with the papilla of each lobe.

Events following the 28th week of gestation result in varying degrees of assimilation of the independent lobes. A reduction in the number of calyces, papillae, and surface lobar clefts follows. Fusion of calyces oc-

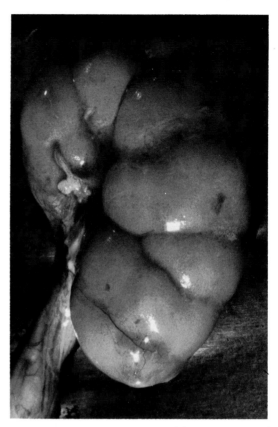

Figure 3–9. Fetal kidney. Note deep clefts delineating margins of each lobe. (Courtesy of H. Z. Klein, M.D., Mt. Zion Hospital and Medical Center of the University of California, San Francisco.)

curs to a greater degree than does fusion of papillae, resulting in a fewer number of individual calyces than papillae by the time of birth. Sykes (1964) reported a mean of 9.0 calyces and 11.4 papillae in a series of kidneys studied at full term. He also noted that the average number of calyces and papillae (respectively, 8.7 and 10.7) was slightly less in the adult, indicating that fusion continues following birth. It is this process of fusion that results in the so-called compound calyx into which two, three, and occasionally more papillae drain. Thus, the calyx loses its one-to-one relationship with an individual lobe and may drain multiple adjacent lobes. The impact of assimilation on the anatomy of the cribriform plate is discussed in the following section, Anatomy of the Papillae.

Another result of lobar fusion is the disappearance of the septal cortex in many areas (Fig. 3–10). Where fusion is most complete, the septal cortex is lost entirely and the medullary portions of adjacent lobes abut each other directly, with no landmarks left to note the site of the previous septal cortex. Where lobar fusion is absent, the septal cortex remains extended into the renal sinus and fuses with the septal cortex of the adjacent lobe and the relationship of single calyx to single papilla remains. Intermediate degrees of fusion also occur, in which the septal cortex persists to varying depths between lobes.

Fusion varies in different parts of the kidney according to a predictable pattern. A greater degree of

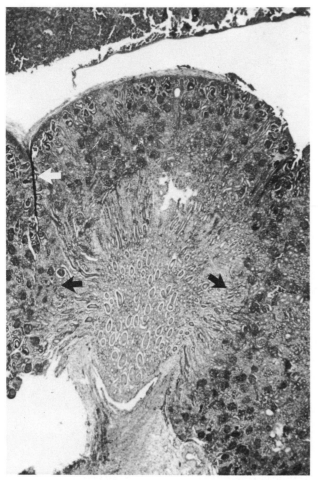

Figure 3–10. Photomicrograph of a lobe from a fetal kidney that has developed beyond the 28th week of gestation. The process of lobar assimilation is manifested by the fusion of the septal cortex of adjacent lobes *(black arrows)* and the obliteration of the deep cleft of connective tissue that previously separated adjacent lobes, a residual portion of which remains *(white arrow)*. The papilla and calyx of the lobe remain unfused.

lobar fusion occurs in the polar regions than in the interpolar region of the kidney. Lobes frequently fuse completely in both the upper and lower poles, and anterior lobes characteristically fuse with posterior lobes. As a result, large compound calyces with absent septal cortex are the rule rather than the exception in the polar regions. This is true to an even greater degree in the superior pole than in the inferior pole. Fusion in the interpolar region of the kidney rarely occurs between anterior and posterior lobes and, as noted previously, is generally less frequent than in the polar regions. Thus, in the middle part of the kidney single calyces are seen frequently during excretory urography, and the septal cortex is visualized regularly on contrast material–enhanced renal images. On the kidney surface, lobar fusion is manifested as a loss of clefts, which for uncertain reasons is most noticeable on the posterior surface.

The renal artery that arises from the aorta is derived from the mesonephric artery. The main branch divides into anterior and posterior parts at a variable point between the aorta and hilum of the kidney. The anterior portion generally perfuses the ventral and upper polar regions, while the posterior portion usually perfuses the dorsal and lower polar regions.

Features of the fused kidney are shown schematically in Figure 3–11.

ANATOMY OF THE PAPILLAE

In the fully developed kidney, papillae have either a simple or a compound form. The shape of the simple papilla is that of a cone whose convex surface projects into the calyceal lumen. This form is unchanged from the embryonic kidney in which each papilla drains urine from a single lobe into a single calyx. The compound papilla has a complex profile with flat, concave, or cleftlike silhouettes projecting into the calyceal lumen. The compound papilla is the result of the partial fusion of lobes, papillae, and calyces that begins after the 28th week of gestation. Urine entering a compound papilla is formed in two or more adjacent, partially assimilated lobes and flows into a compound, or partially assimilated, calyx.

The cribriform plate is the surface of the papilla perforated by the openings of the papillary ducts of Bellini, through which urine passes, normally from collecting ducts into the calyx. There are two basic shapes of papillary duct openings: narrow and slitlike or round and open (Figs. 3–12 and 3–13). The narrow, slitlike opening is seen mainly on simple papillae and on those portions of compound papilla that are least distorted by fusion. The slitlike shape is thought to favor closure of the orifices of the papillary ducts in the presence of elevated intrapelvic pressure, thus

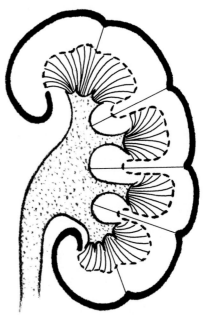

Figure 3–11. Schema of kidney after lobar fusion. Note greater degree of assimilation in both poles, represented by compound calyces and loss of septal cortex. The interpolar region tends to retain individual lobes, septal cortex, and fetal surface lobulation.

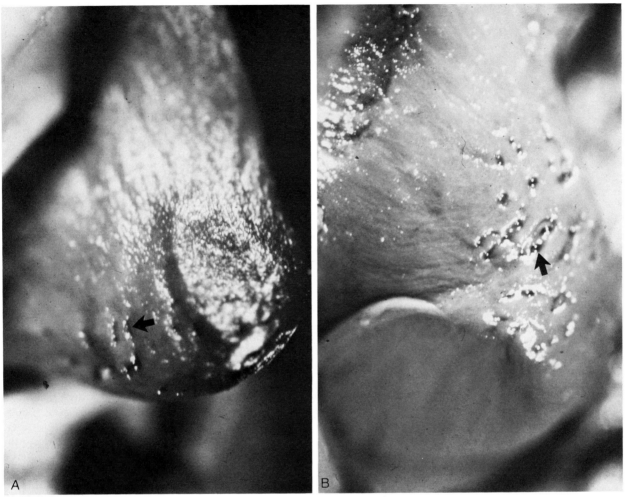

Figure 3–12. Simple and compound normal papillae from human kidney.
A, Simple papilla. The papillary duct orifices *(arrow on one representative example)* are narrow and slitlike.
B, Compound papilla has orifices *(arrow on one representative example)* that are round and open as a result of fusion of adjacent papillae.

Figure 3–13. Schema of papillary duct opening in profile and *en face.* The single cone-shaped pyramid *(A)* has narrow slitlike openings that prevent intrarenal reflux. Compound papillae *(B),* formed as a result of lobar assimilation, have open, round orifices that permit reflux of calyceal urine into the collecting ducts.

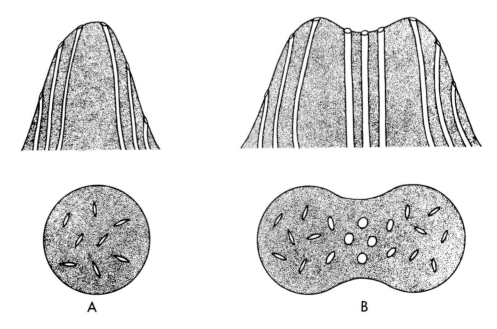

preventing the reflux of urine into the collecting ducts of the medulla.

The round, open type of orifice, on the other hand, is the result of distortion by fusion. In some kidney specimens, these orifices may be open enough to permit direct visualization of the early branches of the collecting duct system. It is generally held that when pelvic pressure is elevated, the round, open-duct orifice is incapable of preventing reflux of urine from the pelvocalyceal system into the collecting ducts and tubules. This is so-called *intrarenal reflux*. It is likely, also, that these orifices provide access for bacteria in pelvocalyceal urine to enter collecting ducts and tubules in the absence of reflux.

It is clear that variations in the shape of papillary duct orifices are related to the embryogenetic process of fusion and that mixtures of shapes are found on both simple and compound papillae. In addition, both papillary profile and orifice shape can be altered by acquired abnormalities, such as recurrent episodes of increased intrapelvic pressure or the development of scars in portions of the lobe. This subject is discussed further in Chapter 5 in relation to the pathogenesis of reflux nephropathy.

Papillae vary in size as well as shape. Large papillae are of no clinical significance (Fig. 3–14).

URORADIOLOGIC LANDMARKS

Ureter

The length and course of the ureter represents ureteral bud growth by elongation during embryogenesis. The proximal two-thirds of the normal ureter is situated in the perirenal space, where it extends from the ureteropelvic junction to the point of its passage through the cone of fused anterior and posterior renal fascia at the caudal margin of the perirenal space (see Chapter 21). Thereafter, the distal one-third of the ureter traverses the extraperitoneal space of the pelvis to its termination at the lateral margin of the interureteric ridge of the bladder.

As the ureter extends distally from the ureteropelvic junction, it lies anteromedial to the medial margin of the lower pole of the kidney and lateral to the superior portion of the psoas muscle. Near the lower pole of the kidney, the ureter moves medially to a position anterior to the psoas muscle. Within the extraperitoneal space of the pelvis, the ureter passes anterior to the common iliac artery in the region of the inferior margin of the sacroiliac joint. From this point, the ureter usually curves in a broad arc that extends laterally to a point near the ischial spine and then medially to its entry into the bladder.

Most proximal ureters are situated within a vertical zone delineated by the lateral margin of the lumbar vertebral pedicles and the tip of a lumbar transverse processes. However, there are marked individual and racial variations in the course of normal ureters, and neither the vertebral pedicle medially nor the transverse process laterally serves as an absolute standard

for normalcy. The position of the ureter is likely to be more medial in individuals of African origin than in those of other races (Adams et al., 1985). The detection of ureteral deviation and its various causes are discussed in Chapters 16, 19, and 21.

Kidney

Many of the anatomic features of the renal lobe are seen best during excretory urography. The opacified calyx and the radiolucent indentation of the papilla mark the apex of the lobe. The cuplike configuration of the calyx, with its acute forniceal angle, is the result of the papillary parenchyma's impression on what was a saclike space in the early embryo. The angle remains sharp as long as the volume of papillary tissue and hydrostatic calyceal pressure are normal. When disease processes reduce the amount of papillary tissue or when urine pressure in the calyx increases, the angle of the fornix widens. The centrilobar cortex of the base of the lobe forms a portion of the border of the kidney. The distance between the papillary tip and the outer margin represents the medulla *and* cortex of the lobe and is a useful representation of the *amount* of renal parenchyma in the lobe.

The radiologist can see this best during the nephrographic phase of the excretory urogram, which depicts the lobar parenchyma (both cortex and medulla) as a homogeneous density, representing contrast material in the lumina of the nephrons and collecting tubules of the lobe. Replacement of lobar parenchyma by abnormal tissue disturbs the homogeneity of the nephrogram. The lateral margins of the lobe are occasionally detectable during excretory urography by a slight notching of the renal contour, termed *fetal lobation*. This represents the point at which the centrilobar cortex of one lobe abuts that of an adjacent lobe. A line drawn from this notch in the renal contour toward the lateral margin of the subservient papilla will approximate the septal cortex of the lobe. In practice, the determination that a renal contour defect is due to fetal lobation, rather than disease-induced scarring, often can be made when the surface indentation is both sharply notched in shape and located between calyces rather than opposite a calyx (Fig. 3–15). A cortical defect opposite a calyx, particularly one that is broad based, represents pathologic loss of lobar tissue. The most direct visualization of the septal cortex occurs during renal angiography, when both the interlobar and arcuate arteries and the cortex itself are selectively opacified (Fig. 3–16).

In the fused adult kidney there is a more or less constant grouping of calyces in each of the three regions of the kidney. Therefore, a group of calyces, often compound, serves each of the two polar regions, and a third group drains the interpolar region of the kidney (Fig. 3–17). This is easily understood, since the calyces, being ureteral bud derivatives, are essential to the formation of their adjacent renal tissue. One should also recognize that not only are there three regional groups of calyces but also that the amount of

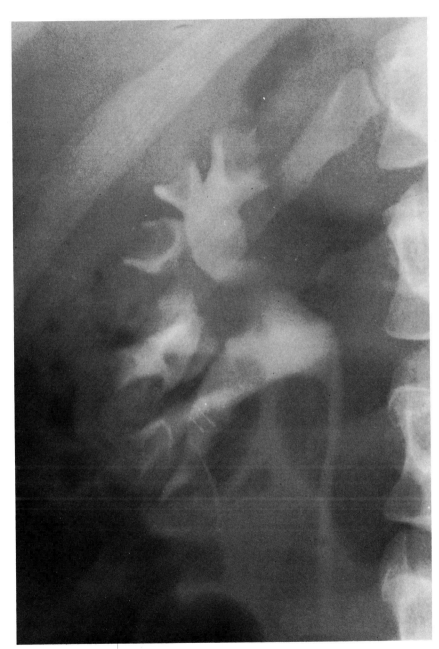

Figure 3–14. Large papillae as a normal variation. The papillae are uniformly large; the calyces are normal. Excretory urogram.

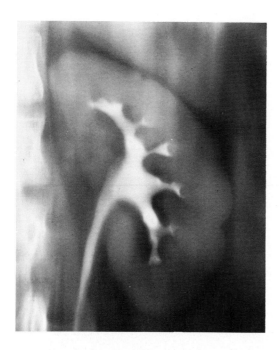

Figure 3–15. Characteristic fetal lobation along lateral margin of kidney. Notches in contour are sharply angulated and occur between two calyces rather than overlying a calyx. These notches represent the lateral margins of adjacent lobes. (Courtesy of Robert R. Hattery, M.D., Mayo Clinic, Rochester, Minnesota.)

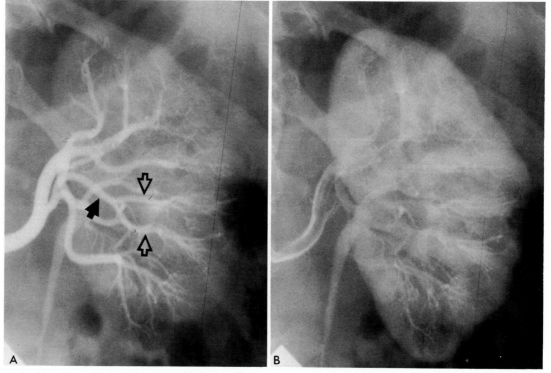

Figure 3–16. Early *(A)* and late *(B)* arterial phase of selective renal arteriogram. In the interpolar region, interlobar arteries branch early into arcuate arteries *(open arrows)*, which run along the corticomedullary interface. In this area, the septal cortex is opacified and surrounds the relatively radiolucent medulla of each lobe. Solid arrow indicates interlobar artery.

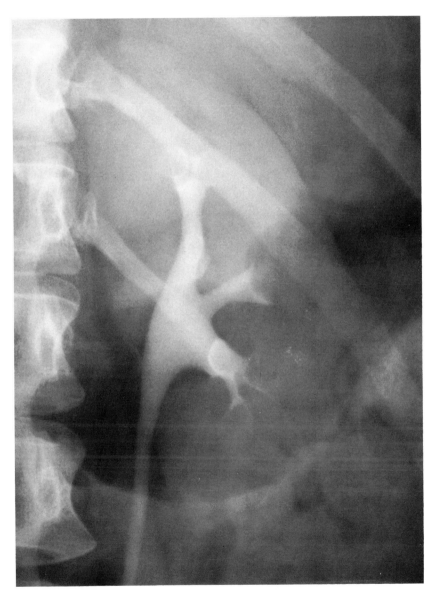

Figure 3–17. Normal pelvocalyceal anatomy illustrating the distribution of calyces into three groups subserving, respectively, the upper polar, interpolar, and lower polar regions. Excretory urogram.

renal tissue drained by each group is proportionate to that in the remainder of the kidney. This is the expected pattern, since all the calyces are derived from the same generation of ureteral bud branches and begin their structural formation at the same time. As a result, calyces and papillae maintain a remarkably constant spatial relationship to each other within the sinus of the kidney. Thus, a line connecting the most peripheral papillae, one to the other, will depict an arc, the *interpapillary line*, which is smooth, conforming in shape to the external contour of the kidney. These features are schematized in Figure 3–18 and illustrated in Figure 3–19.

The interpapillary line was described by Pendergrass in 1943. This measurement is of fundamental importance in the urographic diagnosis of renal disease. In the normal kidney, the thickness of parenchyma lying between the interpapillary line and the outer margin of the kidney is uniform in the interpolar region and expands symmetrically in both poles (Fig. 3–20). Even in the presence of variations in normal contour, such as hepatic or splenic impressions on the renal contour, the arc of the interpapillary line maintains a close parallel relationship with the renal contour, as illustrated in Figures 3–21 and 3–22. Disturbance of this relationship is a sensitive indicator of change in the parenchymal bulk (either gain or loss) and also permits assessment of whether an abnormal process causing such change in bulk is diffuse or focal.

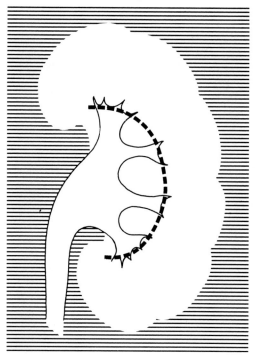

Figure 3–18. Schema of the fused kidney as seen during urography. Note the grouping of calyces for each of three regions (upper and lower polar and interpolar), the symmetry between the interpapillary line and the outer margin of the kidney, and the constancy of renal parenchymal thickness, with widening at both poles.

Opacification of the papillae occurs as an integral part of the nephrogram. Because the countercurrent mechanism concentrating urine is maximal in the papillary region, the papillae are sometimes denser than the remainder of the renal parenchyma. This normal phenomenon is termed *papillary blush*. Occasionally during contrast material–enhanced studies, individual or groups of collecting ducts appear as discrete linear structures radiating from the papillary tips into the medulla for a short distance. This appearance may simulate papillary striations seen in medullary sponge kidney (see Chapter 13). However, in the absence of other evidence for medullary sponge kidney, such as nephrocalcinosis or cysts communicating with collecting ducts, these linear striations are considered normal. Visualization of collecting ducts in papillary tips is seen more frequently with low osmolality contrast material than with high osmolality agents.

The anterior and posterior lobes in the interpolar region do not in fact directly overlie each other. Rather, these two groups are offset, which results in the anterior papillae being situated laterally relative to the posterior papillae. Because of this arrangement, the calyces of the anterior lobes project laterally and are seen in profile on anteroposterior radiographs of the kidney. Those calyces that lie medially in this projection belong to the posterior lobes and usually are seen *en face*. This pattern is shown schematically in Figure 3–23 and illustrated in Figures 3–24 and 3–25. Thus, the reader should keep in mind that urographic landmarks and measurements such as the interpapillary line, parenchymal thickness, and renal contour are usually determined from images of the anterior part of the kidney and are a sampling of a portion of the kidney, not a representation of the whole organ. This limitation, of course, does not apply to cross-sectional images produced by ultrasonography, computed tomography, or magnetic resonance imaging.

Fetal kidneys can be visualized on ultrasound examination as early as 14 menstrual weeks as paired hypoechoic structures on either side of the fetal spine on a cross-sectional image of the abdomen. As the fetus ages, the renal sinus appears as a linear area of echogenicity slightly greater than that of the renal parenchyma. By 30 weeks of gestation, the hyperechoicity of the septal and centrilobar cortex relative to medullary tissue frequently permits differentiation of these two components of the renal parenchyma. Fetal lobation and the pelvocalyceal system are routinely seen at this stage of development as well.

The cortex of the neonatal and infant kidney is often more hyperechoic than the medulla (Fig. 3–26). This reflects the increased size and cellularity of glomeruli during the first few months of life. After 6 months of age, the cortex and the medulla are not consistently different in echo texture.

On renal ultrasound examinations, especially of the right kidney in children, a straight echogenic line between the renal sinus and the ventral surface of the upper portion of the kidney may sometimes be identified. This structure, which often expands at the sur-

Text continued on page 73

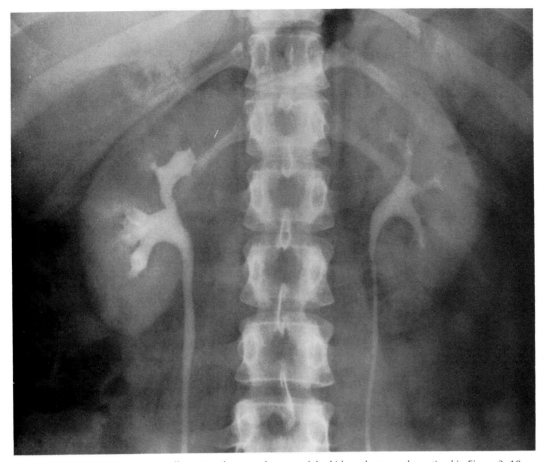

Figure 3–19. Excretory urogram illustrating the same features of the kidney that are schematized in Figure 3–18.

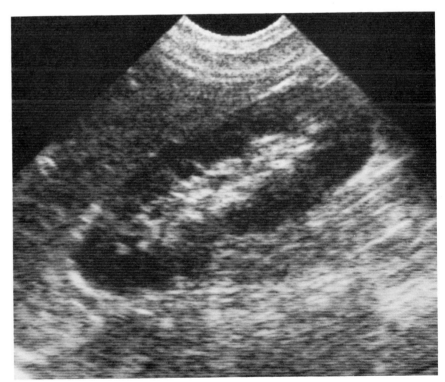

Figure 3–20. The thickness of the renal paren-chyma is uniform throughout the kidney, with slight increases in thickness in the polar regions. Ultrasonogram, longitudinal section.

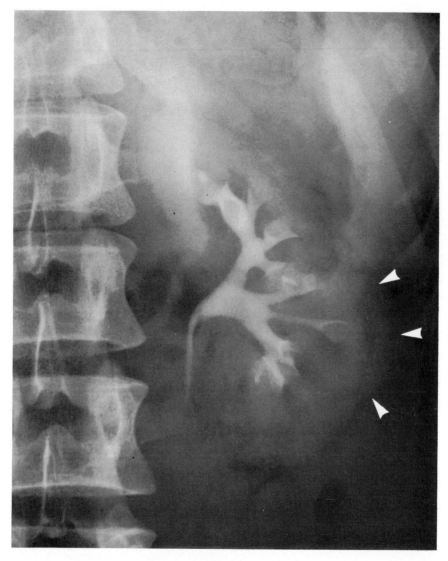

Figure 3–21. The constancy of the relationship of the interpapillary line to the renal contour is illustrated in a case of prominent "dromedary hump" *(arrows)* in which the subservient draining calyx extends outward, so that the thickness of renal parenchyma remains constant in the interpolar region. This finding indicates a normal state rather than a growing mass, which would displace the calyx away from the periphery of the kidney.

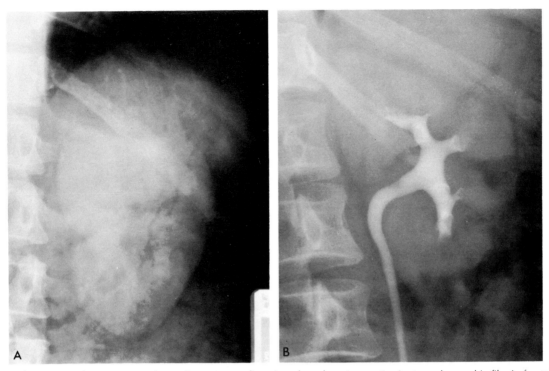

Figure 3–22. Splenic impression on upper pole causing apparent distortion of renal contour on 1-minute nephrographic film in frontal projection *(A)*. A later film in the left posterior oblique projection *(B)* established normal interpapillary line and renal parenchymal thickness. (Courtesy of Department of Diagnostic Radiology, Hammersmith Hospital, London, England.)

Figure 3–23. Schema of transverse section of the interpolar region of the kidney. In the frontal projection, the anterior calyces are lateral to the posterior calyces and are seen in profile. The posterior calyces are seen *en face.* (Modified from Hodson, C. J.: Br. J. Urol., *44:*246, 1972, with kind permission of the author and the *British Journal of Urology.*)

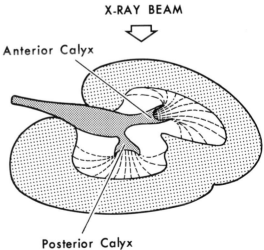
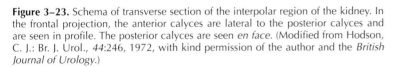

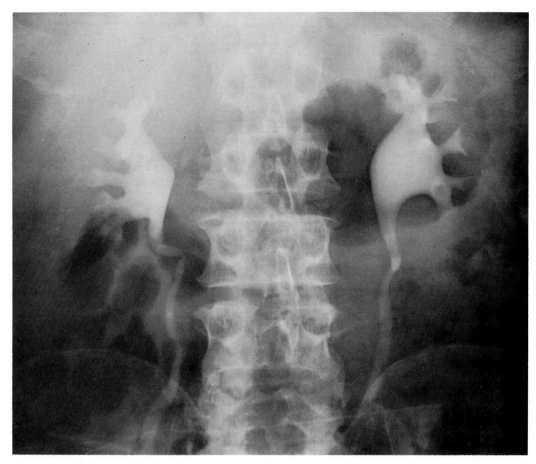

Figure 3–24. Difference in position and projection of anterior and posterior calyces is well illustrated in the left kidney. The lateral calyces seen in profile are anterior; the medial ones seen *en face* are posterior. Because of this relationship, measures of parenchymal thickness and renal contour represent a sampling of anterior lobes.

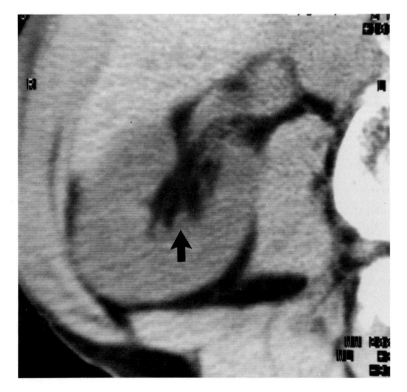

Figure 3–25. Transverse cross section of the right kidney demonstrates the lateral position of the anterior portion of the kidney relative to the posterior lobes. Note also the anterior projection of a papilla from the posterior portion of the kidney *(arrow)* and the anteromedial position of the renal sinus. Computed tomogram, unenhanced.

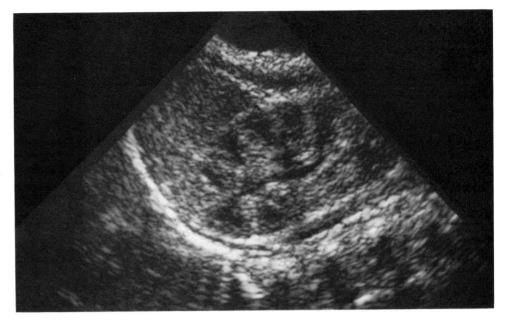

Figure 3–26. Normal neonatal kidney. Ultrasonogram. The cortex is usually more echogenic than the medulla during the first 6 months of life.

face of the kidney into a triangular echogenic focus, has been variably called the *renal parenchymal junctional line*, the *hyperechogenic triangle* and *line*, or the *parenchymal interjunctional line* (Fig. 3–27). Occasionally, the hyperechogenic line runs in a posterior and inferior direction. It is uncommon to identify this structure in the left kidney, in the newborn in whom there is usually a paucity of renal sinus fat, and in adults. It is clear that the hyperechogenic triangle and line represent an extension of fat from the renal sinus to the surface of the kidney. Presumably, this fat is deposited along the interface of adjacent lobes that did not undergo fusion during embryogenesis, perhaps along a plane between the anterior and posterior groups of lobes. The fact that these are infrequently seen in adults may be taken as evidence for continued fusion of lobes after birth.

The position of the kidneys in the retroperitoneum follows a general pattern. The upper pole of the kidney is more medially and posteriorly situated than the lower pole. Because the lower pole calyces are less dependent than the upper pole calyces when the patient is in the supine position, they may not fill well with contrast material, which has a higher specific gravity than urine. This sometimes causes nonopacification of the lower pole calyces and a false assumption of disease. In this case, ureteral compression or prone or upright films are useful means to opacify the lower pole collecting system. Most kidneys are positioned somewhere between the first and third lumbar vertebrae. The pattern for renal position is so variable, however, that meaningful quantification is not possible. Fortunately, the position of the kidney in the retroperitoneum is not of major importance as an aid in the diagnosis of renal disease, although displacement may signal a retroperitoneal mass. (See discussion in Chapter 21.)

RENAL SIZE

Renal size as a clue to the nature of the pathologic process affecting the kidney is one of the major themes of this book. Unfortunately, a basic frustration encountered in adult uroradiology is the absence of valid standards for assessing the significance of a set of measurements in a given individual. The problem is not inherent in the kidneys; in fact, there is close correlation between renal mass and such factors as body build and age. Rather, the problem reflects weaknesses in traditional radiographic methods, such as enlargement of the renal silhouette due to object–film distance and foreshortening of renal length and width caused by rotation of the kidney on both longitudinal and transverse axes as it moves with respiration. Another major problem is that standard radiographic methods permit only two-dimensional measurement of a variably shaped organ. The third dimension, thickness, eludes radiographic imaging of the kidney. Further, true renal size varies with the state of hydration and in response to contrast material. One can readily appreciate the difficult task of determining renal volume from a radiograph.

Another weakness that applies to radiography as well as to ultrasonography, computed tomography, and magnetic resonance imaging is that measurements based on overall length, width, and thickness assume a constant normal ratio between the parenchyma and other internal structures of the kidney such as the pelvocalyceal system and renal sinus fat. Clearly, standards based on measurements of normal kidneys cannot be applied to conditions such as hydronephrosis, cyst, tumor, or proliferation of sinus fat, in which overall bulk is preserved at the expense of renal parenchyma.

The advent of cross-sectional reconstructive tech-

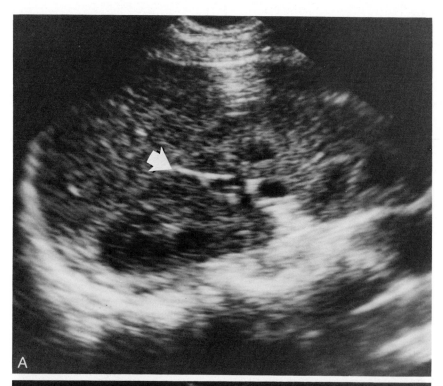

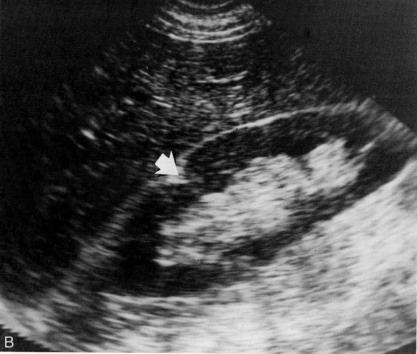

Figure 3–27. Hyperechogenic line and triangle in two normal adult kidneys.

A, A well-defined hyperechogenic line extends from the renal sinus to the anterior surface of the upper pole of the kidney.

B, A hyperechogenic triangle of tissue is present on the anterior surface of the upper portion of the kidney.

(From Dalla Palma, L., et al.: Br. J. Radiol. *63:*680, 1990. Reproduced with kind permission of the author and the *British Journal of Radiology.*)

niques such as ultrasonography, computed tomography, and magnetic resonance imaging has obviated many, although not all, of the aforementioned problems. The following paragraphs discuss the approaches that have been proposed as useful guidelines for the determination of normal renal size in adults. Studies on normal kidney size in infants and children have been more thorough than in the adult. These are discussed at the end of this section.

In 1960, Vuorinen and colleagues attempted to determine an objective measurement of functioning renal parenchyma derived from urographic films by a formula that took into account the product of the height and width of the kidney as a whole and the product of the height and width of the collecting structures within the kidney. A positive correlation between this *renal cortical index* and serum creatinine was found, but the method is cumbersome and has not been validated by experience with large numbers of normal and abnormal subjects. A similar method for measurement of renal substance was reported by Karn in 1962 in a study of a large series of men and women without evidence of renal disease. Karn concluded that the range of measurements of the kidney area is wide and, therefore, a large deviation from the mean was not necessarily an index of disease.

Möel (1956, 1961), on the other hand, made a very thorough study of the problems associated with radiographic measurement of the kidney and came to a more optimistic conclusion. He measured the maximum distance between the outline of the cranial and caudal poles of the kidney—*roentgenographic length*—and the maximum distance between the most lateral and medial parts of the kidney, including the hilar region, at right angles to the roentgenographic length—*roentgenographic width*. The product of these two measurements was called the *measured roentgenographic area of the kidney*, or *T*. Renal mass was calculated as $T^{3/2}$. Using these definitions, Möel studied the radiographs of 100 men and 100 women between 20 and 49 years of age. The data derived from this study have much less variation around the mean than previously cited works and are the most useful available. The data are presented in Tables 3–2 and 3–3.

Table 3–2. RADIOGRAPHIC LENGTH AND WIDTH* OF NORMAL KIDNEYS, MEASURED IN PLAIN RADIOGRAPHS OF 100 MALES AND 100 FEMALES, AGED 20 TO 49

Males				Females			
Right		Left		Right		Left	
Length	Width	Length	Width	Length	Width	Length	Width
12.9	6.2	13.2	6.3	12.3	5.7	12.6	5.9
0.8	0.4	0.8	0.5	0.8	0.5	0.8	0.4

*In centimeters.
From Möel, H.: Acta Radiol. [Diagn.] *46*:640, 1956 and *56* [Suppl. 206]:5, 1961. © 1956, 1961 Munksgaard International Publishers Ltd., Copenhagen, Denmark.

Table 3–3. RADIOGRAPHIC AREA* OF NORMAL KIDNEYS MEASURED IN PLAIN RADIOGRAPHS OF 100 MALES AND 100 FEMALES, AGED 20 TO 49

Males			Females		
Right	Left	Right + Left	Right	Left	Right + Left
79.6	82.7	162.3	70.1	74.1	144.2
8.7	8.3	15.6	8.0	7.3	13.6

*Product of length and width in square centimeters.
From Möel, H.: Acta Radiol. [Diagn.] *46*:640, 1956 and *56* [Suppl. 206]:5, 1961. © 1956, 1961 Munksgaard International Publishers Ltd., Copenhagen, Denmark.

Table 3–4 presents comparisons of the length and width of right and left kidneys in both sexes and illustrates the greater size of the male kidney compared with the female kidney and the usually larger size of the left kidney compared with the right one. Möel also demonstrated that postmortem length, width, and weight can be accurately predicted from the radiograph, once factors producing geometric enlargement and distortion are taken into account. The factors tend to overestimate linear measurements by an average of 17 per cent. In addition, a significant correlation between radiographic area of the kidney and factors relating to body build, such as height, weight, and body surface area, was established. However, the use of these factors in the statistical evaluation of Möel's data did not improve the accuracy of predicting renal mass from the simple direct measurement of kidney area from the radiograph. Ludin (1967) has simplified the estimation of renal weight by computing a set of nomograms based on radiographic measurement of renal length and width. These, too, are of some practical usefulness.

Griffiths and associates (1975) studied the value of estimating renal size from radiographs by correlating the weight of normal kidneys after removal of fat from the renal sinuses with measurements of length,

Table 3–4. COMPARISON BETWEEN RADIOGRAPHIC LENGTH AND WIDTH OF RIGHT AND LEFT KIDNEYS, MEASURED IN PLAIN RADIOGRAPHS OF 100 MALES AND 100 FEMALES, AGED 20 TO 49

Relationship Between Right and Left Kidney	Males	Females	Significance Males	Females
Length:				
Right kidney longer	27	35		
Both kidneys equal	1	5		
Left kidney longer	72	60	+ + +	+
Total number of cases:	100	100		
Width:				
Right kidney wider	36	32		
Both kidneys equal	10	11		
Left kidney wider	54	57		+ +
Total number of cases:	100	100		

From Möel, H.: Acta Radiol. [Diagn.] *46*:640, 1956 and *56* [Suppl. 206]:5, 1961. © 1956, 1961 Munksgaard International Publishers Ltd., Copenhagen, Denmark.

width, depth, and area from radiographs. In this study, radiographic length correlated well with renal weight (r = .85). Radiographic width was found to provide a less accurate index of renal weight (r = .71), and measurement of renal area proved to be no better correlated with weight than length, even when the area occupied by the collecting system was subtracted. These authors concluded that the simplest linear measurements estimated renal size better than the more elaborate methods, which used dimensions measured less reliably and less readily.

Ultrasonography, of all imaging techniques, is particularly applicable to the measurement of renal mass. The ultrasound image is undistorted by magnification and is a true measurement of renal dimension. In addition, views of the kidney can be generated in planes that allow easy measurement of length, width, and thickness. Renal volume can then be determined from these values using the equation for an ellipsoid (Jones et al., 1983) or a modification of it (Hricak and Lieto, 1983). These same theoretical advantages apply to magnetic resonance imaging, although systematic studies have not been reported using this modality.

Computer-based technology has been applied to the planigraphic measurement of renal size using standard excretory urographic images. These determinations correlated well with renal function studies (Ward et al., 1976).

Computed tomographic data on adults relating renal parenchymal thickness, the transverse diameter of the vertebral body, and age have been formulated into a reference table of normal values (Gourtsoyiannis et al., 1990). A decrease in renal parenchymal thickness of about 10 per cent per decade has been found in both men and women throughout adulthood.

Hodson has taken a point of view quite different from those who put considerable credence in the value, accuracy, and practicality of quantitative measurements. In 1960, he reported a number of broad conclusions based on an analysis of 1000 urograms. This work confirmed the observations of others that the kidneys gradually increase in size from birth to the latter part of the second decade, stabilize until the fifth decade, and then gradually decrease in size. Wide variations in size within any given age group were established. The most constant relationship noted in this study was between the radiographic size of the kidney and the total body surface area. Even in this relationship, however, variation was great enough to prevent useful application in any single individual. In addition, Hodson recorded that kidneys of the same radiographic size and shape, as well as kidneys from two individuals of the same age, sex, height, and weight, were subject to variations in real weight of as much as 20 per cent. He believed that this inconsistency was due to individual variation in the anteroposterior dimension of the kidney. Unfortunately, the absence of raw data in Hodson's report makes it difficult to reconcile his conclusions with those of Möel. Most importantly, Hodson emphasized the observation that there is a remarkable tendency

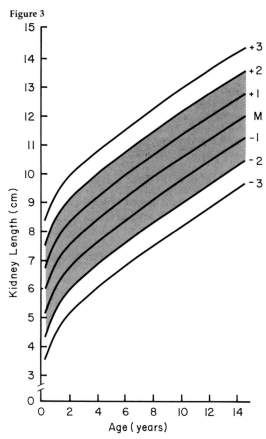

Figure 3–28. Graph of kidney length *versus* age based on excretory urograms in children. The plots include 3 standard deviations above and below the mean. One standard deviation = 0.785 cm. (From Currarino, G., et al.: Radiology *150*:703, 1984. Reproduced with kind permission of the author and *Radiology*.)

toward symmetry in size, shape, and thickness of renal substance between two kidneys within a single individual, keeping in mind the normal tendency of the left kidney to be slightly larger than the right. It is this observation that led Hodson to the precept that "in any individual the two kidneys should be symmetrical in shape, size and thickness and that marked alterations in such symmetry, particularly of the thickness of the renal substance, should be regarded with suspicion."

It is quite obvious that there are a number of approaches to determining normal renal size in the adult. Quantitative data are available and are useful to a certain point. More often than not, however, the qualitative evaluation of renal symmetry and uniformity of parenchymal thickness will be of greatest usefulness in any given individual.

The measurement of normal kidney size in infancy and childhood is subject to fewer vagaries than in the adult. Mean length related to age has been determined for excretory urography by Currarino and colleagues (1984). These data are reproduced in Figure 3–28. Nomograms relating sonographic kidney length to age, height, and weight have been determined by Han and Babcock (1985) and are reproduced in Figure 3–29. Ultrasonographic standards have also been established to relate kidney length to body weight in

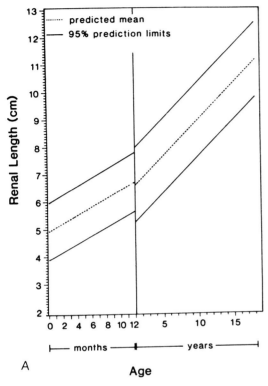

A

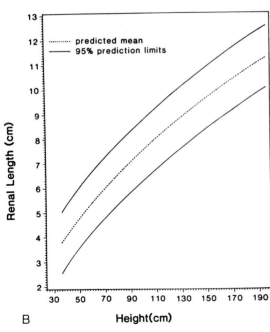

B

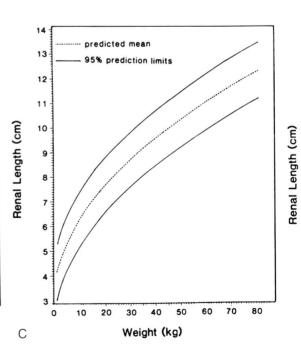

C

Figure 3–29. Graphs of maximum renal length *versus* age *(A)*, height *(B)*, and weight *(C)* based on ultrasonograms in children. (From Han, B. K., and Babcock, D. S.: AJR *145*:611, 1985. Reproduced with kind permission of the authors and the *American Journal of Roentgenology*.)

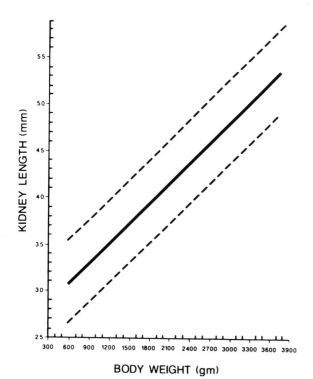

Figure 3–30. Nomogram for kidney length *versus* body weight derived from ultrasonograms in premature infants. The solid line represents the mean and the dotted line the 95 per cent confidence limits. (From Schlesinger, A. E., et al.: Radiology *164*:127, 1987. Reproduced with kind permission of the author and *Radiology.*)

premature infants (Schlesinger et al., 1987; Figure 3–30) and for fetal kidneys (Patten et al., 1990).

ANOMALOUS DEVELOPMENT OF THE KIDNEY AND URETER

Development of a normal kidney and ureter requires formation, elongation, and division of a ureteral bud; simultaneous induction of metanephric blastema into nephrons; dilatation and assimilation of early generations of ureteral bud divisions; and formation of independent renal lobes, most of which eventually fuse. This process begins in the caudal portion of the embryo when each ureteral bud encounters two parasagittal ridges of metanephric tissue situated medial to the umbilical arteries. As nephrogenesis progresses, the two kidneys separate laterally, and the pelvis and proximal ureter of each rotate medially toward the midline from an initial ventral position. However, a disturbance in any of these complex, concurrent developmental steps can produce anomalies in the shape, number, or position of the kidney and/or ureter. This section describes these anomalies. Other developmental abnormalities, such as multicystic dysplastic kidney, calyceal diverticula, megacalyces, ureteropelvic junction obstruction, megaureter, and ureterocele, are discussed in other chapters, in which their presentation is more consistent with the organization of this book.

Anomalies in Renal Form or Position

A disturbance in the separation of the two ridges of the metanephric blastema, in ureteral bud induction of metanephric tissue, or in the ascent and rotation of the kidney results in anomalous renal form or position. This type of anomaly is sometimes associated with anomalies of the ipsilateral genital organ or other organ systems or with genetic disorders such as Turner's syndrome, trisomy in identical twins, Fanconi's anemia, and Laurence-Moon-Biedl syndrome.

Agenesis. In agenesis, absence of a kidney is due to failure of a ureteral bud to form at all, failure of a growing ureteral bud to encounter and induce metanephric tissue, or absence of metanephric blastema. In the first situation, the ipsilateral trigone and ureteral orifice are also absent, a cystoscopic finding also described as hemitrigone. In the latter two situations, which are induction failures, a ureter of varying length ends blindly, usually in association with renal dysgenesis, as discussed below and in Chapter 11. Renal arteries and veins are absent in renal agenesis. With agenesis of the left kidney, the splenic flexure of the colon occupies the renal fossa. Renal agenesis often coexists with other anomalies. In particular, unilateral agenesis may be associated with absence of the ipsilateral adrenal gland and abnormalities of ipsilateral genital structures. In males, these include cyst of the seminal vesicle, absent vas deferens, hypoplastic or absent testes, and hypospadias (Fig. 3–31). In females, renal agenesis may be associated with uterine anomalies (agenesis, hypoplasia, unicornuate, bicornuate) or aplasia of the vagina.

Dysgenesis. Renal dysgenesis or dysplasia is a designation for undifferentiated renal tissue that has no resemblance to either normal kidney or kidney with acquired disease. When dysgenesis exists as an isolated event, the diagnosis is pathologic and does not have a radiologic counterpart. However, dysgenesis is often associated with multiple cysts in the affected kidney and atresia of the ureter, a condition known as *multicystic dysplastic kidney*. Additionally, dysgenesis is sometimes associated with anomalies in contralateral urinary tract structures. This subject is discussed in detail in Chapter 11.

Hypoplasia. The hypoplastic kidney results from a quantitative deficiency in the ureteral bud and metanephric primordia. This anomaly is discussed in Chapter 6 as one of the causes of the unilateral small, smooth kidney.

Ectopia. The position of the kidney and the associated length of the ureter are determined by the extent of ureteral bud elongation. Normally, the kidney is located in the abdomen, adjacent to the upper three lumbar vertebrae. When elongation of the ureteral bud ceases at an earlier than normal stage, the kidney is positioned in the pelvis or at the sacral or lower lumbar levels and the ureter is of appropriate length (Figs. 3–32 through 3–34). On rare occasions, the kidney is intrathoracic. A true intrathoracic kidney occurs on the left side more often than the right side

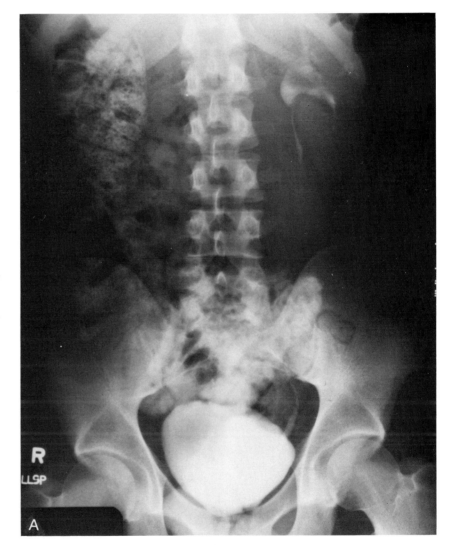

Figure 3–31. Agenesis, right kidney with associated cyst of the ipsilateral seminal vesicle in a 17-year-old boy with rectal pain.

A, Excretory urogram. The right kidney is absent, and there is compensatory hypertrophy of the left kidney. A mass effect is present on the right superolateral aspect of the bladder.

Illustration continued on following page

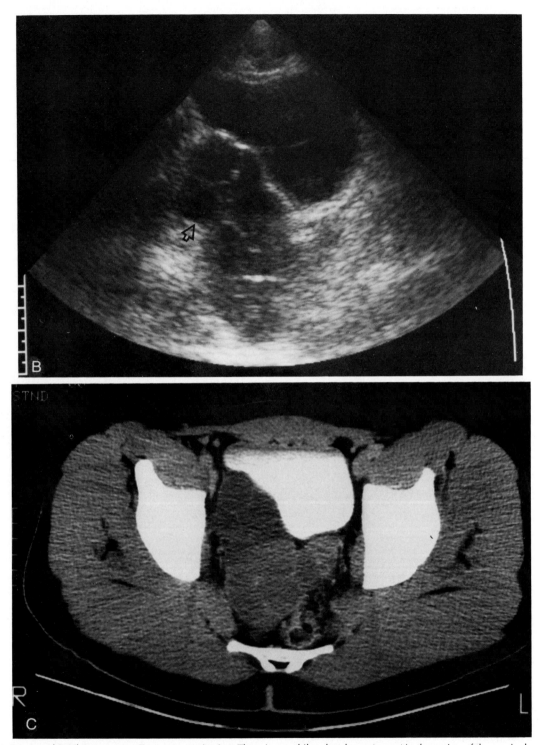

Figure 3–31 *Continued B,* Ultrasonogram. Transverse projection. There is a multiloculated cyst *(arrow)* in the region of the seminal vesicle. *C,* Computed tomogram, contrast material enhanced. The seminal vesicle cyst impresses on the bladder.

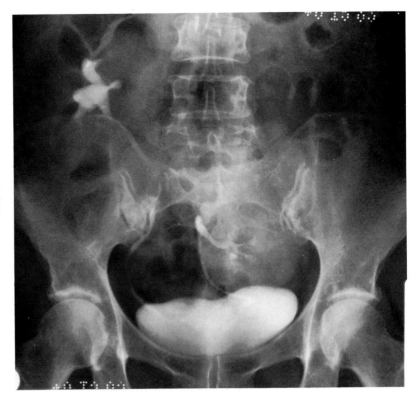

Figure 3–32. Bilateral renal ectopia. The left kidney is situated in the pelvis, whereas the right kidney is at the level of the lower lumbar vertebral segments. Excretory urogram.

and must be distinguished from displacement of the kidney into the thorax through a congenital or acquired diaphragmatic hernia. Ectopic kidneys are perfused by aberrant arteries from the aorta or from iliac arteries.

During elongation a ureteral bud may cross the midline and encounter the contralateral metanephric ridge. Here, the total renal mass becomes situated on one side of the abdomen. In this condition, known as crossed ectopia, the distal ureter inserts into the trigone on the side of origin (Fig. 3–35). Renal tissue in crossed ectopia is usually fused. Rarely are the two kidneys separate from each other. Invariably, ectopia is associated with aberrant renal arteries. Ectopia by itself is of no clinical significance.

Fusion. Fusion anomalies reflect disturbances in the early stage of renal organogenesis when both metanephric ridges lie adjacent to the midline. Presumably, fusion is a failure of separation of the ridges. *Lumps, cakes,* and *discs* are a few of the many terms used to describe the forms of fused kidneys (see Fig. 3–35), with *horseshoe kidney* the most frequently encountered form (Fig. 3–36). Here, the lower poles of both kidneys are joined by either renal or fibrous tissue. Rarely, they are joined at the upper poles. Features of a horseshoe kidney include medial deviation of the lower poles, incomplete ascent (ectopia), and aberrant renal arteries. The fused lower pole is usually situated just caudal to the origin of the inferior mesenteric artery. The collecting systems and proximal ureters of a horseshoe kidney are located more ventral than normal. Occasionally, aberrant arteries cross and obstruct the proximal ureter or ureteropelvic junction on one

or both sides. As a result, infection and stone formation may complicate a horseshoe kidney. The perirenal spaces on both sides of the abdomen communicate with each other in a horseshoe kidney.

Rotation. Failure of medial rotation of the kidney during ascent is the cause of rotational anomalies. Most frequently, the collecting structures remain ventral to the renal parenchyma (Fig. 3–37). Very uncommonly, rotation occurs laterally on the long axis of the kidneys (Fig. 3–38). This results in the renal artery and vein crossing the ventral surface of the kidney. Even more rare is longitudinal axis rotation beyond the medial position. In this circumstance, the pelvocalyceal system is directed toward a dorsal or dorsolateral position, and the renal artery and vein run over the dorsal surface of the kidney. Rotation on the anteroposterior axis of the kidney, although very rare, leads to a transverse position. Anomalies of ectopia, fusion, and rotation frequently coexist.

Anomalies in Number

Abnormality in the number or pattern of division of ureteral buds is the basis of this category of upper urinary tract anomalies.

Supernumerary Kidney. More than two kidneys and ureters form in the presence of an extra number of independent ureteral buds or from multiple early branches of a single ureteral bud. Any of these variations are extremely rare. Supernumerary kidneys are usually, though not invariably, caudal to the normal kidneys and hypoplastic.

Multiplications. Multiple ureteral buds arising in-

Text continued on page 87

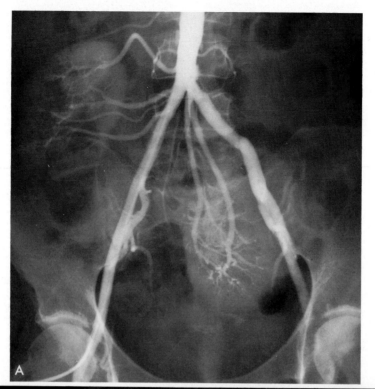

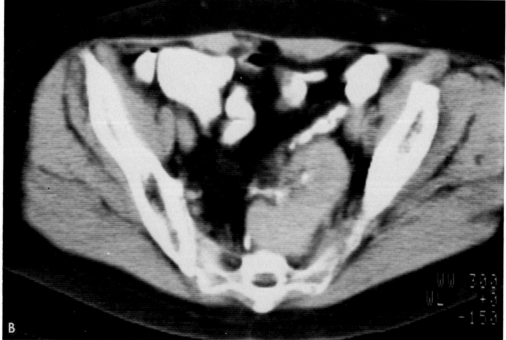

Figure 3–33. Renal ectopia. The left kidney is at the level of the sacrum and derives its arterial supply from a renal artery arising from the distal aorta.
  A, Aortogram. Note multiple aberrant renal arteries to a low-lying right kidney.
  B, Computed tomogram, contrast material enhanced.

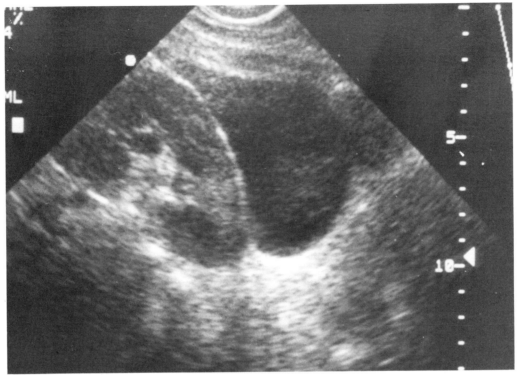

Figure 3–34. Renal ectopia. The kidney is situated in the pelvis cranial and posterior to the bladder. Ultrasonogram, sagittal section.

Figure 3–35. Crossed ectopia. The right ureter crosses the midline at the lower lumbar vertebral level and drains renal tissue fused with the left kidney. Note the orthotopic position of the right distal ureter *(arrow).* Excretory urogram.

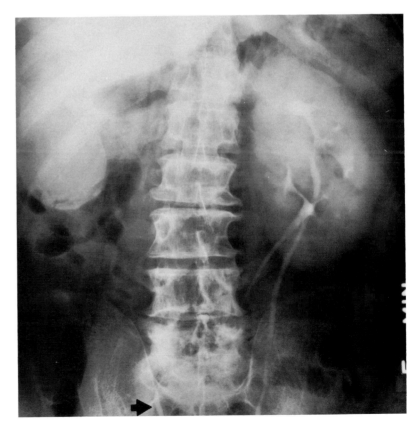

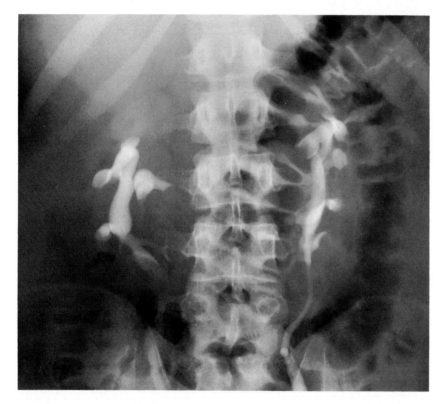

Figure 3–36. Renal fusion. Horseshoe kidney. The lower poles of each kidney are oriented medially, and the pelvis is placed laterally. Excretory urogram.

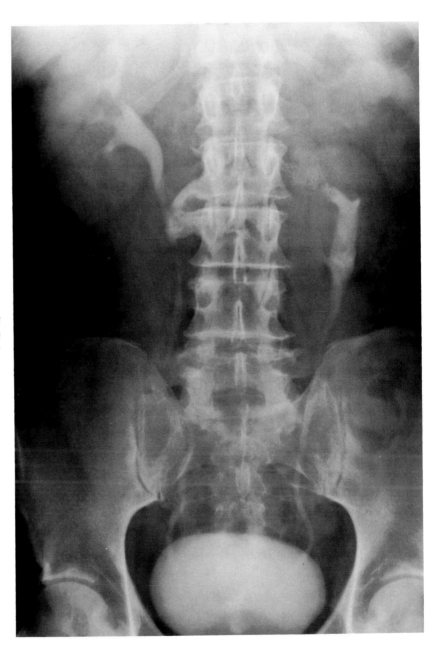

Figure 3–37. Malrotation and incomplete ascent of left kidney. The left renal pelvis remains ventral to the parenchyma, reflecting failure of medial rotation. Excretory urogram.

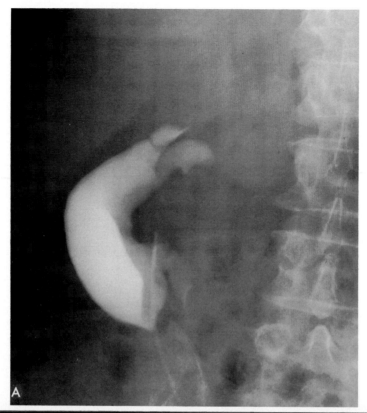

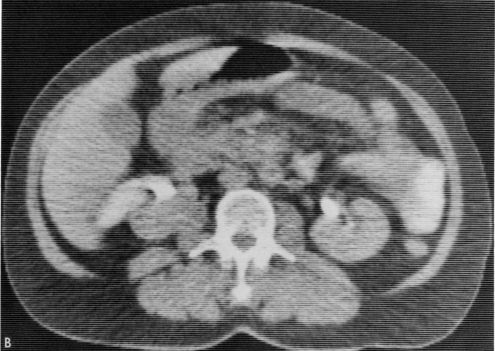

Figure 3–38. Malrotation in lateral direction results in ventrolateral placement of the renal pelvis.
    A, Retrograde pyelogram.
    B, Computed tomogram, contrast material enhanced.

dependently from the mesonephric duct or as early branches of a single ureteral bud are frequently encountered anomalies of the urinary tract. Complete duplication of the ureters draining a single kidney results from two ipsilateral, independent ureteral buds forming simultaneously from the mesonephric duct or very early branching of the ureteral bud with incorporation of each branch into the cloaca as separate structures. The moiety draining the upper pole has an ectopic distal insertion at a point caudal and medial to that of the moiety draining the lower pole. The latter moiety inserts either at the normal, or orthotopic, site in the trigone of the bladder or more cranial and lateral than the normal site, where it is susceptible to vesicoureteral reflux. These relationships are expressed in the Weigert-Meyer law and illustrated schematically in Figure 3–39. The upper pole moiety is susceptible to obstruction either as a complication of the ectopic insertion or by an aberrant artery crossing its ureteropelvic junction. The ectopic ureteral orifice may prolapse into the bladder, a condition known as ectopic ureterocele. The lower pelvocalyceal system moiety drains both the lower pole and the interpolar portion of the kidney and is subject to an increased incidence of vesicoureteral reflux when the intramural segment of its distal ureter is shortened by virtue of a slightly ectopic insertion. A kidney with a duplicated system is larger than normal, reflecting the influence of two ureteral buds in-

ducing metanephric blastema. Kidneys with more than two independent ureters have been reported rarely. Duplication anomalies are discussed further in Chapters 9 and 15.

Partial duplication of a single distal ureter with normal distal insertion into the bladder is the most common of the anomalies associated with ureteral bud division (Fig. 3–40). Here, the first division of the elongating ureteral bud occurs earlier than normal, and the two branches continue to elongate before beginning the series of branches that ultimately lead to formation of the pelvocalyceal system. Early first branching causes duplication of the distal ureter. Late duplication is seen as a bifid pelvis. The most cephalic branch of a duplicated ureter usually drains only the upper pole, whereas the remainder of the kidney is drained by the larger, inferior collecting system. Sometimes, the superior moiety of a duplicated ureter ends abruptly. This represents failure of the ureteral bud to encounter or induce metanephric blastema, a condition known as blind-ending ureter or ureteral diverticulum (Fig. 3–41). Rarely, one encounters more than two branches of a single ureter.

Duplication of a ureter, either complete or incomplete, is a precursor of abnormal placement of renal lobes or lobar dysmorphism. This is discussed in detail at the end of this section.

Abortive Calyx. A blind-ending, short outpouching of the renal pelvis is sometimes seen, usually in kid-

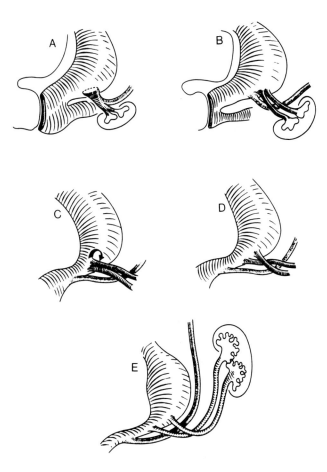

Figure 3–39. Embryologic development of complete duplication of the ureter and pelvocalyceal system.

A, There is early bifurcation of the ureteral bud.

B, The common portion of the distal mesonephric duct and ureteral bud are absorbed into the urogenital sinus such that the orifice of the mesonephric duct is caudal and medial to that of the two ureteral orifices.

C through *E,* There is continued absorption of the ureters into the trigone associated with medial rotation of the ureter draining the upper pole around the ureter draining the lower pole. (From Maizels, M.: Normal development of the urinary tract. *In* Walsh, P. C., Retik, A. B., Stamey, T. A., and Vaughan, E. D., Jr. [eds.]: Campbell's Urology, 6th ed. Philadelphia, W. B. Saunders, 1992, p. 1326.)

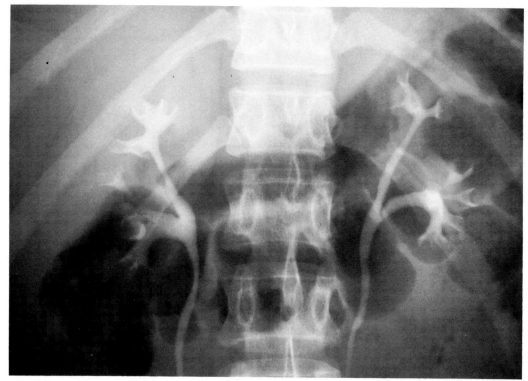

Figure 3–40. Duplication of the pelvocalyceal system. The process is incomplete on the right and complete on the left. Excretory urogram.

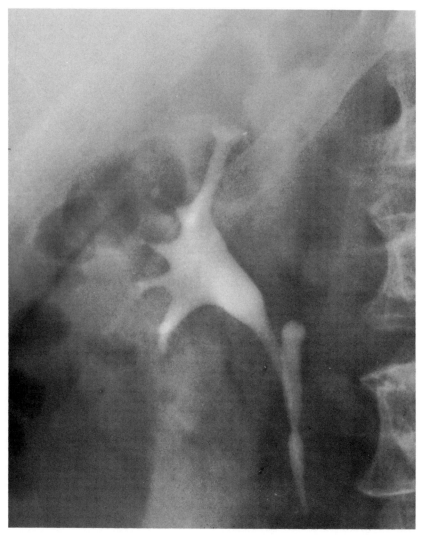

Figure 3–41. Blind-ending ureter. The superior moiety of a duplicated ureter ends abruptly. This represents failure of the ureteral bud to encounter or induce metanephric blastema. This is also known as ureteral diverticulum. Excretory urogram.

neys with a duplex collecting system. This diverticulum-like structure, thought to represent an abortive calyx, occasionally arises from the infundibulum draining the upper pole, rather than directly from the pelvis itself. The direct relationship between this structure and the pelvis, or infundibulum, distinguishes it from a calyceal diverticulum, which arises from a calcyeal fornix. The termination of an abortive calyx is blunt or spiked and is never invaginated by a papilla, as would be seen in a microcalyx or a calyx draining a dysmorphic lobe.

It is likely that an abortive calyx represents a ureteral bud branch that failed to continue to divide. This unusual structure must be distinguished from acquired diseases of an infundibulum or calyx, such as tuberculosis or tumor, that might mimic the appearance of this anomaly.

Unicalyceal (Unipapillary) Kidney. A small number of kidneys have been described as unicalyceal or unipapillary (Fig. 3–42). The hallmark of this anomaly is a single collecting structure, centrally located in the renal sinus and draining the entire kidney. This malformation is sometimes associated with absence of the contralateral kidney, hypertension, proteinuria, azotemia, and anomalies of other organ systems. Histologic study of a limited amount of material has demonstrated reduced numbers of nephrons with enlargement of individual glomeruli and tubules, a condition referred to as *oligomeganephronia*.

It is likely that the single collecting structure represents the renal pelvis, and that calyces and papillae are absent owing to the failure of a complete set of ureteral bud branches in the 6th to 10th generations. In essence, the kidney is a single lobe whose ducts of Bellini drain directly into the pelvis.

Anomalies of Lobar Anatomy (Pseudotumor)

In a previous section of this chapter, the early, orderly arrangement of independent lobes into dorsal and ventral groupings and their subsequent fusion into an adult kidney form was described. During this process, a number of events may occur that distort the prototypical pattern of the kidney. One external cause is pressure from the adjacent spleen that changes the shape of the left kidney. Other distortions are due to the persistence of fetal features, dominance of a part of a lobe, or the aberrant location of an entire lobe—normal variations that may simulate a tumor by causing either a focal bulge in the renal contour or a focal displacement of the pelvocalyceal system. For this reason, these distortions have been designated as renal pseudotumors. It is important to recognize the features that distinguish these normal variants from neoplasia if costly and complex investigations or needless surgery is to be avoided. Usually, differentiation can be achieved by recognizing the characteristic radiologic features that are described below. Doubtful cases can virtually always be resolved by radionuclide imaging, using agents excreted by the renal tubules to

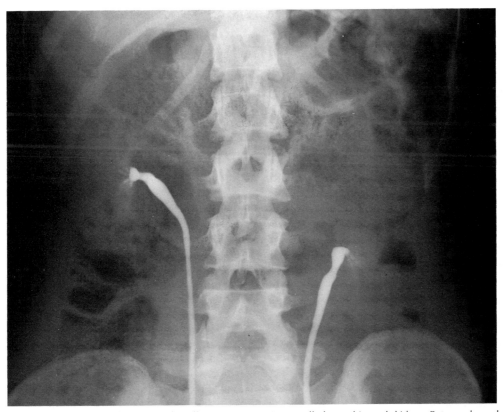

Figure 3–42. Unicalyceal (unipapillary) kidney. A single collecting structure is centrally located in each kidney. Retrograde pyelogram. (Courtesy of Margaret D. Bischel, M.D., Lutheran General Hospital, Park Ridge, Illinois, and JAMA *240*:2467–2468, 1978. Copyright 1978, American Medical Association.)

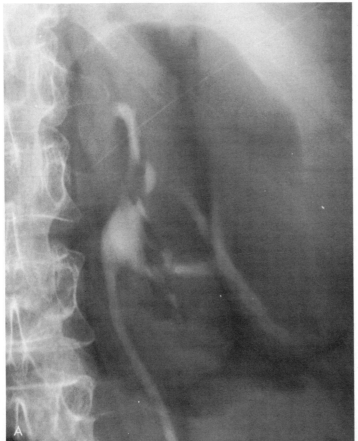

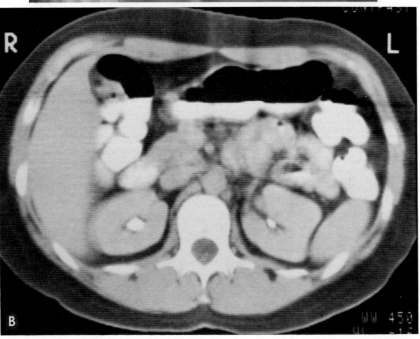

Figure 3–43. Splenic impression. Two different cases in which an enlarged spleen has effaced the lateral margin of the left kidney, producing a pseudotumor.

A, Excretory urogram.

B, Computed tomogram, contrast material enhanced.

demonstrate that the suspected mass is composed of normal tissue.

Splenic Impression. Flattening of the left kidney along its lateral or upper polar margin is frequently present (Fig. 3–43; see Fig. 3–22). Presumably, this impression on the renal contour is made by the spleen during the development of the left kidney. A bulge in the lateral margin of the kidney, just inferior to the flattened splenic impression, is a frequently associated finding that has been referred to as "dromedary hump." The normal nature of this variant shape is affirmed by the uniform thickness of the renal parenchyma between the surface of the kidney and the interpapillary line, particularly in the area of the bulge. Oblique films are often necessary to confirm this.

Fetal Lobation. The adult kidney sometimes retains sharp ridges on its surface, representing the sites where the septal cortices from two adjacent lobes abut (see Fig. 3–15). The centrilobar cortex between these ridges may be prominent and may be confused with neoplasm. This can be avoided by recognition of the characteristic features of fetal lobation, described earlier in this chapter.

Hilar Bulge. The parenchyma that composes the medial part of the kidney just above and below the sinus is often prominent, sometimes to the extent of causing focal displacement of the polar collecting system. This distortion is most frequently encountered in the suprahilar region of the left kidney.

Large Septum or Cloison of Bertin and Lobar Dysmorphism. There is a group of renal pseudotumors that are characterized by focal displacement of the collecting system within a kidney of normal contour. They usually occur in the presence of partial or complete duplication of the pelvocalyceal system, with the mass effect seen most frequently, although not invariably, in the area between the upper and interpolar portions of the kidney. In many instances, what causes the mass effect is normal septal cortex tissue that has persisted during lobar fusion and in the process has become relatively prominent (Figs. 3–44 through 3–46). This situation has been termed *large column of*

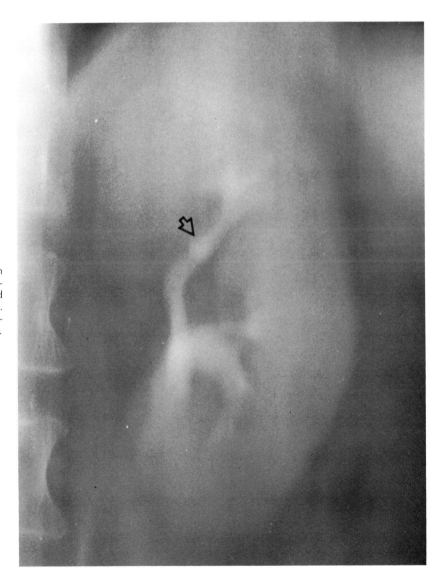

Figure 3–44. Pseudotumor due to large septum (cloison) of Bertin. The renal tissue projects between the moieties of a duplicated system and slightly displaces the upper pole collecting system. Note the characteristic calyx draining into the upper pole infundibulum *(arrow).* Excretory urogram.

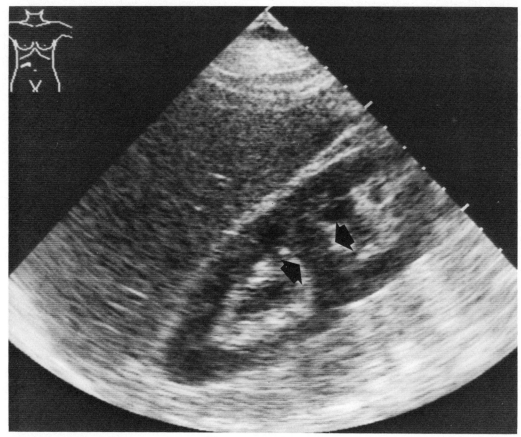

Figure 3–45. Pseudotumor due to a large septum (cloison) of Bertin. The cortical tissue *(arrows)* projects between the two hyperechogenic regions of the renal sinus that contain the duplicated pelvocalyceal system. (From Dalla Palma, L., et al.: Br. J. Radiol. *63*:680, 1990. Reproduced with kind permission of the author and the *British Journal of Radiology.*)

Figure 3–46. Pseudotumor due to large septum (cloison) of Bertin. The pseudotumor *(arrow)* projects into the renal sinus. Computed tomogram, contrast material enhanced. (Courtesy of Michael Federle, M.D., University of Pittsburgh, Pittsburgh, Pennsylvania.)

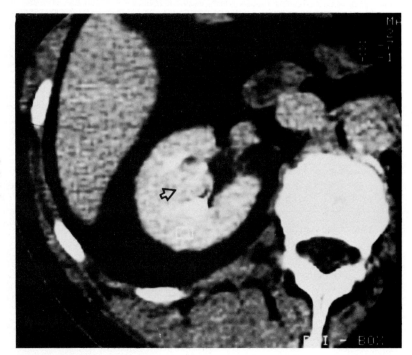

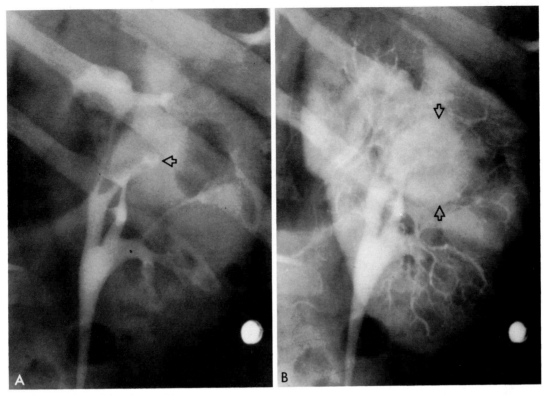

Figure 3–47. Pseudotumor due to lobar dysmorphism.

A, Excretory urogram. A well-formed calyx *(arrow)* and infundibulum extend to the center of the ectopically located renal lobe.

B, Selective renal arteriogram, late arterial phase. The angiographic nephrogram enhances the ring of cortex *(arrows)* surrounding the relatively radiolucent medulla of the ectopic lobe. Note the central position of the papilla and calyx draining this lobe.

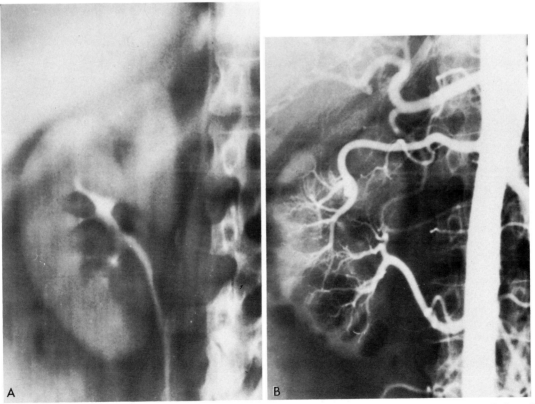

Figure 3–48. Aberrant renal arteries with accessory renal hilus. The kidney is perfused by two renal arteries arising directly from the aorta. The superior vessel enters the upper pole through an accessory hilus.

A, Excretory urogram. Tomogram.

B, Aortogram.

(Courtesy of T. F. Stephenson, M.D., St. Mary's Hospital, Rochester, New York, and AJR *132*:765, 1979.)

Bertin, large cloison, focal cortical hyperplasia, benign cortical rest, cortical island, and *focal renal hypertrophy. Large septum* or *cloison of Bertin* is the most accurate term. In addition to their usual location in a partial or complete duplicated collecting system, these "masses" have a pattern of contrast material enhancement that is characteristic of cortex rather than medulla. Large cloisons are drained by calyces that are connected to the midportion of the pelvis by short infundibula. Sometimes, a papilla arises from the enlarged cortical tissue directly into the pelvis or an infundibulum. This form of aberrant papilla may be confused with a nonopaque filling defect in the collecting system.

Lobar dysmorphism is another form of pseudotumor that is very similar to large cloison (Fig. 3–47). Here, a complete, though diminutive, lobe is situated atypically, deep within the renal substance. As with a large cloison, this occurs in the region of a partial or complete duplication of the collecting system and will focally displace the pelvis or calyces. The presence of a complete lobe, rather than septal tissue alone, is suggested by a well-formed, though diminutive, calyx in the central portion of the "mass." Conclusive evidence of the normal lobar structure is best derived from angiography, which demonstrates early opacification of the septal cortex surrounding a relatively radiolucent medulla, the central location of the microcalyx and papilla, and a set of arcuate arteries serving the diminutive lobe.

Nodular Compensatory Hypertrophy. In the presence of focal renal scarring, areas of unaffected normal tissue will undergo compensatory hypertrophy. This nodular pattern of renal enlargement is seen in severe cases of multifocal reflux nephropathy (see Chapter 5). Focal enlargement of deeply situated septal cortex has also been described in analgesic nephropathy (see Chapter 7). Strictly speaking, these represent renal pseudotumors, but their recognition as a component of a pathologic process should not be difficult.

Anomalies of Renal Arteries

Aberrant renal arteries arise from the aorta between T-11 and L-4 and occur in approximately 25 per cent of all individuals. They are persistent mesonephric vessels and usually perfuse one of the poles. Uncommonly, the aberrant artery may enter the kidney directly in the region perfused through an accessory renal hilus (Fig. 3–48).

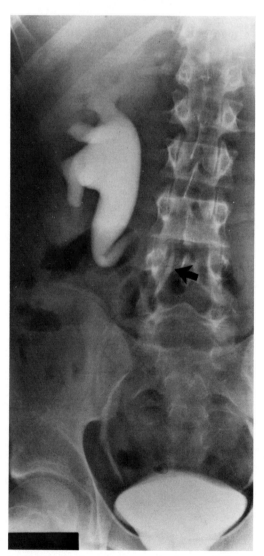

Figure 3–49. Retrocaval ureter. The proximal ureter deviates sharply in a cranial direction and then courses medial to the right pedicle of the fifth lumbar vertebral body *(arrow)* before resuming a normal position at the pelvic brim. Excretory urogram.

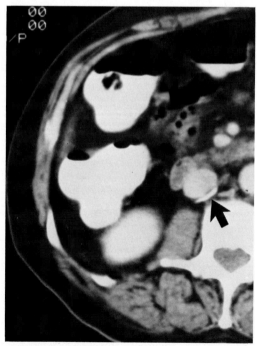

Figure 3–50. Retrocaval ureter. Transverse cross section at the level of the lower pole of the right kidney demonstrates the proximal ureter as it passes posterior to the inferior vena cava *(arrow)*. Computed tomogram, contrast material enhanced.

Retrocaval Ureter

Retrocaval ureter is due to anomalous persistence of the posterior cardinal vein during the development of the inferior vena cava. As a result, the right ureter deviates sharply from its normal position lateral to the inferior vena cava and passes posterior and medial to the inferior vena cava at the level of the third or fourth lumbar vertebral bodies. From this point distally, the ureter partially encircles the vena cava as it moves anterior and then lateral to the vena cava to resume its normal position (Figs. 3–49 and 3–50).

In many instances, retrocaval ureter is asymptomatic. However, obstruction at the site of proximal deviation can cause flank pain or be complicated by urinary tract infection.

Bibliography

Adam, E. J., Desai, S. C., and Lawton, G.: Racial variations in normal ureteric course. Clin. Radiol. 36:373, 1985.

Bischel, M. D., Blustein, W. C., Kinnas, N. C., Valaitis, J., and Rubenstein, M.: Solitary renal calix. JAMA 240:2467, 1978.

Brandt, T. D., Neiman, H. L., Dragowski, M. J., Bulawa, W., and Claykamp, G.: Ultrasound assessment of normal renal dimensions. J. Ultrasound Med. Biol. 1:49, 1982.

Carter, A. R., Horgam, J. G., Jennings, T. A., and Rosenfield, A. T.: The junctional parenchymal defect: A sonographic variant of renal anatomy. Radiology 154:499, 1985.

Cohen, H. L., Cooper, J., Eisenberg, P., Mandel, F. S., Gross, B. R., Goldman, M. A., Barzel, E., and Rawlinson, K. F.: Normal length of fetal kidneys: Sonographic study in 397 obstetric patients. AJR 157:545, 1991.

Cook, W. A., and Stephens, F. D.: Fused kidneys: Morphologic study and theory of embryogenesis. Birth Defects 13:329, 1977.

Cope, J. R., and Trickey, S. E.: Congenital absence of the kidney: Problems in diagnosis and management. J. Urol. 127:10, 1982.

Currarino, G., Williams, B., and Dana, K.: Kidney length correlated with age: Normal values in children. Radiology 150:703, 1984.

Dacie, J. E.: The "central lucency" sign of lobar dysmorphism (pseudotumour of the kidney). Br. J. Radiol. 49:39, 1976.

Dalla Palma, L., Bazzocchi, M., Cressa, C., and Tommasini, G.: Radiological anatomy of the kidney revisited. Br. J. Radiol. 63:680, 1990.

Dinkel, E., Ertel, M., and Dittrick, M.: Kidney size in childhood: Sonographical growth charts for kidney length and volume. Pediatr. Radiol. 15:38, 1985.

Dorph, S., Sovak, M., Talner, L. B., and Rosen, L.: Why does kidney size change during I.V. urography? Invest. Radiol. 12:246, 1977.

Effman, R. L., Ablow, R. C., and Siegel, N. J.: Renal growth. Radiol. Clin. North Am. 15:3, 1977.

Elkin, M.: Radiology of the urinary tract: Some physiological considerations. Radiology 116:259, 1975.

Emamian, S. A., Nielsen, M. B., Pedersen, J. F., and Ytte, L.: Kidney dimensions at sonography: Correlation with age, sex, and habitus in 665 adult volunteers. AJR 160:83, 1993.

Feldman, A. E., Pollack, H. M., Perri, A. J., Jr., Karafin, L., and Kendall, A. R.: Renal pseudotumors: An anatomic-radiologic classification. J. Urol. 120:133, 1978.

Feldman, A. E., Rosenthal, R. S., and Shaw, J. L.: Aberrant renal papilla: A diagnostic dilemma. J. Urol. 114:144, 1975.

Fine, H., and Keen, E. N.: Some observations on the medulla of the kidney. Br. J. Urol. 48:161, 1976.

Friedland, G. W.: Congenital anomalies of the urinary tract. In Friedland, G. W., et al. (eds.): Uroradiology: An Integrated Approach. New York, Churchill Livingstone, 1983, pp. 1349–1519.

Friedland, G. W., and DeVries, P.: Renal ectopia and fusion: Embryologic basis. Urology 5:698, 1975.

Frimann-Dahl, J.: Normal variations of left kidney. Acta Radiol. 55:207, 1961.

Gluer, S., Kluth, D., Reich, P., and Lambrecht, W.: The development of common nephric duct and its significance in upper urinary tract abnormalities. Pediatr. Surg. Int. 8:34, 1993.

Gourtsoyiannis, N., Prassopoulos, P., Cavouras, D., and Pantelidis, N.: The thickness of the renal parenchymal decreases with age: A CT study of 360 patients. AJR 155:541, 1990.

Griffiths, G. J., Cartwright, G., and McLachlan, M. S. F.: Estimation of renal size from radiographs: Is the effort worthwhile? Clin. Radiol. 26:249, 1975.

Han, B. K., and Babcock, D. S.: Sonographic measurements and appearance of normal kidney in children. AJR 145:611, 1985.

Hodson, C. J.: Hypertension of renal origin. In McLaren, J. W. (ed.): Modern Trends in Diagnostic Radiology. New York, Paul B. Hoeber, 1960, pp. 124–134.

Hodson, C. J.: The lobar structure of the kidney. Br. J. Urol. 44:246, 1972.

Hodson, C. J., and Mariani, S.: Large cloisons. AJR 139:327, 1982.

Hoffer, F. A., Hanabongh, A. M., and Teele, R. L.: The interrenicular junction—a mimic of renal scarring on normal paediatric sonograms. AJR 145:1075, 1985.

Hricak, H., and Lieto, R. P.: Sonographic determination of renal volume. Radiology 148:311, 1983.

Jones, T. B., Riddick, L. R., Harpen, M. D., Dubuisson, R. L., and Samuels, D.: Ultrasonic determination of renal mass and renal volume. J. Ultrasound Med. Biol. 2:151, 1983.

Karn, M. N.: Radiographic measurements of kidney section area. Ann. Hum. Genet. 25:379, 1962.

Kasike, B. L., and Umen, A. J.: The influence of age, sex, race and body habitus on kidney weight in humans. Arch. Pathol. Lab. Med. 110:55, 1986.

Kenney, I. J., Wild, S. R.: The renal parenchymal junctional line in children: Ultrasonic frequency and appearances. Br. J. Radiol. 60:865, 1987.

Korenchevsky, V.: Natural relative hypoplasia of organs and process of aging. J. Pathol. 54:13, 1942.

Kunin, M.: The abortive calix: Variations in appearance and differential diagnosis. AJR 139:931, 1982.

Lafortune, M., Constantin, A., Breton, G., and Vallee, C.: Sonography of the hypertrophied column of Bertin. AJR 146:53, 1986.

Leekam, R. N., Matzinger, M. A., Brunelle, M., Gray, R. R., and Grossman, H.: The sonography of renal columnar hypertrophy. J. Clin. Ultrasound 11:491, 1983.

Lewis, E., and Ritchie, W. G. M.: A simple ultrasonic method for assessing renal size. J. Clin. Ultrasound 8:417, 1980.

Ludin, H.: Radiologic estimation of kidney weight. Acta Radiol. (Diagn.) 6:561, 1967.

McCrory, W. W.: Developmental Nephrology. Cambridge, MA, Harvard University Press, 1972.

Möel, H.: Size of normal kidneys. Acta Radiol. (Diagn.) 46:640, 1956.

Möel, H.: Kidney size and its deviation from normal in acute renal failure: A roentgen diagnostic study. Acta Radiol. (Diagn.) 56(Suppl. 206):5, 1961.

Murphy, B. J., Casillas, J., and Becerra, J. L.: Retrocaval ureter: Computed tomography and ultrasound appearance. CT 11:89, 1987.

N'Guessan, G., and Stephens, F. D.: Supernumerary kidney. J. Urol. 130:649, 1983.

Ohlson, L.: Normal collecting ducts and visualization of urography. Radiology 170:33, 1989.

Oliver, J.: Nephrons and Kidneys: A Quantitative Study of Developmental and Evolutionary Mammalian Renal Architectonics. New York, Harper & Row, 1968.

Patriquin, H., Lefaivre, J. F., Lafortune, M., Russo, P., and Boisvert, J.: Fetal lobation: An anatomo-ultrasonographic correlation. J Ultrasound Med. 9:191, 1990.

Patten, R. M., Mack, L. A., Wang, K. Y., and Cyr, D. R.: The fetal genitourinary tract. Radiol. Clin. North Am. 28:115, 1990.

Pendergrass, E. P.: Excretory urography as a test of urinary tract function. Radiology 40:223, 1943.

Peterson, J. E., Pinckney, L. E., Rutledge, J. C., and Currarino, G.: The solitary renal calyx and papilla in human kidneys. Radiology 144:525, 1982.

Pollack, H. M., Edell, S., and Morales, J. D.: Radionuclide imaging in renal pseudotumors. Radiology 111:639, 1974.

Potter, E. L.: Normal and Abnormal Development of the Kidney. Chicago, Year Book Medical Publishers, 1972.

Ransley, P. G.: Intrarenal reflux: anatomical, dynamic and radiological studies—part I. Urol. Res. 5:61, 1977.

Ransley, P. G., and Risdon, R. A.: The renal papilla, intrarenal reflux and chronic pyelonephritis. *In* Hodson, J., and Kincaid-Smith, P. (eds.): Reflux Nephropathy. New York, Masson Publishing, 1979, pp. 126–133.

Ransley, P. G., and Risdon, R. A.: Renal papillary morphology in infants and young children. Urol. Res. 3:111, 1975.

Ransley, P. G., and Risdon, R. A.: Reflux and renal scarring. Br. J. Radiol. Suppl. 14, 1978.

Sarajlic, M., Durst-Zivkovic, B., Svoren, E., Vitkovic, M., Batinic, D., Bradic, I., and Vuckovic, I.: Congenital ureteric diverticula in children and adults: Classification, radiological and clinical features. Br. J. Radiol. 62:551, 1989.

Saxton, H. M.: Opacification of collecting ducts at urography. Radiology 170:16, 1989.

Schlesinger, A. E., Hedlund, G. L., Pierson, W. P., and Null, D. M.: Normal standards for kidney length in premature infants: Determination with US. Radiology 164:127, 1987.

Scott, J. E., Hunter, E. W., Lee, R. E., and Matthews, J. N.: Ultrasound measurement of renal size in newborn infants. Arch. Dis. Child. 65:361, 1990.

Sherwood, T., and Williams, D. I.: Post-obstructive renal atrophy, megacalices, hydrocalices. Conversations Radiol. 1:5, 1973.

Stephenson, T. F., and Paul, G. J.: Accessory renal hilus. AJR 132:765, 1979.

Sykes, D.: The morphology of renal lobulations and calices and their relationship to partial nephrectomy. Br. J. Surg. 51:294, 1964.

Sykes, D.: The correlation between renal vascularization and lobulation of the kidney. Br. J. Urol. 36:549, 1964.

Thomsen, H. S., Larsen, S., and Talner, L. B.: Papillary morphology in adult human kidneys and in body and adult pig kidneys. Eur. Urol. 9:170, 1983.

Thornburn, G. D., Kopald, H. H., Herd, J. A., Hollenberg, M., O'Morchoe, C. C., and Barger, A. C.: Intrarenal distribution of nutrient blood flow determined with krypton[85] in the unanesthetized dog. Circ. Res. 13:290, 1963.

Troell, S., Berg, V., and Johansson, B.: Renal parenchymal volume in children: Normal value assessed by ultrasonography. Acta Radiol. 29:127, 1988.

Vuorinen, P., Pyykönen, L., and Antilla, P.: A renal cortical index obtained from urography films. Br. J. Radiol. 33:622, 1960.

Wald, H.: The weight of normal adult human kidneys and its variability. Arch. Pathol. Lab. Med. 23:493, 1937.

Ward, J. P., Franklin, D. A., and Wickham, J. E. A.: A computer-based technique for measurement of renal parenchymal area on intravenous urograms. Br. J. Radiol. 49:836, 1976.

Webb, J. A. W., Fry, I. K., and Charlton, C. A. C.: An anomalous calyx in the mid-kidney: An anatomical variant. Br. J. Radiol. 48:674, 1975.

Whitehouse, R. W.: High and low-osmolar contrast agents in urography: A comparison of the appearances with respect to pyelotubular opacification and renal length. Clin. Radiol. 37:395, 1986.

Yeh, H. C., Halton, K. P., Shapiro, R. S., Rabinowitz, J. G., and Mitty, H. A.: Junctional parenchyma: Revised definition of hypertrophic column of Bertin. Radiology 185:725, 1992.

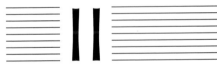

II

RENAL PARENCHYMAL DISEASE

4

A SYSTEMATIC APPROACH TO THE RADIOLOGIC DIAGNOSIS OF PARENCHYMAL DISEASE OF THE KIDNEY

The anatomic information presented in the preceding chapter is but one of two necessary elements in organizing an orderly approach to the radiologic study of renal disease. The other is understanding how the many different pathologic processes that affect the kidney may manifest themselves radiologically. Obviously, some diseases of the kidney produce lesions detectable only by electron or light microscopy; others are best diagnosed by characteristic abnormalities of renal function or urine content. In these circumstances, the radiologist's role, if any, is limited to defining broad categories, such as acute or chronic, or to excluding other disease processes. On the other hand, radiology is unique among the clinical disciplines in its ability to reveal the kidney as a whole *in vivo*. Analysis of kidney size, contour, amount of perfused parenchyma (the nephrogram), calyceal and papillary morphology, and many other features detectable by a variety of imaging modalities may at times provide a more precise clinical diagnosis than can be achieved by microscopic study of needle biopsy tissue or by measurement of various renal function tests.

What is necessary, then, is for the radiologist to organize his or her knowledge of how the kidney responds to various diseases within a framework of what might be detectable by radiologic techniques. This can be accomplished in three ways. First, the impact of a given disease on renal size can be evaluated, since many diseases cause either an increase or a decrease in renal bulk. Second, the appearance of the renal contour can be used as an index of the distribution of lesions within the kidney. Some diseases that produce loss of renal bulk are characteristically confined to the lobe and produce focal scars in the contour of the kidney. Other diseases may cause either an increase or a decrease in renal bulk, but because the lesions are uniformly distributed throughout the whole kidney, the contour retains its normal smoothness. Smooth contour therefore implies global distribution of the pathologic lesion. Still other diseases, particularly some that increase bulk, are regional and may involve one or more separate portions of the kidney, resulting in focal or multifocal expansion of the renal contour. Third, a determination can be made as to whether a given disease characteristically affects the kidney unilaterally or bilaterally. Thus, renal *size, contour*, and *laterality of involvement* provide points of departure for developing an orderly routine for analysis of radiologic images and for establishing an organized categorical framework for the radiologic diagnosis of renal parenchymal disease.

In the sections that follow, pathologic processes are studied in terms of how they alter tissue bulk and what part of the lobar anatomy they involve. These considerations provide the basis for classifying a large number of diseases according to their effect on renal size and contour. These "pathologic-radiologic" categories are refined further by distinguishing diseases that are inherently unilateral from those that are inherently bilateral in their effects. These smaller groups are designated "diagnostic sets." Finally, radiologic features (called "secondary uroradiologic observations") other than size, contour, and laterality of involvement are used to identify individual diseases within each diagnostic set.

Before proceeding, however, it should be pointed out that, in the course of disease, the kidney often will progress from a large size to a small one, inevitably passing through an intermediate period in which its size is within the radiologic limits of normal. Likewise, the development of contour abnormalities, such as scars, is not an overnight phenomenon. The reader should therefore keep in mind that assigning each disease to a radiologic classification based on size, contour, and laterality is perforce somewhat arbitrary and likely to be controversial—but also convenient, efficient, and quite accurate. Assignment of each disease to its diagnostic set has been based either on its most commonly presenting form or on the state of activity during which the radiologist is most likely to encounter it in a clinical setting.

PATHOLOGIC-RADIOLOGIC CONSIDERATIONS

Processes Leading to Loss of Renal Tissue

Reflux Nephropathy (Chronic Atrophic Pyelonephritis). Reflux nephropathy involves extensive tubule atrophy and loss, leukocytic infiltration, and marked fibrosis. The lesion tends to be distributed through the full thickness of all or part of a renal lobe, from centrilobar cortex to papilla. Other areas of the lobe adjacent to the lesion may be normal. The combination of dense fibrosis and full-thickness involvement causes a focal reduction and complete disorganization of the affected renal tissue. Retraction occurs at the external margin of the lobe, at the centrilobar cortex, and at the papillary tip. This is seen radiologically as a focal contour depression overlying a calyx that has become dilated because of papillary retraction and scarring.

The lesion of reflux nephropathy is occasionally limited to a part or the whole of a single lobe, usually in one of the poles of an otherwise normal kidney. Often, however, multiple foci are found in one or both kidneys. In this situation, the disease occurs and progresses independently at each site. So, although reflux nephropathy is inherently a focal disease of a single renal lobe, it may be found at random in many areas of the kidney, producing a radiologic image of multiple contour depressions overlying dilated subservient calyces. Normal tissue occupies intervening areas. This process is illustrated diagrammatically in Figure 4–1.

Lobar Infarction. Lobar infarction also causes tissue loss but in a significantly different manner from that seen in reflux nephropathy. When one or more inter-lobar or arcuate arteries are occluded, infarction develops in the peripheral portion of the lobe, since this part is perfused by fewer vessels than the inner lobe and these vessels are end-arteries. The infarcted area is seen on a cut section of the lobe as a triangular area, with its base on the centrilobar cortex and its apex extending to a variable depth into the medulla. If more than one of the interlobar or arcuate arteries subserving the involved lobe is occluded, the cortical base of the infarct is likely to be situated in the middle of the centrilobar cortex; whereas if only a single vessel is involved, the infarcted area will be eccentrically located on one margin of the centrilobar cortex. Attention to the limited area subserved by each arcuate artery in Figure 3–5 provides an explanation for this pattern.

In addition to the peripheral distribution of the infarct lesion, it is characteristic of infarction to cause tissue loss by a "dropping" out of nephrons without a significant fibrotic response. This is in sharp contrast to the important role of fibroblasts in the production of the reflux nephropathy scar. The scar that forms in lobar infarction, therefore, is a reflection of tissue loss due to the disappearance of the dead tubules, not active retraction secondary to fibrosis. This scarring process, plus the peripheral location of the lesion in the lobe, leaves the papilla undisturbed. Thus, the radiologic hallmark of lobar infarction is a contour defect overlying a normal papilla and calyx. This may occur either singly or at multiple foci, depending on the number of vessels randomly involved. Figure 4–1 schematizes this pattern.

Papillary Necrosis. Papillary necrosis is a pathologic process that occurs in the papillary portion of the medulla. The remainder of the lobe is involved only in a very advanced state of certain forms of the disease. Commonly, multiple papillae in one or both kidneys are abnormal, although the process occasionally may be limited to a single lobe.

Papillary necrosis begins with a stage of necrobiosis of the loops of Henle and the vasa recta at the tip of the papilla. This progresses to frank necrosis with a patchy distribution that eventually involves all elements of the papilla. These stages can be detected radiologically beginning with simple enlargement of an otherwise normal papilla in the earliest period and progressing to include the appearance of fine projections of contrast material extending along the side of the involved papilla, irregularity of the papillary surface, medullary cavitation, and ultimately a complete slough of the papilla. The latter stage is illustrated in Figure 4–1. A late process, only related to the more fulminant forms of papillary necrosis associated with analgesic nephropathy, may involve the entire lobe with fine fibrosis of the interstitial tissue with chronic inflammatory cell infiltrates and tubule loss or atrophy. This stage of chronic interstitial nephritis produces tissue wasting in the whole kidney and presents a radiologic image of global wasting of the kidney since all lobes are involved uniformly. These findings of chronic interstitial nephritis are seen in addition to the usual abnormalities of papillary necrosis.

FOCAL LOSS OF RENAL TISSUE

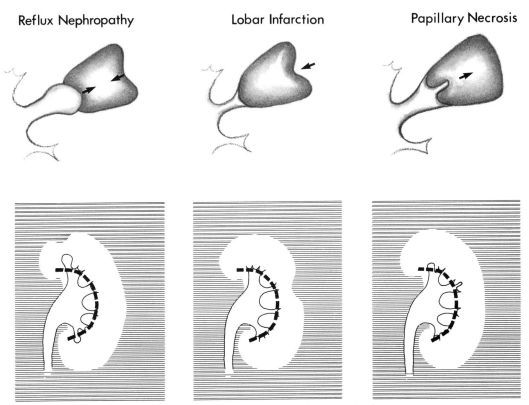

Figure 4–1. Patterns of lobar response to diseases producing focal loss of renal substance. The differences in urographic patterns are illustrated in this pathologic/radiologic category with a schema of the sites of lobar tissue loss in the three entities.

Global Tissue Loss. The global tissue loss category represents a large group of diseases that, apart from their characteristic smallness, lack distinguishing radiologic features. This category is a catchall for a number of specific diseases that vary widely in their histologic appearance, etiology, and clinical significance. One common feature that binds these entities together in a pathologic-radiologic classification is the global distribution of their lesions. Tubule atrophy and a fine interstitial fibrosis account for much of the generalized tissue wasting, regardless of whether the pathologic process primarily involves arterioles, glomeruli, tubules, or the interstitium. Radiologically detectable focal scars and calyceal-papillary distortion are not features of disease in this category.

Table 4–1 includes a list of abnormalities that produce the indeterminate radiologic findings of small kidneys with smooth contours. These include *ischemia due to focal arterial disease, generalized arteriosclerosis, benign* and *malignant nephrosclerosis, atheroembolic renal disease, chronic infarction, chronic glomerulonephritis, radiation nephritis, hereditary nephropathies, congenital hypoplasia, postobstructive atrophy, postinflammatory atrophy, reflux atrophy, amyloidosis (late),* and *arterial hypotension.* Each of these in its usual form will present a radiologic picture of a small kidney with a smooth contour, although variations in this basic pattern do occur in certain diseases. These are discussed specifically in later chapters of this book.

Decreased excretion of contrast material is frequent and reflects the impairment of renal function commonly seen in many of these diseases. Renal parenchyma, as depicted by the interpapillary line, is, of course, thin. An occasional response to parenchymal tissue loss is proliferation of fat around the pelvis, infundibula, and calyces in the renal hilus, causing

Table 4–1. PATHOLOGIC-RADIOLOGIC CLASSIFICATION OF ENTITIES ASSOCIATED WITH BOTH FOCAL AND GLOBAL LOSS OF RENAL TISSUE: NORMAL TO SMALL KIDNEY

Lobar Tissue Loss (Focal Scar)
  Reflux nephropathy (chronic atrophic pyelonephritis)
  Lobar infarction
  Papillary necrosis
Global Tissue Loss (Smooth Contour)
  Ischemia due to focal arterial disease
  Generalized arteriosclerosis
  Benign and malignant nephrosclerosis
  Atheroembolic renal disease
  Chronic infarction
  Chronic glomerulonephritis
  Radiation nephritis
  Hereditary nephropathies
  Congenital hypoplasia
  Postobstructive atrophy
  Postinflammatory atrophy
  Reflux atrophy
  Amyloidosis (late)
  Arterial hypotension

lack of distensibility and attenuation of the collecting system. One exception to these generalizations regarding tissue loss in the indeterminate small kidney is the kidney that shrinks as a result of arterial hypotension and depletion of renal blood volume, rather than loss of parenchyma per se. Radiologic changes seen in the global tissue loss category are schematized in Figure 4–2.

Processes Leading to Increase in Renal Bulk

Processes that increase renal bulk are either diffuse throughout the kidney, causing *global enlargement*, or confined to one or more regions and present as *focal* or *multifocal* enlargement of kidney contour.

Global Tissue Gain. This category, like the global tissue loss group, is an indeterminate pathologic-radiologic category in which the tissue response to disease produces a global enlargement of the organ, with preservation of a smooth contour and, with the single exception of obstructive uropathy, a normal pelvocalyceal-papillary relationship, as shown in Figure 4–3. Many widely varying mechanisms produce this form of diffuse, smooth renal enlargement. They include parenchymal deposition of abnormal proteins (*amyloidosis* and *multiple myeloma*); abnormal collections of fluid in the interstitium, either edema (*acute tubular necrosis, obstructive uropathy*) or blood (*acute arterial infarction, renal vein thrombosis,* or *acute cortical necrosis*); neoplastic (*leukemia*) or inflammatory cell infiltrates (*acute interstitial nephritis* and *acute pyelonephri-*

tis); and proliferative and necrotizing disorders of the glomerulus and microvasculature (the various forms of *acute glomerulonephritis, polyarteritis nodosa* [*microscopic form*], *allergic angiitis, anaphylactoid purpura* [*Schönlein-Henoch syndrome*], *lung hemorrhage* and *glomerulonephritis* [*Goodpasture's syndrome*], *systemic lupus erythematosus, diabetic glomerulosclerosis, thrombotic thrombocytopenic purpura* and *hemolytic-uremic syndrome, Wegener's granulomatosis, focal glomerulonephritis* associated with *subacute bacterial endocarditis,* and *the nephropathy of acquired immunodeficiency syndrome*). *Autosomal recessive (infantile) polycystic kidney disease, acromegaly, duplication of the pelvocalyceal system, compensatory hypertrophy, nephromegaly* associated with *cirrhosis, hyperalimentation, diabetes mellitus,* or *Beckwith-Wiedemann syndrome, acute urate nephropathy, hemophilia, homozygous S disease, Fabry's disease, glycogen storage disease (Type I), paroxysmal nocturnal hemoglobinuria, Bartter's syndrome,* and *physiologic response to contrast material* and *diuretics* are miscellaneous conditions that complete this list. Table 4–2 is a list of all the entities included in this category.

In addition to an enlarged renal silhouette and smooth borders, other radiologic abnormalities found in the global tissue gain category include increased thickness of the renal parenchyma and attenuation or effacement of the calyces, infundibula, and renal pelvis. This occurs when the relatively nondistensible renal capsule can no longer accommodate the increased bulk of cells, fluid, or protein deposits. These changes are presented schematically in Figure 4–3.

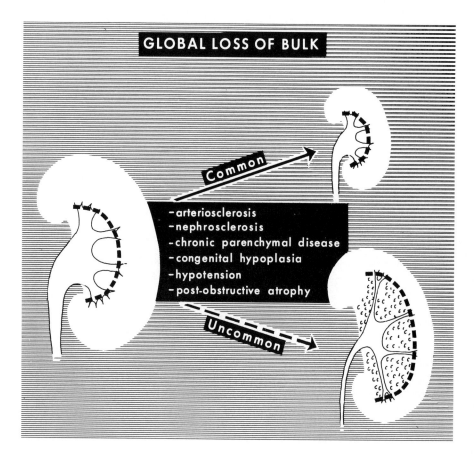

Figure 4–2. Patterns of response to diseases causing global loss of renal bulk. In addition to the decrease in renal size, the smoothness of the renal contour and the normal pelvocalyceal relationships are preserved. Uncommonly, wasted tissue is replaced by central fat deposition, with less decrease in overall renal size.

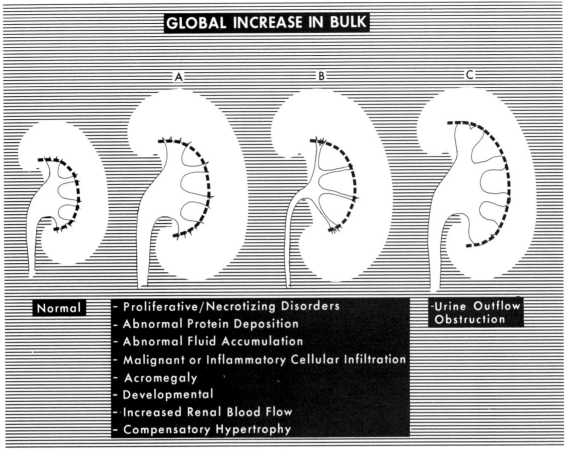

Figure 4–3. Patterns of response to diseases producing generalized increase in renal bulk. Pattern *A* is most common and illustrates the smooth contour, thickened renal parenchyma, and preservation of normal pelvocalyceal relationships. Pattern *B* occurs when the pelvocalyceal system is effaced by surrounding abnormal cells, fluid, or protein deposits. Only in urine outflow obstruction is the pelvocalyceal system dilated, as shown in pattern *C*.

Table 4–2. PATHOLOGIC-RADIOLOGIC CLASSIFICATION OF ENTITIES ASSOCIATED WITH GLOBAL INCREASE IN RENAL BULK: NORMAL TO LARGE KIDNEY

Protein deposition
  Amyloidosis
  Multiple myeloma
Interstitial fluid accumulation
  Acute tubular necrosis
  Obstructive uropathy
  Acute arterial infarction
  Renal vein thrombosis
  Acute cortical necrosis
Malignant cellular infiltration
  Leukemia
Inflammatory cell infiltration
  Acute interstitial nephritis
  Acute pyelonephritis
Proliferative/necrotizing disorders
  Acute glomerulonephritides
  Polyarteritis nodosa (microscopic form)
  Allergic angiitis
  Anaphylactoid purpura (Schönlein-Henoch syndrome)
  Lung hemorrhage and glomerulonephritis (Goodpasture's syndrome)
  Systemic lupus erythematosus

Diabetic glomerulosclerosis
Thrombotic thrombocytopenic purpura and hemolytic-uremic syndrome
Wegener's granulomatosis
Focal glomerulonephritis associated with subacute bacterial endocarditis
Nephropathy of acquired immunodeficiency syndrome
Miscellaneous
  Autosomal recessive (adult) polycystic kidney disease
  Acromegaly
  Duplicated pelvocalyceal system
  Compensatory hypertrophy
  Nephromegaly associated with cirrhosis, hyperalimentation, diabetes mellitus, and Beckwith-Wiedemann syndrome
  Acute urate nephropathy
  Hemophilia
  Homozygous S disease
  Fabry's disease
  Glycogen storage disease (Type I)
  Paroxysmal nocturnal hemoglobinuria
  Bartter's syndrome
  Physiologic response to contrast material and diuretics

Regional Tissue Gain. When a pathologic process arises in a specific component of the lobe but by nature is expansive and perhaps destructive, renal enlargement also occurs. In this situation, the enlargement is regional (polar or interpolar) and sometimes multiple. These diseases are grouped under the category *regional tissue gain* in a pathologic-radiologic classification because they produce single or multiple (focal/multifocal) lobulations in the renal contour. *Simple renal cyst, adenocarcinoma,* and *invasive transitional cell carcinoma* are by far the most frequently encountered masses in adults, while *Wilms' tumor* and *mesoblastic nephroma* account for most cases of neoplastic regional tissue gain in infants and children. Other malignant tumors include *lymphoma, metastases,* and various *sarcomas. Adenoma/oncocytoma, mesoblastic nephroma, angiomyolipoma, multilocular cystic nephroma, juxtaglomerular cell tumor, nephroblastomatosis,* and *mesenchymal tumors* are other benign lesions that produce regional enlargement of the kidney. Focal expansion is also seen in *focal hydronephrosis* and in *abscess* as well as in certain congenital cystic diseases, namely, *autosomal dominant (adult) polycystic kidney disease* and *multicystic dysplastic kidney disease. Acquired cystic kidney disease* and *arteriovenous malformation* complete this list. Table 4–3 lists the entities included in the focal/multifocal large kidney category.

A number of radiologic observations serve to distinguish many of these diseases from each other. Figure 4–4 illustrates the radiologic features that distinguish a cyst, a solid tumor, and an obstructed upper pole infundibulum. These diagnostic features and others are discussed later.

Renal Parenchymal Disease with Normal Size and Contour

Finally, attention must be paid to renal disorders that simply do not fit into a schema for the pathologic-radiologic classification of kidney disease based on

Table 4–3. PATHOLOGIC-RADIOLOGIC CLASSIFICATION OF ENTITIES ASSOCIATED WITH REGIONAL INCREASE IN RENAL BULK: NORMAL TO LARGE KIDNEY

Tumors
  Malignant
    Adenocarcinoma
    Invasive transitional cell carcinoma
    Wilms' tumor
    Lymphoma
    Metastases
    Sarcomas (liposarcoma, fibrosarcoma, myosarcoma, hemangiosarcoma)
  Benign
    Adenoma/oncocytoma
    Mesoblastic nephroma
    Angiomyolipoma
    Multilocular cystic nephroma
    Juxtaglomerular cell tumor
    Nephroblastomatosis
    Mesenchymal (lipoma, fibroma, myoma, hemangioma)
Simple renal cyst
Focal hydronephrosis
Inflammatory mass
  Abscess
  Xanthogranulomatous pyelonephritis
Congenital cystic disease
  Autosomal dominant (adult) polycystic kidney disease
  Multicystic dysplastic kidney
Acquired cystic kidney disease
Arteriovenous malformation

abnormal size and contour. The only radiologic abnormality of one major group is deposition of calcium in the renal parenchyma (i.e., nephrocalcinosis). This process is seen in *primary hyperparathyroidism, milk-alkali syndrome, prolonged immobilization, hypervitaminosis D, sarcoidosis, hyperthyroidism, Cushing's syndrome, renal tubular acidosis,* and *hyperoxaluria;* secondary to *osseous metastatic disease;* or in relation to certain *primary malignant tumors,* notably those of the lung and the kidney. Calcification in cystic dilatations of the distal convoluted tubule occurs in *medullary sponge*

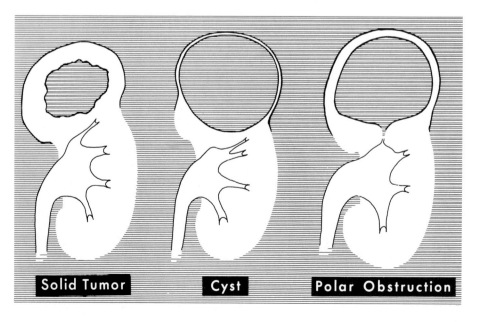

Figure 4–4. Illustrations of radiologic patterns seen with some of the diseases causing focal increases in renal bulk. Also illustrated are the different nephrographic patterns, which allow distinction among these entities. Often a solid tumor has a homogeneous nephrogram.

Solid Tumor   Cyst   Polar Obstruction

kidney without abnormality of renal size or contour. Certain nephrotoxic drugs (e.g., triamterene and amphotericin B) and the diuretic, furosemide, in premature infants produce the same abnormality.

There are still other entities that do not fit naturally into a schema based on size and contour change. Such is the situation with *renal tuberculosis* and *brucellosis*, in which calyceal and papillary ulceration occurs as the earliest manifestation. Only late in the course of these diseases does the radiologist detect the multiplicity of parenchymal abnormalities that may alter size and contour. Thus, it seems appropriate to place renal tuberculosis and brucellosis in the category of diseases that do not affect renal size or contour while recognizing fully that this classification does not apply to advanced cases.

Diabetes insipidus is yet another disorder included in this category, since the abnormally large urine output associated with this abnormality produces marked dilatation of the pelvocalyceal system, often without other radiologic abnormalities.

Table 4–4 lists those entities that according to this approach fall under the category of parenchymal diseases having no effect on renal size or contour.

The overview presented in this section is admittedly unorthodox, for it views pathologic processes through the radiologist's looking glass. Thus, diseases of manifestly dissimilar pathogenesis, and at times distinctive histopathologic appearance, are lumped together in categories based on radiologic expressions held in common. Despite its unorthodoxy, this approach clearly is useful in distinguishing some entities that by other criteria might prove indistinguishable from each other. The next section refines this classification one step further.

URORADIOLOGIC ELEMENTS AND DIAGNOSTIC SETS

In the last analysis, the goal of the radiologist is to establish the correct diagnosis as efficiently as possible

Table 4–4. PATHOLOGIC-RADIOLOGIC CLASSIFICATION OF ENTITIES THAT PRESENT WITH URORADIOLOGIC ABNORMALITIES OTHER THAN ABNORMAL RENAL SIZE OR CONTOUR

Nephrocalcinosis
  Hyperparathyroidism
  Milk-alkali syndrome
  Hypervitaminosis D
  Sarcoidosis
  Hyperthyroidism
  Cushing's syndrome
  Renal tubular acidosis
  Hyperoxaluria
  Primary (lung and kidney) and osseous metastatic carcinoma
  Medullary sponge kidney
  Nephrotoxic drugs
  Furosemide (in premature infants)
Parenchymal diseases seen primarily as calyceal abnormalities
  Tuberculosis
  Brucellosis
  Diabetes insipidus

and in the best interest of the patient. There are many different morphologic and functional aspects of the kidney that can be imaged and evaluated. Two of these, kidney size and contour, have been the criteria used up to this point in the development of a pathologic-radiologic classification of renal disease. Each of the entities listed in Tables 4–1 through 4–4 inherently is either a bilateral or a unilateral process, although on occasion an inherently unilateral process may affect two kidneys more or less by chance. By incorporating the criterion of laterality into the pathologic-radiologic classifications, useful working tools, called "diagnostic sets," can be defined.

Primary Uroradiologic Elements

Renal size, contour, and laterality of involvement become the three *primary uroradiologic elements* on which the following diagnostic sets are based:

> **NORMAL TO SMALL KIDNEY**
> **Small, scarred, unilateral**
> **Small, smooth, unilateral**
> **Small, smooth, bilateral**
>
> **NORMAL TO LARGE KIDNEY**
> **Large, smooth, bilateral**
> **Large, smooth, unilateral**
> **Large, multifocal, bilateral**
> **Large, multifocal, unilateral**
> **Large, unifocal, unilateral**

Diagnostic Sets

Tables 4–5 through 4–12 rearrange diseases listed in the pathologic-radiologic classifications (see Tables 4–1 through 4–4) according to these diagnostic sets. Assignment of each condition is made on the basis of usual rather than invariable forms of presentation. Exceptions do exist and are noted in the classification. In the absence of absolute upper and lower limits of "normal" for renal size, one must always think in terms of "normal to large" or "normal to small." The latter caveat also applies to situations in which diseases are evolving from "large" to "small" as part of their natural history. The reader should also keep in mind that the term *smooth*, when used to describe renal contour, implies a global or generalized distribution of a pathologic process within the renal parenchyma. There are a few situations, such as arteriosclerosis, the hypertensive nephroscleroses, and analgesic nephropathy–associated papillary necrosis with chronic interstitial nephritis, in which focal contour deformities may be superimposed on the basic pattern of a smooth contour. These special situations will be discussed in detail in later chapters.

Table 4–5. DIAGNOSTIC SET: SMALL, SCARRED, UNILATERAL

Reflux nephropathy
(chronic atrophic pyelonephritis)
Lobar infarction

Table 4–6. DIAGNOSTIC SET: SMALL, SMOOTH, UNILATERAL

Ischemia due to focal arterial disease
Chronic infarction
Radiation nephritis
Congenital hypoplasia
Postobstructive atrophy
Postinflammatory atrophy
Reflux atrophy

Table 4–7. DIAGNOSTIC SET: SMALL, SMOOTH, BILATERAL

Generalized arteriosclerosis
Benign and malignant nephrosclerosis
Atheroembolic renal disease
Chronic glomerulonephritis
Papillary necrosis
Hereditary nephropathies
  Hereditary chronic nephritis (Alport's syndrome)
  Medullary cystic disease
Amyloidosis (late)
Arterial hypotension

Table 4–8. DIAGNOSTIC SET: LARGE, SMOOTH, BILATERAL

Proliferative/necrotizing disorders
  Acute glomerulonephritides
  Polyarteritis nodosa (microscopic form)
  Systemic lupus erythematosus
  Wegener's granulomatosis
  Allergic angiitis
  Diabetic glomerulosclerosis
  Lung hemorrhage and glomerulonephritis
    (Goodpasture's syndrome)
  Anaphylactoid purpura (Schönlein–Henoch syndrome)
  Thrombotic thrombocytopenic purpura and hemolytic-uremic syndrome
  Focal glomerulonephritis associated with subacute bacterial endocarditis
  Nephropathy of acquired immunodeficiency syndrome
Amyloidosis
Multiple myeloma
Acute tubular necrosis
Acute cortical necrosis
Leukemia
Acute interstitial nephritis
Autosomal recessive (infantile) polycystic kidney disease
Acute urate nephropathy
Glycogen storage disease (Type I)
Physiologic response to contrast material and diuretics
Homozygous S disease
Paroxysmal nocturnal hemoglobinuria
Hemophilia
Nephromegaly associated with cirrhosis, hyperalimentation, and diabetes
Acromegaly
Fabry's disease
Bartter's syndrome
Beckwith-Wiedemann syndrome

Table 4–9. DIAGNOSTIC SET: LARGE, SMOOTH, UNILATERAL

Renal vein thrombosis
Acute arterial infarction
Obstructive uropathy
Acute pyelonephritis
Compensatory hypertrophy
Duplicated pelvocalyceal system

Table 4–10. DIAGNOSTIC SET: LARGE, MULTIFOCAL, BILATERAL

Autosomal dominant (adult) polycystic kidney disease
Acquired cystic kidney disease
Lymphoma

Table 4–11. DIAGNOSTIC SET: LARGE, MULTIFOCAL, UNILATERAL

Xanthogranulomatous pyelonephritis
Malakoplakia
Multicystic dysplastic kidney

Table 4–12. DIAGNOSTIC SET: LARGE, UNIFOCAL, UNILATERAL

Solid masses
  Malignant neoplasms
    Adenocarcinoma
    Invasive transitional cell carcinoma
    Wilms' tumor
    Metastasis
    Sarcoma
  Benign neoplasms
    Adenoma/oncocytoma
    Angiomyolipoma
    Mesoblastic nephroma
    Nephroblastomatosis
    Juxtaglomerular cell tumor
    Mesenchymal tumor
Fluid-filled masses
  Simple cyst
  Focal hydronephrosis
  Abscess
  Multilocular cystic nephroma
  Arteriovenous malformation

Secondary Uroradiologic Elements

Once having determined which diagnostic set most appropriately matches the primary uroradiologic observations, further distinction among the diseases listed in that set can be made by evaluating additional features, referred to in this text as "secondary uroradiologic elements." These include the following:

Papillae
  Enlarged (global or focal)
  Effaced (global or focal)
  Retracted (global or focal)
  Irregular
  Disrupted (cavity, tract, or slough)
  Cystic dilatations
  Striations
  Decreased number
  Normal

Pelvoinfundibulocalyceal System
Dilated (global or focal)
Attenuated (global or focal)
Irregular
Displaced
Absent
Replaced
Disrupted
Strictured
Notched (including proximal ureter)
Duplicated
Decreased number (calyces)
Opacification time (equal, disparate, or delayed)
Increased density of contrast material
Prolonged retention of contrast material
Normal

Parenchymal Thickness (Distance Between Interpapillary Line and Renal Margin)
Wasted (global or focal)
Expanded (global or focal)
Normal

Nephrogram
Absent
Local replacement
  Margin (smooth or irregular)
  Wall (thin or thick)
  "Beak" deformity
Striated lucencies
Time–density relationship (persistently faint, immediately and persistently dense, or increasingly dense)
Contrast material density (absent, diminished, increased)
Normal

Calcification
Diffuse
Focal
Cortical
Medullary
Papillary
Curvilinear
Peripheral
Nonperipheral
"Tram-line"
Pelvocalyceal stone

Computed Tomographic Attenuation Value/Magnetic Resonance Signal Intensity
Related to renal parenchyma, urine, fat, blood, calcium, urate, iron
Change with time

Unenhanced
Contrast material enhanced (including dynamic sequences)

Echogenicity
Hyperechoic relative to liver (focal, diffuse)
Hypoechoic (focal, diffuse)
Anechoic
Sound transmission (increased, decreased, absent)
Specular interfaces

Miscellaneous
Retroperitoneal space
Kidney mobility
Scoliosis
Baseline focal renal fat lucency
State of contralateral kidney
Doppler flow characteristics

As an example of how this approach is applied, the diagnostic set "large, smooth, unilateral" can be analyzed. Obstructive uropathy is the only one of the six entities included in this set (see Table 4–9) that has the combination of a nephrogram that becomes increasingly dense over time and delayed opacification of a globally dilated collecting system. When the contralateral kidney is small or absent, compensatory hypertrophy is the likely explanation for a kidney that appears entirely normal except for its size. A duplicated pelvocalyceal system is an obvious explanation for smooth renal enlargement. If smooth enlargement is accompanied by global effacement of the collecting system and diminished density of contrast material, abnormal interstitial fluid or cells (as occurs in acute renal venous thrombosis, acute infarction, or acute bacterial nephritis) are suggested. The first of these diagnoses becomes the likely one if the nephrogram becomes increasingly dense over time and contains striae. In this manner, secondary uroradiologic observations lead either to a specific diagnosis or to a narrowing of possible choices within a given set.

The chapters that follow in this part are organized around each of the diagnostic sets. Entities are defined pathologically, and their clinical setting is briefly presented. Radiologic abnormalities are discussed in detail and then summarized in chart form. Each chapter concludes with a differential diagnosis of the conditions discussed. Parenchymal diseases in which renal size and contour remain normal are included in a separate chapter. The emphasis throughout this presentation is on urography, computed tomography, and ultrasonography. Angiographic, radionuclide, and magnetic resonance imaging data are only summarized briefly when applicable.

5

DIAGNOSTIC SET: SMALL, SCARRED, UNILATERAL

REFLUX NEPHROPATHY   DIFFERENTIAL DIAGNOSIS

LOBAR INFARCTION

Two major diseases of the renal parenchyma, reflux nephropathy (chronic atrophic pyelonephritis) and lobar or segmental infarction, are characterized by a focal loss of renal substance that produces surface scars and may eventually reduce kidney size. In both diseases, the abnormality is localized to all or part of a renal lobe. It is for this reason that they are placed in a "unilateral" diagnostic set. It should be realized, however, that these processes occur as random events; therefore, in practice, the classic abnormality described for each of these entities may be detected in multiple sites of one or both kidneys.

REFLUX NEPHROPATHY

Definition

Even though the first comprehensive pathologic and clinical studies of what was originally chronic pyelonephritis were published in the 1930s, a precise definition of this common and serious entity remained uncertain for several decades. Early investigations accurately established the relationship between small, failing kidneys, hypertension, and childhood urinary tract infection, but they also set the stage for the confusion that followed by defining the disease by specific histologic criteria, which have been rigidly adhered to for years. It is now clear that these histologic standards do not distinguish what is now known as reflux nephropathy from a number of other diseases of diverse pathogenesis that develop similar microscopic features. As a result, much of the historic literature on this subject, including the reported frequency of the disease in autopsy series, is inaccurate. It is clear that reflux nephropathy cannot be diagnosed on the basis of histologic features alone. It is also not possible to characterize this disease solely by clinical findings, urine abnormalities, specific tubule or glomerular dysfunctions, or immunologic responses to bacterial infection. To add further confusion, it is known that bacterial infection of the urinary tract is not an invariable finding in reflux nephropathy; that most adult patients with bacterial infection of the urinary tract do not develop morphologic changes in the kidney; that reflux alone may produce tissue wasting; and that the consequence of episodic urinary tract infection first occurring in adulthood is remarkably dissimilar to that first occurring in infancy or childhood.

With bacteriologists, immunologists, nephrologists, pathologists, and radiologists each viewing reflux nephropathy within the context of their own special interests, is there a possibility of agreement on how to identify this entity in a clinical setting? In 1959 while studying this problem, Hodson first suggested an approach, which has gained acceptance over the years. He proposed that the diagnosis of what was then called chronic pyelonephritis be based on features seen in the kidney as a whole rather than on histologic features alone. The gross anatomic features of this disease, he believed, best reflect the marked coarse fibrosis so characteristic of this process, its focal or multifocal distribution with intervening areas of normal tissue, and the fact that the process involves the full thickness of the renal lobe leading to a deep surface scar overlying a deformed calyx.

To emphasize this feature of tissue destruction with involvement of the full thickness of renal parenchyma, Hodson suggested the use of the term *chronic atrophic pyelonephritis*, and it is this nomenclature that prevailed until recently when a new understanding of the pathogenetic mechanisms led to the designation *reflux nephropathy*.

The specific criteria for the diagnosis of reflux nephropathy (chronic atrophic pyelonephritis) are as follows:

1. The disease process is centered in the medulla, with scar formation eventually affecting the whole thickness of the renal substance.
2. There is irregular surface depression over the involved area.

3. Retraction of the subservient papilla with secondary widening of the surrounding calyx occurs.
4. The widened calyx has a smooth margin, although its shape may be variable.
5. The renal tissue adjacent to the involved area is normal or hypertrophied, with a sharp margin between normal and abnormal portions.
6. The distribution of lesions is unifocal or multifocal and involves one or both kidneys.
7. There is reduction in overall size of the involved kidney.

Some of these features are illustrated in Figure 5–1. The validity of these criteria has been supported by experts representing the diverse disciplines concerned with this disease. Although it is clear that these pathologic findings are most commonly associated with reflux nephropathy, they may also develop in the presence of localized obstruction and infection without reflux, particularly the collecting duct obstruction that occurs in renal papillary necrosis or urolithiasis. Under these circumstances, the term *chronic atrophic pyelonephritis* remains appropriate. This chapter, however, focuses on reflux nephropathy.

It should be readily apparent that this definition of reflux nephropathy (chronic atrophic pyelonephritis) assigns an important role to the radiologist in the diagnosis of this disease, since these morphologic criteria are only detectable during life by radiologic means.

Clinical Setting

Advanced cases of reflux nephropathy classically present in young adulthood, most often among women, with symptoms of hypertension and chronic renal failure. Although the majority of these patients are not able to provide a history of urinary tract symptoms before the final illness, the disease seen in the adult is actually the end stage of a process that began in infancy and early childhood. Any discussion on the pathogenesis of reflux nephropathy, therefore, must begin in the early years of life.

Traditionally, it was held that bacterial infection of the kidney parenchyma and pelvocalyceal system was the central element in the production of chronic atrophic pyelonephritis. Gram-negative bacteria, particularly *Escherichia coli*, were most frequently implicated in the infection. Bacteria were considered to ascend in some unidentified manner from the bladder by way of the ureter to the renal pelvis and parenchyma. No other abnormality was considered important in this process, although it was known that urinary tract anomalies predisposed to infection. It is now known that infection of the urine is only one of three elements essential to the development of reflux nephropathy. The other two are vesicoureteral reflux and intrarenal reflux.

Retrograde reflux of urine from the bladder into the ureter has been known since the early cinefluoroscopic examinations of voiding children. Vesicoureteral reflux occurs principally as a function of the length

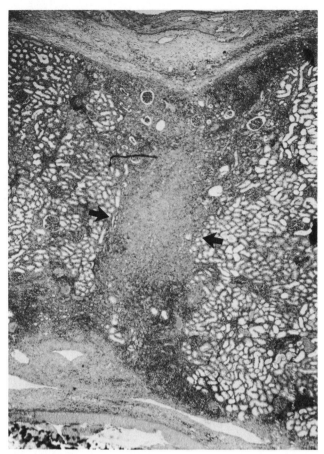

Figure 5–1. Reflux nephropathy (chronic atrophic pyelonephritis). Photomicrograph. A tangential section through a renal lobe demonstrates dense scar *(arrows)* extending from the surface of the kidney above to the pelvocalyceal lining below. The entire thickness of the renal lobe is involved and retracted. Note the sharp margin between normal and abnormal tissue. The scar represents the end stage of a process that began as acute tubulointerstitial nephritis in the collecting ducts comprising one or more medullary rays.

and the angle of insertion of the portion of the distal ureter that passes through the wall of the bladder and tunnels beneath the mucosa before terminating at the trigone. Reflux is more likely to occur when this intramural segment is short and the angle of insertion is wide. Conversely, the longer the submucosal segment and the more acute its angle of insertion, the less likely is reflux to occur. Elongation of this segment as a characteristic of normal growth and development in the infant and young child explains the well-established observation that the frequency of vesicoureteral reflux is inversely related to age. This means that vesicoureteral reflux spontaneously ceases as the intramural portion of the distal ureter lengthens and its angle of insertion becomes more acute during normal growth and development.

Vesicoureteral reflux is a potential source of damage to the renal parenchyma only when it is severe enough to cause the return of a large volume of bladder urine to the renal pelvis under conditions of elevated pressure. This applies to Grade IV or higher reflux using the system of grading outlined in Table 5–1 (see Fig. 5–4). Two forms of renal damage may

Table 5–1. GRADING OF VESICOURETERAL REFLUX

Grade	Description
I	Ureter only
II	Ureter, pelvis, calyces
	No dilatation
	Normal fornices
III	Ureter, pelvis, calyces
	Mild dilatation
	Normal fornices
IV	Ureter, pelvis, calyces
	Moderate dilatation/tortuosity
	Unsharp fornices
	Normal papilla
V	Gross distention
	Effaced papilla

follow. In the first, high-pressure, large-volume reflux *alone* causes varying degrees of pelvocalyceal system dilatation and global renal wasting, a condition termed *reflux atrophy* or *diffuse reflux nephropathy*. (This is discussed in Chapters 6 and 17.) In the second form, major vesicoureteral reflux coexists with infected urine and intrarenal reflux (Fig. 5–2). It is the combi-

nation of these three conditions that initiates the process that will ultimately result in focal parenchymal scars and other pathologic features that characterize focal reflux nephropathy.

Reflux of urine from the collecting system into the renal lobe, known as *intrarenal reflux*, occurs at sites at which the shape of the orifices of Bellini's ducts on the papillae have been deformed by the process of lobar fusion (Fig. 5–3). (See discussion in Chapter 3.) Oval and wide openings allow urine to pass into the collecting ducts that extend through the entire thickness of the renal lobe. Papillary orifices that are narrow and slitlike prevent this passage of urine when elevated pelvocalyceal pressure due to high-volume vesicoureteral reflux is present. Since the duct orifices on any given papilla vary in shape as a function of fusion (compounding), intrarenal reflux may occur in a part, or parts, of a lobe but not necessarily in an entire lobe. The following features explain the pathologic characteristics of reflux nephropathy: full-thickness involvement (reflux into collecting ducts that extend from papillary tip to cortex); partial lobar involvement with adjacent normal tissue (a refluxing

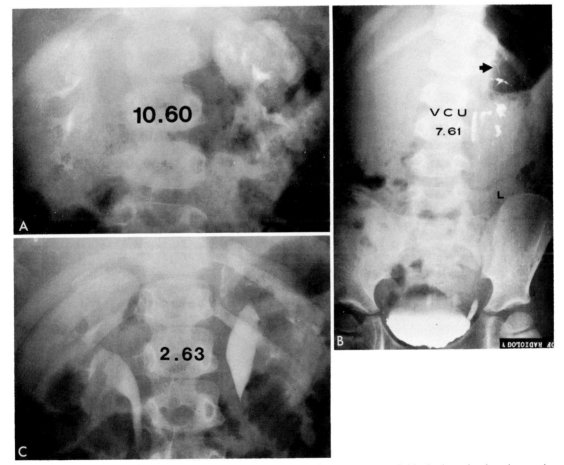

Figure 5–2. Intrarenal reflux of barium into left upper pole during voiding cystourethrogram in a child who later developed parenchymal wasting at the same site.

A, Baseline excretory urogram demonstrates normal parenchymal thickness.

B, Voiding cystourethrogram performed 9 months later demonstrates intrarenal reflux of barium into the upper pole of the left kidney *(arrow)*.

C, Excretory urography 28 months after initial examination demonstrates residual barium and parenchymal wasting at site of intrarenal reflux.

(Courtesy of Gerald Friedland, M.D., Stanford University School of Medicine, Stanford, California.)

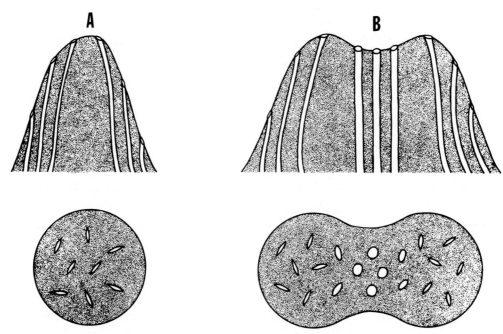

Figure 5–3. Schema of papillary duct opening in profile and *en face*. The single cone-shaped pyramid *(A)* has narrow slitlike openings that prevent intrarenal reflux. Compound papillae *(B)*, formed as a result of lobar assimilation, have open, round orifices that permit intrarenal reflux of calyceal urine into the collecting ducts.

orifice next to a nonrefluxing one, each draining an adjacent set of collecting ducts); and a higher frequency of reflux nephropathy scars in the poles of the kidney than in the interpolar region (more compound papillae in the poles).

Nonrefluxing papillary orifices can convert to refluxing orifices as a result of elevated pressure of calycine urine, as occurs with vesicoureteral reflux, ureteral obstruction, or disordered peristalsis. Thus, the development of intrarenal reflux may be acquired as well as a result of developmental lobar papillary fusion.

It is now generally held that reflux nephropathy is the lesion that follows reflux of infected urine into the collecting ducts of the renal lobe (Fig. 5–4), with an acute tubulointerstitial nephritis in the affected portion of the renal lobe being the earliest response. This reaction has been aptly called *lobar nephronia* and should not be confused with the term that has been inappropriately applied to acute bacterial nephritis in adults, which is a distinctly different entity. The role of sublobar acute tubulointerstitial nephritis in acute infection of the adult kidney is discussed in Chapter 9.

The early acute inflammatory stage of reflux nephropathy, occurring in infancy and childhood, does not alter the radiologic appearance of the renal contour or the papillae. Vascular perfusion and urine formation in the affected portion of the lobe are impaired, however, by the interstitial infiltrate of white blood cells and the accumulation of pus in the collecting ducts that are part of the acute inflammatory response. With persistent or recurrent infection and reflux, the early inflammatory infiltrate is eventually replaced by fibroblasts and scar formation throughout the full thickness of the lobe, as illustrated in Figure

5–1. Retraction of the renal surface and the subjacent papillae follows. (See discussion in Chapter 4.) This process may progress through childhood or arrest at any time in its evolution if either the infection of the urine is eliminated or the vesicoureteral reflux ceases, as a result of normal maturation or surgical intervention. By the midchildhood years, or earlier, the lesions are fully developed and no longer progressive.

The precise genesis of the acute lobar or sublobar tubulointerstitial nephritis of early reflux nephropathy remains controversial. Undoubtedly, both the acute inflammatory response to bacteria in the collecting ducts and the late scar formation represent a complex interplay between bacterial virulence factors and host defense mechanisms. The latter include urodynamic factors, ischemia, extravasation of urine through ruptured fornices, as well as the competency of immune and cellular anti-inflammatory mechanisms. Eventually, glomerulosclerosis develops in the surviving nephrons as a result of hyperfiltration. When enough renal mass is involved, proteinuria and renal failure will follow.

The question of whether reflux nephropathy develops from the combination of vesicoureteral and intrarenal reflux without infection of urine remains unanswered. Most of the clinical and laboratory evidence indicates that infection is essential in producing the fully developed picture of reflux nephropathy. The Ask-Upmark kidney, also known as segmental renal hypoplasia, is possibly a reflection of this uncertainty. The Ask-Upmark kidney has the gross morphologic appearance of reflux nephropathy and similar clinical characteristics. A focal, full-thickness scar overlies a retracted papilla and widened calyx. Its microscopic appearance, however, differs from that of reflux ne-

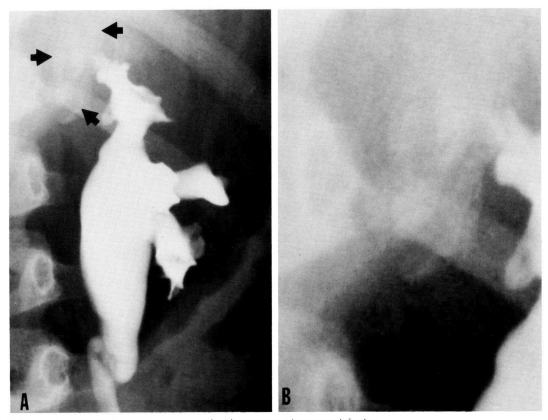

Figure 5–4. Reflux nephropathy. Early stage in a young girl with recurrent urinary tract infection.

A, Voiding cystourethrogram. Vesicoureteral reflux, Grade IV. There is widening of the collecting system and intrarenal reflux into the medial portion of the upper pole *(arrows).*

B, Photographic enlargement of medial portion of upper pole seen in *A.* Fine linear dense striations through the full thickness of the parenchyma represent intrarenal reflux of opacified urine into collecting ducts. Combined with infected urine, this causes an acute tubulointerstitial nephritis, known as lobar nephronia.

(Courtesy of Gerald Friedland, M.D., Stanford University School of Medicine, Stanford, California.)

phropathy. Coarse fibrosis is absent. Glomeruli are few, if present at all. Dilated, colloid-filled tubular structures that resemble thyroid tissue predominate, and there is marked sclerosis of medium-sized arteries. One explanation for this lesion is that it develops from intrarenal reflux of sterile urine, perhaps even during intrauterine development of the kidney. (Aspects of the Ask-Upmark kidney as a form of focal hypoplasia are discussed in the section Congenital Hypoplasia in Chapter 6.)

Clinically, urinary tract infection occurs most frequently in girls and women and, in the first year of life, in uncircumcised male newborns. The combination of urinary tract infection and reflux may express itself by repeated episodes of fever, flank pain, frequency, and dysuria. Often, however, patients have nonlocalizing symptoms such as lethargy and abdominal pain in addition to fever. Of particular importance is the well-documented fact that many young children have bacteriuria, vesicoureteral reflux, and urographic evidence of renal scars, *even though they are asymptomatic.* Three studies of symptomless children in Great Britain have been quoted as showing an incidence of renal scarring in 1 in 200 cases, 1 in 500 cases, and 1 in 180 cases, respectively (Hodson, 1974).

Presumably, these represent occult cases of urinary tract infection and reflux.

Radiologic Findings

It is uncommon to image the lobar or sublobar acute tubulointerstitial nephritis that is the earliest lesion of reflux nephropathy. At this stage, the radiologic findings demonstrate an enlarged, smooth kidney with a sharply defined, deficient nephrogram encompassing the full thickness of the renal parenchyma in one or more portions of the kidney. This corresponds to the infected segments. If multiple sublobar segments are involved, the nephrogram is striated. The nephrogram may be abnormally dense and prolonged in noninvolved portions of the kidney. This probably represents increased interstitial pressure in the acutely inflamed kidney causing an increase in transit time of filtrate through the nephrons. This abnormality is most readily visualized by computed tomography or by radionuclide renography, using ^{99m}Tc-DMSA (Figs. 5–5 and 5–6). Either increased or decreased echoes are present in the kidney at this stage. These findings are identical to those described in Chapter 9 for tubulointerstitial nephritis in acute renal infection begin-

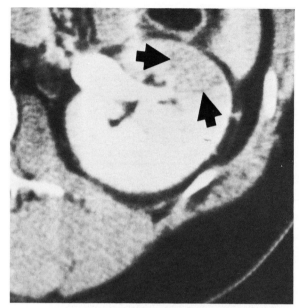

Figure 5–5. Acute tubulointerstitial nephritis in the left kidney of a 23-year-old woman with acute upper urinary tract infection. Computed tomogram, contrast material enhanced. There is a sharply defined, full-thickness nephrographic defect in a lobar distribution in the central portion of the kidney (arrows). This represents diminished perfusion due to acute inflammatory infiltrate.

ning in adulthood. In children, radiologic evaluation is usually initiated at a later stage when the radiologic findings depict inhibition of growth in affected regions of the kidney. This is seen as a reduction in parenchymal thickness (Fig. 5–7) and is most frequently present in the upper renal pole. It can be detected by comparing the area of suspected abnormality with other poles, which normally resemble each other in thickness. Later, particularly after repeated symptomatic attacks of acute infection, destructive deformity of the papilla and surface scarring appear. In Hodson's report (1965) on the development of pyelonephritic scars, the maximum incidence of scar formation occurred between ages 10 and 15, after which new scars did not appear. It is now believed that most scar formation ceases by age 4. This age-related pattern in some way may reflect the spontaneous disappearance of reflux known to occur as children mature. Scar formation can also be arrested by eradication of infection following antibiotic therapy without an antireflux surgical procedure also being performed. Scarring can nonetheless progress after the successful treatment of infection.

The radiologic picture in the adult reflects the severity of the disease in childhood. When the disease process is naturally self-limited, or when successful medical or surgical therapy minimizes damage, the radiologic abnormality is limited to a slight thinning of parenchyma in one area, without cortical scarring or calyceal deformity due to retraction of the papilla. A conclusive radiologic diagnosis of reflux nephropathy based on these minimal findings cannot be made, since this picture is similar to that seen in ischemic or postinfarction states (Fig. 5–8).

Reflux nephropathy can be diagnosed with confidence only when the radiologic pattern reflects "full-thickness" destruction and scarring of all or part of a lobe (i.e., a cortical depression overlying a retracted papilla whose calyx is secondarily dilated). In some individuals, this abnormality will be present at one site (Fig. 5–9); in others, a number of foci in one or both kidneys will be present (Fig. 5–10; see Fig. 5–12.) As stated earlier, these changes, when first detected in adulthood, reflect old disease and are not progressive.

The radiologic abnormalities of reflux nephropathy that have advanced to the intermediate stage of growth inhibition or the mature stage of scar formation are quite distinct from those seen in the large number of patients who in adulthood experience the onset of episodic acute pyelonephritis characterized by significant bacteriuria, pyuria, fever, and flank pain. These individuals do not usually have permanent radiologically detectable renal abnormalities, even though it is known that they may have a functional derangement in the form of diminished concentrating ability. (Acute pyelonephritis in the adult is discussed in Chapter 9.) Focal scar formation of reflux nephropathy (chronic atrophic pyelonephritis) developing *de novo* in the adult points to urinary tract infection coexisting with a complicating factor, such as stone formation, renal papillary necrosis, obstruction, or neuropathic bladder with vesicoureteral reflux (Figs. 5–11 and 5–12).

In the most severe circumstance—a young adult with hypertension, progressive renal failure, and

Text continued on page 121

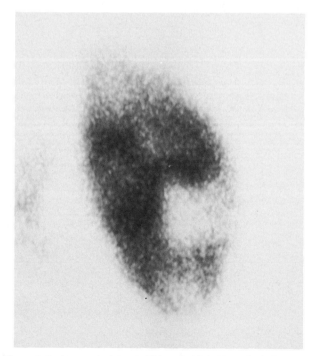

Figure 5–6. Acute tubulointerstitial nephritis in the right kidney of a patient with acute upper urinary tract infection. 99mTc-DMSA radionuclide scan, posterior image. There are sharply defined, full-thickness areas of photopenia. The findings represent acute inflammatory infiltrate in lobar or sublobar sites. (Courtesy of Massoud Majd, M.D., Children's National Medical Center, Washington, DC.)

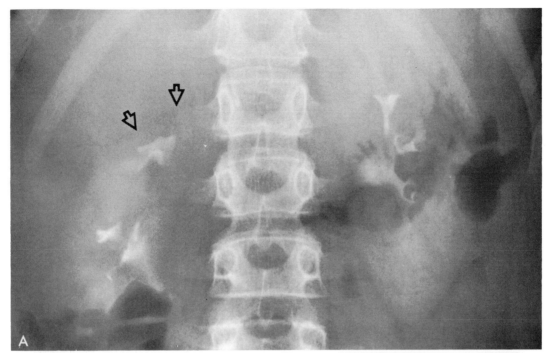

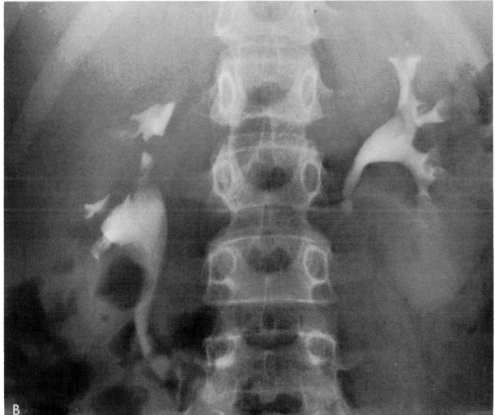

Figure 5–7. Excretory urogram performed on an 11-year-old girl with recurrent urinary tract infections and vesicoureteral reflux into the right pelvocalyceal system. (Same patient illustrated in Fig. 17–14.)

A, There is decreased growth of the right kidney, particularly in the upper pole *(arrows).*

B, Focal contour scars and calyceal dilatation have not yet developed.

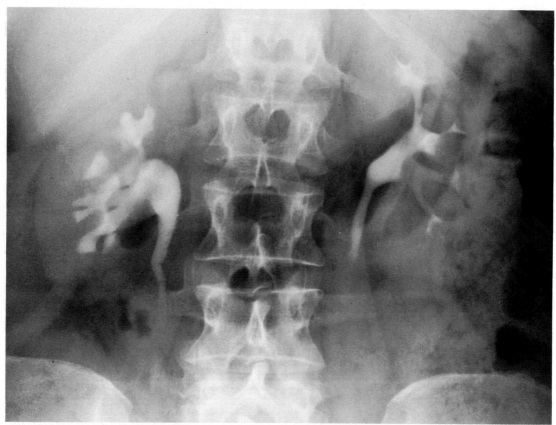

Figure 5–8. Excretory urogram in an infection-free, asymptomatic young adult woman who had a right ureteral implantation during childhood for reflux and infection. The right upper pole is wasted, particularly laterally, but does not have a focal scar. Slight calyceal deformity in the region probably represents atrophy from previous reflux. These findings represent minimal damage from reflux nephropathy in childhood.

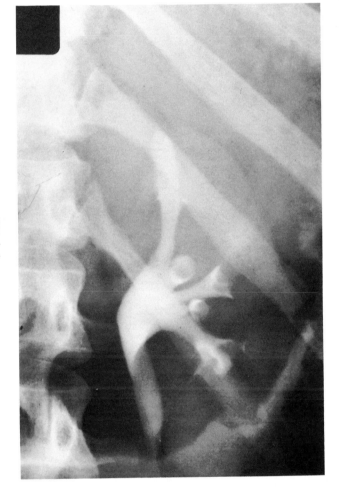

Figure 5–9. Reflux nephropathy in a 26-year-old woman who had a urinary tract infection in childhood. Abnormalities are limited to a focal contour scar overlying a smoothly dilated calyx in the upper pole. (Courtesy of Professor Thomas Sherwood, M.B., University of Cambridge, Cambridge, England.)

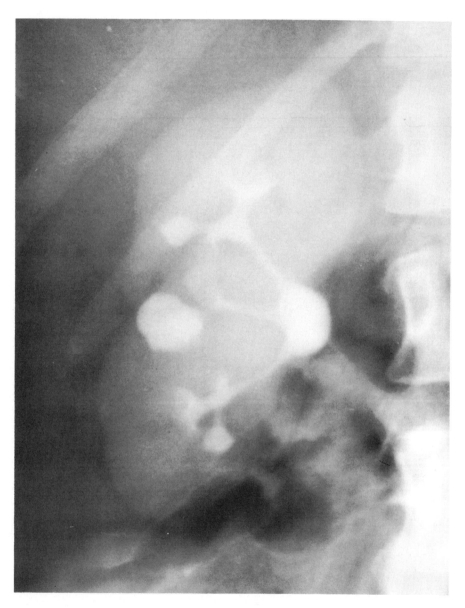

Figure 5–10. Reflux nephropathy. Excretory urogram demonstrates advanced changes in multiple areas of the right kidney. Varying degrees of severity and nonuniform distribution are characteristic of this abnormality.

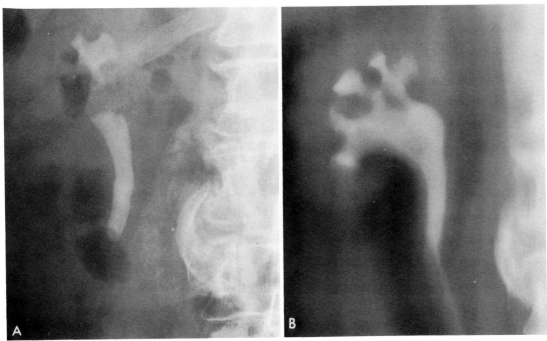

Figure 5–11. Chronic atrophic pyelonephritis in a 62-year-old man with urinary tract infection developing in adulthood in association with stone disease.

A, Preliminary film. A staghorn calculus is present.

B, Excretory urogram. Tomogram. Focal scars and deformed calyces are present.

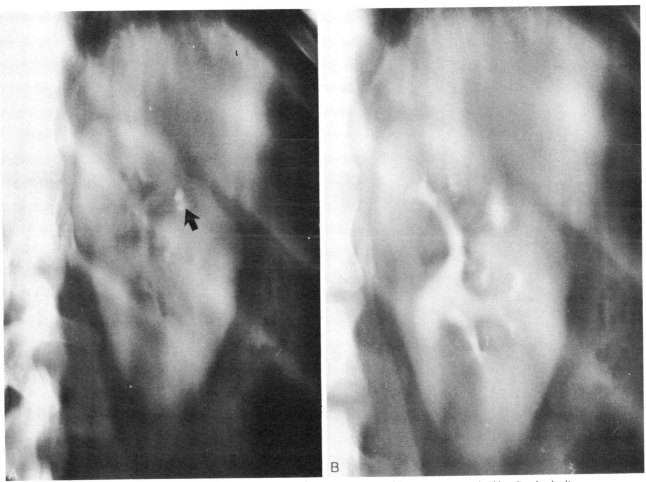

Figure 5–12. Chronic atrophic pyelonephritis developing in a single focus in a 49-year-old woman as a result of localized calculi.

A, Early nephrogram. Tomogram. Two calculi *(arrow)* are clustered in a single calyceal/papillary unit in the upper pole with an overlying parenchymal scar.

B, Excretory urogram. Tomogram. Calyceal dilatation is present. (Courtesy of E. Stephen Amis, M.D., Albert Einstein School of Medicine, New York, New York.)

119

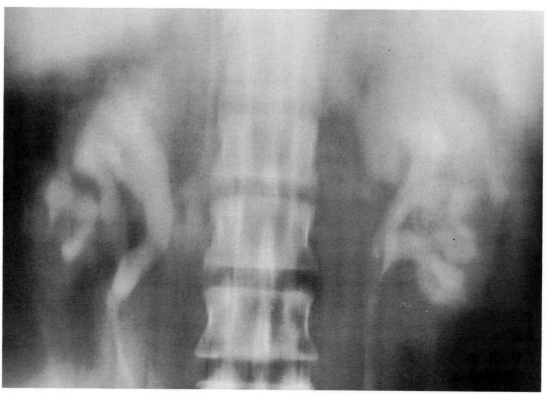

Figure 5–13. Bilateral reflux nephropathy resulting in renal failure. There are small kidneys with multifocal scars and smoothly dilated calyces. The nonuniform pattern of lesion distribution and severity is typical of this disease. Urine volume and density are not diminished, despite renal failure. Excretory urogram. Tomogram.

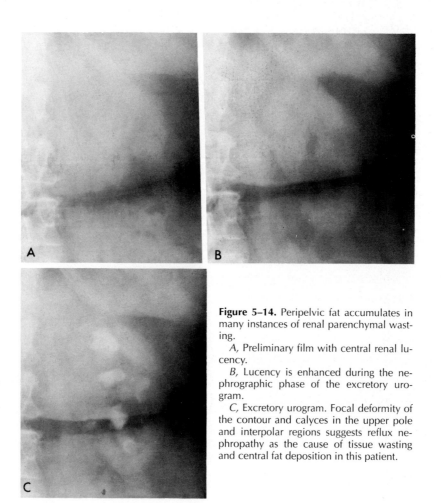

Figure 5–14. Peripelvic fat accumulates in many instances of renal parenchymal wasting.

A, Preliminary film with central renal lucency.

B, Lucency is enhanced during the nephrographic phase of the excretory urogram.

C, Excretory urogram. Focal deformity of the contour and calyces in the upper pole and interpolar regions suggests reflux nephropathy as the cause of tissue wasting and central fat deposition in this patient.

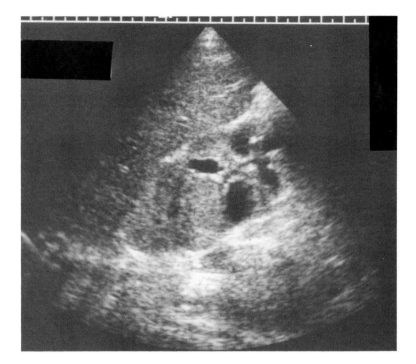

Figure 5–15. Reflux nephropathy, right kidney. Ultrasonogram, sagittal projection. There are multiple foci of scars overlying dilated calyces. (Kindly provided by Ulrike Hamper, M.D., and Sheila Sheth, M.D., The Johns Hopkins University, Baltimore, Maryland.)

renal osteodystrophy—severe bilateral contour defects with corresponding papillary retraction and calyceal widening will be present (Fig. 5–13). Even though this pattern is present in both kidneys, involvement is characteristically asymmetric. The margin of the calyx remains smooth, even when dilatation is advanced, a feature that differentiates reflux nephropathy from calyceal dilatation due to tuberculosis or renal papillary necrosis, in which the margin of the cavity is apt to be irregular.

A few additional miscellaneous observations about advanced reflux nephropathy should be noted. Occasionally, marked peripelvic sinus fat accumulates as destruction of renal tissue advances. This may be detectable as central renal lucency on a preliminary film or a computed tomogram or as increased echogenicity of the central sinus complex on an ultrasonogram

(Fig. 5–14). When advanced reflux nephropathy affects only one kidney, contralateral compensatory hypertrophy is present. Focal areas of compensatory hypertrophy of unaffected parenchyma may develop as pseudotumors adjacent to scars. Although microscopic nephrocalcinosis is commonly seen in reflux nephropathy, its radiologic detection is unusual. Finally, it is unusual to detect abnormalities in either contrast material density or urine volume, even in patients with severe functional impairment due to advanced disease.

Ultrasonography demonstrates the focal retraction of the renal surface and underlying dilated calyx, as does excretory urography and computed tomography (Fig. 5–15). In addition, increased parenchymal echogenicity is present in the area of scar formation.

The radiologic evaluation of a child for reflux ne-

SUMMARY OF ABNORMAL URORADIOLOGIC FINDINGS
REFLUX NEPHROPATHY

Primary Uroradiologic Elements
    Size—normal to small
    Contour—normal (early, intermediate)
          —focal scar (late; may be multifocal)
    Lesion distribution—unilateral (may be bilateral)
Secondary Uroradiologic Elements
    Papillae—normal (early, intermediate)
          —retracted (late; focal)
    Calyces—normal (early, intermediate)
          —widened (late; focal)
    Parenchymal thickness—normal (early)
                  —wasted (intermediate, late; focal)
                  —focal compensatory hypertrophy
    Nephrogram—deficient enhancement (lobar, sublobar; full-thickness; may be striated)
    Echogenicity—increased (focal)
                 —increased central sinus complex

phropathy has the double objective of detecting significant vesicoureteral reflux and assessing the renal parenchyma for retarded growth or scar formation. The additional obligation of follow-up is imposed if either is present. Vesicoureteral reflux can be investigated by either voiding cystourethrography or radionuclide cystography. Kidney structure can be assessed by excretory urography, ultrasonography, or radionuclide techniques. Each of these methods has specific advantages and disadvantages. The specific protocol chosen varies among institutions.

LOBAR INFARCTION

Definition

Each of the three diagnostic sets for small kidneys discussed in this and the following two chapters includes entities arising from abnormalities of blood flow. The specific diagnostic set to which each of these is assigned depends first on whether the interruption of blood supply is partial (ischemic) or complete (infarctive) and second on what amount of tissue is affected. Many combinations are possible. When the vascular abnormality is generalized in the small vessels, both kidneys are affected diffusely. (See Chapter 7 on bilaterally small, smooth kidneys.) On the other hand, when a major renal artery stenosis causes ischemia, or when infarction of the entire kidney occurs, wasting is global but limited to one kidney (see Chapter 6 on unilaterally small, smooth kidneys).

The discussion in this chapter focuses on those circulatory abnormalities that follow thrombosis or embolization of one or a group of related interlobar or arcuate arteries. The infarction that results is limited to a portion of a lobe, a whole lobe, or neighboring parts of adjacent lobes, depending on the number and the size of arteries involved. If all the arteries perfusing a single lobe are occluded, the entire lobe will shrink, and a surface scar in the area of the centrilobar cortex and peripheral part of the medulla will be produced. Since each interlobar artery usually divides into arcuate arteries running to adjoining portions of two adjacent lobes, scar formation is rarely limited to a single lobe. Instead, a scar bridging adjacent portions of each lobe is usually the minimal result of an interlobar artery occlusion. (Refer to Fig. 3–5 to better understand the anatomic basis for scar distributions in lobar infarction.)

The sequence of events that occur following interruption of blood supply to a portion of the kidney has been studied most thoroughly in experimental animals; these parallel the changes that occur in humans. The earliest abnormality is venous and capillary hyperemia, seen within an hour after segmental arterial obstruction as a triangular reddish region, with its base in the subcapsular area and its apex pointing toward the medulla (Fig. 5–16). Owing to hyperemia, the area bulges above the surface of the rest of the kidney. Within 7 days the lesion begins to decrease in volume. After approximately 28 days, a pronounced surface depression forms as dead tubules and other

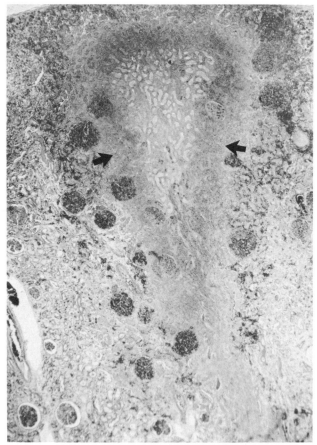

Figure 5–16. Acute lobar infarction. Photomicrograph. There is a triangular-shaped area of infarcted kidney surrounded by a zone of hyperemia *(arrows)*. The base of the triangle is at the periphery of the kidney. At this stage, imaging studies demonstrate only the absence of perfusion and urine formation in the affected region and no contour defect.

cellular elements disappear (Fig. 5–17). Unlike reflux nephropathy, fibroblasts are not a prominent feature of this process, and scar formation is due to a "falling out" of dead tissue rather than retraction by fibrosis. The deformity is thereby limited to the area of actual tissue death, namely, the peripheral portion of the lobe. The papilla is usually not involved in lobar infarction because of the multiplicity of vessels, including the spiral arteries, that perfuse it. Even when infarcted, the papilla usually retains its normal shape. Thus, a cut section through a kidney with a mature lobar infarction reveals a deep surface scar limited to the area supplied by the interrupted vessel, obliteration of the corticomedullary junction, preservation of the papilla of the involved lobe, and normal adjacent tissue.

Clinical Setting

Lobar infarction is due either to embolism or to thrombosis at the site of arteriosclerotic plaque or aneurysm. Of these, embolism is by far the more common cause. Among patients with renal infarcts, 75 to 95 per cent have had embolic phenomena secondary

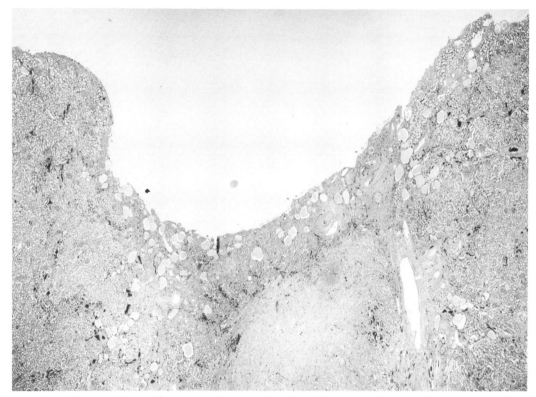

Figure 5–17. Mature lobar infarction. Photomicrograph. At this stage, the infarcted tissue has disappeared, leaving a broad-based defect on the surface of the kidney.

to cardiac lesions, particularly rheumatic heart disease with arrhythmia. Other cardiac sources of renal arterial emboli are recent myocardial infarction, prosthetic valves, myocardial trauma, intracardiac catheters, and myocardial tumors. Renal infarcts secondary to emboli have been reported in as many as 25 per cent of patients with subacute bacterial endocarditis. Less common causes of lobar infarcts are arteriosclerosis, thromboangiitis obliterans, polyarteritis nodosa, syphilitic cardiovascular disease, and aneurysm of the aorta or renal artery.

Small renal infarcts often produce neither symptoms nor abnormal physical or laboratory findings. Diagnosis, therefore, is frequently based on incidental observations made during urography, computed tomography, angiography, surgery, or autopsy. In one autopsy study of the clinical and pathologic features of renal infarction, 205 cases were culled from over 14,000 autopsies, an incidence of 1.4 per cent (Hoxie and Coggin, 1940). Of these cases, only two were diagnosed before death. Symptoms include the abrupt onset of abdominal or flank pain (35 to 50 per cent of patients), fever (32 to 67 per cent of patients), and nausea with vomiting (approximately 50 per cent of patients). Albuminuria, often heavy, is present more frequently (approximately one-half of all patients) than hematuria (one-third of all patients). Hematuria is usually microscopic and only occasionally gross, but urinalysis is normal in one-third of the patients with renal infarction. Leukocytosis and elevation of serum lactic dehydrogenase level may occur within the first 24 hours after infarction and reflect responses to tissue death. In many patients with renal infarction, symptoms are vague and do not suggest the correct diagnosis. Laboratory evidence of functional impairment of the kidney is not a feature of small, focal renal infarcts unless these are numerous and superimposed on kidneys already compromised by pre-existing disease.

Radiologic Findings

The radiologic findings in lobar or segmental infarction vary with the age of the lesion. Within the first week, renal size and contour remain normal, since there is essentially no tissue loss during this period. Other abnormalities may be present early, however. Shortly after the onset of infarction, a nephrographic defect may be detected by contrast material–enhanced or radionuclide imaging techniques. This defect corresponds to the infarct itself and reflects the lack of perfusion of the involved area by blood containing contrast material. The defect is likely to be triangular, with the base situated on the outer margin of the kidney. The scar that forms later occurs at the same site (Fig. 5–18). The calyx and infundibulum may become attenuated or displaced by hyperemic tissue swelling (Fig. 5–19). Obviously, nonopacification of the calyx is more a result of local tissue pressure surrounding the calyx than of lobar nonfunction, since the calyx otherwise would passively fill with contrast material excreted by other parts of the kidney.

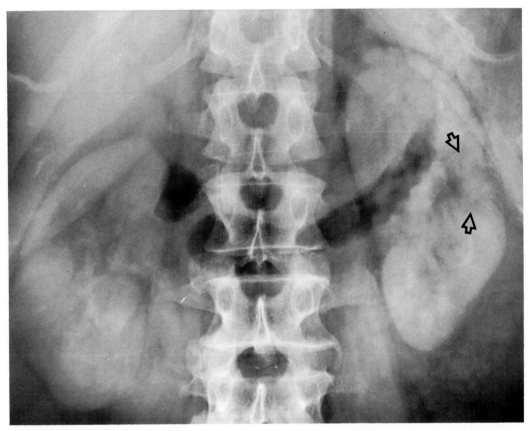

Figure 5–18. Lobar infarction in a 61-year-old man who experienced sudden left groin and flank pain accompanied by microscopic hematuria. Excretory urography was performed 3 days later. A triangular radiolucent nephrographic defect with its base on the renal margin is present in the interpolar region *(arrows)*. (Same patient illustrated in Fig. 23–15.) Excretory urogram, early film. (Kindly provided by Ira Kanter, M.D., Peralta Hospital, Oakland, California.)

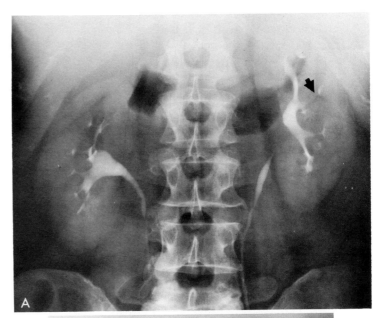

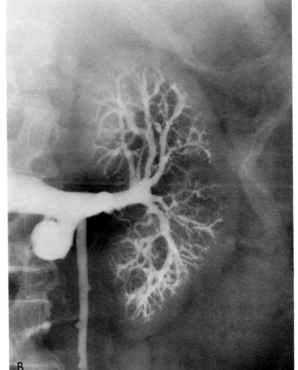

Figure 5–19. Lobar infarction. (Same patient as described in Figures 5–18 and 5–20.)

A, The uppermost calyx and infundibulum *(arrow)* in the left interpolar region are attenuated and the midportion of the pelvis is displaced medially.

B, Retrograde venogram. Marked attenuation of interlobar, arcuate, and interlobular veins in involved area illustrates the effect of localized hyperemic tissue swelling, which also produces the deformities in the pelvo-infundibulocalyceal system seen during excretory urography.

(Kindly provided by Ira Kanter, M.D., Peralta Hospital, Oakland, California.)

Nonenhancement of the entire kidney is a feature usually associated with main renal artery occlusion and total infarction. It may occasionally be present, however, when infarction involves a much smaller amount of renal tissue, as in lobar infarction. The exact physiologic basis for this phenomenon is unclear. Speculation has centered on a neural reflex mechanism causing generalized spasm of the renal vascular bed. Whatever the cause, this phenomenon is usually transitory, and repeat imaging studies reveal restored enhancement within a short time.

Selective renal angiography can provide important information in the early diagnosis of lobar renal infarction. The embolus itself may be seen as an intraluminal filling defect or as an abrupt termination of an interlobar or arcuate artery. The involved vessels may not opacify, or they may retain contrast material longer than normal vessels of similar size in other parts of the kidney. This reflects downstream obstruction. A nephrographic defect is readily apparent in the nonperfused area (Figs. 5–20 and 5–21).

With maturation of the infarct after approximately 4 weeks, the urographic or computed tomographic findings become quite specific: A wide-based depression in the renal contour at the site of infarction develops, while the underlying papillae remain normal (Figs. 5–22 and 5–23).

As a result, focal thinning of the renal parenchyma occurs. This can be identified easily by drawing the interpapillary line, which remains normal, and an outline of the renal contour, which indents at the site of the infarct (Fig. 5–24). Occasionally, the amount of lobar tissue loss will be so extensive that some papillary distortion occurs. This is always minimal relative to the deformity that develops in the remainder of the lobe and does not approximate that seen in reflux nephropathy (Fig. 5–25). Sometimes, numerous small infarcts cause multiple focal scars in one or both kidneys without a detectable decrease in renal length or width (Figs. 5–26 and 5–27).

Histopathologically, nephrocalcinosis occurs more frequently in infarcted kidneys than in those from a general autopsy population. The radiologic detection of these calcific deposits is unusual, however.

Text continued on page 133

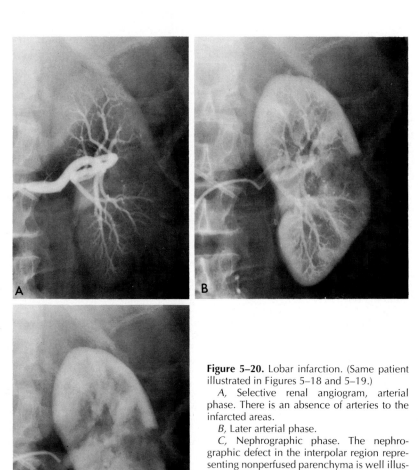

Figure 5–20. Lobar infarction. (Same patient illustrated in Figures 5–18 and 5–19.)

A, Selective renal angiogram, arterial phase. There is an absence of arteries to the infarcted areas.

B, Later arterial phase.

C, Nephrographic phase. The nephrographic defect in the interpolar region representing nonperfused parenchyma is well illustrated.

(Kindly provided by Ira Kanter, M.D., Peralta Hospital, Oakland, California.)

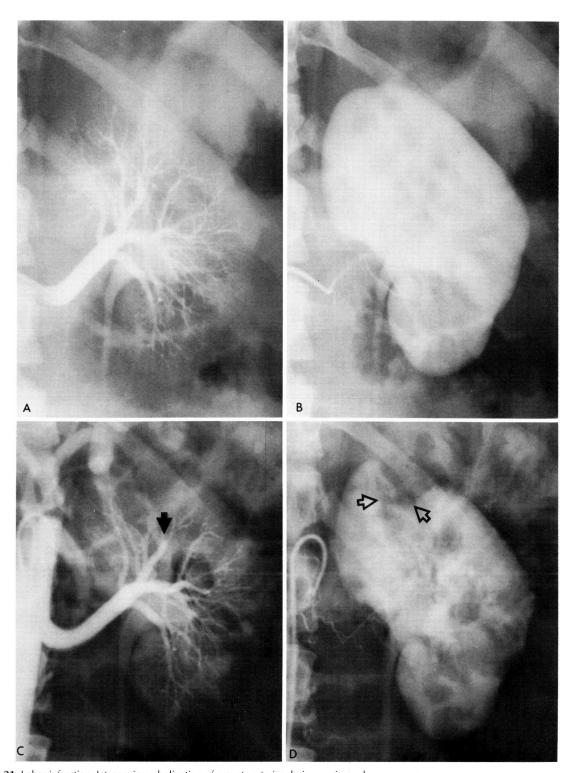

Figure 5–21. Lobar infarction. Iatrogenic embolization of arcuate arteries during angiography.

A and *B,* Initial selective renal arteriogram demonstrates normal arteries and angiographic nephrogram.

C, A few minutes later, a midstream aortogram reveals complete occlusion of some arcuate arteries to an upper pole lobe *(arrow),* presumably due to embolization during selective catheterization.

D, Prominent nephrographic defect *(arrows)* in area perfused by occluded vessels.

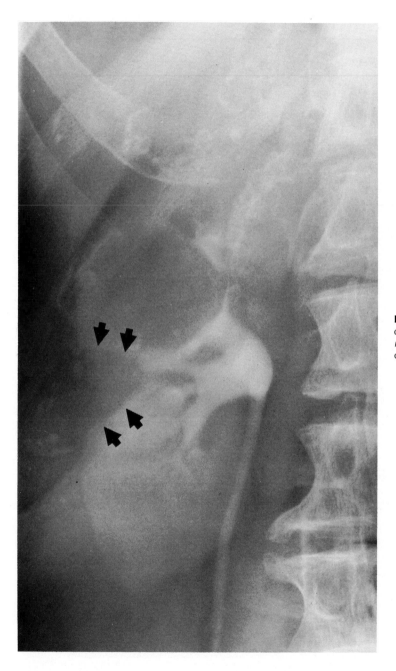

Figure 5–22. Mature lobar infarct seen as a deep focal depression of the renal contour in the interpolar region *(arrows)*. The underlying papillae remain normal. Simple renal cysts are present just above the infarct and in the lower pole.

Figure 5–23. Mature lobar infarct involving lobes on the posterior surface of the left kidney. The deep focal depression of the renal contour extends to the underlying calyx. Computed tomogram, contrast material enhanced. (Courtesy of J. Price, M.D., Alta Bates Hospital, Berkeley, California.)

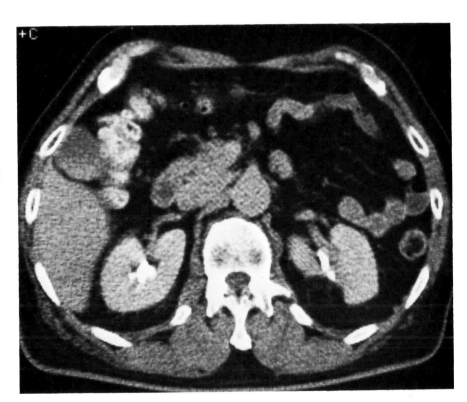

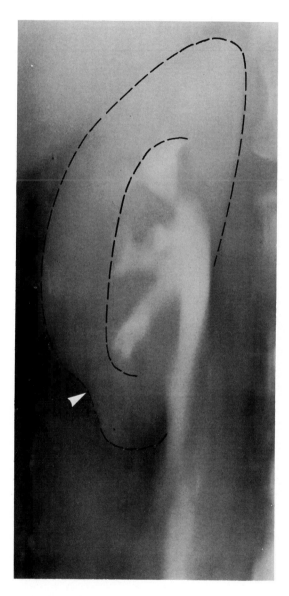

Figure 5–24. Mature lobar infarct. The interpapillary line remains normal, whereas the renal contour indents focally at the site of infarction *(arrow).*

Figure 5–25. Mature lobar infarct in lateral aspect of lower pole extensive enough to cause slight papillary deformity *(arrows)*. Papillary abnormalities are uncommon in lobar infarction and are always minimal compared with those seen in reflux nephropathy. (Same patient illustrated in Fig. 5–28.) (Courtesy of Robert Clark, M.D., St. Francis Memorial Hospital, San Francisco, California.)

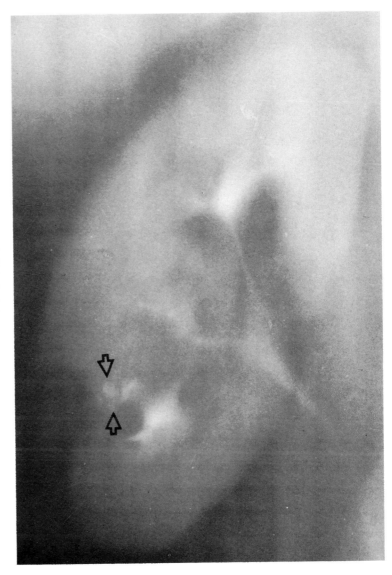

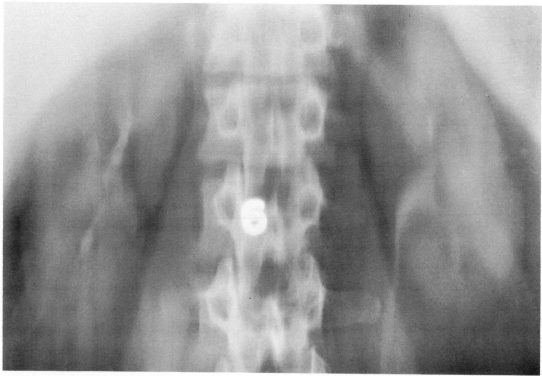

Figure 5–26. Bilateral lobar infarcts in a 54-year-old man with hypertension. Multiple focal contour scars have formed, whereas kidney size remains within normal limits. Excretory urogram. Tomogram. (Same patient illustrated in Fig. 5–27.)

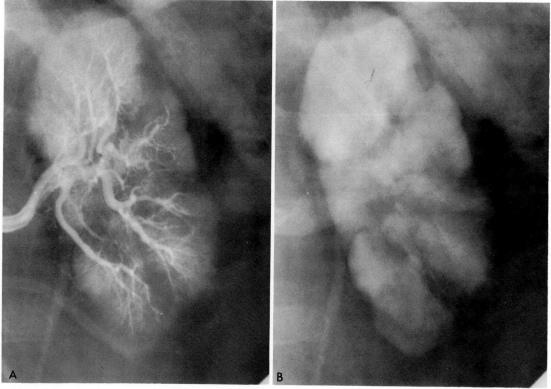

Figure 5–27. Multiple lobar infarcts. (Same patient illustrated in Fig. 5–26.)
   A, Selective arteriogram. Arterial phase shows arteriosclerotic narrowing and dilatation of many arcuate arteries and absence of branching vessels.
   B, Nephrographic phase. Several lobar infarcts are readily apparent.

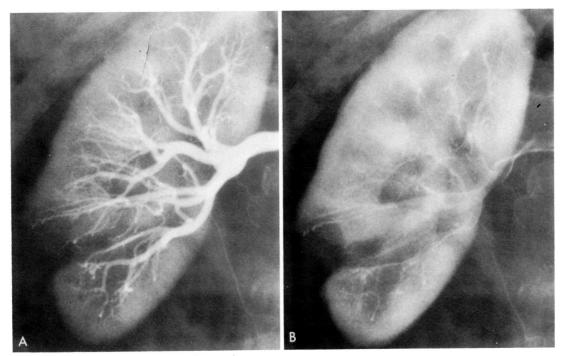

Figure 5–28. Mature lobar infarction. (Same patient illustrated in Fig. 5–25.)
    A, Selective arteriogram, early arterial phase. There is absence of arcuate arteries in the infarcted area and tortuosity of vessels adjacent to the infarct.
    B, Late arterial phase. There is retention of contrast material in the tortuous vessels, indicating reduced flow. The broad-based contour defect is well demonstrated.

Selective renal angiography performed 3 to 4 weeks after lobar infarction may demonstrate irregular narrowing, prolonged retention of contrast material, or nonopacification of the affected vessel. The embolus itself will no longer be visible by this time. Scar formation on the margin of the kidney is usually well seen during the angiographic nephrogram (Fig. 5–28).

Ultrasonography is not useful for the diagnosis of early lobar infarction. As the infarct matures, increased echogenicity occurs at the site of the contour deformity. This is due to perirenal fat filling in the space left by the disappearance of the infarcted renal tissue (Fig. 5–29). This finding may be present whenever focal loss of renal tissue has occurred, including postsurgical scars, and is not specific for lobar infarction.

Retrograde pyelography may be necessary in establishing the early diagnosis of lobar renal infarction when excretory urography, computed tomography, or radionuclide studies fail to visualize the kidney or show an obliterated group of calyces. Characteristically, retrograde pyelography demonstrates normal

---

SUMMARY OF ABNORMAL URORADIOLOGIC FINDINGS
LOBAR INFARCTION

Early (within 4 weeks)
  Primary Uroradiologic Elements
    Size—normal
    Contour—normal
    Lesion distribution—unilateral (may be bilateral)
  Secondary Uroradiologic Elements
    Pelvoinfundibulocalyceal system—attenuated (focal, occasional)
    Nephrogram—absent (focal, occasional; global, rarely)
Late (after 4 weeks)
  Primary Uroradiologic Elements
    Size—normal to small
    Contour—focal scar (may be multifocal)
    Lesion distribution—unilateral (may be bilateral)
  Secondary Uroradiologic Elements
    Parenchymal thickness—wasted (focal) with normal interpapillary line
    Echogenicity—increased (focal)

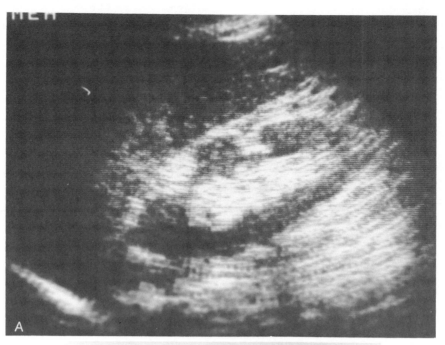

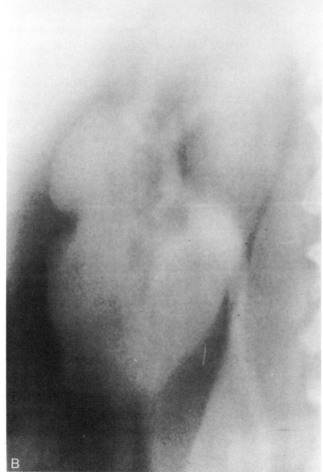

Figure 5–29. Mature lobar infarction in the right kidney of a 47-year-old asymptomatic man.
   A, Ultrasonogram, longitudinal section. Hyperechoic perirenal fat fills the surface defects at the sites of infarction.
   B, Excretory urogram. Tomogram. Two surface scars overlying normal calyces are apparent. These correspond to the hyperechoic foci demonstrated on ultrasonography.

calyces and papillae in both early and late stages, although calyceal effacement in the involved area might be present early on.

DIFFERENTIAL DIAGNOSIS

When the lesions of reflux nephropathy and lobar infarction are fully developed, their radiologic patterns are quite specific. In the former, a focal contour scar overlies a smoothly dilated calyx, whereas in the latter, a broadly based contour depression exists over a normal papilla. Both diseases, occurring as random events, may be multifocal, bilateral, or both.

Cases of minimal reflux nephropathy in which arrest of growth results in slight reduction in parenchymal thickness, usually in one pole, without contour or papillary deformity are radiologically indistinguishable from changes seen in ischemia or late infarction of a region of the kidney. Usually, the clinical history in these patients is not helpful in discriminating between these disorders, and a specific diagnosis cannot be made by the radiologist.

Diseases that produce radiologic abnormalities of the papillae or calyces must be considered in the differential diagnosis of reflux nephropathy. Papillary necrosis is one of these. Features of papillary necrosis not seen in reflux nephropathy include irregularity of the dilated calyx at the site of papillary slough, papillary calcification, and cavitation within attached papillae. In renal tuberculosis, focal papillary deformities and calyceal dilatation can be similar to those seen in reflux nephropathy, but cortical scarring tends to occur late in the course of the disease, when other features characteristic of tuberculosis are also present. These include inflammatory parenchymal masses, calcification, and dilatation of all or part of the pelvoinfundibulocalyceal system and ureter, which also have focal structures. Finally, focal obstruction confined to one calyx will cause papillary effacement and calyceal dilatation. A focal scar in the kidney contour overlying this site will not be present in this situation unless infection supervenes, in which case the lesion will take on the radiologic pattern of reflux nephropathy.

Attenuation of a calyx or a group of related calyces occasionally present in early lobar infarction may also occur in inflammatory lesions such as acute pyelonephritis, in early tuberculosis, in small focal abscess, or in localized hemorrhage. Differentiation of these entities from lobar infarction is unlikely unless the nephrographic defect of early lobar infarction is also present. Infiltrating uroepithelial carcinoma can also obliterate a calyx. Retrograde pyelography may be useful in demonstrating other features of tumor, such as mucosal irregularity or collecting system filling defects, in these cases.

When lobar infarction results in nonopacification of the whole kidney, differential diagnosis includes main renal artery occlusion and congenital or surgical absence of the kidney. Nonopacification is transitory when caused by lobar infarction and either permanent or associated with slow recovery when resulting from main renal artery occlusion. Renal angiography, computed tomography, retrograde pyelography, and radionuclide and Doppler ultrasound flow studies are important adjunctive studies in the differentiation of these lesions.

Bibliography

Reflux Nephropathy

Allen, T. D., Arant, B. S., and Roberts, J. A.: Commentary: Vesicoureteral reflux—1992. J. Urol. 148:1758, 1992.

Alon, U., Berant, M., and Pery, M.: Intravenous pyelography in children with urinary tract infection and vesicoureteral reflux. Pediatrics 83:332, 1989.

Angel, J. R., Smith, T. W., Jr., and Roberts, J. A.: The hydrodynamics of pyelorenal reflux. J. Urol. 122:20, 1979.

Arant, B. S., Jr., Sotelo-Avila, C., and Bernstein, J.: Segmental "hypoplasia" of the kidney (Ask-Upmark). J. Pediatr. 95:931, 1979.

Arima, M., Matsui, T., Ogino, T., Shimada, K., Hosokawa, S., Mori, Y., and Ikoma, F.: Vesicoureteral reflux in infants under one-year-old: Follow-up study and consideration on development of renal scarring. Urology 41:372, 1993.

Bailey, R. R.: The relationship of vesico-ureteric reflux to urinary tract infection and chronic pyelonephritis. Clin. Nephrol. 1:132, 1973.

Becker, J. A., Butt, K., and Lipkowitz, G.: Segmental infarction of the renal allograft: Ultrasound/MRI observations. Urol. Radiol. 11:109, 1989.

Bernstein, J., and Arant, B. S.: Morphological characteristics of segmental renal scarring in vesicoureteral reflux. J. Urol. 148:1712, 1992.

Bisset, G. S., and Strife, J. L.: The duplex collecting system in girls with urinary tract infection: Prevalence and significance. AJR 148:497, 1987.

Bisset, G., Strife, J. L., and Dunbar, J. S.: Urography and voiding cystourethrography: Findings in girls with urinary tract infection. AJR 148:479, 1987.

Cardiff-Oxford Bacteriuria Study Group: Sequelae of covert bacteriuria in schoolgirls: A four-year follow-up study. Lancet 1:889, 1978.

Cardiff-Oxford Bacteriuria Study Group: Long-term effects of bacteriuria on the urinary tract in school girls. Radiology 132:343, 1979.

Chapman, S. J., Chantler, C., Haycock, G. B., Maisey, M. N., and Saxton, H. M.: Radionuclide cystography in vesicoureteral reflux. Arch. Dis. Child. 63:650, 1988.

Claësson, I., and Lindberg, U.: Asymptomatic bacteriuria in schoolgirls. Radiology 124:179, 1977.

Claësson, I., Jacobsson, B., Jodal, U., and Winberg, J.: Early detection of nephropathy in childhood urinary tract infection. Acta Radiol. (Diagn.) 22:315, 1981.

Cremin, B. J.: Observations on vesico-ureteric reflux and intrarenal reflux: A review and survey of material. Clin. Radiol. 30:607, 1979.

Edwards, D., Normand, I. C. S., Prescod, N., and Smellie, J. M.: Disappearance of vesicoureteric reflux during long-term prophylaxis of urinary tract infection in children. Br. Med. J. 2:285, 1977.

Elison, B. S., Taylor, D., Van der Wall, H., Pereira, J. K., Cahill, S., Rosenberg, A. R., Farnsworth, R. H., and Murray, I. P. C.: Comparison of DMSA scintigraphy with intravenous urography for the detection of renal scarring and its correlation with vesicoureteral reflux. Br. J. Urol. 69:294, 1992.

Farmer, E., and Heptinstall, R.: Chronic non-obstructive pyelonephritis—a re-appraisal. In Kincaid-Smith, P., and Fairley, K. F. (eds.): Renal Infection and Renal Scarring. Proceedings of the International Symposium on Pyelonephritis, Vesicoureteric Reflux and Renal Papillary Necrosis. Melbourne, Mercedes Publishing Co., 1970.

Farnsworth, R. H., Rossleigh, M., Leighton, D. M., Bass, S. J., and Rosenberg, A. R.: The detection of reflux nephropathy in infants by [99m]technetium dimercaptosuccinic acid studies. J. Urol. 145:542, 1991.

Fay, R., Winter, R., Cohen, A., Brosman, S. A., and Bennett, C.: Segmental renal hypoplasia and hypertension. J. Urol. *113*:561, 1975.

Filly, R. A., Friedland, G. W., Govan, D. E., and Fair, W. R.: Urinary tract infections in children: II. Roentgenologic aspects. West. J. Med. *121*:374, 1974.

Freedman, L. R.: Chronic pyelonephritis at autopsy. Ann. Intern. Med. *66*:697, 1967.

Gillenwater, J. Y., Harrison, R. B., and Kunin, C. M.: Natural history of bacteriuria in schoolgirls: A long-term case-control study. N. Engl. J. Med. *301*:396, 1979.

Ginalski, J. M., Michaud, A., and Genton, N.: Renal growth retardation in children: Sign suggestive of vesicoureteral reflux? AJR *145*:617, 1985.

Ginsburg, C. M., and McCraken, G. H.: Urinary tract infections in young infants. Pediatrics *69*:409, 1982.

Govan, D. E., Fair, W. R., Friedland, G. W., and Filly, R. A.: Urinary tract infections in children: III. Treatment of ureterovesical reflux. West. J. Med. *121*:382, 1974.

Gross, G. W., and Lebowitz, R. L.: Infection does not cause reflux. AJR *137*:929, 1981.

Hannerz, L., Wikstad, I., Johansson, L., Broberger, O., and Aperia, A.: Distribution of renal scars and intrarenal reflux in children with past history of urinary tract infection. Acta Radiol. *28*:443, 1987.

Hellström, M., Jacobsson, B., Mårild, S., and Jodal, U.: Voiding cystourethrography as a predictor of reflux nephropathy in children with urinary tract infection. AJR *152*:801, 1989.

Heptinstall, R. H.: The enigma of chronic pyelonephritis. J. Infect. Dis. *120*:104, 1969.

Heptinstall, R. H.: Pathology of the Kidney. 4th ed. Boston, Little, Brown & Co., 1992.

Hill, G. S. (ed.): Uropathology. New York, Churchill Livingstone, 1989.

Himmelfarb, E., Rabinowitz, J. G., Parvey, L., Gammill, S., and Arant, B.: The Ask-Upmark kidney: Roentgenographic and pathological features. Am. J. Dis. Child. *129*:1440, 1975.

Hodson, C. J.: The radiological diagnosis of pyelonephritis. Proc. R. Soc. Med. *52*:669, 1959.

Hodson, C. J.: Coarse pyelonephritic scarring or atrophic pyelonephritis. Proc. R. Soc. Med. *58*:785, 1965.

Hodson, C. J. and Wilson, S.: Natural history of chronic pyelonephritic scarring. Br. Med J. *2*:191, 1965.

Hodson, C. J.: The radiological contribution toward the diagnosis of chronic pyelonephritis. Radiology *88*:857, 1967.

Hodson, C. J.: Radiological diagnosis of renal involvement. *In* O'Grady, F., and Brumfitt, W. (eds.): Urinary Tract Infection. London, Oxford University Press, 1968, pp. 108–112.

Hodson, C. J.: The mechanism of scar formation in chronic pyelonephritis. *In* Kincaid-Smith, P., and Fairley, K. F. (eds.): Renal Infection and Renal Scarring. Proceedings of the International Symposium on Pyelonephritis, Vesicoureteral Reflux and Renal Papillary Necrosis. Melbourne, Mercedes Publishing Co., 1970.

Hodson, C. J.: Letter to the editor. Br. J. Radiol. *47*:153, 1974.

Hodson, C. J., Mailing, T. M. J., McManamon, P. J., and Lewis, M. G.: The pathogenesis of reflux nephropathy (chronic atrophic pyelonephritis). Br. J. Radiol. Supplement 13, 1975.

Hodson, C. J., and Kincaid-Smith, P. (eds.): Reflux Nephropathy. New York, Masson Publishing USA, 1979.

Hodson, C. J.: Reflux nephropathy: A personal historical review. AJR *137*:451, 1981.

Hugosson, C. O., Chrispin, A. R., and Wolverson, M. K.: The advent of the pyelonephritic scar. Ann. Radiol. *19*:1, 1976.

Huland, H., Busch, R., and Riebel, T.: Renal scarring after symptomatic and asymptomatic upper urinary tract infection: A prospective study. J. Urol. *128*:682, 1982.

International Reflux Study Committee: Medical versus surgical treatment of primary vesicoureteral reflux: A prospective international reflux study in children. J. Urol. *125*:277, 1981.

Johnston, J. H., and Mix, L. W.: The Ask-Upmark kidney: A form of ascending pyelonephritis? Br. J. Urol. *48*:393, 1976.

Kass, E. H., and Zinner, S. H.: Bacteriuria and renal disease. J. Infect. Dis. *120*:27, 1969.

Kay, C. J., Rosenfield, A. T., Taylor, K. J. W., and Rosenberg, M. A.: Ultrasonic characteristics of chronic atrophic pyelonephritis. AJR *132*:47, 1979.

Kincaid-Smith, P.: Reflux nephropathy. Br. Med. J. *286*:2002, 1983.

Kogan, S. J., Sigler, L., Levitt, S. B., Reda, E. F., Weiss, R., and Greifer, I.: Elusive vesicoureteral reflux in children with normal contrast cystograms. J. Urol. *136*:325, 1986.

Lapides, J.: Mechanisms of urinary tract infection. Urology *14*:217, 1979.

Lebowitz, R. L., and Mandell, J.: Urinary tract infection in children: Putting radiology in its place. Radiology *165*:1, 1987.

Lebowitz, R. L.: Neonatal vesicoureteral reflux: What do we know? Radiology *187*:17, 1993.

Lerner, G. R., Fleischmann, L. E., and Perlmutter, A. D.: Reflux nephropathy. Pediatr. Clin. North Am. *34*:747, 1987.

Longcope, W. T., and Winkenwerder, W. L.: Clinical features of the contracted kidney due to pyelonephritis. Bull. Johns Hopkins Hosp. *53*:255, 1933.

Losse, H., Asscher, A. W., and Lison, A. E. (eds.): Pyelonephritis. Vol. IV. Urinary Tract Infections. New York, Thieme-Stratton, 1980.

MacGregor, M.: Pyelonephritis lenta: Consideration of childhood urinary infection as the forerunner of renal insufficiency in later life. Arch. Dis. Child. *45*:159, 1970.

McCurdy, F. A., and Vernier, R. L.: Unique consequences of kidney infections in infants and children: Pathogenesis, early recognition and prevention of scarring. Am. J. Nephrol. *1*:184, 1981.

Miller, T., and Phillips, S.: Pyelonephritis: The relationship between infection, renal scarring and antimicrobial therapy. Kidney Int. *19*:654, 1981.

Moreau, J.-F., Grenier, P., Grünfeld, J.-P., and Brabant, J.: Renal clubbing and scarring in adults: A retrospective study of 110 cases. Urol. Radiol. *1*:129, 1980.

Morgan, M., Asscher, A. W., and Moffat, D. B.: The role of vesicoureteric (V-U) reflux in the pathogenesis of kidney scars in the rat. Nephron *17*:8, 1976.

Newhouse, J. H., and Amis, E. S., Jr.: The relationship between renal scarring and stone disease. AJR *151*:1153, 1988.

Olbing, H., Claësson, I., Ebel, K. D., Seppänen, U., Smellie, J. M., Tamminenmobius, T., and Wikstad, I.: Renal scars and parenchymal thinning in children with vesicoureteral reflux: A 5-year report of the International Reflux Study in Children (European branch). J. Urol. *148*:1653, 1992.

Ransley, P. G., and Risdon, R. A.: Renal papillae and intrarenal reflux in the pig. Lancet *2*:1114, 1974.

Ransley, P. G., and Risdon, R. A.: Renal papillary morphology and intrarenal reflux in the young pig. Urol. Res. *3*:105, 1975.

Ransley, P. G., and Risdon, R. A.: Renal papillary morphology in infants and young children. Urol. Res. *3*:111, 1975.

Ransley, P. G.: Intrarenal reflux: Anatomical, dynamic and radiological studies: I. Urol. Res. *5*:61, 1977.

Ransley, P. G., and Risdon, R. A.: Reflux and renal scarring. Br. J. Radiol. Supplement 14, 1978.

Ridson, R. A.: The small scarred kidney in childhood. Pediatr. Nephrol. *7*:361, 1993.

Roberts, J. A.: Pathogenesis of pyelonephritis. J. Urol. *129*:1102, 1983.

Rolleston, G. L., Maling, T. M. J., and Hodson, C. J.: Intrarenal reflux and the scarred kidney. Arch. Dis. Child. *49*:531, 1974.

Ronald, A. R., and Simonsen, J. N.: Infections of the upper urinary tract. *In* Schrier, R. W., Gottschalk, C. W. (eds.): Diseases of the Kidney. 4th ed. Boston, Little, Brown & Co., 1988, pp. 1065–2208.

Rosenberg, A. R., Rossleigh, M. A., Brydon, M. P., Bass, S. J., Leighton, D. M., and Farnsworth, R. H.: Evaluation of acute urinary tract infection in children by dimercaptosuccinic acid scintigraphy: A prospective study. J. Urol. *148*:1746, 1992.

Rubin, R. H., Tolkoff-Rubin, N. E., and Cotran, R. S.: Urinary tract infection, pyelonephritis and reflux nephropathy. *In* Brenner, B. M., and Rector, F. C., Jr. (eds.): The Kidney. 4th ed. Philadelphia, W. B. Saunders, 1991, p. 1369.

Rushton, H. G., Winberg, J., Jodal, U., Roberts, J. A., and O'Hanley, P.: Pyelonephritis: Pathogenesis and management update. Dialogues Pediatr. Urol. *13*:2, 1990.

Rushton, H. G., and Majd, M.: Dimercaptosuccinic acid renal scintigraphy for the evaluation of pyelonephritis and scarring: A review of experimental and clinical sutdies. J. Urol. *148*:1726, 1992.

Senekjian, H. O., and Suki, W. N.: Vesicoureteral reflux and reflux nephropathy. Am. J. Nephrol. 2:245, 1982.

Shanon, A., Feldman, W., McDonald, P., Martin, D. J., Matzinger, M. A., Shillinger, J. F., McLaine, P. N., and Wolfish, N.: Evaluation of renal scars by technetium-labelled dimercaptosuccinic acid scan, intravenous urography and ultrasonography: A comparative study. J. Pediatr. 120:399, 1992.

Shapiro, E., Slovis, T. L., Perlmutter, A. D., and Kohns, L. R.: Optimal use of 99mtechnetium-glucoheptonate scintigraphy in the detection of pyelonephritis scarring in children: A preliminary report. J. Urol. 140:1175, 1988.

Sherwood, T.: Radiology now: Ureteric reflux (editorial). Br. J. Radiol. 46: 653, 1973.

Shimada, K., Matsui, T., Ogino, T., Arima, M., Mori, Y., and Ikoma, F.: Renal growth and progression of reflux nephropathy in children with vesicoureteral reflux. J. Urol. 140:1097, 1988.

Smith, J. F.: The diagnosis of the scars of chronic pyelonephritis. J. Clin. Pathol. 15:522, 1962.

South Bedfordshire Practitioners' Group: Development of renal scars in children: Missed opportunities in management. Br. Med. J. 301:1082, 1990.

Spencer, J. R., and Schaeffer, A. J.: Pediatric urinary tract infection. Urol. Clin. North Am. 13:661, 1986.

Stamey, T. A., and Pfau, A.: Urinary infections: A selective review and some observations. Calif. Med. 113:16, 1970.

Stoller, M. L., and Kogan, B. A.: Sensitivity of 99mtechnetium-dimercaptosuccinic acid for the diagnosis of chronic pyelonephritis: Clinical and theoretical considerations. J. Urol. 135:977, 1986.

Sty, J. R., Wells, R. G., Schroeder, B. A., and Starshak, R. J.: Diagnostic imaging in pediatric renal inflammatory disease. JAMA 256:895, 1986.

Sty, J. R., Wells, R. G., Starshak, R. J., and Schroeder, B. A.: Imaging in acute renal infection in children. AJR 148:471, 1987.

Tamminen, T. E., and Kaprio, E. A.: The relation of the shape of renal papillae and of collecting duct openings to intrarenal reflux. Br. J. Urol. 49:345, 1977.

Thomsen, H. S., Talner, L. B., and Higgins, C. B.: Intrarenal backflow during retrograde pyelography with graded intrapelvic pressure: A radiologic study. Invest. Radiol. 17:593, 1982.

Torres, V. E., Velosa, J. A., Holley, K. E., Kelalis, P. P., Stickler, G. B., and Kurtz, S. B.: The progression of vesicoureteral reflux nephropathy. Ann. Intern. Med. 92:776, 1980.

Vaisrub, S.: Reflux nephropathy. JAMA. 245:2430, 1981.

Van den Abbeele, A. D., Treves, S. T., Lebowitz, R. L., Baver, S., Davis, R. T., Retik, A., and Colodny, A.: Vesicoureteral reflux in asymptomatic siblings of patients with known reflux: Radionuclide cystography. Pediatrics 79:147, 1987.

Vargas, A., Evans, K., Ransley, P., Rosenberg, A. R., Rothwell, D., Sherwood, T., Williams, D. I., Barratt, T. M., and Carter, C. O.: A family study of vesicoureteric reflux. J. Med. Genet. 15:85, 1978.

Verber, I. G., Strodley, M. R., and Meller, S. T.: 99Tc-dimercaptosuccinic acid (DMSA) scan as first investigation of urinary tract infection. Arch. Dis. Child. 63:1320, 1988.

Weiss, S., and Parker, F.: Pyelonephritis: Its relation to vascular lesions and to arterial hypertension. Medicine (Baltimore) 18:221, 1939.

White, R. H. R.: Vesicoureteral reflux and renal scarring. Arch. Dis. Child. 64:407, 1989.

Whitworth, J. A., Fairley, K. F., O'Keefe, G. M., and Johnson, W.: The site of renal infection: Pyelitis or pyelonephritis? Clin. Nephrol. 2:9, 1974.

Wikstad, I., Aperia, A., Broberger, O., and Ekengren, K.: Vesicoureteric reflux and pyelonephritis: Long time effect on area of renal parenchyma. Acta Radiol. (Diagn.) 20:252, 1979.

Wikstad, I., Aperia, A., Broberger, O., and Löhr, G.: Long-time effect of large vesicoureteral reflux with or without urinary tract infection. Acta Radiol. (Diagn.) 22:325, 1981.

Winberg, J.: Progressive renal damage from infection with or without reflux: Commentary. J. Urol. 148:1733, 1992.

Wiswell, T. E., Smith, F. R., and Bass, J. W.: Decreased incidence of urinary tract infection in circumcised male infants. Pediatrics 75:901, 1985.

Woodard, J. R., and Rushton, H. G.: Reflux uropathy. Pediatr. Clin. North Am. 34:1349, 1987.

Zerin, J. M., Ritchey, M. L., and Chang, A. C. H.: Incidental vesicoureteral reflux in neonates with antenatally detected hydronephrosis and other renal abnormalities. Radiology 187:157, 1993.

Zuchelli, P., and Gaggi, R.: Reflux nephropathy in adults. Nephron 57:2, 1991.

Lobar Infarction

Barney, J. D., and Mintz, E. R.: Infarcts of the kidney. JAMA. 100:1, 1933.

Belt, A. E., and Joelson, J. J.: The effect of ligation of branches of the renal artery. Arch. Surg. 10:117, 1925.

Edwards, E.: Acute renal calcification: An experimental and clinicopathologic study. J. Urol. 80:161, 1958.

Elkin, M.: Radiology of the urinary tract: Some physiological considerations. Radiology 116:259, 1975.

Erwin, B. C., Carroll, B. A., Walter, J. F., and Sommer, F. G.: Renal infarction appearing as an echogenic mass. AJR 138:759, 1982.

Halpern, M.: Acute renal artery embolus: A concept of diagnosis and treatment. J. Urol. 98:552, 1967.

Heitzman, E. R., and Perchik, L.: Radiographic features of renal infarction: Review of 13 cases. Radiology 76:39, 1961.

Hilton, S., Bosniak, M. A., Ragharendra, B. N., Subramanyam, B. R., Rothberg, M., and Megibow, A. J.: CT findings in acute renal infarction. Urol. Radiol. 6:158, 1984.

Hodson, C. J.: The effects of disturbance of flow on the kidney. J. Infect. Dis. 120:54, 1969.

Hodson, C. J. The lobar structure of the kidney. Br. J. Urol. 44:246, 1972.

Hoxie, H. J., and Coggin, C. B.: Renal infarction: Statistical study of 205 cases and detailed report of an unusual case. Arch. Intern. Med. 65:587, 1940.

Janower, M. L., and Weber, A. L.: Radiologic evaluation of acute renal infarction. AJR 95:309, 1965.

Karsner, H. T., and Austin, J. H.: Studies in infarction: Experimental bland infarction of the kidney and spleen. JAMA 57:951, 1911.

Kelly, K. M., Craven, J. D., Jorgens, J., and Barenfus, M.: Experimental renal artery thromboembolism. Invest. Radiol. 11:88, 1976.

Lang, E. K.: Arteriographic diagnosis of renal infarcts. Radiology 88:1110, 1967.

Lang, E. K., Mertz, J. H. D., and Nourse, M.: Renal arteriography in the assessment of renal infarction. J. Urol. 99:506, 1968.

MacNider, W. deB.: The pathological changes which develop in the kidney as a result of occlusion, by ligature, of one branch of the renal artery. J. Med. Res. 22:91, 1910.

Naidich, J. B., Naidich, T. P., Pudlowski, R. M., Waldbaum, R. S., Hyman, R. A., and Stein, H. L.: Angiographic patterns of post-traumatic renal scarring. AJR 128:729, 1977.

Papanicolaou, N., Habory, O. L., and Pfister, R. C.: Fat-filled postoperative renal cortical defects: Sonographic and CT appearance. AJR 151:503, 1988.

Parker, J. M., and Lord, J. D.: Renal artery embolism: A case report with return of complete function of the involved kidney following anticoagulant therapy. J. Urol. 106:339, 1971.

Regan, F. C., and Crabtree, E. G.: Renal infarction: Clinical and possible surgical entity. J. Urol. 59:981, 1948.

Sheehan, H. L., and Davis, J. C.: Complete permanent renal ischaemia. J. Pathol. 76:569, 1958.

Siegelman, S. S., and Caplan, L. H.: Acute segmental renal artery embolism: A distinctive urographic and arteriographic complex. Radiology 88:509, 1967.

Solez, K.: Acute renal failure (acute tubular necrosis, infarction and cortical necrosis). In Heptinstall, R. H. (ed.): Pathology of the Kidney. 4th ed. Boston, Little, Brown & Co., 1992.

Wisoff, C. P., and Chambers, D. E.: Subtotal renal infarction. AJR 98:63, 1966.

6

DIAGNOSTIC SET: SMALL, SMOOTH, UNILATERAL

ISCHEMIA SECONDARY TO FOCAL ARTERIAL DISEASE

CHRONIC RENAL INFARCTION

RADIATION NEPHRITIS

CONGENITAL HYPOPLASIA

POSTOBSTRUCTIVE ATROPHY

POSTINFLAMMATORY ATROPHY

REFLUX ATROPHY

DIFFERENTIAL DIAGNOSIS

Generalized, that is, global, decrease in the size of one kidney with preservation of normal pelvocalyceal relationships characterizes the radiologic appearance of the entities discussed in this chapter. This pattern is the one common bond among these processes, which otherwise are widely dissimilar in their pathogenesis.

It will be noted that several of the entities included in the "small, smooth, unilateral" diagnostic set represent late stages of pathologic processes that initially produced unilateral enlargement of the kidney. Among these processes are infarction of all or large amounts of kidney tissue and obstructive uropathy. It is hoped that this order of presentation—late changes before acute ones —will not confuse the reader.

This is the first chapter to include diseases with "smallness" as the only radiologic abnormality. The reader should refer to Chapter 3 for a discussion of renal measurements. Unfortunately, no accurate, practical, quantitative yardstick is available to establish "normal" renal size. In this subjective setting, one should keep in mind that apparent smallness may be erroneously suggested by abnormal enlargement of the contralateral kidney and that a kidney that may measure within normal limits actually was normally larger at an earlier time.

ISCHEMIA SECONDARY TO FOCAL ARTERIAL DISEASE

Definition

When nutrient renal blood flow is inadequate for normal cell metabolism, there is a global decrease in renal bulk primarily due to tubule atrophy. The proximal convoluted segment in particular becomes smaller in diameter. This process is noted also in the glomeruli, which become crowded together, smaller in size, and hyalinized. These changes develop when stenosing lesions of the renal arterial tree become advanced. The number and size of the renal arteries involved determine the pattern of wasting. If arteriosclerosis is generalized in the interlobar and arcuate arteries, both kidneys will shrink uniformly. (See discussion in Chapter 7.) The pattern discussed in this chapter, global shrinkage of one kidney, occurs when a single focus of narrowing develops in the main renal artery.

In the general population, focal narrowing of the main renal artery is usually due to an atheromatous lesion in the proximal 2 cm of the vessel. Less frequently, the distal main artery or its early branches are the site of stenosis, particularly at points of bifurcation. The atherosclerotic plaque is most often eccentrically placed in the arterial lumen. Narrowing results from both growth of the plaque and from intermittent bleeding into the plaque wall.

Other forms of arterial disease, particularly in children and in women, also can result in ischemia and renal wasting. In one study of angiograms of 884 hypertensive patients with renovascular disease, 63 per cent of patients had atherosclerotic lesions while 32 per cent had renal arterial dysplasia (Bookstein et al., 1972). This latter group is called "fibromuscular hyperplasia" by some; others identify angiographic-pathologic subtypes including "intimal fibroplasia," "fibromuscular hyperplasia," "medial fibroplasia," and "subadventitial fibroplasia." Dysplastic lesions result from abnormal accumulation of collagen, hyperplasia of smooth muscle and fibrous tissue cells, disruption or thinning of the elastica interna, and development of fibrous rings. Each subtype has a distinctive combination of these features distributed in different portions of the arterial wall. Although subtyping may provide some discriminatory clinical and prognostic information, these diagnoses are usually grouped into the single category "fibromuscular hyperplasia."

Lesions other than atherosclerosis and dysplasia that can produce ischemia and a small kidney are quite uncommon. These include renal artery aneurysm, renal arteriovenous fistula, Takayasu's disease, thromboangiitis obliterans, syphilitic arteritis, dissecting aortic aneurysm, post–radiation renal artery stenosis, and extrinsic pressure on the renal artery from a lesion in the kidney hilus, such as tumor, fibrous bands, or parapelvic cyst.

Clinical Setting

The development of ischemic atrophy becomes clinically important only when it is associated with hypertension. The focal arterial lesion that produces a small kidney in a person who remains normotensive is of no particular consequence except insofar as it may lead to renal insufficiency when it is bilateral or occurs in a solitary kidney. Indeed, moderate-to-severe renal artery narrowing occurs often in older, normotensive patients and in patients with essential (i.e., nonrenovascular) hypertension.

The pathophysiology of the ischemic kidney and of renovascular hypertension has been the subject of extensive laboratory and clinical investigation. Studies show that a drop in glomerular filtration rate follows the decrease in renal perfusion pressure caused by renal artery stenosis. As a result, the volume of glomerular filtrate decreases. In addition, a greater percentage of the filtrate is reabsorbed owing to complex osmotic and humoral factors. The renin-angiotensin-aldosterone mechanism plays an important role in the development of these changes, as well as in the production of hypertension. The net result of the renal response to arterial stenosis is hyperreninemic hypertension and an increase in the concentration of filtered, nonreabsorbable substances, including urographic contrast material, diminished urine volume, and decreased urine flow rate on the affected side as compared with the nonischemic contralateral kidney.

The histologic nature of the stenosing lesion varies with age and sex. Males older than age 50 are likely to have atherosclerotic lesions, whereas females in younger age groups (mean age of 38) more frequently develop dysplastic arterial disease. Both atherosclerotic and dysplastic lesions can be progressive and bilateral. This fact is of obvious importance in evaluating therapeutic choices for these patients.

One of the major clinical challenges in setting diagnostic strategies for the hypertensive population at large is to identify patients who have renovascular hypertension, that is, those with renal artery stenosis, that if corrected will mitigate or cure high blood pressure. These patients, who comprise less than 3 per cent of the hypertensive population, need to be distinguished from those whose hypertension is due to other causes. Historically, a modification of the excretory urogram, known as the "hypertensive" or "rapid sequence" urogram was used as a primary screen of

the hypertensive population to identify patients with curable hypertension. This experience, analyzed by the Cooperative Study of Renovascular Hypertension, provided a vivid example of how the excretory urogram reflects renal pathophysiology (Bookstein et al., 1972). Critical assessment of the modified excretory urogram as a screening test of the general hypertensive population for a renovascular cause, however, has demonstrated its low positive predictive value, reflecting both the poor sensitivity of the test and the low prevalence of renovascular hypertension. The same considerations have limited the usefulness of traditional radionuclide renography. As a result, emphasis has shifted to using clinical features as the initial criteria for selecting the hypertensive patient who should be subjected to the definitive test of renal angiography. These clinical features encompass patients, especially women, younger than the age of 45 whose diastolic pressure persists at about 100 mm Hg or more despite careful medical management and older patients with pre-existing hypertension that abruptly accelerates. Other clinical features that increase the probability of a renovascular cause for hypertension include failure of moderate hypertension to respond to medical treatment and an abdominal bruit. Patients selected by these criteria are then studied with arteriography using either film-screen or digital techniques. Angioplasty can be performed at the same time when a suitable renal artery stenosis is discovered. Sampling of renal veins for renin assay, Doppler measurement of renal artery blood flow, and magnetic resonance angiography comprise other methodologies whose efficacy is either disputed or yet to be proven. The methodology and the diagnostic role of captopril radionuclide renography are discussed in detail in Chapter 2.

Radiologic Findings

Calcification in a renal artery aneurysm or in the wall of a severely atheromatous renal artery may be present (Figs. 6–1 and 6–2). However, most abnormal findings are found in the excretory urogram and the renal angiogram.

Length. Information from the Cooperative Study of Renovascular Hypertension (Bookstein et al., 1972) has provided quantitative data for the use of renal length as a discriminatory factor in differentiating patients whose hypertension is due to renovascular disease from those with essential hypertension (Fig. 6–3). This study demonstrated that the number of misclassifications of these two categories could be minimized by considering all right-sided kidneys that were more than 2.0 cm shorter than the left and all left-sided kidneys that were more than 1.5 cm shorter than the right to be indicative of renovascular hypertension. These figures take into account the fact that the right kidney is normally shorter than the left. In some patients, however, renal length may be normal even in the presence of severe, functionally significant stenosis. (See Figs. 6–1 and 6–5.)

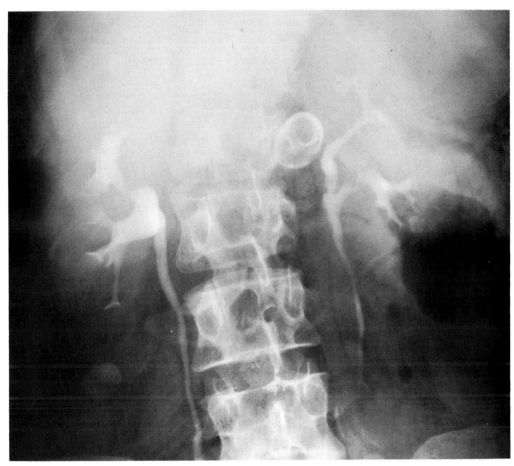

Figure 6–1. Ischemia due to focal arterial disease. Five-minute film during excretory urography in a middle-aged hypertensive woman. There is calcification of a left renal artery aneurysm. Diminished urine volume and pelvoureteral notching due to arterial collaterals are present on the involved side. Renal length is within normal limits. (Same patient illustrated in Figs. 6–2, 6–4A, and 6–6.)

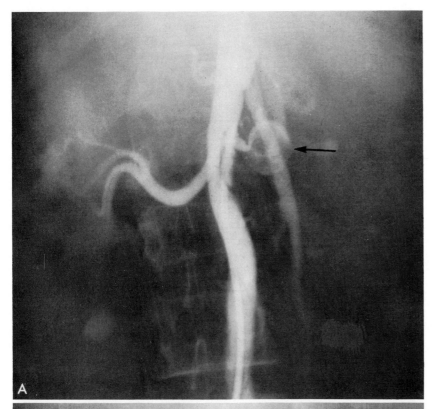

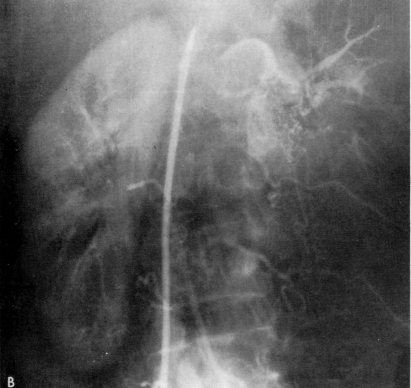

Figure 6–2. Aortogram of patient illustrated in Figures 6–1, 6–4A, and 6–6.

A, Early arterial phase, anteroposterior projection. High-grade obstruction caused by a calcified left main renal artery aneurysm *(arrow)* is present.

B, Delayed film, right posterior oblique projection. Peripelvic and periureteric collaterals and intrarenal arteries are now opacified.

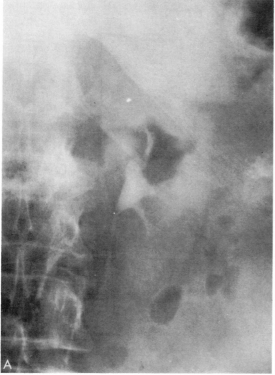

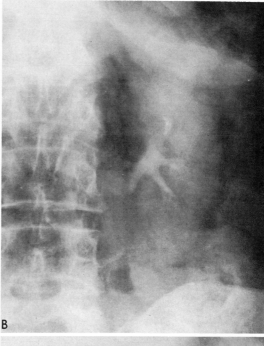

Figure 6–3. Ischemia due to focal arterial disease. Progressive global decrease in left kidney length in a middle-aged hypertensive woman with angiographically proven left main renal artery stenosis.

    A, 1966. Left kidney length = 10.5 cm.

    B, 1967. Left kidney length = 9.5 cm.

    C, 1970. Left kidney length = 8.0 cm.

    Note preservation of smooth margin. Patient was treated with antihypertensive medication.

Contour. The ischemic kidney maintains a smooth contour despite a decrease in size (see Fig. 6–3). When renal artery stenosis with ischemia is bilateral, urographic evaluation becomes less precise because many of the abnormal signs of renovascular hypertension are dependent on comparisons between a normal kidney on one side and an ischemic kidney on the other. In this situation, radiologic diagnosis is far more dependent on angiographic than on urographic findings.

Appearance Time. Of all the radiologic signs evaluated in the cooperative study, delay in appearance time of contrast material in the calyces on the involved side, either alone or in combination with other abnormalities, was found to be the single most reliable feature in distinguishing essential from renovas-

cular hypertension. This finding was present in 59 per cent of patients with renovascular hypertension and in only 2 per cent of those with essential hypertension (Fig. 6–4). This abnormality is a direct expression of the decrease in glomerular filtration rate that follows reduction in perfusion pressure of the kidney. For each unit of time, fewer molecules of iodine-bearing contrast material are cleared from the plasma on the affected side than from the contralateral nonischemic kidney. As a result, there is a period of time after injection of contrast material when the number of atoms of iodine present in the calyces of the normal kidney allows radiographic detection, while the amount of iodine cleared on the ischemic side is insufficient for radiographic visualization.

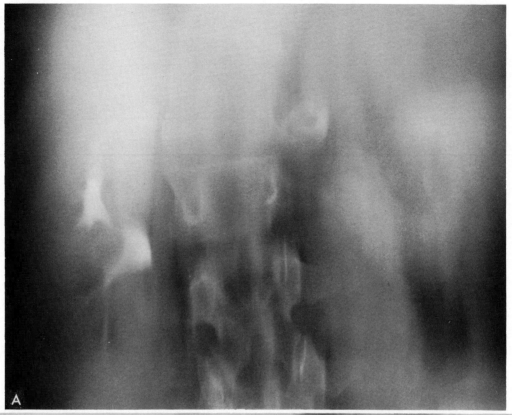

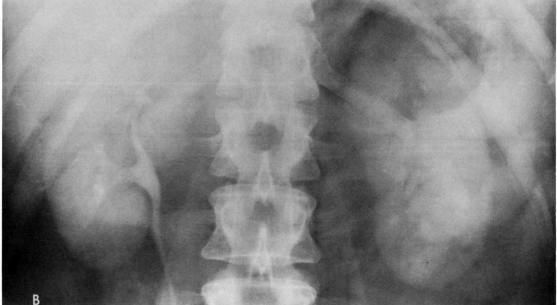

Figure 6–4. Ischemia due to focal arterial disease. Delayed calyceal opacification.

A, Tomogram approximately 3 minutes after contrast material injection shows no calyceal opacification on the left, while the right system is opacified. (Same patient illustrated in Figs. 6–1, 6–2, and 6–6.)

B, The same finding is illustrated in a different patient with bilateral renal arterial dysplasia with radiologic evidence of greater functional impairment on the left. (Same patient illustrated in Fig. 6–5.)

(Fig. 6–4*B* courtesy of J. Shanser, M.D., St. Francis Memorial Hospital, San Francisco, California, and M. Korobkin, M.D., University of Michigan, Ann Arbor, Michigan.)

The rapid sequence hypertensive urogram is a modification of the standard urogram that increases the likelihood of detecting differences in calyceal opacification time by obtaining films at frequent intervals during the first few minutes following contrast material injection. A film taken immediately on completion of a rapid injection of contrast material is followed by films at 1-minute intervals up to 5 minutes. Abdominal compression is not used during this period, to avoid urine stasis from ureteral obstruction, which might depress glomerular filtration rate and cause a false-positive sign.

When the minute-sequence urogram was first introduced, it was suggested that a difference in the density of the nephrogram on early films was the most sensitive indicator of unilaterally diminished perfusion pressure. Experience has shown that this observation is imprecise, because differences in baseline density are usually present on the preliminary film in the kidney area. Differential calyceal opacification, rather than differential nephrographic density, is the feature to be evaluated in the early stages of the rapid sequence urogram.

Urine Volume and Density. Because salt and water reabsorption are enhanced in the ischemic kidney, the volume of urine it forms in any given time period is less than the amount the normal side forms. This phenomenon is manifested as a lack of distention of the pelvocalyceal and ureteral structures on the involved side (Fig. 6–5; see Fig. 6–1). Increased density of contrast material in the collecting structures is also due to

increased water reabsorption, causing hyperconcentration in the urine of nonreabsorbable solutes (see Fig. 6–5). Caution must be used in evaluating urine opacity, however, as a large collecting structure will appear denser than a small one, even when the concentration of contrast material is equal, because a greater number of atoms of iodine stand in the way of the x-ray beam. Therefore, comparison of density must be made in segments of the collecting system that are roughly equal in volume. In practice, this is often difficult; equivocal signs should not be weighed too heavily in arriving at a final diagnosis.

Urine Transit Time. Another physiologic consequence of reduced perfusion pressure and glomerular filtration rate is prolonged transit of urine through the tubules and down the ureter. This is detected in late urographic films (usually after 30 minutes) by the persistent opacification of the pelvocalyceal system and ureter of the ischemic kidney at a time when the normal kidney shows "washing out" of contrast material. This sign can be enhanced by the infusion of an osmotic diuretic, such as urea or mannitol (Fig. 6–6). This modification has not proved worthwhile, considering the added expense and time.

Ureteral Notching. Another of the classic urographic abnormalities of ischemia is ureteral notching. This occurs as a result of enlargement of the collateral arteries that carry blood around the obstructing lesion (Fig. 6–7; see Figs. 6–1 and 6–2). Although there are many potential collateral arteries, the periureteric and peripelvic vessels are particularly important because

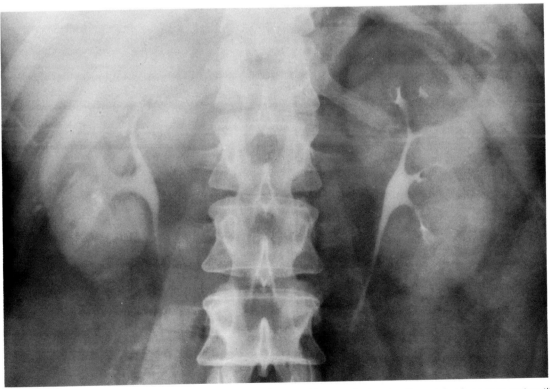

Figure 6–5. Ischemia due to focal arterial disease. Diminished urine volume and increased urine density on left side in same patient illustrated in Figure 6–4*B*. Calyceal volume appears diminished on the left compared with the right. Note normal kidney length. (Courtesy of J. Shanser, M.D., St. Francis Memorial Hospital, San Francisco, California, and M. Korobkin, M.D., University of Michigan, Ann Arbor, Michigan.)

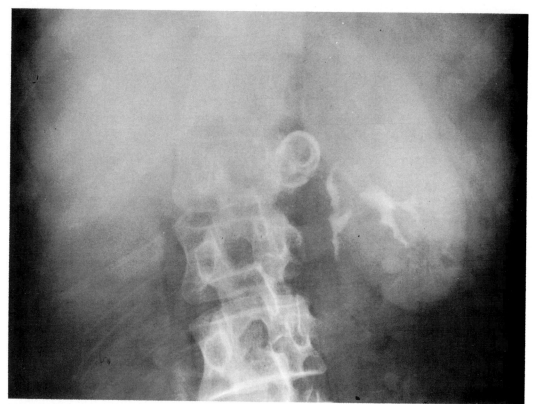

Figure 6–6. Ischemia due to focal arterial disease. Delayed "washout" of contrast material from left kidney 10 minutes after infusion of urea. Contrast material has been removed from the normal right kidney by the urea-induced diuresis. (Same patient as illustrated in Figs. 6–1, 6–2, and 6–4A.)

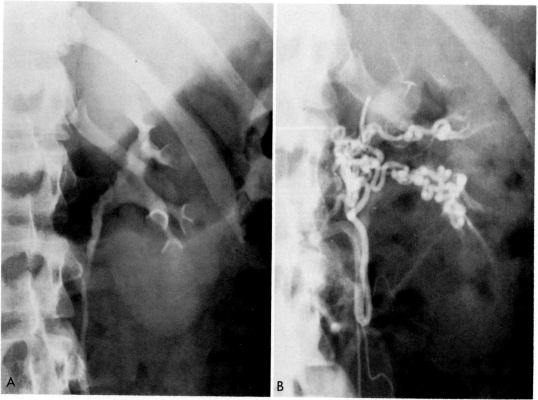

Figure 6–7. Ischemia due to focal arterial disease. Ureteral and pelvic notching in a 16-year-old girl with severe hyperreninemic hypertension due to surgically proven intimal fibroplasia of left renal artery.

A, Excretory urogram. Indentations on margin of pelvis and ureter are present.

B, Lumbar arteriogram. There are dilated tortuous periureteric and peripelvic collateral arteries, which correspond to the abnormalities depicted in *A.* (Same patient illustrated in Figures 16–18 and 16–21.)

(Courtesy of Janet Dacie, M.B., St. Bartholomew's Hospital, London, England.)

**SUMMARY OF ABNORMAL URORADIOLOGIC FINDINGS
ISCHEMIA SECONDARY TO FOCAL ARTERIAL DISEASE**

Primary Uroradiologic Elements
   Size—normal to decreased (may have less than normal increase in renal
      surface area in response to contrast material or diuretics
   Contour—smooth (global)
   Lesion distribution—unilateral
Secondary Uroradiologic Elements
   Pelvoinfundibulocalyceal system—
      Attenuated (global)
      Notched (proximal ureter)
      Delayed opacification time
      Increased density of contrast material
      Delayed washout of contrast material
   Parenchymal thickness—wasted (global)
   Calcification—linear (aneurysmal or atherosclerotic in renal hilus)
   Arteries—stenotic, aneurysmal, collateralized

---

they impress on structures visualized during urography and are seen as multiple mural notches in the proximal ureter and the pelvis.

Change in Renal Size. One final observation may be made during excretory urography. The normal kidney increases in size when exposed to contrast material either alone or in combination with certain diuretic drugs. It has been shown that the degree of enlargement is less than normal in a kidney with significant renal artery stenosis. The surface area of a normal kidney, measured by planimetry, increases 5 to 10 per cent over a 15-minute period following use of contrast material and ethacrynic acid or urea. Under similar conditions, the surface area increase is usually less than 5 per cent in patients with renovascular hypertension. The details of "vasodilated excretory urography" are available in the literature. This test, however, is not useful in the evaluation of the hypertensive patient.

In renovascular ischemia, the contralateral kidney is usually normal in size. Occasionally, compensatory hypertrophy is seen when the ischemic process is severe.

The data from the Cooperative Study of Renovascular Hypertension revealed that as the severity of stenosis (judged by arteriography) increased, the frequency of urographic abnormalities, singly or in combination, increased. With 80 to 99 per cent reduction in luminal diameter, 83 per cent of the patients had an abnormal urogram. However, the false-positive rate of over 20 per cent reduces the value of the rapid sequence urogram as a sensitive screening test for renovascular hypertension. A normal urogram in the presence of clinical features suggestive of renovascular hypertension (e.g., abdominal bruit, young age, recent onset of high blood pressure) should not deter one from performing an angiogram or renal vein renin assay.

Renal Angiogram. Renal angiography has a historic role in the evaluation of the ischemic kidney. This technique precisely identifies the site, nature, and extent of the arterial lesion and is indispensable in establishing the diagnosis and planning a therapeutic approach, by either surgery or percutaneous transluminal angioplasty. In addition, useful hemodynamic data can be derived from the thoroughly performed angiogram by observing factors such as the presence of collaterals, dilution defects in opacified extrarenal vessels during pharmacologic manipulation of renal blood flow, and spillover of contrast material into the aorta following selective injection at a constant, known rate. In some patients, digital subtraction angiography provides an adequate display of arterial anatomy. Other aspects of the angiograpic evaluation of the ischemic kidney, including renal vein sampling for renin levels, are beyond the scope of this text and are the subject of numerous articles cited in the bibliography at the end of this chapter.

CHRONIC RENAL INFARCTION

Definition

The kidney that has undergone complete infarction eventually becomes globally small and is enhanced minimally or not at all during excretory urography or computed tomography. The sequence of histologic events is the same as described for lobar infarction in Chapter 5. All elements of the kidney atrophy, and interstitial fibrosis with obliteration of the vessels develops. Some perfusion of the renal tissue may persist through capsular, pelvic, and ureteric collateral arteries not affected by the occlusive process. This does not necessarily represent nutrient perfusion to functioning tissue, however.

There are times when infarction affects a major portion, but not all, of the kidney. In this situation an entire pole or the dorsal or ventral part of the organ becomes atrophic, while the noninvolved portion continues to function. Since infarction in these cases involves much more than the lobe, the pattern of wasting leaves a smooth margin.

**SUMMARY OF ABNORMAL URORADIOLOGIC FINDINGS
CHRONIC RENAL INFARCTION**

Primary Uroradiologic Elements
  Size—normal to small
  Contour—smooth (global)
  Lesion distribution—unilateral
Secondary Uroradiologic Elements*
  Parenchymal thickness—wasted (global, occasionally regional)
  Nephrogram—diminished to absent contrast material density
  Echogenicity—increased

*Functional abnormalities seen in the ischemic kidney (see pages 143–147) may also be present in incomplete forms of chronic infarction.

Clinical Setting

Total or major segmental renal infarction is very uncommon when compared with the frequency of lobar infarction. Infarction may be due to embolization, thrombosis, or traumatic avulsion of the main renal artery or one of its major divisions. Blunt trauma to the kidney and renal venous thrombosis are two other situations that can produce major renal infarction leading to global atrophy.

The late stage of complete infarction is clinically silent. Total infarction rarely is associated with sustained hypertension or with any other renal symptomatology if the contralateral kidney is adequate to maintain renal function. When infarction does not involve the whole kidney or when the process eventually resolves, the affected renal tissue may atrophy.

Radiologic Findings

The classic radiologic appearance of late total renal infarction includes global shrinkage of the kidney, absent opacification during excretory urography or computed tomography, and a normal pelvocalyceal system shown on a retrograde pyelogram (Fig. 6–8). Decrease in renal size can be detected within 2 weeks after the onset of infarction and reaches maximal extent by 5 weeks. The contralateral kidney enlarges in individuals young enough to provide this reserve.

Contrast material excreted by uninvolved parts of the kidney in cases of partial infarction is distributed passively into the morphologically normal calyces serving the nonfunctioning portions of the kidney. The involved area in these cases can be identified only by regional thinning of the renal parenchyma (Figs. 6–9 and 6–10). With excretory urography this is detectable most readily in the polar regions and is very difficult to define when the ventral or dorsal parts of the kidney are involved, because of the difficulty in obtaining steep lateral profile projections in these areas. Cross-sectional imaging techniques, especially computed tomography, clearly demonstrate these regions.

Global atrophy may follow a total infarction that resolves early enough to preserve organ viability (Fig.

6–11). In some cases, ischemia persists, and the same functional urographic abnormalities seen in main renal artery narrowing are present.

The infarcted kidney produces greater than normal echogenicity. Ultrasonography also well demonstrates the wasting of renal parenchyma and the preservation of a smooth renal contour.

The angiographic findings in late renal infarction range from failure to demonstrate any arteries (see Fig. 6–8C) to the nonopacification of major regional branches (see Fig. 6–9B) or an accessory renal artery (see Fig. 6–10B). In kidneys that have undergone resolution of an infarctive process, the findings will vary and include normal to decreased numbers of vessels, diminished density of the nephrogram, and thinned parenchyma.

RADIATION NEPHRITIS
Definition

Radiation nephritis occurs as a result of the kidneys being included within a therapeutic field of radiation beyond a certain dose. Other sources of radiation, such as radioactive isotopes, diagnostic x-rays, and atomic explosions, have not been shown to produce this abnormality in humans.

Pathologically, all elements of renal tissue are affected. Interstitial fibrosis, tubule atrophy, glomerular sclerosis, sclerosis of arteries of all sizes, hyalinization of afferent arterioles, and thickening of the renal capsule are present in varying degrees.

The amount of tissue involved is determined by the radiation field. Radiation nephritis is usually limited to one kidney; obviously both may be involved under appropriate conditions.

Clinical Setting

The threshold dose for the induction of nephritis in humans appears to be 2300 R administered over a 5-week period. Clinically, both acute and chronic forms have been described. The chronic form may follow a period of clinically apparent acute disease or appear *de novo* without any prior evidence of radiation-in-

Text continued on page 154

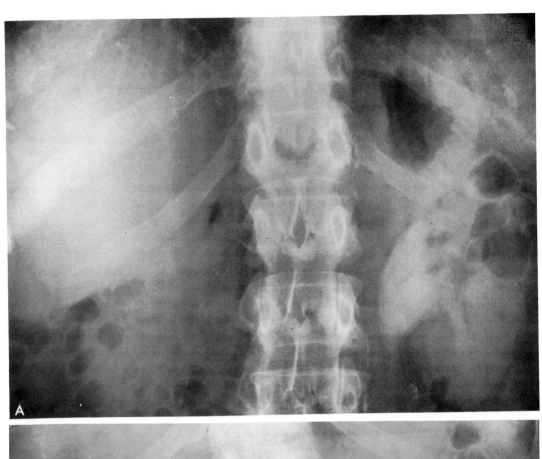

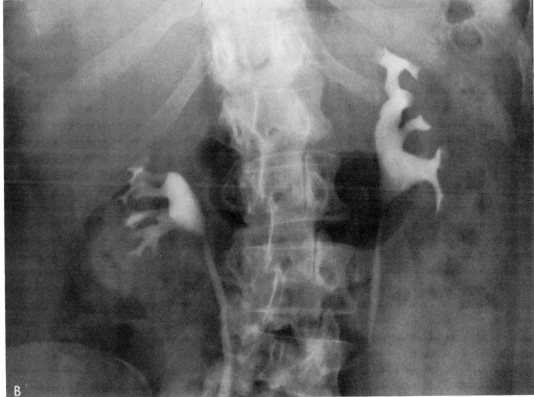

Figure 6–8. Chronic total infarction of the right kidney.
A, No right renal substance is opacified at any time during excretory urography.
B, Bilateral retrograde pyelography demonstrates normal papillae and calyces. Crowding of the right-sided structures suggests smallness of the kidney.

Illustration continued on the following page

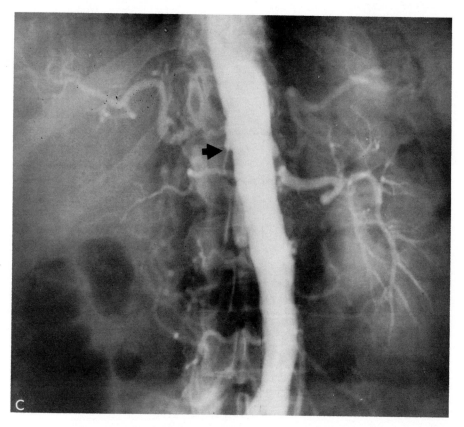

Figure 6–8 *Continued C,* Aortogram demonstrates complete occlusion of right renal artery *(arrow)* and no collateral flow. Autopsy revealed a small, smooth kidney due to old infarction from a thrombosis in the proximal main renal artery.

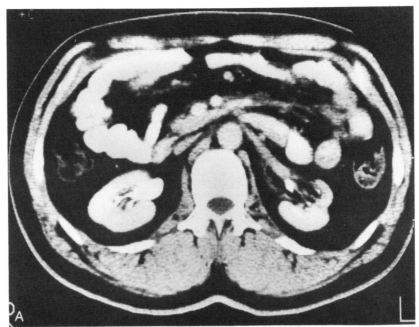

Figure 6–9. Chronic infarction of the ventral portion of the left kidney in a 41-year-old hypertensive woman. There has been occlusion of the major anterior branch of the renal artery caused by arterial dysplasia.

A, Computed tomogram, contrast material enhanced. Global wasting of the ventral portion of the left kidney parenchyma has occurred.

B, Selective renal arteriogram. Subtraction technique. There is complete occlusion of the major branch of the renal artery to the ventral portion of the kidney *(arrow).*

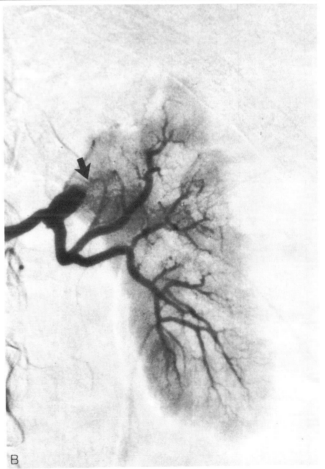

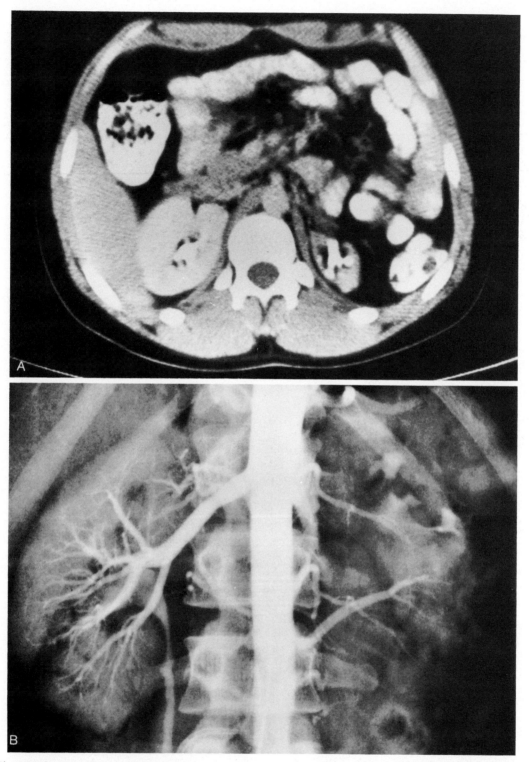

Figure 6–10. Chronic infarction of the upper half of a left kidney perfused by two renal arteries. The superior artery had been transected as a result of previous blunt abdominal trauma.

   A, Computed tomogram, contrast material enhanced. The global wasting of the upper pole is so marked that there is associated dilatation of underlying calyces.

   B, Aortogram. The artery to the upper half of the left kidney is missing. The lower half of the kidney is perfused by a renal artery arising at the level of the superior plate of the L-3 vertebral body.

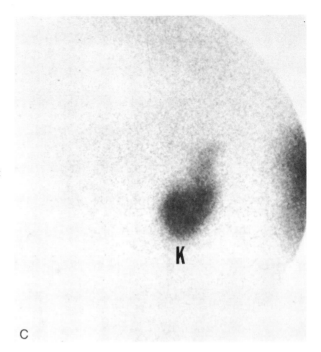

Figure 6–10 *Continued C,* Radionuclide scan. The upper half of the left kidney (K) is globally wasted.

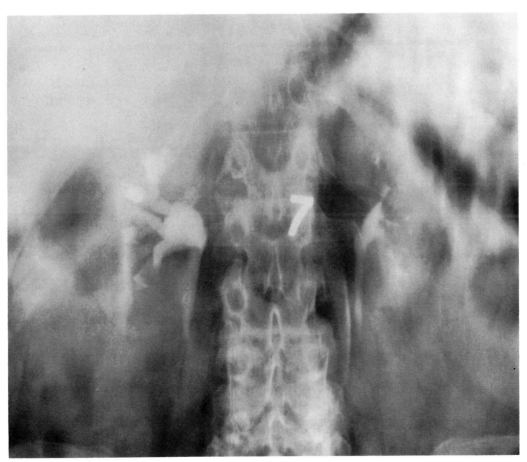

Figure 6–11. Chronic renal infarction. Unilateral global atrophy of left kidney with preservation of function 30 months after acute infarction complicating colon surgery. Infarction apparently resolved early enough to preserve organ viability. Despite atrophy, hypertension did not develop. Radiologic studies obtained in this patient during the acute episode are illustrated in Figure 9–7.

SUMMARY OF ABNORMAL URORADIOLOGIC FINDINGS
RADIATION NEPHRITIS

Primary Uroradiologic Elements
    Size—normal to small
    Contour—smooth (global)
    Lesion distribution—consistent with radiation field
Secondary Uroradiologic Elements*
    Parenchymal thickness—wasted (global, related to radiation field)
    Nephrogram—diminished density of contrast material

*Functional abnormalities seen in the ischemic kidney (see pages 143–147) may also be present in unilateral cases of radiation nephritis.

---

duced renal disease. This often occurs at a later time, perhaps 2 years or more after the initial exposure to radiation.

Radiation nephritis is associated with anemia, proteinuria, hyposthenuria, and azotemia. Granular epithelial and hyaline casts are seen in the urinary sediment. Moderate to malignant hypertension is present in half of the patients. This may be due to renin-angiotensin factors. In many respects the clinical picture is similar to that of chronic glomerulonephritis. However, radiation nephritis may be compatible with long life, even in the presence of progressive reduction in renal size.

Deterioration of renal function and clinical findings are most likely related to glomerular damage. The basic mediating factor in the pathogenesis of this disease, however, is radiation-induced damage to the small vessels of the kidney.

Radiologic Findings

There is nothing specific about the radiologic appearance of the kidney in radiation nephritis. In some patients, renal size remains normal; in others, the kidney becomes profoundly small. A smooth contour and a normal pelvocalyceal system are preserved. Atrophy is limited to those portions of the kidney included in the radiation field (Fig. 6–12).

In unilateral disease, the same radiologic abnormalities of ischemia seen in renal artery stenosis may also be present. The contralateral kidney is likely to undergo compensatory hypertrophy, particularly when radiation nephritis develops in younger patients. Depending on the size and shape of the radiation field, both kidneys may be involved.

CONGENITAL HYPOPLASIA

Definition

A hypoplastic kidney is underdeveloped because of a quantitative deficiency in its ureteric and metanephric primordia. As a result, there is miniaturization of the kidney due to a reduction in both the number of renal lobes and the amount of nephrons contained in each lobe. The number of calyces and papillae are fewer than normal. Function persists in those nephrons that

do develop. The microscopic anatomy of the hypoplastic kidney, uncomplicated by any superimposed process, is characterized by smallness of cell size and occasional hyaline degeneration of the glomeruli.

The *Ask-Upmark kidney* is considered by some to be an important variant of true renal hypoplasia in which nephrogenesis is arrested in one or several adjacent lobes following the formation of juxtamedullary nephrons. The Ask-Upmark kidney is also referred to as *aglomerular focal hypoplasia* in the European literature. Urographically, a focal area of renal wasting is associated with ectasia of the corresponding calyces. There are many who consider the Ask-Upmark kidney to be nothing more than a kidney with a single focus of reflux nephropathy. Certainly, the radiologic features are compatible with this diagnosis, and the absence of a history of urinary tract infection does not dissuade one from adopting this point of view. (This is expanded on in Chapter 5.) The issue remains unresolved, however. The basis for the deep transverse groove on the cortical surface described in some case reports of Ask-Upmark kidney has not been established.

The diagnosis of renal hypoplasia is imprecise unless strict morphologic criteria are applied. The literature has been confused by the inclusion of many acquired diseases that produce small kidneys and because the true hypoplastic kidney often acquires disease, especially infection. If this diagnosis is to be made with accuracy, particular emphasis must be placed on finding five or fewer calyces in a small kidney—a very rare occurrence.

Clinical Setting

In unilateral renal hypoplasia, the contralateral kidney becomes hypertrophied and normal renal function is maintained. Clinical concern in this situation is limited to the preservation of the dominant kidney. On the other hand, bilateral hypoplasia leads to renal failure, the intensity of which varies with the amount of tissue present. Failure to thrive, renal osteodystrophy, and other stigmata of impaired renal function appear during childhood, usually before the end of the first decade. Death occurs before age 20 in most cases. Thus, renal hypoplasia in the adult is unilateral.

Figure 6–12. Radiation-induced atrophy.

A, Normal excretory urogram in an 11-year-old boy with Hodgkin's disease before para-aortic nodal radiation. Arrows point to the margin of the kidneys in those areas that eventually atrophy.

B, Excretory urogram 5 years later. Radiation field included medial aspect of the right kidney and upper pole of the left kidney. Arrows point to the margins of the kidney where atrophy can be detected by their proximity to adjacent calyces. Margins remain smooth.

(Courtesy of the late A. J. Palubinskas, M.D., University of California, San Francisco.)

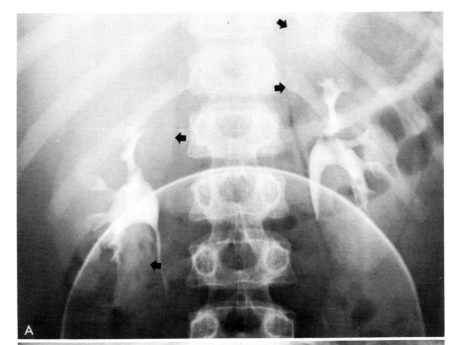

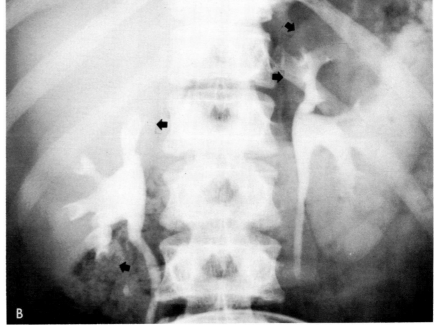

SUMMARY OF ABNORMAL URORADIOLOGIC FINDINGS
CONGENITAL HYPOPLASIA

Primary Uroradiologic Elements
Size—decreased
Contour—smooth (global)
Lesion distribution—unilateral
Secondary Uroradiologic Elements
Papillae—decreased number
Calyces—decreased number

Radiologic Findings

The single, small, smooth kidney with five or fewer calyces and an enlarged contralateral kidney provides the basis for the radiologic diagnosis of renal hypoplasia (Fig. 6–13). Associated urogenital anomalies, such as ectopia and ureteral duplication, are common but of little value in distinguishing hypoplasia from other causes of the small kidney because of their common occurrence in general. The hypoplastic kidney usually has sufficient functioning nephrons for opacification of the pelvocalyceal system.

POSTOBSTRUCTIVE ATROPHY

Definition

Generalized papillary atrophy associated with a variable amount of caliectasis and global thinning of the renal parenchyma are changes that occasionally follow correction of urinary obstruction. Usually the kidney shrinks as well, but there are some cases in which renal length remains normal or even increases as the volume of the dilated pelvocalyceal system increases. Also included in this category are those unusual cases

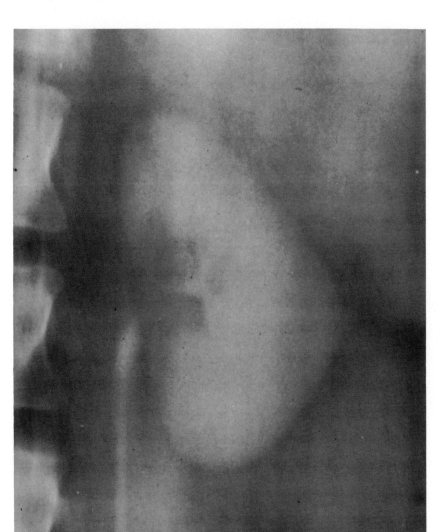

Figure 6–13. Congenital hypoplasia. The small, smooth left kidney has fewer than five identifiable calyces. Excretory urogram. Tomogram. (Courtesy of Professor L. Dalla Palma, University of Trieste, Trieste, Italy.)

in which the kidney undergoes rather rapid parenchymal wasting, with little, if any, calyceal dilatation following relief of a limited period of urinary obstruction.

Clinical Setting

Atrophy of tissue due to urinary tract obstruction is thought to result from the direct effect of increased hydrostatic pressure on renal tissue and ischemia from compression of intrarenal arteries and veins. Presumably, progressive atrophy following relief of obstruction, particularly of a mild degree and moderate duration, is primarily due to ischemia. Experimental work in the pig indicates that direct pressure from obstruction causes tubule rupture, cell atrophy, and loss of bulk of the renal pyramids. This mechanism, rather than ischemia, may be dominant when the residual effect of relieved obstruction is clubbed calyces as well as global parenchymal atrophy.

Most patients with postobstructive atrophy have a proven history of obstruction or at least prior symptoms of renal colic. A significant number of the cases originally reported by Hodson and Craven (1966), however, had no such history, and the existence of previous obstruction was presumed by these authors.

Why some patients respond to relieved obstruction in this manner, whereas others in apparently identical circumstances do not, is not known.

Radiologic Findings

The radiologic findings can be predicted from the definition given earlier in this section. An essential feature of postobstructive atrophy is the uniformity with which the entire kidney is involved. This, of course, is the expected response, since the hydrostatic effects of a "downstream" obstruction are directed equally to all parts of the kidney.

The postobstructive atrophic kidney is usually, but not invariably, a small kidney. Regardless of size, all kidneys with this condition are included in this diagnostic set because they all have undergone loss of renal tissue. Dilatation of the collecting structures is found in those situations in which renal size is preserved or increased (Fig. 6–14).

The small, smooth kidney with little or no papillary wasting or calyceal dilation is the least common presentation of postobstructive atrophy (Fig. 6–15). It is also more of an engima than the other forms, in view of the absence of radiologic evidence for increased hydrostatic pressure, namely, collecting system dilatation. The progression of atrophy in these cases can be documented by serial urography, ultrasonography, or computed tomography and occurs rather rapidly over a 6- to 12-week period following relief of obstruction of moderate duration.

Compensatory hypertrophy of the contralateral kidney may be present, depending on the age of the

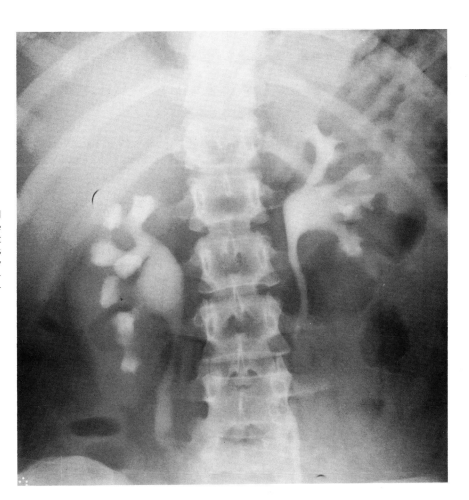

Figure 6–14. Nonobstructive caliectasis and global parenchymal atrophy involving the right kidney of a 26-year-old woman without a prior history of urinary tract disease. This pattern is associated either with previously reversed urinary tract obstruction or with vesicoureteral reflux. Kidney length may be normal, as in this case, reduced, or increased.

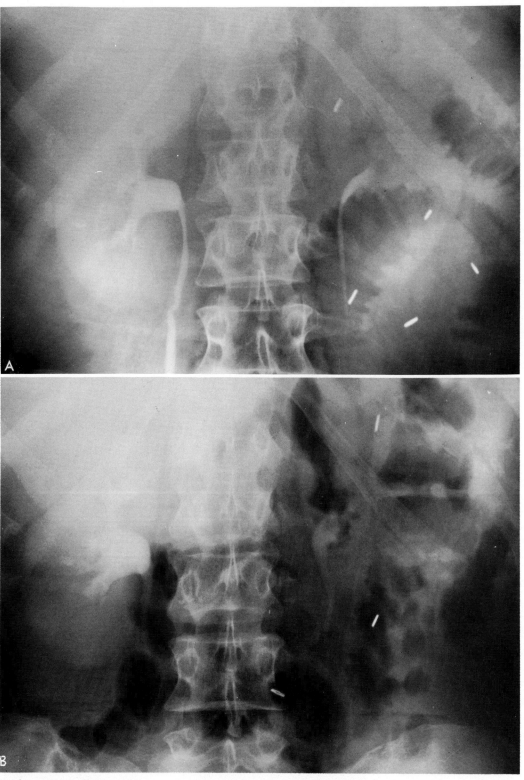

Figure 6–15. Postobstructive atrophy.
  A, Normal baseline urogram in a patient with malignant lymphoma. Left kidney measures 11.5 cm.
  B, Excretory urogram 5 years later after an episode of treated left hydronephrosis. Kidney now measures 7.4 cm and is smooth in outline. Papillary and calyceal architecture remains normal. No radiation therapy was given to the left kidney, and the patient was normotensive.

**SUMMARY OF ABNORMAL URORADIOLOGIC FINDINGS
POSTOBSTRUCTIVE ATROPHY**

Primary Uroradiologic Elements
    Size—small (normal or enlarged in minority of cases)
    Contour—smooth (global)
    Lesion distribution—unilateral
Secondary Uroradiologic Elements
    Papillae—effaced (global), may be normal in uncommon form
    Pelvoinfundibulocalyceal system—calyces dilated (global, may be normal in uncommon form
    Parenchymal thickness—wasted (global)

---

patient, duration of the process, and severity of functional impairment in the involved kidney.

POSTINFLAMMATORY ATROPHY

An unusual form of severe acute pyelonephritis occurs in some adult patients who have altered host resistance due to diabetes mellitus or other underlying conditions. During the acute phase of this infection, the kidney becomes smoothly enlarged, with marked impairment of contrast material excretion. This condition is termed *acute bacterial nephritis* and is discussed in Chapter 9.

The rapid return of function following appropriate antibiotic therapy that characterizes this disorder has been interpreted as evidence that the acutely infected kidney is rendered ischemic by inflammatory infiltrates surrounding and occluding the interlobular arteries in the cortex. This concept is supported by laboratory investigations of acute infection in the rabbit kidney (Hill and Clark, 1972). Another possible cause of ischemia is effacement of medium-sized renal arteries by generalized swelling of the kidney or by vasospasm.

Generalized wasting of the renal parenchyma, a sequela to treated acute bacterial nephritis, occurs within a few weeks after the initiation of appropriate antibiotic therapy. The loss of renal tissue is global, with preservation of a smooth or minimally irregular contour. Focal scars of the reflux nephropathy type do not occur in these patients.

Renal papillary necrosis is also a result of acute bacterial nephritis, but it may go unrecognized during the acute phase because of the severely impaired ex-

cretion of contrast material. All of these changes may develop after only a single episode of infection.

Clinical Setting

No specific clinical abnormalities have been consistently associated with the late treated stage of acute bacterial nephritis, although the possibility exists that hyperreninemic hypertension may result from ischemic atrophy of the formerly infected kidney. The clinical manifestations of the acute phase are described in Chapter 9.

Radiologic Findings

In successfully treated acute bacterial nephritis, global wasting of the kidney leads to a uniform decrease in renal size with a smooth or minimally irregular contour (Fig. 6–16). The change in renal size occurs over the few weeks after initiation of appropriate antibiotic therapy. Renal papillary necrosis is probably a feature of the acute phase of bacterial nephritis, but it goes unrecognized because of severely impaired contrast material excretion early in the course of the infection. It is only after the kidney recovers its function and can be opacified that this abnormality is detected (Fig. 6–17).

REFLUX ATROPHY
Definition

Vesicoureteral reflux severe enough to drive a large volume of urine under high pressure from the bladder to the pelvocalyceal system causes structural damage

---

**SUMMARY OF ABNORMAL URORADIOLOGIC FINDINGS
POSTINFLAMMATORY ATROPHY**

Primary Uroradiologic Elements
    Size—small
    Contour—smooth (global)
    Lesion distribution—unilateral
Secondary Uroradiologic Elements
    Papillae—disrupted
    Parenchymal thickness—wasted (global)

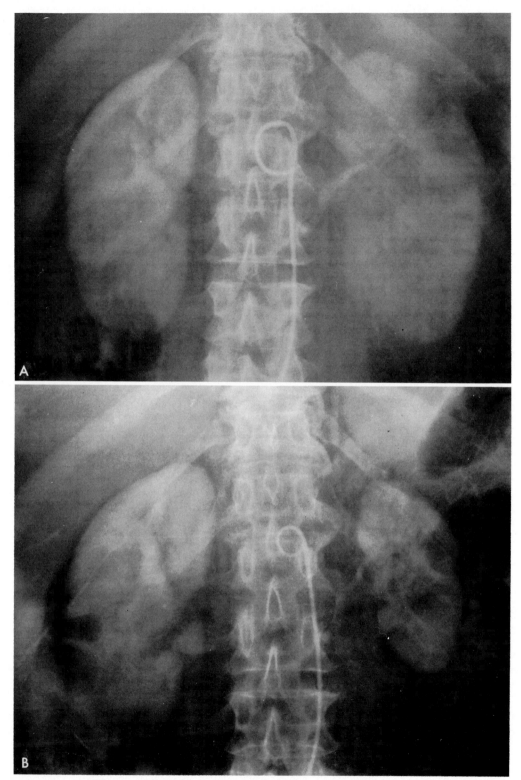

Figure 6–16. Postinflammatory atrophy developing in a 57-year-old woman with previously undiagnosed diabetes mellitus and acute bacterial nephritis.

 A, Nephrographic phase of aortogram performed during acute illness illustrates enlarged smooth left kidney (length = 15.7 cm) that did not excrete contrast material during urography.

 B, Nephrographic phase of aortogram 12 months later shows global atrophy of left kidney (length = 10.3 cm). Faint pelvocalyceal opacification occurred during urography at this time.

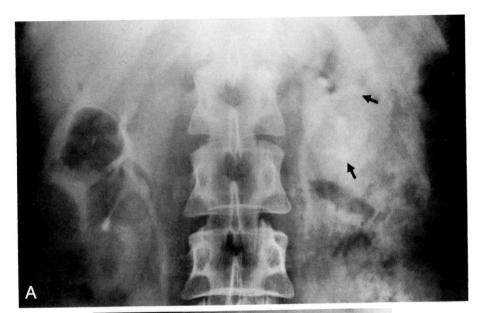

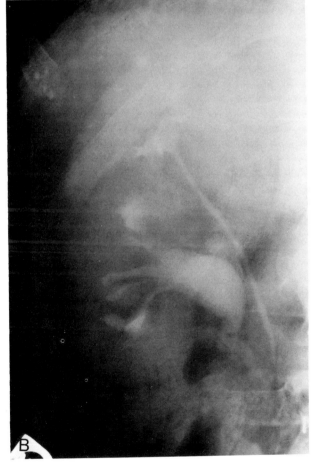

Figure 6–17. Postinflammatory atrophy illustrating global wasting and papillary necrosis in two patients.

A, Excretory urogram. Small, smooth left kidney with clubbed calyces *(arrows)* 3 years after an episode of acute bacterial nephritis.

B, Excretory urogram. Global atrophy and papillary necrosis in the lower moiety of a completely duplicated system. Acute bacterial nephritis was limited to this portion of the kidney. The superior moiety is normal.

(Fig. 6–17*A* courtesy of T. Freed, M. D., Marin General Hospital, Greenbrae, California.)

SUMMARY OF ABNORMAL URORADIOLOGIC FINDINGS
REFLUX ATROPHY

Primary Uroradiologic Elements
  Size—small
  Contour—smooth (global)
  Lesion distribution—unilateral
Secondary Uroradiologic Elements
  Papillae—effaced (global)
  Pelvoinfundibulocalyceal system—dilated; longitudinal striations may be seen when collapsed
  Parenchymal thickness—wasted (global)

---

to the kidney characterized by generalized, uniform wasting of the renal parenchyma, with flattening of papillae and dilatation of the pelvocalyceal system.

This condition, known as reflux atrophy, differs fundamentally from that other form of renal damage associated with severe vesicoureteral reflux, namely, reflux nephropathy; neither infection nor intrarenal reflux need be present, and focal scars do not develop. (Reflux nephropathy is discussed in Chapter 5.)

The exact pathogenesis of reflux atrophy has not been elucidated. Undoubtedly, increased hydrostatic pressure of pelvocalyceal urine is a principal factor. Atrophy follows as a result of direct pressure on the nephrons and collecting ducts or impairment of the drainage of the nephrons or, indirectly, through ischemia. In experimental animals, reflux atrophy evolves over a period of a few weeks following the development of severe vesicoureteral reflux.

Clinical Setting

Reflux atrophy itself produces no clinical signs or symptoms. Symptom-producing urinary tract infection may develop incidentally. When reflux atrophy develops in both kidneys, loss of renal parenchyma can be severe enough to cause renal failure.

Reflux atrophy persists after the spontaneous or surgical resolution of vesicoureteral reflux. Thus, an exact cause may never be established in adult patients who are discovered to have global atrophy and a dilated pelvocalyceal system, as discussed in the section Differential Diagnosis.

Radiologic Findings

Overall reduction in renal size with preservation of a smooth contour, generalized flattening or retraction of papillae, and dilatation of the collecting system and ureter constitute the radiologic findings of reflux atrophy (Fig. 6–18). When the pelvocalyceal system is not fully distended, as in dehydration and other causes of oliguria, longitudinal striations may be seen as regular lucent bands in the pelvis or ureter (Fig. 6–19). These represent redundant mucosa and disappear when the collecting system is distended. This is discussed further in Chapter 15. Active vesicoureteral reflux is usually absent when this condition is discovered in the adult.

DIFFERENTIAL DIAGNOSIS

In the unilaterally small, smooth kidney, functional radiologic abnormalities such as delayed calyceal opacification time, diminished urine volume, increased urine opacity, and delayed washout of opacified urine (as compared with the normal contralateral kidney) indicate ischemia. These findings are usually due to *focal arterial disease* narrowing the main renal artery, but *chronic incomplete infarction* and *radiation nephritis* also can cause identical abnormalities. Ureteral notching is not associated with the latter two and, when present, is evidence for focal arterial narrowing. Angiography, of course, leads to a definitive diagnosis.

When functional radiologic abnormalities are absent, using radiologic techniques to make a distinction among the several causes of unilaterally small, smooth kidney with normal calyces and papillae is difficult, if not impossible. This is true not only for focal arterial disease, postinfarctive states, and radiation nephritis but also for the uncommon form of *postobstructive atrophy* (with normal papillae and calyces) and *postinflammatory atrophy* as well, unless accompanied by papillary necrosis.

Postinflammatory atrophy causes both global atrophy and renal papillary necrosis. This combination of abnormalities is also found in advanced forms of analgesic nephropathy in which chronic interstitial fibrosis reduces kidney size. Analgesic nephropathy, however, is always bilateral, whereas postinflammatory atrophy is usually, although not invariably, unilateral.

Total infarction eventually produces a small, smooth kidney that does not opacify during excretory urography. Retrograde pyelography is necessary to demonstrate the papillae and pelvocalyceal system, which are normal. This combination of urographic and pyelographic findings is unique to *chronic renal infarction.*

An appropriate clinical history of exposure to therapeutic radiation is often the only way to identify *radiation nephritis* as the cause of a small, smooth kidney. Abnormalities of the lumbar spine and pelvis, including disturbance of growth and maturation, are helpful observations when present.

A reduction in the number of calyces and papillae is basic to the diagnosis of *renal hypoplasia*. There is

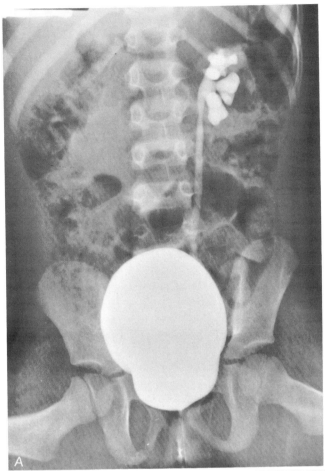

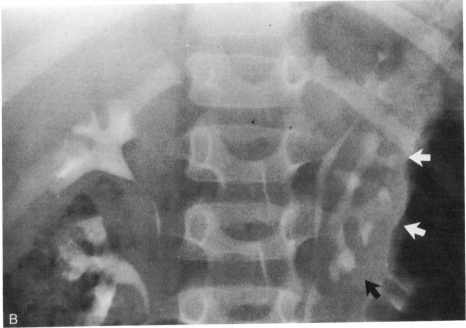

Figure 6–18. Reflux atrophy in the lower pole moiety of the left kidney with a completely duplicated collecting system.
A, Voiding cystourethrogram. Grade V vesicoureteral reflux into the lower pole moiety of the left kidney is present.
B, Excretory urogram. There is global wasting of that portion of the parenchyma affected by vesicoureteral reflux *(arrows).*

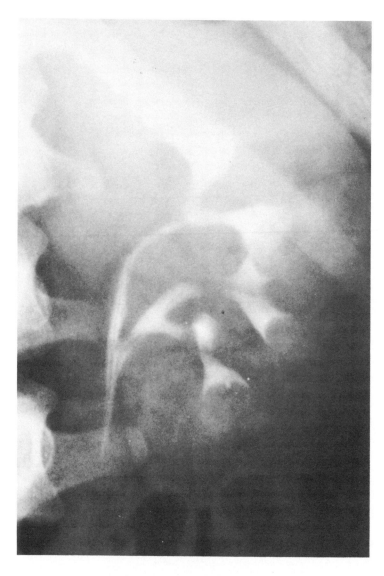

Figure 6–19. Longitudinal striations in the mucosa of the left renal pelvis in a patient with vesicoureteral reflux. Excretory urogram. The striations represent redundancy of the mucosa in a nondistended system.

scant room for confusing this entity with others in the same diagnostic set if this criterion is strictly applied. Enlargement of the contralateral kidney should invariably be present, since the process is lifelong. On the other hand, contralateral enlargement develops inconstantly as a function of age at onset when acquired disease results in a unilaterally small kidney.

Papillary effacement and calyceal dilatation in the absence of urinary tract infection are distinctive features of *postobstructive atrophy* and *reflux atrophy*. The global distribution of these findings and the preservation of a smooth outline distinguish these entities from reflux nephropathy, tuberculosis, and most forms of renal papillary necrosis. Postobstructive atrophy and reflux atrophy are radiologically indistinguishable. In fact, these entities probably have a common pathophysiologic basis, namely, increased hydrostatic pressure diffusely applied to the kidney parenchyma.

Bibliography

Ischemia Secondary to Focal Arterial Disease

Amplatz, K.: Two radiographic tests for assessment of renovascular hypertension. Radiology 79:807, 1962.

Andersson, I.: Unilateral renal artery stenosis and hypertension: I. Angiography. Acta Radiol. (Diagn.) 20:878, 1979.

Andersson, I., Bergentz, S.-E., Ericsson, B. F., Dymling, J. F., Hansson, B.-G., and Hökfelt, B.: Unilateral renal artery stenosis and hypertension: II. Angiographic findings correlated with blood pressure response after surgery. Acta Radiol. (Diagn.) 20:895, 1979.

Berland, L. L., Koslin, D. B., Routh, W. O., and Keller, F. S.: Renal artery stenosis and prospective evaluation of diagnosis with color duplex US compared with angiography. Radiology 174:421, 1990.

Berman, L. B., and Vertes, V.: The pathophysiology of renin. Clin. Symp. 25:3, 1973.

Bookstein, J. J.: Appraisal of arteriography in estimating hemodynamic significance of renal artery stenosis. Invest. Radiol. 1:281, 1966.

Bookstein, J. J., Abrams, H. L., Buenger, R. E., Lecky, J., Franklin, S. S., Reiss, M. D., Bleifer, K. H., Klatte, E. C., and Maxwell, M. H.: Radiologic aspects of renovascular hypertension: I. Aims and methods of the Radiology Study Group. JAMA 220:1218, 1972.

Bookstein, J. J., Abrams, H. L., Buenger, R. E., Lecky, J., Franklin, S. S., Reiss, M. D., Bleifer, K. H., Klatte, E. C., Varady, P. O., and Maxwell, M. H.: Radiologic aspects of renovascular hypertension: II. The role of urography in unilateral renovascular disease. JAMA 220:1225, 1972.

Bookstein, J. J., Abrams, H. L., Buenger, R. E., Lecky, J., Franklin, S. S., Reiss, M. D., Bleifer, K. H., Klatte, E. C., and Maxwell, M. H.: Radiologic aspects of renovascular hypertension: III. Appraisal of arteriography. JAMA 221:368, 1972.

Bookstein, J. J., and Ernst, C. B.: Vasodilatory and vasoconstrictive pharmacoangiographic manipulation of renal collateral flow. Radiology 108:55, 1973.

Bookstein, J. J., and Walter, J. F.: The role of abdominal radiography in hypertension secondary to renal or adrenal disease. Med. Clin. North Am. 59:169, 1975.

Bookstein, J. J., Maxwell, M. H., Abrams, H. L., Buenger, R. E., Lecky, J., and Franklin, S. S.: Cooperative study of radiologic aspects of renovascular hypertension: Bilateral renovascular disease. JAMA 237:1706, 1977.

Cho, K. J.: Renal angiography in renovascular hypertension. Urol. Radiol. 3:213, 1981–1982.

Chuang, V. P., Ernst, C. B., and Kotchen, T. A.: Effects of furosemide on renal venous plasma renin activity. Radiology 130:613, 1979.

Cordonnier, J. J.: Unilateral renal artery disease with hypertension. J. Urol. 82:1, 1959.

Cragg, A. H., Smith, T. P., Thompson, B. H., Marone, T. P., Stanson, A. W., Shaw, G. T., Hunter, D. W., and Cochran, S. T.: Incidental fibromuscular dysplasia in potential renal changes: Long-term clinical follow-up. Radiology 172:145, 1989.

Desberg, A. L., Paushter, D. M., Lammert, G. K., Hale, J. C., Troy, R. B., Novick, A. C., Nally, J. V., Jr., and Weltevreden, A. M.: Renal artery stenosis: Evaluation with color Doppler flow imaging. Radiology 177:749, 1990.

DeWardener, H. E.: Control of sodium reabsorption. Br. Med. J. 3:611 and 676, 1969.

Dondi, M., Fanti, S., Defabritiis, A., Zuccala, A., Gaggi, R., Mirelli, M., Stella, A., Marengo, M., Losinno, F., and Monetti, N.: Prognostic value of captopril renal scintigraphy in renovascular hypertension. J. Nucl. Med. 33:11, 1992.

Dorph, S., and Øigaard, A.: Variations in size of the normal kidney following intravenous administration of water-soluble contrast medium and urea. Br. J. Radiol. 46:183, 1973.

Dorph, S., and Øigaard, A.: Variations in renal size in the diagnosis of renovascular hypertension. Br. J. Radiol. 46:187, 1973.

Dorph, S., Hegedüs, V., and Palbøl, J.: Kidney distention during I.V. urography in normal rats and in rats with artificial unilateral renal artery stenosis. Br. J. Radiol. 52:461, 1979.

Dunnick, N. R., Svetkey, L. P., Cohan, R. H., Newman, G. E., Braun, S. D., Himmelstein, S., Bollinger, R. R., McCann, R. L., Wilkinson, R. H., and Klotman, P. E.: Intravenous digital subtraction renal angiography: Use in screening for renovascular hypertension. Radiology 171:219, 1989.

Dunnick, N. R., and Sfakianakis, G. N.: Screening for renovascular hypertension. Radiol. Clin. North Am. 29:497, 1991.

Dustan, H. P., Humphries, A. W., deWolf, V. G., and Page, I. H.: Normal arterial pressure in patients with renal arterial stenosis. JAMA 187:1028, 1964.

Dustan, H. P.: Physiologic consequences of renal arterial stenosis. N. Engl. J. Med. 281:1348, 1969.

Erbslöh-Möller, B., Dumas, A., Roth, D., Sfakianakis, G. N., and Bourgoignie, J. J.: Furosemide–131I-Hippuran renography after angiotensin-converting enzyme inhibition for the diagnosis of renovascular hypertension. Am. J. Med. 90:23, 1991.

Eyler, W. R., Clark, M. D., Garman, J. E., Rian, R. L., and Meininger, D. E.: Angiography of the renal areas including a comparative study of renal artery stenosis in patients with and without hypertension. Radiology 78:879, 1962.

Fine, E. J., and Sarkar, S.: Differential diagnosis and management of renovascular hypertension through nuclear medicine techniques. Semin. Nucl. Med. 19:101, 1989.

Gerlock, A. J., Goncharenko, V. A., and Ekelund, L.: Radiation-induced stenosis of the renal artery causing hypertension: A case report. J. Urol. 118:1064, 1977.

Gersten, B. E., Stegman, C. J., and Bookstein, J. J.: Antegrade flow in extrarenal arteries arising distal to renal artery stenosis. Radiology 98:93, 1971.

Goncharenko, V., Gerlock, A. J., Shaff, M. I., and Hollifield, J. W.: Progression of renal artery fibromuscular dysplasia in 42 patients as seen on angiography. Radiology 139:45, 1981.

Halpern, M., and Evans, J. A.: Coarctation of the renal artery with "notching" of the ureter: A roentgenologic sign of unilateral renal disease as a cause of hypertension. AJR 88:159, 1962.

Hegedüs, V., Faarup, P., Nørgaard, T., and Lonholdt, C.: Volume changes in the rat renal cortex during uropathy, Br. J. Radiol. 51:793, 1978.

Heptinstall, R. H.: Hypertension II: Secondary forms. In Heptinstall, R. H. (ed.): Pathology of the Kidney. 4th ed. Boston, Little, Brown & Co., 1992, pp. 1029–1096.

Hietala, S. O., Zelenak, J. J., Beachley, M. C., and Tisnado, J.: Influence of contrast material on renal venous renin activity. AJR 132:429, 1979.

Hill, S.: Renal vascular lesions. In Hill, G. S. (ed.): Uropathology. New York, Churchill Livingston, 1989, pp. 189–234.

Hillman, B. J.: Renovascular hypertension: Diagnosis of renal artery stenosis by digital video subtraction angiography. Urol. Radiol. 3:219, 1981–82.

Hillman, B. J.: Imaging advances in the diagnosis of renovascular hypertension. AJR 153:5, 1989.

Holley, K. E., Hunt, J. C., Brown, A. L., Jr., Kincaid, O. W., and Sheps, S. G.: Renal artery stenosis: A clinical-pathologic study in normotensive and hypertensive patients. Am. J. Med. 37:14, 1964.

Jones, E. O. P., Wilkinson, R., and Taylor, R. M. R.: Contralateral renal artery fibromuscular dysplasia after nephrectomy for renal artery stenosis. Br. Med. J. 1:825, 1978.

Kirkendall, W. M., and Overtorf, M.: Plasma renin activity and systemic arterial hypertension. Mod. Concepts Cardiovasc. Dis. 42:47, 1973.

Lewin, A., Blaufox, D., Castle, H., Entwisle, G., and Langdorf, H.: Apparent prevalence of curable hypertension in the hypertension, detection and follow-up program. Arch. Intern. Med. 145:424, 1985.

Luke, R. G.: Nephrosclerosis. In Schrier, R. W., and Gottschalk, C. W. (eds.): Diseases of the Kidney. 4th ed. Boston, Little, Brown & Co., 1988, pp. 1573–1596.

Mann, S. J., Pickering, T. G., Sos, T. A., Uzzo, R. G., Sarkar, S., Friend, K., Rackson, M. E., and Laragh, J. H.: Captopril renography in the diagnosis of renal artery stenosis: Accuracy and limitations. Am. J. Med. 90:30, 1991.

Mann, S. J., and Pickering, T. G.: Detection of renovascular hypertension—state of art—1992. Ann. Intern. Med. 117:10, 1992.

Maxwell, M. H.: Reversible renal hypertension: Clinical characteristics and predictive tests. Am. J. Cardiol. 9:126, 1962.

Oparil, S., and Harber, E.: The renin-angiotensin system. N. Engl. J. Med. 291:399 and 446, 1974.

Paul, R. E., Ettinger, A., Faisinger, M. H., Callow, A. D., Kahn, P. C., and Inker, L. H.: Angiographic visualization of renal collateral circulation as a means of detecting and delineating renal ischemia. Radiology 84:1013, 1965.

Peart, W. S.: Hypertension and the kidney: I. Clinical, pathological and functional disorders, especially in man. Br. Med. J. 2:1353, 1959.

Pickering, T. G.: Renovascular hypertension: Etiology and pathophysiology. Semin. Nucl. Med. 19:79, 1989.

Pickering, T. G., Laragh, J. H., and Sos, T. A.: Renovascular hypertension. In Schrier, R. W., and Gottschalk, C. W. (eds.): Diseases of the Kidney. 4th ed. Boston, Little, Brown & Co., 1988, pp. 1597–1622.

Plantureux, P., and Plainfossé, M. C.: Should complete intravenous urography still be performed systematically in all cases of arterial hypertension? Remarks on 1,500 cases. Ann. Radiol. 20:545, 1977.

Poutasse, R. F., and Dustan, H. P.: Arteriosclerosis and renal hypertension: Indications for aortography in hypertensive patients and results of treatment of obstructive lesions of renal artery. JAMA 165:1521, 1957.

Raust, J., Michel, J. R., Bacques, O., Affre, J., and Moreau, J.-F.: A critical review of the variations in size of the kidney caused by increased diuresis in hypertensive patients. J. Radiol. 60:283, 1979.

Schreiber, M. J., Pohl, M. A., Novick, A. C.: The natural history of atherosclerotic and fibrous renal artery disease. Urol. Clin. North Am. 11:383, 1984.

Schwarten, D. E.: Transluminal angioplasty of renal artery stenosis: 70 experiences. AJR 135:969, 1980.

Sherwood, T.: Finding and dilating renal artery stenosis for hypertension: Clin. Radiol. 39:359, 1988.

Sos, T. A., Vaughan, E. D., Jr., Pickering, T. G., Case, D. B., Sniderman, K. W., Sealey, J., and Laragh, J. H.: Diagnosis of renovascular hypertension and evaluation of "surgical" curability. Urol. Radiol. 3:199, 1981–1982.

Stanley, J. C.: Renovascular hypertension: Surgical treatment. Urol. Radiol. 3:205, 1981–1982.

Stewart, B. H., Dustan, H. P., Kiser, W. S., Meaney, T. F., Straffon, R. A., and McCormack, L. J.: Correlation of angiography and natural history in evaluation of patients with renovascular hypertension. J. Urol. 104:231, 1970.

Tack, C., and Sos, T. A.: Radiologic diagnosis of renovascular hypertension and percutaneous transluminal renal angioplasty. Semin. Nucl. Med. 19:89, 1989.

Talner, L. B., Stone, R. A., Coel, M. N., Levy, S. B., and Emarine, C. W.: Furosemide-augmented intravenous urography: Results in essential hypertension. AJR 130:257, 1978.

Thornbury, J. R., Stanley, J. C., and Fryback, D. G.: Hypertensive Urogram: A nondiscriminating test for renovascular hypertension. AJR 138:43, 1982.

Thornbury, J. R., Stanley, J. C., and Fryback, D. G.: Limited use of hypertensive excretory urography. Urol. Radiol. 3:209, 1981–1982.

Thornbury, J. R., Stanley, J. C., and Fryback, D. G.: Optimizing work-up of adult hypertensive patient for renal artery stenosis: Observations about hypertensive urography, digital subtraction angiography, and patient selection. Radiol. Clin. North Am. 22:333, 1984.

Webb, J. A. W., and Talner, L. B.: The role of intravenous urography in hypertension. Radiol. Clin. North Am.:17:187, 1979.

Wicks, J. D., and Mettler, F. A., Jr.: Use of ultrasound in renal hypertension. Urol. Radiol. 5:37, 1983.

Wolf, G. L., and Wilson, W. J.: Vasodilated excretory urography: An improved screening test for renal arterial stenosis? AJR 114:684, 1972.

Wolf, G. L.: Rationale and use of vasodilated excretory urography in screening for renovascular hypertension. AJR 119:692, 1973.

Chronic Renal Infarction

Clark, R. E., Teplick, S. K., and Long, J. M.: Small atrophic kidney secondary to renal vein thrombosis: Report of a case diagnosed arteriographically. J. Urol. 114:457, 1975.

Erwin, B. C., Carroll, B. A., Walter, J. F., and Sommer, F. G.: Renal infarction appearing as an echogenic mass. AJR 138:759, 1982.

Glazer, G. M., Francis, I. R., Brady, T. M., and Teng, S. S.: Computed tomography of renal infarction: Clinical and experimental observations. AJR 139:721, 1983.

Glazer, G. M., Saddekni, S., Sniderman, K. W., Weiner, M., Beinart, C., Pickering, T. G., Case, D. B., Vaughan, E. D., Jr., and Laragh, J. H.: Renal artery angioplasty: Techniques and early results. Urol. Radiol. 3:223, 1981–1982.

Heitzman, E. R., and Perchik, L.: Radiographic features of renal infarction: Review of 13 cases. Radiology 76:39, 1961.

Hoxie, H. J., and Coggin, C. B.: Renal infarction: Statistical study of 205 cases and detailed report of an unusual case. Arch. Intern. Med. 65:587, 1940.

Janower, M. L., and Weber, A. L.: Radiologic evaluation of acute renal infarction. AJR 95:309, 1965.

Lang, E. K.: Arteriographic diagnosis of renal infarcts. Radiology 88:1110, 1967.

Solez, K.: Acute renal failure (acute tubular necrosis, infarction and cortical necrosis). In Heptinstall, R. H. (ed.): Pathology of the Kidney. 4th ed. Boston, Little, Brown & Co., 1992, pp. 1235–1314.

Teplick, J. G., and Yarrow, M. W.: Arterial infarction of kidney. Ann. Intern. Med. 42:1041, 1955.

Radiation Nephritis

Aron, B. S., and Schlesinger, A.: Complications of radiation therapy: The genitourinary tract. Semin. Roentgenol. 9:65, 1974.

Crummy, A. B., Hellman, S., Stansel, H. C., Jr., and Hukill, P. B.: Renal hypertension secondary to unilateral radiation damage relieved by nephrectomy. Radiology 84:108, 1965.

Heptinstall, R. H.: Irradiation injury and effects of heavy metals. In Heptinstall, R. H. (ed.): Pathology of the Kidney. 4th ed. Boston, Little, Brown & Co., 1992, pp. 2085–2111.

Keane, W. F., Crosson, J. T., and Shapiro, F.: Ultrastructural abnormalities in radiation-induced renal disease. Abstract #283 in Abstracts of Free Communications. VIth International Congress of Nephrology, Florence, Italy, 1975.

Keane, W. F., Crosson, J. T., Staley, N. A., Anderson, W. R., and Shapiro, F. L.: Radiation-induced renal disease: A clinicopathologic study. Am. J. Med. 60:127, 1976.

Madrazo, A., Schwarz, G., and Churg, J.: Radiation nephritis: A review. J. Urol. 114:822, 1975.

Moore, L., Curry, N. S., and Jenrette, J. M.: Computed tomography of acute radiation nephritis. Urol. Radiol. 8:89, 1986.

Nolan, C. R., III, and Linas, S. L.: Accelerated and malignant hypertension. In Schrier, R. W., and Gottschalk, C. W. (eds.): Diseases of the Kidney. 4th ed. Boston, Little, Brown & Co., 1988, pp. 1703–1826.

Shapiro, A. P., Cavallo, T., Cooper, W., Lapenas, D., Bron, K., and Berg, G.: Hypertension in radiation nephritis. Arch. Intern. Med. 137:848, 1977.

Vidt, D. G.: Hypertension induced by irradiation to the kidney. Arch. Intern. Med. 137:840, 1977.

Congenital Hypoplasia

Boissant, P.: What to call the hypoplastic kidney? Arch. Dis. Child. 37:142, 1962.

Risdon, R. A., Young, L. W., and Chrispin, A. R.: Renal hypoplasia and dysplasia: A radiological and pathological correlation. Pediatr. Radiol. 3:213, 1975.

Risdon, R. A.: Development, developmental defects, and cystic diseases of the kidney. In Heptinstall, R. H. (ed.): Pathology of the Kidney. 4th ed. Boston, Little, Brown & Co., 1992, pp. 93–168.

Templeton, A. W., and Thompson, I. M.: Aortographic differentiation of congenital and acquired small kidneys. Arch. Surg. 97:114, 1968.

Postobstructive Atrophy

Craven, J. D., and Lecky, J. W.: The natural history of postobstructive renal atrophy shown by sequential urograms. Radiology 101:555, 1971.

Craven, J. D., Hodson, C. J., and Lecky, J. W.: An atypical response on the kidney to a period of ureteric obstruction. Radiology 105:39, 1972.

Hodson, C. J., and Craven, J. D.: The radiology of obstructive atrophy of the kidney. Clin. Radiol. 17:305, 1966.

Hodson, C. J., Craven, J. D., Lewis, D. G., Matz, L. R., Clarke, R. J., and Ross, E. J.: Experimental obstructive nephropathy in the pig. Br. J. Urol. 41 (Suppl.):5, 1969.

Hodson, C. J.: Post-obstructive renal atrophy (nephropathy). Br. Med. Bull. 28:237, 1972.

Postinflammatory Atrophy

Bailey, R. R., Little, P. J., and Rolleston, G. L.: Renal damage after acute pyelonephritis. Br. Med. J. 1:550, 1969.

Davidson, A. J., and Talner, L. B.: Urographic and angiographic abnormalities in adult-onset acute bacterial nephritis. Radiology 106:249, 1973.

Davidson, A. J., and Talner, L. B.: Late sequelae of adult-onset acute bacterial nephritis. Radiology 127:367, 1978.

Hill, G. S., and Clark, R. L.: A comparative angiographic, microangiographic, and histologic study of experimental pyelonephritis. Invest. Radiol. 7:33, 1972.

Lilienfield, R. M., and Lande, A.: Acute adult onset bacterial nephritis: Long-term urographic and angiographic follow-up. J. Urol. 114:14, 1975.

Reflux Atrophy

Hodson, C. J.: The diffuse form of reflux nephropathy. In Losse, H., Asscher, A. W., and Lison, A. E. (eds.): Pyelonephritis. Vol. IV. Urinary Tract Infections. New York, Thieme-Stratton, 1980, pp. 84–90.

7

DIAGNOSTIC SET: SMALL, SMOOTH, BILATERAL

GENERALIZED ARTERIOSCLEROSIS	HEREDITARY NEPHROPATHIES
	Hereditary Chronic Nephritis (Alport's
NEPHROSCLEROSIS (BENIGN AND	Syndrome)
MALIGNANT)	Medullary Cystic Disease
ATHEROEMBOLIC RENAL DISEASE	AMYLOIDOSIS (LATE)
CHRONIC GLOMERULONEPHRITIS	ARTERIAL HYPOTENSION
RENAL PAPILLARY NECROSIS	DIFFERENTIAL DIAGNOSIS

Bilaterally small, smooth kidneys are the result of diseases that affect all renal tissue either exclusively as a primary process or as part of a generalized, multisystemic disorder. Chronic glomerulonephritis, renal papillary necrosis, hereditary chronic nephritis, and medullary cystic disease are examples of the former; and arteriosclerosis, nephrosclerosis and the late stage of amyloidosis illustrate the latter group. Both kidneys can also become small and smooth when they are the target of an "upstream" shower of atheromatous emboli, an uncommon condition known as *atheroembolic renal disease*. Hypotension may cause the same change transiently by reducing the volume of intrarenal blood and urine that normally distends the kidneys.

Chronic interstitial nephritis is not treated as a separate category in this diagnostic set, even though kidneys with this histologic picture are uniformly wasted. Most authorities now believe that this term is simply a description of a histologic pattern reflecting a variety of etiologies, some yet to be defined, that can lead to small kidneys and renal failure.

Except in renal papillary necrosis, the calyces and papillae remain normal in diseases included in this diagnostic set. The preservation of a smooth contour as the kidney shrinks reflects the generalized, or global, nature of tissue loss inherent in these abnormalities. A smooth contour, however, is not invariably maintained in arteriosclerosis, nephrosclerosis, or renal papillary necrosis, exceptions that will be discussed in detail in the appropriate following sections.

Abnormalities in the echogenicity of the renal parenchyma occur frequently in the varied chronic wasting disorders that cause both kidneys to become small and smooth. These abnormalities take several forms.

A generalized increase in parenchymal echoes, which often become greater in intensity than those of the liver, may be noted (Fig. 7–1). Additionally, an increased prominence of central sinus echoes occurs when sinus fat proliferation accompanies parenchymal wasting (Fig. 7–2). Obliteration of differences in cortical and medullary echogenicity has been reported, but these differences are often not present even in normal kidneys. The presence of any of these abnormalities in ultrasonograms may denote parenchymal disease, but they are neither specific to any given entity or group of diseases nor indicative of particular prognoses.

Many of the diseases included in the small, smooth, bilateral diagnostic set lead to end-stage renal disease and necessitate chronic dialysis. During long-term dialysis, chronically failed kidneys may undergo cystic degeneration that transforms their radiologic appearance. This condition, known as *acquired cystic disease* of the kidney, is discussed in Chapter 10.

GENERALIZED ARTERIOSCLEROSIS

Definition

When arteriosclerosis involves most of the interlobar and arcuate arteries, the kidneys become wasted owing to insufficient nutrient blood flow for sustenance of the renal parenchyma. Unlike focal narrowing of the main renal artery, discussed in Chapter 6, the process is disseminated, and uniform shrinkage of both kidneys occurs.

Arteriosclerosis can reduce the kidney to one-half its normal weight. The degree of wasting is variable and depends on the extent of involvement of medium-sized arteries. Frequently, narrowing of vessels

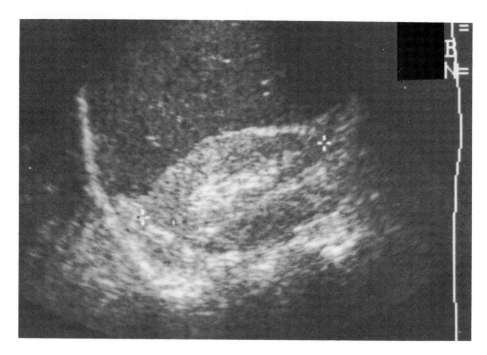

Figure 7–1. End-stage renal failure causing an increase in the echogenicity of kidney parenchyma relative to that of the liver. This pattern is not specific to any particular disease or group of diseases. Ultrasonography also demonstrates the small size and smooth contour of the kidneys. Ultrasonogram, longitudinal section.

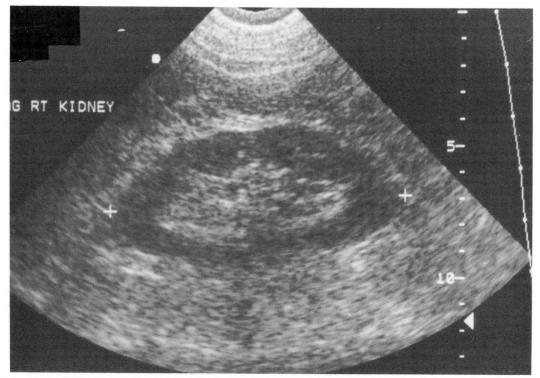

Figure 7–2. End-stage renal failure with increased prominence of central sinus echoes due to proliferation of sinus fat. Ultrasonogram, longitudinal section.

progresses to complete occlusion and focal infarction. As a result, the smooth surface of the arteriosclerotic kidney becomes punctuated with shallow scars, which are variable in number and random in distribution. The papillae and calyces remain normal. Occasionally, fat proliferates in the renal hilus and replaces the parenchyma lost in the central part of the kidney.

The histologic appearance of the arteriosclerotic kidney is nonspecific and difficult to distinguish from other entities that cause wasting of renal tissue. Medium-sized arteries develop multiple sites of atheromatous thickening, with fraying of the internal elastic lamina and calcification. The glomeruli vary from normal to sclerotic. The tubules, particularly proximal convoluted tubules, become atrophic and have thickened basement membranes. Interstitial fibrosis occurs, but it is finer than that seen in reflux nephropathy.

Small, smooth kidneys develop in patients with scleroderma or chronic tophaceous gout. It is generally held that this is due, at least in part, to premature or accelerated development of atherosclerosis in medium- and small-sized arteries. Other parenchymal changes seen in chronic gouty nephropathy are deposition of uric acid and urate in the tubules and interstitial tissue, interstitial fibrosis, and nephron atrophy.

Patients with the classic form of polyarteritis nodosa, in whom necrotizing vascular lesions occasionally occlude medium-sized renal arteries, also develop small, smooth kidneys as a result of diffuse ischemia.

Clinical Setting

Arteriosclerotic disease of the kidneys is a part of the generalized atherosclerosis associated with aging. Most authorities agree that ischemia resulting from vascular narrowing causes reduction of renal mass and a slowly progressive decrease in renal function. The possibility does exist, however, that these changes occur as part of an independent cellular involutional process unrelated to atherosclerosis.

By definition, arteriosclerosis of the kidney is associated with normal arterial blood pressure and has little, if any, clinical importance. Renal plasma flow, glomerular filtration rate, and various tubule functions measurably deteriorate over a long period of time, but clinical manifestations are not seen. If hypertension develops, the situation is reclassified as benign or malignant nephrosclerosis.

The clinical features of scleroderma, chronic tophaceous gout, or polyarteritis nodosa obviously predominate when the accelerated atherosclerotic or necrotizing arterial lesions associated with these diseases produce small, smooth kidneys.

Radiologic Findings

Reduction in renal size due to uncomplicated arteriosclerosis is usually not detected before the sixth decade and becomes more apparent with advancing age. Both kidneys are affected more or less equally. Calcification of medium-sized intrarenal arteries may be noted on a preliminary film (Fig. 7–3). Since wasting is global, the kidneys often have a smooth contour (Fig. 7–4). However, shallow focal scars may be present at sites where arterial narrowing has progressed to infarction (Fig. 7–5; see Fig. 7–8B). Uniform narrowing of the distance between the interpapillary line and outer margin of the kidney reflects parenchymal loss (see Fig. 7–5). The nephrogram, papillae, and pelvocalyceal system are normal (see Fig. 7–4) or reflect renal sinus fat proliferation, which often accompanies diffuse parenchymal wasting. This is seen as a radiolucency in the central portion of the kidney that is accentuated during urography (see Fig. 7–5) or as sinus tissue of negative attenuation value in computed tomography (Fig. 7–6). An increase in the volume of echoes in the central sinus complex is the ultrasound image of this condition (see Fig. 7–2). Lack of distensibility of the pelvocalyceal system may occur when sinus fat proliferation is marked. Renal sinus lipomatosis, discussed in detail in Chapter 16, may occur in any wasting process, in either one or both kidneys, and is thus nonspecific.

The radiologic findings in scleroderma, chronic gouty nephropathy, and the classic form of polyarteritis nodosa are the same as those seen in uncomplicated arteriosclerosis (Fig. 7–7).

Renal angiography can clearly demonstrate arteriosclerotic disease of the interlobar- and arcuate-sized

---

**SUMMARY OF ABNORMAL URORADIOLOGIC FINDINGS
GENERALIZED ARTERIOSCLEROSIS**

Primary Uroradiologic Elements
  Size—normal to small
  Contour—smooth (global); may have random, shallow scars
  Lesion distribution—bilateral
Secondary Uroradiologic Elements
  Parenchymal thickness—wasted (global)
  Attenuation value—sinus fat increased
  Echogenicity—may be increased in the parenchyma or central sinus

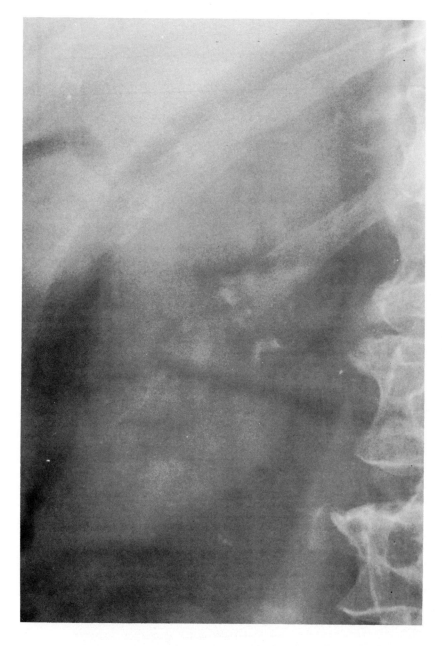

Figure 7–3. Arteriosclerotic calcification of intra-renal arterial branches in the right kidney of a 71-year-old normotensive male. Preliminary film. Calcification is extrapelvic, as demonstrated on subsequent urographic films.

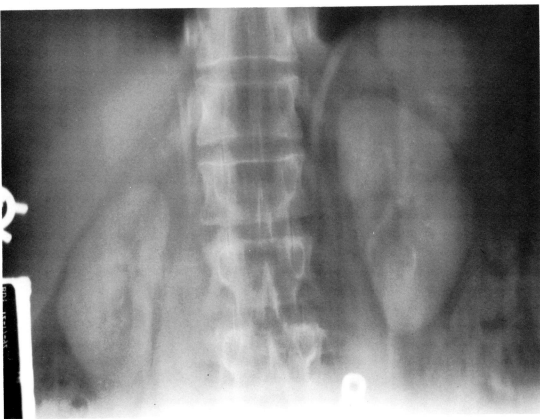

Figure 7–4. Arteriosclerosis. Global wasting of both kidneys with preservation of a smooth contour in an 80-year-old normotensive woman with normal blood urea nitrogen value. The pelvocalyceal system is normal. Tomogram. Right kidney length = 9.3 cm; left kidney length = 10.8 cm.

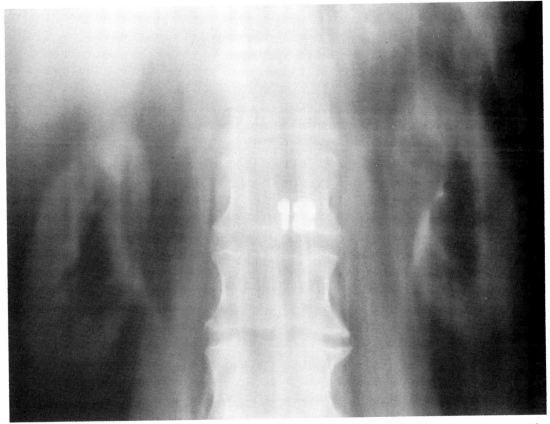

Figure 7–5. Arteriosclerosis. Shallow focal scars superimposed on globally wasted kidneys in an elderly normotensive woman without azotemia. Scars occur at random sites where arterial narrowing progresses to infarction. Uniform thinning of renal parenchyma is highlighted by marked renal sinus lipomatosis effacing the pelvocalyceal system. Tomogram. Right kidney length = 11.4 cm; left kidney length = 12.0 cm.

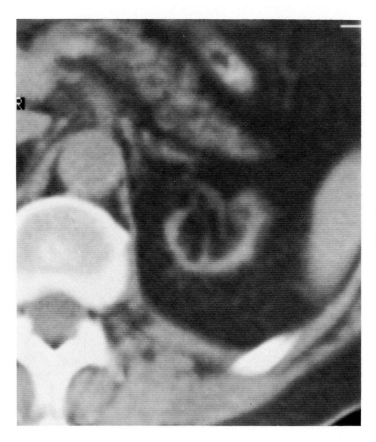

Figure 7–6. Renal sinus fat proliferation in global renal wasting is seen as increased sinus tissue with negative attenuation value. This often causes effacement of the pelvocalyceal system. Note general wasting of the parenchyma. Computed tomogram, contrast material enhanced.

vessels (Fig. 7–8). In addition to focal narrowing of these vessels, particularly at points of bifurcation, there is loss of normal arterial tapering, decrease in number of branching vessels, increased tortuosity, and abrupt change in the caliber of the distal arcuate arteries in advanced cases. These abnormalities are nonspecific and can be seen in most other forms of chronic renal disease. The similarity between normal patterns of vascular aging and patterns seen in chronic acquired diseases limits the usefulness of angiography in the diagnosis of parenchymal disease of the kidney. This is discussed further in Chapter 26. Angiography is rarely indicated in the diagnosis of arteriosclerotic disease of the kidneys.

In advanced cases of arteriosclerotic wasting, the echogenicity of the renal parenchyma may be increased in a diffuse, but nonspecific, pattern. The central sinus echo complex may also become more prominent with sinus fat proliferation.

NEPHROSCLEROSIS (BENIGN AND MALIGNANT)

Definition

Patients with arterial hypertension develop thickening and subendothelial hyalinization of the afferent arterioles in addition to arteriosclerosis of the medium and small-sized arteries. These changes constitute the histologic picture of benign nephrosclerosis.

The development of accelerated or malignant hypertension produces proliferative endarteritis of afferent arterioles and interlobular arteries, necrotizing arteriolitis, and necrotizing glomerulitis. Arteriolar rupture may occur as a result of these changes. Pronounced atrophy of tubules and fine interstitial fibrosis with chronic inflammatory cell infiltrate also contribute to the smallness of these kidneys.

Generalized reduction in kidney size, with smooth contour and normal pelvocalyceal and papillary structures, occurs in both benign and malignant nephrosclerosis. Superimposed scars of lobar infarction may be present. In malignant nephrosclerosis, intrarenal or subcapsular hemorrhage occasionally develops as a result of rupture of necrotic arterioles.

Clinical Setting

Hypertension is a basic clinical feature of nephrosclerosis. Whether elevated blood pressure is a cause or a result of the afferent arteriolar lesion is a historical controversy. The onset of hypertension usually occurs before 50 years of age. Even when hypertension exists for many years, serious renal functional impairment does not develop in the benign form of nephrosclerosis. Many patients do have some reduction in renal plasma flow and tubule function, slight proteinuria, and hyaline or granular casts in their urine, but these are rarely of clinical consequence.

The clinical situation in malignant hypertension is more serious than in benign hypertension. In the ma-

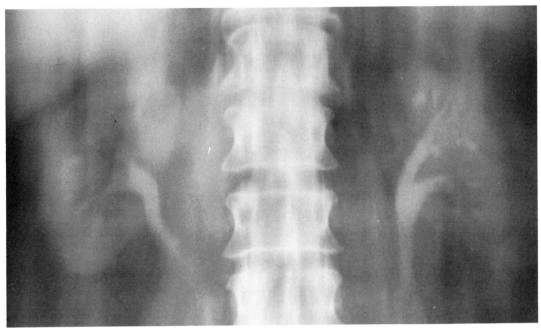

Figure 7–7. Gouty nephropathy. Bilaterally small kidneys in a 71-year-old normotensive man with severe chronic tophaceous gout and mild azotemia. Shallow focal scars are seen in several areas of the right kidney. Renal wasting in this situation is presumably due to severe arteriosclerosis and chronic interstitial fibrosis. Tomogram. Right kidney length = 10.4 cm; left kidney length = 9.9 cm.

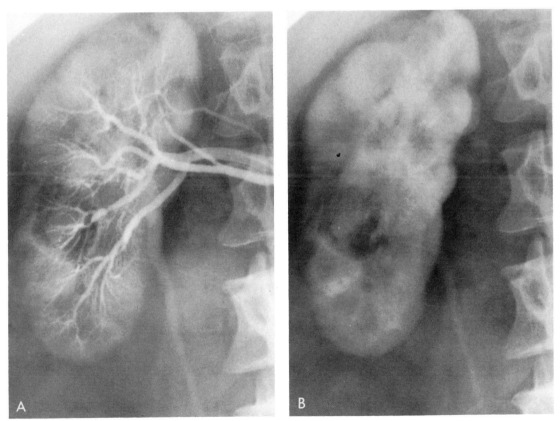

Figure 7–8. Arteriosclerosis of interlobar and arcuate arteries.
 A, Arterial phase of selective arteriogram. Note irregular narrowing and dilatation of arteries, especially at bifurcations.
 B, Shallow scars due to infarction are well illustrated during nephrographic phase.

**SUMMARY OF ABNORMAL URORADIOLOGIC FINDINGS
NEPHROSCLEROSIS (BENIGN AND MALIGNANT)**

Primary Uroradiologic Elements
    Size—normal to small
    Contour—smooth (global); may have random, shallow scars
    Lesion distribution—bilateral
Secondary Uroradiologic Elements
    Parenchymal thickness—wasted (global)
    Nephrogram—diminished contrast material density (malignant form)
    Attenuation value—focal high values in parenchyma (malignant, nonenhanced scan)
    Echogenicity—may be increased in the parenchyma or central sinus
    Retroperitoneal space—subcapsular, perirenal blood (attenuation value changes with time)

---

lignant form, rapid deterioration of renal function occurs in association with headache, weight loss, dizziness, and impaired vision. Papilledema with fundal hemorrhage and exudate develops. Gross hematuria and heavy proteinuria are common. Some patients die of renal failure or as a result of complications in other organ systems, particularly the heart and the brain.

Radiologic Findings

The radiologic findings in benign nephrosclerosis overlap those of arteriosclerotic kidney disease. The kidneys are symmetrically reduced in size, and their contour remains smooth except for occasional, random, shallow infarct scars in some patients. The pelvocalyceal and papillary structures are remarkable only for the surrounding fatty deposition sometimes present. The kidney opacifies normally (Fig. 7–9).

Malignant nephrosclerosis differs from renal arteriosclerosis and benign nephrosclerosis in that enhancement of the kidney by contrast material is invariably diminished, usually to a marked degree (Fig. 7–10). In other respects, the radiologic findings are the same. It seems reasonable to expect small kidneys and sinus fat accumulation more often in patients whose malignant stage was preceded by a relatively long period of benign nephrosclerosis. When malignant nephrosclerosis arises *de novo*, as sometimes happens, the kidneys may be normal in size. This holds true only for a limited period of time before progressive reduction of renal mass occurs.

Parenchymal hemorrhage due to necrotizing arteriolitis is usually petechial and cannot be detected with the poor opacification achieved during urography but might be apparent as focal areas of high attenuation in computed tomograms performed without contrast material enhancement. Occasionally, bleeding extends to the subcapsular surface of the kidney or the perirenal space. This results in a concave, inward displacement of the nephrogram and adjacent calyces, occasional extension of blood into the perinephric space, and displacement of the capsular artery, seen during angiography. (See discussion in Chapter 21.)

As stated earlier, renal parenchymal and central

sinus echogenicity may be increased in chronic parenchymal disease such as nephrosclerosis. Subcapsular and perirenal hemorrhages are detectable by ultrasonography as hypoechoic or echo-free collections and as high attenuation tissue by computed tomography, as described in further detail in Chapter 21.

ATHEROEMBOLIC RENAL DISEASE
Definition

Atheroembolic renal disease results from the dislodgement from the aorta of multiple atheromatous emboli that occlude intrarenal arteries, from arcuate-sized vessels down to the afferent arterioles. The appearance of the kidneys depends on the amount of time that has passed following such an event. Shortly after the embolic episode, the affected arteries are packed with cholesterol crystals and amorphous debris. Eventually, this leads to the production of foreign body giant cells. Finally, focal areas of concentric fibrosis develop at points where emboli initially were situated, usually at arterial bifurcations. The net result of these changes is diffuse patches of ischemia in which atrophy predominates over infarction.

Because this disorder occurs only when the aorta is severely atherosclerotic, the kidneys may already be somewhat reduced in size as a result of age or coexisting hypertension. Atheroembolic disease itself reduces renal mass, although this is not seen for some time following embolization. Infarct scars are often superimposed on the fine granular scars of ischemia. As is true in other vascular disorders previously described in this chapter, papillary and pelvocalyceal structures retain their normal appearance.

Clinical Setting

Dislodgement of atheromatous debris from the aorta above the renal arteries may result from external trauma or direct insult to the aorta during surgery or catheter manipulation. Spontaneous embolization is also thought to occur. As many as 15 to 30 per cent of patients with severe erosive atherosclerotic disease of the aorta have atherosclerotic emboli in the kidneys.

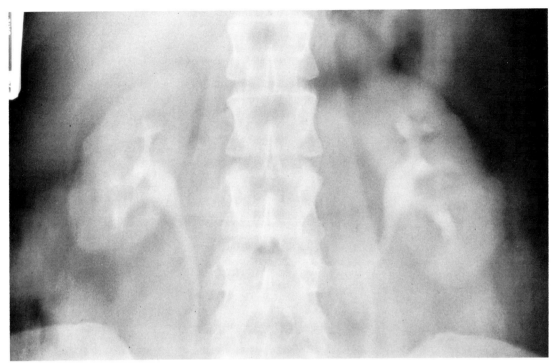

Figure 7–9. Benign nephrosclerosis. Excretory urogram in a 46-year-old woman with essential hypertension. Both kidneys are globally wasted, with several shallow infarct scars. The pelvocalyceal system and renal opacification are normal. (Courtesy of Department of Diagnostic Radiology, Hammersmith Hospital, Royal Postgraduate Medical School, London, England.)

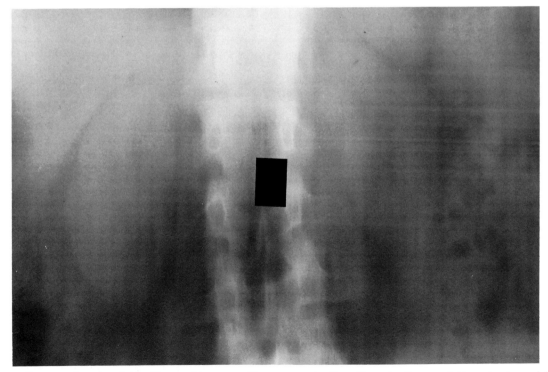

Figure 7–10. Malignant nephrosclerosis in a 69-year-old woman with recent acceleration of long-standing essential hypertension and development of azotemia. Excretory urogram. Tomogram taken 105 minutes after injection of contrast material. Kidneys are small, smooth, and only slightly opacified. Right kidney length = 10.6 cm; left kidney length = 10.6 cm.

SUMMARY OF ABNORMAL URORADIOLOGIC FINDINGS
ATHEROEMBOLIC RENAL DISEASE

Primary Uroradiologic Elements
   Size—normal to small
   Contour—smooth (global); may have random, shallow scars
   Lesion distribution—bilateral
Secondary Uroradiologic Elements
   Parenchymal thickness—wasted (global)
   Nephrogram—diminished contrast material density (excretory urogram)
            —patchy distribution (computed tomogram)
   Arteries—embolic occlusion (arteriogram)

Massive embolization leads to oliguria or anuria and uremia after a relatively short time. In most cases the course is more indolent, although renal failure eventually ensues. Hypertension is often present, occasionally in the accelerated form. Protein and occasional hyaline or granular casts are present in the urine, whereas hematuria and red cell casts are an uncommon finding in renal atheroembolism.

Radiologic Findings

No comprehensive study of the radiologic features of atheroembolic renal disease has been published. Nevertheless, pathologic and clinical evidence is abundant and suggests that the radiologic picture should show the kidneys to be normal to small, bilaterally involved, and smooth. Shallow infarct scars occur inconstantly. There is impaired opacification of the kidney, reflecting the deficiency in renal perfusion. This would be most readily apparent as a patchy nephrogram by computed tomography. Normal renal size in the early stage of this process is to be expected.

Cholesterol emboli large enough to occlude interlobar or arcuate-sized arteries have been demonstrated by angiography. These filling defects are indistinguishable from other types of emboli.

CHRONIC GLOMERULONEPHRITIS

Definition

When the many types of acute glomerulonephritis progress to the chronic stage, they assume a common final form in which loss of renal substance reflects the combined effects of both the nephritis and the secondary hypertension.

In chronic glomerulonephritis, reduction in kidney size is global, symmetric, and often profound. The lobular or idiopathic membranous forms of chronic glomerulonephritis may have normal-sized kidneys. A fine granularity of the subcapsular surface is noted on direct examination of the kidney, but this is not detectable radiologically. The cut surface of the chronic glomerulonephritic kidney reveals an evenly thinned parenchyma and normal papillae. Common to all situations in which wasting occurs over a long period, an excess of peripelvic fat is often present.

The majority of glomeruli have hyalinized tufts and collagen deposition internal to Bowman's capsule. The more extensive the glomerular damage, the greater the reduction in renal weight. Such profound tubule atrophy occurs that tubules may completely disappear. Where tubules persist, hyaline droplet degeneration is seen, with frequent casts, red blood cells, and polymorphonuclear leukocytes in the lumina. A uniform, fine fibrosis of the interstitial tissues occurs in association with infiltrates of lymphocytes and plasma cells. The changes in the arteries and arterioles are those associated with hypertension.

Clinical Setting

Chronic glomerulonephritis develops over a period of weeks to months following an episode of acute glomerulonephritis. Not all cases result from acute poststreptococcal glomerulonephritis. Some may develop without a prior clinically apparent acute phase or from forms of acute glomerulonephritis unrelated to streptococcal infection. In any event, this disease occurs more frequently in the male than in the female and is most prevalent between the second and fifth decades.

Patients with chronic glomerulonephritis usually present with insidious onset of peripheral edema associated with proteinuria. Occasionally, massive edema appears rapidly, along with other stigmata of the nephrotic syndrome. It is estimated that 50 per cent of patients with chronic glomerulonephritis eventually develop the nephrotic syndrome. Hypertension is present and progresses with advancing renal failure. Urinalysis reveals protein, red blood cells, leukocytes, renal epithelial cells, and hyaline and granular casts. Oval fat bodies are seen when the nephrotic syndrome is present.

The terminal stage of untreated chronic glomerulonephritis is characterized by cardiac decompensation, severe hypertension, anemia, marked impairment of renal function producing isosthenuria and polyuria, hyperphosphatemia, and hypocalcemia.

Radiologic Findings

There is nothing unique about the radiologic picture of chronic glomerulonephritis. Both kidneys become

---

SUMMARY OF ABNORMAL URORADIOLOGIC FINDINGS
CHRONIC GLOMERULONEPHRITIS

Primary Uroradiologic Elements
  Size—small
  Contour—smooth (global)
  Lesion distribution—bilateral
Secondary Uroradiologic Elements
  Parenchymal thickness—wasted (global)
  Nephrogram—diminished contrast material density
  Calcification—cortical (uncommon)
  Attenuation value—sinus fat increased
  Echogenicity—increased in the parenchyma
             —may be increased in the central sinus

---

globally small and have smooth contours, normal calyces and papillae, and occasional peripelvic fat proliferation. Density of the nephrogram and pelvo-calyceal system varies with severity of the disease (Figs. 7–11 and 7–12). Calcification in the renal cortex is sometimes present (Fig. 7–13).

Increased echogenicity of the renal parenchyma relative to the liver and increased prominence of the central sinus complex are nonspecific findings in chronic glomerulonephritis.

Angiography in chronic glomerulonephritis reveals arterial tortuosity, loss of branches, and lack of normal tapering of the arteries. These changes are the same as those seen in both arteriosclerosis (aging) and nephrosclerosis; thus angiography is of no value in the diagnosis of chronic glomerulonephritis.

RENAL PAPILLARY NECROSIS

Definition

Necrosis of the renal papilla has several causes and a number of clinical, pathologic, and radiologic forms. In mild to moderate cases, renal size and function are normal and structural changes are limited to one, several, or all papillae. In advanced states, the kidneys

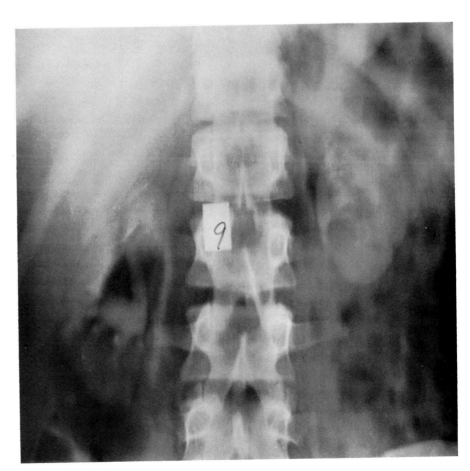

Figure 7–11. Chronic glomerulonephritis. A 5-minute tomogram illustrates bilaterally small, smooth kidneys with moderate opacification of a normal pelvocalyceal system in a 20-year-old woman. Uniform reduction in parenchymal thickness is particularly apparent in the right kidney. Right kidney length = 10.9 cm; left kidney length = 10.7 cm.

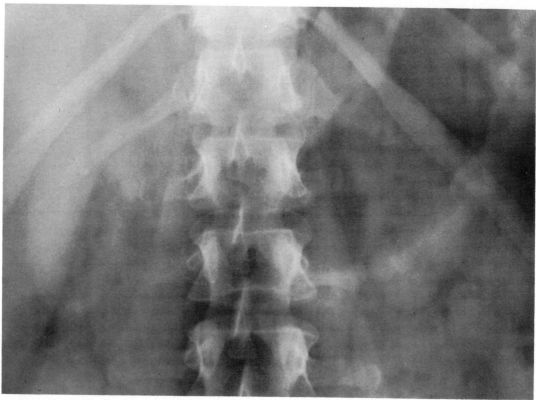

Figure 7–12. Chronic glomerulonephritis in a 37-year-old woman with anemia, proteinuria, and creatinine clearance of 3 ml/min. Marked impairment of contrast material excretion reflects advanced stage of disease. Ten-minute film. (Same patient illustrated in Fig. 23–17.) Right kidney length = 9.4 cm; left kidney length = 9.0 cm.

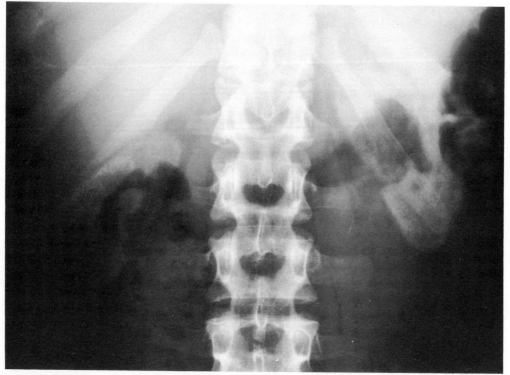

Figure 7–13. Diffuse cortical nephrocalcinosis associated with chronic glomerulonephritis is seen on a standard radiograph of the abdomen. Both kidneys are uniformly involved, and the medullae are spared. (Courtesy of the Department of Radiology, University of Ottawa, Ottawa, Canada.)

become globally shrunken and have impaired function. Therefore, renal papillary necrosis is included in the diagnostic set of bilaterally small kidneys with a global pattern of shrinkage.

This discussion is focused on renal papillary necrosis associated with analgesic use, since this form has been most comprehensively studied and is most prevalent in North America, Europe, and Australia. Differences between analgesic nephropathy and other causes of papillary necrosis, such as diabetes mellitus, urinary tract infection, renal vein thrombosis, prolonged hypotension, urinary tract obstruction, dehydration, S hemoglobinopathy, nonsteroidal anti-inflammatory drugs, hemophilia, and Christmas disease will be commented on in each section.

Medullary ischemia is the central finding in experimental analgesic nephropathy. Necrobiosis of the loops of Henle and of the vasa recta in the papillary tip are early abnormalities. Patchy necrosis of the papilla with overall survival of the collecting tubules occurs at an intermediate stage of severity. Frank necrosis of all elements of the papilla and formation of a clear line of demarcation between the necrotic and the viable portions of the papillary tissue characterize the most advanced stage. These observations suggest that initial damage occurs at the loop of Henle and the vasa recta.

In humans, severity of pathologic change varies directly with the amount of analgesic drugs ingested and closely parallels the sequence of events seen in the experimental animal. The precise pathogenesis of papillary necrosis is unknown. A combination of direct tubule toxicity by metabolites of phenacetin and medullary ischemia due to prostaglandin synthetase inhibition is a likely explanation. In any case, a high concentration of the toxic material occurs in the loop of Henle region of the papilla where the initial and maximal damage occurs. Early change is represented by a yellowish-appearing papilla, with necrosis of the epithelium of the loops of Henle and occasional foci of calcification but no disruption of papillary integrity. As damage progresses, there may be total loss of the loops of Henle, while the collecting duct epithelium remains intact. At this stage the endothelium of the vasa recta is also destroyed and calcium accumulates in many areas of the papilla. In the most advanced form there is diffuse fibrosis and chronic inflammatory cell infiltration in the interstitium as well as tubule atrophy and glomerular hyalinization. These changes, representing chronic interstitial fibrosis, are "end stage" and account for a decrease in renal size and function. In general, the collecting ducts draining the nephrons of the septal cortex at the margin of the lobe better maintain their viability than the ducts located centrally in the lobe, probably because they are not obstructed by necrosis at the papillary tip. As a result, tubule atrophy is predominantly centrilobar and is associated with an increased prominence (either relative or due to true hypertrophy) of the septal cortex drained by the more intact peripheral collecting tubules. These changes produce an uneven pattern of atrophy on the surface of the kidney in which broad, flat, depressed areas of centrilobar cortex are bordered by raised ridges of preserved or hypertrophic septal cortex.

Most investigators interested in this disorder take the position that chronic interstitial inflammation is due to obstruction of the collecting tubules by necrosis of the papilla. Some, however, believe that global shrinkage and renal failure are the result of a direct effect of toxic material on the renal parenchyma. Infection does not appear to be a major factor in causing papillary necrosis in analgesic nephropathy.

Changes in the gross appearance of the papilla parallel the severity of the histologic damage. Initially, the papilla enlarges slightly. Patchy disruption of the integrity of the papilla follows, with the development of tracts communicating with the calyceal system. Cavitation of the papillary substance, with or without complete separation of the papilla from the remainder of the medulla, is a late finding. Occasionally, the necrotic papilla remains *in situ*, where it may calcify or ossify.

It is not uncommon to observe marked papillary necrosis in kidneys that are normal in size and smooth in contour. This simply reflects the very important point that shrinkage of size occurs only in the advanced state, when chronic interstitial fibrosis and tubule atrophy occur. Wasting may occur rapidly, however, once it begins.

Other etiologies may produce patterns that are different from those seen with analgesic abuse. Fulminant papillary necrosis is produced by urinary tract obstruction and infection, with or without diabetes mellitus, and was the first type of papillary necrosis to be described. Acute inflammation, extensive papillary sloughing, and enlarged kidneys are seen in these cases. At the other extreme, papillary necrosis associated with heterozygous-S hemoglobinopathy is very minimal, and progression to small kidneys and renal failure has not been noted. In some circumstances, papillary necrosis affects only one kidney, as may be seen in ureteral obstruction, acute bacterial nephritis, tuberculosis, and renal vein thrombosis. It should be apparent, therefore, that the presentation of papillary necrosis depends on the clinical setting in which it occurs.

Clinical Setting

The diagnosis of analgesic nephropathy is made most often in middle-aged and elderly women who give a history, sometimes difficult to elicit, of ingestion of large amounts of analgesic drugs over a long period of time. This disorder can be particularly severe in hot, dry climates, suggesting that dehydration enhances the effect of the toxic material, presumably by increasing its concentration in the interstitium of the papilla. Symptoms closely resemble those of acute urinary tract infection and include recurrent attacks of fever, dysuria, headache, and malaise. Passage of necrotic papillae or stones produces urinary tract obstruction and colic. Heavy pyuria and fragments of papillae are seen on microscopic examination of the urine. Eventually, sometimes over a short period, these changes may lead to small kidneys with impaired function, anemia, and uremia. Rarely, analgesic nephropathy presents as acute oliguric failure with large kidneys and intact papillae. Transitional cell carcinoma of the kidney is more common in patients with analgesic nephropathy than in the general population. It is important for the radiologist to assess the urograms of these individuals with this complication in mind. (See discussion in Chapter 15.)

The association of renal papillary necrosis with diabetes mellitus has not been investigated as thoroughly as analgesic nephropathy. A combination of ischemia and infection has been considered the basis for this relationship. Fulminating disease with severe infection and azotemia frequently leading to death was once the most common presentation of renal papillary necrosis in the diabetic patient. This is rarely encountered now, presumably because of advances in the management of both diabetes and urinary tract infection. Papillary necrosis is also found in some diabetic patients with chronic or recurrent infection of the urinary tract and moderate impairment of renal function. These patients have hematuria, pyuria, bac-

teriuria, and proteinuria in addition to glycosuria. Papillary necrosis developing in patients with diabetes mellitus uncomplicated by urinary tract infection or obstruction is alluded to in the literature but remains undocumented.

Patients with S hemoglobinopathy also develop papillary necrosis. When the affected red blood cells enter the hypertonic and hypoxic area of the medulla, sickling occurs and causes blockage of the vasa recta perfusing the papillary region. In the homozygous-S state, papillary necrosis can be part of a more complex disorder of the kidneys, which includes glomerular microinfarcts, glomerulopathy, lobar infarcts, obliteration of tubules, and fibrosis. Because symptoms from other organ systems usually predominate in sickle cell disease (homozygous-S), contrast material–enhanced studies of the kidneys are not often performed on these patients. In patients with heterozygous-S hemoglobinopathy, particularly those with SA hemoglobin, minimal papillary necrosis develops without specific signs or symptoms. This abnormality is nonprogressive and not associated with renal failure.

Rarely, papillary necrosis is associated with noninfected urinary tract obstruction, renal vein thrombosis, or trauma. Here, papillary necrosis would likely be unilateral, and the clinical findings would be dom-

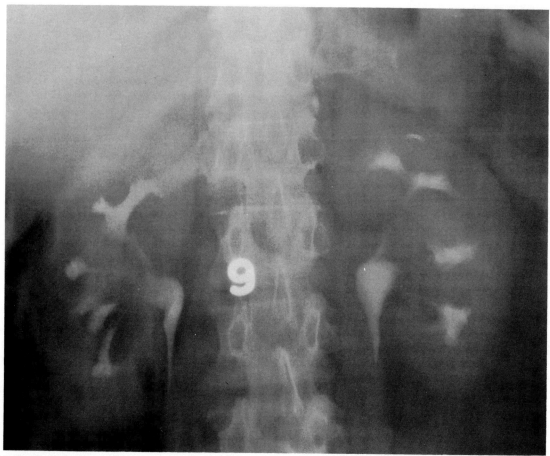

Figure 7–14. Renal papillary necrosis with normal-sized kidneys in a 54-year-old alcoholic, diabetic, and analgesic-abusing woman. Uniform thinning of renal parenchyma has occurred, with multiple papillary abnormalities. Tomogram. (Same patient illustrated in Fig. 7–23.) Right kidney length = 13.8 cm; left kidney length = 13.3 cm.

inated by the underlying disease. Similarly, renal tuberculosis often includes a necrotizing papillitis as one of its many manifestations, and this is sometimes limited to one kidney or a part of one kidney. Papillary necrosis also occurs in infants in association with shock from a variety of disorders and has been reported in hemophilia and Christmas disease. Nonsteroidal anti-inflammatory agents that have in common, along with aspirin and phenacetin, the ability to inhibit prostaglandin synthetase activity also cause papillary necrosis. Finally, a relationship between hepatic cirrhosis and renal papillary necrosis has been proposed but because of the sparse, available evidence must be considered tentative.

Radiologic Findings

The radiologic appearance of papillary necrosis has been studied extensively and is best demonstrated by excretory urography. Renal size is normal in most cases of analgesic nephropathy, although in some patients both kidneys shrink as the abnormality progresses (Figs. 7–14 and 7–15). Kidney contour remains smooth except in some advanced cases in which a "wavy" appearance develops owing to the prominence of septal cortex surrounding atrophic areas of centrilobar cortex (Fig. 7–16). Small kidneys have not been reported in S hemoglobinopathy or in uncomplicated diabetes. The fulminant form of renal papillary necrosis (see Fig. 14–22) with smooth renal enlargement and decreased function is very uncommon and is associated with urinary tract obstruction and infection, uncontrolled diabetes mellitus and severe infection, acute bacterial nephritis, renal vein thrombosis, homozygous-S hemoglobinopathy, and, only rarely, analgesic nephropathy. In some of these disorders, the papillary necrosis may be limited to one kidney. In most instances, the kidney size is normal to small and the outline is smooth.

In an early stage of the disease, papillary swelling may be the only radiologic abnormality present. This may be difficult to distinguish from the normal kidney. Necrosis of the papilla and disruption of its uroepithelial lining takes several radiologic forms. Figure 7–17 presents examples of tract formation, which is an early manifestation of necrosis. These appear as faint streaks of density oriented parallel to the long axis of the papilla, usually extending from the fornix. This pattern is commonly seen in heterozygous-S hemoglobinopathies and less commonly in mild diabetes mellitus. Tract formation can be easily overlooked unless careful attention is given to technical details

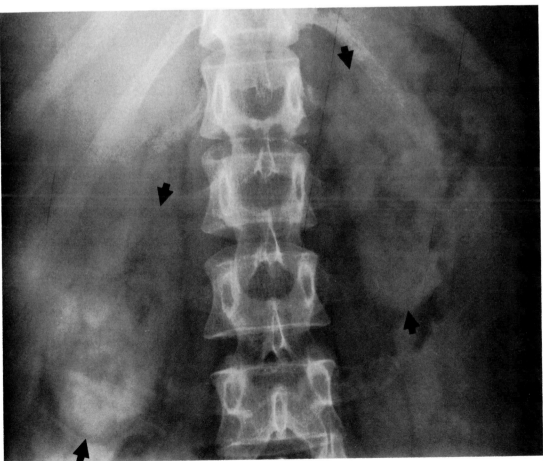

Figure 7–15. Renal papillary necrosis with global wasting of both kidneys and azotemia in a 38-year-old woman with a history of heavy use of analgesic drugs for headache. Smooth renal contours persist. Three-minute film for nephrogram. Arrows indicate renal length. (Same patient illustrated in Fig. 7–26.) Right kidney length = 9.4 cm; left kidney length = 9.5 cm.

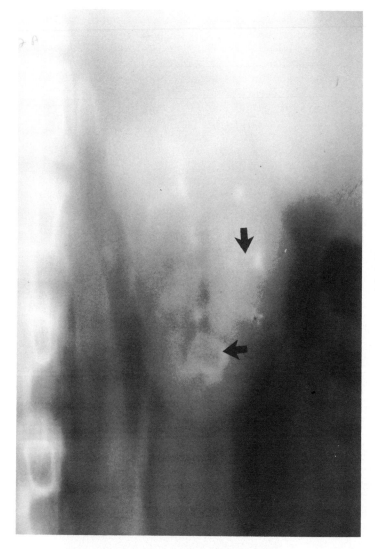

Figure 7–16. Renal papillary necrosis with "wavy" contour superimposed on global wasting of the kidney. Analgesic nephropathy in a 44-year-old man. All papillae are involved, and there are nonopaque filling defects representing sloughed papillae in two calyces (*arrows*). Tomogram. (Same patient illustrated in Fig. 7–24.)

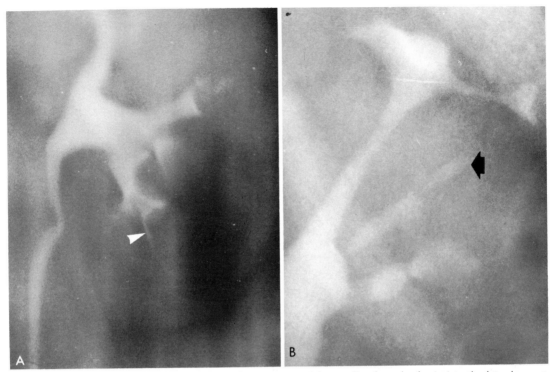

Figure 7–17. Renal papillary necrosis represented by tracts of contrast material extending from the fornix into the lateral aspects of medulla *(arrows).*

A, A 51-year-old woman with mild diabetes mellitus and normal-sized kidneys. (Same patient illustrated in Fig. 7–27.)

B, Similar finding in a patient with SA hemoglobinopathy. (From Eckert, D.E., et al.: Radiology *113:*59, 1974. Reproduced with kind permission of the authors and *Radiology.)*

such as proper collimation, oblique views, and adequate calyceal distention. Conclusive evidence of tract formation requires identification on more than one film and the absence of excessive calyceal distention, either from obstruction or abdominal compression.

Papillary necrosis is readily detectable when there is cavitation of the central portion of the papilla or complete sloughing of the papillary tip. The cavitating form has been called "medullary" or "partial papillary slough," while detachment of the whole papilla has been labeled "papillary" or "total papillary sloughing." Medullary cavitation is often central but may also be eccentric. The long axis of the cavity parallels the long axis of the papilla. The shape of the cavity varies from long and thin to short and bulbous. Some cavities have sharp margins; others are irregular (Figs. 7–18 through 7–20). A total papillary slough can be identified by a band of density across the base of the papilla. As the papillary tip separates farther from its medullary base, the band of density widens. With complete separation, the sloughed tissue is seen as a triangular radiolucent filling defect in the opacified calyx (Fig. 7–21; see Fig. 7–16). Margins at the point of separation are initially rough but later become smooth. Necrotic tissue may pass into the renal pelvis and beyond, causing obstruction. The remaining calyx has a round or saccular shape and smooth margins (Fig. 7–22).

There is a form of papillary necrosis that is difficult to diagnose because the necrotic tissue does not slough and the silhouette of the papilla is preserved.

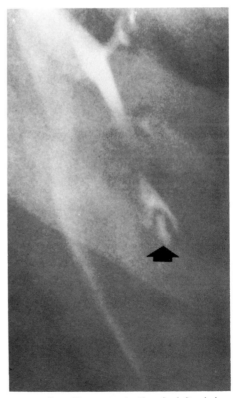

Figure 7–18. Renal papillary necrosis. Sharply defined elongated cavity *(arrow)* in center of papilla in a patient with SA hemoglobinopathy represents the "medullary" form of papillary necrosis. (From Eckert, D.E., et al.: Radiology *113:*59, 1974. Reproduced with kind permission of the authors and *Radiology.)*

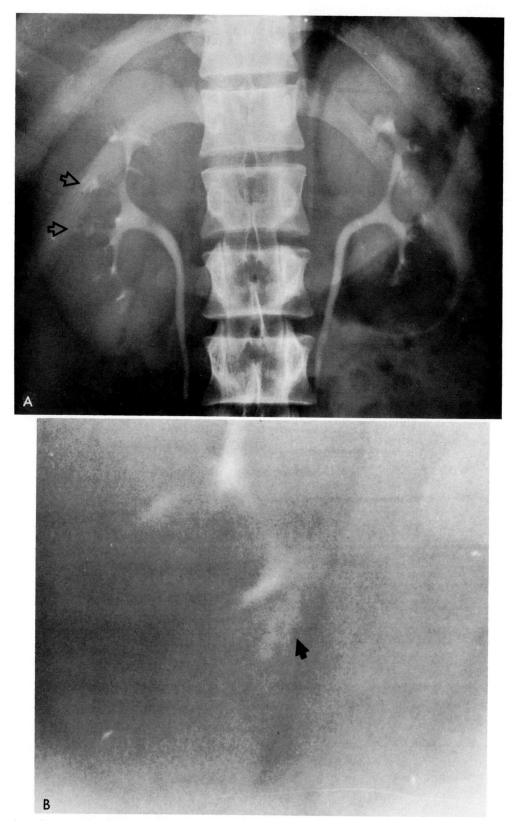

Figure 7–19. Renal papillary necrosis with various forms of cavitation in a 33-year-old man with SC hemoglobinopathy and hematuria.
    A, Kidneys are normal sized and smooth in contour. Central cavitation is present in many papillae, particularly in right interpolar areas *(arrows).*
Right lower and left upper poles are magnified in *B* and *C.*
    B, Ill-defined smudge *(arrow)* represents early cavitation. Lucent oblique line is psoas margin, not medial border of kidney.

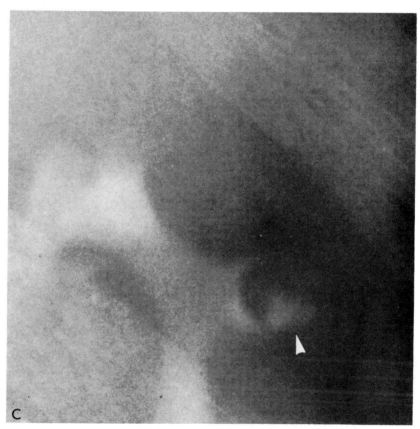

Figure 7–19 *Continued C,* Eccentric, irregular cavity near forniceal angle *(arrow).*

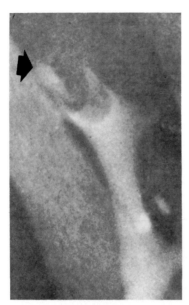

Figure 7–20. Renal papillary necrosis. Elongated cavity situated eccentrically in the papilla of a patient with SA hemoglobinopathy. (From Eckert, D.E., et al.: Radiology *113*:59, 1974. Reproduced with kind permission of the authors and *Radiology*.)

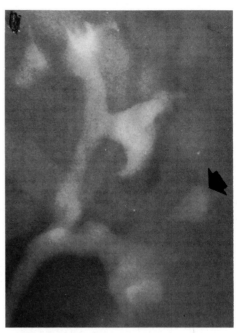

Figure 7–22. Renal papillary necrosis. Loss of papillary tip, either by sloughing or atrophy, leaves smooth-margined saccular calyx *(arrow)* without overlying focal contour scar in a patient with SA hemoglobinopathy. (From Eckert, D.E., et al.: Radiology *113*:59, 1974. Reproduced with kind permission of the authors and *Radiology*.)

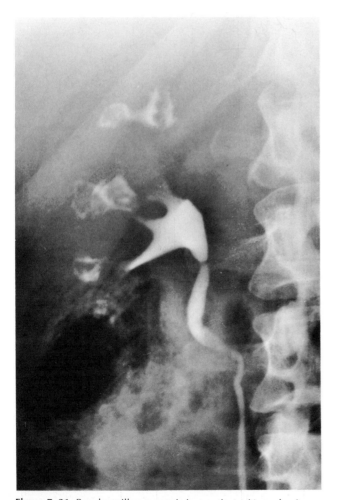

Figure 7–21. Renal papillary necrosis in a patient with analgesic nephropathy. Each of the papillae has separated and forms nonopaque calyceal filling defects, many of which have triangular shapes. This represents the "papillary" form of papillary necrosis.

This form has been termed *necrosis in situ.* These papillae may shrink slightly over time, and some calcify or ossify. A confident radiologic diagnosis of papillary necrosis in this form requires supportive clinical evidence or other specific coexisting radiologic abnormalities, such as cavities or sloughing.

Calcification in papillary tissue (nephrocalcinosis) is common in analgesic nephropathy but has not been reported in papillary necrosis due to heterozygous-S hemoglobinopathy. Presumably, this difference reflects greater tissue damage from analgesic drugs. Nephrocalcinosis may be seen either in papillae that have no other radiologic abnormality or in those that have cavitated. In most instances, foci of calcification are round, homogeneous, and arranged in a semilunar arc that corresponds to the positions of the papillary tips (Figs. 7–23 and 7–24). This appearance is indistinguishable from that of nephrocalcinosis due to causes other than papillary necrosis. On the other hand, a ring-shaped, triangular pattern of calcification is unique to papillary necrosis (Fig. 7–25). Here, calcium outlines the periphery of a necrotic papilla, which may be sloughed and moving down the urinary tract. Calcification or ossification may be the only radiologic abnormality in the *necrosis in situ* form of papillary necrosis.

Enlargement of the septum of Bertin may centrally displace an adjacent calyx or infundibulum. This can create the impression of a mass (Fig. 7–26). A radionuclide scan may be necessary to identify this deformity as a pseudotumor.

An abnormally dense and persistent nephrogram has been reported in papillary necrosis in experimen-

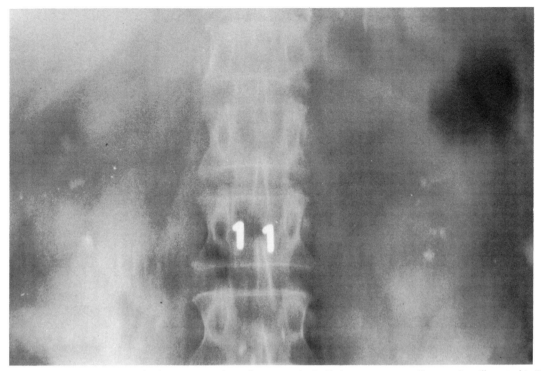

Figure 7–23. Papillary calcification at multiple sites in renal papillary necrosis. Preliminary tomogram. (Same patient illustrated in Fig. 7–14.)

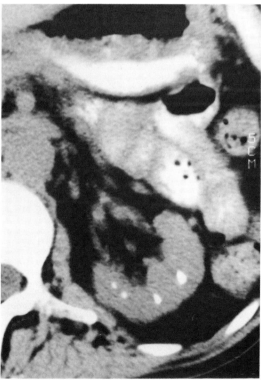

Figure 7–24. A semilunar arc of calcification in the tips of multiple papillae is illustrated in a patient with renal papillary necrosis. Computed tomogram, unenhanced. (Same patient illustrated in Fig. 7–16.)

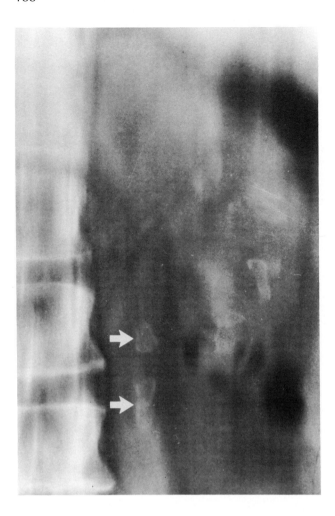

Figure 7–25. Calcification in a triangular ring pattern is unique to renal papillary necrosis. In this example, several sloughed papillae are located in the proximal ureter (*arrows*) in addition to the calyces.

SUMMARY OF ABNORMAL URORADIOLOGIC FINDINGS
RENAL PAPILLARY NECROSIS

Primary Uroradiologic Elements
    Size—normal to small (small form limited to analgesic nephropathy; large in acute fulminant form)
    Contour—smooth (global) ("wavy" contour in some cases of advanced analgesic nephropathy)
    Lesion distribution—bilateral (may be unilateral when due to obstruction, renal vein thrombosis,
        acute bacterial nephritis, tuberculosis)
Secondary Uroradiologic Elements
    Papillae
        Enlarged (early)
        Disrupted (cavity, tracts, or slough)
        Retracted
    Pelvoinfundibulocalyceal system
        Dilated (focal, calyx)
        Displaced (secondary to enlarged septal cortex—occasional)
        Intraluminal filling defects (opaque or nonopaque)
    Parenchymal thickness
        Wasted (global)—in analgesic nephropathy
    Calcification
        Papillary
        Curvilinear—ring-shaped and triangular in sloughed papilla
    Nephrogram
        Contrast material density diminished (some cases of advanced analgesic nephropathy)
        Increasingly dense (rare)

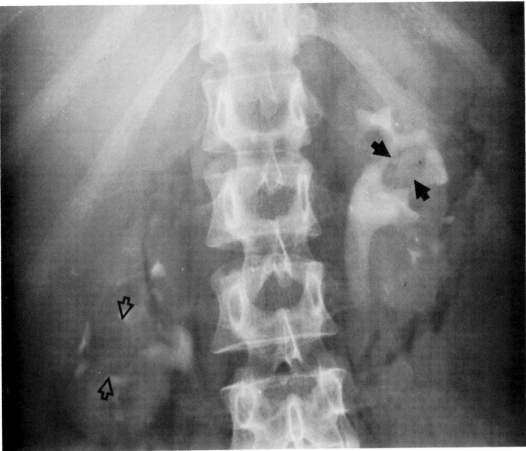

Figure 7–26. Focal masslike displacement of pelvocalyceal systems bilaterally. (Same patient illustrated in Fig. 7–15.) This type of deformity is sometimes seen in advanced analgesic nephropathy due to hypertrophy of the septal cortex.

tal animals, in infants with shocklike states, and rarely in adults. Although rare, such a nephrogram should alert the radiologist to the possibility of papillary necrosis. Presumably, this finding is due to tubule obstruction by necrosis of papillary tips.

Necrotic tissue passing down the pelvocalyceal system and the ureter produces the radiologic picture of obstruction. The obstructing material is often nonopaque. When recovered in the urine, its tissue origin can usually be established by pathologic examination. Blood clots may act similarly (Fig. 7–27).

Even though histologic damage may be present in all papillae, radiologically detectable lesions may be spotty or unilateral. Usually, multiple sites of involvement are present bilaterally, although the pattern of lesions may be mixed.

Diminished excretion of contrast material, reflecting renal failure, occurs in advanced stages of analgesic nephropathy but is not seen with other causes of *chronic* papillary necrosis. This usually occurs in patients with small kidneys and a long history of analgesic abuse. Impaired contrast material density is also seen with large kidneys in *acute* analgesic nephropathy, in papillary necrosis due to overwhelming urinary tract infection in the obstructed or diabetic patient, and in sickle cell nephropathy with impaired concentration of urine.

Only a few studies of ultrasonography in papillary necrosis have been reported. Sloughed papillae might be imaged as material within the collecting system lumen. These may have the sound-reflecting characteristics of stones, if calcified, or exhibit an echo pattern similar to that of renal parenchyma, if uncalcified. Calyces may be dilated at the site of a disgorged papilla, or the entire collecting system may be dilated when obstruction supervenes. Overall, the poor spatial resolution of ultrasonography limits its usefulness in the assessment of papillary necrosis.

HEREDITARY NEPHROPATHIES

Hereditary chronic nephritis (Alport's syndrome) and medullary cystic disease are two hereditary diseases of the kidney that produce small kidneys and renal failure. These entities are dissimilar and discussed separately in this section. Other radiologically detectable forms of hereditary disease produce large kidneys (autosomal dominant and recessive polycystic diseases), result in nephrocalcinosis (primary hyperoxaluria, and renal tubular acidosis), or involve the kidneys secondarily (renal amyloidosis secondary to familial Mediterranean fever). These disorders are discussed in other chapters.

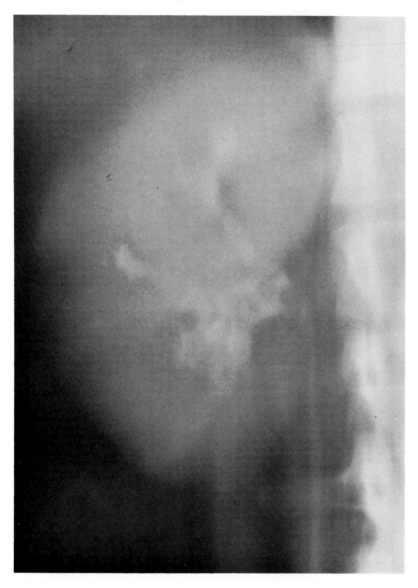

Figure 7–27. Multiple radiolucent filling defects in the pelvis of the right kidney, which caused intermittent obstruction. These represent either blood clots, sloughed papillary tissue, or a combination of both. Obstruction and hematuria are common complications of renal papillary necrosis. (Same patient illustrated in Fig. 7–17A.)

SUMMARY OF ABNORMAL URORADIOLOGIC FINDINGS
HEREDITARY CHRONIC NEPHRITIS

Primary Uroradiologic Elements
Size—small
Contour—smooth (global)
Lesion distribution—bilateral
Secondary Uroradiologic Elements
Parenchymal thickness—wasted (global)
Nephrogram—contrast material density diminished

Hereditary Chronic Nephritis (Alport's Syndrome)

Definition

The kidneys in hereditary chronic nephritis are invariably decreased in size, often to a marked degree, but remain smooth.

The most distinctive histologic feature of hereditary chronic nephritis is the presence of fat-filled macrophages, "foam cells." These are particularly abundant in the corticomedullary junction. Otherwise, the microscopic anatomy in this disorder is nonspecific. Diffuse fibrosis and chronic inflammatory cells are found in the interstitial tissue. Abnormalities in the glomeruli, when present, are identical to those of glomerulonephritis. Varying degrees of tubule atrophy and dilatation resemble the histologic pattern seen in reflux nephropathy (chronic atrophic pyelonephritis).

Clinical Setting

The form of genetic transmission of hereditary chronic nephritis has yet to be precisely established. Cases have been reported in which families follow the pattern of autosomal dominant inheritance, but the many exceptions to this indicate a more complex genetic basis.

Males are affected with a more severe form of renal disease than females. Symptoms, usually episodic hematuria, begin in childhood. This is often preceded by upper respiratory tract infections. The urine also contains white blood cells, casts, and protein. Renal insufficiency is progressive, with few males living beyond the fifth decade without dialysis. In females, the disease is usually nonprogressive, and death due to chronic nephritis is uncommon. One striking feature in both sexes is the absence of hypertension as a prominent aspect of the disease.

In addition to renal abnormalities, most patients also have nerve deafness and a variety of ocular abnormalities, including congenital cataracts, nystagmus, myopia, and spherophakia. The presence of hearing or visual abnormalities is not essential to the diagnosis of hereditary chronic nephritis, however.

Radiologic Findings

Small, smooth kidneys with impaired excretion of contrast material are the radiologic abnormalities of hereditary chronic nephritis (Fig. 7–28). Obviously, this diagnosis is dependent on clinical features in addition to radiologic findings.

Reports of renal angiographic findings in Alport's syndrome indicate that vascular changes are nonspecific.

Medullary Cystic Disease

Definition

Medullary cystic disease is the second of the heritable causes of renal failure associated with normal-sized to small kidneys with smooth outlines.

A variable number of cysts, found for the most part in the corticomedullary and medullary areas of the kidney, are seen in the cut section of these kidneys. The cysts range in size from less than 100 μm to 1 cm or more in diameter. The usual sharp demarcation between cortex and medulla is obliterated. Most cysts are too small to distort the pelvocalyceal system or the renal contour.

A flattened or low cuboidal tubule epithelium is seen on microscopy. Except for cysts, other findings are nonspecific and mimic many other "small kidney" disorders. These include hyalinization of glomeruli, periglomerular fibrosis, fibrosis and chronic inflammatory cell infiltration of the interstitium, and tubule atrophy.

It is generally accepted that medullary cystic disease is the same disease as familial juvenile nephronophthisis. However, another point of view holds that nephronophthisis is distinguishable by age at onset and by pattern of inheritance.

Clinical Setting

Medullary cystic disease is inherited as either an autosomal dominant or an autosomal recessive trait. Disease presenting in the first two decades is usually transmitted as an autosomal recessive inheritance, whereas autosomal dominant patterns characterize those that appear in third or subsequent decades.

The onset of symptoms (usually polydipsia, polyuria, and nocturia) is insidious. Hypertension is not a prominent feature of medullary cystic disease and may not appear at all until late in the course of the disease. A normochromic, normocytic anemia secondary to chronic uremia is a universal finding in symptomatic patients. Characteristically, these patients have hyposthenuria and are salt-wasters. Apart from

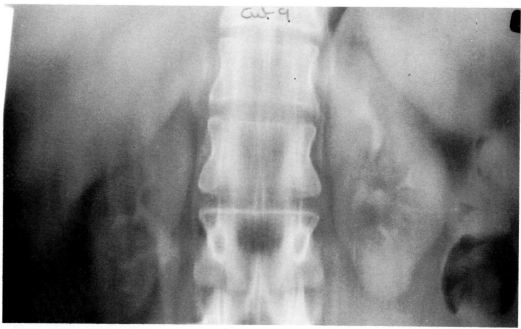

Figure 7–28. Hereditary chronic nephritis (Alport's syndrome). Bilaterally small, smooth kidneys with normal pelvocalyceal system in a 52-year-old woman with mild intermittent hypertension, proteinuria, and slight azotemia. One of her sons died of "nephritis," and another had renal function and auditory and ocular abnormalities. Tomogram. (Courtesy of Department of Diagnostic Radiology, Hammersmith Hospital, Royal Postgraduate Medical School, London, England.)

a loss of concentrating ability, abnormalities in the urine are usually absent. Death due to uremia usually occurs in the third decade, although a few patients have been known to survive into the seventh decade.

Radiologic Findings

Normal-sized to small kidneys, smooth contour, and impaired excretion of contrast material are the common features of medullary cystic disease. In many patients, these are the only findings, and the radiologic examination is nonspecific. In some patients, sharply defined radiolucent nephrographic defects may be observed when the medullary cysts are large. A striated, late-appearing, and persistent nephrogram limited to the medullary portions of the parenchyma has also been described (Fig. 7–29). This corresponds to urine stasis in dilated tubules and collecting ducts. Detection of nephrographic abnormalities during excretory urography in medullary cystic disease re-

quires an optimal dose of contrast material and the use of tomography. Because cysts are usually small, pelvocalyceal displacement and lobulation of the renal contour are uncommon.

Computed tomography is more sensitive than excretory urography in detecting the cysts of medullary cystic disease (Fig. 7–30A). In other respects, the abnormalities demonstrable by computed tomography are the same as those described above for excretory urography. Likewise, ultrasonography is also more sensitive than excretory urography for demonstrating medullary cystic disease (Fig. 7–30B). High-resolution, precisely focused images of the kidney define small, fluid-filled cysts as well as small, smooth hyperechoic kidneys.

Angiographic findings in medullary cystic disease have been reported on a number of occasions. The angiographic nephrogram with its intense stain permits visualization of the cysts, particularly when they

---

SUMMARY OF ABNORMAL URORADIOLOGIC FINDINGS
MEDULLARY CYSTIC DISEASE

Primary Uroradiologic Elements
    Size—normal to small
    Contour—smooth (global)
    Lesion distribution—bilateral
Secondary Uroradiologic Elements
    Parenchymal thickness—wasted (global)
    Nephrogram—contrast material density diminished; replaced occasionally by focal, sharply defined, multiple, thin-walled radiolucencies of varying size; delayed, persistent medullary striations
    Echogenicity—increased; fluid-filled medullary or corticomedullary masses

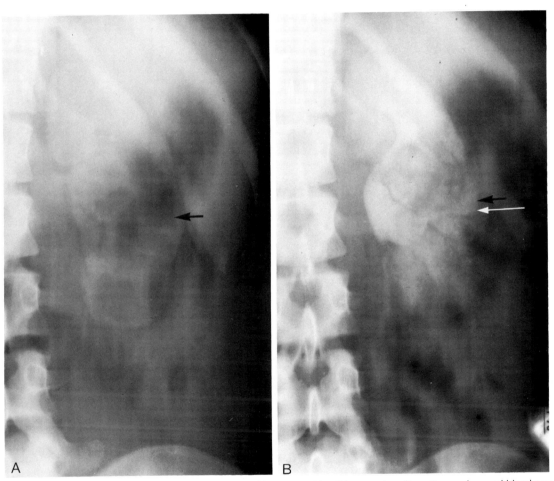

Figure 7–29. Medullary cystic disease in an asymptomatic 26-year-old woman with mild azotemia, salt wasting, and normal blood pressure.
  A, Excretory urogram, 15-second tomogram. Angiographic nephrogram demonstrates slight thinning of the cortex and a slightly enlarged medulla *(arrow)* that remains normally radiolucent.
  B, Excretory urogram. Tomogram. A 30-minute delayed film reveals loss of opacification of the cortex and a persistent, dense nephrogram limited to the medulla *(large arrow)*, representing stasis in tubules and collecting ducts. Small cysts are represented by round radiolucencies *(small arrow)*.
  (Courtesy of Daniel P. Link, M.D., University of California, Davis, and American Journal of Roentgenology *133*:303, 1979.)

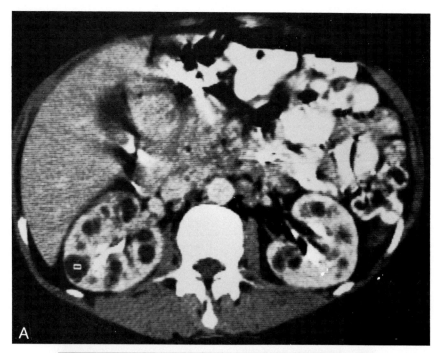

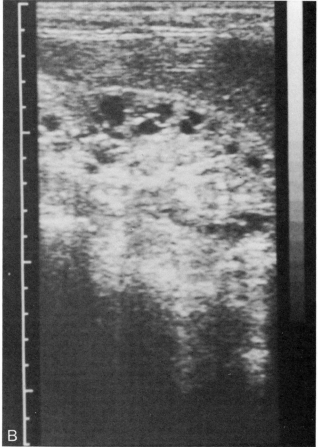

Figure 7–30. Medullary cystic disease in a 55-year-old man with salt-losing nephropathy.

A, Computed tomogram, contrast material enhanced. Fluid-filled cysts of varying size are in the medulla and corticomedullary region. Characteristically, they are not of sufficient size to distort the contour or enlarge the size of the kidneys.

B, The same abnormalities demonstrated by computed tomography are seen by ultrasonography. Note also the nonspecific increase in renal parenchymal echogenicity.

(Courtesy of John D. Rego, M.D., et al., San Francisco General Hospital, San Francisco, California, and *J. Ultrasound Med. 2:*433, 1983.)

are very small. Angiography, however, offers no advantage over other modalities.

AMYLOIDOSIS (LATE)

Amyloidosis of the kidneys causes smooth enlargement of both kidneys; this is discussed in detail in Chapter 8. With time, however, amyloid kidneys become small, with preservation of a normal contour and pelvocalyceal relationships. Presumably, this occurs as a result of ischemic atrophy of nephrons induced by involvement of the renal arteries by amyloid deposits. These changes occur consistently. Thus, amyloidosis must be considered in the differential diagnosis of bilaterally small, as well as large, smooth kidneys.

ARTERIAL HYPOTENSION

Definition

Under normal circumstances, the kidney is distended by blood filling the vascular bed and urine filling the tubules and pelvocalyceal system. When arterial hypotension occurs, intrarenal hypovolemia, primary vasoconstriction, and depletion of intratubular urine volume brought on by reduced glomerular filtration follow. The net consequence of these events can be seen radiologically as a reduction in renal size and an abnormal nephrogram.

Clinical Setting

Reduced renal size due to hypotension was first described in patients undergoing aortography under general anesthesia. In modern practice, hypotension is usually encountered as an adverse response to contrast material during the performance of an excretory urogram, computed tomogram, or arteriogram. The condition can go unsuspected because the patient may be free of pallor, diaphoresis, and lightheadedness. Sometimes the first indication of hypotension is the radiologist's observation that the kidneys are smaller on early films of the urogram than on the preliminary film and that the calyces fail to opacify despite the presence of a distinct nephrogram. With appropriate intravascular volume replacement therapy these abnormalities disappear.

Radiologic Findings

Because hypotension is systemic, shrinkage is global and bilateral. Since this finding is usually seen as a reaction to contrast material, the acuteness of this process often can be documented by comparing renal size on post– and pre–contrast material images.

Two abnormal nephrographic patterns have been described. In the more common one, the nephrogram becomes progressively dense over time, while in the other, the nephrogram persists unchanged. It has been postulated that in the first instance decreased perfusion pressure reduces glomerular filtration and causes stasis of filtrate in the tubules. At the same time, hypoperfusion of the kidney leads to increased sodium and water reabsorption, which acts to promote further filtration by depleting intratubular volume. An increased accumulation of contrast material in the tubules results. Since overall filtration remains impaired, there is no effective forward flow of filtrate down the tubules; thus, the nephrogram becomes increasingly dense. Why some patients exhibit the second nephrographic pattern of persistent, unchanging density is not certain. This may be a function of a large initial dose of contrast material and the degree of hypotension.

Once hypotension is reversed, the nephrogram characteristically reverts to normal and there is progressive opacification of the collecting system (Fig. 7–31).

DIFFERENTIAL DIAGNOSIS

The radiologic pictures of *generalized arteriosclerosis* and *benign nephrosclerosis* are identical. Distinction between these two depends on clinical information, specifically normal blood pressure and advanced age (sixth decade and older) in the former and arterial hypertension and an onset before age 50 in the latter. Renal opacification is normal in both disorders.

In *malignant nephrosclerosis, atheroembolic renal disease, chronic glomerulonephritis,* and the *hereditary nephropathies,* depressed renal function impairs contrast material enhancement, sometimes to a very marked degree. Arterial hypertension is a significant problem in all these disorders except the hereditary nephropathies. These patients also have distinctive clinical features, such as a family history of renal disease, ocular

---

SUMMARY OF ABNORMAL URORADIOLOGIC FINDINGS*
ARTERIAL HYPOTENSION

Primary Uroradiologic Elements
    Size—small (compared to size on pre–contrast material image)
    Contour—smooth (global)
    Lesion distribution—bilateral
Secondary Uroradiologic Elements
    Pelvoinfundibulocalyceal system—absent opacification
    Nephrogram—increasingly dense (common); persistently dense (uncommon)

*All findings revert to normal with correction of hypotension.

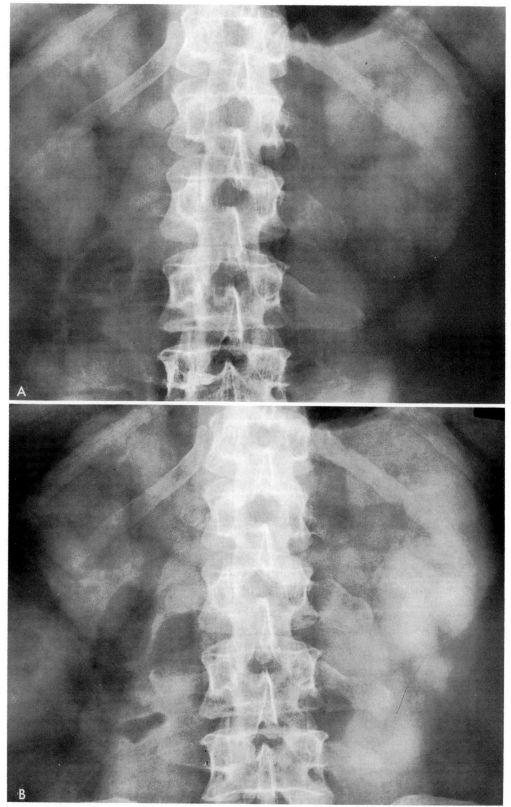

Figure 7–31. Renal shrinkage and abnormal nephrogram due to arterial hypotension associated with adverse response to contrast material. *A,* Five-minute film showing slight increase in nephrographic density with no pelvocalyceal opacification. *B,* Ten-minute film. Right kidney length = 13.4 cm; left kidney length = 13.2 cm.

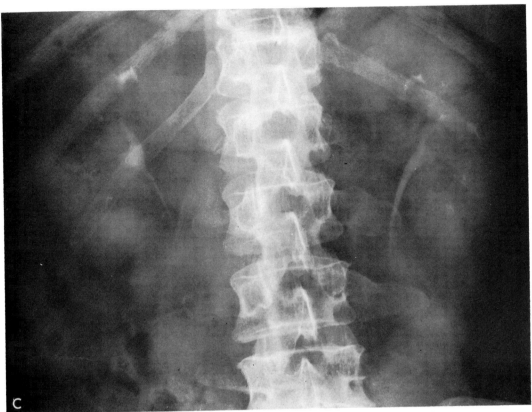

Figure 7–31 *Continued C,* Forty-five-minute film following successful treatment of hypotension. Pelvocalyceal systems are now opacified and the nephrogram is of normal density. Kidneys have increased 1 cm. in length. Right kidney length = 14.4 cm; left kidney length = 14.2 cm. (Same patient illustrated in Fig. 23–19.)

and hearing disorders in hereditary chronic nephritis, or salt-wasting in medullary cystic disease. The demonstration of medullary or corticomedullary cysts in bilaterally small, smooth kidneys in the appropriate clinical setting supports the diagnosis of medullary cystic disease. This radiologic finding, however, may also be seen in acquired renal cystic disease that develops in end-stage renal disease patients who have undergone a prolonged period of dialysis. This entity is discussed in detail in Chapter 10.

Disorders that produce bilaterally small, smooth kidneys as a result of primary disease of the arterial bed occasionally demonstrate randomly placed, small infarct scars representing sites where the arterial lesion has progressed to complete occlusion. These are seen in generalized arteriosclerosis, benign and malignant nephrosclerosis, and atheroembolic renal disease, but not in the other entities of this diagnostic set.

Arterial hypotension as a cause of small, smooth kidneys is distinguishable by the transient nature of the abnormalities and by the abnormal time–density relationship of the nephrogram.

Renal papillary necrosis is easily distinguished from other entities in this diagnostic set as the only one with papillary abnormalities. Also, global wasting is limited to some cases of advanced analgesic nephropathy and is not seen with the same regularity as in other "bilaterally small, smooth" kidney diseases. Renal papillary necrosis due to analgesic nephropathy must be distinguished from renal papillary necrosis due to other etiologies. In general, papillary necrosis limited to one kidney is associated with urinary tract obstruction, renal vein thrombosis, acute bacterial nephritis, or tuberculosis. Papillary necrosis that is unifocal (i.e., involving one, or possibly, two papillae) suggests tuberculosis or an excavating pyogenic abscess as the underlying etiology. In addition to analgesic nephropathy, papillary-calyceal deformity with or without parenchymal loss can be seen in medullary sponge kidney, reflux nephropathy, and postobstructive or postinflammatory atrophy.

Cavitation of the papilla is often the first radiologic manifestation of renal tuberculosis. This may occur in one or more foci and can be indistinguishable from the other entities discussed in this chapter that also produce papillary necrosis. In the early stages, tuberculosis produces a smudged, ill-defined collection of contrast material in the papillary or peripapillary region associated with a swollen papillary tip. This may extend into the medulla. This pattern can be identical with those produced by analgesic nephropathy, S hemoglobinopathy, and diabetes mellitus. Advanced tuberculosis, with extensive areas of tissue destruction and calcification, focal scars, and inflammatory masses, is quite dissimilar from the late changes of renal papillary necrosis. Tuberculosis is discussed further in Chapter 13.

Papillary calcification occurs in medullary sponge kidney, in renal papillary necrosis due to analgesic nephropathy, and in a variety of other causes associated with nephrocalcinosis, as discussed in Chapter 13. Usually the pattern of calcification is punctate but otherwise nonspecific. However, when the papillary calcification is ring shaped, renal papillary necrosis can be uniquely considered as the etiology. In medullary sponge kidney, the discrete foci of calcification that are defined on the preliminary film characteristically become obscured during excretory urography as contrast material enters the cystic cavities that communicate with the collecting ducts and surrounds the calculi that are located there. This phenomenon does not occur in the other forms of nephrocalcinosis, including renal papillary necrosis. Likewise, opacification of the dilated spaces in the papillae of the sponge kidney during excretory urography creates a pattern of multiple, circumscribed punctate densities. In renal papillary necrosis, the cavity is usually single. Characteristically, but not invariably, the dilated spaces of sponge kidney do not fill during retrograde pyelography; the opposite is true for the cavity of papillary necrosis. Finally, medullary sponge kidney is unassociated with decrease in renal size at any stage in its natural history. (Chapter 13 includes a detailed discussion of medullary sponge kidney.)

Papillary and calyceal abnormalities of reflux nephropathy may be identical to those of renal papillary necrosis. However, reflux nephropathy can be distinguished by a focal contour scar overlying the papillary deformity, whereas wasting, when it does occur in papillary necrosis, is global. Also, papillary calcification is rare in reflux nephropathy and common in papillary necrosis.

Postobstructive atrophy affecting both kidneys has a number of features in common with papillary necrosis. Papillae disappear, and the kidney undergoes global shrinkage. Both the distribution and the severity of papillary abnormalities are more uniform in postobstructive atrophy than in papillary necrosis. In addition, a mixture of cavitation and atrophy is seen in papillary necrosis, whereas atrophy alone follows relief of obstruction.

In advanced analgesic nephropathy with severe renal failure, opacification of the kidneys may be so impaired that only a small, smooth outline can be identified during excretory urography. Retrograde pyelography can demonstrate the papillary abnormalities that distinguish papillary necrosis from other forms of small, smooth kidney failure, such as chronic glomerulonephritis and malignant nephrosclerosis in which the papillae remain intact.

Papillary necrosis presenting as acute renal failure with enlarged, smooth kidneys may be impossible to distinguish from the many other causes of bilaterally enlarged, failed kidneys (discussed in Chapter 8), based on radiologic data alone. To make matters more difficult, evolution of papillary abnormalities may be delayed in these conditions, and a number of retrograde pyelograms may be required before characteristic papillary deformities are demonstrated.

Bibliography

General

Ambos, M. A., Bosniak, M. A., Gordon, R., and Madayag, M. D.: Replacement lipomatosis of the kidney. AJR 130:1087, 1978.
Brenner, B. M., and Rector, F. C. (eds.): The Kidney. 4th ed. Philadelphia, W. B. Saunders, 1991.
Heptinstall, R. H. (ed.): Pathology of the Kidney. 4th ed. Boston, Little, Brown & Co., 1992.
Hricak, H., Cruz, C., Romanski, R., Uniewski, M. H., Levin, N. W., Madrazo, B. L., Sandler, M. A., and Eyler, W. R.: Renal parenchymal disease: Sonographic-histologic correlation. Radiology 144:141, 1982.
Murray, T., and Goldberg, M.: Chronic interstitial nephritis: Etiologic factors. Ann. Intern. Med. 82:453, 1975.
Platt, J. F., Rubin, J. M., Bowerman, R. A., and Marn, C. S.: The inability to detect kidney disease on the basis of echogenicity. AJR 151:317, 1988.
Rosenfield, A. T., and Siegel, N. J.: Renal parenchymal disease: Histologic-sonographic correlation. AJR 137:793, 1981.
Schrier, R. W., and Gottschalk, C. W. (eds.): Diseases of the Kidney. 4th ed. Boston, Little, Brown & Co., 1988.

Generalized Arteriosclerosis

Barlow, K. A., and Beilin, L. J.: Renal disease in primary gout. Q. J. Med. 37:79, 1968.
Bell, E. T.: Renal Disease. Philadelphia, Lea & Febiger, 1946.
Case records of the Massachusetts General Hospital: Case 34–1978. Scleroderma involving skin and kidneys. N. Engl. J. Med. 299:466, 1978.
Griffiths, G. J., Robinson, K. B., Cartwright, G. O., and McLachlan, M. S. F.: Loss of renal tissue in the elderly. Br. J. Radiol. 49:111, 1976.
Heptinstall, R. H. (ed.): Pathology of the Kidney. 4th ed. Boston, Little, Brown & Co., 1992.
Hill, G. S.: Renal vascular lesions. In Hill, G. S. (ed.): Uropathology. New York, Churchill Livingstone, 1989, pp. 189–234.
Ives, H. E., and Paniel, T. O.: Vascular diseases of the kidney. In Brenner, B. M., and Rector, F. C. (eds.): The Kidney. 4th ed. Philadelphia, W. B. Saunders, 1991.
Luke, R. G.: Nephrosclerosis. In Schrier, R. W., and Gottschalk, C. W. (eds.): Diseases of the Kidney. 4th ed. Boston, Little, Brown & Co., 1988, pp. 1573–1596.
McLachlan, M., and Wasserman, P.: Changes in sizes and distensibility of the ageing kidney. Br. J. Radiol. 54:488, 1981.
Murray, T., and Goldberg, M.: Chronic interstitial nephritis: Etiologic factors. Ann. Intern. Med. 82:453, 1975.
Oliver, J. A., and Cannon, P. J.: The kidney in scleroderma. Nephron 18:141, 1977.
Talbott, J. H., and Terplan, K. L.: The kidney in gout. Medicine (Baltimore) 39:405, 1960.
Tyler, F. H.: Urate nephropathy. In Strauss, M. B., and Welt, L. G. (eds.): Diseases of the Kidney. 2nd ed. Boston, Little, Brown & Co., 1971, pp. 891–901.

Nephrosclerosis (Benign and Malignant)

Heptinstall, R. H.: Hypertension I: Essential hypertension. In Heptinstall, R. H. (ed.): Pathology of the Kidney. 4th ed. Boston, Little, Brown & Co., 1992, pp. 951–1028.
Luke, R. G.: Nephrosclerosis. In Schrier, R. W., Gottschalk, C. W. (eds.): Diseases of the Kidney. 4th ed. Boston, Little, Brown & Co., 1988, pp. 1573–1596.
Nolan, C. R., III, and Linas, S. L.: Accelerated and malignant hypertension. In Schrier, R. W., Gottschalk, C. W. (eds.): Diseases of the Kidney, 4th ed. Boston, Little, Brown & Co., 1988, pp. 1703–1826.

Atheroembolic Renal Disease

Case records of the Massachusetts General Hospital: Case 50–1977. Atheromatous emboli to kidneys. N. Engl. J. Med. 297:1337, 1977.

Case records of the Massachusetts General Hospital: Case 4–1984. Atheroembolic renal disease. N. Engl. J. Med. 310:244, 1984.

Case records of the Massachusetts General Hospital: Case 2–1991. Renal cholesterol embolism. N. Engl. J. Med. 324:113, 1991.

Dahlberg, P. J., Frecentese, D. F., and Gobbill, T. H.: Cholesterol embolism: Experience with 22 histologically proven cases. Surgery 105:737, 1989.

Fine, M. J., Kapoor, W., and Falonga, V.: Cholesterol crystal embolization: A review of 221 cases in the English literature. Angiology 38:769, 1987.

Harrington, J. T., Sommers, S. C., and Kassirer, J. P.: Atheromatous emboli with progressive renal failure: Renal arteriography as the probable inciting factor. Ann. Intern. Med. 68:152, 1968.

Kassirer, J. P.: Atheroembolic renal disease. N. Engl. J. Med. 280:812, 1969.

Lie, J. T.: Cholesterol atheromatous embolism: The great masquerader revisited. In Rosen, P. P., and Fechner, R. E. (eds.): Annual 1992, Pt 2 (Series: Pathology Annual 27). Norwalk, CT, Appleton & Lange, 1992, pp. 17–50.

Palmer, F. J., and Warren, B. A.: Multiple cholesterol emboli syndrome complicating angiographic techniques. Clin. Radiol. 39:519, 1988.

Chronic Glomerulonephritis

Arons, W. L., Christensen, W. G., and Sosman, M. C.: Nephrocalcinosis visible by x-ray associated with chronic glomerulonephritis. Ann. Intern. Med. 42:260, 1955.

Cohen, H. L., Kassner, E. G., and Haller, J. D.: Nephrocalcinosis in chronic glomerulonephritis: Report of the youngest patient. Urol. Radiol. 2:51, 1980.

Heptinstall, R. H.: Pathology of the Kidney. 4th ed. Boston, Little, Brown & Co., 1992.

Mena, E., Bookstein, J. J., and Gikas, P. W.: Angiographic diagnosis of renal parenchymal disease: Chronic glomerulonephritis, chronic pyelonephritis, and arteriolonephrosclerosis. Radiology 108:523, 1973.

Schrier, R. W., and Gottschalk, C. W. (eds.): Diseases of the Kidney. 4th ed. Boston, Little, Brown & Co., 1988.

Renal Papillary Necrosis

Abdulhayoglu, S., and Marble, A.: Necrotizing renal papillitis (papillary necrosis) in diabetes mellitus. Am. J. Med. Sci. 248:623, 1964.

Abel, J. A.: Analgesic nephropathy—a review of the literature, 1967–70. Clin. Pharmacol. Ther. 12:583, 1971.

Abrahams, C.: More on the pathology of analgesic abuse. N. Engl. J. Med. 301:437, 1979.

Adams, F. G., and Murray, R. M.: The radiologic diagnosis of analgesic nephropathy. Clin. Radiol. 26:417, 1975.

Bengtsson, U., Angervall, L., Ekman, H., and Lehmann, L.: Transitional cell tumors of the renal pelvis in analgesic abusers. Scand. J. Urol. Nephrol. 2:145, 1968.

Bengtsson, U., Johansson, S., and Angervall, L.: Malignancies of the urinary tract and their relation to analgesic abuse. Kidney Int. 13:107, 1978.

Berman, L. B.: Sickle cell nephropathy. JAMA 228:1279, 1974.

Berning, H., Orellana, K., and Selberg, W.: Nierenpapillenekrosen, Klinische Pathologie von 238 Beobachtungen. Dtsch. Med. Wochenschr. 99:1749, 1974.

Braden, G. L., Kozinn, D. R., Hampf, F. E., Parker, T. H., and Germain, M. J.: Ultrasound diagnosis of early renal papillary necrosis. J. Ultrasound Med. 10:401, 1991.

Brezin, J. H., Katz, S. M., Schwartz, A. B., and Chinitz, J. L.: Reversible renal failure and nephrotic syndrome associated with nonsteroidal anti-inflammatory drugs. N. Engl. J. Med. 301:1271, 1979.

Burry, A. F.: The evolution of analgesic nephropathy. Nephron 5:185, 1968.

Burry, A. F.: The pathology and pathogenesis of renal papillary necrosis, renal infection and renal scarring. In Kincaid-Smith, P., and Fairley, K. F. (eds.): Renal Infection and Renal Scarring. Proceedings of the International Symposium on Pyelonephritis, Vesico-ureteral Reflux and Renal Papillary Necrosis. Melbourne, Mercedes Publishing Co., 1971.

Burry, A.: Pathology of analgesic nephropathy: Australian experience. Kidney Int. 13:34, 1978.

Chrispin A. R.: Medullary necrosis in infancy. Br. Med. Bull. 28:233, 1972.

Cuttino, J. T., Jr., Herman, P. G., and Mellins, H. W.: The renal collecting system after medullary damage. Invest. Radiol. 12:241, 1977.

Duggin, G. G.: Mechanisms in the development of analgesic nephropathy. Kidney Int. 18:553, 1980.

Eckert, D. E., Jonutis, A. J., and Davidson, A. J.: The incidence and manifestations of urographic papillary abnormalities in patients with S-hemoglobinopathies. Radiology 113:59, 1974.

Editorial, Analgesic nephropathy or phenacetin poisoning. Br. Med. J. 1:588, 1974.

Fairley, K. F., and Kincaid-Smith, P.: Renal papillary necrosis with a normal pyelogram. Br. Med. J. 1:156, 1968.

Gaakeer, H. A., and DeRuiter, H. J.: Carcinoma of the renal pelvis following the abuse of phenacetin-containing analgesic drugs. Br. J. Urol. 51:188, 1979.

Gloor, F. J.: Changing concepts in pathogenesis and morphology of analgesic nephropathy as seen in Europe. Kidney Int. 13:27, 1978.

Handa, S. P., and Tewari, H. D.: Urinary tract carcinoma in patients with analgesic nephropathy. Nephron 28:62, 1981.

Hare, W. S. C.: The radiology of analgesic nephropathy. In Kincaid-Smith, P., and Fairley, K. F. (eds.): Renal Infection and Renal Scarring. Proceedings of the International Symposium on Pyelonephritis, Vesico-ureteral Reflux and Renal Papillary Necrosis. Melbourne, Mercedes Publishing Co., 1971.

Hare, W. S. C., and Poynter, J. D.: The radiology of renal papillary necrosis as seen in analgesic nephropathy. Clin. Radiol. 25:423, 1974.

Harrow, B. R., Sloane, J. A., and Liebman, N. C.: Roentgenologic demonstration of renal papillary necrosis in sickle-cell trait. N. Engl. J. Med. 268:969, 1963.

Harrow, B. R.: Nephropathy of diabetes with emphasis on papillary necrosis. Postgrad. Med. 37:A63, 1965.

Harrow, B. R.: Renal papillary necrosis: A critique of pathogenesis. J. Urol. 97:203, 1967.

Hartman, G. W., Torres, V. E., Leago, G. F., Williamson, B., Jr., and Hattery, R. R.: Analgesic-associated nephropathy: Pathophysiological and radiological correlation. JAMA 251:1734, 1984.

Henrich, W. L.: Nephrotoxicity of nonsteroidal anti-inflammatory agents. In Schrier, R. W., and Gottschalk, C. W. (eds.): Diseases of the Kidney. 4th ed. Boston, Little, Brown & Co., 1988, pp. 1319–1336.

Heptinstall, R. H. (ed.): Pathology of the Kidney. 4th ed. Boston, Little, Brown & Co., 1992.

Hodson, C. J.: Differential diagnosis between atrophic pyelonephritis and analgesic nephropathy. In Kincaid-Smith, P., and Fairley, K. F. (eds.): Renal Infection and Renal Scarring. Proceedings of the International Symposium on Pyelonephritis, Vesico-ureteral Reflux and Renal Papillary Necrosis. Melbourne, Mercedes Publishing Co., 1971.

Hoffman, J. C., Schnur, M. J., and Koenigsberg, M.: Demonstration of renal papillary necrosis by sonography. Radiology 145:785, 1982.

Husserl, F. E., Lange, R. K., and Kantrow, C. M., Jr.: Renal papillary necrosis and pyelonephritis accompanying fenoprofen therapy. JAMA 242:1896, 1979.

Johansson, S., Angervall, L., Bengtsson, U., and Wahlqvist, L.: Uroepithelial tumors of the renal pelvis associated with abuse of phenacetin-containing analgesics. Cancer 33:743, 1974.

Kincaid-Smith, P.: Pathogenesis of the renal lesion associated with the abuse of analgesics. Lancet 1:859, 1967.

Kincaid-Smith, P.: Analgesic nephropathy. Kidney Int. 13:1, 1978.

Kincaid-Smith, P., and Nanra, R.S.: Lithium-induced and analgesic-induced renal diseases. *In* Schrier, R. W., and Gottschalk, C. W. (eds.): Diseases of the Kidney. 4th ed. Boston, Little, Brown & Co., 1988, pp. 1197–1228.

Levine, E., and Bernard, D.: Analgesic nephropathy: A clinicoradiological study. S. Afr. Med. J. *47:*2439, 1973.

Lindvall, N.: Renal papillary necrosis, a roentgenographic study of 155 cases. Acta Radiol. (Suppl.) *192,* 1960.

Lindvall, N.: Radiological changes of renal papillary necrosis. Kidney Int. *13:*93, 1978.

Longacre, A. M., and Popky, G. L.: Papillary necrosis in patients with cirrhosis: A study of 102 patients. J. Urol. *99:*391, 1968.

Lourie, S. H., Denman, S. J., and Schroeder, E. T.: Association of renal papillary necrosis and ankylosing spondylitis. Arthritis Rheum. *20:*917, 1977.

McCall, I. W., Moule, N., Desai, P., and Serjeant, G. R.: Urographic findings in homozygous sickle cell disease. Radiology *126:*99, 1978.

McCredie, M., Coates, M. S., Ford, J. M., Disney, A. P. S., Auld, J. J., and Stewart, J. H.: Geographic distribution of cancers of the kidney and urinary tract and analgesic nephropathy in Australia and New Zealand. Aust. N. Z. J. Med. *20:*684, 1990.

Mellins, H. Z.: Chronic pyelonephritis and renal medullary necrosis. Semin. Roentgenol. *6:*292, 1971.

Molland, E. A.: Experimental renal papillary necrosis. Kidney Int. *13:*5, 1978.

Murray, G., Wyllie, R. G., Hill, G. S., Ramsden, P. W., and Heptinstall, R. H.: Experimental papillary necrosis of the kidney: I. Morphologic and functional data. Am. J. Pathol. *68:*285, 1972.

Murray, T. G., and Goldberg, M.: Analgesic-associated nephropathy in the U.S.A.: Epidemiologic, clinical and pathogenetic features. Kidney Int. *13:*64, 1978.

Nanra, R. S., Chirawong, P., and Kincaid-Smith, P.: Medullary nephropathy—the pathogenesis of renal papillary necrosis. Aust. N.Z. J. Med. *3:*580, 1973.

Nanra, R. S.: Analgesic nephropathy. Med. J. Aust. *1:*745, 1976.

Pandya, K. K., Koshy, M., Brown, N., and Presman, D.: Renal papillary necrosis in sickle cell hemoglobinopathies. J. Urol. *115:*497, 1976.

Perillie, P. E., and Epstein, F. H.: Sickling phenomenon produced by hypertonic solutions: A possible explanation for the hyposthenuria of sicklemia. J. Clin. Invest. *42:*570, 1963.

Poynter, J. D., and Hare, W. S. C.: Necrosis *in situ:* A form of renal papillary necrosis seen in analgesic nephropathy. Radiology *111:*69, 1974.

Puvaneswary, M., and Segasothy, M.: Analgesic nephropathy: Ultrasonic features. Aust. Radiol. *32:*247, 1988.

Roberts, G. M., Evans, K. T., Bloom, A. L., and Al-Gailani, F.: Renal papillary necrosis in haemophilia and Christmas disease. Clin. Radiol. *34:*201, 1983.

Sandler, D. P., Burr, R., and Weinberg, C.R.: Nonsteroidal anti-inflammatory drugs and the risk for chronic renal disease. Ann. Intern. Med. *115:*165, 1991.

Sherwood, T., Swales, J. D., and Tange, J. D.: Experimental renal papillary necrosis: Progressive changes on intravenous urography. Invest. Radiol. *6:*239, 1971.

Sherwood, T., Doyle, F. H., Boulton-Jones, M., Joekes, A. M., Peters, D. K., and Sissons, P.: The intravenous urogram in acute renal failure. Br. J. Radiol. *47:*368, 1974.

Talner, L. B., Webb, J. A. W., and Dail, D. H.: Lacunae: A urographic finding in chronic obstructive uropathy. AJR *156:*985, 1991.

Ulreich, S.: Ultrasound in the evaluation of renal papillary necrosis. Radiology *148:*864, 1983.

Van Eps, L. W. S., Pinedo-Veels, C., deVries, G. H., and deKoning, J.: Nature of concentrating defect in sickle-cell nephropathy: Microradioangiographic studies. Lancet *1:*450, 1970.

Wagner, E. H.: Nonsteroidal anti-inflammatory drugs and renal disease—still unsettled (editorial). Ann. Intern. Med. *115:*227, 1991.

Weber, M., Braun, B., and Kohler, H.: Ultrasonic findings in analgesic nephropathy. Nephron *39:*216, 1985.

Whelton, A., and Hamilton, C. W.: Nonsteroidal anti-inflammatory drugs: Effects on kidney function. J. Clin. Pharmacol. *31:*588, 1991.

Zwergel, U. E., Zwergel, T. B. H., Neisius, D. A., and Ziegler, M.: Effects of prostaglandin synthetase inhibitors on the upper urinary tract. Urol. Res. *18:*429, 1990.

Hereditary Chronic Nephritis

Atkin, C. L., Gregory, M. C., and Border, W. A.: Alport syndrome. *In* Schrier, R. W., and Gottschalk, C. W. (eds.) Diseases of the Kidney. 4th ed. Boston, Little, Brown & Co., 1988, pp. 617–643.

Chuang, V. P., and Reuter, S. R.: Angiographic features of Alport's syndrome: Hereditary nephritis. AJR *121:*593, 1974.

Demetropoulos, K. C., Hoskins, P., and Rapp, R.: Angiographic study of hereditary nephritis (Alport's syndrome). Radiology *108:*539, 1973.

Kashtan, C. E., and Michael, A. F.: Hereditary nephritis. Semin. Nephrol. *9:*135, 1989.

Perkoff, G. T.: The hereditary renal diseases. N. Engl. J. Med. *277:*79, 1967.

Purriel, P., Drets, M., Cestau, R. S., Borras, A., Ferreira, W. A., De Lucca, A., and Fernandez, L.: Familial hereditary nephropathy (Alport's syndrome). Am. J. Med. *49:*753, 1970.

Medullary Cystic Disease

Burgener, F. A., and Spataro, R. F.: Early medullary cystic disease: A urographic diagnosis? Radiology *130:*321, 1979.

Cantani, A., Bamonte, G., Ceccoli, D., Biribicchi G., and Farinella, F.: Familial juvenile nephronophthisis: A review and differential diagnosis. Clin. Pediatr. *25:*90, 1986.

Case records of the Massachusetts General Hospital: Case 15–1970. Medullary cystic disease. N. Engl. J. Med. *282:*799, 1970.

Fanconi, G., Hanhart, V. E., Albertini, A., Uhlinger, E., Dolivo, G., and Prader, A.: Die familiäre juvenile Nephronopthise. Die idiopatische parenchymatöse Schrumpfeniere. Helv. Paediatr. Acta *6:*1, 1951.

Gardner, K. D., Jr.: Evolution of clinical signs in adult-onset cystic disease of the renal medulla. Ann. Intern. Med. *74:*47, 1971.

Gardner, K. D., Jr.: Medullary and miscellaneous renal cystic disorders. *In* Schrier, R. W., and Gottschalk, C. W. (eds.): Diseases of the Kidney. 4th ed. Boston, Little, Brown & Co., 1988, pp. 559–572.

Gardner, K. D., Jr., and Bernstein, J. (eds.): The Cystic Kidney. Boston, Kluwer Academic Publishers, 1990.

Giangiacomo, J., Monteleone, P. L., and Witzleben, C. L.: Medullary cystic disease vs. nephronophthisis: A valid distinction? JAMA *232:*629, 1975.

Link, D. P., Hansen, S., and Palmer, J.: High dose excretory urography and medullary cystic disease of the kidney. AJR *133:*303, 1979.

Mena, E., Bookstein, J. J., McDonald, F. D., and Gikas, P. W.: Angiographic findings in renal medullary cystic disease. Radiology *110:*277, 1973.

Mongsau, J. G., and Worthen, H. G.: Nephronophthisis and medullary cystic disease. Am. J. Med. *43:*345, 1967.

Olsen, A., Hojhus, J. H., and Steffensen, G.: Renal medullary cystic disease: Findings at urography and ultrasonography. Acta Radiol. *29:*527, 1988.

Rego, J. D., Jr., Laing, F. C., and Jeffrey, R. B.: Ultrasonic diagnosis of medullary cystic disease. J. Ultrasound Med. *2:*433, 1983.

Risdon, R. A.: Development, developmental defects, and cystic diseases of the kidney. *In* Heptinstall, R. H. (ed.): Pathology of the Kidney. 4th ed. Boston, Little, Brown & Co., 1992, pp. 93–168.

Rosenfield, A. T., Siegel, N. J., and Kappelman, N. B.: Gray scale ultrasonography in medullary cystic disease of the kidney and congenital hepatic fibrosis with tubular ectasia: New observations. AJR *129:*297, 1977.

Spicer, R. D., Ogg, C. S., Saxton, H. M., and Cameron, J. S.: Renal medullary cystic disease. Br. Med. J. *1:*824, 1969.

Steele, B. T., Lirenman, D. S., and Beattie, C. W.: Nephronophthisis. Am. J. Med. *68:*531, 1980.

Swenson, R. S., Kempson, R. L., and Friedland, G. W.: Cystic disease of the renal medulla in the elderly. JAMA *228:*1401, 1974.

Wood, B. P.: Renal cystic disease in infants and children. Urol. Radiol. *14:*284, 1992.

Arterial Hypotension

Fry, I. K., and Cattell, W. R.: Nephrogram pattern during excretion urography. Br. Med. Bull. 28:227, 1972.

Haber, K.: Changes in renal size as related to blood pressure during an idiosyncratic reaction to radiographic contrast. J. Urol. 111:288, 1974.

Hodson, C. J.: Physiological changes in size of the human kidney. Clin. Radiol. 12:91, 1961.

Katzberg, R. W., and Schabel, S. T.: Bilaterally small kidneys in shock. JAMA 235:2213, 1976.

Korobkin, M. T., Kirkwood, R., and Minagi, H.: The nephrogram of hypotension. Radiology 98:129, 1971.

Korobkin, M.: The nephrogram of hemorrhagic hypotension. AJR 114:673, 1972.

Korobkin, M., Shanser, J. D., and Carlson, E. L.: The nephrogram of normovolemic, renal artery hypotension. Invest. Radiol. 11:71, 1976.

Wickbom, I.: The influence of the blood pressure in urographic examination (preliminary report). Acta Radiol. 34:1, 1950.

8

DIAGNOSTIC SET: LARGE, SMOOTH, BILATERAL

PROLIFERATIVE/NECROTIZING
DISORDERS

ABNORMAL PROTEIN DEPOSITION
  Amyloidosis
  Multiple Myeloma

ABNORMAL FLUID ACCUMULATION
  Acute Tubular Necrosis
  Acute Cortical Necrosis

NEOPLASTIC CELL INFILTRATION
  Leukemia

INFLAMMATORY CELL INFILTRATION
  Acute Interstitial Nephritis

AUTOSOMAL RECESSIVE (INFANTILE)
POLYCYSTIC KIDNEY DISEASE

MISCELLANEOUS CONDITIONS
  Acute Urate Nephropathy
  Glycogen Storage Disease, Type I (Von
    Gierke's Disease)
  Physiologic Response to Contrast Material
    and Diuretics
  Homozygous-S Disease
  Paroxysmal Nocturnal Hemoglobinuria
  Hemophilia
  Nephromegaly Associated with Cirrhosis,
    Hyperalimentation, and Diabetes
    Mellitus
  Acromegaly
  Fabry's Disease
  Bartter's Syndrome
  Beckwith-Weidemann Syndrome

DIFFERENTIAL DIAGNOSIS

Most of the diseases discussed in this chapter present as renal failure that has been apparent for only a short time. The value of performing radiologic studies on patients with these diseases lies in the demonstration of bilaterally enlarged, smooth, nonobstructed kidneys. The collecting structures are either normal or generally effaced by the swollen kidneys. When these findings are present, it can be surmised that the disease is parenchymal, of recent onset, and possibly reversible. Once this is established, the nephrologist usually turns to the study of needle biopsy tissue by light and electron microscopy and by immunologic techniques for a more specific diagnosis, since clinical, laboratory, and radiologic features overlap and are nonspecific in acute renal failure.

On the other hand, there are some diseases or conditions in the diagnostic set, "large, smooth, bilateral," that are of long standing and not associated with acute renal failure. In addition to autosomal recessive (infantile) polycystic kidney disease, these include a miscellaneous group that have clinical and/or radiologic features that distinguish them from the more commonly encountered causes of acute renal failure.

It is important for the radiologist to have some grasp of the varied diseases that cause global enlargement of both kidneys, even though most of these cannot be specifically diagnosed by radiologic techniques. The organization of this chapter is based for the most part on the mechanism of renal enlargement, namely, excessive cellular infiltration or proliferation, abnormal deposition of proteins, or increased accumulation of interstitial edema or blood. With this approach, diseases are grouped under the following categories: proliferative/necrotizing disorders, abnormal protein deposition, abnormal fluid accumulation, neoplastic infiltration, and inflammatory infiltration. The final sections include autosomal recessive (infantile) polycystic kidney disease and a miscellaneous group of unrelated diseases and physiologic states in which both kidneys enlarge.

PROLIFERATIVE/NECROTIZING DISORDERS
Definition

In general, the proliferative and necrotizing diseases that cause smooth enlargement of the total renal mass fall into two groups: those that affect the kidneys alone and those that affect the kidneys as part of a multisystemic disorder. In both cases, the glomerulus is the principal site of abnormalities, which include proliferation or necrosis of cellular elements, increased lobulation, and enlargement of epithelial cells. Fibrinous and proteinaceous deposits may be found in the capsular space. The morphologic diagnosis of a specific disease within this group is dependent on integrating light, electron, and immunofluorescent microscopic patterns of glomerular involvement with other clinical or laboratory abnormalities.

These various disorders also affect other structural components of the kidney, particularly the blood vessels and the interstitium, but in a nonspecific way. The interlobular arteries may show collagenous intimal thickening, and in some of these diseases there are necrotizing cellular changes and thrombosis of small arteries, arterioles, and capillaries. Edema, scattered foci of round cells, and a fine fibrosis are frequently seen in the interstitial space.

The net effect of these abnormalities is an increase in renal bulk and an impairment of renal function, particularly glomerular filtration. Both of these features produce radiologic abnormalities.

Clinical Setting

The proliferative/necrotizing disorders that affect the kidney alone are those of the acute glomerulonephritides. These include *acute (post-streptococcal) glomerulonephritis, rapidly progressive glomerulonephritis, idiopathic membranous glomerulonephritis, membranoproliferative glomerulonephritis, IgA nephropathy glomerulosclerosis, glomerulosclerosis related to heroin abuse,* and *lobular glomerulonephritis.* All are characterized by enlargement of both kidneys during the early phase of the illness. Some, like acute (post-streptococcal) glomerulonephritis, cause kidneys to become globally small with chronic renal failure after a considerable period of time if resolution does not occur. In others, such as idiopathic membranous glomerulonephritis, kidneys may remain normal to slightly enlarged even after a protracted period of clinical disease. When the disease is rapid and unrelenting, such as often occurs in rapidly progressive glomerulonephritis, the kidneys will remain large throughout the course of the illness.

Patients with these diseases of the kidney have smoky urine, periorbital and peripheral edema, and cardiovascular symptoms related to salt and water retention and hypertension. The nephrotic syndrome is often present, as are nitrogen retention and hematuria. Red blood cell, granular, and leukocyte casts are found in the urine. At times, a normochromic, normocytic anemia develops. There is considerable overlap in signs and symptoms among all the acute glomerulonephritides.

Proliferative and necrotizing abnormalities of the glomerulus also occur in multisystemic diseases. These include *polyarteritis nodosa* (microscopic form), *systemic lupus erythematosus, Wegener's granulomatosis, allergic angiitis, diabetic glomerulosclerosis, lung hemorrhage* and *glomerulonephritis (Goodpasture's syndrome), anaphylactoid purpura (Schönlein-Henoch syndrome), thrombotic thrombocytopenic purpura* in adults and *hemolytic-uremic syndrome* in infants and children, *focal glomerulonephritis associated with subacute bacterial endocarditis,* and the *nephropathy of acquired immunodeficiency syndrome.* In these diseases, clinical features that are more disease specific are superimposed on features generally found in isolated acute glomerular disease. For example, fever, arthritis, abdominal pain, polyneuritis, leukocytosis, and eosinophilia occur in addition to nitrogen retention, hematuria, proteinuria, and cylindruria in patients with the "microscopic" form of polyarteritis nodosa and systemic lupus erythematosus.

Some diseases in this group have more specific patterns. Granulomatous lesions with vascular necrosis are found in the kidney, lungs, and upper respiratory tract in Wegener's granulomatosis. Granulomatous foci occur in many organs in allergic angiitis, a syndrome that also includes asthma, fever, and eosinophilia in addition to the signs and symptoms produced by the renal lesion. Goodpasture's syndrome is a combination of glomerular disease and necrotizing alveolitis producing lung hemorrhage. Hemoptysis, dyspnea, and anemia appear during a rapidly progressive course of renal failure, which usually leads to death after a short time. In Schönlein-Henoch syndrome, purpuric skin lesions, intestinal colic, intussusception, joint pains, and gastrointestinal bleeding reflect involvement of the skin, gastrointestinal tract, and joints, whereas hematuria and proteinuria represent the glomerular disease seen in most of these patients. Thrombotic thrombocytopenic purpura is characterized by hemolytic anemia, hemorrhage, oliguric or anuric renal failure, gastrointestinal bleeding, and central nervous system dysfunction in adults. This results from erythrocyte fragmentation, thrombocytopenia, and intravascular coagulation. The same condition is known as the hemolytic-uremic syndrome when it occurs in infants and children. Acute cortical necrosis may be a component of the hemolytic-uremic syndrome and result in chronic renal failure.

Acute glomerular lesions and enlarged kidneys are present only in the "microscopic" form of polyarteritis nodosa. The other mode of presentation, bilaterally small kidneys, is seen in the "classic" form, which is discussed in Chapter 7.

Immunologic mechanisms have been established for some of the acute disorders of glomeruli, whereas in others the pathogenesis remains obscure. A variety of glomerular abnormalities causing acute renal failure have been described in some cases of acquired immunodeficiency syndrome. The reader is referred to sources cited in the bibliography for a more thorough background on each of these diseases.

Radiologic Findings

Invariably, both kidneys are involved in the proliferative and necrotizing disorders of the glomerulus, although asymmetry has been reported. Renal size varies from normal to markedly enlarged. Because involvement is global, parenchymal thickening is equal throughout and the contour remains smooth.

Ultrasonography is the most efficacious test for the demonstration of the radiologic findings that are characteristic of necrotizing and proliferative disorders of the glomerulus: bilaterally large, smooth kidneys; a homogeneous pattern of normal to increased (relative to the liver) echo intensity; and the absence of pelvo-calyceal dilatation (Fig. 8–1). These findings indicate that the renal failure is acute and not due to obstruction of both kidneys ("postrenal failure") but give no indication of either the specific nature or the severity of the disease. Diagnostic evaluation thereafter is directed to renal biopsy. Unique within this group of diseases, hemolytic-uremic syndrome characteristically produces selective hyperechoicity of the cortex relative to the medulla (Fig. 8–2). This pattern probably is due to platelet aggregation and fibrin thrombi within the microvasculature of the cortex in addition to swelling of endothelial and mesangial cells of the glomeruli. The degree of cortical hyperechoicity correlates well with the severity of renal impairment in the hemolytic-uremic syndrome but does not predict outcome (Choyke et al., 1988).

When ultrasonography is not available, excretory urography can be used to determine the presence of bilaterally enlarged, smooth, nonobstructed kidneys (Figs. 8–3 through 8–5). Glomerular functional impairment is often severe enough to require both high doses of contrast material (up to 750 mg of iodine per kilogram of body weight) and tomography to evaluate the nephrogram and visualize the pelvocalyceal system. Alerted by adequate clinical information regarding the state of renal function *before* the examination, the radiologist should obtain tomograms before injecting contrast material. These preliminary films allow for any necessary adjustments of radiographic technique and provide baseline data for detecting

minimal degrees of parenchymal opacification. To take advantage of the period during which the plasma level of contrast material is highest, tomograms should be exposed between 10 and 30 minutes after the contrast material is injected. This is quite different from obstructive uropathy, in which delayed opacification occurs. The nephrogram is homogeneous, and its density varies from normal to faint. During the course of a radiologic study using contrast material, the density of the nephrogram may persist unchanged or may become increasingly opaque. Pelvocalyceal opacification varies from normal to only a faint calyceal outline discerned on standard or computed tomograms (Fig. 8–6).

Extrarenal excretion of contrast material by the intestinal mucosa and hepatobiliary system is seen occasionally in these patients as an opacification of the colon on films taken 1 or 2 days after excretory urography (Fig. 8–7).

The radiologist should insist that *the patient always be examined in an appropriately hydrated state. Contrast material should not be administered to a patient with renal failure who has been dehydrated.* Chapters 1 and 24 present a more detailed discussion of the radiologic examination of patients in renal failure.

Angiographic findings in the renal arterial bed are quite nonspecific in the proliferative and necrotizing diseases of the glomerulus. Aneurysms of medium-sized vessels associated with polyarteritis nodosa are seen in the "classic" form of this disease, which is associated with small kidneys.

Text continued on page 211

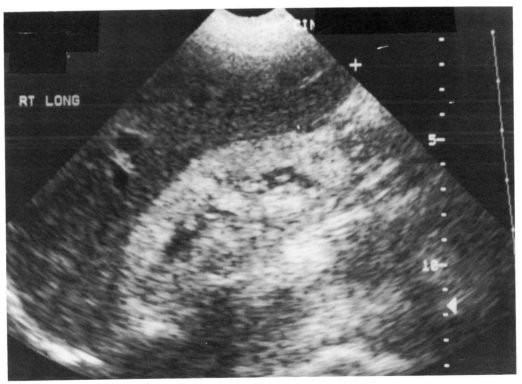

Figure 8–1. Lupus nephritis in a 28-year-old woman. Ultrasonogram in a longitudinal section demonstrates a right kidney that is smooth in contour and enlarged for a person of small stature. There is diffuse hyperechoicity relative to the liver. The left kidney had similar characteristics. (Kindly provided by Wendelin S. Hayes, D.O., Department of Radiologic Pathology, Armed Forces Institute of Pathology, Washington, D.C.)

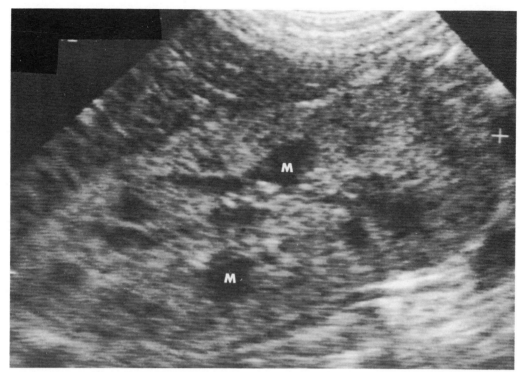

Figure 8–2. Hemolytic-uremic syndrome in a 5-year-old girl with azotemia, oliguria, diarrhea, and dehydration. Ultrasonogram of the enlarged right kidney demonstrates a hyperechoic cortex relative to the liver and hypoechoic medullae (M). (Kindly provided by Peter Choyke, M.D., Department of Radiology, National Institutes of Health, Bethesda, Maryland.)

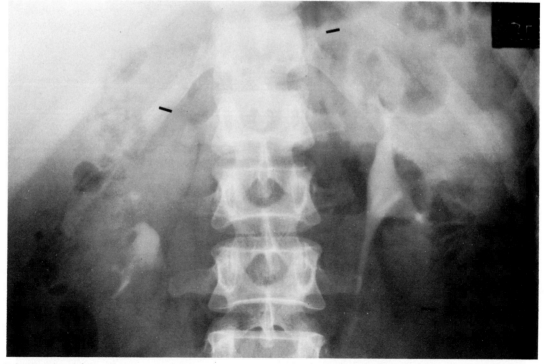

Figure 8–3. Polyarteritis nodosa (microscopic form) in a middle-aged man with fever, arthralgia, and renal failure. The diseases in the diagnostic set "large, smooth, bilateral" cause kidney length to vary from the upper range of normal, as in this case, to marked elongation.
  Right kidney length = 12.5 cm; left kidney length = 14.0 cm. (Courtesy of Department of Diagnostic Radiology, Hammersmith Hospital, Royal Postgraduate Medical School, London, England.)

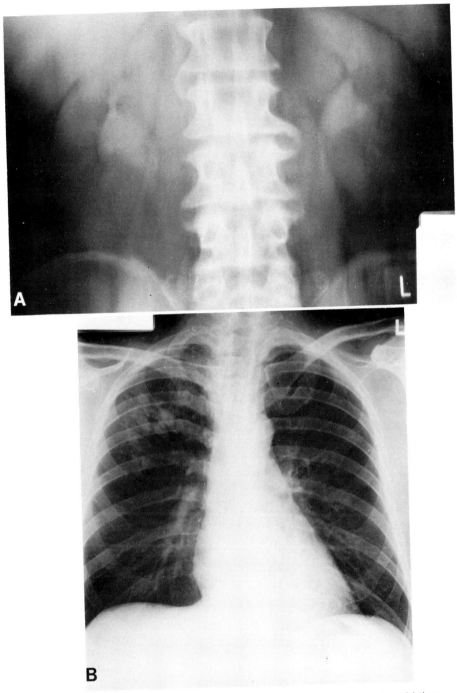

Figure 8–4. Goodpasture's syndrome in a 54-year-old man with hemoptysis, microscopic hematuria, and renal failure.
A, Tomogram during excretory urography. The kidneys are moderately enlarged, with smooth contours and impaired contrast material excretion. Right kidney length = 14.0 cm; left kidney length = 14.5 cm.
B, Chest film demonstrates abnormal densities in right upper lung field, representing pulmonary bleeding.
(Courtesy of Department of Diagnostic Radiology, Hammersmith Hospital, Royal Postgraduate Medical School, London, England.)

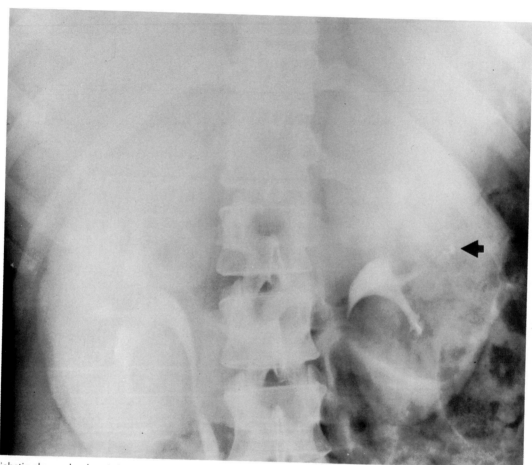

Figure 8–5. Diabetic glomerulosclerosis in a 26-year-old woman with severe juvenile diabetes mellitus. A focus of papillary necrosis is present in the left kidney *(arrow)*.
  Right kidney length = 15.4 cm; left kidney length = 15.5 cm.

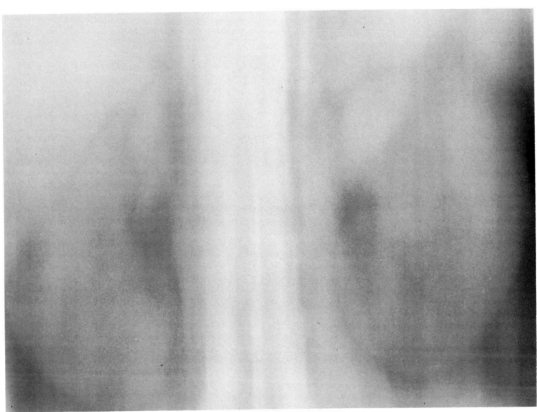

Figure 8–6. Rapidly progressive glomerulonephritis in a 42-year-old man. Tomogram obtained 10 minutes after injection of 37.5 gm of iodine (125 ml of sodium diatrizoate 50%). Nephrographic density, always faint, was maximal at this time. Calyces were never visualized. Absence of an increasingly dense nephrogram and no collecting system opacification at 24 hours is strong evidence of a renal, rather than postrenal, cause of kidney failure. Right kidney length = 20.7 cm; left kidney length = 20.0 cm.

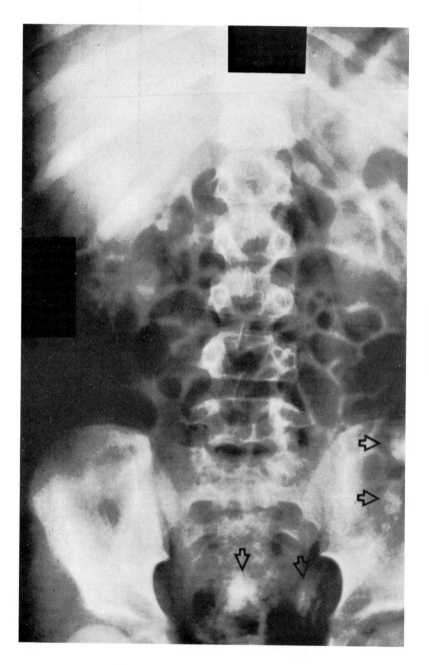

Figure 8–7. Extrarenal excretion of contrast material in a youth with acute glomerulonephritis and blood urea nitrogen of 160 mg/dl. Opacification of distal descending and sigmoid colon is present on a film taken 32 hours after intravenous injection of contrast material *(arrows)*. A faint nephrogram persists.

**SUMMARY OF ABNORMAL URORADIOLOGIC FINDINGS
PROLIFERATIVE/NECROTIZING DISORDERS**

Primary Uroradiologic Elements
  Size—normal to large
  Contour—smooth (global)
  Lesion distribution—bilateral
Secondary Uroradiologic Elements
  Pelvoinfundibulocalyceal system—attenuated (global) occasionally
  Parenchymal thickness—expanded (global)
  Nephrogram—contrast material density diminished; increasingly dense (uncommon)
  Echogenicity—normal to increased (diffuse); increased (cortex) in hemolytic-uremic
    syndrome

ABNORMAL PROTEIN DEPOSITION

Amyloidosis

Definition

Amyloidosis is characterized by the accumulation of extracellular eosinophilic protein substances in various organs of the body. The kidneys are involved in over 80 per cent of cases of amyloidosis secondary to chronic suppurative or inflammatory disease. Renal involvement is found in approximately 35 per cent of patients with primary amyloidosis in which the breast, alimentary tract, tongue, spleen, and connective tissue may also be affected.

The glomerulus is the principal site of amyloid deposition. The interstitium and the media and the adventitia of the interlobular arteries are frequently also involved. Round cell accumulation and a fine fibrosis develop in the interstitium, while the tubules become atrophic and actually may disappear in advanced disease.

Amyloid accumulation initially produces bilaterally enlarged, smooth kidneys. With time, however, the kidney in amyloidosis becomes diffusely wasted. This presumably reflects ischemic changes caused by amyloid involvement of arteries over a long period of time. Similarly, ischemia probably accounts for the tubule atrophy and interstitial fibrosis seen in this disease.

Clinical Setting

Renal amyloidosis occurs either in the primary form or in association with chronic suppurative or inflammatory diseases such as tuberculosis, osteomyelitis, bronchiectasis, ulcerative colitis, and rheumatoid arthritis. Amyloid deposition is also seen in the kidneys of patients with multiple myeloma and Waldenström's macroglobulinemia. In familial Mediterranean fever, amyloidosis is common and often severe enough to cause renal failure.

Although some patients may be asymptomatic and show no signs of renal impairment, proteinuria is present in most cases and may be part of the nephrotic syndrome. Nitrogen retention occurs but is usually not advanced until late in the disease. Hypertension is either absent or not as severe as in other forms of chronic renal failure. Renal vein thrombosis is a well-recognized complication of renal amyloidosis and may transform a patient with mild chronic renal failure into one with acute oliguric failure.

Radiologic Findings

In the early stage of renal amyloidosis, the kidneys are enlarged and smooth in contour, with normal to impaired opacification and normal collecting systems (Fig. 8–8). With time, the kidneys decrease in size and eventually become small (Fig. 8–9).

When renal vein thrombosis complicates amyloi-

**SUMMARY OF ABNORMAL URORADIOLOGIC FINDINGS
AMYLOIDOSIS**

Primary Uroradiologic Elements
  Size—normal to large (becomes small with time)
  Contour—smooth (global)
  Lesion distribution—bilateral
Secondary Uroradiologic Elements
  Pelvoinfundibulocalyceal system—attenuated (global) occasionally
  Parenchymal thickness—expanded (global); becomes wasted with time
  Nephrogram—contrast material density normal to diminished
  Echogenicity—normal to increased
  Renal vein—thrombus (occasionally)

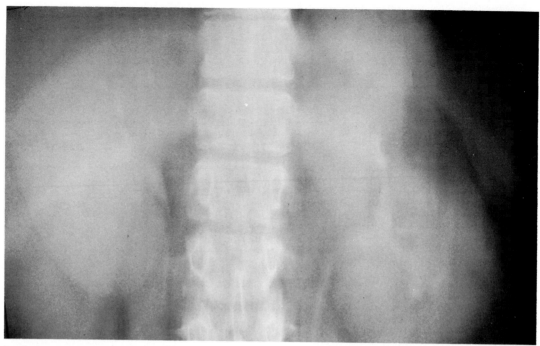

Figure 8–8. Amyloidosis in a 28-year-old man with proteinuria and a history of Still's disease, diagnosed 23 years earlier. Bilateral global renal enlargement, impaired contrast material excretion, and normal pelvocalyceal systems are noted. Right kidney length = 14.2 cm; left kidney length = 14.3 cm. (Courtesy of Department of Diagnostic Radiology, Hammersmith Hospital, Royal Postgraduate Medical School, London, England.)

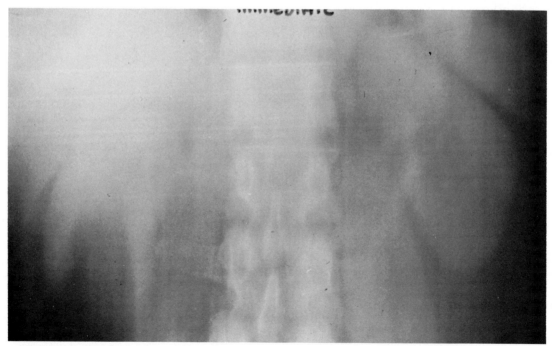

Figure 8–9. Amyloidosis presenting as bilaterally small, smooth kidneys and renal failure in a 34-year-old drug addict with chronic leg infection. Small kidneys may be the result of ischemia following amyloid involvement of the blood vessels. Right kidney length = 10.2 cm; left kidney length = 11.7 cm. (Courtesy of Department of Diagnostic Radiology, Hammersmith Hospital, Royal Postgraduate Medical School, London, England.)

dosis, renal function is acutely impaired. This can be demonstrated radiologically by decreased kidney opacification. Renal vein thrombosis can be confirmed by venography, ultrasonography, computed tomography, or magnetic resonance imaging.

The echogenicity of the renal parenchyma is normal to increased in a nonspecific pattern in renal amyloidosis. Ultrasonography effectively documents the change in renal size and also the smooth contour.

Renal angiography in the amyloid kidney demonstrates normal main renal arteries but excessive narrowing of peripheral arteries, which may become irregular and incompletely filled. Aneurysms sometimes form in small vessels, which may rupture. Loss of corticomedullary demarcation may be seen during the angiographic nephrogram phase. These vascular abnormalities are nonspecific, and there is no basis for the use of angiography to diagnose renal amyloidosis.

Multiple Myeloma

Definition

Multiple myeloma causes renal insufficiency in 30 to 50 per cent of cases as a result of precipitation of abnormal proteins in the tubule lumina. Renal function may also be compromised by impaired renal blood flow due to increased blood viscosity, by nephrocalcinosis resulting from hypercalcemia, by Bence Jones protein toxicity on the tubules, and by amyloidosis. Diffuse infiltration of plasma cells per se occurs uncommonly and is usually not associated with a clinically recognizable disturbance in renal function.

Casts of albumin, fibrinogen, IgG, and Bence Jones proteins obstruct distal convoluted tubules and collecting ducts and are surrounded by varying degrees of giant cell reaction. Intratubular obstruction is followed by atrophy of affected nephrons. Lymphocytic infiltration and a fine fibrosis are present in the interstitium. When acute renal failure develops, the interstitium becomes edematous as well. Glomeruli are either normal or show evidence of ischemia and amyloid deposition.

Most myelomatous kidneys are enlarged. As in amyloidosis, some kidneys eventually become small. Because involvement is global, the pelvocalyceal rela-

tionships remain normal, and the kidney surface is smooth. Enlargement is most marked when acute renal failure supervenes.

Clinical Setting

Multiple myeloma is characterized by the presence of abnormal proteins in serum and urine. These are derived from the proliferation of abnormal plasma cells. Symptoms are insidious in onset and include progressive weakness, weight loss, anorexia, nausea and vomiting, and bone pain.

Proteinuria is present in more than 50 per cent of myeloma patients. Renal failure may be chronic or may present acutely as oliguria or anuria.

Radiologic Findings

Radiologically, myelomatous kidneys are smooth and often markedly enlarged. Ultrasonographic echo patterns vary from normal to increased. Reduced opacification reflects impaired renal function (Fig. 8–10). The pelvoinfundibulocalyceal relationships are normal, but these structures may become diffusely attenuated when the kidneys are swollen owing to large amounts of intratubular protein deposition, causing tubule blockage and interstitial edema. This results in acute oliguric failure and an increasingly dense nephrogram. The distance between the interpapillary line and the outer margin of the kidney, the parenchymal thickness, is increased.

The administration of contrast material in patients with multiple myeloma requires an awareness of potential hazards. It is essential that dehydration be avoided if the risk of complications is to be minimized. These concerns are dealt with in Chapter 1.

ABNORMAL FLUID ACCUMULATION

Acute Tubular Necrosis

Definition

Acute tubular necrosis is a state of reversible renal failure with or without oliguria that follows exposure of the kidney either to certain toxic agents or to a period of prolonged, severe ischemia.

Microscopically, the tubules vary from normal to dilated and are filled with cellular debris. Necrosis of

---

SUMMARY OF ABNORMAL URORADIOLOGIC FINDINGS
MULTIPLE MYELOMA

Primary Uroradiologic Elements
    Size—normal to large (may become small with time)
    Contour—smooth (global)
    Lesion distribution—bilateral
Secondary Uroradiologic Elements
    Pelvoinfundibulocalyceal system—attenuated (global) occasionally
    Parenchymal thickness—expanded (global)
    Nephrogram—contrast material density normal to diminished; increasingly dense (acute oliguric
        failure)
    Echogenicity—normal to increased

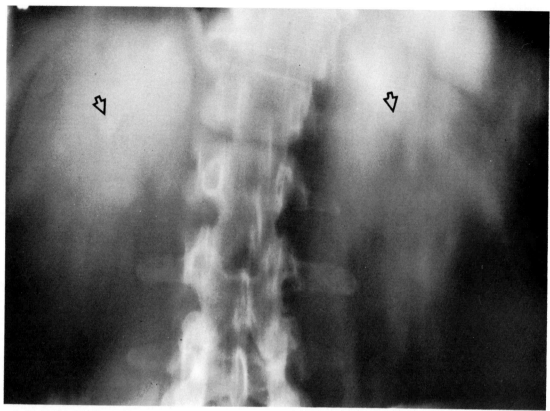

Figure 8–10. Multiple myeloma with severe renal failure in an elderly man. Bilateral global renal enlargement. Faint opacification of nondilated calyces seen by tomography at 10 minutes *(arrows)* excludes the diagnosis of obstructive uropathy. The serum creatinine value of 30.0 mg/dl at the time of this examination illustrates the efficacy of high-dose urography and tomography regardless of the severity of renal failure. The need for this modality to exclude a diagnosis of obstructive uropathy is eliminated when ultrasonography is available.

the epithelium of the renal tubules occurs. In some situations, particularly when nephrotoxins are the cause, the basement membrane is spared. At other times, such as following ischemia, the basement membrane becomes fragmented. Acute tubular necrosis affects all portions of the nephron in a patchy distribution. Interstitial edema is pronounced and accompanied by infiltrates of lymphocytes, mononuclear cells, and plasma cells.

The kidneys are enlarged primarily as a result of interstitial edema. The surface remains smooth, and the parenchyma is uniformly increased in thickness.

The pathogenesis of acute tubular necrosis is the subject of considerable controversy. One theory holds that tubule damage is the primary event and causes tubule obstruction. In this scheme, the immediate cause of acute renal failure is passive backflow leakage of filtrate into the interstitium. Supporters of this theory continue to use the term *acute tubular necrosis*. An alternate name, *vasomotor nephropathy*, has been proposed by those who believe that the primary event is always preglomerular ischemia. In this concept, oliguria reflects failure of filtration at the glomerular level, not leakage of filtrate across damaged tubules. No final conclusion about the pathogenesis of acute tubular necrosis has evolved. It is likely that both tubular and vascular mechanisms are interdependent.

Clinical Setting

Bichloride of mercury, ethylene glycol, carbon tetrachloride, bismuth, arsenic, and uranium can produce acute tubular necrosis. Urographic contrast material is also nephrotoxic, particularly when administered to a patient with pre-existing renal disease who has been dehydrated. Ischemic causes of acute tubular necrosis include shock from any cause, crush injuries, burns, transfusion reactions, and severe dehydration. Surgical procedures such as renal transplantation or aortic resection are associated with a high incidence of acute tubular necrosis as a result of temporary interruption of renal blood flow.

Oliguria (urine output of 500 ml or less per day) or anuria becomes evident shortly after the initiating incident and usually lasts for 10 to 20 days. During this time the urine darkens and contains protein. Isosthenuria is present. Dialysis during oliguria or anuria is often required. In some patients, urine volume is normal.

Recovery is signaled by the onset of the diuretic phase characterized by an increase in urine output and a decrease in blood urea nitrogen. With time, tubule function returns, and the kidney once again regains its ability to concentrate the glomerular filtrate. Recovery is then complete.

Radiologic Findings

Usually, both kidneys are enlarged and smooth in outline. The time–density pattern of the nephrogram during the urographic or computed tomographic examination is a useful diagnostic feature. Most patients with acute tubular necrosis have a nephrogram that becomes dense immediately following contrast material injection and remains so for a prolonged time (Fig. 8–11). A second time–density pattern, seen in approximately 25 per cent of patients, is the nephrogram that becomes increasingly dense during the contrast material–enhanced study (Fig. 8–12). A feeble or absent nephrogram is very uncommon in acute tubular necrosis and should suggest a complicating perfusion problem, such as acute cortical necrosis.

Despite a large amount of contrast material in the kidney substance, seen as a dense nephrogram that may persist beyond 24 hours, the pelvocalyceal system may opacify faintly or not at all. This is not surprising, since the tubules often are blocked by debris, and much of the contrast material may have leaked through damaged tubules into the interstitium. Opacification of the pelvocalyceal system might indicate a lesser degree of renal damage than in cases in which the pelvis and calyces do not opacify. Usually, the collecting systems are globally effaced by surrounding interstitial edema.

Following recovery from acute tubular necrosis due to mercury, uranium nitrite, or acetazolamide, calcium may be deposited in the necrotic proximal convoluted

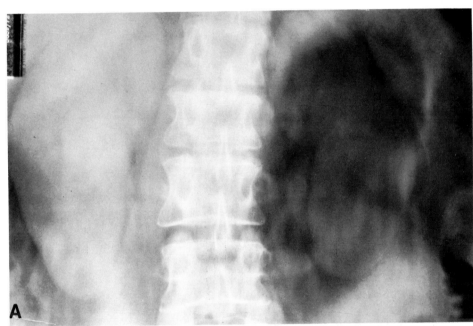

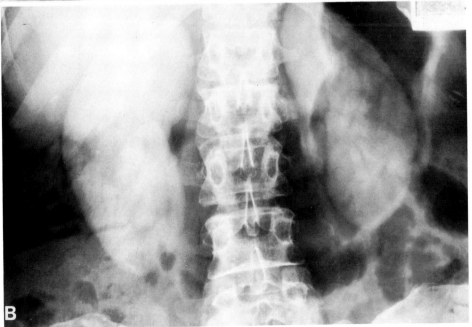

Figure 8–11. Acute tubular necrosis in a 30-year-old woman with anuria. Immediately dense, persistent nephrogram.

A, Two-minute tomogram reveals immediately dense nephrogram with global enlargement of both kidneys.

B, Sixteen-hour film reveals persistent nephrographic density without substantial change from A. No collecting system opacification.

Right kidney length = 15.8 cm; left kidney length = 15.2 cm.

(Courtesy of Professor Thomas Sherwood, M. B., University of Cambridge, Cambridge, England.) (Same patient illustrated in Fig. 23–23.)

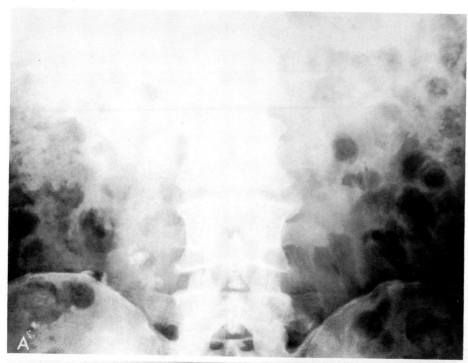

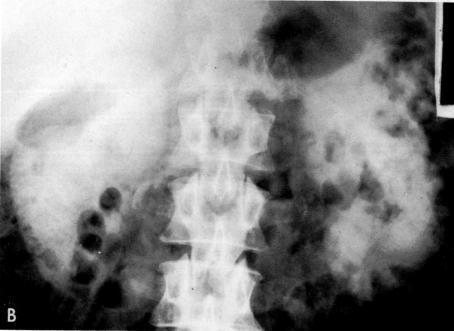

Figure 8–12. Acute tubular necrosis in a 60-year-old man who developed oliguric renal failure following severe trauma. Increasingly dense nephrogram.

A, Preliminary film.

B, Thirty minutes after injection of contrast material.

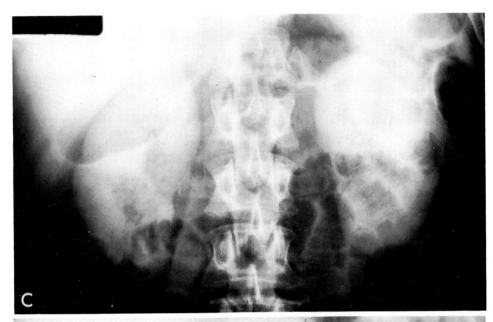

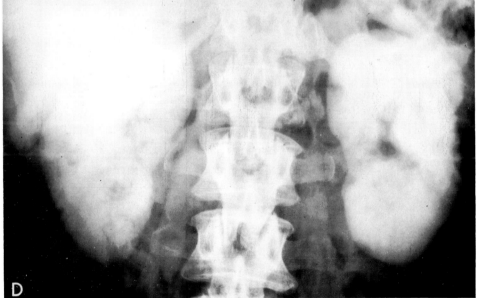

Figure 8–12 *Continued*

C, Film at 5.5 hours.

D, Film at 18 hours. In addition, the kidneys are globally enlarged and smooth and the pelvocalyceal system does not opacify.

Right kidney length = 15.0 cm; left kidney length = 14.3 cm.

(Courtesy of Professor Thomas Sherwood, M. B., University of Cambridge, Cambridge, England.) (Same patient illustrated in Fig. 23–21.)

**SUMMARY OF ABNORMAL URORADIOLOGIC FINDINGS
ACUTE TUBULAR NECROSIS**

Primary Uroradiologic Elements
    Size—large
    Contour—smooth (global)
    Lesion distribution—bilateral
Secondary Uroradiologic Elements
    Pelvoinfundibulocalyceal system—attenuated (global); opacification diminished or absent
    Parenchymal thickness—expanded (global)
    Nephrogram—immediately and persistently dense (approximately 75 per cent of patients); increas-
        ingly dense and persistent (approximately 25 per cent of patients); persistently faint (rare and
        suggests complications)
    Calcification—diffuse (rare)
    Echogenicity—normal to diminished (medulla); normal to increased (cortex)

---

tubules and be detectable by radiography, computed tomography, or ultrasonography.

Ultrasonography of the kidney is of primary value in acute tubular necrosis to document renal size and bilateral involvement and to eliminate obstruction as a cause of oliguria or anuria. The echogenicity of renal parenchyma has been reported as normal but might actually be hypoechoic (compared with a baseline study) because of interstitial edema in the medulla.

Selective renal arteriography has been performed in patients with acute tubular necrosis, mainly on an investigative basis. These studies have shown reduction in caliber and accentuated tapering of the interlobar and arcuate arteries. The arterial walls, however, remain smooth. The arcuate arteries have been described as attenuated; the arteries of the renal cortex are not discernible. Transit time of contrast material is prolonged. The normally sharp line between cortex and medulla is absent, and the renal vein poorly visualized. It is claimed that these angiographic findings can be used to distinguish acute tubular necrosis from other causes of acute oliguric renal failure. A diagnostic approach based on the clinical history, urinalysis, ultrasonography (to exclude obstruction), and renal biopsy is simpler and less expensive. Renal angiography is not necessary to establish this diagnosis.

Acute Cortical Necrosis

Definition

Acute cortical necrosis is a very uncommon form of acute renal failure in which there is death of the renal cortex and sparing of the medulla. When all cortical tissue is involved, renal failure is permanent, and life can be maintained only by dialysis or transplantation. Sometimes necrosis occurs in a patchy distribution, and enough viable cortex remains to support life, although with moderate renal failure.

The full extent of the microscopic changes of acute cortical necrosis is apparent between 36 and 72 hours after the process begins. Glomerular capillaries become distended with dehemoglobinized red blood cells. Tubule cells in the cortex undergo coagulation

necrosis and are stripped away from the basement membrane. There is increased interstitial fluid in the area of necrosis and leukocytic infiltrates along the margin of the infarct. Thrombi in afferent arterioles extending into the glomerular capillaries and back into interlobular arteries are occasional findings. The medulla is normal except for vascular congestion.

A thin rim of subcapsular tissue on the external surface of the cortex and a thin rim of juxtamedullary cortex are often preserved. Presumably, this occurs because these areas are perfused by arteries not involved in the process leading to infarction. These fine rims of viable cortex separate the necrotic cortex from the renal capsule externally and from the medulla internally. Dense calcification occurs at these interfaces, giving rise to the so-called tram-line calcification discussed in the section on radiologic findings. Calcium is deposited in tubules, glomeruli, and interstitium and can be detected microscopically as early as 6 days after the onset of acute cortical necrosis.

Grossly, the kidneys are large and smooth. On a cut section, the cortex forms a distinct pale band around the medulla. After 2 to 3 weeks, a generalized decrease in size occurs, eventually leaving small, smooth kidneys.

Clinical Setting

Acute cortical necrosis occurs most often in obstetric patients who have premature separation of the placenta with concealed hemorrhage, septic abortion, or placenta previa. Children with dehydration and fever, infections, and transfusion reactions also have an increased risk of developing acute cortical necrosis. In infants, the hemolytic-uremic syndrome combines features of acute cortical necrosis and an acute glomerulopathy and is described in a preceding section (see Fig. 8–2). In the adult, this condition is associated with sepsis, dehydration, shock, myocardial failure, burns, and snakebite and occurs as a complication of abdominal aortic surgery.

There is no agreement about what pathophysiologic mechanisms lead to acute cortical necrosis in these diverse clinical situations. Theories advanced to ex-

---

SUMMARY OF ABNORMAL URORADIOLOGIC FINDINGS
ACUTE CORTICAL NECROSIS

Primary Uroradiologic Elements
    Size—large (becomes small within a few months)
    Contour—smooth (global)
    Lesion distribution—bilateral
Secondary Uroradiologic Elements
    Pelvoinfundibulocalyceal system—absent to faint opacification; effaced
    Parenchymal thickness—expanded (global)
    Nephrogram—absent cortical nephrogram; selective enhancement of medulla
    Calcification—cortical (diffuse or "tramline")
    Echogenicity—cortex hypoechoic (early); hyperechoic with acoustic shadows after calcium deposi-
        tion

---

plain this condition have been based on concepts of ischemia due to vasospasm of small vessels, toxic damage to glomerular capillary endothelium, and primary intravascular thrombosis following excessive release of thromboplastin.

The onset of renal cortical necrosis is manifested by anuria, slight fever, leukocytosis, and few specific physical findings. When a sample of urine is available for analysis, protein and red blood cells are found. When all the renal cortex is involved, uremia develops rapidly and follows an unrelenting course to death, unless modified by dialysis or transplantation. With patchy cortical necrosis, survival is likely.

Radiologic Findings

At the earliest stage of acute cortical necrosis, the kidneys are diffusely enlarged and smooth. Early reports of urography in patients with total cortical involvement indicated that the nephrogram was absent. However, using a large dose of contrast material and standard or computed tomography, a distinctive nephrographic pattern characterized by a thin zone of nonenhanced cortex between a rim of opacified outer cortex and a faint enhancement of the remainder of the renal parenchyma (inner cortex and medulla) is seen. With patchy cortical necrosis, faint opacification of the parenchyma and pelvocalyceal system is possible. Global shrinkage of the kidneys occurs within a few months, eventually leading to very small, smooth kidneys (Fig. 8–13).

The distinctive radiologic feature of acute cortical necrosis is the development of calcification in the cortex, including the septal cortex. Radiographically detectable calcification has been reported as early as 24 days after the onset of the disease at a time when the kidneys are still enlarged. The pattern of calcium deposition is either punctate or linear in the form of two thin, parallel tracks. The latter pattern, referred to as "tram-line" calcification, reflects the interfaces made by the central zone of dead cortex with the viable subcapsular and juxtamedullary cortex on either side.

Computed tomography demonstrates the predominant contrast enhancement of the medulla and the distinctive low attenuation zone of cortical necrosis more readily than excretory urography (Fig. 8–14).

Similarly, the greater density discrimination of computed tomography compared with radiography permits earlier detection of cortical calcification.

Ultrasonography of the patient with acute cortical necrosis demonstrates enlargement of both kidneys and documents the absence of obstruction. A circumferential hypoechoic zone corresponding to the area of cortical necrosis may be seen. Ultrasound evaluation is particularly well suited for following the change in renal size from large to small. Deposition of cortical calcium causes dense cortical echoes and acoustic shadowing.

Selective renal arteriography shows prolongation of transit time in the renal arteries, nonopacification of interlobular arteries, and a disturbed cortical nephrogram (Fig. 8–15). Of these three findings, the cortical nephrogram provides the most useful and specific information. When cortical necrosis is total, a thin rim of nonopacifying tissue is noted. Patchy cortical necrosis, which carries the probability of at least partial clinical recovery, is seen angiographically as a nonhomogeneous cortical nephrogram, with alternating radiolucent and densely stained areas.

NEOPLASTIC CELL INFILTRATION

Leukemia

Definition

Leukemia is the most common malignant cause of bilateral global renal enlargement. Hodgkin's disease and malignant lymphoma occasionally produce this condition but more commonly cause multifocal renal enlargement. (See discussion in Chapter 10.) Multiple myeloma infrequently enlarges the kidney because of myeloma cell infiltration.

The leukemic cells infiltrate the interstitial tissue and crowd out normal structures. The tubules are replaced, rather than obstructed, and are more frequently involved than the glomeruli. All portions of the kidney parenchyma are involved, however. Rarely, leukemia causes a unifocal renal mass due to a chloroma, myeloblastoma, or a myeloblastic sarcoma.

The kidneys are often two to three times enlarged and maintain smooth surfaces. At times, enlarged and

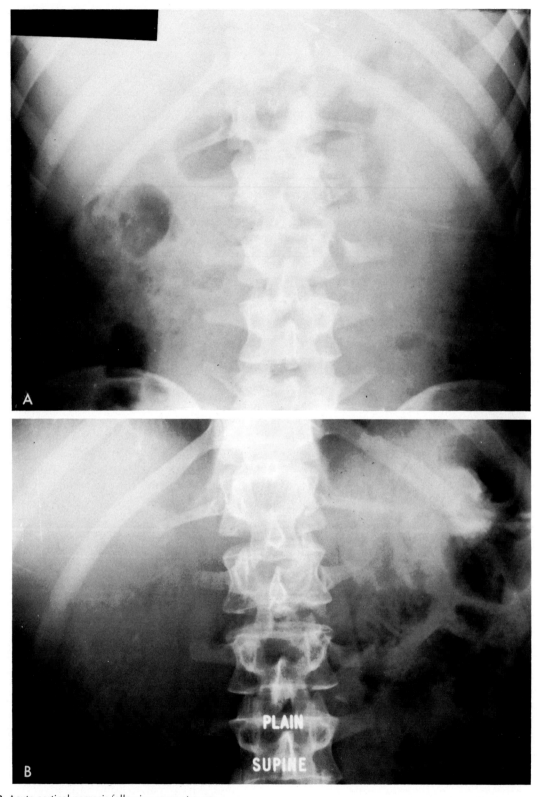

Figure 8–13. Acute cortical necrosis following severe trauma.
  A, Film of abdomen at the time of injury. Multiple fractures. The kidney outlines are not well defined but appear to be diffusely enlarged.
  B, Film taken 3 weeks after *A*. Kidneys are of normal size and smooth and contain faint calcification in a cortical distribution.

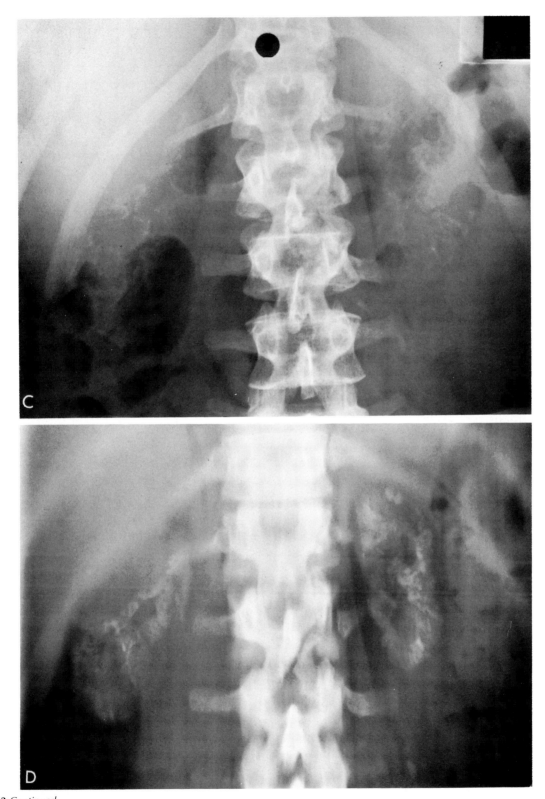

Figure 8–13 *Continued*
C, Film taken 6 weeks after *A*. Extension of linear calcification throughout cortices of both kidneys.
D, Tomogram, 1 year after *A*. Marked global wasting and cortical calcification of both kidneys. Patient was maintained by long-term dialysis.
(Courtesy of Professor Thomas Sherwood, M. B., University of Cambridge, Cambridge, England.)

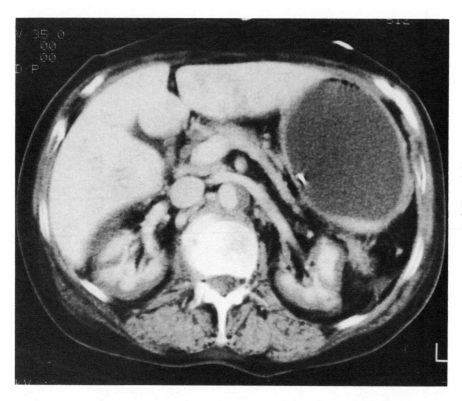

Figure 8–14. Acute cortical necrosis in a 74-year-old woman with recent surgery for thoracic and abdominal aortic dissection. Computed tomogram with contrast material enhancement demonstrates absence of enhancement of the cortex and selective enhancement of the medullae of both kidneys.

smooth kidneys occur in leukemic patients without leukemic infiltration of the kidneys. Some of these patients have acute urate nephropathy; another group shows no demonstrable histologic cause for nephromegaly.

Clinical Setting

Lymphocytic rather than granulocytic forms of leukemia are more frequently associated with renal enlargement. Children with acute leukemia are more likely to develop nephromegaly, but this occurrence is not uncommon in an adult patient with leukemia. Interestingly, renal leukemic infiltrate is unrelated to the peripheral white blood cell count, which can be normal or depleted at the time the kidneys are involved.

Varying degrees of renal failure accompany leukemic infiltration. Renal failure may be due to acute uric acid nephropathy, intrarenal hemorrhage, or obstructive uropathy from uric acid stone or blood clot, rather than cellular infiltration itself.

Radiologic Findings

The kidneys are symmetrically enlarged, and the contour is smooth with leukemic involvement. Nephrographic and pelvocalyceal density varies from normal to markedly depressed. Because of the added bulk produced by the abnormal white blood cells, the collecting systems may be attenuated and nondistensible.

Hemorrhage complicating leukemic kidney disease can appear as a focal mass or masses, subcapsular collections of blood, or obstructive or nonobstructive clots in the renal pelvis or ureters. The latter must be distinguished from uric acid stones, which also occur as a metabolic complication of high cell turnover in leukemic patients.

SUMMARY OF ABNORMAL URORADIOLOGIC FINDINGS
LEUKEMIA

Primary Uroradiologic Elements
  Size—large
  Contour—smooth (global)
  Lesion distribution—bilateral
Secondary Uroradiologic Elements
  Pelvoinfundibulocalyceal system—attenuated (global) occasionally; nonopaque filling defects (blood clot or uric acid stones)
  Parenchymal thickness—expanded (global)
  Nephrogram—contrast material density normal to diminished.
  Echogenicity—normal to increased.

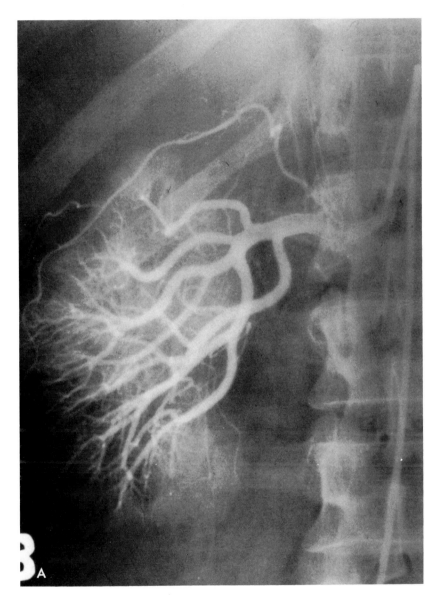

Figure 8–15. Acute cortical necrosis. Selective renal arteriogram.

A, Arterial phase. Interlobar and arcuate vessels are patent.

Illustration continued on following page

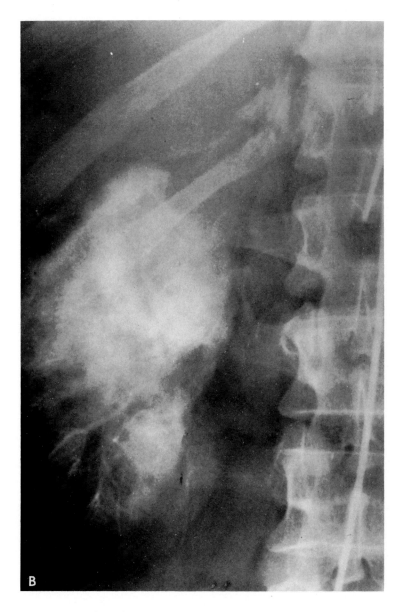

Figure 8–15 *Continued*
  B, Nephrographic phase. Obliteration of the cortical microvasculature leads to an absent nephrogram in the periphery of the kidney.
  (Courtesy of R. J. Tuttle, M. D., Burlington, Ontario, Canada.)

INFLAMMATORY CELL INFILTRATION

Acute Interstitial Nephritis

Definition

Acute interstitial nephritis is characterized histologically by infiltration of the interstitium by lymphocytes, plasma cells, eosinophils, and a few polymorphonuclear leukocytes. Interstitial edema is prominent. Fibrosis is absent, reflecting the transitory nature of this disorder. Tubular necrosis or atrophy occurs while the glomeruli and blood vessels are uninvolved, an important feature that distinguishes this entity from similar interstitial changes seen in patients with polyarteritis, the acute glomerulonephritides, and arteriosclerosis.

Paradoxically, the type of cells found in this disease are those usually associated with chronic processes. The designation "acute" is based on clinical features, not on the nature of the cells.

The infiltrating inflammatory cells and interstitial edema produce bilateral global renal enlargement.

Clinical Setting

Acute interstitial nephritis is a complication of exposure to certain drugs. These most notably include antibiotics (methicillin, ampicillin, cephalothin, and penicillin), sulfonamides, nonsteroidal anti-inflammatory drugs and analgesics (fenoprofen, naproxen, ibuprofen), the anticonvulsive phenytoin, the antihistamine cimetidine, and the anticoagulant phenindione. Numerous other drugs have been reported in isolated cases. In general, it is held that acute interstitial nephritis is mediated through immunologic, rather than nephrotoxic, mechanisms.

Cases associated with drug reaction usually evolve between 5 days and 5 weeks of the exposure. Fever, eosinophilia, and a rash are associated with hematuria, proteinuria, and varying levels of azotemia. Recovery occurs with withdrawal of the offending drug.

Radiologic Findings

Bilaterally enlarged, smooth kidneys with normal to diminished opacification are seen in cases of acute interstitial nephritis. In severe cases, effacement of the collecting systems can be expected (Fig. 8–16). Echogenicity is normal to increased.

AUTOSOMAL RECESSIVE (INFANTILE) POLYCYSTIC KIDNEY DISEASE

Definition

Autosomal recessive, or infantile, polycystic kidney disease is characterized pathologically by dilatation of renal collecting tubules, cystic dilatation of biliary radicles, and periportal fibrosis. Variable degrees of renal failure and portal hypertension are the clinical correlates of this heritable disorder, which occurs in between 1:6,000 and 1:14,000 births. In all respects, including the mode of genetic transmission, autosomal recessive polycystic kidney disease is distinct from autosomal dominant (adult) polycystic kidney disease.

Although the term *autosomal recessive polycystic kidney disease* is preferred, this condition has also been referred to as *infantile* or *Type I polycystic kidney disease, polycystic disease of the newborn, hamartomatous form of polycystic kidney disease, microcystic kidney, tubular gigantism,* and *sponge kidney.* The last term has been used almost exclusively in Europe.

The pathogenesis of autosomal recessive polycystic kidney disease has not been firmly established. Using microdissection techniques, Osathanondh and Potter (1964) found fusiform sacculation and cystic diverticula of the collecting tubules that communicated freely with functioning nephrons (Fig. 8–17). The earliest developing, most distal collecting tubules were more severely affected than were the later developing, more proximal collecting tubules. This finding suggested to these investigators that the pathologic alterations occurred after induction of the metanephric blastema and attachment of nephrons. They postulated that hyperplasia of the interstitial portion of the collecting tubule was the cause of autosomal recessive polycystic kidney disease and that this hyperplasia began distally and progressed proximally. Within this concept, mild forms of medullary tubular ectasia seen in autosomal recessive polycystic kidney disease presenting at a later age represent quantitatively lesser degrees of collecting tubule hyperplasia.

The etiology of the hepatic pathology is, likewise, not clearly defined. Lieberman and colleagues (1971) demonstrated that the bile duct abnormality occurs at a specific level of the duct system, just as does the

---

SUMMARY OF ABNORMAL URORADIOLOGIC FINDINGS
ACUTE INTERSTITIAL NEPHRITIS

Primary Uroradiologic Elements
   Size—large
   Contour—smooth (global)
   Lesion distribution—bilateral
Secondary Uroradiologic Elements
   Pelvoinfundibulocalyceal system—attenuated (global) occasionally
   Parenchymal thickness—expanded (global)
   Nephrogram—contrast material density normal to diminished
   Echogenicity—normal to increased

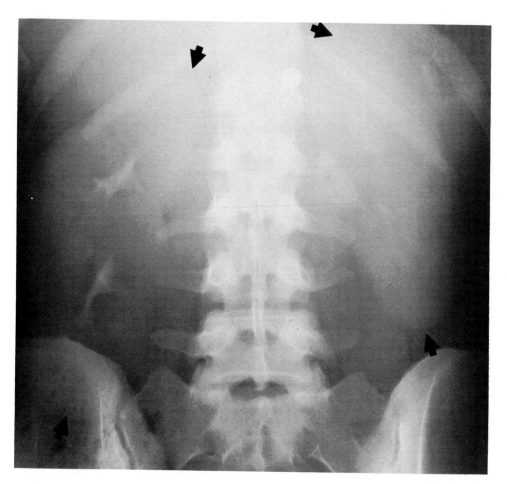

Figure 8–16. Acute interstitial nephritis due to methicillin toxicity in a 25-year-old heroin addict being treated for presumed subacute bacterial endocarditis that later was not substantiated. After 10 days of methicillin, flank pain, proteinuria, azotemia, and eosinophilia developed. Excretory urography at this time revealed smooth enlargement of both kidneys, with effacement of poorly opacified collecting structures. Abnormal findings were reversed by methicillin withdrawal. Right kidney length = 20.7 cm; left kidney length = 17.5 cm.

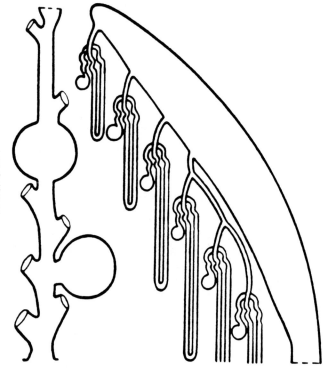

Figure 8–17. Schematic diagram of nephron dissection in autosomal recessive polycystic kidney disease. Fusiform dilatation of the terminal branch of a collecting duct with normal nephrons is illustrated on the right. Diverticular and saccular enlargements of a distal collecting duct from the medulla are represented on the left. (From Potter E. L.: Normal and Abnormal Development of the Kidney, 1972. Reproduced with kind permission of the author and Year Book Medical Publishers.)

renal collecting duct abnormality. This suggests a developmental abnormality occurring between the 12th and 20th generation of branching of the biliary epithelial bud. It is likely that a common mechanism exists in both kidney and liver.

Autosomal recessive polycystic kidney disease is expressed within a spectrum that varies from predominant renal and minimal (subclinical) hepatic involvement that first becomes apparent in the newborn and infant to predominant hepatic and minimal (subclinical) renal involvement that is first encountered clinically in middle and late childhood. In the discussion that follows the two extremes are classified as "neonatal" and "juvenile," respectively. The reader, however, should understand that this entity may present at any point in a time continuum with clinical features that combine elements of both extremes.

Neonatal. In its most severe, neonatal form, autosomal recessive polycystic kidney disease is characterized by massive enlargement of the kidneys, with each kidney weighing up to several hundred grams. The renal surface is smooth, and the kidneys maintain a reniform shape with fetal lobation. Small opalescent "cysts," which actually represent very dilated collecting tubules seen end on stud the subcapsular surface. These measure 1 to 8 mm, although a few are occasionally larger. The dilated, radially arranged collecting tubules that extend from papillary tips to renal cortex give the cut surface of the kidney the appearance of a sponge and obscure the corticomedullary junction. The fluid within the dilated tubules and cysts is clear, light yellow urine; if hemorrhage has occurred, however, the color may be light brown. The collecting tubules open into the papillae through a normal number of dilated orifices or papillary ducts. Microscopically, the dilated tubules are lined by focal areas of hyperplastic low columnar or cuboidal epithelium. Microdissection of the dilated tubules demonstrates their communication with functioning, though compressed, nephrons. Interstitial tissue is moderately increased. Glomeruli are widely spaced but normal in appearance and probably normal in number.

Patients with the neonatal form of autosomal recessive polycystic kidney disease have some form of associated hepatic pathology. The predominant findings are microscopic: a disordered proliferation and ectasia of bile ducts and an increase in portobiliary connective tissue. Both small and medium-sized interlobular bile ducts and septal bile ducts may be dilated. Bulbar protrusion of the duct wall occurs, apparently caused by an overgrowth of connective tissue into the lumen, and bridge formation occurs across duct walls. These findings create extensive irregularity along the course of the ectatic bile ducts. The hepatic lobular architecture is well preserved, and the parenchymal cells are normal.

Juvenile. When autosomal recessive polycystic kidney disease presents in older children, hepatic disease predominates over renal impairment. Periportal fibrosis is marked and causes focal dilatation of the biliary tree. Portal hypertension, hepatofugal blood flow, splenomegaly, and gastric and esophageal varices often dominate the clinical picture. This form of autosomal recessive polycystic kidney disease has been termed *congenital hepatic fibrosis* by some investigators. It is not clear, however, whether all children with congenital hepatic fibrosis have autosomal recessive polycystic kidney disease. In an older child, cystic dilatation of renal tubules and associated renal enlargement is less pronounced than in an infant. In some patients, there is marked focal cystic dilatation of ducts and increased mature interstitial fibrosis. This advanced stage may be mistaken for autosomal dominant polycystic kidney disease.

Caroli's disease has been described as segmental saccular dilatation of hepatic bile ducts and periportal fibrosis. Caroli's disease may, in fact, be an expression of the same disorder as autosomal recessive polycystic kidney disease.

Clinical Setting

Neonatal. In the more common neonatal form of autosomal recessive polycystic kidney disease, massive renal enlargement and severe renal failure dominate the clinical picture. Nephromegaly may be so severe as to cause dystocia. Diminished urine output *in utero* leads to marked oligohydramnios and development of Potter's facies. Secondary pulmonary hypoplasia develops due to oligohydramnios and compression of the thoracic contents by massive nephromegaly; the infant exhibits severe respiratory distress at birth. Recurrent pneumothoraces and pneumomediastinum may complicate efforts to ventilate the hypoplastic lungs. Death most frequently occurs from a combination of renal failure and pulmonary hypoplasia. The occasional infant who survives a neonatal presentation of autosomal recessive polycystic kidney disease develops systemic hypertension and has persistent renal insufficiency with inability to concentrate urine.

Juvenile. Beyond the immediate period of birth, a more variable course is encountered in children with autosomal recessive polycystic kidney disease. In general, the earlier the presentation the more severe the renal insufficiency and systemic arterial hypertension, while the older the infant or child is at the time of diagnosis, the more dominant are the hepatic manifestations. Children with intermediate forms of the disease present first with functionally impaired kidneys. With the passage of time, renal insufficiency persists and portal hypertension from congenital hepatic fibrosis emerges as a major clinical problem. Portal hypertension should be anticipated as a complication of autosomal recessive polycystic kidney disease in all patients with long-term survival.

Congenital hepatic fibrosis with hepatosplenomegaly and variceal bleeding are the typical presentations of older children with autosomal recessive polycystic kidney disease. In this type of patient, renal involvement is usually limited to mild nephromegaly and medullary tubular ectasia. Infrequently, patients who present with congenital hepatic fibrosis later develop renal insufficiency. Progression of portal hypertension is variable. In the majority of cases, a portocaval shunt will be necessary within several years.

Rarely, autosomal recessive polycystic kidney disease is first detected in adulthood in association with mild portal hypertension and renal failure.

Radiologic Findings

Neonatal. Abdominal enlargement due to large kidneys is evident on an abdominal film in the newborn with autosomal recessive polycystic kidney disease. A small malformed thorax, pneumothorax, and pneumomediastinum are commonly seen on the chest radiograph.

Excretory urography demonstrates diminished renal enhancement, massively enlarged kidneys, and a striated nephrogram reflecting contrast material in dilated collecting tubules. Striations are radial and extend throughout the kidney, from cortex to medulla (Fig. 8–18). These findings are pathognomonic of autosomal recessive polycystic kidney disease. Renal

function is usually so impaired that retention of contrast material in the tubules may persist for days.

Ultrasonography usually demonstrates enlarged, hyperechoic kidneys with obliteration of the distinction between cortex and medulla (Fig. 8–19). Reniform shape is preserved. The renal parenchyma may be as echogenic as the central sinus complex and more so than the liver. Increased echogenicity represents changes in acoustic impedance at the cyst lumen–cyst wall interface. In some cases, the cortex is hypoechoic relative to the medulla, which is the reversal of the normal neonatal pattern (Fig. 8–20). This reversal of the normal echo texture represents the fact that the peripheral collecting tubules in the cortex are more dilated and, thus, have a greater fluid volume than the collecting tubules of the medulla, which are more compressed. Occasionally, a few macroscopic cysts are present. In the newborn period, the liver may appear normal by ultrasonography or may show increased echogenicity and early bile duct ectasia or cysts. A presumptive prenatal diagnosis of autosomal recessive polycystic kidney disease can be made when bilateral large echogenic kidneys and oligohydramnios are demonstrated *in utero*. Although the ultrasono-

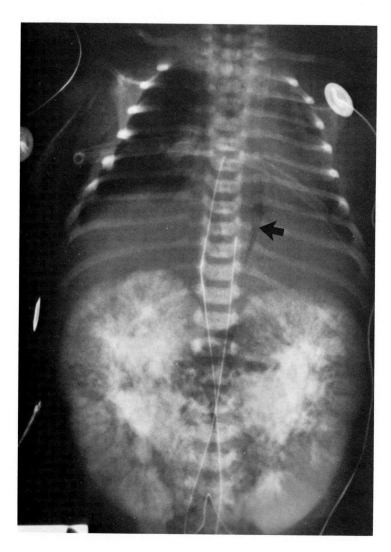

Figure 8–18. Autosomal recessive polycystic kidney disease. Neonatal form. Excretory urogram. A film obtained 2 hours after contrast material administration demonstrates large, smooth kidneys with delayed excretion and a striated nephrogram representing accumulation of contrast material in dilated collecting ducts. Air along the aorta *(arrow)* is secondary to pneumothorax and pneumomediastinum.

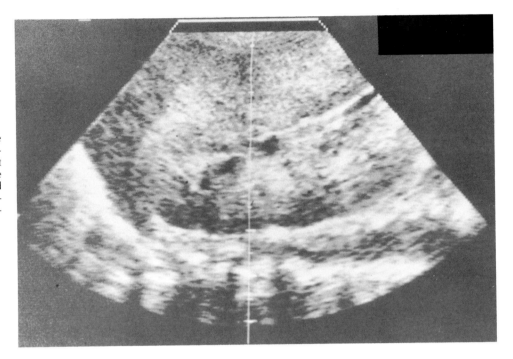

Figure 8–19. Autosomal recessive polycystic kidney disease. Neonatal form. Ultrasonogram of the right kidney in longitudinal section. The renal margin is poorly defined, and demarcation from the liver is indistinct. The kidney is large and diffusely increased in echogenicity.

graphic features of autosomal recessive polycystic kidney disease can be detected as early as the late second trimester, some affected fetuses appear normal well into the third trimester.

Unenhanced computed tomography demonstrates bilateral nephromegaly and kidney attenuation values near that of water, representing the large proportion of the renal mass that is composed of urine in dilated tubules (Fig. 8–21A). Contrast material–enhanced computed tomograms demonstrate delayed, but prolonged, renal opacification, and a striated nephrogram

that is especially prominent in the medulla (see Fig. 8–21B). The liver may demonstrate nonsegmental low density linear bands that correspond to areas of either hepatic fibrosis or bile duct dilatation.

Juvenile. An abdominal radiograph in the older child with autosomal recessive polycystic kidney disease may be normal or may demonstrate hepatosplenomegaly, nephromegaly with or without nephrocalcinosis, or both. Esophageal varices due to portal hypertension may be seen on upper gastrointestinal studies. Excretory urography usually demonstrates

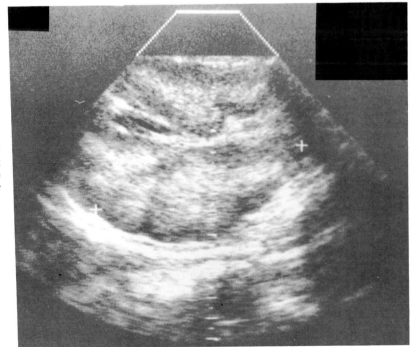

Figure 8–20. Autosomal recessive polycystic kidney disease. Neonatal form. Ultrasonogram of the right kidney in longitudinal section. The kidney is smooth and large. The cortex is hypoechoic relative to the medullae.

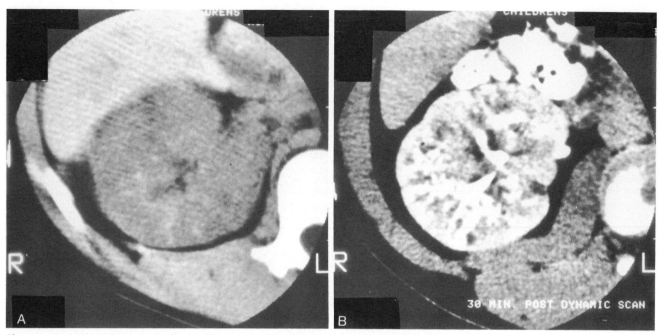

Figure 8–21. Autosomal recessive polycystic kidney disease. Neonatal form. Computed tomogram.
   A, Unenhanced scan. The kidneys are large but maintain their reniform shape. The overall attenuation value is less than soft tissue owing to the large volume of urine in the dilated tubules.
   B, Scan obtained 15 minutes after contrast material administration. Striations are prominent. There is persistent cortical enhancement.

normal opacification of the kidneys. A striated accumulation of contrast material in the papillae corresponding to slightly dilated distal collecting ducts has the same appearance as medullary sponge kidney (Fig. 8–22). (See Chapter 13.)

Abdominal ultrasonographic findings include hepatomegaly, splenomegaly, increased hepatic echogenicity, and biliary ectasia (Fig. 8–23). Intraluminal bulbar protrusions, bridge formations across dilated lumina, and portal radicles partially or completely

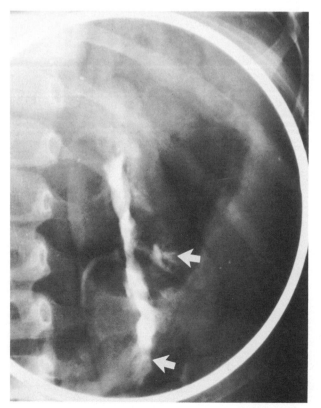

Figure 8–22. Autosomal recessive polycystic kidney disease. Juvenile form. Excretory urogram. There are linear collections of contrast material within papillae (*arrows*) in a pattern that is indistinguishable from medullary sponge kidney. The kidney is enlarged.

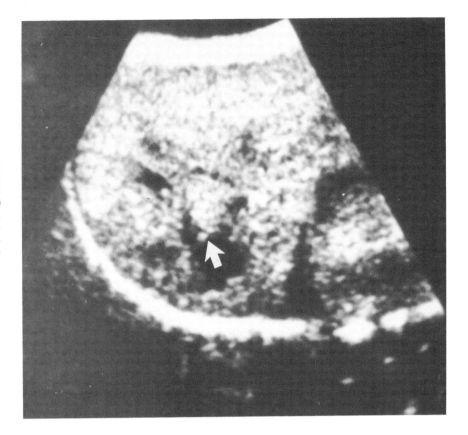

Figure 8–23. Autosomal recessive polycystic kidney disease. Juvenile form. Ultrasonogram of the liver. Focal dilatations of the biliary tract with intraluminal wall protrusion *(arrow)* are present. These bridges occasionally contain branches of the portal vein and its surrounding connective tissue core. The echogenicity of the hepatic parenchyma is increased.

surrounded by bile ducts may also be seen. When liver disease is complicated by cholangitis, ultrasonography may detect associated choledocholithiasis. Ultrasonography of the kidney may be normal in the juvenile form, although moderate nephromegaly, increased parenchymal echogenicity (especially in the medullary pyramid), and loss of corticomedullary differentiation is sometimes present. Discrete cysts cor-

responding to dilated collecting ducts may also be identified within the medulla.

Computed tomography of the abdomen in the juvenile form of autosomal recessive polycystic kidney disease frequently demonstrates hepatosplenomegaly (Fig. 8–24). Discrete cysts in the liver corresponding to focal bile duct dilatation may be identified and confirmed by the use of intravenous cholangiographic

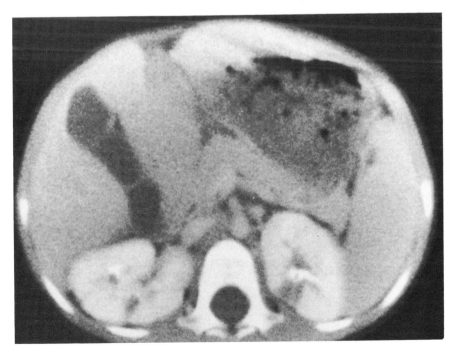

Figure 8–24. Autosomal recessive polycystic kidney disease. Juvenile form. Contrast material–enhanced computed tomogram demonstrates hepatosplenomegaly and slight nephromegaly. Several low-density areas in the kidney represent dilated collecting ducts. The kidneys are, however, minimally involved.

SUMMARY OF ABNORMAL URORADIOLOGIC FINDINGS
AUTOSOMAL RECESSIVE (INFANTILE) POLYCYSTIC KIDNEY DISEASE

Primary Uroradiologic Elements
  Size—large
  Contour—smooth (global)
  Lesion distribution—bilateral
Secondary Uroradiologic Elements
Neonatal form:
  Pelvoinfundibulocalyceal system—attenuated (global)
  Parenchymal thickness—expanded (global)
  Nephrogram—contrast material density diminished; striated
  Attenuation value—less than soft tissue (unenhanced)
  Echogenicity—increased (diffuse); loss of corticomedullary differentiation; decreased cortex and
      increased medulla (occasional)
Juvenile form:
  Nephrogram—striated (papillae, common; diffuse, rare)
  Calcification—nephrocalcinosis (papillae)
  Echogenicity—increased (papillae)
  Miscellaneous—hepatosplenomegaly, varices, dilated bile ducts, increased hepatic echogenicity

---

contrast material. The portal and splenic veins may be enlarged as a result of portal hypertension and hepatofugal flow. Computed tomography of the kidney may demonstrate renal enlargement; the nephrocalcinosis pattern of medullary sponge kidney; multiple, discrete, cortical, and medullary cysts; and a striated nephrogram in papillary tips (see Fig. 8–24).

Liver–spleen radionuclide scans demonstrate hepatosplenomegaly and numerous well-circumscribed photopenic regions in the liver when technetium 99m sulfur colloid is utilized. These same photopenic areas will accumulate radioactivity when a technetium 99m–labeled hepatobiliary agent is used. Transhepatic, intravenous, or retrograde cholangiography also demonstrates focal biliary dilatation.

MISCELLANEOUS CONDITIONS

Acute Urate Nephropathy

When nephrons are flooded with large amounts of uric acid, minute biurate crystals form and become deposited in the collecting tubules and interstitium. Acute oliguric renal failure follows from intratubular obstruction. Although this may occur in any patient with a very high serum uric acid level, it is seen most commonly during therapy for cancer, particularly leukemia, Hodgkin's disease and malignant lymphoma, myeloproliferative disorders, and polycythemia vera. In these patients, the cytotoxic agents release large amounts of nucleoprotein, which are metabolized to uric acid.

There is scant radiologic literature on acute urate nephropathy. From what is known pathologically, the kidneys are globally enlarged and have normal collecting systems. The nephrographic pattern shows increasing density with time. This relationship reflects continued glomerular filtration and retention of filtered contrast material in the obstructed tubules. Delayed opacification of the pelvocalyceal system does not occur because of the tubule blockage (Fig. 8–25).

The radiologist must undertake excretory urography or computed tomography with considerable caution in the severely hyperuricemic patient because of the uricosuric effect of contrast material. Alkaline diuresis, a large fluid intake, and the use of allopurinol should be instituted before the administration of contrast material if the risk of causing acute urate nephropathy is to be minimized.

Glycogen Storage Disease, Type I (von Gierke's Disease)

Nephromegaly to a marked degree occurs in children and young adults with glycogen storage disease, Type I, because of accumulation of glycogen in the epithelium of proximal convoluted tubules. Renal failure is not invariably present but develops mainly in older patients who have not had optimal therapy. Kidneys may be normal in size when patients are under good metabolic control. Other features of this genetically transmitted disorder that may produce radiologic abnormalities are growth retardation, hepatomegaly, hepatic adenoma and adenocarcinoma, gouty arthritis, and uric acid stones.

Physiologic Response to Urographic Contrast Material and Diuretics

Agents that cause vasodilatation and/or diuresis may increase renal size, presumably because of volume expansion of the vascular tree, the tubule lumina, and the interstitial fluid space. Increases of up to 35 per cent of the renal area have been reported. The mean increase, however, is close to 5 per cent. This degree of enlargement does not produce kidney images that necessarily fall into the abnormally large category. In addition to urographic contrast material, this phenomenon is also seen with urea, glucose, ethacrynic acid, furosemide, acetylchlorine, and prostaglandins.

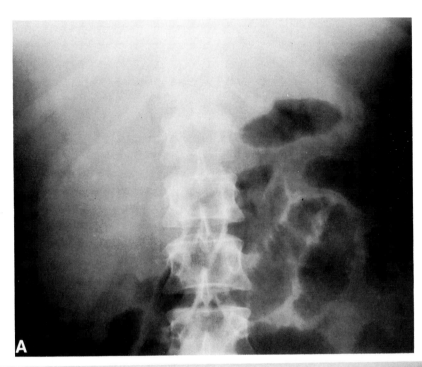

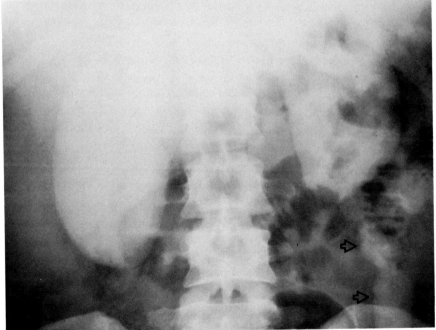

Figure 8–25. Acute urate nephropathy in a 31-year-old woman with extensive hepatic metastases from a poorly differentiated carcinoma thought to be gastrointestinal in origin. Serum uric acid = 25 mg/dl. Patient developed oliguria while dehydrated. Anuria ensued, despite correction of fluid balance. Excretory urogram performed at this time demonstrates globally enlarged kidneys with a progressive increase in density of the nephrogram over 2 days. Excretory urography should be avoided in a situation such as this.

A, Ten-minute film. Homogeneous nephrogram.

B, Sixty-four hour film. Persistent nephrogram. Extrarenal excretion of contrast material opacifies descending sigmoid colon *(arrows)*.

Right kidney length = 16.0 cm; left kidney length = 15.2 cm.

(Same patient illustrated in Fig. 23–22.)

Homozygous-S Disease

Both kidneys may enlarge in homozygous-S (sickle cell) disease, owing to vascular dilatation, engorgement of vessels, glomerular enlargement, and interstitial edema (Fig. 8–26). Increased renal blood flow may also be a factor. Other radiologic abnormalities in homozygous-S disease are lobar infarction, impaired density of contrast material, and dilated pelvocalyceal systems and ureters. The latter reflect defective water concentrating ability. Papillary necrosis may also be seen in homozygous-S disease but is more common in heterozygous-S states. (See Chapter 7.) Decreased cortical signal intensity, most evident on T2-weighted magnetic resonance images, has been reported. Because of the sharply reduced life expectancy of patients with sickle cell disease, these changes usually are seen only in young persons.

Paroxysmal Nocturnal Hemoglobinuria

This rare, acquired hemolytic disorder results from complement-mediated membrane damage to erythrocytes, granulocytes, and platelets that have been derived from an abnormal clone of stem cells. Young adults are most frequently affected with clinical manifestations of fever, abdominal and back pain, and the effects of venous thrombosis of both peripheral and viscera-draining veins (portal and hepatic, cerebral, mesenteric, and renal). Chronic hemolysis causes anemia, hemoglobinuria, and hemosiderinuria. Repeated microvascular thromboses in the kidney produce nephromegaly, lobar infarcts, and papillary necrosis. These findings are similar to those of homozygous-S disease described in the preceding section. In addition, massive deposition of ferric iron–containing hemosiderin in proximal convoluted tubules causes markedly decreased magnetic resonance signal intensity of the renal cortex, most notably on gradient-echo sequences (Fig. 8–27). This is a reversal of the normal signal relationship of cortex to medulla.

Hemophilia

In a series of 12 patients with hemophilia, four had global enlargement of both kidneys that otherwise were normal (Dalinka et al., 1975). All of the patients were adults, and none had obstruction of the urinary tract. Apart from enlargement of the glomeruli seen in biopsy specimens of two of these patients, no explanation is available for the nephromegaly associated with this disorder. Papillary necrosis in hemophilia has also been described, as discussed in Chapter 7.

Nephromegaly Associated with Cirrhosis, Hyperalimentation, and Diabetes Mellitus

Nephromegaly has been reported in cases of hepatic cirrhosis, regardless of the cause. Renal enlargement is particularly prominent in patients with marked fatty changes in the liver. The basis for this relationship is unknown. Renal tissue fluid, proteins, lipids,

and carbohydrates are normal. Hyperplasia and hypertrophy of renal cells are thought to account for the increased kidney bulk.

Smooth enlargement of both kidneys as a response to hyperalimentation (total parenteral nutrition) has been well documented. This is most likely due to an increase in the fluid compartments of the kidney related to hyperosmolality of the administered solutions. Renal enlargement reverses promptly following cessation of this form of nutritional therapy.

Bilateral nephromegaly also occurs in some patients with insulin-dependent diabetes mellitus early in the course of their illness and in the absence of diabetic glomerulosclerosis. This is often associated with an increase in glomerular filtration rate as well as renal plasma flow. Possible explanations for this well-documented occurrence include nephron hypertrophy and glycosuric osmotic diuresis. Transient nephromegaly in newborns born of diabetic mothers also occurs.

Acromegaly

The kidneys are part of the generalized organomegaly seen in acromegaly. Renal function and structure are otherwise normal.

Fabry's Disease

Smooth enlargement of both kidneys has been reported in young adults with Fabry's disease or angiokeratoma corporis diffusum universale. Nephromegaly develops in the stage of the disease before the onset of renal failure. Thereafter, the kidneys become small. Presumably, renal enlargement is due to lipid deposition in the parenchyma.

Bartter's Syndrome

Bartter's syndrome is a metabolic disorder that leads to growth retardation, distinctive craniofacial features, and muscle weakness. Hypercalciuria, hypokalemia, hyperaldosteronism, and increased plasma renin levels are also present. Paradoxically, blood pressure is normal despite elevated plasma renin. Children and young adults are most often affected, but there are variants of the syndrome that present in the neonatal period. Kidney enlargement, when present, probably reflects either hyperplasia of the juxtaglomerular apparatus, which is the principal morphologic abnormality found in the kidney, or polyuria, or both. Radiologic findings that may be present in Bartter's syndrome, in addition to nephromegaly, include dilatation of the pelvocalyceal system and ureter from polyuria, hyperechoicity of the renal medulla due to nephrocalcinosis, and diffuse increase in renal parenchymal echo intensity with loss of corticomedullary distinction, a nonspecific finding.

Beckwith-Wiedemann Syndrome

Bilateral global enlargement of the kidneys is one feature of Beckwith-Wiedemann syndrome, an uncom-

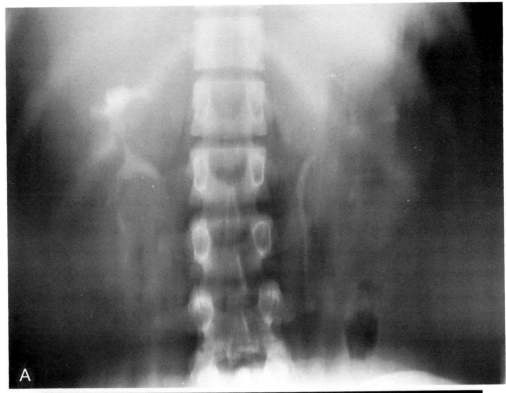

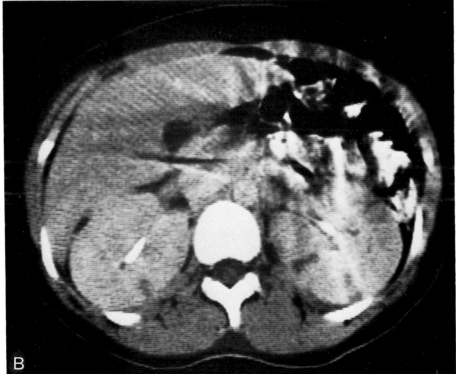

Figure 8–26. Homozygous-S disease with bilateral, smooth renal enlargement.

A, Excretory urogram. Tomogram. Note absence of several papillae due to papillary necrosis.

B, Computed tomogram, contrast material enhanced.

Focal areas of nonenhanced parenchyma represent small lobar infarcts. (Courtesy of M. Federle, M. D., University of Pittsburgh, Pittsburgh, Pennsylvania.)

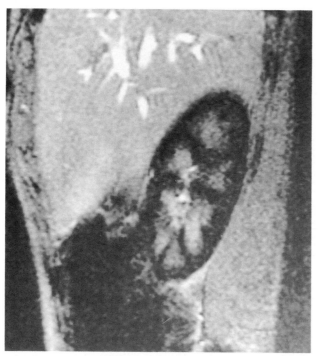

Figure 8–27. Paroxysmal nocturnal hemoglobinuria in a 16-year-old boy with three episodes of fever, abdominal pain, brown urine, and jaundice over a 3-year period. Gradient-echo sequence magnetic resonance image in the sagittal plane. There is marked decrease in the signal intensity in the cortex and normal signal intensity in the medullae. (Kindly provided by the Department of Radiology and Radiological Sciences, The Johns Hopkins University, Baltimore, Maryland.)

monly encountered set of abnormalities found in infants. In addition to nephromegaly, other findings include large body size, macroglossia, hemihypertrophy (including unilateral renal enlargement), advanced skeletal maturation, omphalocele, diastasis recti or umbilical hernia, hepatomegaly, mild microcephaly, earlobe deformities, and facial nevi. Neonatal hypoglycemia may dominate the clinical presentation, and polycythemia may be present. Macroglossia and macrosomia become less apparent with age.

As many as 10 per cent of patients with Beckwith-Wiedemann syndrome develop an abdominal malignancy involving liver (hepatoblastoma or hepatocarcinoma), kidney (Wilms' tumor), gonad (gonadoblastoma), or adrenal (carcinoma). Other kidney abnormalities associated with Beckwith-Wiedemann syndrome include medullary sponge kidney, medullary dysplasia, and pyelocalyceal diverticulum.

DIFFERENTIAL DIAGNOSIS

Except for *autosomal recessive (infantile) polycystic kidney disease*, *hemolytic-uremic syndrome*, and *paroxysmal nocturnal hemoglobinuria*, there are no radiologic findings that specifically distinguish any one of the disorders from another in the diagnostic set "large, smooth, bilateral." Clinical and laboratory findings, histologic and immunologic studies, and clinical course must be relied on for establishing a diagnosis in most cases.

Evaluation of the time–density aspects of the nephrogram may be of some help in grouping these entities, however. The nephrogram usually remains faint in the *proliferative/necrotizing disorders* and either absent or faint in *acute cortical necrosis*. An immediately dense and persistent nephrogram is most commonly associated with *acute tubular necrosis* but is also seen in some cases of *acute glomerulonephritis*, *"acute-on-chronic" renal failure*, and *acute bacterial nephritis*. A progressively dense nephrogram is associated with *acute urate nephropathy, multiple myeloma, amyloidosis*, and some cases of *acute tubular necrosis*. This same pattern is often seen in bilateral *postrenal obstruction*. In this latter instance, the correct diagnosis is established either by ultrasonography or delayed opacification of dilated collecting structures within the first 24 hours of the urographic examination. In the other entities, the collecting systems are collapsed and often not opacified at all.

Some of the diseases that produce enlarged, smooth kidneys can be distinguished from each other by their association with abnormalities in other organs. *Goodpasture's syndrome, Wegener's granulomatosis, Schönlein-Henoch syndrome, thrombotic thrombocytopenic purpura and hemolytic-uremic syndrome, amyloidosis, multiple myeloma, leukemia, glycogen storage disease Type I*, and *Beckwith-Wiedemann syndrome* fall into this category.

The radiologic findings in *acute cortical necrosis* are not specific early in the course of the illness except when a cortical rim nephrographic defect or hypoechoic zone is identified. The appearance of calcification in a cortical distribution and rapid global wasting of the kidneys are features unique to acute cortical necrosis, but these findings require a few weeks' lapse of time before they become detectable.

Hemolytic-uremic syndrome characteristically causes intense hyperechoicity of the cortex relative to the medulla. Likewise, reversal of the normal signal relationship between cortex and medulla on magnetic resonance images of the kidney is a hallmark of *paroxysmal nocturnal hemoglobinuria*.

In the newborn and infant, radiologic studies, particularly those using contrast material enhancement and demonstrating a striated nephrogram, leave little doubt about the diagnosis of *autosomal recessive (infantile) polycystic kidney disease*. The ultrasonographic finding of hyperechoic, enlarged, smooth kidneys may also be present in *autosomal dominant (adult) polycystic kidney disease* presenting in the newborn or infant. Here, an accurate diagnosis requires pathologic examination of tissue. In the juvenile form, autosomal recessive polycystic kidney disease may be confused with *medullary sponge kidney* (see Chapter 13). The latter, however, is uncommon in childhood and not associated with nephromegaly or liver disease.

Multiple fluid-filled renal cysts of varying size are found in numerous syndromes of developmental or genetic origin. These are known variably as *glomerulocystic, microcystic*, or *pluricystic disorders of the kidney*. Bilateral, smooth renal enlargement and a diffuse increase in echogenicity may make these disorders indistinguishable from the neonatal form of autosomal recessive (infantile) polycystic kidney disease, autosomal dominant (adult) polycystic kidney disease presenting in infancy, or acute tubular necrosis in the newborn. Other clinical stigmata, which are almost always present in the glomerulocystic/microcystic/pluricystic syndromes, permit an accurate diagnosis.

Occasionally, autosomal dominant (adult) polycystic kidney disease discovered in adulthood is associated with smooth renal enlargement, normal opacification, and nondisplaced collecting structures. This is discussed and illustrated in Chapter 10. Careful evaluation of the nephrogram in these patients will always reveal sharply defined radiolucent defects quite unlike the homogeneous nephrogram found in the disorders presented in this chapter. Both ultrasonography and computed tomography invariably yield a specific pattern in these patients.

Bibliography

General

Brenbridge, A. N., Cheralier, R. L., El-Dahr, S., and Kaiser, D. L.: Pathologic significance of nephromegaly in pediatric disease. Am. J. Dis. Child. 141:652, 1987.

Brezis, M., Rosen, S., and Epstein, F. H.: Acute renal failure. In Brenner, B. M., and Rector, F. C. (eds.): The Kidney. 4th ed. Philadelphia, W. B. Saunders, 1991, pp. 993–1061.

Fitch, S. J., and Stapleton, F. B.: Ultrasonographic features of glomerulocystic disease in infancy: Similarity to infantile polycystic disease. Pediatr. Radiol. 16:400, 1986.

Fredericks, B. J., de Campos, M., Chow, C. W., and Powell, H. R.: Glomerulocystic renal disease: Ultrasound appearances, Pediatr. Radiol. 19:184, 1989.

Heptinstall, R. H. (ed.): Pathology of the Kidney. 4th ed. Boston, Little, Brown & Co., 1992.

Hricak, H., Cruz, C., Romanski, R., Uniewiski, M. H., Levin, N. W., Madrazo, B. L., Sandler, M. A., and Eyler, W. R.: Renal parenchymal disease: Sonographic-histologic correlation. Radiology 144:141, 1982.

Jeffrey, R. B., and Federle, M. P.: CT and ultrasonography of acute renal abnormalities. Radiol. Clin. North Am. 21:515, 1983.

Platt, J.F., Rubin, J. M., Bowerman, R. A., and Marn, C. S.: The inability to detect kidney diseases on the basis of echogenicity. AJR 151:317, 1988.

Rosenfield, A. T., Siegel, N. J.: Renal parenchymal disease: Histopathologic-sonographic correlation. AJR 137:793, 1981.

Taxy, J. B., and Filmer, R. B.: Glomerulocystic kidney: Report of a case. Arch. Pathol. Lab. Med. 100:186, 1976.

Weese-Mayer, D. E., Smith, K. M., Reddy, K. J., Slafsky, J., and Posnanski, A. K.: Computerized tomography and ultrasound in the diagnosis of cerebro-hepato-renal syndrome of Zellweger. Pediatr. Radiol. 17:170, 1987.

Proliferative/Necrotizing Disorders

Amorosi, E. L., and Ultmann, J. E.: Thrombotic thrombocytopenic purpura: Report of 16 cases and review of the literature. Medicine (Baltimore) 45:139, 1966.

Atkins, R. C., and Thomson, N.: Rapidly progressive glomerulonephritis. In Schrier, R. W., and Gottschalk, C. W. (eds.): Diseases of the Kidney. 4th ed. Boston, Little, Brown & Co., 1988, pp. 1903–1938.

Balow, J. E., and Fauci, A. S.: Vasculitic diseases of the kidney: Polyarteritis nodosa, Wegener's granulomatosis, allergic angiitis, and granulomatosis and other disorders. In Schrier, R. W., and Gottschalk, C. W. (eds.): Diseases of the Kidney. 4th ed. Boston, Little, Brown & Co., 1988, pp. 2335–2360.

Bell, D. S. H.: Diabetic nephropathy: Changing concepts of pathogenesis and treatment. Am. J. Med. Sci. 301:195, 1991.

Benoit, F. L., Rulon, D. B., Theil, G. B., Doolan, P. D., and Watten, R. H.: Goodpasture's syndrome: A clinicopathologic entity. Am. J. Med. 37:424, 1964.

Boyd, R. M., Warren, L., and Garrow, D. G.: Renal size in various nephropathies. AJR 119:723, 1973.

Bradley, G. E., Gailey, R. R., McGiven, A. R., and Day, W. A.: IgA nephropathy: A report of three cases. N. Z. Med. J. 83:219, 1976.

Brezis, M., Rosen, S., and Epstein, F. H.: Acute renal failure. In Brenner, B. M., and Rector, F. C. (eds.): The Kidney. 4th ed. Philadelphia, W. B. Saunders, 1991.

Case records of the Massachusetts General Hospital: Case 17–1978. Goodpasture's syndrome. N. Engl. J. Med. 298:1014, 1978.

Case records of the Massachusetts General Hospital: Case 24–1979. Wegener's granulomatosis. N. Engl. J. Med. 300:1378, 1979.

Chesney, R. W., O'Regan, S., Kaplan, B. S., and Nogrady, M. B.: Asymmetric renal enlargement in acute glomerulonephritis. Radiology 122:431, 1977.

Choyke, P. L., Grant, E. G., Hoffer, F. A., Tina, L., and Korec, S.: Cortical echogenicity in the hemolytic-uremic syndrome: Clinical correlation. J. Ultrasound Med. 7:439, 1988.

Connor, E., Gupta, S., and Joshi, V.: Acquired immunodeficiency syndrome: Associated renal disease in children. J. Pediatr. 113:39, 1988.

Cunningham, E. E., Brentjens, J. R., Zielezny, M. A., Andres, G. A., and Venuto, R. C.: Heroin nephropathy: A clinicopathologic and epidemiologic study. Am. J. Med. 68:47, 1980.

Davson, J., Ball, J., and Platt, R.: Kidney in periarteritis nodosa. Q. J. Med. 17:175, 1948.

Duncan, D. A., Drummond, K. N., Midrach, A. F., and Vermier, R. L.: Pulmonary hemorrhage and glomerulonephritis. Ann. Intern. Med. 62:920, 1965.

Ekelund, L., and Lindholm, T.: Angiography in collagenous disease of the kidney. Acta Radiol. (Diagn.) 15:413, 1974.

Falkoff, G. E., Rigsby, C. M., and Rosenfield, A. T.: Partial, combined cortical and medullary nephrocalcinosis: US and CT patterns in AIDS-associated MAI Infection Radiology 162:343, 1987.

Fry, I. K., and Cattell, W. R.: The nephrographic pattern during excretion urography. Br. Med. Bull. 28:227, 1972.

Gardenswartz, M. H., and Tapper, M. L.: Renal disease in acquired immune-deficiency syndrome. In Schrier, R. W., Gottschalk, C. W. (eds.): Diseases of the Kidney. 4th ed. Boston, Little, Brown & Co., 1988, pp. 2615–2628.

Glassock, R. J., Cohen, A. H., Adler, S. G., and Ward, H. J.: Primary glomerular diseases. In Brenner, B. M., and Rector, F. C. (eds.): The Kidney. 4th ed. Philadelphia, W. B. Saunders, 1991, pp. 1182–1279.

Glassock, R.J., Cohen, A.H., Adler, S.G., and Ward, H.J.: Secondary glomerular diseases. In Brenner, B.M., and Rector, F.C. (eds.): The Kidney. 4th ed. Philadelphia, W. B. Saunders, 1991, pp. 1280–1368.

Graif, M., Shohet, I., Strauss, S., Yahar, J., and Itzchok, Y.: Hemolytic-uremic syndrome: Sonographic-clinical correlation. J. Ultrasound Med. 3:563, 1984.

Hamper, U. M., and Golblum, L. E., and Hutchins, G. M.: Renal involvement in AIDS: Sonographic-pathologic correlation. AJR 150:1321, 1988.

Heptinstall, R. H.: Classification of glomerulonephritis; focal, and mesangial proliferative forms of glomerulonephritis; recurrent hematuria. In Heptinstall, R. H. (ed.): Pathology of the Kidney. 4th ed. Boston, Little, Brown & Co., 1992, pp. 261–296.

Heptinstall, R. H.: Polyarteritis (periarteritis) nodosa, Wegener's syndrome, and other forms of vasculitis. In Heptinstall, R. H., (ed.): Pathology of the Kidney. 4th ed. Boston, Little, Brown & Co., 1992, pp. 1097–1162.

Heptinstall, R. H.: Hemolytic-uremic syndrome, thrombotic thrombocytopenic purpura, and systemic sclerosis (systemic scleroderma). In Heptinstall, R. H. (ed.): Pathology of the Kidney. 4th ed. Boston, Little, Brown & Co., 1992, pp. 1163–1234.

Herman, P. G., Balikian, J. P., Seltzer, S. E., and Ehrie, M.: The pulmonary-renal syndrome. AJR 130:1141, 1978.

Hostetter, T. H.: Diabetic nephropathy. In Brenner, B. M., and Rector, F. C. (eds.): The Kidney. 4th ed. Philadelphia, W. B. Saunders, 1991, pp. 1695–1727.

Kenney, P. J., Brinsko, R. E., Patel, D. V., Spitzer, R. E., and Farrar, F. M. Sonography of the kidneys in hemolytic-uremic syndrome. Invest. Radiol. 21:547, 1986.

Lalli, A. F.: Renal enlargement. Radiology 84: 688, 1965.

Levitt, L. M., and Burbank, B.: Glomerulonephritis as a complication of Schönlein-Henoch syndrome. N. Engl. J. Med. 248:530, 1953.

Llach, F., Descoeudres, C., and Massry, S. G.: Heroin associated nephropathy: Clinical and histological studies in 19 patients. Clin. Nephrol. 11:7, 1979.

McCluskey, R. T.: Immunologic aspects of renal disease. In Heptinstall, R. H. (ed.): Pathology of the Kidney. 4th ed. Boston, Little, Brown & Co., 1992.

Miller, F. H., Parikh, S., Gore, R. M., Nemcek, A. A. J., Fitzgerald, S. W., and Vogelzand, R. L.: Renal manifestations of AIDS. Radiographics 13:587, 1993.

Neild, G. H.: Haemolytic uraemic syndrome. Nephrology Grand Rounds. Clinical issues in nephrology. Nephron 59:194, 1991.

Rao, T. K. S., Friedman, E. A., and Nicastri, A. D.: The types of renal disease in acquired immunodeficiency syndrome. N. Engl. J. Med. 316:1062, 1987.

Remuzzi, G., and Bertani, T.: Thrombotic thrombocytopenic purpura, hemolytic uremic syndrome and acute cortical necrosis. In Schrier, R. W., and Gottschalk, C. W. (eds.): Diseases of the Kidney. 4th ed. Boston, Little, Brown & Co., 1988, pp. 2301–2334.

Rodríguez-Iturbe, B.: Acute poststreptococcal glomerulonephritis. In Schrier, R. W., and Gottschalk, C. W. (eds.): Diseases of the Kidney. 4th ed. Boston, Little, Brown & Co., 1988, pp. 1929–1948.

Rose, G. A.: The natural history of polyarteritis. Br. Med. J. 2:1148, 1957.

Rose, G. A., and Spencer, H.: Polyarteritis nodosa. Q. J. Med. 26:43, 1957.

Rousseau, E., Russo, P., and Lapointe, N.: Renal complications of acquired immunodeficiency syndrome in children. Am. J. Kidney Dis. 11:48, 1988.

Rothfield, N., McCluskey, R. T., and Baldwin, D. S.: Renal disease in systemic lupus erythematosus. N. Engl. J. Med. 269:537, 1963.

Schwartz, E. E., Teplick, J. G., Onesti, G., and Schwartz, A. B.: Pulmonary hemorrhage in renal disease: Goodpasture's syndrome and other causes. Radiology 122:39, 1977.

Sherwood, T., Doyle, F. H., Boulton-Jones, M., Joekes, A. M., Peters, D. K., and Sissons, P.: The intravenous urogram in acute renal failure. Br. J. Radiol. 47:368, 1974.

Silveira, E., Levin, N. W., Cortes, P., and Rubenstein, A. H.: Increased renal growth in diabetes mellitus. Abstract. No. 535. In Abstracts of Free Communication, VIth International Congress of Nephrology. Florence, Italy, 1975.

Slovis, T. L., Sty, J. R., and Haller, J. O.: Imaging of the Pediatric Urinary Tract. Philadelphia, W. B. Saunders, 1989.

Strauss, J., Abitol, C., Zillervelo, G., Scott, G., Parades, A., Malaga, S., Montane, B., Mitchell, C., Parks, W., and Pardo, V.: Renal disease in children with acquired immunodeficiency syndrome. N. Engl. J. Med. 321:625, 1989.

Teague, C. A., Doak, P. B., Simpson, I. J., Rainer, S. P., and Herdson, P. B.: Goodpasture's syndrome: An analysis of 29 cases. Kidney Int. 13:492, 1978.

Deposition of Abnormal Proteins

Auerbach, O., and Stemmerman, M. G.: Renal amyloidosis. Arch. Intern. Med. 74:244, 1944.

Berdon, W. E., Schwartz, R. H., Becker, J., and Baker, D. H.: Tamm-Horsfall proteinuria: Its relationship to prolonged nephrogram in infants and children and to renal failure following intravenous urography in adults with multiple myeloma. Radiology 92:714, 1969.

Brandt, K., Catcart, E. S., and Cohen, A. S.: A clinical analysis of the course prognosis of forty-two patients with amyloidosis. Am. J. Med. 44:955, 1968.

Case records of the Massachusetts General Hospital: Case 18–1976. Multiple myeloma. N. Engl. J. Med. 294:998, 1976.

Case records of the Massachusetts General Hospital: Case 5–1980. Amyloidosis. N. Engl. J. Med. 302:336, 1980.

Cohen, A. S.: Amyloidosis. N. Engl. J. Med. 277:574 and 628, 1967.

Cwynarski, M. T., and Saxton, H. M.: Urography in myelomatosis. Br. Med. J. 1:486, 1969.

Dixon, H. M.: Renal amyloidosis in relation to renal insufficiency. Am. J. Med. Sci. 187:401, 1934.

Ekelund, L., and Lindholm, T.: Angiography in collagenous disease of the kidney. Acta Radiol. (Diagn.) 15:394, 1974.

Ekelund, L.: Radiologic findings in renal amyloidosis. AJR 129:851, 1977.

Forsell, A., and Isaksson, B.: Nephroangiography in amyloidosis. Acta Radiol. (Diagn.) 17:797, 1976.

Fry, I. K., and Cattell, W. R.: The nephrographic pattern during excretion urography. Br. Med. Bull. 28:227, 1972.

Jones, N. F.: Renal amyloidosis: Pathogenesis and therapy. Clin. Nephrol. 6:459, 1976.

Kyle, R. A., and Bayrd, E. D.: Amyloidosis: Review of 236 cases. Medicine (Baltimore) 54:271, 1975.

Lasser, E. C., Lang, J. H., and Zawadzki, Z. A.: Contrast media: Myeloma protein precipitates in urography. JAMA 198:945, 1966.

McCormick, T. L., and Cho, K. J.: Angiographic findings in renal amyloidosis. AJR 129:855, 1977.

McIntyre, O. R.: Current concepts in cancer: Multiple myeloma. N. Engl. J. Med. 301:193, 1979.

Medical staff conference. University of California, San Francisco: The kidney in multiple myeloma. West. J. Med. 129:41, 1978.

Myers, G. H., Jr., and Witten, D. M.: Acute renal failure after excretory urography in multiple myeloma. AJR 113:583, 1971.

Pear, B. L.: Radiographic manifestations of amyloidosis. AJR 111:821, 1971.

Subramanyam, B. R.: Renal amyloidosis in juvenile rheumatoid arthritis: Sonographic features. AJR 136:411, 1981.

Vaamonde, C. A., and Pardo, V: Multiple myeloma and amyloidosis. In Schrier, R. W., and Gottschalk, C. W. (eds.): Diseases of the Kidney. 4th ed. Boston, Little, Brown & Co., 1988, pp. 2439–2480.

Vix, V. A.: Intravenous pyelography in multiple myeloma. Radiology 87:896, 1966.

Wang, C. C., and Robbins, L. L.: Amyloid disease: Its roentgen manifestations. Radiology 66:489, 1956.

Abnormal Fluid Accumulation

Berman, L. B.: Vasomotor nephropathy. JAMA 231:1067, 1975.

Bowley, N. B.: Renal opacification during intravenous urography in acute cortical necrosis (the nephrogram in cortical necrosis). Br. J. Radiol. 54:524, 1981.

Deutsch, V., Frankl, O., Drory, Y., Eliahon, H., and Braf, S. F.: Bilateral renal cortical necrosis with survival through the acute phase with a note on the value of selective renal nephro-angiography. Am. J. Med. 50:828, 1971.

Feldman, H. A., Goldfarb, S., and McCurdy, D. K.: Recurrent radiographic dye-induced renal failure. JAMA 229:72, 1974.

Fry, I. K., and Cattell, W. R.: The nephrographic pattern during excretion urography. Br. Med. Bull. 28:227, 1972.

Goergen, T. G., Lindstrom, R. R., Tan, H., and Lilley, J. J.: CT appearance of acute renal cortical necrosis. AJR 137:176, 1981.

Hollenberg, N. K., Adams, D. F., Merrill, J. P., and Abrams, H. L.: Acute renal failure due to nephrotoxins: Renal hemodynamics and angiographic studies in man. N. Engl. J. Med. 282:1329, 1970.

Kleinknecht, D., Grünfeld, J.-P., Gomez, P. C., Moreau, J.-F., and Garcia-Torres, R.: Diagnostic procedures and long-term prognosis in bilateral renal cortical necrosis. Kidney. Int. 4:390, 1973.

Levinsky, N. G.: Pathophysiology of acute renal failure. N. Engl. J. Med. 296:1453, 1977.

Lloyd-Thomas, H. G., Balme, R. H., and Key, J. J.: Tramline calcification in renal cortical necrosis. Br. Med. J. 1:909, 1962.

McAlister, W. H., and Nedelman, S. H.: The roentgen manifestations of bilateral renal cortical necrosis. AJR 86:129, 1961.

Möell, H.: Gross bilateral renal cortical necrosis during long periods of oliguria-anuria: Roentgenologic observations in two cases. Acta Radiol. (Diagn.) 48:355, 1957.

Moreau, J.-F., Kleinknecht, D., Grünfeld, J. P., Reboul, F., Sabto, J., and Michel, J. R.: Aspects artériographiques des nécroses corticales rénales. J. Radiol. 55:1, 1974.

Nomura, G., Kinoshita, E., Yamagata, Y., and Koga, N.: Usefulness of ultrasonography for assessment of severity and course of acute tubular necrosis. J. Clin. Ultrasound 12:135, 1984.

Oken, D. E.: Nosologic considerations in the nomenclature of acute renal failure. Nephron 8:505, 1971.

Older, R. A., Korobkin, M., Cleeve, D. M., Schaaf, R., and Thompson, W.: Contrast-induced acute renal failure: Persistent nephrogram as clue to early detection. AJR 134:339, 1980.

Robinson, P. J. A., Gaunt, A., and McLachlan, M. S. F.: Nephrographic density and renal diatrizoate content in experimental acute renal failure. Br. J. Radiol. 49:321, 1976.

Rosenberg, H. K., Gefter, W. B., Lebowitz, R. L., Mahboubi, S., and Rosenberg, H.: Prolonged dense nephrograms in battered children. Urology 221:325, 1983.

Sefczek, R. J., Beckman, I., Lupetin, A. R. and Dash, N.: Sonography of acute cortical necrosis. AJR 142:553, 1984.

Sherwood, T., Doyle, F. H., Boulton-Jones, M., Joekes, A. M., Peters, D. K., and Sissons, P.: The intravenous urogram in acute renal failure. Br. J. Radiol. 47:368, 1974.

Sherwood, T., and Evans, D. J.: Intravenous urography in experimental acute renal failure: Nephrograms and pyelograms in saline-loaded rats. Nephron 22:577, 1978.

Smolens, P., and Stein, J. H.: Pathophysiology of acute renal failure. Am. J. Med. 70:479, 1981.

Sty, J. R., Starshak, R. J., and Hubbard, A. M.: Acute renal cortical necrosis in hemolytic uremic syndrome. JCU 11:175, 1983.

Whelan, J. G., Jr., Ling, J. T., and Davis, L. A.: Antemortem roentgen manifestations of bilateral renal cortical necrosis. Radiology 89:682, 1967.

Neoplastic Infiltration

Amromin, G. O.: Pathology of Leukemia. New York, Hoeber, 1968, p. 251.

Besse, B. E., Jr., Lieberman, J. E., and Lusted, L. B.: Kidney size in acute leukemia. AJR 80:611, 1958.

Wewerka-Lutz, Y.: Renal involvement in malignant lymphoma. Schweiz. Med. Wochenschr. 102:689, 1972.

Inflammatory Cell Infiltration

Appel, G. B.: A decade of penicillin-related acute interstitial nephritis—more questions than answers. Clin. Nephrol. 13:151, 1980.

Baker, S. B., and Williams, R. T.: Acute interstitial nephritis due to drug sensitivity. Br. Med. J. 1:1655, 1963.

Baldwin, D. S., Levine, B. B., McCloskey, R. T., and Gallo, G. R.: Renal failure and interstitial nephritis due to penicillin and methicillin. N. Engl. J. Med. 279:1245, 1968.

Cogan, M. G.: Tubulo-interstitial nephropathies: A pathophysiologic approach. West. J. Med. 132:134, 1980.

Grüfeld, J.-P., Kleinecht, D., and Droz, D.: Acute interstitial nephritis. In Schrier, R. W., and Gottschalk, C. W. (eds.): Diseases of the Kidney. 4th ed. Boston, Little, Brown & Co., 1988, pp. 1461–1488.

Heptinstall, R. H.: Interstitial nephritis. In Heptinstall, R. H. (ed.): Pathology of the Kidney. 4th ed. Boston, Little, Brown & Co., 1992, pp. 1315–1368.

Autosomal Recessive (Infantile) Polycystic Kidney Disease

Alvarez, F., Bernard, O., Brunelle, F., and Hadchuoel, M.: Congenital hepatic fibrosis in children. J. Pediatr. 99:370, 1981.

Argubright, K. F., and Wicks, J. D.: Third trimester ultrasonic presentation of infantile polycystic kidney disease. Am. J. Perinatol. 4:1, 1987.

Bernstein, J.: Heritable cystic disorders of the kidneys: The mythology of polycystic disease. Pediatr. Clin. North Am. 18:435, 1971.

Bernstein, J.: The classification of renal cysts. Nephron 2:91, 1973.

Blyth, H., and Ockenden, B.: Polycystic disease of kidneys and liver presenting in childhood. J. Med. Genet. 8:257, 1971.

Boal, D., and Teele, R.: Sonography of infantile polycystic kidney disease. AJR 135:575, 1980.

Cuarrarino, G., Stannard, M. W., and Rutledge, J. C.: The sonolucent cortical rim in infantile polycystic kidneys: Histologic correlation. J. Ultrasound Med. 8:571, 1989.

Davies, C. H., Stringer, D. A., Whyte, H., Daneman, A., and Mancer, K.: Congenital hepatic fibrosis with saccular dilatation of intra-

hepatic bile ducts and infantile polycystic kidneys. Pediatr. Radiol. 16:302, 1986.

Eggli, K. H., and Hartman, D. S.: Autosomal recessive polycystic kidney disease. In Hartman, D. S. (ed.): Renal Cystic Disease, fascicle I of the Atlas of Radiologic Pathologic Correlation. Washington, D. C., Armed Forces Institute of Pathology, 1989.

Fitch, S. J. and Stapleton, F. B.: Ultrasonographic features of glomerulocystic disease in infancy: Similarity to infantile polycystic kidney disease. Pediatr. Radiol. 16:400, 1986.

Fredericks, B. J., de Campo, M., Chow, C. W., and Powell, H. R.: Glomerulocystic disease: Ultrasound appearances. Pediatr. Radiol. 19:184, 1989.

Glassberg, K. I., and Filmer, R. B.: Renal dysplasia, renal hypoplasia, and cystic disease of the kidney. In Kelalis, P., King, L., and Belman, A. B. (eds.): Clinical Pediatric Urology. 2nd ed. Philadelphia, W. B. Saunders, 1985, p. 922.

Grantham, J. J., and Gabow, P.: Polycystic kidney diseases. In Schrier, R. W., Gottschalk, C. W. (eds.): Diseases of the Kidney. 4th ed. Boston, Little, Brown & Co., 1988, pp. 583–616.

Grossman, H., Winchester, P. H., and Chisari, F. V.: Roentgenographic classifications of renal cystic disease. AJR 10:319, 1968.

Gwinn, J., and Landing, B.: Cystic diseases of the kidneys in infants and children. Radiol. Clin. North Am. 6:191, 1968.

Hayden, C. K., Swischuk, L. E., Smith, T. H., and Armstrong, E. A.: Renal cystic disease in childhood. Radiographics 6:97, 1986.

Howie, J. L., and Nicholson, R. L.: CT evaluation of infantile polycystic disease. J. Can. Assoc. Radiol. 31:202, 1980.

Hussman, K. L., Friedwald, J. P., Gollub, M. J., and Melamed, J.: Caroli's disease associated with infantile polycystic kidney disease. J. Ultrasound Med. 10:235, 1991.

Jorgensen, M. J.: The ductal plate malformation. Acta Pathol. Microbiol. Immunol. Scand. (Suppl.) 257:1, 1977.

Kääriäinen, H., Jääskeläinen, J., Kivisaan, L., Koskimies, O., and Norio, R.: Dominant and recessive polycystic kidney disease in children: Classification by intravenous pyelography, ultrasound, and computed tomography. Pediatr. Radiol. 18:45, 1988.

Kaiser, J. A., Mall, J.C., Salmen, B. J., and Parker, J. J.: Diagnosis of Caroli's disease by computed tomography: Report of two cases. Radiology 132:661, 1979.

Kogutt, M. S., Robichaux, W. H., Boineau, F. G., Drake, G. K., and Simonton, S. C.: Asymmetric renal size in autosomal recessive polycystic kidney disease: A unique presentation. AJR 160:835, 1993.

Kuhn, J. P., and Berger, P. E.: Computed tomography of the kidney in infancy and childhood. Radiol. Clin. North Am. 19:445, 1981.

Lieberman, E., Salinas-Madrigal, L., Gwinn, J., Brennan, L. P., Fine, R. N., and Landing, B. H.: Infantile polycystic disease of the kidneys and liver: Clinical, pathological and radiological correlations and comparison with congenital hepatic fibrosis. Medicine 50:277, 1971.

Luthy, D. A., and Hirsch, J. H.: Infantile polycystic kidney disease: Observations from attempts at prenatal diagnosis. Am. J. Med. Genet. 20:505, 1985.

Madewell, J. E., Hartman, D. S., and Lichtenstein, J. E.: Radiologic-pathologic correlations in cystic disease of the kidney. Radiol. Clin. North Am. 17:261, 1979.

Mall, J. C., Ghahremani, G. G., and Bayer, J. L.: Caroli's disease associated with congenital hepatic fibrosis and renal tubular ectasia. Gastroenterology 66:1029, 1974.

Marchal, G. J., Desmet, V. J., Proesmans, W. C., et al.: Caroli disease: High-frequency US and pathologic findings. Radiology 158:507, 1986.

McGonigle, R., Mowat, A., and Benwick, M.: Congenital hepatic fibrosis and polycystic kidney disease: Role of portacaval shunt and transplantation in three patients. Q. J. Med. 50:269, 1981.

Melson, G. L., Shackelford, G. D., Cole, B. R., et al.: The spectrum of sonographic findings in infantile polycystic kidney disease with urographic and clinical correlations. JCU 13:113, 1985.

Mittelstaedt, C. A., Volberg, F. M., Fischer, G. J., and McArtney, W. H.: Caroli's disease: Sonographic findings. AJR 134:585, 1980.

Moreno, A. J., Parker, A. L., Spicer, M. J., et al.: Scintigraphic and radiographic findings in Caroli's disease. Am. J. Gastroenterol 79:299, 1984.

Mujahed, Z., Glenn, F., and Evans, J. A.: Communicating cavernous ectasia of the intrahepatic ducts (Caroli's disease). AJR 113:21, 1971.

Nakanuma, Y., Terada, T., Ohta, G., Kurachi, M., and Matsubara, F.: Caroli's disease in congenital hepatic fibrosis and infantile polycystic disease. Liver 2:346, 1982.

Osathanondh, V., and Potter, E. L.: Pathogenesis of polycystic kidneys. Arch. Pathol. 77:461, 1964.

Patriquin, H. B., and O'Regan, S.: Medullary sponge kidney in childhood. AJR 145:315, 1985.

Potter, E. L.: Normal and Abnormal Development of the Kidney, Chicago, Year Book Medical Publishers, 1972.

Premkumar, A., Berdon, W. E., Levy, J., Amondio, J., Abramson, S. J., and Newhouse, J. H.: The emergence of hepatic fibrosis and portal hypertension in infants and children with autosomal polycystic kidney disease. Pediatr. Radiol. 18:123, 1988.

Rabinowitz R., Segal, A., Rao, H. K,. and Pathak, A.: Computed tomography in diagnosis of infantile polycystic kidney disease. J. Urol. 120:616, 1978.

Rosenfield, A. T., Siegel, N. J., Kappelman, N. B., and Taylor, K. J. W.: Gray scale ultrasonography in medullary cystic disease of the kidney and congenital hepatic fibrosis with tubular ectasia: New observations. AJR 129:297, 1977.

Six, R., Oliphant, M., and Grossman, H.: A spectrum of renal tubular ectasia and hepatic fibrosis. Radiology 117:117, 1975.

Stapleton, F. B., Magill, H. L., and Kelly, D. R.: Infantile polycystic kidney disease: An imaging dilemma. Urol. Radiol. 5:89, 1983.

Sztriha, L., Gyurkovits, K., Ormos, J., and Monus, Z.: Congenital hepatic fibrosis with polycystic disease of the kidneys. Hepatogastroenterology 29:259, 1982.

Taxy, J. B., and Filmer, R. B.: Glomerulocystic kidney. Arch. Pathol. Lab. Med. 100:186, 1976.

Thaler, M., Ogata, E., Goodman, J., Piel, C. F., and Korobkin, M. T.: Congenital fibrosis and polycystic disease of liver and kidneys. Am. J. Dis. Child. 126:374, 1973.

Unite, I., Maitem, A., Bagnasco, F., and Irwin, G. A.: Congenital hepatic fibrosis associated with renal tubular ectasia. Radiology 109:565, 1973.

Weese-Mayer, D. E., Smith, K. M., Reddy, J. K., Salafsky, I., Poznanski, A. K.: Computerized tomography and ultrasound in the diagnosis of cerebro-hepato-renal syndrome of Zellinger. Pediatr. Radiol. 17:170, 1987.

Wernecke, K., Heckemann, R., Bachmann, H., and Peters, P. E.: Sonography of infantile polycystic kidney disease. Urol. Radiol. 7:138, 1985.

Wood, B. P.: Renal cystic disease in infants and children. Urol. Radiol. 14:284, 1992.

Acute Urate Nephropathy

Fry, I. K., and Cattell, W. R.: The nephrographic pattern during excretion urography. Br. Med. Bull. 28:227, 1972.

Kelley, W. M.: Uricosuria and x-ray contrast agents. N. Engl. J. Med. 284:975, 1971.

Martin, D. J., and Jaffe, N.: Prolonged nephrogram due to hyperuricaemia. Br. J. Radiol. 44:806, 1971.

Postlethwaite, A. E., and Kelley, W. M.: Uricosuric effect of radiocontrast agents: A study in man of four commonly used preparations. Ann. Intern. Med. 74:845, 1971.

Robinson, R. R., and Yarger, W. E.: Acute uric acid nephropathy. Arch. Intern. Med. 137:839, 1977.

Glycogen Storage Disease, Type I

Chen, Y.-T., Feinstein, K. A., Coleman, R. A., and Effmann, E. L.: Variability of renal length in Type I glycogen storage disease. J. Inherit. Metab. Dis. 13:259, 1990.

Chen, Y.-T.: Type I glycogen storage disease: Kidney involvement, pathogenesis and its treatment. Pediatr. Nephrol. 5:71, 1991.

Chen, Y.-T., Coleman, R. A., Sheinman, J. L., Kolbeck, P. C., and Sidury, J. B.: Renal disease in Type I glycogen storage disease. N. Engl. J. Med. 318:7, 1988.

Miller, J. H., Stanley, P., and Gates, G. F.: Radiography of glycogen storage disease. AJR 132:379, 1979.

Slovis, T. L., Sty, J. R., and Haller, J. O.: Imaging of the Pediatric Urinary Tract. Philadelphia, W. B. Saunders, 1989.

Verani, R., and Bernstein, J.: Renal glomerular and tubular abnormalities in glycogen storage disease Type I. Arch. Pathol. Lab. Med. 112:271, 1988.

Response to Urographic Contrast Material and Diuretics

Dorph, S., and Øigaard, A.: Variations in size of the normal kidney following intravenous administration of water-soluble contrast medium and urea. Br. J. Radiol. 46:183, 1973.

Dorph, S., and Øigaard, A.: Renal distention in response to water-soluble contrast medium and various diuretics: A comparative study. Scand. J. Urol. Nephrol. 9:114, 1975.

Vuorinen, P., and Wegelius, U.: Changes of renal size after drinking and intravenous glucose infusion. Br. J. Radiol. 38:673, 1965.

Wolf, G. L.: Rationale and use of vasodilated excretory urography in screening for renovascular hypertension. AJR 119:692, 1973.

Wolpert, S. M.: Variation in kidney length during intravenous pyelography. Br. J. Radiol. 38:100, 1965.

Homozygous-S Disease

Addae, S. K.: The kidney in sickle cell disease: V. Clinical manifestations. Ghana Med. J. 12:352, 1973.

Berman, L. B.: Sickle cell nephropathy. JAMA 228:1279, 1974.

Buckalew, V. M., and Someren, A.: Renal manifestations of sickle cell disease. Arch. Intern. Med. 133:660, 1974.

Karayalcin, G., Dorfman, J., Rosner, F., and Aballi, A. J.: Radiological changes in 127 patients with sickle cell anemia. Am. J. Med. Sci. 271:132, 1976.

Lande, J. M., Glazer, G. M., Sarnaik, S., Aisen, A., Rucknagle, D., Martel, W.: Sickle cell nephropathy: MR imaging. Radiology 158:379, 1986.

McCall, I. W., Moule, N., Desai, P., and Serjeant, G. R.: Urographic findings in homozygous sickle cell disease. Radiology 126:99, 1978.

Mostofi, F. K., Bruegge, C. F. V., and Diggs, L. W.: Lesions in kidneys removed for unilateral hematuria in sickle cell disease. Arch. Pathol. 63:336, 1957.

Statius van Eps, L. W., and de Jong, P. E.: Sickle cell disease. In Schrier, R. W., and Gottschalk, C. W. (eds.): Diseases of the Kidney. 4th ed. Boston, Little, Brown & Co., 1988, pp. 2561–2582.

Paroxysmal Nocturnal Hemoglobinuria

Braren, V., Butler, S. A., Hartmann, R. C., and Jenkins, D. E., Jr.: Urologic manifestations of paroxysmal nocturnal hemoglobinuria. J. Urol. 114:430, 1975.

Clark, D.A., Butler, S. A., Braren, V., Hartmann, R. C., and Jenkins, D. E.: The kidneys in paroxysmal nocturnal hemoglobinuria. Blood 57:83, 1981.

Kaplan, M. E.: Acquired hemolytic disorders. In Wyngaarden, J. B., and Smith, L. H., Jr. (eds.): Cecil's Textbook of Medicine. Philadelphia, W. B. Saunders, 1988, p. 922.

Lupetin, A. R.: Magnetic resonance appearance of the kidneys in paroxysmal nocturnal hemoglobinuria. Urol. Radiol. 8:101, 1986.

Hemophilia

Dalinka, M. K., Lally, J. F., Rancier, L. F., and Mata, J.: Nephromegaly in hemophilia. Radiology 115:337, 1975.

Roberts, G. M., Evans, K. T., Bloom, A. L., and Al-Gailani, F.: Renal papillary necrosis in haemophilia and Christmas disease. Clin. Radiol. 34:201, 1983.

Cirrhosis, Hyperalimentation, and Diabetes Mellitus

Christiansen, J. S., Gammelgaard, J., Tronier, B., Svendsen, P. A., and Parving, H.-H.: Kidney function and size in diabetes before and during initial insulin treatment. Kidney Int. 21:638, 1982.

Cochran, S. T., Pagani, J. J., and Barbaric, Z. L.: Nephromegaly in hyperalimentation. Radiology 130:603, 1979.

Laube, H., Norris, H. T., and Robbins, S. L.: The nephromegaly of chronic alcoholics with liver disease. Arch. Pathol. Lab. Med. 84:290, 1967.

Mauer, S. M., Steffes, M. W., and Brown, D. M.: The kidney in diabetes. Am. J. Med. 70:603, 1981.

Mogensen, C. E., and Andersen, M. J. F.: Increased kidney size and glomerular filtration rate in early juvenile diabetes. Diabetes 22:706, 1973.

Osterby, R., and Gundersen, H. J. G.: Glomerular size and structure in diabetes mellitus: I. Early abnormalities. Diabetologia 11:225, 1975.

Fabry's Disease

Case records of the Massachusetts General Hospital: Case 2–1984. Fabry's disease. N. Engl. J. Med. 310:106, 1984.

Novello, A. C., and Bennett, W. M.: Fabry's disease and nail-patella syndrome. In Schrier, R. W., Gottschalk, C. W. (eds.): Diseases of the Kidney. 4th ed. Boston, Little, Brown & Co., 1988, pp. 643–662.

Stiennon, M., and Goldberg, M. E.: Renal size in Fabry's Disease. Urol. Radiol. 2:17, 1980.

Bartter's Syndrome

Cogan, M. G., and Rector, F. C., Jr.: Acid base disorders. In Brenner, B. M., and Rector, F. C. (eds.): The Kidney. 4th ed. Philadelphia, W. B. Saunders, 1991, pp. 737–804.

Garel, L., Filiatrault, D., and Robitaille, P.: Nephrocalcinosis in Bartter's syndrome. Pediatr. Nephrol. 2:315, 1988.

Matsumoto, J., Han, B. K., Rovetto, C. R., and Welch, T. R.: Hypercalciuric Bartter syndrome: Resolution of nephrocalcinosis with indomethacin. AJR 152:1251, 1989.

Strause, S., Robinson, G., Lotan, D., and Itzechak, Y.: Renal sonography in Bartter syndrome. J. Ultrasound Med. 6:205, 1987.

Taybi, H.: Radiology of Syndromes and Metabolic Disorders. 2nd ed. Chicago, Year Book Medical Publishers, 1983, p. 32.

Beckwith-Wiedemann Syndrome

Beckwith, J. B.: Macroglossia, omphalocele, adrenal cytomegaly, gigantism and hyperplastic visceromegaly. Birth Defects 5:188, 1969.

Bronk, J. B., and Parker, B. R.: Pyelocalyceal diverticula in the Beckwith-Wiedemann syndrome. Pediatr. Radiol. 17:80, 1987.

Chesney, R. W., Kaufman, R., Stapleton, F. B., and Rivas, M. L.: Association of medullary sponge kidney and medullary dysplasia in Beckwith-Wiedemann Syndrome. J. Pediatr. 115:761, 1989.

Lee, F. A.: Radiology of the Beckwith-Wiedemann syndrome. Radiol. Clin. North Am. 10:261, 1972.

McCarten, K. M., Cleveland, R. H., Simeone, J. F., and Aretz, T.: Renal ultrasonography in Beckwith-Wiedemann syndrome. Pediatr. Radiol. 11:46, 1981.

9

DIAGNOSTIC SET: LARGE, SMOOTH, UNILATERAL

Diseases discussed in this chapter classically involve one kidney only. This is not to say that both kidneys are never involved in renal vein thrombosis, acute hemorrhagic infarction, obstructive uropathy, acute pyelonephritis, or duplication of the pelvocalyceal system. When bilateral involvement does occur, however, it is a chance phenomenon, not a natural feature of the disease process itself.

RENAL VEIN THROMBOSIS

Definition

The rapidity with which renal vein occlusion occurs partially determines the pattern of response in the kidney. At one extreme, sudden, total occlusion produces hemorrhagic infarction, permanent loss of function, and eventual shrinkage of the kidney. At the other, gradual onset of venous occlusion allows time for collateral channels to develop, leaving normal renal anatomy and function undisturbed. The appearance of the kidney depends not only on the rapidity with which occlusion occurs, but also on the completeness of the occlusion, the amount of collateral channel development, and the degree to which the thrombosis eventually recanalizes. In addition, venous thrombosis in the adult is usually a complication of a primary renal disease that itself will alter the appearance of the kidney.

When renal vein occlusion is sudden, there is no time for effective development of collateral pathways. The interstices of the kidney swell with blood from ruptured venules and capillaries. The organ becomes generally enlarged and tense, and urine formation ceases. Eventually, fibrous tissue replaces necrotic nephrons, resulting in a globally wasted, nonfunctioning kidney. The pattern is the same as that seen in acute infarction due to main renal artery occlusion or severe trauma to the kidney.

There are times when venous occlusion develops rapidly and extensively—yet irreversible changes leading to renal atrophy do not follow because collateral drainage develops to some degree. In this circumstance, interstitial edema and congested intrarenal vessels cause global enlargement of the kidney. Function, although impaired, continues. Either these changes persist in a steady state or complete resolution occurs as recanalization of the thrombus or further expansion of collateral venous pathways provides adequate venous drainage. In these cases, there is thickening of basement membranes, interstitial edema, and polymorphonuclear leukocyte margination in capillaries. Mild tubule atrophy and interstitial fibrosis may eventually develop.

Finally, the process of venous obstruction can be so indolent as not to alter gross renal morphology. Cases of this type may present as the nephrotic syndrome even when the process is unilateral. A glomerular lesion similar to that of membranous glomerulonephritis has been described in these patients.

Clinical Setting

Renal vein thrombosis in the newborn is usually associated with dehydration, birth asphyxia, hypotension, sepsis, or maternal diabetes mellitus. In the older child, severe dehydration is sometimes complicated by renal vein thrombosis. In the adult, thrombosis is most often a complication of another renal disease, such as amyloidosis, membranous glomerulonephritis, or other conditions that cause the nephrotic syndrome. Thrombosis of the inferior vena cava with retrograde propagation of clot into the renal vein, extrinsic pressure by tumor on the inferior vena cava or renal vein, extension of a kidney tumor into the renal vein, and trauma are other conditions that predispose to renal vein thrombosis.

243

A sudden, major occlusion causes sharp flank pain and tenderness, and the kidney often becomes palpable. Fever and leukocytosis develop. Gross or microscopic hematuria may be present, but a normal urinalysis is not uncommon when urine formation ceases on the involved side.

When the degree of occlusion is less acute, unilateral global renal enlargement will be accompanied by deteriorating function of the involved kidney. This may progress or may reverse, depending on the extent of recanalization of the thrombus, the lysis of clot by therapy, or the opening up of collateral venous drainage.

Patients with slowly developing chronic occlusion may be asymptomatic or may present with the nephrotic syndrome (edema, hyperlipidemia, hypoproteinemia, and massive proteinuria) representing a predisposing condition.

Radiologic Findings

Kidney enlargement can be striking in acute renal vein thrombosis. Experimental and clinical studies have shown that the flow of contrast material into the kidney is very much reduced or even absent. When this occurs, a very large, smooth renal mass with little or no opacification is seen during contrast material—enhanced studies such as excretory urography or computed tomography (Fig. 9–1). If unresolved, this form of venous occlusion produces renal infarction and eventually causes a small, smooth, nonfunctioning renal outline on late follow-up studies. This transition may occur over a period of 2 months. Deposition of calcium in a fine reticular pattern within the renal substance has been reported as a late sequela of renal vein thrombosis in infants. This is thought to represent calcium deposition in intrarenal veins and might also occur in adults.

When venous occlusion is partial or accompanied by adequate collateral formation, or when resolution of a previously more acute and complete occlusion takes place, the kidney is large and smooth, but some degree of contrast material excretion can be expected. The collecting system has a normal distribution within the renal substance but is usually attenuated by the surrounding swollen kidney. In a few cases, the nephrogram has been described as increasingly dense with time (Fig. 9–2A and B). This undoubtedly represents continued arterial perfusion to a kidney unable to eliminate the accumulating contrast material through usual venous or urinary pathways. Alternating radiolucent and radiopaque nephrographic striations, thought to represent contrast material in dilated tubules in the medullary rays, have been described in both excretory urograms and angiograms. A cortical rim sign, usually associated with acute arterial infarc-

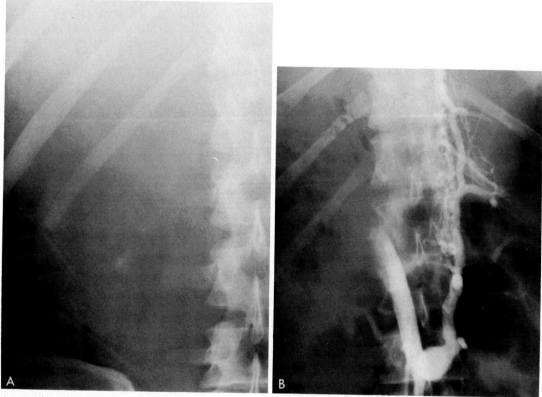

Figure 9–1. Acute right renal vein occlusion following trauma in a young man with congenital absence of the left kidney.
  A, Excretory urogram. The kidney is enlarged and poorly outlined. A small collection of contrast material is present in a lower pole calyx. The remainder of the collecting system is effaced.
  B, Inferior vena cavagram. Renal vein obstruction is secondary to a large retroperitoneal hematoma displacing and occluding the inferior vena cava. Collateral drainage is through the azygous system.

tion, has also been associated with renal vein thrombosis.

Enlargement of collateral pathways for renal venous outflow is an important sequel to occlusion of the renal vein. Gonadal, ureteric, lumbar, adrenal, and capsular veins participate. Both the enlarged gonadal and the ureteric veins produce easily identified indentations on a well-distended, opacified pelvis and ureter. These may resemble ureteritis or pyelitis cystica (Fig. 9–3). If contrast material excretion is insufficient for visualization of the pelvis and ureter, retrograde pyelography is necessary to demonstrate these findings. In addition a feathery mucosal pattern may be seen in the pelvis and the proximal ureter. This appearance, representing either distended submucosal veins, mural edema, or hemorrhage, often disappears when the pelvis is distended during retrograde pyelography or following effective ureteral compression (see Fig. 9–2C).

Patients with renal vein thrombosis, including cases associated with the nephrotic syndrome, may have entirely normal radiologic studies. This suggests an incomplete occlusion from the onset, the recanalization or lysis of an earlier thrombus, or the presence of collaterals adequate in volume to carry the renal venous efflux.

Computed tomographic findings include those described for excretory urography. Additional features may include prolonged corticomedullary differentia-

tion, distended collateral veins in the renal sinus, focal zones of nonenhanced parenchyma in areas of infarction, retroperitoneal hemorrhage, and enlargement of the renal vein in which there is low attenuation thrombus (Fig. 9–4 through 9–6). Fine linear densities radiating from the kidney into the perirenal space have been described as characteristic, although not pathognomonic, of renal vein thrombus. These structures, which enhance with contrast material, most likely represent collateral renal veins traversing the perirenal space.

Ultrasonography demonstrates smooth enlargement of the kidney, with increased parenchymal thickness and a variable echo pattern (Figs. 9–5 and 9–6). Within the first 2 to 3 weeks of the onset of thrombosis, the echogenicity of the kidney diminishes, presumably owing to interstitial fluid accumulation. Thereafter, echogenicity increases as fibrosis causes global wasting of the kidney. Hyperechoic areas may be present at the site of lobar infarction. The renal vein is enlarged, and thrombus may be demonstrated as intraluminal echogenic tissue that extends into the inferior vena cava, giving rise to the same findings seen with tumor extension into the renal vein (see Fig. 12–28). Doppler ultrasound scanning detects reduction or absence of venous blood flow. Ultrasonography also detects perirenal hemorrhage when acute renal vein thrombosis causes rupture of the kidney.

Magnetic resonance imaging of the inferior vena

Text continued on page 252

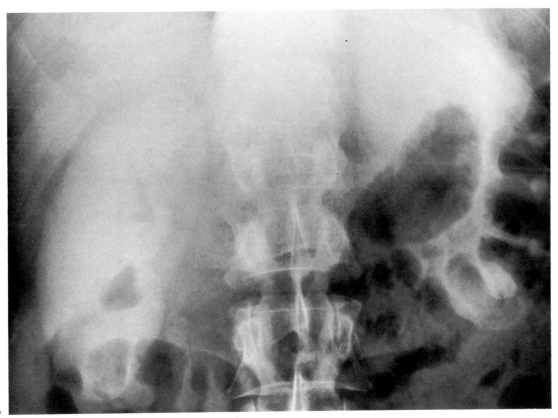

A

Figure 9–2. Left renal vein thrombosis in a 60-year-old man with nephrotic syndrome.
A, Film taken 1 minute after contrast material injection demonstrates a large left kidney (length = 16.9 cm) with a denser nephrogram than seen on the right kidney.

Illustration continued on following page

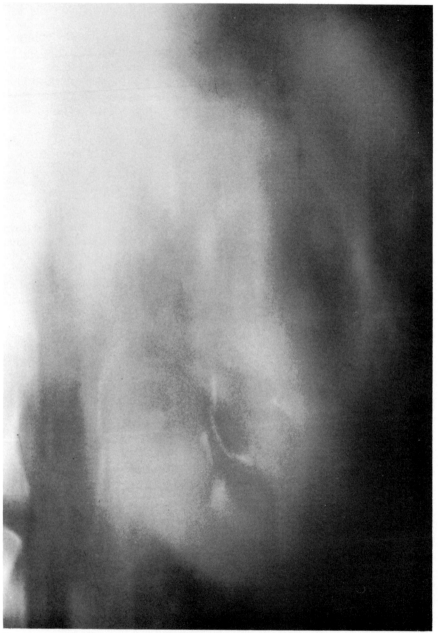

Figure 9–2 *Continued B,* Tomogram during excretory urography. The collecting system is normally distributed within the kidney substance but is effaced by surrounding interstitial edema.

B

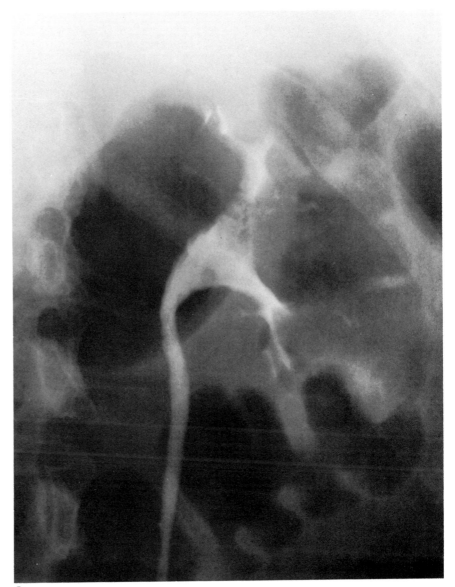

Figure 9–2 *Continued C,* Retrograde pyelogram. Nodular defects and a feathery mucosal pattern are seen in the pelvis, presumably reflecting distended submucosal veins, mural edema, or hemorrhage.

Illustration continued on following page

C

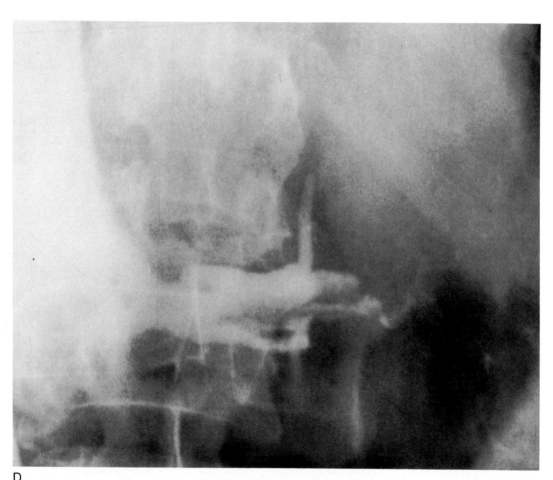

D

Figure 9–2 *Continued D,* Left retrograde renal venogram. The proximal part of the renal vein contains a large thrombus.

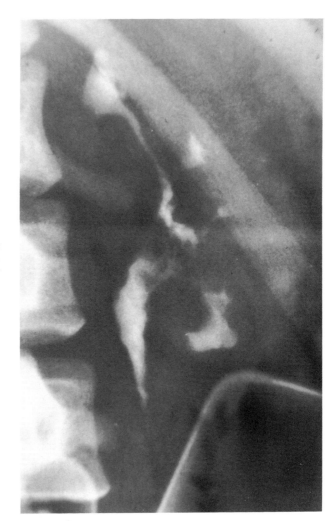

Figure 9–3. Renal vein thrombosis, left kidney. Excretory urogram with compression. There are multiple mural notches deforming the pelvis, which does not distend normally. The notches represent distended collateral veins.

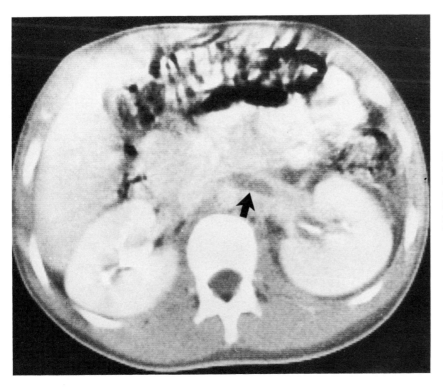

Figure 9–4. Renal vein thrombosis, left kidney. Computed tomogram, contrast material enhanced. The left kidney is enlarged and smooth, and the pelvocalyceal system is attenuated. Enhancing soft tissue representing venous collateral pathways surrounds the thrombosed left renal vein, which is unenhanced *(arrow)*.

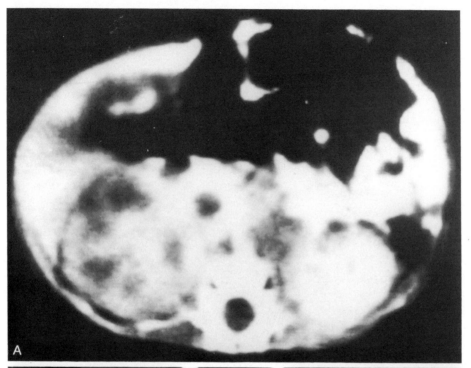

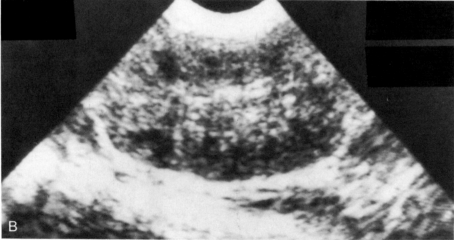

Figure 9–5. Renal vein thrombosis, right kidney, in a newborn with a palpable mass in the right upper quadrant of the abdomen.

A, Computed tomogram, contrast material enhanced. The right kidney is enlarged, and there is persistent corticomedullary differentiation indicating prolonged circulation time through the kidney.

B, Ultrasonogram, longitudinal section, demonstrates smooth enlargement and increased cortical echogenicity relative to the medullae, a normal finding in the newborn.

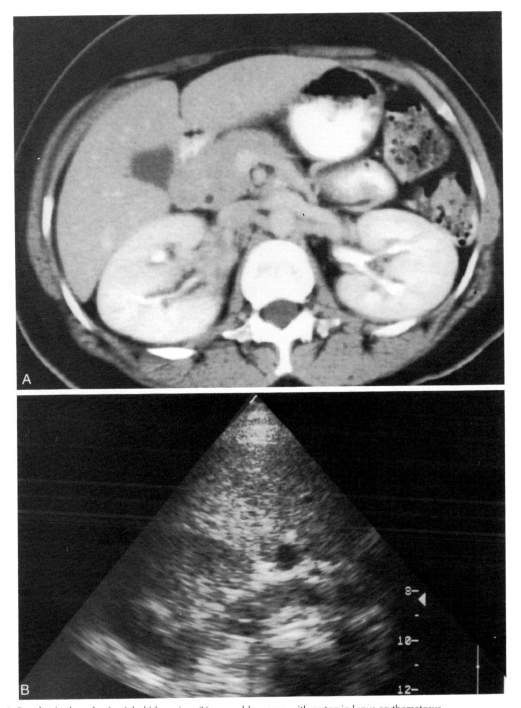

Figure 9–6. Renal vein thrombosis, right kidney, in a 26-year-old woman with systemic lupus erythematosus.
   A, Computed tomogram, contrast material enhanced. Abnormal soft tissue structures in the right renal sinus represent collateral veins.
   B, Ultrasonogram, transverse section. There is increased soft tissue in the right renal sinus and an absence of a normal renal vein.

Illustration continued on following page

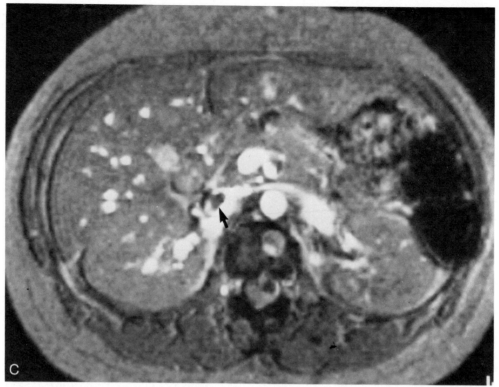

Figure 9–6 *Continued C,* Magnetic resonance image, gradient-echo sequence. There is a flow void at the confluence of the right renal vein and the inferior vena cava representing thrombus *(arrow).*
(Kindly supplied by Wendelin Hayes, D. O., Armed Forces Institute of Pathology, Washington, D.C.)

cava, main renal vein, and intrarenal branches provides a means for directly confirming the presence of thrombus (Fig. 9–6). Angiography, usually venography, also provides similar information (see Fig. 9–2D). It is prudent first to perform an inferior vena cavogram with a catheter placed well below the renal veins to evaluate the inferior vena cava for diseases that might be the cause of secondary renal venous occlusion. Clots extending into the vena cava from the renal veins can also be identified during cavography. Cautious selective catheterization of the renal vein can then follow if caval disease is absent. Retrograde injection of contrast material into interlobar and arcuate

veins is necessary to detect thrombi limited to these vessels. This can be accomplished by placing the catheter tip well into the renal vein and injecting contrast material while the patient performs the Valsalva maneuver. Some authors advocate arterial injection of epinephrine through a selective renal artery catheter to decrease renal blood flow and thereby allow enhanced opacification of the venous tree when contrast material is injected retrograde through a venous catheter. Careful interpretation is necessary to avoid confusing normal renal vein valves with thrombotic occlusion.

Renal arteriography in renal vein thrombosis shows

SUMMARY OF ABNORMAL URORADIOLOGIC FINDINGS
RENAL VEIN THROMBOSIS

Primary Uroradiologic Elements
    Size—normal to large (may become small in late stage)
    Contour—smooth (global)
    Lesion distribution—unilateral
Secondary Uroradiologic Elements
    Pelvoinfundibulocalyceal system—attenuated (global); mucosal irregularity; notching; often opacified only by retrograde pyelography
    Parenchymal thickness—expanded (global)
    Nephrogram—contrast material density absent, diminished or normal; increasingly dense (occasional); striated (rare); focal infarction; prolonged corticomedullary differentiation
    Echogenicity—diminished (early); increased (late)
    Renal veins—dilated; intraluminal thrombus; diminished to absent flow
    Retroperitoneum—dilated collaterals; hemorrhage

stretching of intrarenal arteries, increased circulation time, and diminished or absent venous opacification. The angiographic nephrogram may stain more intensely than normal, and the corticomedullary border is disrupted. A striated nephrogram has been reported. These findings are not specific, however. Occasionally, venous collaterals will opacify.

ACUTE ARTERIAL INFARCTION

Definition

Acute hemorrhagic infarction of the kidney follows embolic or thrombotic renal artery occlusion, blunt abdominal trauma, or sudden, complete renal venous occlusion. In this section, the early changes of infarction following arterial occlusion or blunt trauma are discussed; renal vein occlusion is presented in the preceding section, and a comprehensive discussion of renal trauma is presented in Chapter 27.

When infarction involves most or all of the kidney, there is marked hyperemia of the glomeruli and capillaries. The interstitial spaces, too, become filled with blood, owing to altered capillary permeability. The source of the blood is subsidiary arterial channels, such as capsular arteries, retrograde flow from veins, or continued main arterial perfusion in the case of renal vein occlusion. With time, the hemorrhage and necrotic tissue become surrounded with leukocytes and the cellular elements lose their identifying features.

The infarcted kidney is large and tense, with red discoloration. After 2 to 3 weeks the kidney begins to shrink as a result of autolysis of cells, resorption of free hemoglobin, and development of interstitial fibrosis.

Clinical Setting

Only a small number of cases of renal infarction involve the whole (or even a major segment of) kidney. The majority are either lobar or regional and are discussed in Chapters 5 and 6. Main renal artery occlusion is usually due to an embolus from the heart with rheumatic valvular disease and arrhythmia, subacute bacterial endocarditis, left atrial mural thrombus or tumor, myocardial trauma, or prosthetic valves. In only a minority of cases is the occlusion due to primary arterial disease, such as atherosclerosis, thromboangiitis obliterans, polyarteritis nodosa, or aneurysm.

The kidney is the organ most likely to suffer damage in blunt abdominal trauma. This most often takes the form of parenchymal contusion. Avulsion of the vascular pedicle, fracture of the renal capsule and parenchyma, subcapsular or perirenal hematoma, and laceration of the pelvocalyceal system and ureter also occur. Generalized and extensive contusion is the same as hemorrhagic infarction of the parenchyma, the point of concern in this section.

Signs and symptoms of acute renal infarction vary from none to abrupt onset of severe abdominal or flank pain, with nausea, vomiting, hematuria, and albuminuria. Fever and leukocytosis may be present. An enlarged, tender renal mass can occasionally be palpated. It is important to note that urinalysis may be completely normal when damage to the kidney is severe enough to prevent urine formation. In traumatic infarction due to avulsion of the renal artery, shock may be the dominant clinical finding.

Radiologic Findings

A nonopacified kidney of normal to enlarged size with a normal pelvocalyceal system demonstrated by retrograde pyelography is characteristic of renal artery occlusion due to embolus or thrombosis (Fig. 9–7). The same finding is seen in avulsion of the renal artery, in which case other evidence of trauma, such as fractures or retroperitoneal hematoma, will be noted on the plain film examination of the abdomen. When renal trauma or venous occlusion is the cause of renal infarction, interstitial hemorrhage is the dominant feature. Under these circumstances, the kidney is enlarged, and contrast material accumulation occurs at diminished levels of density. The pelvocalyceal system, when opacified, is effaced and attenuated by the surrounding swollen interstitial fluid. Blood clots may form filling defects in the collecting system.

A cortical rim nephrogram is a distinctive abnormality that occurs in nearly one-half of patients with infarction of either the entire kidney or of the major ventral or dorsal segments (Fig. 9–8; see Fig. 9–10C). This thin rim of contrast material–enhanced tissue represents peripheral cortex that continues to be perfused by capsular collateral arteries. Following administration of contrast material, this region is distinguishable from the nonperfused, and thus nonenhanced, underlying parenchyma. A "cortical rim" sign is best identified by computed tomography, but it can also be demonstrated by excretory urography with tomography. The same finding has also been described in renal vein thrombosis, probably due to renal ischemia or infarction. Nephrographic striations are another abnormality that has been described in renal contusion due to blunt trauma.

In renal infarction, computed tomography demonstrates the above-described abnormalities better than excretory urography. Subcapsular collections of blood and thickening of the renal fascia are additional abnormalities that are well demonstrated by computed tomography.

Ultrasonography in acute renal infarction documents the global increase in renal size and is useful in eliminating obstructive uropathy as a cause of unilateral, smooth renal enlargement. The echogenicity of the acutely infarcted kidney may be diminished as a reflection of interstitial fluid accumulation. With time, this pattern will reverse, as fibrosis develops and causes renal wasting. Doppler ultrasonography will show that renal arterial and venous blood flow is absent.

Angiography provides specific diagnostic informa-

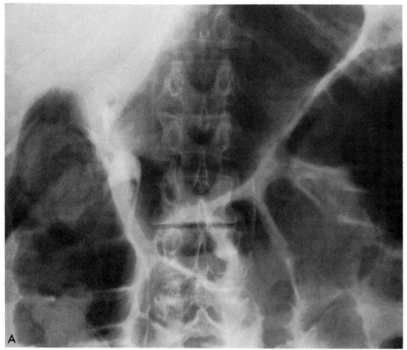

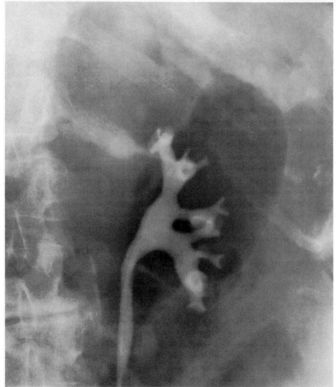

Figure 9–7. Acute left renal infarction in a 78-year-old woman who developed left flank pain and slight leukocytosis following colon surgery. Urinalysis was normal. Radionuclide scan revealed markedly diminished left kidney flow.

A, Excretory urogram. The left kidney did not opacify over a 24-hour period. The right kidney is normal.

B, Left retrograde pyelogram performed to exclude obstructive uropathy. The pelvocalyceal system is normal.

Thirty months later, excretory urography showed that function had returned and global atrophy had developed. (See Fig. 6–11.)

SUMMARY OF ABNORMAL URORADIOLOGIC FINDINGS
ACUTE ARTERIAL INFARCTION

Primary Uroradiologic Elements
    Size—normal to large (may become small in late stage)
    Contour—smooth (global)
    Lesion distribution—unilateral
Secondary Uroradiologic Elements
    Pelvoinfundibulocalyceal system—normal to attenuated (global); often opacified only by retrograde
      pyelography
    Parenchymal thickness—normal to expanded (global)
    Nephrogram—contrast material density absent to diminished; cortical rim enhancement; striations
      (rare)
    Echogenicity—normal to diminished (may increase in late stage)
    Renal artery—intraluminal thrombus, occlusion; absent flow

---

tion in renal infarction by identifying an avulsion injury of the renal artery or an embolus or thrombus in the main renal artery or its major branches (Figs. 9–9 and 9–10). When infarction is due to blunt trauma or venous thrombosis, the findings are nonspecific and reflect swelling of the interstitum. This is seen as attenuation of arteries, decreased number of branches, increased circulation time, and a disrupted corticomedullary junction. With severe trauma, extravasation may occur intrarenally or extrarenally. Other angiographic findings that follow blunt injury to the kidney are arteriovenous fistulas, pseudoaneurysms, and the development of collateral veins.

The magnetic resonance appearance of acute renal infarction has not been studied thoroughly. Limited experience suggests prolongation of T1 relaxation time, low signal intensity, and a loss of corticomedullary differentiation.

Partial or complete recovery of renal infarction from any cause is always possible. The severity of the initiating event will determine the speed of resolution, which is usually in the range of a few weeks to a few months. If recovery is not complete, the kidney eventually wastes, which is discussed in Chapter 6 (see Fig. 6–11).

OBSTRUCTIVE UROPATHY

Obstruction of the urinary tract is discussed in this section in the context of the diagnostic set "large, smooth, unilateral." Other aspects of the subject are presented in Chapter 11, in which the relationship between *in utero* urinary tract obstruction and multicystic dysplastic kidney disease is presented, in Chapter 15, in which congenital ureteropelvic junction obstruction is discussed in detail, and in Chapter 17, in which obstruction is considered as one of several causes of dilatation of the pelvocalyceal system.

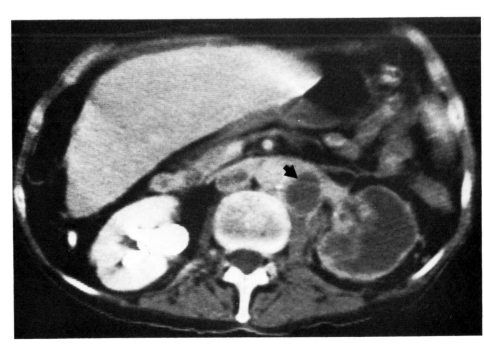

Figure 9–8. Occlusion of left main renal artery by metastatic deposit from lung carcinoma. Computed tomogram, contrast material enhanced. The low-density metastasis *(arrow)* occluded the left renal artery, causing smooth enlargement of the kidney and an absent nephrogram. A rim nephrogram develops where collateral circulation continues to perfuse the cortex. (Courtesy of Stuart London, M. D., Oakland, California.) (Same patient illustrated in Fig. 23–12.)

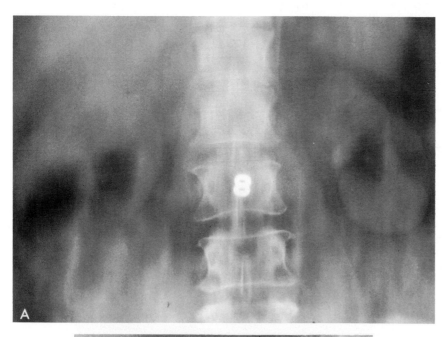

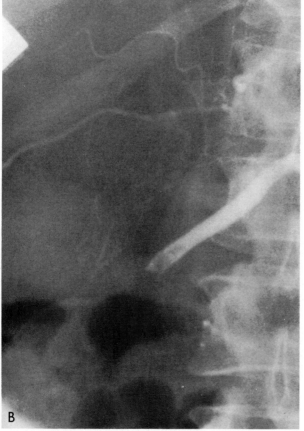

Figure 9–9. Acute embolus to main right renal artery in a woman with rheumatic heart disease and atrial fibrillation.

A, Excretory urogram. Tomogram obtained at 30 minutes. The right kidney is enlarged (length = 14.5 cm) and has a faint nephrogram. The left kidney has evidence of old and recent lobar infarctions.

B, Selective right renal arteriogram demonstrates complete occlusion of the main renal artery.

(Same patient illustrated in Fig. 23–11.)

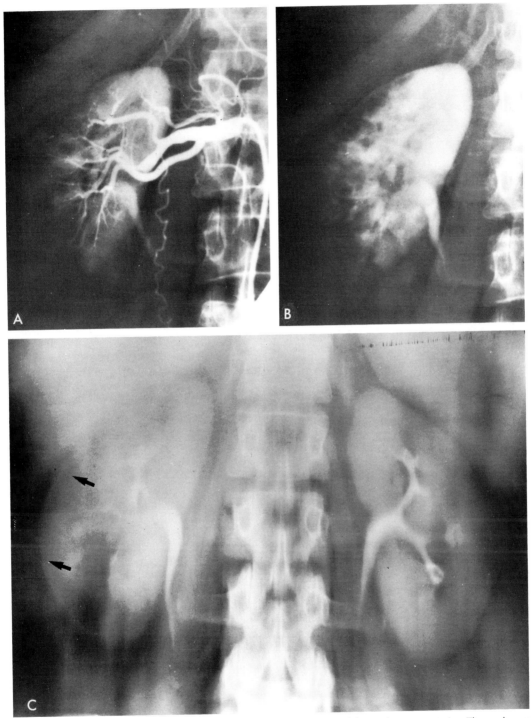

Figure 9–10. Segmental renal artery occlusion. Multiple emboli have occluded both interlobar and arcuate arteries. The nephrogram is absent in those portions of the kidney served by the occluded vessels. Collateral blood flow causes a rim of nephrographic density in the cortex.

A, Selective right renal arteriogram, arterial phase. There are numerous points of occlusion.

B, Selective right renal arteriogram, nephrographic phase. The distribution of the perfusion abnormality is well visualized.

C, Excretory urogram. Tomogram. The nephrogram is absent in the lateral portion of the right kidney, except at the rim of the cortex (*arrows*).

(Courtesy of Professor César Pedrosa and E. Ramirez, M. D., Hospital Clinico de San Carlos, Madrid, Spain.) (Same patient illustrated in Fig. 23–13.)

Definition

Urinary tract obstruction produces anatomic and functional changes that vary with the rapidity of onset, the degree of occlusion, and the distance between the kidney and the obstructing lesion. The anatomy of the involved renal pelvis, particularly whether its location is intrarenal or extrarenal, is an important additional variable. Some authorities distinguish between an obstruction that produces dilatation of the collecting structures without functional deficit, terming this *hydronephrosis* or *obstructive uropathy,* and an obstruction in which renal functional impairment accompanies dilatation of the urinary conduit, calling this *obstructive nephropathy.*

Urinary tract obstruction has a broad range of characteristics. When obstruction is acute, it is usually due to an easily reversible condition and only transient functional abnormalities without major structural change develop. Ureteral stone is the prototypical example of this form, in which slight global enlargement of the kidney occurs as a result of interstitial edema and dilatation of renal tubules, principally the distal tubules and the collecting ducts. At the other end of the spectrum, obstruction develops insidiously and silently. By the time of discovery there may be marked structural damage and profound functional derangement. This form of obstruction is seen with congenital narrowing of the ureter, slow-growing ureteral tumors, or retroperitoneal disease. In these cases, the kidney is globally enlarged, often extremely so, owing to marked dilatation of the pelvis and infundibulocalyceal system. Atrophy and fibrosis of the surrounding renal parenchyma occur as a result of pressure from the dilated collecting system and ischemia from a decrease in the size and number of arteries and arterioles.

Clinical Setting

Acute urinary obstruction is most commonly associated with the passage of a calculus or a blood clot. Ureteral colic dominates the clinical picture. Hematuria is usually microscopic in calculus disease and macroscopic when a blood clot is present. With gross hematuria, carcinoma, renal arteriovenous malformation, trauma, or excessive anticoagulant therapy must be considered as causative factors arising in the upper urinary tract. Surgical trauma, either an inadvertent suture on the ureter or ureteral edema following instrumentation, is a cause of acute obstruction that may be clinically silent.

Urinary tract obstruction can develop insidiously with few, if any, clinical symptoms in a variety of conditions. These include benign and malignant tumors of the ureter and inflammatory strictures and retroperitoneal diseases, usually tumor or fibrosis. Ureteropelvic junction obstruction and ureteral valves are congenital disorders that produce obstructive uropathy.

Regardless of the cause, hydrostatic pressure is increased proximal to an obstruction as long as the kidney produces a normal volume of urine. Rather quickly, however, the increased pressure in the tubule lumina approaches filtration pressure in the glomerular capillaries, and glomerular filtration and urine volume diminish. However, complete cessation of urine formation does not occur because a number of factors operate to partially compensate for the elevated hydrostatic pressure, thereby favoring continued glomerular filtration. These include continued urine flow beyond the site of obstruction, continued water reabsorption by the tubules, distention of the pelvis and ureters (whose muscular contractions eventually diminish when a certain degree of dilatation is reached), increased lymphatic uptake of urine, and leakage of urine into interstitial and vascular spaces following spontaneous rupture of the collecting system at the calyceal fornices. Despite these compensating factors, hydrostatic pressure remains elevated throughout the nephrons, collecting tubules, and the extrarenal collecting system to the point of obstruction. This is reversible if the obstruction is relieved. Over time, however, the increased hydrostatic pressure of persistent obstruction causes atrophy of nephrons and an irreversible decrease in the volume of urine formed by the kidney. At this point the thickness of renal parenchyma decreases uniformly while dilatation of the collecting system causes progressive overall enlargement of the kidney. When nephron atrophy reduces the volume of urine formed by the obstructed kidney to an amount equal to that which can pass through the obstruction, the pressure proximal to the obstruction becomes normal and parenchymal atrophy ceases. Input-output equilibrium may occur at any point along a continuum of severity. Thus, patients with intermediate degrees of obstruction develop moderate parenchymal atrophy and collecting system dilatation that does not progress beyond a certain point while patients with severe obstruction develop nearly total atrophy of nephrons, loss of function, and striking dilatation of the pelvocalyceal system.

Infection is a particularly serious complication of a chronically obstructed collecting system that requires early recognition and treatment. *Pyonephrosis,* as this condition is known, presents as sepsis in an individual whose urinary tract obstruction has often gone undiagnosed. Purulent exudate collects in the dilated pelvocalyceal system, giving rise to characteristic ultrasonographic features. Renal function, if previously present at all, deteriorates rapidly. Without prompt intervention, the kidney will be destroyed.

Radiologic Findings

The predominant radiologic findings in acute urinary tract obstruction reveal diminished filtration of contrast material rather than the structural effect of obstruction. Delayed parenchymal opacification compared with the nonobstructed kidney, progressive increase in the density of the nephrogram with time, and delayed opacification of the collecting system are sometimes recognized more easily than subtle dilatation of the calyces, pelvis, or ureter (Fig. 9–11). The nephrogram reflects continued accumulation of io-

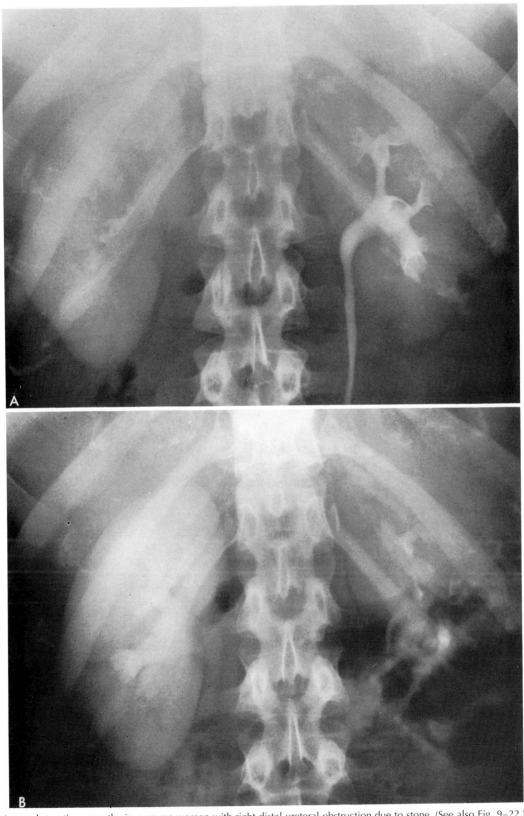

Figure 9–11. Acute obstructive uropathy in a young woman with right distal ureteral obstruction due to stone. (See also Fig. 9–22.) (Same patient illustrated in Fig. 23–18.)
   A, Excretory urogram, 10-minute film. There is delayed parenchymal and collecting system opacification compared with the normal left kidney.
   B, Excretory urogram, 4-hour film. The nephrogram has become increasingly dense, and the slightly dilated collecting system is opacified.

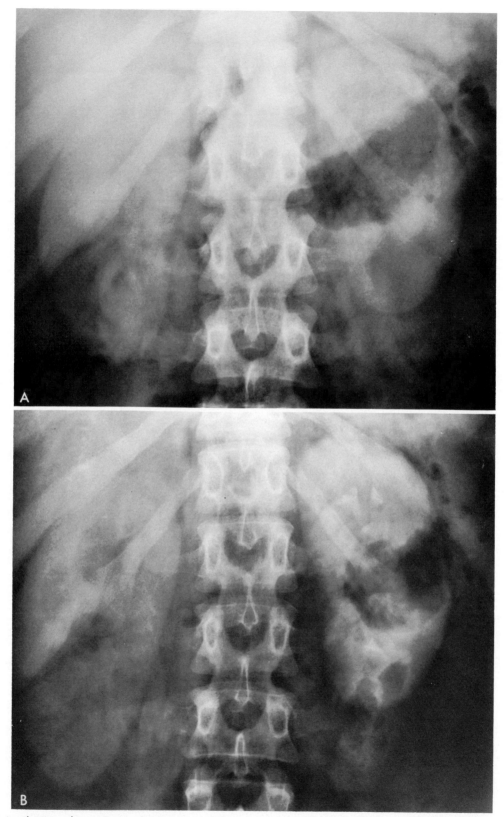

Figure 9–12. Obstructive uropathy causing renal enlargement in a 36-year-old woman who developed a vesicovaginal fistula following radiation therapy for carcinoma of the cervix. Bilateral ureteral obstruction, more severe on the right side, developed after a ureteroileostomy was performed because of the fistula.

  A, Excretory urogram, 1-minute film before radiation therapy. Right kidney length = 12.0 cm; left kidney length = 11.0 cm.

  B, Excretory urogram, 1-minute film, 2 years after ureteroileostomy. Obstruction is present bilaterally, and both kidneys have enlarged. A negative pyelogram is present on the more severely obstructed right side. Right kidney length = 14.3 cm; left kidney length = 12.3 cm.

dine-bearing molecules in the tubule lumina and the sluggish or absent forward flow of urine. As obstruction becomes chronic, the radiologic picture is dominated by ureteral and/or pelvic dilatation and renal parenchymal loss in addition to delayed opacification. The nephrogram, no longer progressively dense, becomes faint as the number of nephrons is reduced through pressure atrophy. Global enlargement of the kidney outline occurs in both acute and chronic obstruction (Fig. 9–12). In some cases of long-standing, unrelieved obstruction, however, the kidney eventually shrinks (Fig. 9–13).

Rupture of the calyceal fornix as a result of rapid calyceal dilatation provides one of the more dramatic urographic findings in acute obstructive uropathy (Figs. 9–14 and 9–15). When this occurs, opacified urine can be seen in the renal sinus extending around the renal pelvis and ureters or in the lymphatics or veins. Forniceal rupture may occur spontaneously.

Sometimes it is associated with the urographic procedure itself when the contrast material–induced diuresis produces a sudden increase in urine volume or when abdominal compression is used. Forniceal rupture is more likely to occur in the kidney whose pelvis is surrounded by parenchymal tissue ("intrarenal" pelvis) than in the one whose pelvis is predominantly external to the kidney tissue ("extrarenal" pelvis). The lack of distensibility of the intrarenal pelvis in the face of increased hydrostatic pressure makes the fornix of each calyx more susceptible to rupture. Chronic leakage into the perirenal space leads to the formation of a uriniferous perirenal pseudocyst or urinoma, which is discussed in Chapter 21.

Acute urinary tract obstruction is associated with two additional findings, which are both uncommon. The first is alternating radiolucent and radiopaque striae in the nephrogram (Fig. 9–16). They are oriented perpendicular to the surface of the kidney and

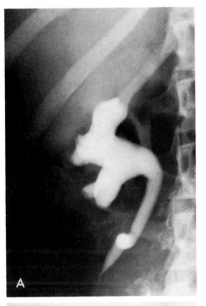
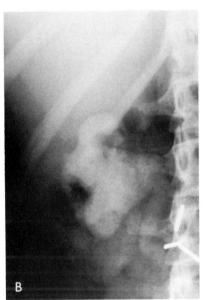
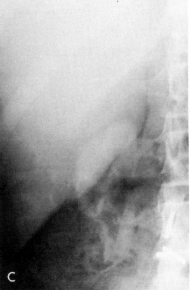

Figure 9–13. Obstructive uropathy leading to atrophy in an 18-year-old woman with choriosarcoma of the ovary metastatic to the right periaortic lymph nodes.

A, Initial excretory urogram. Metastatic nodes, opacified following lymphangiography, displace and obstruct the proximal ureter. Kidney length = 12.4 cm.

B, Excretory urogram 5 months later. Obstruction has not been relieved by intervening surgery. Kidney length = 12.1 cm.

C, Excretory urogram 2 years after initial study. Right kidney function is severely impaired. Kidney length = 5.8 cm.

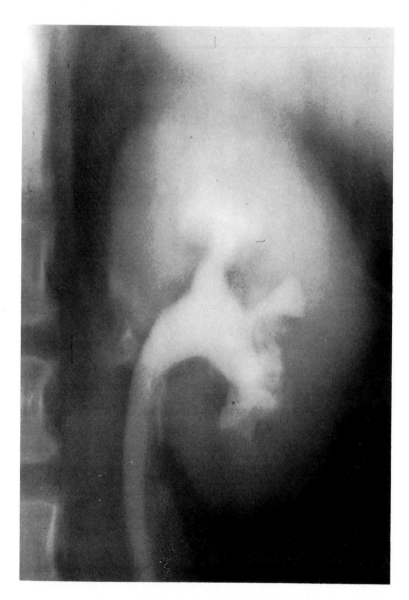

Figure 9–14. Acute obstructive uropathy complicated by forniceal rupture and by leakage of contrast material into the renal sinus. Contrast material is seen in tissue between the calyces and outside the pelvis and the proximal ureter. This complication occurs more frequently in kidneys with "intrarenal" location of the pelvis, as illustrated in this patient.

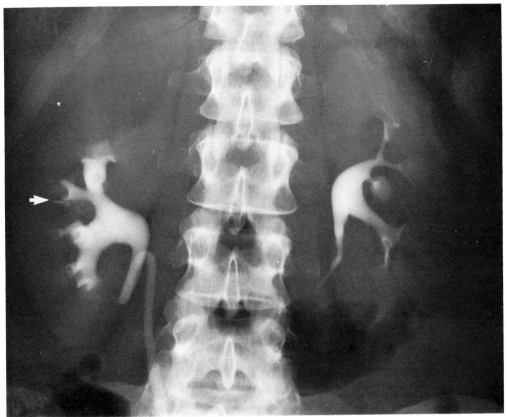

Figure 9–15. Acute obstructive uropathy due to stone in the right distal ureter. There is minimal enlargement of the pelvocalyceal system. Dilatation of the forniceal angles and leakage of contrast material into the sinus *(arrow)* through a ruptured fornix reflect elevated hydrostatic pressure in the pelvis of the kidney. Excretory urogram, 20-minute film. (Same patient illustrated in Fig. 17–4.)

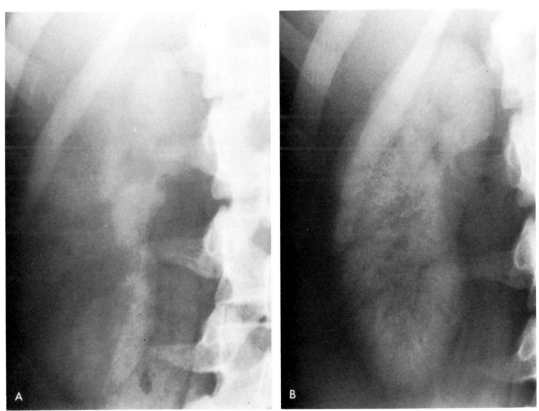

Figure 9–16. Acute obstructive uropathy associated with a striated nephrogram thought to represent contrast material in dilated tubules in the medullary rays. (Same patient illustrated in Fig. 23–24.)

A, Excretory urogram, 5-minute film. Delayed opacification.

B, Excretory urogram, 45-minute film. Striae are well illustrated.

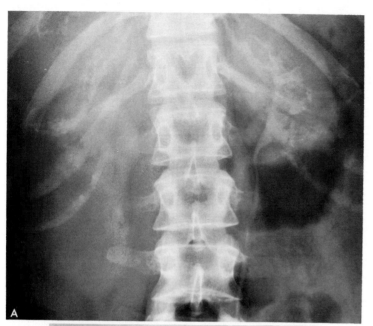

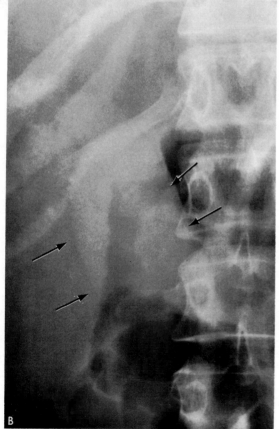

Figure 9–17. Gallbladder opacification following excretory urography in a 33-year-old woman with acute obstructive uropathy due to right ureteral stone.

A, Excretory urogram, 5-minute film. Delayed right-sided opacification. Normal left kidney.

B, Twenty-four-hour film of the abdomen. The faintly opacified gallbladder is to the right of the first and second lumbar vertebrae *(arrows).*

are seen in some cases of acute obstruction due to ureteral calculus. Striae are believed to represent contrast material in dilated tubules and collecting ducts in the medullary rays. The second uncommon urographic finding is opacification of the gallbladder late in the course of the urographic examination in patients with acute unilateral obstruction due to ureteral stone and a normal contralateral kidney (Fig. 9–17). This phenomenon is related to increased hepatic excretion of contrast material due to prolonged plasma disappearance time. Gallbladder opacification in this circumstance is detected on radiographs of the abdomen obtained 8 to 24 hours after administration of contrast material.

When urinary tract obstruction has been present for an extended period of time, the radiologic findings are dominated by dilatation of the pelvocalyceal system and ureter proximal to the obstruction. The silhouette of the calyces usually produces a multilobulated sac, but in extreme cases only a single dilated structure is all that remains of the entire pelvoinfundibulocalyceal system. Contrast material enhancement of the compressed and atrophic renal parenchyma surrounding dilated calyces produces the "rim" sign of chronic obstruction (Fig. 9–18). This sign must be kept separate from the "cortical rim" sign of complete or major segmental acute arterial infarction that was discussed in the previous section. Opacification of this tissue is slower and less dense than that of tissue on the contralateral side. The pattern of increasing nephrographic density over time that is seen in acute obstructive uropathy is absent, representing nephron loss through atrophy, a reduction in the volume of urine being formed, and the resulting normalization of hydrostatic pressure in the collecting system (Fig. 9–19). On early urographic films, the nephrogram of the compressed parenchyma outlines the nonopacified dilated collecting systems, producing a "negative pyelogram" (Fig. 9–20; see Fig. 9–18). Delayed films will eventually demonstrate opacification of the dilated collecting system itself as contrast material passes downward from nephrons into the large reservoir of unopacified urine. The demonstration of the pelvocalyceal system may require films as late as 24 hours after injection of contrast material. Upright films in which contrast material accumulates in dependent portions of the dilated system may facilitate earlier visualization (Fig. 9–21). In chronic obstruction of intermediate severity, a narrow, semilunar band of marked radiodensity at the interface between renal parenchyma and a dilated calyx may be seen during contrast material–enhanced studies of the kidney (see Fig. 9–21A). This observation, the "calyceal crescent" sign, represents concentrated contrast material in the distal portion of collecting ducts that have become oriented parallel rather than perpendicular to the calyx as a result of atrophy of the papillae and dilatation of the calyces.

The radiologist should attempt to demonstrate the point of obstruction and thereby eliminate the need

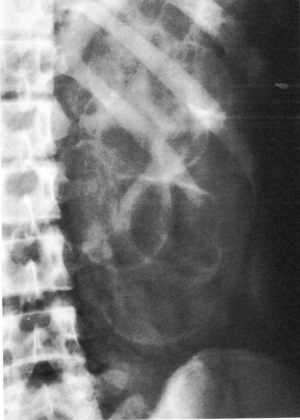

Figure 9–18. Chronic obstructive uropathy of the left kidney. Excretory urogram. The kidney is enlarged, smooth, and composed of very thin bands of atrophic renal parenchyma surrounding very dilated calyces. Opacification of the atrophied bands of parenchyma constitute the "rim" sign of chronic obstruction. The nonopacified, dilated collecting structures are called the "negative pyelogram." (Same patient illustrated in Fig. 9–25.)

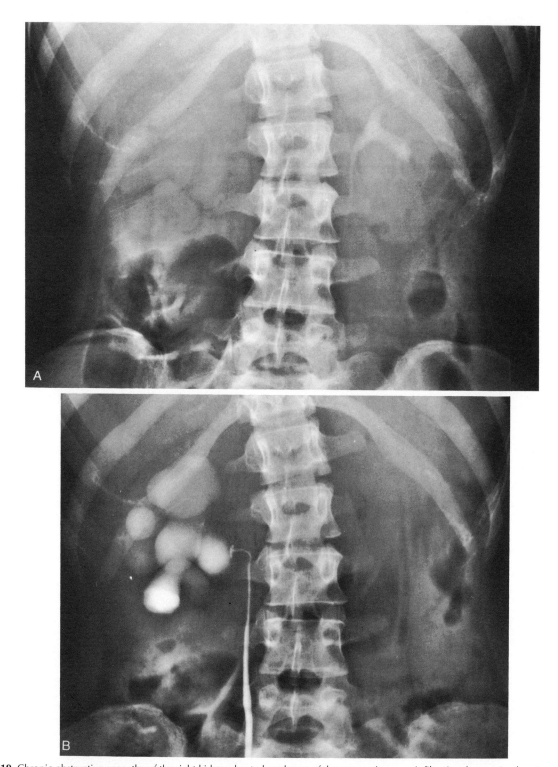

Figure 9–19. Chronic obstructive uropathy of the right kidney due to lymphoma of the retroperitoneum infiltrating the proximal ureter.
   A, Excretory urogram, 10-minute film. The nephrogram is barely perceived even at its maximum. There is faint opacification of dilated calyces.
   B, Retrograde pyelogram. A narrowed proximal ureter and the dilated collecting system are identified.

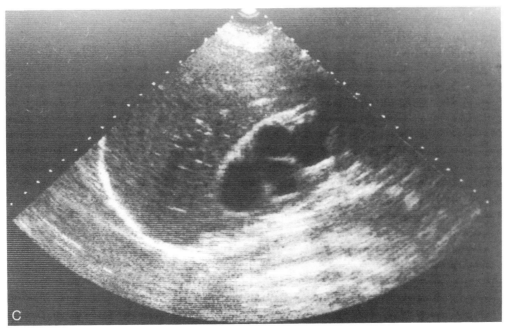

Figure 9–19 *Continued C,* Ultrasonogram, longitudinal section. The anechoic, dilated collecting system confirms the diagnosis.

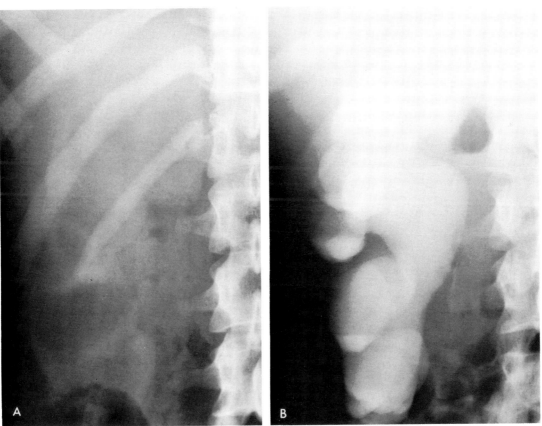

Figure 9–20. Chronic obstructive uropathy in a 27-year-old woman with long-standing ureteropelvic junction obstruction. Kidney length = 16.3 cm. (Same patient illustrated in Fig. 17–8.)

A, Excretory urogram. Early film demonstrates the nephrogram of compressed parenchyma (the "rim" sign) surrounding the nonopacified dilated calyces—the "negative pyelogram."

B, Excretory urogram. The previously radiolucent dilated calyces are opacified on a delayed upright film.

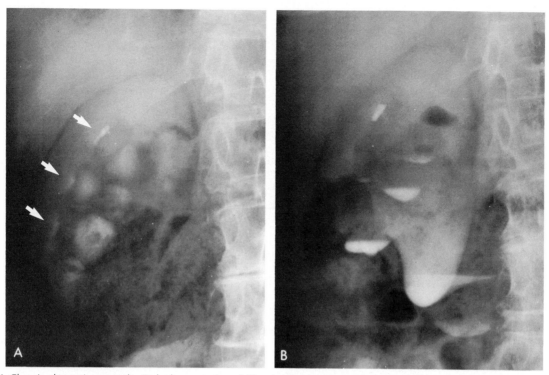

Figure 9–21. Chronic obstructive uropathy. Early demonstration of dilated collecting system on an upright film.
A, Excretory urogram, supine film. Narrow, semilunar bands of contrast material *(arrows)* called "calyceal crescents" are present at the interface between renal parenchyma and the faintly opacified dilated calyces.
B, Excretory urogram, upright film. Layering of contrast material facilitates visualization of dilated calyces.

for retrograde instrumentation. This can be achieved in many obstructed patients by using an appropriately large dose of contrast material and by obtaining delayed films (Fig. 9–22). Positioning the patient upright or prone encourages the high specific gravity contrast material to settle into the distal portions of the urinary collecting system. Antegrade pyelography performed through a catheter or a needle placed percutaneously through the flank and into the dilated

system is a valuable technique in the demonstration of the point of obstruction.

A balanced state between the volume of urine formed and the volume of urine that passes beyond an incomplete obstruction produces urographic findings of moderate parenchymal thinning, collecting system dilatation, and renal enlargement (Fig. 9–23). The nephrogram may be diminished in peak density compared with the nonobstructed contralateral kid-

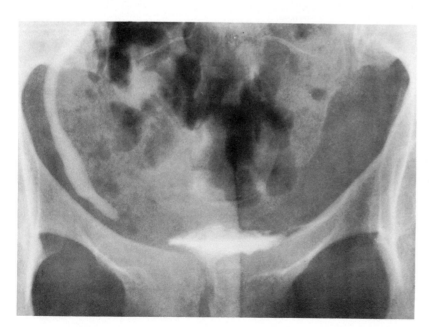

Figure 9–22. Distal ureteral obstruction secondary to stone. In obstructive uropathy, delayed upright or prone films are usually required to identify the point of obstruction. (Same case illustrated in Figs. 9–11 and 23–18.)

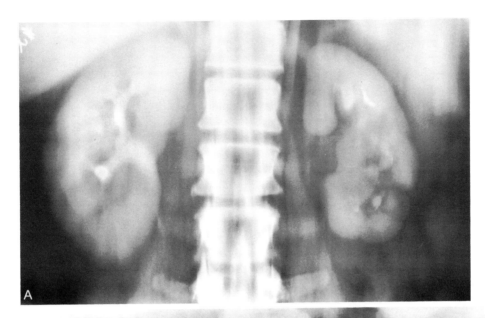

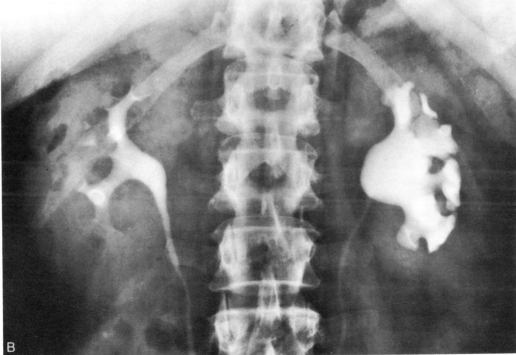

Figure 9–23. Chronic obstructive uropathy of the left kidney, intermediate grade. There is moderate parenchymal thinning and collecting system dilatation, but the time–density pattern of the nephrogram is normal, indicating a stable state.
  A, Excretory urogram, 3-minute tomogram.
  B, Excretory urogram, 10-minute film.

ney, but the time–density curve follows a normal rather than an increasingly dense pattern (see Chapter 23). These abnormalities do not progress unless the severity of the obstruction progresses.

The radiologic findings in obstructive uropathy are not always straightforward, particularly in cases in which the severity or the duration of the abnormality is intermediate, or the obstruction is intermittent. Provocative tests, such as diuresis urography or diuresis renography, have been developed for these problems. Further discussion of these, as well as direct pressure–flow studies of the pelvocalyceal system are included in Chapters 2, 15, and 17.

The computed tomographic findings of acute and chronic obstruction parallel those of excretory urography. Computed tomography demonstrates prolonged selective enhancement of the cortex relative to the medulla in acute obstruction, an observation not seen during excretory urography because of the superimposition of cortex and medulla on standard radiography of the kidney. The urine-filled, dilated pelvocalyceal system yields an attenuation value close to that of water and is readily distinguished from the higher values of the unenhanced renal parenchyma (Fig. 9–24). Parapelvic cysts (discussed in Chapter 16) have an appearance on unenhanced computed tomograms that may be identical to that of hydronephrosis. Distinction between these two entities requires the use of contrast material to demonstrate enhancement of the obstructed system or the absence of enhancement in the case of the parapelvic cyst (Fig. 9–25; see Fig. 16–4). In pyonephrosis, the attenuation value of the pus-filled hydronephrotic collecting system is greater than that of water.

The sensitivity of ultrasonography in the diagnosis of obstructive uropathy is dependent on the degree of dilatation of the pelvocalyceal system. Since dilatation of the collecting structure is not a major feature of acute obstructive uropathy, ultrasonography is of limited value in establishing this diagnosis. Here, excretory urography remains the most sensitive test. With subacute or chronic obstruction, on the other hand, dilatation is the predominant feature and is readily detectable as a central, fluid-filled, branching structure (see Fig. 9–19C). Consequently, the sensitivity of ultrasonography is approximately 98 per cent in the diagnosis of obstruction beyond the acute stage. This subject, including causes of false-positive and false-negative results, is discussed in detail in Chapter 17. Ultrasonography is particularly valuable in establishing the diagnosis of pyonephrosis. In this condition, the dilated, fluid-filled collecting system will also contain echogenic material representing pus, stones, and cellular debris (Fig. 9–26). This echo pattern may be limited to the dependent part of the pelvis and form a fluid–debris level that shifts with changes in the position of the patient. Other ultrasonographic patterns of pyonephrosis are dense peripheral echoes caused by bubbles of gas and diminished sound transmission with diffuse echoes throughout the collecting system. Stones are strongly echogenic and cause acoustic shadows.

Attenuated, sparse, displaced arteries with prolonged circulation time and dense opacification of rims of atrophied parenchyma are distinctive angiographic features of chronic obstructive uropathy. However, angiography is no longer used to diagnose obstructive uropathy.

SUMMARY OF ABNORMAL URORADIOLOGIC FINDINGS
OBSTRUCTIVE UROPATHY

Acute Obstructive Uropathy
Primary Uroradiologic Elements
    Size—normal to large
    Contour—smooth (global)
    Lesion distribution—unilateral
Secondary Uroradiologic Elements
    Pelvoinfundibulocalyceal system—opacification time delayed; dilated (minimal); disrupted (occasional focal forniceal tear)
    Nephrogram—increasingly dense; striae (uncommon)
    Gallbladder opacification—uncommon
Chronic Obstructive Uropathy
Primary Uroradiologic Elements
    Size—large (may become small in late stage)
    Contour—smooth (global)
    Lesion distribution—unilateral
Secondary Uroradiologic Elements
    Pelvoinfundibulocalyceal system—opacification time delayed ("negative pyelogram"); dilated (moderate to marked); attenuation value equal to water
    Parenchymal thickness—wasted (global)
    Nephrogram—contrast material density diminished; thick walls ("rim" sign); "calyceal crescent" sign
    Echogenicity—anechoic, dilated collecting system

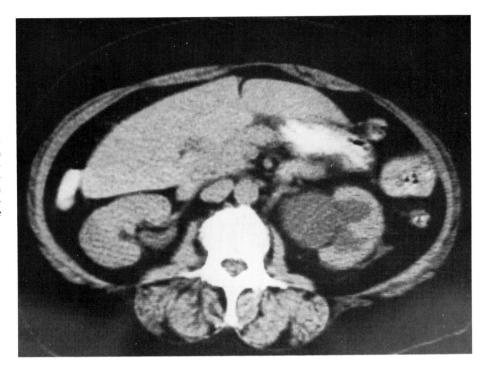

Figure 9–24. Chronic obstructive uropathy of the left kidney. The attenuation value of the dilated pelvocalyceal system equals that of water. Note the wasting of the renal parenchyma, which is a feature of chronic obstruction. Computed tomogram, unenhanced. (Same patient illustrated in Fig. 17–12.)

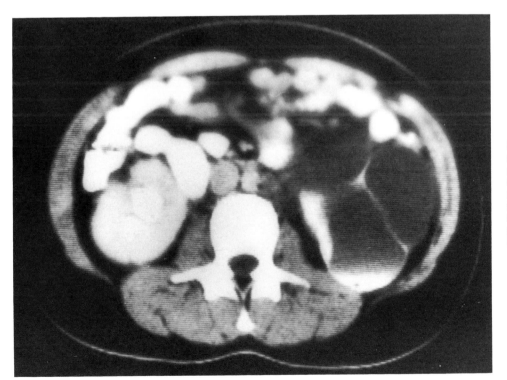

Figure 9–25. Chronic obstructive uropathy of the left kidney. Computed tomogram, contrast material enhanced. The severely atrophied renal parenchyma is enhanced ("rim" sign), and there is layering of contrast material in the dilated collecting system. (Same patient illustrated in Fig. 9–18.)

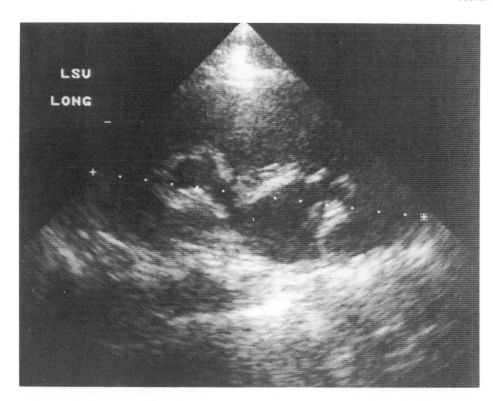

Figure 9–26. Pyonephrosis of a chronically obstructed left kidney. Ultrasonogram, longitudinal section. The dilated pelvocalyceal system separates the central sinus complex and contains diffuse faint echoes caused by inflammatory debris. (Kindly provided by Sheila Sheth, M. D., and Ulrike Hamper, M. D., The Johns Hopkins University, Baltimore, Maryland.)

ACUTE PYELONEPHRITIS

Definition

Acute upper urinary tract infection, characterized by fever, flank pain, bacteriuria, and pyuria, is a cause of unilateral global renal enlargement. Acute pyelonephritis develops from pathogenic coliform bacteria that initially enter the bladder from perineal or vaginal colonies by way of the urethra. A short urethra explains the prevalence of urinary tract infections in females, whereas both the greater length of the urethra and antibacterial properties of prostatic secretions have a protective effect against urinary tract infection from coliform bacteria in males. In older children and adults, pathogenic bacteria usually move from the bladder into the upper tract against the direction of urine flow by virtue of their ability to adhere to ureteral epithelium and certain motility characteristics. This is, of course, different from the situation in newborns and infants, in whom vesicoureteral reflux is a more common mechanism for infecting the upper tract.

Acute pyelonephritis develops when bacteria pass from pelvocalyceal urine through papillary duct orifices and provoke an acute tubulointerstitial nephritis along the course of the medullary rays (see Chapter 3). From a gross morphologic view, this inflammatory response involves the full thickness of a renal lobe or a part of a lobe, extending from the tip of the papilla to the surface of the kidney. There is a sharp line of demarcation between the area of inflammation and adjacent portions of normal parenchyma. Inflammatory exudate fills and obstructs collecting tubules and ducts, and the acute inflammatory cell infiltrate diminishes urine formation in the affected nephrons by obliterating the microvasculature of the affected tissue.

Lobar or sublobar acute tubulointerstitial nephritis involving the medullary rays, then, is the elemental pathologic process present in the earliest stages of reflux nephropathy (see Chapter 5); in acute pyelonephritis, acute bacterial nephritis and emphysematous pyelonephritis (discussed in this section); and in the evolution of renal abscess secondary to ascending infections (see Chapter 12). These entities differ from each other by virtue of differences in the cellular, humoral, or immunologic factors that constitute the host response of any given individual. Thus, scarring in the newborn (reflux nephropathy), early resolution without structural damage to the kidney in the older child or adult (acute pyelonephritis), overwhelming involvement of the kidney with late structural damage (acute bacterial nephritis or emphysematous pyelonephritis), and liquefaction and encapsulation (abscess) reflect the influence of patient age, use of antiinflammatory or immunosuppressive drugs, or coexistent diseases (diabetes mellitus, autoimmune deficiency syndrome, drug abuse) on the form and adequacy of the host response to the common element of acute tubulointerstitial nephritis.

Renal parenchymal involvement may not be present in all cases of uncomplicated acute pyelonephritis. The limited nature of the clinical syndrome and the lack of structural or functional damage to the kidney over time suggests that the clinical syndrome may sometimes be due to pyelitis rather than pyelonephritis. However, there is a substantial anecdotal radiologic experience that suggests parenchymal involvement, in at least some, if not most, patients.

Clinical Setting

Acute pyelonephritis, thus defined, predominantly affects girls and women to approximately age 40. The infecting organism is most commonly *Escherichia coli.* Recurrent episodes may involve different serotypes of the same genus or other gram-negative bacteria, such as *Enterobacter* species, *Klebsiella* species, *Pseudomonas aeruginosa,* or *Proteus mirabilis.* It is generally accepted that these organisms ascend to the upper urinary tract by way of the ureter, rather than following lymphatic or hematogenous routes.

The sudden onset of fever, chills, flank pain, frequency, and dysuria is the usual clinical pattern of acute pyelonephritis. Leukocytosis is present. Urinalysis reveals bacteria, leukocytes, leukocyte casts, and red blood cells. Bacteriuria is considered "significant" if quantitative culture of a cleanly voided urine specimen reveals more than 100,000 bacteria per milliliter of urine.

This disorder may be limited to a single episode or may follow a pattern of recurrent attacks. In the interval between acute symptomatic episodes, some patients have sterile urine; others have bacteriuria without symptoms. Unlike kidney infection in the infant and young child, structural damage in the form of focal kidney scars overlying dilated calyces does not usually occur as a consequence of recurrent acute pyelonephritis originating in older children and adults unless there is underlying obstruction or neuropathic disease leading to reflux.

Acute bacterial nephritis is a particularly severe form of pyelonephritis that causes both functional and structural damage to the affected kidney, with distinctive radiologic abnormalities. This disorder occurs in patients with altered host resistance, most often due to diabetes mellitus but also associated with immunosuppression, long-term corticosteroid therapy, intravenous drug abuse, or acquired immunodeficiency syndrome. Cases of women with diabetes mellitus, often previously undiagnosed, and without a prior history of urinary tract infection have been the predominant ones reported. The acute infection of the parenchyma may be diffuse and generalized or may have a patchy or multifocal distribution. In some patients, a regional pattern of involvement is demonstrated by radiologic studies, principally computed tomography. Involvement of both kidneys leading to acute renal failure has been reported. Patients with acute bacterial nephritis present with fever or septicemia and often do not have localized physical findings. *Escherichia coli* is the predominant infecting organism. Appropriate antibiotic therapy usually produces favorable results when the infection is recognized promptly. Unlike uncomplicated acute pyelonephritis in older children and adults, acute bacterial nephritis may lead to global renal atrophy and papillary necrosis. Other terms used to describe acute bacterial nephritis are *acute suppurative pyelonephritis, adult-onset acute bacterial nephritis, acute focal bacterial nephritis, segmental bacterial nephritis,* and *lobar nephronia.* The latter term is more accurately applied to lobar or sublobar acute interstitial nephritis, the elemental inflammatory response common to reflux nephropathy, as well as to acute pyelonephritis, acute bacterial nephritis, and the early stages of renal abscess.

Emphysematous pyelonephritis is the most severe form of acute pyelonephritis, representing a stage of acute bacterial nephritis that includes the formation of gas in the pelvocalyceal system, the interstices of renal parenchyma, as well as in the subcapsular and perirenal space. This develops in patients with altered host response, most commonly due to diabetes mellitus. Septicemia and shock dominate the clinical picture. Mortality in this condition, which also has distinctive radiologic features, is greater than 50 per cent.

Radiologic investigations are usually not performed in older girls and adult women who develop acute pyelonephritis that responds rapidly to treatment. Imaging studies are performed in those patients who either fail to respond to therapy or who have relapses involving the same serotype organism. Here, a careful assessment is required to exclude underlying papillary necrosis, congenital anomalies, obstruction, urolithiasis, medullary sponge kidney, or evidence of vesicoureteral reflux. On the other hand, excretory urography is usually indicated in males who develop acute pyelonephritis for the first time, even when response to therapy is rapid.

Radiologic Findings

The likelihood of detecting radiologic abnormalities in uncomplicated acute pyelonephritis depends on how soon after the onset of symptoms the examination is performed. Abnormal findings can be expected in nearly one-half of the patients who are examined within the first 24 hours of the onset of symptoms. This number diminishes rapidly following successful antibiotic therapy.

Global enlargement of the kidney on the symptomatic side, or occasionally of both kidneys, even though symptoms are unilateral, is the most frequent abnormal finding. Decreased density of contrast material, delayed calyceal opacification, pelviectasis and caliectasis, focal polar swelling, and focal calyceal compression are additional excretory urographic abnormalities found in these patients (Fig. 9–27; see Fig. 9–30). The same abnormalities are demonstrable by computed tomography, whose greater contrast resolution and cross-sectional anatomic display result in more readily detectable nephrographic abnormalities. These are characterized by sharply defined wedge-shaped zones of diminished enhancement that radiate from the collecting system to the renal surface and enhance only slightly after contrast material is administered. These features reflect lobar or sublobar acute tubulointerstitial nephritis in the distribution of medullary rays. Striations within these wedge-shaped, low-density zones may be present (Figs. 9–28 and 9–29). In some patients, the nephrographic defects are patchy and less sharply defined. All of these areas are

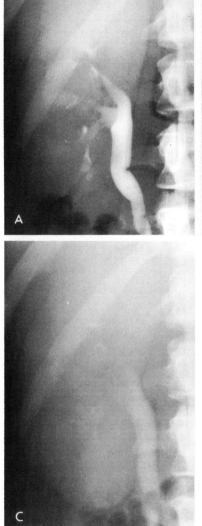

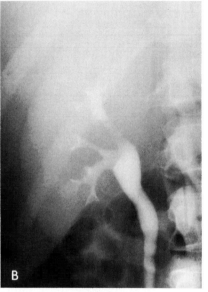

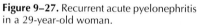

Figure 9–27. Recurrent acute pyelonephritis in a 29-year-old woman.

A, Excretory urogram during an acute episode of pyelonephritis. There is some enlargement of the kidney and calycealinfundibular effacement. Kidney length = 13.3 cm.

B, Normal excretory urogram 2 years after the initial examination taken when the patient was asymptomatic. Kidney length = 12.9 cm.

C, Excretory urogram during another acute episode of pyelonephritis 3 years after the first study. There is impaired excretion of contrast material, smooth enlargement of the kidney, and an effaced pelvocalyceal system. Note the absence of focal scars. Kidney length = 13.9 cm.

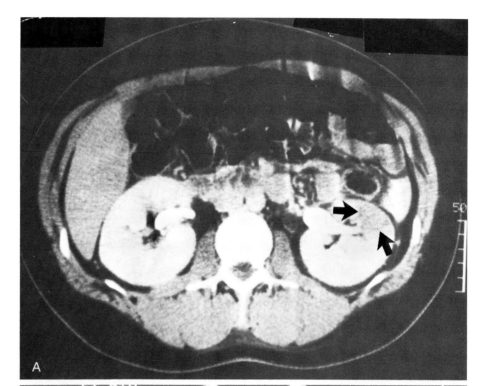

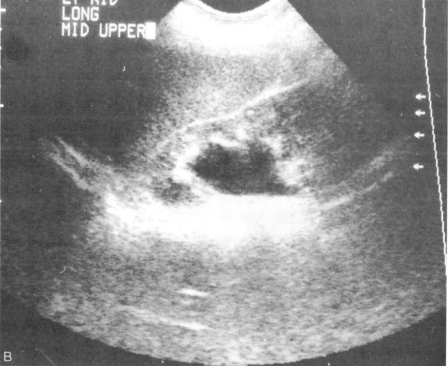

Figure 9–28. Acute pyelonephritis of the left kidney.

A, Computed tomogram, contrast material enhanced. There is a wedge-shaped, sharply marginated, full-thickness area of diminished enhancement (arrows).

B, Ultrasonogram, longitudinal section. The lower half of the left kidney is enlarged and diminished in echogenicity compared with the upper half, which was not involved and had an incidentally discovered duplicated and obstructed pelvocalyceal system.

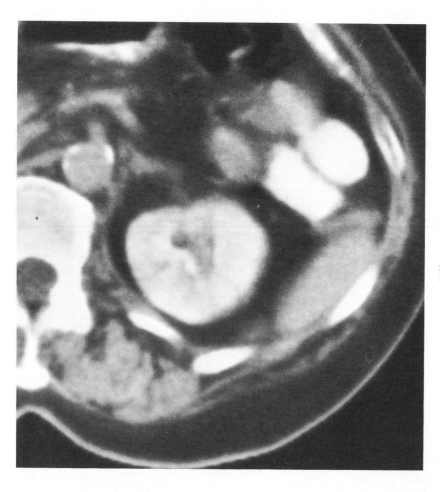

Figure 9–29. Acute pyelonephritis of the left kidney. There are fine linear striations and sharply marginated, wedge-shaped areas of diminished enhancement adjacent to areas of normal nephrogram. Computed tomogram, contrast material enhanced.

isodense with normal parenchyma before contrast material is administered.

Ultrasonography in uncomplicated acute pyelonephritis may demonstrate smooth renal enlargement. Diminished parenchymal echogenicity may be either generalized or regional (Fig. 9–30).

The radiologic findings of acute bacterial nephritis, previously described as a particularly severe form of renal infection that occurs in patients with a modified immune status, reflect an extreme expression of the spectrum of abnormalities of uncomplicated acute pyelonephritis. In these patients, there is a marked reduction in renal function seen on contrast material–enhanced images as a diminished to absent nephrogram and collecting system opacification (Fig. 9–31). Some cases have been reported in which the nephrogram has been immediately dense and persistent or striated, but this has not been common. The kidney is markedly enlarged and smooth in outline. Computed tomography demonstrates the nephrographic defects particularly well, and they may be patchy or involve the entire kidney uniformly (Fig. 9–32). When advanced, acute bacterial nephritis leads to multifocal areas of suppuration and liquefaction (Fig. 9–33). These abscesses cause mass effects on the collecting structures and produce the same radiologic findings as a simple, unifocal abscess, which is described in

Chapter 12. The abscesses may rupture through the subcapsular space into the perinephric space.

Acute bacterial nephritis appears as a large, smooth kidney and produces diminished echogenicity in ultrasonographic studies. Anechoic focal masses in areas where abscess formation has developed may be seen. Ultrasonography does not have the sensitivity of computed tomography in detecting the abnormalities of acute bacterial nephritis, but it is useful in eliminating the suspicion of urinary tract obstruction in the initial clinical assessment of the patient.

The most distinctive angiographic finding in acute bacterial nephritis is a pattern of alternating radiolucent and radiodense striations in the periphery of the kidney during the nephrographic phase (Fig. 9–34). These probably represent obliteration of interlobular arteries in the cortex by perivascular inflammatory cells. Other angiographic findings reflect decreased perfusion of the involved kidney and, in advanced cases, stretching of vessels by inflammatory masses.

Characteristically, the severe radiologic and functional abnormalities of acute bacterial nephritis return to normal shortly after the start of the appropriate antibiotic therapy (Fig. 9–35). However, unlike resolved, uncomplicated acute pyelonephritis, permanent structural damage is often present. Papillary necrosis is apparent as soon as the kidney is able to

Text continued on page 282

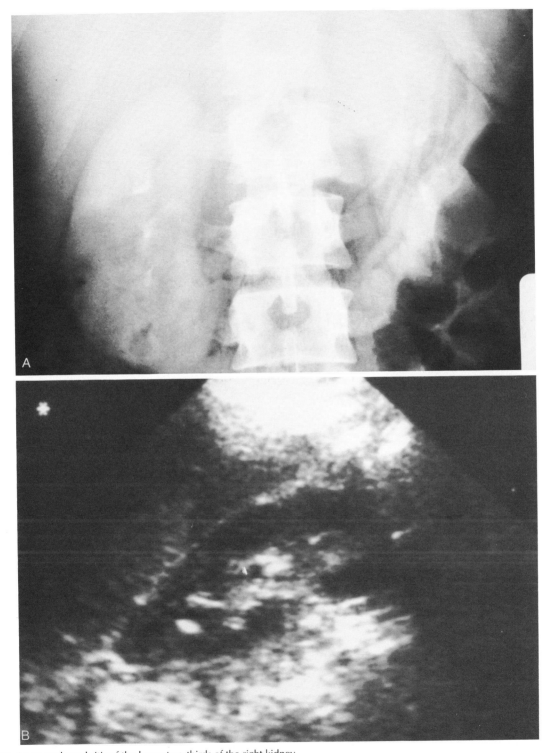

Figure 9–30. Acute pyelonephritis of the lower two-thirds of the right kidney.

A, Excretory urogram, 2-minute film. The involved portion of the kidney is enlarged and smooth and has a diminished nephrogram and effaced calyces compared with the upper, uninvolved pole.

B, Ultrasonogram, longitudinal section. Smooth enlargement and diminished echogenicity is demonstrated.

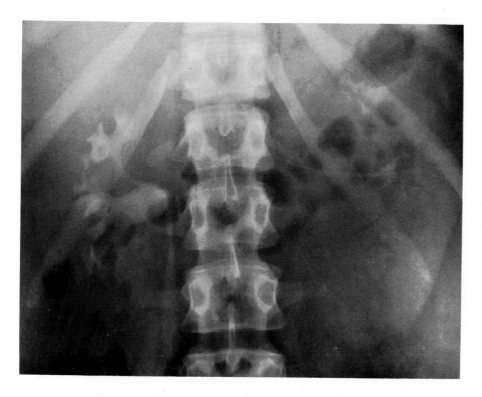

Figure 9–31. Acute bacterial nephritis in a 23-year-old woman. Excretory urogram reveals enlarged left kidney, persistent nephrogram of diminished density, and faint opacification of nondilated calyces. (Same case illustrated in Figs. 9–34 and 9–35.) (Reproduced from Radiology *106*:249, 1973, with permission.)

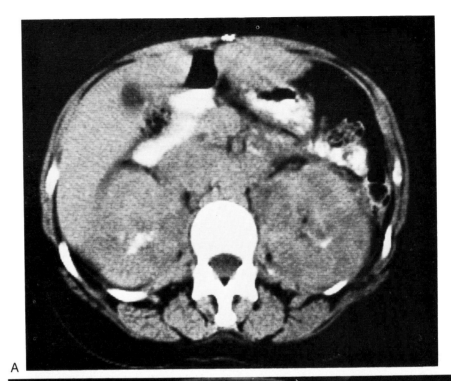

Figure 9–32. Acute bacterial nephritis involving both kidneys in a drug addict with acute renal failure. Computed tomogram, contrast material enhanced.

A, Section through the superior part of the kidneys demonstrates smooth, global enlargement and patchy nephrograms.

B, Section obtained through the lower parts of the kidneys demonstrates homogeneous, though diminished nephrograms and effaced collecting systems.

(Courtesy of H. Hricak, M. D., University of California, San Francisco.)

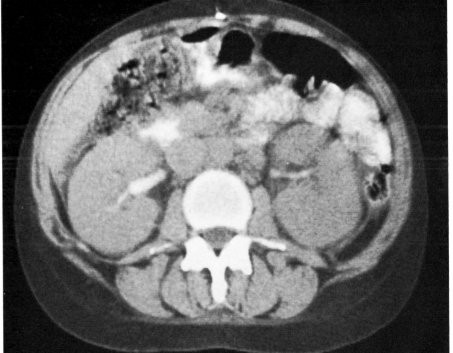

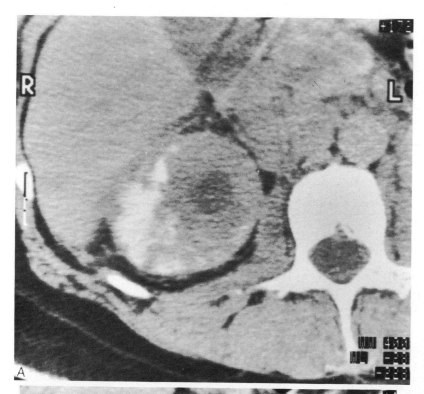

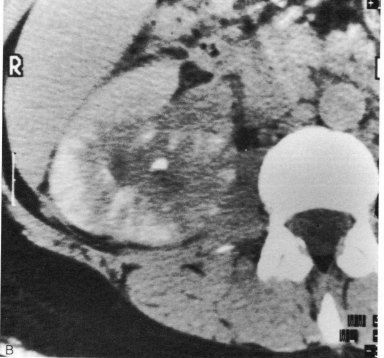

Figure 9–33. Acute bacterial nephritis of the right kidney. Computed tomogram, contrast material enhanced.

A, Section through upper pole demonstrates confluent area of diminished enhancement with a central, low-density area of suppuration.

B, Section through the mid kidney demonstrates areas of diminished enhancement that are both striated and confluent.

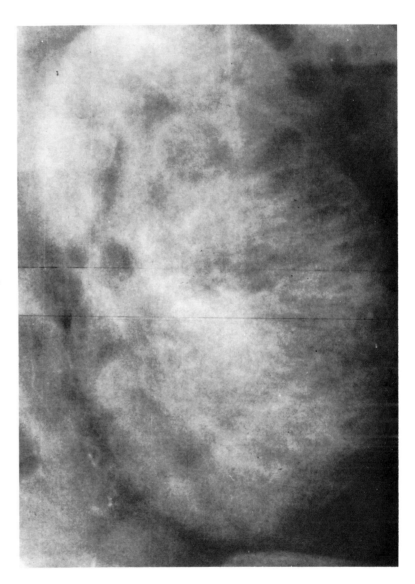

Figure 9–34. Acute bacterial nephritis. Nephrographic phase of selective renal arteriogram performed during an acute phase in the same patient illustrated in Figures 9–31 and 9–35. Characteristic linear stripes are present. (Reproduced from Radiology *106*:249, 1973, with permission.)

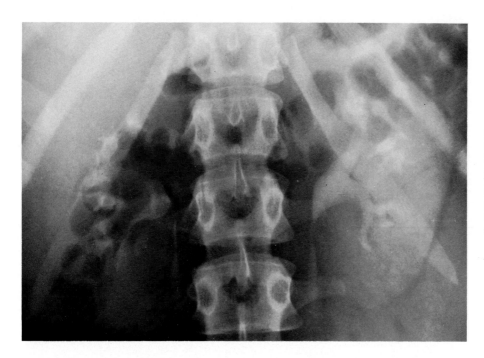

Figure 9–35. Acute bacterial nephritis. Excretory urogram 7 days after initial examination during the course of appropriate antibiotic therapy. Kidney size is smaller. The calyces opacify promptly and are no longer effaced. (Same case illustrated in Figs. 9–31 and 9–34.) (Reproduced from Radiology *106*:249, 1973, with permission.)

excrete enough contrast material to opacify the collecting system. In fact, it is likely that papillary necrosis is present in the earliest stage of acute bacterial nephritis but goes undetected because visualization of the calyces is not possible. Within a few weeks to months, global wasting of the recovered kidney will become apparent. (See Figs. 6–16 and 6–17.) Thus, postinflammatory atrophy enters the differential diagnosis of the unilateral, small, smooth kidney. (See discussion in Chapter 6.)

Radiolucent gas in and around an enlarged, nonopacified kidney characterizes the radiologic findings in a gas-forming infection of the kidney, known as *emphysematous pyelonephritis* (Figs. 9–36 and 9–37). In this serious condition, gas is present in the pelvocalyceal system, interstitial tissue, and perirenal space. Gas-attenuated sound causes a featureless image on ultrasonography.

MISCELLANEOUS CONDITIONS

Compensatory hypertrophy and duplication of the pelvocalyceal system are two situations in which a normal kidney becomes globally enlarged. Both of these conditions must be considered in the differential diagnosis of the unilaterally large, smooth kidney.

Compensatory Hypertrophy

When a kidney is congenitally absent, is surgically removed, or becomes diseased to the point that its excretory workload falls below a certain point, the functional capabilities and size of the normal contralateral kidney increase by virtue of an increase in the size of individual nephrons (Fig. 9–38). In cases of renal aplasia or severe hypoplasia, the functioning kidney will be large from birth, whereas growth oc-

---

SUMMARY OF ABNORMAL URORADIOLOGIC FINDINGS
ACUTE PYELONEPHRITIS*

Primary Uroradiologic Elements
    Size—normal to large
    Contour—smooth (global)
    Lesion distribution—unilateral (enlargement may be bilateral even with unilateral symptoms)
Secondary Uroradiologic Elements
    Pelvoinfundibulocalyceal system—opacification time delayed; dilated; attenuated; contains gas (emphysematous pyelonephritis)
    Nephrogram—contrast material density diminished (global, wedge-shaped, or patchy); immediately dense, persistent; striated (rare); interstitial gas (emphysematous pyelonephritis)
    Echogenicity—normal to decreased (global, regional, or focal); impaired sound transmission (emphysematous pyelonephritis)

*Note: Abnormalities vary with severity of infection and host response from none to intermediate (acute pyelonephritis) to severe (acute bacterial nephritis) to extreme (emphysematous pyelonephritis).

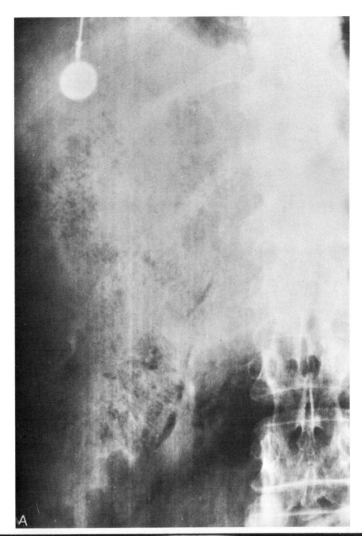

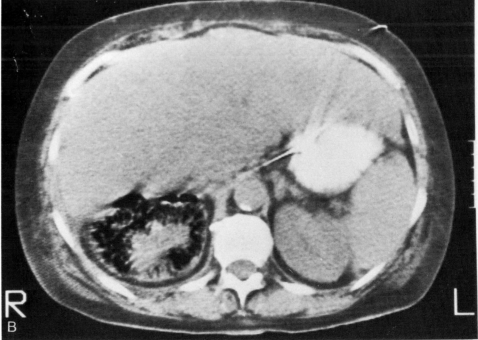

Figure 9–36. Emphysematous pyelonephritis of the right kidney. Gas is present in the interstitium of the kidney and the medial and ventral perirenal space.

A, Radiograph of the abdomen.

B, Computed tomogram, unenhanced.

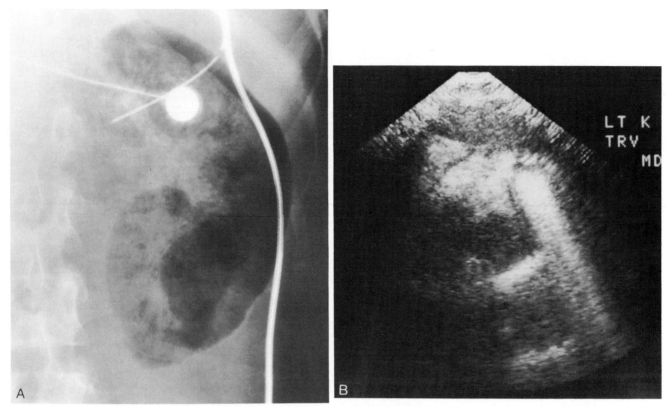

Figure 9–37. Emphysematous pyelonephritis of the left kidney. Gas is present in the interstitium of the kidney and the perirenal space.
A, Radiograph of the abdomen.
B, Ultrasonogram, longitudinal section. The gas reflects sound transmission, resulting in a hyperechoic appearance with acoustic shadowing.

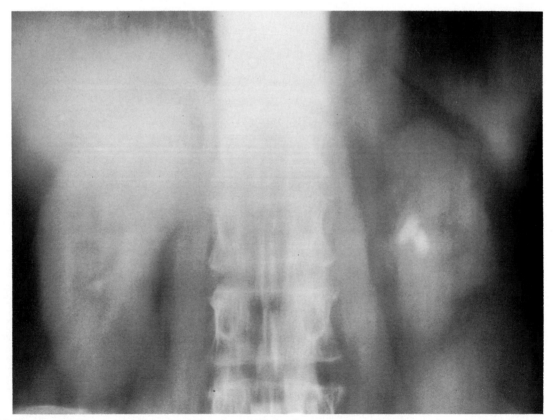

Figure 9–38. Compensatory hypertrophy of the right kidney in a middle-aged woman with severe reflux nephropathy of the left kidney. The right kidney is large but otherwise normal. Right kidney length = 14.2 cm; left kidney length = 10.3 cm.

curs slowly over years when function of the diseased kidney deteriorates gradually. Even though compensatory hypertrophy following surgical removal of the opposite kidney has been shown to begin within a few days in experimental animals, it is not detectable by clinical tests of renal function in humans for several weeks. Maximum increase in size is reached in approximately 6 months.

It is known that renal function and size decrease gradually as a function of age. It therefore might be expected that the ability of the kidney to undergo compensatory hypertrophy would also diminish with age. In fact, it has been claimed by some that compensatory hypertrophy does not occur at all after contralateral nephrectomy in patients older than 30 years. This is clearly not accurate, as evidenced by other studies that have shown that enlargement may occur at any age, although a greater degree of hypertrophy occurs in children than in adults (Fig. 9–39).

Radiologically, the hypertrophied kidney is normal in all respects except for its size and the thickness of the renal parenchyma. Since the urine flow rate from this kidney is twice normal, the pelvocalyceal system and ureter may appear more distended than usual.

Duplicated Pelvocalyceal System

In Chapter 3 it was noted that the metanephric blastema differentiates into nephrons under the inductive influence of the advancing point of the ureteric bud, which itself contributes collecting tubules to the renal parenchyma. Duplication of the renal pelvis represents earlier than normal dichotomous branching of the ureteral bud. The two branches encounter a greater mass of metanephric blastema than otherwise would have occurred. This is the basis for the larger than normal amount of renal parenchyma associated with a duplex collecting system (Fig. 9–40).

Of the two pelvocalyceal systems, the larger is usually the inferior one, which combines both interpolar and lower polar calyces. The renal lobes draining into the two systems do not assimilate with each other to the degree that occurs in a single system. As a result, an excessive amount of renal parenchyma, including cortex, may lie between the two sets of collecting structures and cause a masslike effect on adjacent calyces and infundibula. This commonly occurs both in complete and partial forms of duplications and has been described under such terms as *heterotopic cortex*,

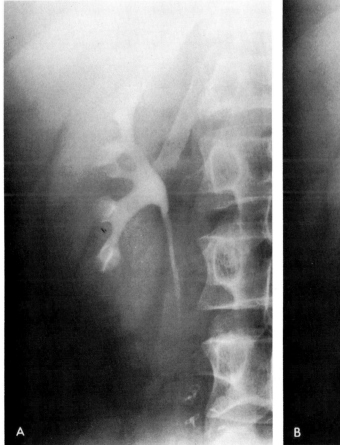
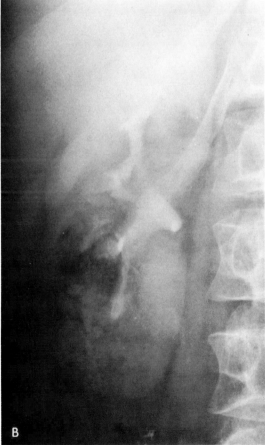

Figure 9–39. Compensatory hypertrophy of the right kidney following left nephrectomy in a 76-year-old man.
   A, Excretory urogram performed at age 70. Normal examination. Kidney length = 14.8 cm.
   B, Excretory urogram at age 76. Contralateral nephrectomy had been performed 2 years earlier. The right kidney has enlarged but is otherwise normal. Kidney length = 18.0 cm.

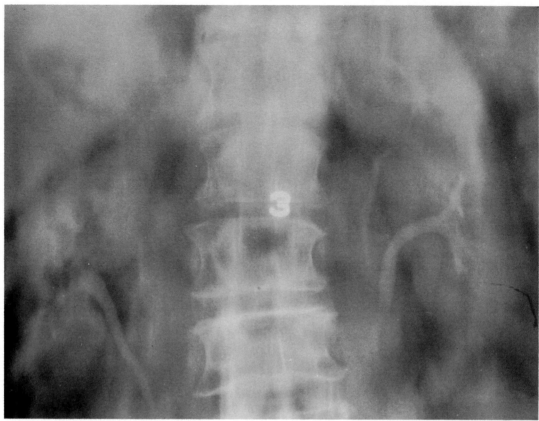

Figure 9–40. Duplicated collecting system causing smooth enlargement of the left kidney. Tomogram during excretory urography. Right kidney length = 13.9 cm; left kidney length = 17.8 cm.

lobar dysmorphism, ectopic cortex, cortical island, hypertrophied column of Bertin, and *renal pseudotumor.* This is a normal variant and should not be confused with a neoplasm or cyst, as discussed in detail in Chapter 3.

DIFFERENTIAL DIAGNOSIS

The radiologic features of the diseases discussed in this chapter overlap to a great extent. All produce enlargement of one kidney and are often associated with diminished opacification.

Obstructive uropathy is the only abnormality in this diagnostic set in which the collecting structure dilates. This finding, particularly when coupled with an increasingly dense nephrogram, firmly establishes the diagnosis. When obstructive uropathy is bilateral, an increasingly dense nephrogram may be confused with hypotension, acute tubular necrosis, intratubular block, or acute bilateral renal vein thrombosis. None of these disorders has a dilated collecting system, however. Diabetes insipidus, discussed in Chapter 17, produces a dilated collecting system owing to excessive urine volume, but there is no delayed opacification, nephrographic abnormality, or demonstrable point of obstruction in this uncommon disease.

The specific diagnosis of diseases in this diagnostic set, other than obstructive uropathy, often requires specialized procedures, such as Doppler ultrasonography, computed tomography, magnetic resonance imaging, or renal venography to define renal vein thrombosis or Doppler ultrasonography, radionuclide renography, or arteriography to confirm renal artery occlusion as a cause of kidney infarction. Acute pyelonephritis has no specific radiologic abnormality, except in the acute bacterial nephritis form in which computed tomographic findings and angiographic striations are characteristic.

Bibliography

Renal Vein Thrombosis

Abeshouse, B. S.: Thrombosis and thrombophlebitis of the renal veins. Urol. Cut. Rev. *49*:661, 1945.

Baum, N. H., Moriel, E., and Carlton, C. E., Jr.: Renal vein thrombosis, J. Urol. *119*:443, 1978.

Beckmann, C. F., and Abrams, H. L.: Renal venography: Anatomy, technique, application, analysis of 132 venograms, and a review of the literature. Cardiovasc. Interven. Radiol. *3*:45, 1980.

Beckmann, C. F., and Abrams, H. L.: Idiopathic renal vein varices: Incidence and significance. Radiology *143*:649, 1982.

Beinart, C., Sniderman, K. W., Saddekhi, S., Weiner, M., Vaughan, E. D., Jr., and Sos, T. A.: Left renal vein hypertension: A cause of occult hematuria. Radiology *145*:647, 1982.

Belman, A. B.: Renal vein thrombosis in infancy and childhood: A contemporary survey. Clin. Pediatr. *15*:1033, 1976.

Bidgood, W. D., Cuttino, J. T., Jr., Clark, R. L., and Volberg, F. M.: Pyelovenous and pyelolymphatic backflow during retrograde pyelography in renal vein thrombosis. Invest. Radiol. *16*:13, 1981.

Bigongiari, L. R., Patel, S. K., Appelman, H., and Thornbury, J. R.: Medullary rays: Visualization during excretory urography. AJR *125*:795, 1975.

Braun, B., Wellemann, L. S., and Weigand, W.: Ultrasonographic demonstration of renal vein thrombosis. Radiology 138:157, 1981.

Chait, A., Stoane, L., Moskowitz, H., and Mellins, H. Z.: Renal vein thrombosis. Radiology 90:886, 1968.

Clark, R. A., Wyatt, G. M., and Colley, D. P.: Renal vein thrombosis: An underdiagnosed complication of multiple renal abnormalities. Radiology 132:43, 1979.

Coel, M. N., and Talner, L. B.: Obstructive nephrogram due to renal vein thrombosis. Radiology 101:573, 1971.

Crummy, A. B., and Hipona, F. A.: The roentgen diagnosis of renal vein thrombosis: Experimental aspects. AJR 93:898, 1965.

DeTroyer, A., Paduart, P., Shockert, J., and Parmentier, R.: Unilateral renal vein thrombosis and nephrotic syndrome. Br. Med. J. 4:730, 1975.

Duncan, A. W., Schorr, W., Clark, F., and Kerr, D. N. S.: Unilateral renal vein thrombosis and nephrotic syndrome. J. Urol. 104:502, 1970.

Gatewood, O. M. B., Fishman, E. K., Burrow, C. R., Walker, W. G., Goldman, S. M., and Siegelman, S. S.: Renal vein thrombosis in patients with nephrotic syndrome: CT diagnosis. Radiology 159:117, 1986.

Glazer, G. M., Francis, I. R., Gross, B. H., and Amendola, M. A.: Computed tomography of renal vein thrombosis. J. Comput. Assist. Tomogr. 8:288, 1984.

Greene, A., Cromie, W. J., and Goldman, M.: Computerized body tomography in neonatal renal vein thrombosis. Urology 20:213, 1962.

Hricak, H., Sandler, M. A., Madrazo, B. L., Eyler, W. R., and Sy, G. S.: Sonographic manifestation of acute renal vein thrombosis: An experimental study. Invest. Radiol. 16:30, 1981.

Keating, M. A., and Althausen, A. F.: The clinical spectrum of renal vein thrombosis. J. Urol. 133:938, 1985.

Llach, F.: Acute renal vein thrombosis. In Schrier, R. W., and Gottschalk, C. W. (eds.): Diseases of the Kidney. 4th ed. Boston, Little, Brown & Co., 1988, pp. 1447–1460.

Llach, F., Papper, S., and Massry, S. G.: The clinical spectrum of renal vein thrombosis: Acute and chronic. Am. J. Med. 69:819, 1980.

McCarthy, L. J., Titus, J. L., and Dougherty, G. W.: Bilateral renal vein thrombosis and the nephrotic syndrome in adults. Ann. Intern. Med. 58:837, 1963.

McDonald, P. T., and Hutton, J. E., Jr.: Renal vein valve. JAMA 238:2303, 1977.

Mulhern, C. B., Arger, P. H., Miller, W. T., and Chait, A.: The specificity of renal vein thrombosis. AJR 125:291, 1975.

O'Dea, M. J., Malek, R. S., Tucker, R. M., and Fulton, R. E.: Renal vein thrombosis. J. Urol. 116:410, 1976.

Olin, T. B., and Reuter, S. R.: A pharmacoangiographic method for improving nephrophlebography. Radiology 85:1036, 1965.

Pollak, V. E., Kanter, A., and Zaltzman, S.: Renal vein thrombosis. Postgrad. Medicine 40:282, 1966.

Rosenberg, E. R., Trought, W. S., Kirks, D. R., Sumner, T. E., and Grossman, H.: Ultrasonic diagnosis of renal vein thrombosis in neonates. AJR 134:35, 1980.

Rosenfield, A. T., Zeman, R. K., Cronan, J. J., and Taylor, K. J. W.: ultrasound in experimental and clinical renal vein thrombosis. Radiology 137:735, 1980.

Sutton, T. J., Leblanc, A., Gauthier, N., and Hassan, M.: Radiological manifestations of neonatal renal vein thrombosis on follow-up examinations. Radiology 122:435. 1977.

Trew, P. A., Biava, D. G., Jacobs, R. P., and Hopper, J., Fr.: Renal vein thrombosis in membranous glomerulopathy: Incidence and association. Medicine (Baltimore) 57:69, 1978.

Weiner, P. L., Lim, M. S., Knudson, D. H and Semerdjian, H. S.: Retrograde pyelography in renal vein thrombosis. Radiology 111:77, 1974.

Wicks, J. D., Bigongiari, L. R., Foley, W. D., and Walter, J.: Parenchymal striations in renal vein thrombosis: Arteriographic demonstration. AJR 129:95, 1977.

Winfield, A. C., Gerlock, A. J., Jr., and Shaff, M. I.: Perirenal cobwebs: A CT sign of renal vein thrombosis. J. Comput. Assist. Tomogr. 5:405, 1981.

Zheutlin, N., Hughes, D., and O'Loughlin, B. J.: Radiographic findings in renal vein thrombosis. Radiology 73:884, 1959.

Acute Arterial Infarction

Duggan, M. L.: Acute renal infarction. J. Urol. 90:669, 1963.

Fishman, M. C., Naidich, J. B., and Stein, H. L.: Vascular magnetic resonance imaging. Radiol. Clin. North Am. 24:485, 1986.

Gasparini, M., Hofmann, R., and Stoller, M.: Renal artery embolism: Clinical features and therapeutic options. J. Urol. 147:567, 1992.

Glazer, G. M., and London, S. S.: CT appearance of global renal infarction, J. Comput. Assist. Tomogr. 5:847, 1981.

Glazer, G. M., Francis, I. R., Brady, T. M., and Teng, S. S.: Computed tomography of renal infarction: Clinical and experimental observations. AJR 140:721, 1983.

Halpern, M.: Acute renal artery embolus: A concept of diagnosis and treatment. J. Urol. 98:552, 1967.

Hann, L., and Pfister, R. C.: Renal subcapsular rim sign: New etiologies and pathogenesis. AJR 138:51, 1982.

Heitzman, E. R., and Perchik, L.: Radiographic features of renal infarction: Review of 13 cases. Radiology 76:39, 1961.

Hessel, S. J., and Smith, E. H.: Renal trauma: A comprehensive review and radiologic assessment. CRC Crit. Rev. Diagn. Imaging 5:251, 1974.

Hoxie, H. J., and Coggin, C. B.: Renal infarction: Statistical study of 205 cases and detailed report of an unusual case. Arch. Intern. Med. 65:587, 1940.

Ishikawa, I., Masuzaki, S., Saito, T., Yuri, T., Shinoda, A., and Tsujigiwa, M.: Magnetic resonance imaging in renal infarction and ischemia. Nephron 51:99, 1989.

Ives, H. E., and Daniel, T. O.: Vascular diseases of the kidney, In Brenner, B. M., and Rector, F. C. (eds.): The Kidney. 4th ed. Philadelphia, W.B. Saunders, 1991, pp. 1497–1550.

Janower, M. L., and Weber, A. L.: Radiologic evaluation of acute renal infarction. AJR 95:309, 1965.

Lang, E. K.: Arteriographic diagnosis of renal infarcts. Radiology 88:1110, 1967.

Lang, E. K., Mertz, J. H. O., and Nourse, M.: Renal arteriography in the assessment of renal infarct. J. Urol. 99:506, 1968.

Lessman, R. K., Johnson, S. F., Coburn, J. W., and Kaufman, J. J.: Renal artery embolism: Clinical features and long-term follow-up of 17 cases. Ann. Intern. Med. 89:477, 1978.

Martin, K. W., McAlister, W. H., and Schakelford, G. O.: Acute renal infarction: Diagnosis by Doppler ultrasound. Pediatr. Radiol. 18:373, 1988.

Parker, J. M., and Lord, J. D.: Renal artery embolism: A case report with return of complete function of the involved kidney following anticoagulant therapy. J. Urol. 106:339, 1971.

Paul, G. J., and Stephenson, T. F.: The cortical rim sign in renal infarction. Radiology 122:338, 1977.

Regan, F. C., and Crabtree, E. G.: Renal infarction: Clinical and possible surgical entity. J. Urol. 59:981, 1948.

Rubin, B. E., and Schliftman, R.: The striated nephrogram in renal contusion. Urol. Radiol. 1:119, 1979.

Sheehan, H. L., and Davis, J. C.: Complete permanent renal ischaemia. J. Pathol. 76:569, 1958.

Solez, K.: Acute renal failure (acute tubular necrosis, infarction, and cortical necrosis. In Heptinstall, R. H. (ed.): Pathology of the Kidney. 4th ed. Boston, Little, Brown & Co., 1992, pp. 1235–1314.

Teplick, J. G., and Yarrow, M. W.: Arterial infarction of kidney. Ann. Intern. Med. 42:1041, 1955.

Wise, H. M., Jr.: Hypertension resulting from hydronephrosis. JAMA 231:491, 1975.

Wong, W., Moss, A. A., Federle, M. P., Cochran, S. T., and London, S. S.: Renal infarction: CT diagnosis and correlation between CT findings and etiologies. Radiology 150:201, 1984.

Obstructive Uropathy

Amis, E. S., Jr., Cronan, J. J., and Pfister, R. C.: Pseudohydronephrosis on non-contrast computed tomography. J. Comput. Assist. Tomogr. 6:511, 1982.

Bigongiari, L. R., Davis, R. M., Novak, W. G., Wicks, J. D., Kass, E., and Thornbury, J. R.: Visualization of medullary rays on excretory urography in experimental ureteric obstruction. AJR 129:89, 1977.

Bigongiari, L. R., Patel, S. K., Appelman, H., and Thornbury, J. R.: Medullary rays: Visualization during excretory urography. AJR 125:795, 1975.

Bretland, P. M.: Acute ureteric obstruction—clinical and radiological aspects. Proc. R. Soc. Med. 67:1215, 1974.

Choyke, P. L.: The urogram: Are rumors of its death premature? Radiology 184:33, 1992.

Coleman, B. G., Arger, P. H., Mulhern, C. B., Jr., Pollack, H. M., and Banner, M. P.: Pyelonephrosis: Sonography in the diagnosis and management. AJR 137:939, 1981.

Cooke, G. M., and Bartucz, J. P.: Spontaneous extravasation of contrast medium during intravenous urography: Report of fourteen cases and a review of the literature. Clin. Radiol. 25:87, 1974.

Cremin, B. J.: Urinary ascites and obstructive uropathy. Br. J. Radiol. 48:113, 1975.

Cronan, J. J.: Contemporary concepts in imaging urinary tract obstruction. Radiol. Clin. North Am. 29:527, 1991.

Dalla Palma, L., Bazzocchi, M., Pozzi-Mucelli, R. S., Stacul, F., Rossi, M., and Agostini, R.: Ultrasonography in the diagnosis of hydronephrosis in patients with normal renal function. Urol. Radiol. 5:221, 1983.

Dyer, R. B., Gilpin, J. W., Zagona, R. J., Chen, M. Y. M., and Case, L. D.: Vicarious contrast material excretion in patients with acute unilateral ureteral obstruction. Radiology 177:739, 1990.

Elkin, M.: Obstructive uropathy and uremia. Radiol. Clin. North Am. 10:447, 1972.

Ellenbogen, P. H., Scheible, F. W., Talner, L. B., and Leopold, G. R.: Sensitivity of grey scale ultrasound in detecting urinary tract obstruction. AJR 130:731, 1978.

Erwin, B. C., Carroll, B. A., and Sommer, F. G.: Renal colic: The role of ultrasound in initial evaluation. Radiology 152:147, 1984.

Fernbach, S. K.: The dilated urinary tract in children. Urol. Radiol. 14:34, 1992.

Gillenwater, J. Y.: The pathophysiology of urinary tract obstruction. In Walsh, P. C., Retik, A. B., Stamey, T. A., and Vaughan, E. D., Jr. (eds.): Campbell's Urology. 6th ed. Philadelphia, W.B. Saunders, 1992, pp. 499–532.

Haddad, M. C., Sharif, H. S., Abomelha, M. S., Riley, P. J., Sammak, B. M., and Shahed, M. S.: Management of renal colic: Redefining the role of the urogram? Radiology 184:35, 1992.

Haddad, M. C., Sharif, H. S., Shahed, M. S., Mutaiery, M. A., Samihan, A. M., Sammak, B. M., Southcombe, L. A., and Crawford, A. D.: Renal colic: Diagnosis and outcome. Radiology 184:83, 1992.

Hill, G. S.: Basic physiology and morphology of hydronephrosis. In Hill, G. S. (ed.): Uropathology. New York, Churchill Livingstone, 1989, pp. 467–516.

Lee, J. K. T., Baron, R. L., Nelson, G. L., McClennan, B. L., and Weyman, P. J.: Can real-time ultrasonography replace state B scanning in the diagnosis of renal obstruction? Radiology 139:161, 1981.

Parkhouse, H. F., and Barratt, T. M.: Investigation of the dilated urinary tract. Pediatr. Nephrol. 2:43, 1988.

Pillay, V. K. G., and Dunea, G.: Clinical aspects of obstructive uropathy. Med. Clin. North Am. 55:1417, 1971.

Ramsey, E. W., Jarzylo, S. V., and Bruce, A. W.: Spontaneous extravasation of urine from the renal pelvis and ureter. J. Urol. 110:507, 1973.

Saxton, H. M., Ogg, C. S., and Cameron, J. S.: Needle nephrostomy. Br. Med. Bull. 28:210, 1972.

Sokoloff, J., and Talner, L. B.: The heterotopic excretion of sodium iothalamate. Br. J. Radiol. 46:571, 1973.

Subramanyam, B. R., Raghavendra, N. G., Bosniak, M. A., Lefleur, R. S., Rosen, R. J., and Horii, S. C.: Sonography of pyelonephrosis: A prospective study. AJR 140:991, 1983.

Talner, L. B., Scheible, W., Ellenbogen, P. H., Beck, C. H., and Gosink, B. B.: How accurate is ultrasonography in detecting hydronephrosis in uremic patients? Urol. Radiol. 3:1, 1981.

Talner, L. B.: Urinary obstruction. In Pollack, H. M. (ed.): Clinical Urography. Philadelphia, W.B. Saunders, 1990, pp. 1535–1629.

Tanagho, E. A.: Mechanics of ureteral dilatation. Can. J. Surg. 15:4, 1972.

Umerak, B.: The layered pyelogram in hydronephrosis. Br. J. Radiol. 48:982, 1975.

Wilson, D. R.: Urinary tract obstruction. In Schrier, R. W., and Gottschalk, C. W. (eds.): Diseases of the Kidney. 4th ed. Boston, Little, Brown & Co., 1988, pp. 715–746.

Wise, H. M., Jr.: Hypertension resulting from hydronephrosis. JAMA 231:491, 1975.

Yarger, W. E.: Urinary tract obstruction. In Brenner, B. M., and Rector, F. C. (eds.): The Kidney. 4th ed. Philadelphia, W.B. Saunders, 1991, pp. 1768–1808.

Yoder, I. C., Pfister, R. C., Lindfor, K. K., and Newhouse, J. H.: Pyelonephrosis: Imaging and intervention. AJR 141:735, 1983.

Acute Pyelonephritis

Adler, S. N.: Nonobstructive pyelonephritis initially seen as acute renal failure. Arch. Intern. Med. 138:816, 1978.

Andriole, V. T.: Urinary tract infections: Recent developments. J. Infect. Dis. 156:865, 1987.

Bailey, R. R., Little, P. J., and Rolleston, G. L.: Renal damage after acute pyelonephritis. Br. Med. J. 1:550, 1969.

Berliner, L., and Bosniak, M. A.: The striated nephrogram in acute pyelonephritis. Urol. Radiol. 4:41, 1982.

Björgivinsson, E., Majd, M., and Eggli, K. D.: Diagnosis of acute pyelonephritis in children: Comparison of sonography and Tc-DMSA scintigraphy. AJR 157:539, 1991.

Davidson, A. J., and Talner, L. B.: Urographic and angiographic abnormalities in adult-onset acute bacterial nephritis. Radiology 106:249, 1973.

Davidson, A. J., and Talner, L. B.: Late sequelae of adult-onset acute bacterial nephritis. Radiology 127:367, 1978.

DeLange, E. E., and Jones, B.: Unnecessary intravenous urography in young women with recurrent urinary tract infections. Clin. Radiol. 34:551, 1983.

Eggli, D. F., and Tulchinsky, M.: Scintigraph evaluation of pediatric urinary tract infection. Semin. Nucl. Med. 23:199, 1993.

Evanhoff, G. V., Thompson, C. S., Foley, R., and Weinman, E. J.: Spectrum of gas within the kidney. Am. J. Med. 83:149, 1987.

Fierer, J.: Acute pyelonephritis. Urol. Clin. North Am. 14:251, 1987.

Gold, R. P., McClennan, B. L., and Rottenberg, R. R.: CT appearance of acute inflammatory disease of the renal interstitium. AJR 141:343, 1983.

Greenhill, A. H., Norman, M. E., Cornfield, D., Chatten, J., Buck, B., and Witzleben, C. L.: Acute renal failure secondary to acute pyelonephritis. Clin. Nephrol. 8:400, 1977.

Heptinstall, R. H.: Urinary tract infection and clinical features of pyelonephritis. In Heptinstall, R. H. (ed.): Pathology of the Kidney. 4th ed. Boston, Little, Brown and Co., 1992, pp. 1433–1488.

Heptinstall, R. H.: Pyelonephritis: Pathologic features. In Heptinstall, R. H. (ed.): Pathology of the Kidney. 4th ed. Boston, Little, Brown & Co., 1992, pp. 1489–1562.

Hill, G. S., and Clark, R. L.: A comparative angiographic, microangiographic and histologic study of experimental pyelonephritis. Invest. Radiol. 7:33, 1972.

Hill, G. S.: Urinary tract infections: General considerations. In Hill, G. S. (ed.): Uropathology. New York, Churchill Livingstone, 1989, pp. 279–332.

Hill, G. S.: Renal infection. In Hill, G. S. (ed.): Uropathology. New York, Churchill Livingstone, 1989, pp. 333–430.

Hoddick, W., Jeffrey, R. B., Goldberg, H. I., Federle, M. P., and Laing, F. C.: CT and sonography of severe renal and perirenal infections. AJR 140:517, 1983.

Hodson, C. J.: The effects of disturbance of flow on the kidney. J. Infect. Dis. 120:54, 1969.

Hodson, C. J.: The mechanism of scar formation in chronic pyelonephritis. In Kincaid-Smith, P., and Fairley, K. F. (eds.): Renal Infection and Renal Scarring. Proceedings of the International Symposium on Pyelonephritis, Vesicoureteric Reflux and Renal Papillary Necrosis. Melbourne, Mercedes Publishing Co., 1970.

Hoffman, E. P., Mindelzun, R. E., and Anderson, R. V.: Computed tomography in acute pyelonephritis associated with diabetes. Radiology 135:691, 1980.

Huang, J. J., Sung, J. M., Chen, K. W., Ruaan, M. K., Shu, G. H. F., and Chuang, Y. C.: Acute bacterial nephritis: A clinicoradiologic correlation based on computed tomography. Am. J. Med. 93:289, 1992.

Huland, H., Busch, R., and Riebel, T.: Renal scanning after symptomatic and asymptomatic upper urinary tract infection: A prospective study. J. Urol. 128:682, 1982.

Johnson, J. R., Vincent, L. M., Wang, K., Roberts, P. L., and Stamm, W. E.: Renal ultrasonographic correlates of acute pyelonephritis. Clin. Infect. Dis. 14:15, 1992.

June, C. H., Browning, M. D., Smith, P., Wenzel, D. J., Pyatt, R. S., Checchio, L. M., and Amis, E. S., Jr.: Ultrasonography and computed tomography in severe urinary tract infection. Arch. Intern. Med. 145:841, 1985.

Kanel, K. T., Kroboth, F. J., Schwentker, F. N., and Lecky, J. W.: The intravenous pyelogram in acute pyelonephritis. Arch. Intern. Med. 148:2144, 1988.

Kass, E. H., and Zinner, S. H.: Bacteriuria and renal disease. J. Infect. Dis. 120:27, 1969.

Kellett, M. J.: Urinary tract infections in adults. Br. J. Radiol. 53:1106, 1980.

Lautin, E. M., Gordon, P. M., Friedman, A. C., Dourmashkin, L., and Fromowitz, F.: Emphysematous pyelonephritis: Optimal diagnosis and treatment. Urol. Radiol. 1:93, 1979.

Lebowitz, R. L., and Mandell, J.: Urinary tract infection in children: Putting radiology in its place. Radiology 165: 1, 1987.

Lee, J. K. T., McClennan, B. L., Melson, G. L., and Stanley, R. J.: Acute focal bacterial nephritis: Emphasis on gray scale sonography and computed tomography. AJR 135:87, 1980.

Lee, S. E., Yoon, D. K., and Kim, Y. K.: Emphysematous pyelonephritis. J. Urol. 118:916, 1977.

Little, P. J., McPherson, D. R., and deWardener, H. E.: The appearance of the intravenous pyelogram during and after acute pyelonephritis. Lancet 1:1186, 1965.

Majd, M., and Rushton, H. G.: Renal cortical scintigraphy in the diagnosis of acute pyelonephritis. Semin. Nucl. Med. 22:98, 1992.

Measley, R. E., Jr., and Levison, M. E.: Host defense mechanisms in the pathogenesis of urinary tract infection. Med. Clin. North Am. 75:275, 1991.

Moseley, I. F., McIntosh, C. S., Fry, I. K., and Cattell, W. R.: In Cameron, J. S. (ed.): Proceedings of the European Dialysis Transplant. Assoc., Berlin, 1971, Volume 8. London, Pitman Medical, 1971, pp. 537–541.

Parsons, C. L.: Pathogenesis of urinary tract infection: Bacterial adherence, bladder defense mechanisms. Urol. Clin. North Am. 13:563, 1986.

Rauschkolb, E. N., Sandler, C. M., Patel, S., and Childs, T. L.: Computed tomography of renal inflammatory disease. J. Comput. Assist. Tomogr. 6:502, 1982.

Richie, J. P., Nicholson, T. C., Hunting, D., and Brosman, S. A.: Radiographic abnormalities in acute pyelonephritis. J. Urol. 119:832, 1978.

Roberts, J. A.: Pathogenesis of pyelonephritis. J. Urol. 129:1102, 1983.

Roberts, J. A.: Etiology and pathophysiology of pyelonephritis. Am. J. Kidney Dis. 17:1, 1991.

Ronald, A. R., and Simonsen, N.: Infections of the upper urinary tract in diseases of the kidney. In Schrier, R. W., Gottschalk, C. W. (eds.): Diseases of the Kidney. 4th ed. Boston, Little, Brown and Co., 1988.

Rosenfield, A. T., Glickman, M. G., Taylor, K. J. W., Crade, M., and Hodson, J.: Acute focal bacterial nephritis (acute lobar nephronia). Radiology 132:553, 1979.

Rubin, R. H., Tolkoff, N. E., and Cotran, R. S.: Urinary Tract Infection, Pyelonephritis and Reflux Nephropathy. In Brenner, B. M., and Rector, F. C. (eds.): The Kidney. 4th ed. Philadelphia, W.B. Saunders, 1991, pp. 1369–1430.

Rushton, H. G.: Pyelonephritis: Pathogenesis and management update. Dialogues in Pediatr. Urol. 13:1, 1990.

Rushton, H. G., Majd, M., Jantausch, B., Wiedermann, B. L., and Belman, A. B.: Renal scarring following reflux and nonreflux pyelonephritis in children: Evaluation with technetium-99m-dimercaptosuccinic acid scintigraphy. J. Urol. 147:1327, 1992.

Schainuck, L. I., Fouty, R., and Cutler, R. E.: Emphysematous pyelonephritis: A new case and review of previous observations. Am. J. Med. 44:134, 1968.

Shortliffe, L. M. D.: Urinary tract infections in infants and children. In Walsh, P. C., Retik, A. B., Stamey, T. A., and Vaughan, E. D., Jr. (eds.): Campbell's Urology. 6th ed. Philadelphia, W. B. Saunders, 1992, pp. 1669–1686.

Silver, T. M., Kass, E. J., Thornbury, J. R., Konnak, J. W., and Wolfman, M. G.: The radiological spectrum of acute pyelonephritis in adults and adolescents. Radiology 118:65, 1976.

Smith, J. W.: Southwestern Internal Medicine Conference: Prognosis in pyelonephritis: Promise or progress? Am. J. Med. Sci. 297:54, 1989.

Sobel, J. D.: Bacterial etiologic agents in the pathogenesis of urinary tract infection. Med. Clin. North Am. 75:253, 1991.

Sobel, J. D., and Kaye, D.: Host defense mechanisms in urinary tract infections. In Schrier, R. W., and Gottschalk, C. W. (eds.): Diseases of the Kidney. 4th ed. Little, Brown & Co., 1988, pp. 967–992.

Soulen, M. C., Fishman, F. K., Goldman, S. M., and Gatewood, O. M. B.: Bacterial renal infection: Role of CT. Radiology 171:703, 1989.

Svanborg, C., deMan, P., and Sandberg, T.: Renal involvement in urinary tract infection. Kidney Int. 39:541, 1991.

Teplick, J. G., Teplick, S. K., Berinson, H., and Haskin, M. E.: Urographic and angiographic changes in acute unilateral pyelonephritis. Clin. Radiol. 30:59, 1978.

Tsugaya, M., Hirao, N., Sakagami, H., Ontagurao, K., and Washida, H.: Renal cortical scarring in acute pyelonephritis. Br. J. Urol. 69:245, 1992.

Whitworth, J. A., Fairley, K. F., O'Keefe, C. M., and Johnson, W.: The site of renal infection: Pyelitis or pyelonephritis? Clin. Nephrol. 2:9, 1974.

Compensatory Hypertrophy

Boner, G., Sherry, J., and Rieselbach, R. E.: Hypertrophy of the normal human kidney following contralateral nephrectomy. Nephron 9:364, 1972.

Dossetor, R. S.: Renal compensatory hypertrophy in the adult. Br. J. Radiol. 48:993, 1975.

Ekelund, L., and Gothlin, J.: Compensatory renal enlargement in older patients. AJR 127:713, 1976.

Heideman, H. D., and Rosenbaum, H. D.: A study of renal size after contralateral nephrectomy. Radiology 94:599, 1970.

Malt, R. A.: Compensatory growth of the kidney. N. Engl. J. Med. 280:1446, 1969.

Ogden, D. A.: Donor and recipient function 2 to 4 years after renal homotransplantation: A paired study of 28 cases. Ann. Intern. Med. 67:998, 1967.

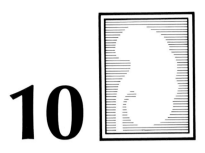

10

DIAGNOSTIC SET: LARGE, MULTIFOCAL, BILATERAL

AUTOSOMAL DOMINANT (ADULT)
POLYCYSTIC KIDNEY DISEASE

ACQUIRED CYSTIC KIDNEY DISEASE

LYMPHOMA

DIFFERENTIAL DIAGNOSIS

Enlargement of the kidney and distortion of the renal contour by multiple mass lesions occur in almost all cases of autosomal dominant polycystic kidney disease and in many instances of acquired cystic kidney disease. The same pattern is commonly, but not invariably, present when lymphoma involves the kidney. Together, these diseases constitute the diagnostic set "large, multifocal, bilateral."

AUTOSOMAL DOMINANT (ADULT) POLYCYSTIC KIDNEY DISEASE

Definition

The adult form of polycystic kidney disease is an autosomal dominant heritable disorder that results in a large number of cysts of varying size in the kidney. Progressive azotemia usually develops at some point in the natural history of this disease.

The most commonly accepted explanation for this disorder is based on the microdissection studies of Osathanondh and Potter (1964), who classified this as Type III in the Potter classification of cystic disease of the kidney. These studies demonstrated that the cysts of autosomal dominant polycystic kidney disease arise from any part of the nephron and the collecting duct and maintain their continuity to these structures. Most often the cysts arise from the tip of Henle's loop, Bowman's space, and the proximal convoluted tubules. This finding, illustrated schematically in Figure 10–1, is in contradistinction to autosomal recessive (infantile) polycystic kidney disease in which the cystic dilatation is limited to the collecting ducts and the nephrons are uninvolved. (See Chapter 8 and Fig. 8–17.)

Flattened or cuboidal epithelium characterizes the lining of cysts in autosomal dominant polycystic kidney disease. Stromal changes are those of end-stage kidney disease with tubule atrophy and vascular and glomerular scleroses. Dystrophic calcification is common.

The gross pathologic findings vary with the number and size of cysts. With minimal disease, the kidney is normal in size and its surface is smooth; cysts are discovered only on cut section. As the size and number of cysts increase, they enlarge the kidney, although they do not necessarily distort the renal contour. Increase in renal volume usually precedes impaired renal function. In early stages of autosomal dominant polycystic kidney disease, there may also be marked asymmetry in the volume of the two kidneys. As the cysts continue to enlarge, they project beyond the renal margin, causing the renal contour to become bosselated. Although the pelvis and calyces are intrinsically normal, they are usually deformed by the expanding cysts. With advanced disease, the parenchyma is almost completely replaced by innumerable cysts. Cyst size varies from barely visible to several centimeters in diameter, and involvement may be quite asymmetric. Uncomplicated cysts contain clear, yellow fluid with electrolyte and urea levels similar to urine, in contrast to simple renal cyst fluid, which is chemically similar to plasma. Hemorrhage, however, is common. Infected cysts contain purulent material. The cysts of autosomal dominant polycystic kidney disease presenting in the newborn or infant may be macroscopic but usually are so small as to be microscopic or just barely visible to the unaided eye.

Although reports of unilateral "polycystic kidney disease" exist, it is unlikely that these actually represent the disorder described here since the genetic nature of autosomal dominant polycystic kidney disease implies involvement of both organs. Cases of so-called unilateral polycystic kidney disease probably are examples either of multiple simple cysts involving only one kidney or are, in fact, autosomal dominant polycystic kidney disease with marked asymmetry and with the "normal" kidney containing cysts too small

291

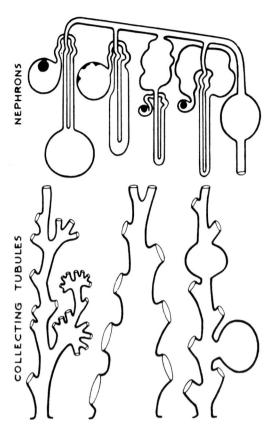

Figure 10–1. Schematic diagram of nephron dissection in autosomal dominant polycystic kidney disease. Localized or diffuse saccular and fusiform dilatations of any segment of nephrons and collecting ducts are illustrated. (From Potter, E. L.: Normal and Abnormal Development of the Kidney, 1972. Reproduced with kind permission of the author and Year Book Medical Publishers.)

for detection radiologically. For similar reasons, multiple simple cysts localized to one portion of the kidney, known as localized cystic disease, are neither genetically transmitted nor associated with renal failure and should not be considered a form of autosomal dominant polycystic kidney disease.

Liver cysts are found in up to 60 per cent of patients with autosomal dominant polycystic kidney disease. These are usually spherical, unilocular, and occasionally large enough to cause hepatomegaly. Pancreatic cysts are found in approximately 10 per cent and splenic cysts are found in up to 5 per cent of these patients. Cysts of thyroid, ovary, endometrium, seminal vesicles, lung, brain, pituitary gland, breasts, peritoneum, parathyroid, pineal, and epididymis have also been reported.

Cerebral aneurysms occur in approximately 15 per cent of patients with autosomal dominant polycystic kidney disease as discovered in autopsy series. This prevalence may be underestimated, however, since one clinical study in which aneurysms were searched for by complete cerebral angiography reported a detection rate of 40 per cent (Wakabayashi et al., 1983). An association between autosomal dominant polycystic kidney disease and cerebral arteriovenous malformation has been suggested (Proesmans et al., 1982).

It is unclear as to whether there is an associated incidence of renal carcinoma in patients with autosomal dominant polycystic kidney disease. Some of the cases reported in support of such a relationship have been of cystic kidneys that were part of von Hippel-Lindau disease or tuberous sclerosis. Although some authorities doubt an increased incidence of carcinoma in polycystic kidneys, others posit a relationship between autosomal dominant polycystic kidney disease, epithelial hyperplasia, and renal neoplasia.

Clinical Setting

Autosomal dominant polycystic kidney disease is the most common of the hereditary renal diseases, accounting for up to 12 per cent of all patients on long-term hemodialysis in the United States. Because the disease may be clinically silent, the reported prevalence in autopsy series is somewhat higher than in clinical series. There is no sex predilection.

The disease is transmitted as an autosomal dominant trait with nearly 100 per cent penetrance, if the carrier lives long enough. Because the disease is characterized by variable expressivity and because some cases may represent spontaneous mutation, as many as 50 per cent of affected patients have no family history of renal disease.

The morphologic changes of autosomal dominant polycystic kidney disease probably begin *in utero* in most patients, as suggested by prenatal sonographic studies. Rarely, the severity of the disease is sufficient to cause renal failure *in utero,* in which case the pregnancy is complicated by oligohydramnios and the infant may demonstrate the findings of Potter's syndrome. Otherwise, clinical manifestations are very uncommon in children. Most patients become symptomatic in the fourth or fifth decade. Rarely, the disease is uncovered as late as the ninth decade. As ultrasonographic or computed tomographic screening of patients at risk increases, the mean age of discovery will surely diminish. It is generally held that if cysts are not identified by age 30 in a screening ultrasonogram of a patient with a positive family history for autosomal dominant polycystic kidney disease, there is little likelihood that the patient has the disease.

Palpable mass, hypertension, abdominal pain, hematuria, and urinary tract infection are common. Hypertension may antedate renal impairment. The absence of hypertension at the time of diagnosis may be a favorable prognostic sign. Proteinuria and hematuria are often present. Polycythemia occurs secondary to erythropoietin production by the affected kidneys. As the cysts enlarge, more renal parenchyma is destroyed and azotemia worsens. In most patients, renal failure occurs by the age of 60.

Infection, hemorrhage, stone formation, cyst rupture, and obstruction are complications of autosomal dominant polycystic kidney disease. Urinary tract infections may accelerate deterioration of renal function. Experimental evidence suggests that cystic kidneys are more easily infected than noncystic kidneys and that bacteria may play a role in the formation or enlargement of cysts. Infected cysts may be asymptomatic and detected only through their aspiration or through an incidental finding at surgery or autopsy. Urinary tract instrumentation often induces infection with considerable morbidity and mortality. Hemorrhage is intracystic or retroperitoneal or into the collecting system, with resultant hematuria. Occasionally, bleeding is massive and requires nephrectomy. Calculi form, presumably as a result of urine stasis in partially obstructed collecting structures. Before the availability of hemodialysis and transplantation, untreated patients died of renal failure and its complications within 10 years of the onset of clinical symptoms.

Extrarenal cysts seldom cause symptoms. There is no correlation between the severity of renal cystic disease and severity of hepatic cysts. Hepatic function and portal pressure are usually normal, although prolonged survival may lead to morbidity and mortality from impaired hepatic function.

A variety of cardiac and aortic lesions have been described in patients with polycystic kidney disease. These include aortic root dilatation, aortic regurgitation, bicuspid aortic valve, aortic coarctation, mitral valve prolapse, and abdominal aortic aneurysm. Colonic diverticula have also been described as more frequent in patients with autosomal dominant polycystic kidney disease than in the general population.

Death due to rupture of a cerebral aneurysm into the brain and subarachnoid space occurs in approximately 10 per cent of patients with autosomal dominant polycystic kidney disease. This complication of cerebral aneurysm rupture may increase as survival is prolonged by dialysis and transplantation.

Radiologic Findings

The abdominal film is normal in the early stage of autosomal dominant polycystic kidney disease. As the disease progresses, the enlarged kidneys may become recognizable as soft tissue masses. It is often not possible to identify the entire renal outline on an abdominal radiograph in patients with autosomal dominant polycystic kidney disease, whereas this is usually accomplished readily in patients with other causes of renal enlargement. Enlargement is frequently asymmetric and may result in displacement of the duodenum, the flexures of the colon, and other intraperitoneal and extraperitoneal structures. Extrinsic scalloping of the posterior wall of the stomach may be seen on upper gastrointestinal studies. The psoas muscles may be obscured. Dystrophic calcification has variable patterns, including thin or thick curvilinear densities or scattered amorphous plaques (Fig. 10–2). Renal calculi often signify superimposed infection.

The nephrogram is characterized by numerous sharply marginated radiolucencies throughout the parenchyma of both kidneys, best demonstrated by tomography. Young, asymptomatic patients frequently have enlarged kidneys with smooth outlines and normal collecting structures, although the nephrogram

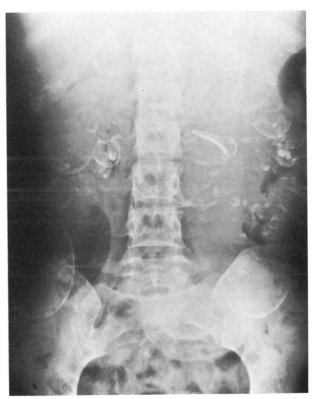

Figure 10–2. Autosomal dominant polycystic kidney disease. Abdominal radiograph. The kidneys fill the upper and midabdomen and displace intestine into the pelvis. Psoas margins are obscure. There is calcium deposited in a curvilinear pattern in the walls of a large number of cysts. (Courtesy of Stanford M. Goldman, M.D., The Johns Hopkins University, Baltimore, Maryland.) (Same patient illustrated in Fig. 10–10.)

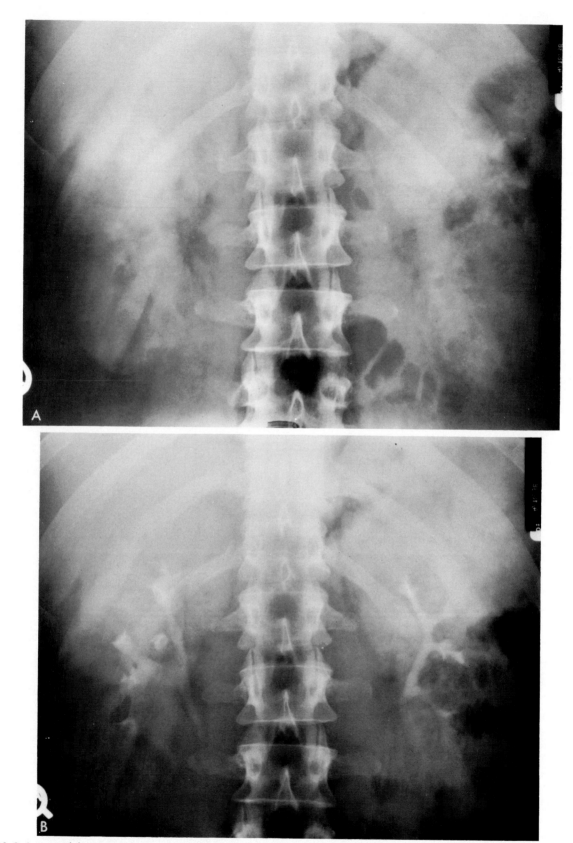

Figure 10–3. Autosomal dominant polycystic kidney disease in a 38-year-old man with hypertension and bilaterally large, smooth kidneys. *A,* Excretory urogram, 2-minute film. Characteristic multiple radiolucencies of varying size are present in the nephrogram. Right kidney length = 17.5 cm; left kidney length = 18.0 cm. *B,* Excretory urogram, 5-minute film. There is no distortion of the pelvocalyceal system.

will be abnormal even at this stage (Fig. 10–3). As the disease progresses, however, the contour becomes bosselated. The larger cysts will elongate, efface, and displace the calyces (Fig. 10–4). Occasionally, a large cyst will obstruct one or more calyces. Cysts that have ruptured into the collecting system may fill with contrast material during excretory urography or retrograde pyelography. In advanced disease with diminished renal function, tomography is often necessary to identify the cystic nephrogram. Occasionally, hepatic cysts may also be identified on tomographic sections obtained during excretory urography.

Ultrasonography may detect minimal disease as small echo-free masses in slightly large but otherwise normal kidneys. As the disease progresses, the kidneys enlarge, the contour becomes bosselated, and numerous cysts are visualized (Figs. 10–5 and 10–6). Marked variation in the size of the cysts is common. The central sinus echo complex is distorted by the larger cysts. Cysts complicated by hemorrhage or infection have internal echoes, fluid–debris levels, and thick walls. Differentiation between hemorrhage and infection is impossible by ultrasonography alone. Calcification (dystrophic or nephrolithiasis) is very echogenic and causes acoustic shadows.

Ultrasonography may detect autosomal dominant polycystic kidney disease *in utero* as enlarged kidneys, ascites, hepatomegaly, and renal cysts. In the newborn, the ultrasonographic features of autosomal dominant polycystic kidney disease may be indistinguishable from the nephromegaly and diffuse increased echogenicity of autosomal recessive polycystic kidney disease, although in some instances small cysts are visible as well (Fig. 10–7). In older children, the pattern is similar to that seen in adults. Ultrasonography may reveal nephromegaly and cysts in asymptomatic children of parents with known disease and, thus, is an excellent modality for screening (Fig. 10–8).

Cysts of the liver, pancreas, or spleen appear as echo-free masses with increased through-sound transmission. Their detection helps confirm the diagnosis of autosomal dominant polycystic kidney disease. When these extrarenal cysts are prominent, it is often difficult to assess the boundaries of contiguous organs.

Computed tomography demonstrates multiple round to oval cysts that are variable in size and scattered throughout the cortex and medulla (Fig. 10–9). Uncomplicated cysts have attenuation values near that of water and do not enhance. Because of the dense parenchymal blush of uninvolved surrounding renal parenchyma, cysts are accentuated on contrast material–enhanced scans. With advanced disease, unenhanced scans often demonstrate curvilinear or amorphous dystrophic calcifications within cyst walls

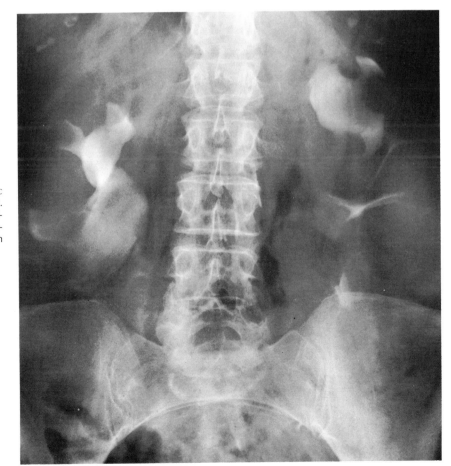

Figure 10–4. Autosomal dominant polycystic kidney disease in a 74-year-old woman. Marked multifocal enlargement of both kidneys, focal displacement of the collecting structures, and normal opacification are common urographic features of this disease.

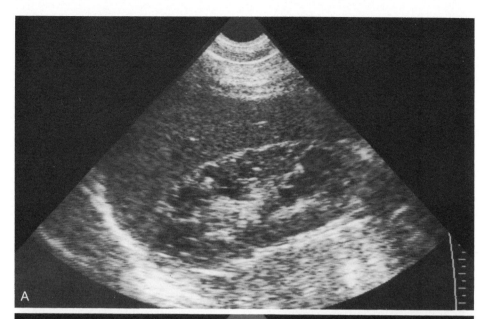

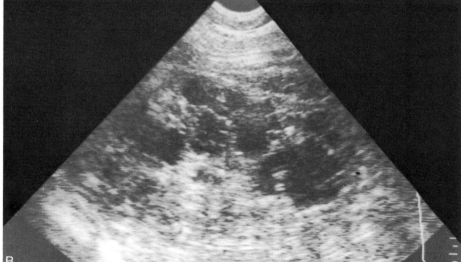

Figure 10–5. Autosomal dominant polycystic kidney disease increasing in size over a 4-year interval. The kidney also changes from a smooth to a bosselated contour in the same interval. Ultrasonograms of the right kidney in longitudinal section.

A, 1983. Length = 9 cm.
B, 1987. Length = 13 cm.

(Kindly provided by Brian Garra, M.D., Georgetown University, Washington, D.C.)

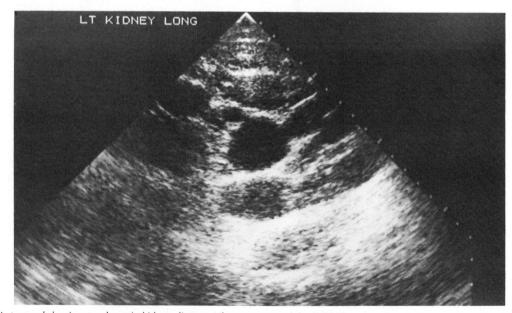

Figure 10–6. Autosomal dominant polycystic kidney disease. Ultrasonogram of the left kidney in a longitudinal section. The kidney is enlarged and bosselated by numerous, varying-sized cysts containing uncomplicated fluid.

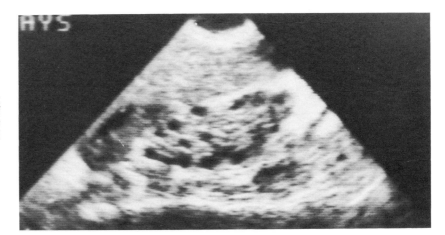

Figure 10–7. Autosomal dominant polycystic kidney disease in a newborn. Ultrasonogram of the right kidney, longitudinal section. The kidney is smooth and hyperechoic and contains a small number of detectable cysts.

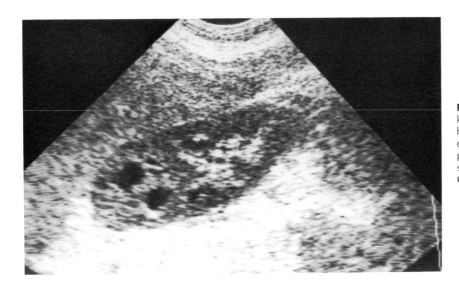

Figure 10–8. Autosomal dominant polycystic kidney disease in an asymptomatic 14-year-old boy with a positive family history. Ultrasonogram of the right kidney in a longitudinal section. Hyperechoicity and several cysts indicate a carrier state. (Kindly provided by Brian Garra, M.D., Georgetown University, Washington, D.C.)

Figure 10–9. Autosomal dominant polycystic kidney disease. Computed tomogram, contrast material enhanced. The large kidneys, with multiple masses of varying size, are well demonstrated in this 35-year-old hypertensive man with mild azotemia. The masses have a water attenuation value and do not enhance after contrast material is injected. Note distorted and compressed collecting structures.

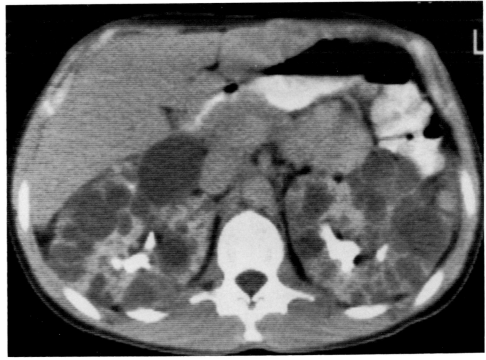

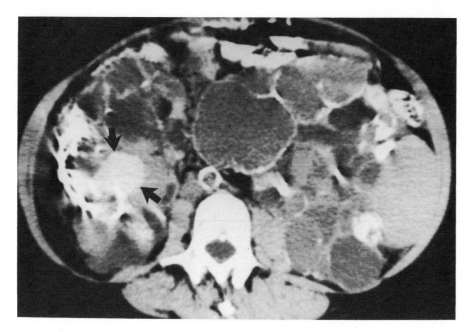

Figure 10–10. Autosomal dominant poly-cystic kidney disease with extensive, thick calcification of cyst walls bilaterally. One cyst in the right kidney *(arrows)* has a high attenuation value representing hemorrhage. Computed tomogram, contrast material enhanced. (Kindly provided by Stanford M. Goldman, M.D., The Johns Hopkins University, Baltimore, Maryland.) (Same patient illustrated in Fig. 10–2.)

or compressed atrophic parenchyma and acute hemorrhage into cysts recognized as a well-defined hyperdense mass on an unenhanced scan (Fig. 10–10). These high density cysts are common especially in patients with marked renal enlargement and flank pain. They are often multiple and subcapsular or perirenal. With time, the computed tomographic density of a hemorrhagic cyst diminishes.

An infected cyst may also have a thick, irregular wall that calcifies. The attenuation value of an infected cyst is slightly higher than that of water and may be variable within a single cyst. Localized thickening of Gerota's fascia is a nonspecific finding sometimes seen with infection. Gas within an infected cyst is easily detected with computed tomography. A perinephric abscess may also develop in conjunction with infection of the cystic kidney.

Cysts are frequently identified in the liver and, occasionally, in the pancreas and spleen (Fig. 10–11). There is no relationship between the number of cysts recognized in the liver and their frequency in the kidney.

Intrarenal arteries are stretched and displaced by the numerous cysts in the medulla and cortex. Angiography demonstrates well the multiple, sharply defined, variable sized nephrographic defects caused by the cysts. Cysts complicated by hemorrhage or infection may have abnormal vessels that simulate those usually associated with neoplasia. Hepatic and splenic cysts appear as avascular masses on selective visceral injections.

Magnetic resonance imaging demonstrates the number and size of the cysts, the size of the kidneys, the contents of the cysts, and the extent of extrarenal disease. Uncomplicated cysts are homogeneous and low intensity on T1-weighted images and homogeneous and high intensity on T2-weighted images, just as are simple cysts. Cysts complicated by hemorrhage are usually hyperintense, but the appearance varies with the amount of time since the bleeding episode. Layering may be present in cysts with recent hemorrhage. Infected cysts and cysts with high protein content are intermediate between the two extremes of uncomplicated and complicated cysts.

SUMMARY OF ABNORMAL URORADIOLOGIC FINDINGS
AUTOSOMAL DOMINANT (ADULT) POLYCYSTIC KIDNEY DISEASE

Primary Uroradiologic Elements
    Size—large
    Contour—multifocal masses (smooth—rarely)
    Lesion distribution—bilateral (may be asymmetric)
Secondary Uroradiologic Elements
    Pelvoinfundibulocalyceal system—displaced and attenuated (normal—rarely)
    Nephrogram—replaced (multiple masses with smooth margins, varying size; radiolucent with urography or angiography; water density/intensity and nonenhancing with computed tomography/magnetic resonance)
    Echogenicity—multiple, fluid-filled masses (may be diffusely echogenic when cysts are small)

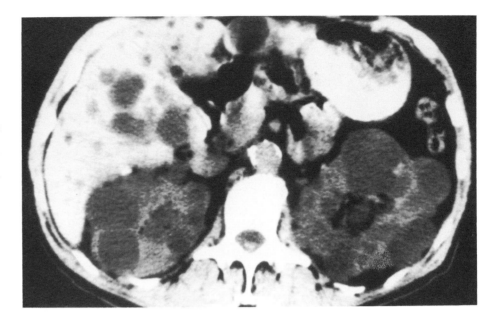

Figure 10–11. Autosomal dominant polycystic kidney disease. Computed tomogram, unenhanced. Multiple hepatic cysts of varying size are present. Note the asymmetry of renal involvement.

ACQUIRED CYSTIC KIDNEY DISEASE

Definition

Multiple cyst formation occurs in chronically failed kidneys, especially in patients undergoing long-term hemodialysis or peritoneal dialysis. This condition, known as *acquired cystic kidney disease,* causes enlargement of the small, smooth, failed kidneys. Sometimes, the degree of enlargement approximates that of the large bulk usually associated with autosomal dominant (adult) polycystic kidney disease. The etiology of this disorder has not been established, although a direct relationship between the prevalence of acquired cystic kidney disease and the duration of dialysis has been demonstrated. Some degree of remission following successful transplantation has been reported.

The cysts of uncomplicated acquired cystic kidney disease are filled with clear fluid and vary from microscopic to 3.0 cm in diameter. They may be as few as five but are most commonly multiple and cause multifocal enlargement of the renal contour. Bleeding into cysts is common. Most cysts are lined by a single layer of cuboidal or columnar epithelium and are in continuity with the tubule lumen. Commonly, however, atypical, hyperplastic, multilayered epithelium with papillary projections is present. This may represent a stage in the development of adenoma or carcinoma, which develops more frequently in patients with acquired cystic kidney disease than in the general population. Calcium may be found in the cyst wall.

Severe sclerosis occurs in the medium-and small-sized arteries of kidneys with acquired cystic disease. These vessels, which are unsupported by surrounding solid parenchyma, become markedly tortuous and project into the cavities of the cysts.

Clinical Setting

Acquired cystic kidney disease occurs during the course of long-term dialysis for the treatment of end-stage renal disease and, less frequently, in patients with chronic renal failure that does not require dialysis. Longitudinal studies have demonstrated that renal volume may diminish in the first 3 years after the start of treatment. Thereafter, cyst formation develops and progresses and kidney bulk increases. Up to 80 per cent of patients are affected after 7 or more years of dialysis.

Acquired cystic disease of the kidney by itself is clinically silent. Clinical concern centers on the high prevalence of carcinoma in these kidneys and the risk of major hemorrhage from spontaneous arterial rupture. Adenomatous tumors that are both benign and malignant cytologically occur frequently. Malignant tumors occur more frequently than in the general population; their lethality in terms of mortality rates appears to be similar to adenocarcinoma of the kidney that develops spontaneously. Hemorrhage due to spontaneous arterial rupture is often major and life threatening when bleeding extends into the kidney tissue and perirenal space. Hypovolemic hypotension and severe pain may be the result. Minor bleeding into the cysts also occurs.

Radiologic Findings

Acquired cystic kidney disease is best detected and followed by computed tomography. Because of severe renal functional impairment and other limitations, excretory urography is of no value.

Renal size varies directly with the duration of hemodialysis. Early in the development of cysts, the kidneys remain small (Fig. 10–12). With time, kidney volume increases, often exceeding normal (Fig. 10–13). Cysts are sharply marginated and have attenuation values of water unless bleeding has caused an increase in this value. Despite severe renal failure, the renal parenchyma enhances slightly. Both adenomas and carcinomas demonstrate soft tissue attenuation values and are sharply defined (see Fig. 10–12). These

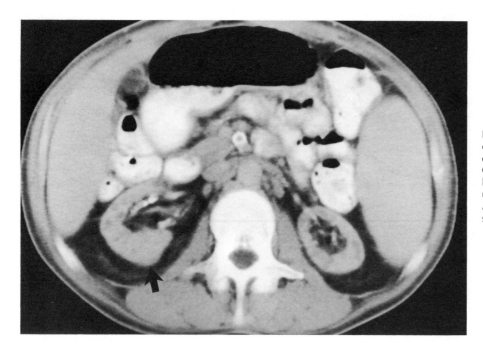

Figure 10–12. Acquired cystic kidney disease in a patient with end-stage renal disease maintained on hemodialysis. Computed tomogram, unenhanced. The kidneys contain several small, low attenuation cysts but remain small and smooth. An adenocarcinoma is present on the dorsal aspect of the right kidney (*arrow*).

solid masses, which may project into the fluid-filled cysts, enhance in a homogeneous pattern after contrast material is administered. With major hemorrhage due to a ruptured intrarenal artery aneurysm, computed tomography demonstrates fresh blood with a high attenuation value within and surrounding the kidney.

The fluid-filled nature of the multiple cysts is well demonstrated by ultrasonography. The anechoic masses are surrounded by highly echogenic tissue representing the chronically diseased kidney. Carci-

noma and adenoma can be detected by ultrasonography as echogenic masses, but computed tomography detects them more effectively.

Angiography may be used to evaluate the patient with major hemorrhage or to assess a tumor. Marked tortuosity of severely sclerotic vessels, with aneurysmal dilatation, lack of tapering, and few branches are characteristic of this disorder (Fig. 10–14). With major bleeding, the nephrogram will be disordered and the arteries will be displaced by blood in the perirenal space.

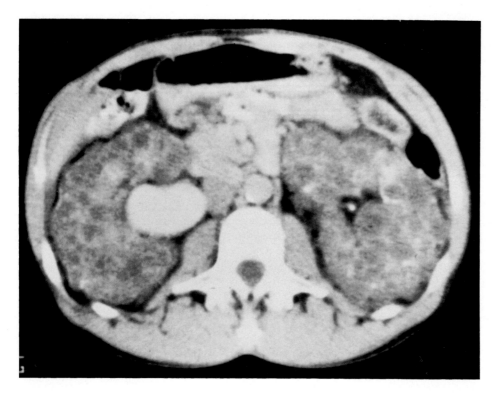

Figure 10–13. Acquired cystic kidney disease. Computed tomogram, contrast material enhanced. Multiple fluid-filled masses of varying sizes enlarge the kidneys and create a multilobulated contour. (Courtesy of G. Friedland, M.D., Stanford University, Stanford, California.)

**SUMMARY OF ABNORMAL URORADIOLOGIC FINDINGS
ACQUIRED CYSTIC KIDNEY DISEASE**

Primary Uroradiologic Elements
    Size—small (early); large (late)
    Contour—multifocal masses
    Lesion distribution—bilateral
Secondary Uroradiologic Elements
    Nephrogram—replaced (multiple masses with smooth margins; varying size; radiolucent with angi-
       ography; water density and nonenhancing with computed tomography)
    Echogenicity—multiple, fluid-filled masses

LYMPHOMA

Definition

All forms of lymphoma have similar patterns of renal involvement, although each has distinctive pathologic, clinical, and prognostic features. In one autopsy series of 690 patients with lymphoma, renal involvement occurred in one-third (Richmond et al., 1962). Bilateral involvement occurred three times more often than unilateral disease. Of all the cases, multiple nodules were present in 61 per cent, although some were too small for detection on radiographs. Eleven per cent had invasion from perirenal disease, 7 per cent had a single, bulky tumor, and 7 per cent had a small,

solitary nodule. Diffuse infiltration occurred in 6 per cent, and microscopic disease was found in only 7 per cent. Most other series reporting renal involvement in lymphoma confirm this pattern of lesion distribution.

Renal involvement occurs most frequently with non-Hodgkin's lymphoma and least often with Hodgkin's disease. Leukemia, which is quite separate from malignant lymphoma, causes bilateral, diffuse infiltration of the kidneys and is discussed in Chapter 8.

Lymphoid tissue is not native to the kidney. Renal lymphoma, therefore, always represents either blood-borne metastases or direct invasion by tumor growing in the perirenal space. Hematogenous metastases most commonly produce multiple, bilateral nodules.

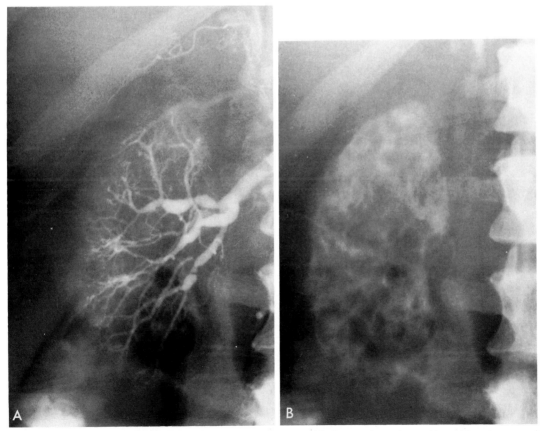

Figure 10–14. Acquired cystic kidney disease. The renal arteries are tortuous and lack normal tapering and branching. Aneurysmal dilatations in medium-sized vessels are common. Selective right renal arteriogram.
   A, Arterial phase.
   B, Nephrographic phase. Note the persistent small size of the kidney and multiple radiolucencies due to cysts.

Because lymphoma grows by infiltration, the interface between lymphomatous deposits and normal parenchyma is not sharp. As the kidney enlarges, the reniform or bean shape is preserved, at least initially. Eventually, the lymphomatous masses become so large that they appear expansile, or ball shaped. (See discussion of patterns of tumor growth in Chapter 12.) Direct invasion of the kidney by lymphoma in the perirenal space occurs either through the renal sinus from tumor medial to the kidney (transsinus spread), or across the renal capsule from tumor in the perirenal space lateral to the kidney (transcapsular spread). Transsinus spread is often associated with obstructive uropathy as a result of involvement of the ureter or renal pelvis. When tumor surrounds the pelvis, caliectasis without pelviectasis is seen.

Clinical Setting

Lymphoma of the kidneys does not commonly produce clinical findings referable to the urinary tract. Uremia is rare. Renal parenchymal nodules may produce flank pain or tenderness, a palpable mass, or hematuria. Masses in the region of the renal hilus can produce hypertension or renal vein occlusion as a result of pressure on the renal pedicle. Obstructive uropathy may directly follow retroperitoneal involvement of ureters or indirectly from retroperitoneal fibrosis.

Proteinuria, cylindruria, elevated blood urea nitrogen levels, and hypercalcemia are often present. Hypercalcemia may be severe enough to cause nephropathy. Complications of irradiation or chemotherapy that may be manifest in the urinary tract are uric acid nephropathy (see Chapter 8) and radiation nephritis (see Chapter 6). Renal amyloidosis is a complication of Hodgkin's disease in a few patients.

Radiologic Findings

Urography is often normal or reveals minimal nephrographic defects in cases in which metastatic lymphoma nodules are present in the kidneys but not large enough to displace the collecting structures or distort the renal contour. At this stage, reniform shape is preserved. With growth, these masses produce bilaterally enlarged kidneys, multifocal bulges of the renal contour, and displacement of the collecting system (Fig. 10–15). At times, a single mass in one kidney will be the only finding. Opacification of the kidney progressively diminishes as lymphomatous masses grow, coalesce, and replace nephrons. Lymphoma invading the kidney from the perirenal space, either by a transsinus or a transcapsular route, produces a large, retroperitoneal soft tissue mass and displacement of the kidney. The nephrogram is deficient and poorly marginated wherever the parenchyma has been invaded. With transsinus invasion, the kidney is displaced laterally and the pelvis is surrounded by tumor. In this situation, the pelvis is obstructed but

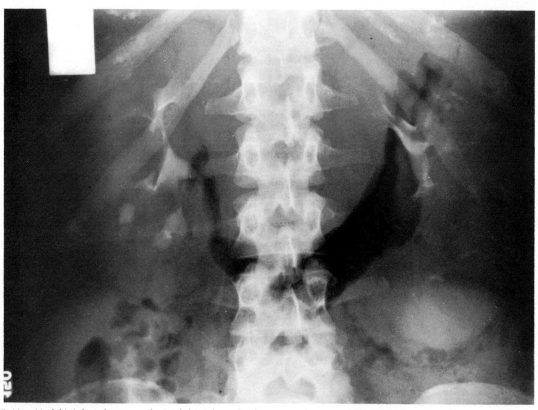

Figure 10–15. Non-Hodgkin's lymphoma producing bilateral renal enlargement due to multifocal masses. The collecting systems are displaced at several sites. Excretory urogram.

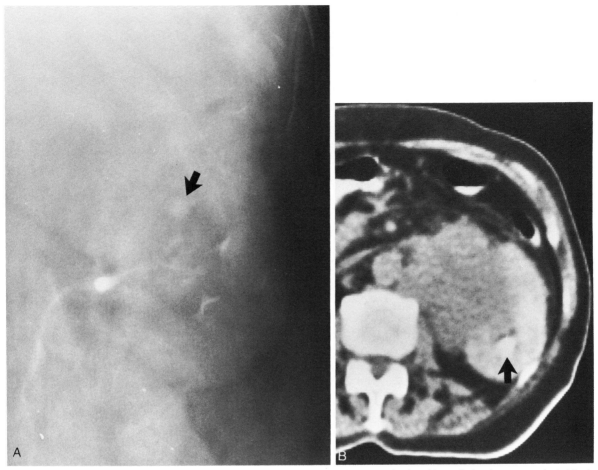

Figure 10–16. Lymphoma invading the left kidney by the "trans-sinus" route. The kidney is displaced laterally by the tumor, which fills the renal sinus and perirenal space medial to the kidney. As a result, the pelvis is obstructed but cannot dilate, but there is some caliectasis *(arrows).*
   A, Excretory urogram.
   B, Computed tomogram, contrast material enhanced.

not necessarily dilated. Caliectasis, however, is usually present (Fig. 10–16). Obstructive uropathy may also result from ureteral encasement by lymphomatous tissue more caudal in the retroperitoneum.

Computed tomography identifies the lymphomatous mass or masses more often than excretory urography or ultrasonography (Fig. 10–17). These masses are nonencapsulated and have irregular margins. Be-

fore contrast material administration, the attenuation value of lymphomatous tissue is slightly less than normal parenchyma. Contrast material enhancement is minimal, always less than that of the renal parenchyma, and usually homogeneous. Transsinus and transcapsular invasion of lymphoma from the perirenal space and lymphomatous involvement of other organs and lymph nodes are well demonstrated by

---

**SUMMARY OF ABNORMAL URORADIOLOGIC FINDINGS
LYMPHOMA**

Primary Uroradiologic Elements
   Size—normal to large
   Contour—normal to multifocal masses (smooth—early; expansile—late)
   Lesion distribution—bilateral (occasionally unilateral; rarely unifocal)
Secondary Uroradiologic Elements
   Pelvoinfundibulocalyceal system—normal to displaced (focal); caliectasis without pelviectasis (transsinus invasion)
   Parenchymal thickness—normal to expanded (focal)
   Nephrogram—multifocal masses (attenuation valve less than normal tissue; minimal enhancement with contrast material)
   Echogenicity—multifocal hypoechoic masses with poor sound transmission

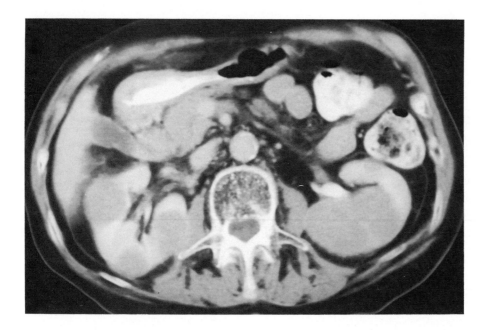

Figure 10–17. Lymphoma causing multifocal enlargement of both kidneys. Computed tomogram, contrast material enhanced. Three discrete, ball-shaped masses are present in the right kidney. The pattern of involvement of the left kidney is infiltrative and preserves reniform shape. Note, also, multiple periaortic lymph nodes.

computed tomography (Figs. 10–18 and 10–19; see Fig. 10–16).

Lymphomatous kidney and perirenal space masses are identified by ultrasonography as hypoechoic structures, with poor sound transmission and a pattern of fine internal echoes (Fig. 10–20). The central sinus echoes of the kidney may be diminished or disappear when sinus fat is replaced by lymphomatous tissue.

Uncommon radiologic findings in renal lymphoma include global enlargement of both kidneys, with smooth contours, ureteral displacement, and retroperitoneal fibrosis. Renal vein occlusion may be associated with renal sinus tumor.

Most lymphomatous renal masses are hypovascular; very few are hypervascular. Medium-sized arteries are displaced by the tumors, and neovascularity may be present. Early venous filling has been reported but is rare. The angiographic findings of lymphoma in the kidney overlap those of renal carcinoma

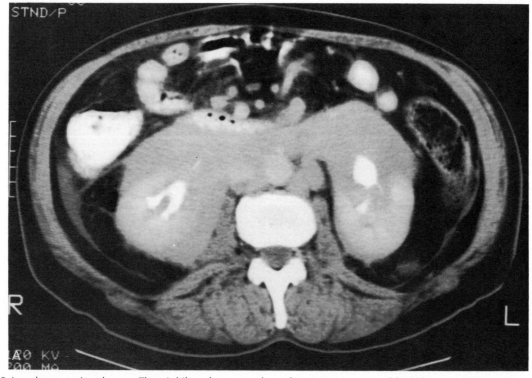

Figure 10–18. Lymphoma, perirenal space. There is bilateral transcapsular and transsinus invasion of the kidney, as well as a para-aortic mass. *A,* Computed tomogram, contrast material enhanced.

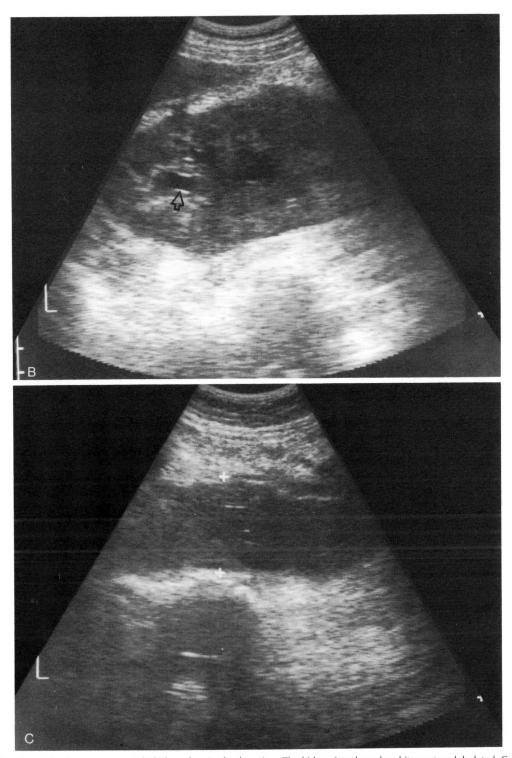

Figure 10–18 *Continued B,* Ultrasonogram, right kidney, longitudinal section. The kidney is enlarged and its contour lobulated. Caliectasis *(arrow)* is present.
    C, Ultrasonogram, midline, transverse section. A periaortic mass *(cursors)* is present.

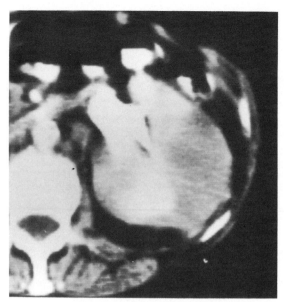

Figure 10–19. Lymphoma invading the kidney from the lateral perirenal space, the "transcapsular" route. Computed tomogram, contrast material enhanced.

and of other solid tumors and inflammatory masses. Angiography offers no useful information in the assessment of this disease.

DIFFERENTIAL DIAGNOSIS

The differential diagnosis of diseases within this diagnostic set is guided by the determination of whether the lesions are fluid-filled cysts, solid tumors, or a combination of the two, and by the clinical setting. The distinction between fluid-filled and solid masses is best accomplished by ultrasonography or

computed tomography, using the criteria described in Chapters 12 and 25.

If the lesions producing bilateral, multifocal enlargement of the kidneys are filled with fluid, the differential diagnosis, in addition to autosomal dominant polycystic kidney disease or acquired cystic kidney disease, includes multiple simple cysts of both kidneys and chronic, severe, bilateral obstructive uropathy with marked caliectasis. Multiple simple cysts are fewer and more uniform than those seen in polycystic kidney disease. Further, they occur in patients who do not necessarily have hypertension, renal failure, or a family history of renal disease. These considerations also apply to multiple bilateral renal cysts that develop as part of von Hippel-Lindau disease or tuberous sclerosis in which, additionally, other characteristic features are present. The demonstration of communication among multiple dilated fluid-filled spaces by ultrasonography or computed tomography distinguishes chronic obstructive uropathy from cystic disease of the kidney. This distinction can also be made by the conversion of radiolucent areas to radiodense ones on late films during excretory urography. A history of long-term dialysis serves to distinguish acquired cystic kidney disease from autosomal dominant polycystic kidney disease, both of which can lead to identical radiologic findings. Finally, multiple fluid-filled renal cysts are found in numerous syndromes that are known variably as glomerulocystic, microcystic, or pluricystic disorders of the kidney. Here, too, clinical findings help to clarify the diagnosis. These are discussed briefly in Chapter 8.

When masses in both kidneys are solid, lymphoma is the most likely diagnosis, although masses composed of erythroid and myeloid cells in agnogenic myeloid metaplasia and extramedullary hematopoiesis can cause identical radiologic abnormalities. Occa-

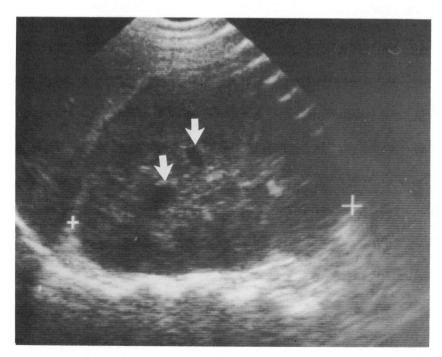

Figure 10–20. Lymphoma of the kidney causing multifocal enlargement of the right kidney. Ultrasonogram, longitudinal section. Multiple hypoechoic masses are present. Dilated, fluid-filled central structures *(arrows)* represent calyces obstructed by the adjacent tumors. The opposite kidney was similarly involved.

sionally, metastatic deposits are bilateral and multiple and must be included in this differential diagnosis. Multiple, bilateral solid masses representing angiomyolipomas may dominate the appearance of the kidneys in patients with tuberous sclerosis. This diagnosis is established by the demonstration of fat as one of the soft tissue components of the renal masses, by the stigmata of tuberous sclerosis in other organs, and by a characteristic clinical history. (See discussion in Chapter 12.) In infants and children, large kidneys with multifocal and bilateral solid masses suggest the diagnosis of Wilms' tumor in association with nephroblastomatosis or other predisposing conditions. This is also discussed in Chapter 12.

Occasionally, both solid tumors and cysts are the cause of kidney enlargement by multiple and bilateral masses. This combination may be seen in acquired cystic kidney disease (cysts, adenomas, and adenocarcinomas), von Hippel-Lindau disease (cysts and adenocarcinomas) or tuberous sclerosis (cysts and angiomyolipomas). As discussed earlier, each of these have additional radiologic and clinical features that permit accurate diagnosis.

Bibliography

Autosomal Dominant (Adult) Polycystic Kidney Disease

Barbaric, Z. L., Spataro, R. F., and Segal, A. J.: Urinary tract obstruction in polycystic renal disease. Radiology 125:627, 1977.

Bennett, W. M.: Diagnostic considerations in autosominal dominant polycystic kidney disease. Semin. Nephrol. 10:552, 1990.

Billing, L.: The roentgen diagnosis of polycystic kidneys. Acta Radiol. 41:305, 1954.

Blyth, H., and Ockenden, B. G.: Polycystic disease of kidneys and liver presenting in childhood. J. Med. Genet. 8:257, 1971.

Bosniak, M. A., and Ambos, M. A.: Polycystic kidney disease. Semin. Roentgenol. 10:133, 1975.

Cornell, S. H.: Angiography in polycystic disease of the kidney. J. Urol. 103:24, 1970.

Elkin, M., and Bernstein, J.: Cystic diseases of the kidney: Radiological and pathological considerations. Clin. Radiol. 20:65, 1969.

Elkin, M.: Renal cysts and abscesses. Curr. Probl. Radiol. 5:14, 1975.

Elkin, M.: Renal cystic disease—an overview. Semin. Roentgenol. 10:99, 1975.

Fick, G. M., Johnson, A. M., Strain, J. D., et al.: Characteristics of very early onset autosomal dominant polycystic kidney disease. J. Am. Soc. Nephrol. 3:1863, 1993.

Gabow, P. A.: Autosomal dominant polycystic kidney disease. In Gardner, K. D., Jr., and Bernstein, J. (eds.): The Cystic Kidney. Dordrecht, Kluwer Academic Publishers, 1990, pp. 295–326.

Gabow, P. A.: Autosomal dominant polycystic kidney disease—more than a renal disease. Am. J. Kidney Dis. 16:403, 1990.

Gabow, P. A.: Polycystic kidney disease: Clues to pathogenesis. Kidney Int. 40:989, 1991.

Gabow, P. A.: Medical progress—autosomal dominant polycystic kidney disease. N. Engl. J. Med. 329:332, 1993.

Gardner, K. P., Jr., and Evan, A. P.: Cystic kidneys: An enigma evolves. Am. J. Kidney Dis. 3:403, 1984.

Goldman, S. M., and Hartman, D. S.: Autosomal dominant polycystic kidney disease. In Hartman, D. S. (ed.): Renal Cystic Disease. Philadelphia, W.B. Saunders, 1989, pp. 88–107.

Gonzalo, A., Rivera, M., Quereda, C., and Ortuno, J.: Clinical features and prognosis of adult polycystic kidney disease. Am. J. Nephrol. 10:470, 1990.

Grantham, J. J.: Polycystic kidney disease—an old problem in a new context. N. Engl. J. Med. 319:944, 1988.

Granthan, J. J., and Gabow, P. A.: Polycystic kidney disease. In

Schrier, R. W. and Gottchalls, C. W. (eds.): Diseases of the Kidney. Boston, Little Brown & Co., 1988, pp. 583–615.

Gregoire, J. R., Torres, V. E., Holley, K. E., and Farrow, G. M.: Renal epithelial hyperplastic and neoplastic proliferation in autosomal dominant polycystic kidney disease. Am. J. Kidney Dis. 9:27, 1987.

Grossman, H., Rosenberg, E. R., Bowie, J. D., et al.: Sonographic diagnosis of renal cystic diseases. AJR 140:81, 1983.

Halpern, M., Dalyrymple, B., and Young, J.: The nephrogram in polycystic disease. J. Urol. 103:21, 1970.

Hatfield, P. M., and Pfister, R. C.: Adult polycystic disease of kidneys (Potter Type 3). JAMA 222:1527, 1972.

Huston, J., Torres, V. E., Sullivan, P. P., et al.: Value of magnetic resonance angiography for the detection of intracranial aneurysm in autosomal dominant polycystic kidney disease. J. Am. Soc. Nephrol. 3:1871, 1993.

Kääriäinen, H., Jääskeläinen, J., Kivisaari, L., Koskimies, O., and Norio, R.: Dominant and recessive polycystic kidney disease in children: Classification by intravenous pyelography, ultrasound, and computed tomography. Pediatr. Radiol. 18:45, 1988.

Kutcher, R., Schneider, M., and Gordon, D. H.: Calcification in polycystic disease. Radiology 122:77, 1977.

Lalli, A. F., and Poirier, V. C.: Urographic analysis of the development of polycystic kidney disease. AJR 119:705, 1973.

Lee, J. K. T., McClennan, B. L., and Kissane, J. M.: Unilateral polycystic kidney disease. AJR 130:1165, 1978.

Levine, E., and Grantham, J. J.: Perinephric hemorrhage in autosomal dominant polycystic kidney disease: CT and MR findings. J. Comput. Assist. Tomogr. 11:108, 1987.

Lieske, J. C., and Toback, F. G.: Autosomal dominant polycystic kidney disease. J. Am. Soc. Nephrol. 3:1442, 1993.

McFarland, W. L., Wallace, S., and Johnson, D. E.: Renal carcinoma and polycystic disease. J. Urol. 107:530, 1972.

McHugo, J. M., Shafi, M. I., Rowlands, D., and Weaver, J. B.: Prenatal diagnosis of adult polycystic kidney disease. Br. J. Radiol. 61:1072, 1988.

Osathanondh, V., and Potter, E. L.: Pathogenesis of polycystic kidneys: Type 3 due to multiple abnormalities of development. Lab. Med. Arch. Pathol. 77:485, 1964.

Parfrey, P. S., Bear, J. C., Morgan, J., et al.: The diagnosis and prognosis of autosomal dominant polycystic kidney disease. N. Engl. J. Med. 323:1085, 1990.

Potter, E. L.: Normal and Abnormal Development of the Kidney. Chicago, Year Book Medical Publishers, 1972.

Proesmans, W., Van Damme, B., Casaer, P., and Marchal, G.: Autosomal dominant polycystic kidney disease in the neonatal period: Association with a cerebral arteriovenous malformation. Pediatrics 70:971, 1982.

Regan, R. J., Abercrombie, G. F., and Lee, H. A.: Polycystic renal disease—occurrence of malignant change and role of nephrectomy in potential transplant recipients. Br. J. Urol. 49:85, 1977.

Renal cystic disease: Medical Staff Conference, University of California, San Francisco. Calif. Med. 119:36, 1973.

Risdon, R. A.: Development, developmental defects, and cystic diseases of the kidney. In Heptinstall, R. H. (ed.): Pathology of the kidney. 4th ed. Boston, Little, Brown & Co., 1992, pp. 93–167.

Rosenfield, A. T., Lipson, M. H., Wolf, B., et al.: Ultrasonography and nephrotomography in the presymptomatic diagnosis of dominantly inherited (adult-onset) polycystic kidney disease. Radiology 135:423, 1980.

Seagal, A. J., Spataro, R. F., and Barbaric, Z. L.: Adult polycystic kidney disease: A review of 100 cases. J. Urol. 118:711, 1977.

Strand, W. R., Rushton, H. G., Markle, B. M., and Kapur, S.: Autosomal dominant polycystic kidney disease in infants: Asymmetric disease mimicking a unilateral renal mass. J. Urol. 141:1151, 1989.

Tegtmeyer, C. J., Cail, W., Wyker, A. W., Jr., and Gillenwater, J. Y.: Angiographic diagnosis of renal tumors associated with polycystic disease. Radiology 126:105, 1978.

Wakabayashi, T., Fujita, S., Ohbora, Y., Suyama, T., Tamuki, N., and Matsumoto, S.: Polycystic kidney disease and intracranial aneurysms. J. Neurosurg. 58:488, 1983.

Welling, L. W., and Granthan, J. J.: Cystic and developmental diseases of the kidney. In Brenner, B. M., Rector, F. C. (eds.): The Kidney. 4th ed. Philadelphia, W.B. Saunders, 1991, pp. 1657–1694.

Acquired Cystic Kidney Disease

Andersen, B. L., Curry, N. S., and Gobien, R. P.: Sonography of evolving renal cystic transformation associated with hemodialysis. AJR 141:1003, 1983.

Basile, J. J., McCullough, D. L., Harrison, L. H., and Dyer, R. B.: End-stage renal disease associated with acquired cystic disease and neoplasia. J. Urol. 140:938, 1988.

Brennan, J. F., Stilmant, M. M., Babayan, R. K., and Siroky, M. B.: Acquired renal cystic disease: Implications for the urologist. Br. J. Urol. 67:342, 1991.

Chandhoke, P. S., Torrence, R. J., Clayman, R. V., and Rothstein, M.: Acquired cystic disease of the kidney: A management dilemma. J. Urol. 147:969, 1992.

Chung-Park, M., Parveen, T., and Lam, M.: Acquired cystic disease of the kidneys and renal cell carcinoma in chronic renal insufficiency without dialysis treatment. Nephron 53:157, 1989.

Dunnill, M. S., Millard, P. R., and Oliver, D.: Acquired cystic disease of the kidneys: A hazard of long-term intermittent maintenance haemodialysis. J. Clin. Pathol. 30:868, 1977.

Feiner, H. D., Katz, L. A., and Gallo, G. R.: Acquired cystic disease of kidney in chronic dialysis patients. Urology 17:260, 1981.

Grantham, J. J.: Acquired cystic kidney disease. Kidney Int. 40:143, 1991.

Heptinstall, R. H.: End-stage renal disease. In Heptinstall, R. H. (ed.): Pathology of the Kidney. 4th ed. Boston, Little, Brown & Co., 1992, pp. 749–753.

Hogg, R. J.: Acquired renal cystic disease in children prior to the start of dialysis. Pediatr. Nephrol. 6:176, 1992.

Ishikawa, I., Saito, Y., Onouchi, Z., et al.: Development of acquired cystic disease and adenocarcinoma of the kidney in glomerulonephritis chronic hemodialysis patients. Clin. Nephrol. 14:1, 1980.

Ishikawa, I., Yuri, T., Kitada, H., Hirohisa, S., and Shinoda, A.: Regression of acquired cystic disease of the kidney after successful renal transplantation. Am. J. Nephrol. 3:310, 1983.

Ishikawa, I.: Acquired renal cystic disease. In Gardner, K. D., Jr., and Bernstein, J. (eds.): The Cystic Kidney. Dordrecht, Kluwer Academic Publishers, 1990, pp. 351–378.

Ishikawa, I., Saito, Y., Shikura, N., et al.: Ten-year prospective study on the development of renal cell carcinoma in dialysis patients. Am. J. Kidney Dis. 5:452, 1990.

Ishikawa, I.: Uremic acquired renal cystic disease: Natural history and complications. Nephron 58:257, 1991.

Ishikawa, I., Shikura, N., and Shinoda, A.: Cystic transformation in native kidneys in renal allograft recipients with long-standing good function. Am. J. Nephrol. 11:217, 1991.

Jabour, B. A., Ralls, P. W., Tang, W. W., et al.: Acquired cystic disease of the kidneys: Computed tomography and ultrasonography appraisal in patients on peritoneal and hemodialysis. Invest. Radiol. 22:728, 1987.

Katz, A., Sombolos, K., and Oreopoulos, D. G.: Acquired cystic disease of the kidney in association with chronic ambulatory peritoneal dialysis. Am. J. Kidney Dis. 9:426, 1987.

Kutcher, R., Amodio, J. B., and Rosenblatt, R.: Uremic renal cystic disease: Value of sonographic screening. Radiology 147:833, 1983.

Leichter, H. E., Dietrich, R., Salusky, I. B., et al.: Acquired cystic kidney disease in children undergoing long-term dialysis. Pediatr. Nephrol. 2:8, 1988.

Levine, E., Grantham, J. J., Slusher, S. L., Greathouse, J. L., and Krohn, B. P.: CT of acquired cystic kidney disease and renal tumors in long-term dialysis patients. AJR 142:125, 1984.

Levine, E., Grantham, J. J., and MacDougall, M. L.: Spontaneous subcapsular and perinephric hemorrhage in end-stage kidney disease: Clinical and CT findings. AJR 148:755, 1987.

Levine, E., Hartman, D. S., and Smirniotopolous, J. G.: Renal cystic diseases associated with renal neoplasms. In Hartman, D. S. (ed.): Renal Cystic Disease. Philadelphia, W. B. Saunders, 1989, pp. 38–72.

Levine, E., Slusher, S. L., Grantham, J. J., and Wetzel, L. H.: Natural history of acquired renal cystic disease in dialysis patients: A prospective longitudinal CT study. AJR 156:501, 1991.

Matson, M. A., and Cohen, E. P.: Acquired cystic kidney disease: Occurrence, prevalence and renal cancers. Medicine 69:217, 1990.

Sasagawa, I., Terasawa, Y., Imai, K., Sekino, H., and Takahashi, H.: Acquired cystic disease of the kidney and renal carcinoma in hemodialysis patients: Ultrasonographic evaluation. Br. J. Urol. 70:236, 1992.

Scanlon, M. H., and Karasick, S. R.: Acquired renal cystic disease and neoplasia: Complications of chronic hemodialysis. Radiology 147:837, 1983.

Taylor, A. J., Cohen, E. P., Erickson, S. J., Olson, D. L., and Folley, W. D.: Renal imaging in long-term dialysis patients: A comparison of CT and sonography. AJR 153:765, 1989.

Lymphoma

Case records of Massachusetts General Hospital. Case 51–1978. Renal lymphoma. N. Engl. J. Med. 299:1456, 1978.

Chilcote, W. A., and Borkowski, G. P.: Computed tomography in renal lymphoma. J. Comput. Assist. Tomogr. 7:439, 1983.

Cohan, R. H., Dunnick, N. R., Leder, R. A., and Baker, M. E.: Computed tomography of renal lymphoma. J. Comput. Assist. Tomogr. 14:933, 1990.

Ellman, L., Davis, J., and Lichtenstein, N. S.: Uremia due to occult lymphomatous infiltration of the kidneys. Cancer 33:203, 1974.

Hahn, F. J. Y., and Peterson, N.: Renal lymphoma simulating adult polycystic disease. Radiology 122:655, 1977.

Hartman, D. S., Davis, C. J., Jr., Goldman, S. M., Friedman, A. C., and Fritzsche, P.,: Renal lymphoma: Radiologic-pathologic correlation of 21 cases. Radiology 144:759, 1982.

Heiken, J. P., Gold, R. P., Schnur, M. J., King, D. L., Bashist, B., and Glazer, H. S.: Computed tomography of renal lymphoma with ultrasound correlation. J. Comput. Assist. Tomogr. 7:245, 1983.

Horii, S. C., Bosniak, M. A., Megibow, A. J., et al.: Correlation of CT and ultrasound in the evaluation of renal lymphoma. Urol. Radiol. 5:69, 1983.

Jafri, S. Z. H., Bree, R. L., Amendola, M. A., et al.: CT of renal and perirenal non-Hodgkin lymphoma. AJR 138:1101, 1982.

Kiely, J. M., Wagoner, R. D., and Holley, K. F.: Renal complications of lymphoma. Ann. Intern. Med. 71:1159, 1969.

Krudy, A. G., Dunnick, N. R., Magrath, I. T., et al.: CT of American Burkitt lymphoma. AJR 136:747, 1981.

Kursh, E. D., and Persky, L.: Selective renal arteriography in renal lymphoma. J. Urol. 105:772, 1971.

Kyaw, M., and Koehler, P. R.: Renal and perirenal lymphoma: Arteriographic findings. Radiology 93:1055, 1969.

Lalli, A. F.: Lymphoma and the urinary tract. Radiology 93:1051, 1969.

Martinez-Maldonado, M., and Ramirez de Arellano, G. A.: Renal involvement in malignant lymphomas: A survey of 49 cases. J. Urol. 95:485, 1966.

Pick, R. A., Castellino, R. A., and Seltzer, R. A.: Arteriographic findings in renal lymphomas. AJR 111:530, 1971.

Redlin, L., Francis, R. S., and Orlando, M. M.: Renal abnormalities in agnogenic myeloid metaplasia. Radiology 121:605, 1976.

Reznek, R. H., Mootoosamy, I., Webb, J. A. W., and Richards, M. A.: CT in renal and perirenal lymphoma: A further look. Clin. Radiol. 42:233, 1990.

Richmond, J., Sherman, R. S., Diamond, N. D., and Craver, L. F.: Renal lesions associated with malignant lymphomas. Am. J. Med. 32:184, 1962.

Ruchman, R. B., Yeh, H. C., Mitty, H. A., et al.: Ultrasonographic and computed tomographic features of renal sinus lymphoma. JCU 16:35, 1988.

Seltzer, R. A., and Wenlund, D. E.: Renal lymphoma, arteriographic studies. AJR 101:692, 1967.

Shapiro, J. H., Ramsay, C. G., Jacobson, H. G., et al.: Renal involvement in lymphomas and leukemias in adults. AJR 88:928, 1962.

Townsend, R. R., Laing, F. C., Jeffrey, R. B., and Bottles, K.: Abdominal lymphoma in AIDS: Evaluation with US. Radiology 171:719, 1989.

Weinberger, E., Rosenbaum, D. M., and Pendergrass, T. W.: Renal involvement in children with lymphoma: Comparison of CT with sonography. AJR 155:347, 1990.

Wentzell, R. A., and Berkheiser, S. W.: Malignant lymphomatosis of kidneys. J. Urol. 74:177, 1955.

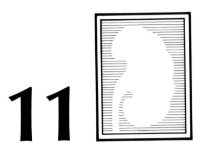

11

DIAGNOSTIC SET: LARGE, MULTIFOCAL, UNILATERAL

XANTHOGRANULOMATOUS PYELONEPHRITIS	MULTICYSTIC DYSPLASTIC KIDNEY DISEASE
MALAKOPLAKIA	DIFFERENTIAL DIAGNOSIS

Three diseases characteristically appear as a multilobulated enlargement of a single kidney. In two, xanthogranulomatous pyelonephritis and malakoplakia, chronic infection is associated with multiple inflammatory masses. The third, multicystic dysplastic kidney disease, is a congenital disorder leading to multiple cystic masses. All of these are quite uncommon.

XANTHOGRANULOMATOUS PYELONEPHRITIS

Definition

Xanthogranulomatous pyelonephritis is a chronic renal infection that in its most common form leads to a scarred, contracted renal pelvis, dilated calyces, and diffuse infiltration of the renal parenchyma by plasma cells and lipid-laden macrophages, which may form multiple yellow-colored masses. Less often, this disease process is unifocal and affects a single infundibulum and calyx and the corresponding parenchyma. The term *xanthogranulomatous* describes the yellow color imparted to the renal parenchyma and inflammatory masses by the high lipid content of the macrophages. Calculus in the pelvis of xanthogranulomatous kidneys occurs in over 75 per cent of cases. Calculus usually assumes a staghorn shape and is composed of struvite. The dilated calyces, whose walls are thickened by inflammation, are filled with pus. Extension of the inflammatory process into the psoas muscle and perirenal and pararenal spaces occurs frequently. Parenchymal calcification is uncommon.

It is generally held that xanthogranulomatous pyelonephritis develops as a complication of chronic infection in a collecting system that has a long-standing partial obstruction caused by stones, stricture, or uroepithelial tumor. The characteristic histologic response is thought to result from the liberation of lipid from tissue destroyed through bacterial action. The possibility that an undefined metabolic defect plays a role in the genesis of this unusual disorder has also been proposed.

Clinical Setting

Xanthogranulomatous pyelonephritis occurs predominantly in females and affects all age groups from children to the elderly. Chronic, undiagnosed illness for several months usually precedes the diagnosis. Signs and symptoms include abdominal and flank pain, low-grade fever, weight loss, and malaise. Many patients have no lower urinary tract symptoms. A renal mass may be palpable. Anemia, leukocytosis, pyuria, and albuminuria may be present. Bacteria are cultured from the urine in approximately two-thirds of patients. *Proteus mirabilis* and *Escherichia coli* are the organisms most likely to be found. *Pseudomonas aeruginosa* and *Enterobacter aerogenes* are isolated less frequently.

Radiologic Findings

Xanthogranulomatous pyelonephritis is most commonly encountered in its diffuse form. In this situation, a radiopaque calculus is present in the renal pelvis of an enlarged, multilobulated kidney that fails to opacify or has diminished opacification during excretory urography. Thickening of the renal fascia may be identified with standard or computed tomograms (Figs. 11–1 and 11–2). On retrograde pyelography, irregular filling defects in a contracted pelvis and marked caliectasis are demonstrated (Fig. 11–3).

In the diffuse form of xanthogranulomatous pyelonephritis, ultrasonography demonstrates well the multifocal enlargement of the kidney. The dominant finding reflects the markedly dilated calyces that are filled with the products of inflammation and are seen as multiple, uniformly aligned hypoechoic structures

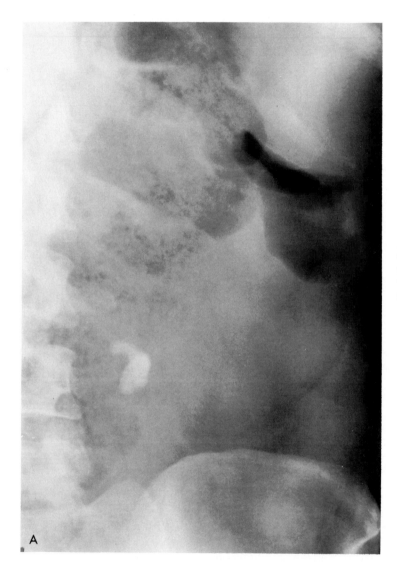

Figure 11–1. Xanthogranulomatous pyelonephritis (diffuse form) in a 40-year-old woman with a 6-year history of urinary tract infection, 6 months of left flank pain, and a tender left flank mass palpable for 2 weeks. Hematuria and pyuria were present, and the urine was infected with *Escherichia coli.*

A, Preliminary film. A large radiopaque calculus is present in the region of the renal pelvis. The kidney outline is enlarged.

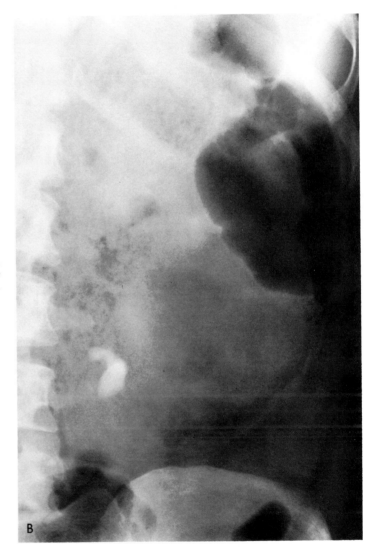

Figure 11–1 *Continued B,* Excretory urogram, 10-minute film. There is no apparent accumulation of contrast material. (Same case illustrated in Fig. 11–3.) (Courtesy of Lee B. Talner, M. D., University of California, San Diego.)

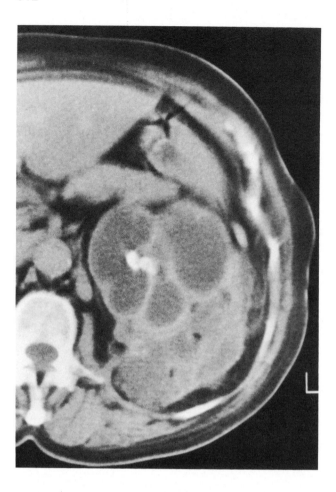

Figure 11–2. Xanthogranulomatous pyelonephritis with perinephric extension in a 66-year-old woman with a 3-month history of left flank pain and weight loss. Computed tomogram, unenhanced. There is extension of the inflammatory process into the perirenal and posterior pararenal spaces. A portion of a staghorn calculus is seen in the contracted pelvis.

with an internal pattern of fine echoes. The calyces may be surrounded by a thin zone of increased echogenicity that probably represents the surrounding inflammatory reaction. The frequently present pelvic calculus causes a highly reflective image with acoustic shadowing (Fig. 11–4). Parenchymal xanthogranulomatous masses cause focal zones of echogenicity similar to that of the renal parenchyma. Extension of inflammation into the retroperitoneum and psoas muscle may be identified by ultrasonography.

Computed tomography demonstrates the multifocal nature of renal enlargement in diffuse xanthogranulomatous pyelonephritis (Fig. 11–5). With this modality, the calyces appear as dilated structures with attenuation values that are in the range of water. Calculus in the pelvis is readily identified as a radiopaque structure. Characteristically, there is intense enhancement of tissue surrounding the dilated calyces. This presumably reflects the inflammatory tissue in the calyceal wall and renal parenchyma. Computed tomography is particularly valuable in identifying extension of the xanthogranulomatous infection into the psoas muscle and perirenal and pararenal spaces (see Fig. 11–2).

Angiography in xanthogranulomatous pyelonephritis reveals a lack of normal arborization of the intrarenal arteries, displacement of vessels around dilated calyces or granulomatous masses, and attenua-

---

SUMMARY OF ABNORMAL URORADIOLOGIC FINDINGS
XANTHOGRANULOMATOUS PYELONEPHRITIS

Primary Uroradiologic Elements
    Size—large
    Contour—multifocal masses (unifocal mass or smooth contour uncommon)
    Lesion distribution—unilateral
Secondary Uroradiologic Elements
    Pelvoinfundibulocalyceal system—pelvis contracted and calyces dilated; attenuation values slightly
        less to slightly greater than water; rim enhancement (diffuse form); displaced (focal form)
    Nephrogram—absent (diffuse form); focal replacement (focal form)
    Echogenicity—calyces (hypoechoic with echogenic rim); parenchymal masses (echoic)
    Calcification—calculus in pelvis (common); parenchymal calcification (uncommon)

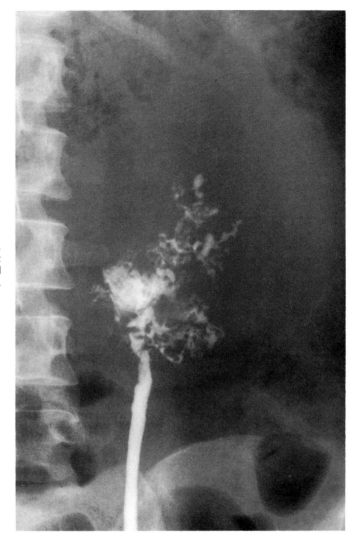

Figure 11–3. Xanthogranulomatous pyelonephritis (diffuse form). Retrograde pyelogram. There is obstruction of the ureteropelvic junction. The multiple filling defects seen throughout the dilated calyces are caused by xanthogranulomas projecting into the lumen. (Same case illustrated in Fig. 11–1.)

tion of arterial caliber. Neovascularity indistinguishable from that of neoplastic processes, nephrographic defects, and enlargement of capsular arteries have been described. None of these angiographic findings is specific.

The radiologic findings in the focal form of xanthogranulomatous pyelonephritis are similar to those for the diffuse type but are limited to the calyces and the parenchyma of a portion of the kidney, often in association with an obstructive calyceal stone or an obstructed duplicated pelvocalyceal system (Figs. 11–6 and 11–7). In focal forms, the renal pelvis may be involved only to the extent of being displaced by the limited inflammatory mass. Here, the uninvolved portion of the kidney is functionally and structurally normal. Xanthogranulomatous pyelonephritis of a duplicated collecting system involves the entire hemipelvis.

MALAKOPLAKIA

Definition

Malakoplakia of the renal parenchyma is a very uncommon inflammation characterized by cortical and medullary granulomatous masses that contain large mononuclear cells with abundant cytoplasm. These cells, called Hansemann macrophages, contain large intracytoplasmic inclusion bodies composed of calcium and iron-laden lysosomal material. Known as Michaelis-Gutmann bodies, these inclusions are probably phagocytized bacilli in various stages of defective digestion. Michaelis-Gutmann bodies can also be found in an extracellular location. Electron microscopy suggests what is considered the likely cause of malakoplakia—namely an intracellular abnormality of the macrophage, probably occurring at the level of the phagolysosomes. Malakoplakia is usually associated with *Escherichia coli* infections, although *Klebsiella* species have also been involved.

The granulomas of renal parenchymal malakoplakia are sharply demarcated, soft, yellow-brown masses situated in the cortex and the medulla. Approximately 75 per cent of reported cases have been multifocal and 50 per cent bilateral. Unifocal masses occur in about 25 per cent of cases. Extension of the inflammatory process into the renal sinus and perirenal space and renal vein thrombosis has been noted in many instances.

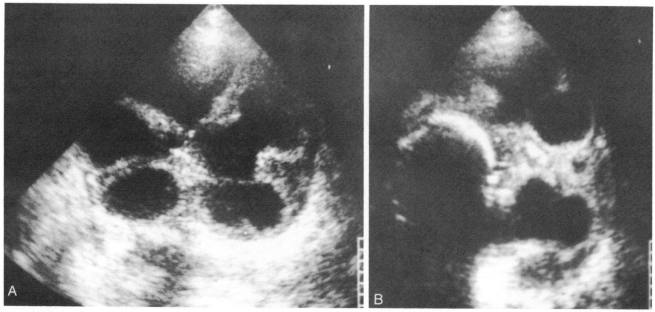

Figure 11–4. Xanthogranulomatous pyelonephritis, diffuse form, left kidney. Ultrasonogram.
   A, Longitudinal section. The uniformly dilated calyces contain faint echoes caused by the products of inflammation. There is a surrounding, thin zone of hyperechoicity representing the xanthomatous inflammatory reaction.
   B, Transverse section. The staghorn calculus within a contracted pelvis causes specular echoes and shadowing.

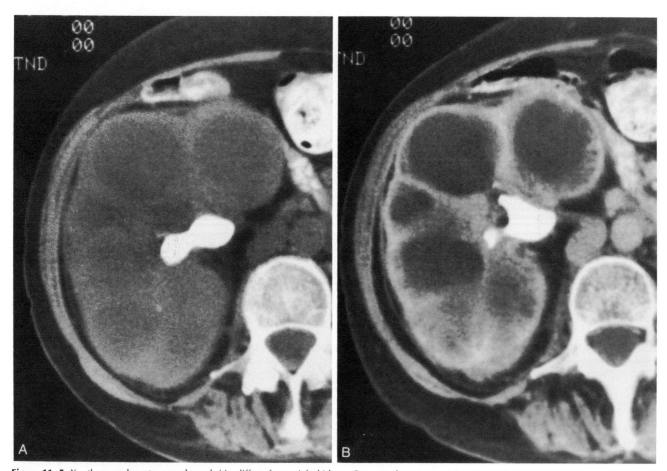

Figure 11–5. Xanthogranulomatous pyelonephritis, diffuse form, right kidney. Computed tomogram.
   A, Unenhanced scan. The kidney is massively enlarged by multiple uniform masses of slightly lower attenuation than the surrounding parenchyma. A staghorn calculus is present in a contracted pelvis.
   B, Enhanced scan. The inflammatory reaction in the parenchyma surrounding the dilated calyces causes marked enhancement.

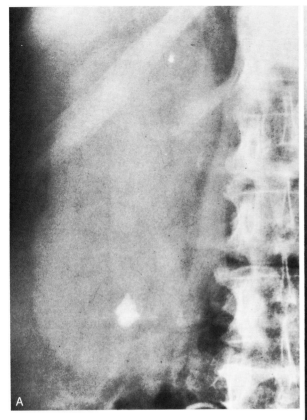

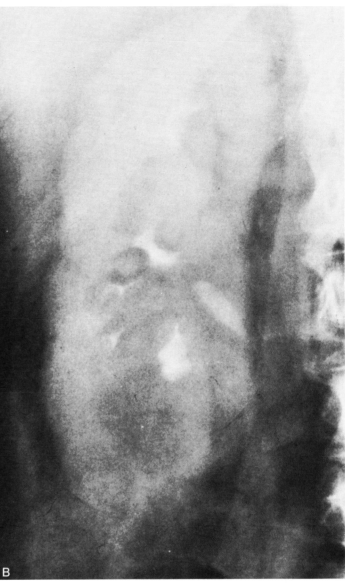

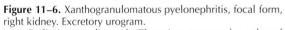

Figure 11–6. Xanthogranulomatous pyelonephritis, focal form, right kidney. Excretory urogram.

A, Preliminary radiograph. There is a mass and a calyceal calculus in the lower pole.

B, Ten-minute radiograph. The lower pole mass enhances less than the surrounding parenchyma. The calculus is located at the apex of the mass.

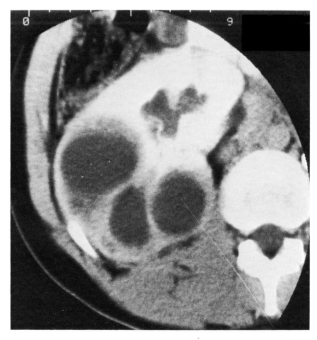

Figure 11–7. Xanthogranulomatous pyelonephritis, focal form, right kidney. Computed tomogram, contrast material enhanced. The characteristic abnormality is limited to the dorsal portion of the kidney.

Megalocytic interstitial nephritis is a term that has been used to describe a pathologic process that differs from malakoplakia only in that the granulomas are limited to the renal cortex. In all other respects this process is identical to malakoplakia, and the two terms should probably be considered synonymous.

Malakoplakia of the urinary tract most commonly affects the bladder. Involvement of the prostate, testes, ureter, renal pelvis, and parenchyma is much less frequent. The radiologic appearance of malakoplakia of the pelvocalyceal system and ureter is described in Chapter 15 and that of the bladder is described in Chapter 19.

Clinical Setting

Middle-aged women with a history of urinary tract infection are the usual group affected by renal parenchymal malakoplakia. Infants and children are affected rarely. Clinical features include dysuria, fever, anemia, leukocytosis, pyuria, and bacteriuria. A renal mass may be palpable, especially with retroperitoneal extension. Malakoplakia may cause renal failure either by bilateral renal parenchymal involvement or by obstructive uropathy due to bladder or bilateral ureteropelvocalyceal involvement.

Radiologic Findings

Malakoplakia of the renal parenchyma causes multifocal enlargement of the kidney without pelvocalyceal obstruction or calcification (Fig. 11–8). Contrast material excretion is diminished to absent. The multiple granulomas cause a mass effect on the pelvocalyceal system and a lobulated contour. Uncommonly, the radiologic findings are those of a unifocal mass indistinguishable from those discussed in Chapter 12.

Ultrasonography defines well the multifocal enlargement of the kidney and the absence of obstruction. Malakoplakia granulomas distort the central sinus echoes by their mass effect, contain low-amplitude internal echoes, and have poorly defined margins.

Computed tomography of this rare form of renal infection shows multiple soft tissue masses that enhance less than the renal parenchyma following contrast material administration. Computed tomography is particularly valuable in detecting extension of the inflammatory process into the retroperitoneum.

Angiographic findings in renal malakoplakia include hypovascular masses, displacement and stretching of intrarenal arteries around the granulomas, and occasional encasement of arteries. Lack of normal branching and the presence of neovascularity have been described. The angiographic nephrogram is inhomogeneous, owing to replacement of the nephrons by multiple granulomas. Renal vein thrombosis may be present.

MULTICYSTIC DYSPLASTIC KIDNEY DISEASE

Definition

Multicystic dysplastic kidney is a nonhereditary developmental anomaly characterized by cysts and varying amounts of dysplastic tissue with little or no discernible renal parenchyma. Common synonyms include renal dysplasia, renal dysgenesis, multicystic kidney, and Potter Type II renal cystic disease. Multicystic dysplastic kidney is usually unilateral and involves the entire kidney. Uncommonly, it is bilateral and fatal or limited to just one region of the kidney.

Multicystic dysplastic kidney disease takes two forms: the pelvoinfundibular atretic type and the hy-

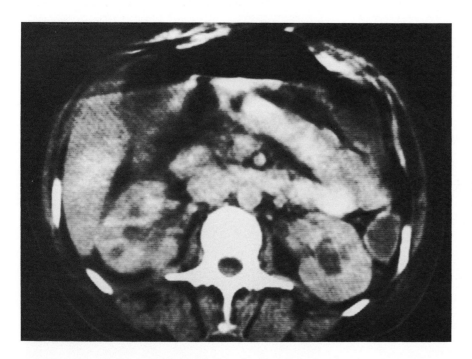

Figure 11–8. Malakoplakia involving both kidneys of a 56-year-old woman with chronic urinary tract infection. The kidneys are enlarged by multiple focal granulomas that are seen as nephrographic defects. Computed tomogram, contrast material enhanced.

SUMMARY OF ABNORMAL URORADIOLOGIC FINDINGS
MALAKOPLAKIA

Primary Uroradiologic Elements
    Size—large
    Contour—multifocal masses (unifocal uncommon)
    Lesion distribution—unilateral (bilateral in up to 50 per cent of cases)
Secondary Uroradiologic Elements
    Pelvoinfundibulocalyceal system—displaced (multifocal)
    Nephrogram—diminished to absent opacification; replaced (multifocal)
    Echogenicity—hypoechoic masses; distorted central sinus complex

---

dronephrotic type. Each represents a disorder in the interaction between the ampullary tips of ureteral buds and the metanephric blastema during formation of the renal parenchyma. (See Chapter 3 for a discussion of the normal embryonic development of the kidney.) The two forms differ as to the point during embryogenesis of the kidney that the disorder begins.

In the pelvoinfundibular atretic form of multicystic kidney, the failure of the ureteral bud branches to induce metanephric blastema occurs early in fetal life. Very few nephrons develop, no urine is formed, and the ureter and renal artery are atretic. The few branches of the ureteral bud that do develop terminate in cysts. Thus, the "kidney" lacks a reniform shape and is composed of only a cluster of thin-walled cysts of varying size and number (Fig. 11–9). These cysts are held together by connective tissue. Microscopically, a few widely scattered glomeruli with or without aggregates of tubules can be identified. The dominant tissue is dysplastic and consists of collagen, vascular channels, nerve trunks, cartilage, and, most characteristically, primitive ducts derived from ureteral buds. These are lined by cuboidal or low columnar epithelium and are circumscribed by undifferentiated spindle cells. Large cysts have a flattened or destroyed epithelium and an acellular, collagenous wall. With time, these cyst walls may calcify, or, alternatively, the entire conglomerate of cysts may regress, leaving a mass of solid dysplastic tissue. Uncommonly, the pelvoinfundibular atretic form of multicystic kidney disease occurs bilaterally or is segmental and limited to one portion of an otherwise normal kidney. The pelvoinfundibular atretic form of multicystic kidney disease is classified as Type II in the Potter classification of renal cystic disease. The characteristic abnormality as seen in nephron dissection is schematized in Figure 11–10.

In the hydronephrotic form of multicystic kidney, severe urinary tract obstruction develops at some point in fetal life *after* an initial period of normal organogenesis. This congenital obstruction is usually at the ureteropelvic or the ureterovesical junction or due to posterior urethral valves. The effect of obstruction on the kidney is twofold: both hydronephrosis and

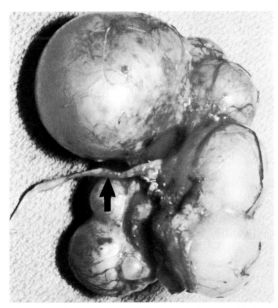

Figure 11–9. Multicystic dysplastic kidney, pelvoinfundibular atretic type. Gross specimen. The lesion is a grapelike aggregate of cysts with no renal pelvis. The ureter *(arrow)* is atretic.

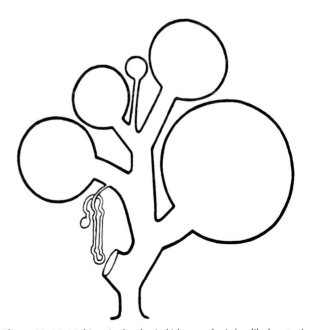

Figure 11–10. Multicystic dysplastic kidney, pelvoinfundibular atretic type. Schematic nephron demonstrates enlarged collecting ducts that are sparsely branched and terminate in cysts. Only one abnormal nephron connected to a collecting duct is present. (From Potter, E. L.: Normal and Abnormal Development of the Kidney, 1972. Reproduced with kind permission of the author and Year Book Medical Publishers.)

dysplasia are superimposed on a kidney that has already undergone a period of normal differentiation before the onset of the obstruction. In the hydronephrotic form of multicystic kidney, the kidney retains its reniform shape. Dilatation of the pelvis or of the pelvis and ureter proximal to the site of obstruction is present. This may be bilateral in cases of posterior urethral valve. The cysts that form are peripheral in the renal parenchyma and project from the surface of the kidney (Fig. 11–11). These communicate with the dilated pelvocalyceal system. Microscopically, normal nephrons are numerous and coexist with dysplastic tissue composed of primitive ducts with mesenchymal collars arranged in aggregates resembling renal medullary tissue. Islands of cartilage are occasionally present. The hydronephrotic form of multicystic kidney thus represents a combination of normal organogenesis, hydronephrosis, and cystic dysplasia. The severity of the hydronephrotic form of cystic dysplasia correlates with the degree of obstruction and the stage at which it occurs. A severe obstruction occurring very early in fetal life results in a pathologic appearance similar to the multicystic dysplastic kidney of the pelvoinfundibular atretic type with the added, unique feature of dilatation of the pelvis. In the mildest form, partial urinary tract obstruction develops late in gestation after formation of most of the renal parenchyma has been completed. On this mild end only small cysts involving the last one to two generations of nephrons adjacent to the renal capsule are found. This corresponds to the Potter Type IV cystic kidney. Hydronephrotic cystic dysplasia as seen in nephron dissection is schematized in Figure 11–12. Hydronephrotic cystic dysplasia may be segmental in association with a completely duplicated, obstructed ureter, or it may be bilateral as a result of a posterior urethral valve or prune-belly syndrome. When cysts

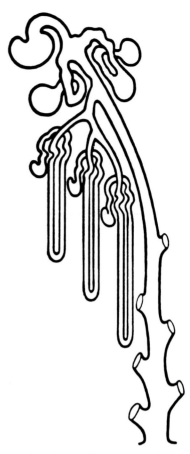

Figure 11–12. Multicystic dysplastic kidney, hydronephrotic type. Schematized diagram demonstrates three early generations of normal nephrons, cystic dilatation and dysplasia of more peripheral, later-forming generations of nephrons and the terminal portions of the collecting ducts into which they drain. (From Potter, E. L.: Normal and Abnormal Development of the Kidney, 1972. Reproduced with kind permission of the author and Year Book Medical Publishers.)

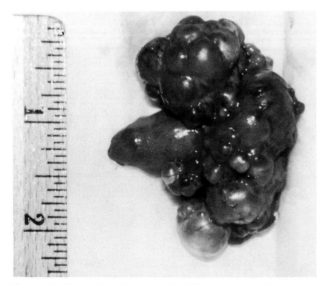

Figure 11–11. Multicystic dysplastic kidney, hydronephrotic type. Gross specimen. The kidney is grossly distorted by cysts aggregated on the surface of the kidney but retains its reniform shape. The renal pelvis is dilated as a result of a congenital ureteropelvic junction obstruction.

are microscopic or barely macroscopic, the gross pathology and corresponding radiologic images are dominated by the findings of hydronephrosis and dysplastic solid tissue with a diminished cystic component.

Clinical Setting

The clinical features of pelvoinfundibular atretic and severe hydronephrotic multicystic kidney are similar. It is commonly stated that males and females are equally affected and that there is no predilection for one side of involvement over the other. However, an extensive review of the literature reveals a preponderance of males and left-sided lesions (Piel, 1990). The pelvoinfundibular atretic form of multicystic dysplastic kidney is usually encountered as a large abdominal mass in an otherwise asymptomatic newborn. Once discovered, the most important clinical consideration is the search for a coexistent anomaly that might pose a risk of damage to the contralateral kidney. This occurs in 30 to 40 per cent of cases, usually in the form of a ureteropelvic junction obstruction, renal agenesis, or hypoplasia.

The pelvoinfundibular atretic form of multicystic dysplastic kidney is sometimes discovered in the older child or in an adult. In most of these cases, the malformed kidney is small or of normal size and is detected as an incidental radiologic finding, usually in the form of ring calcification or a mass of nonenhancing solid or cystic tissue in the renal fossa. Because the risk of malignant change in the pelvoinfundibular atretic form of multicystic kidney is exceedingly low, the need for removal is usually limited to those infants in whom symptoms develop as a result of the large size of the mass. In many instances, however, a large cystic mass regresses into a smaller mass of predominant solid tissue during the first few months of life.

The clinical features of the hydronephrotic form of multicystic kidney reflect the underlying hydronephrosis rather than the cystic dysplastic component of the abnormality. These include a hydronephrotic mass and urinary tract infection.

Neither the pelvoinfundibular atretic nor the severe hydronephrotic forms of multicystic kidney disease are compatible with life when both kidneys are involved. In this circumstance the fetus or newborn demonstrates the stigmata of Potter's syndrome reflecting anuria or severe oliguria *in utero*. These include oligohydramnios, pulmonary hypoplasia and thoracic underdevelopment, wide-set eyes, low-set ears, a beaked nose, and a deep palmar crease.

Radiologic Findings

The radiologic findings of multicystic dysplastic kidney disease vary with the age of the patient, the type (pelvoinfundibular atretic or hydronephrotic), and whether involvement is unilateral or bilateral and segmental or total.

In the newborn, abdominal radiography demonstrates a large, noncalcified abdominal mass that displaces bowel gas and frequently crosses the midline (Fig. 11–13). Contrast enhancement does not occur in the pelvoinfundibular atretic form, whereas demonstrable enhancement of compressed parenchyma and delayed accumulation of contrast material in cysts is seen in the hydronephrotic form. Bilateral involvement is detected as abdominal distention and pulmonary hypoplasia.

Multicystic dysplastic kidney discovered in the older child or in the adult has one or more ring calcifications and no evidence of function (Fig. 11–14). Compensatory hypertrophy of the contralateral kidney is present.

Segmental multicystic dysplasia is most commonly the result of obstruction of the upper pole of a duplicated collecting system. This appears as a focal mass with some degree of delayed enhancement and dilatation of the collecting system and ureter to the point of obstruction, usually an ectopic ureterocele. In the rare instance of segmental atretic type of multicystic kidney, the nonfunctioning mass of cysts and/or dysplastic tissue is limited to a portion of the kidney.

The ultrasonographic findings of multicystic dysplastic kidney with pelvoinfundibular atresia include cysts that vary in size and shape, with the largest cyst being peripheral in location; absent communication between adjacent cysts; absent renal parenchyma between cysts; absent central sonolucency corresponding to a renal pelvis; and echogenic areas representing primitive mesenchyme or tiny cysts in an eccentric location. The proportion of cysts to dysplastic tissue

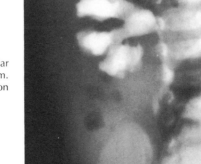

Figure 11–13. Multicystic dysplastic kidney, pelvoinfundibular atretic type, left kidney in a male newborn. Excretory urogram. The left kidney is not seen. There is a ureteropelvic junction obstruction on the right side.

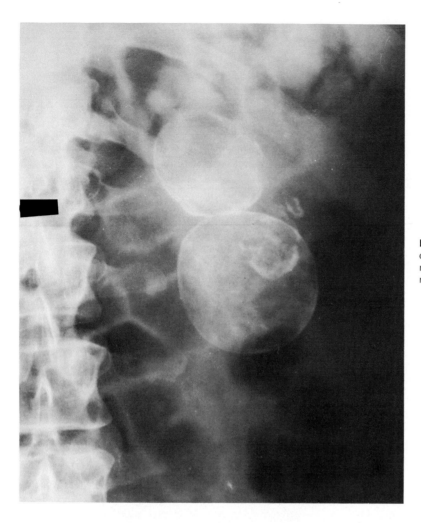

Figure 11–14. Multicystic dysplastic kidney, pelvoinfundibular atretic type, left kidney in an adult. Abdominal radiograph. Multiple calcified cysts are present. The right kidney exhibited compensatory hypertrophy.

may be quite variable (Fig. 11–15). Hydronephrotic multicystic kidney demonstrates numerous peripheral cysts and a large medial fluid-filled structure corresponding to the dilated renal pelvis. The peripheral cysts may communicate with each other or with the renal pelvis. A reniform shape is preserved to some extent.

In many cases there may be considerable difficulty in distinguishing by ultrasonography severe hydronephrosis without renal dysplasia from the hydronephrotic form of multicystic dysplastic kidney. Similarly, ultrasonographic differentiation between hydronephrotic multicystic kidney and pelvoinfundibular atresia can be difficult when the renal pelvis is small and obscured by peripheral cysts.

Ultrasonography is useful in detecting bilateral disease and contralateral anomalies, especially hydronephrosis. Serial ultrasonographic examinations have demonstrated marked reduction in the size of cysts and the eventual complete disappearance of cysts in multicystic dysplastic kidney (Fig. 11–16). When this process is complete, differentiation from renal agenesis may be impossible without documentation by serial examination. Surgical findings in such cases show no trace of a kidney, artery, or ureter or a very small multicystic dysplastic kidney.

In the adult, ultrasonography usually reveals one or more cystic masses in the renal fossa. The multicystic kidney is often not large, and cyst wall calcification is easily recognized by acoustic shadowing.

Segmental multicystic dysplastic kidney may present as a focal multiloculated mass. When the cysts are very small, the multicystic segment may be echogenic.

Multicystic dysplastic kidney is often detected prenatally by maternal ultrasonography. Precise differentiation between the pelvoinfundibular atretic type, the hydronephrotic type, and uncomplicated hydronephrosis may, however, be extremely difficult *in utero.* Maternal ultrasonography is also helpful in detecting contralateral renal anomalies, which can be detected in about 30 per cent of fetuses with unilateral multicystic kidney (see Fig. 11–13). Contralateral, mild fetal pyelectasis is found in about 15 per cent of fetuses with multicystic dysplastic kidney and is not clinically significant.

By computed tomography, multicystic dysplastic kidney appears as a nonreniform mass that replaces the normal kidney. The aggregate is made up of numerous, variably sized, smaller masses of water density. Septa may be visible and enhance with contrast medium. Less commonly, only one cystic mass is pre-

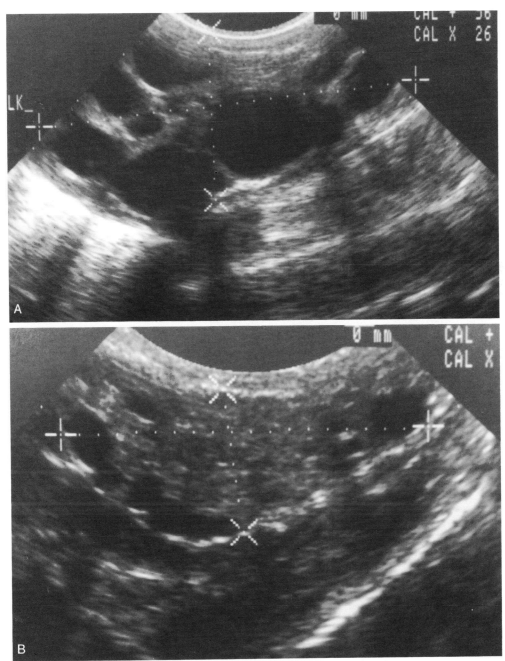

Figure 11–15. Multicystic dysplastic kidney, pelvoinfundibular atretic type, involving both kidneys in a newborn. Ultrasonograms, longitudinal sections, demonstrate asymmetric findings.
  A, Left kidney. Multiple cysts of varying size are the prominent finding. Dysplastic tissue is represented by thick septa between cysts.
  B, Right kidney. The dominant finding is the echogenic mass of dysplastic tissue, with a few small scattered cysts.

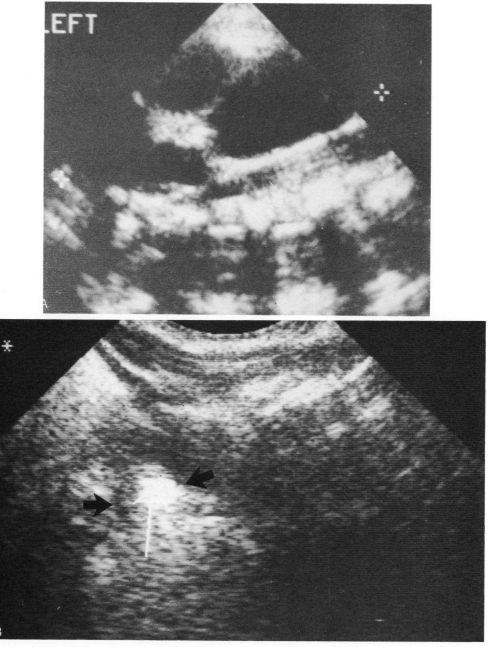

Figure 11–16. Multicystic dysplastic kidney, pelvoinfundibular atretic form, left kidney, demonstrating involution over 6 months. Ultrasonograms, longitudinal section.

A, At birth, multiple cysts and thick bands of dysplastic tissue constitute a mass in the renal fossa.

B, Six months later, the findings have involuted and only a small amount of dysplastic tissue remains *(arrows).*

sent. No function is seen in the pelvoinfundibular atresia form. In the hydronephrotic form of multicystic kidney, computed tomography is more sensitive than urography in demonstrating calyceal crescents and contrast medium puddling in cysts and the collecting system. In the adult, cyst wall calcification or a small amount of residual dysplastic tissue may be seen. Abnormalities of the vascular pedicle in adults with sufficient retroperitoneal fat may also be demonstrated. Segmental multicystic dysplastic kidney may present as a focal multicystic or multiloculated mass.

Radionuclide imaging provides functional and morphologic information about the multicystic kidney. Visualization depends on the presence of normal glomeruli and tubules within the cystic kidney and is, thus, limited to the hydronephrotic form. In cases of pelvoinfundibular atresia, radionuclide studies demonstrate a photon-deficient mass in the renal fossa reflecting absent perfusion. With segmental multicystic dysplastic kidney, activity will be decreased or absent in the involved portion of the kidney.

Angiography demonstrates absence or hyperplasia of the ipsilateral renal artery in the pelvoinfundibular atresia form of multicystic dysplasia. A nephrogram is absent, and no renal vein is seen during the venous phase of the study. A focal avascular or hypovascular mass without neovascularity is found in segmental involvement.

In cases of pelvoinfundibular atresia, retrograde pyelography demonstrates a small caliber ureter that ends blindly (Fig. 11–17). Sacculations or pseudodiverticula are frequently present. Retrograde studies performed on a hydronephrotic multicystic kidney demonstrate communication of the collecting system with dysplastic ducts and cysts.

Cyst puncture in pelvoinfundibular atresia usually demonstrates noncommunication of the punctured cyst with the other cysts. The hydronephrotic form of multicystic kidney often shows communication of the cysts with dilated calyces and pelvis. In equivocal cases, cyst puncture is extremely useful in differentiating hydronephrotic multicystic kidney from that associated with atresia.

DIFFERENTIAL DIAGNOSIS

A large, multilobulated kidney containing calculi and opacifying poorly or not at all suggests the diagnosis of *xanthogranulomatous pyelonephritis*, although staghorn calculus leading to epidermoid (squamous cell) carcinoma of the pelvis can create the same radiologic appearance. When the kidney contains multiple masses, functions, and does not contain pelvic calculi,

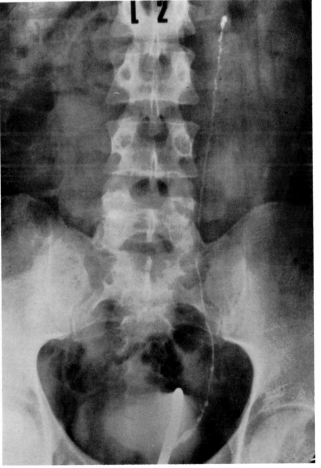

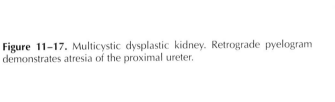

Figure 11–17. Multicystic dysplastic kidney. Retrograde pyelogram demonstrates atresia of the proximal ureter.

SUMMARY OF ABNORMAL URORADIOLOGIC FINDINGS
MULTICYSTIC DYSPLASTIC KIDNEY

Primary Uroradiologic Elements
  Size—large (may become normal to small with time)
  Contour—multifocal masses (unifocal in segmental)
  Lesion distribution—unilateral
Secondary Uroradiologic Elements
  Pelvoinfundibulocalyceal system
    Atretic form—absent (including absent or atretic proximal ureter)
    Hydronephrotic form—dilated (including ureter) to level of obstruction
  Nephrogram
    Atretic form—enhancement absent
    Hydronephrotic form—faint, delayed rims
  Calcification—curvilinear (occasional)
  Echogenicity
    Atretic form—nonreniform anechoic masses; echogenic septa; largest cyst not medial; no communications; central sinus complex absent
    Hydronephrotic form—reniform, dilated pelvis, cysts peripheral and may communicate
  Cyst puncture
    Atretic form—smooth walled, noncommunicating
    Hydronephrotic form—smooth walled; communicate with collecting system.

---

additional considerations must include *malakoplakia* as well as unusual presentations of other diseases, such as multiple angiomyolipomas or adenocarcinomas, metastatic deposits, and lymphoma. Ultrasonography and computed tomography may be helpful when they yield characteristic findings, such as calyceal rim enhancement in xanthogranulomatous pyelonephritis. Angiography might be a useful adjunct in difficult problems of differential diagnosis. Here, a highly vascular mass would strengthen the likelihood of angiomyolipoma or carcinoma. Avascular or hypovascular lesions, on the other hand, are encountered in each of the diagnostic possibilities considered.

Multicystic dysplastic kidney in the adult must be distinguished from chronic obstructive uropathy and tuberculous autonephrectomy, especially when the latter contains curvilinear calcifications. This distinction is easily made by ultrasonography, with the demonstration of characteristic fluid-filled masses. Similarly, ultrasonography also distinquishes multicystic dysplastic kidney from other causes of multifocal enlargement of one kidney, such as xanthogranulomatous pyelonephritis, malakoplakia, multiple angiomyolipomas multiple metastatic deposits, and cystic degeneration of a large carcinoma. Demonstration of an atretic ureter and of absence or hypoplasia of the renal artery firmly establishes the diagnosis of multicystic dysplastic kidney.

Bibliography

Xanthogranulomatous Pyelonephritis

Anhalt, M. A., Cawood, C. D., and Scott, R., Jr.: Xanthogranulomatous pyelonephritis: A comprehensive review with report of 4 additional cases. J. Urol. *105*:10, 1971.

Antonakopoulos, G. N., Chapple, C. R., Newman, J., Crocker, J., Tudway, D. C., O'Brien, J. M., and Considine, J.: Xanthogranulomatous pyelonephritis: A reappraisal and immunohistochemical study. Arch. Pathol. Lab. Med. *112*:275, 1988.

Avni, E. F., Thoua, Y., Lalmand, B., and Didier, F.: Multicystic dysplastic kidney: Natural history from in utero diagnosis and postnatal followup. J. Urol. *138*:1420, 1987.

Becker, J. A.: Xanthogranulomatous pyelonephritis: A case report with angiographic findings. Acta Radiol. (Diagn.) *4*:139, 1966.

Clark, R. I., McAllister, H. A., and Harrell, J. E.: Case of the month from the AFIP. Radiology *92*:597, 1969.

Cohen, M. S.: Granulomatous nephritis. Urol. Clin. North Am. *13*:647, 1986.

Fagerholm, M.: Case of the autumn season (xanthogranulomatous pyelonephritis). Semin. Ultrasound *4*:145, 1983.

Goldman, S. M., Hartman, D. S., Fishman, E. K., Finizio, J., Gatewood, O. M. B., and Siegelman, S. S.: CT of xanthogranulomatous pyelonephritis: Radiologic-pathologic correlation. AJR *141*:963, 1984.

Goodman, M., Curry, T., and Russell, T.: Xanthogranulomatous pyelonephritis (XGP): A local disease with systemic manifestations: Report of 23 patients and review of the literature. Medicine *58*:171, 1979.

Grainger, R. G., and Longstaff, A. J.: Xanthogranulomatous pyelonephritis: A reappraisal. Lancet *1*:1398, 1982.

Hartman, D. S., Davis, C. J., Jr., Goldman, S. M., Isbister, S. S., and Sanders, R. C.: Xanthogranulomatous pyelonephritis: Sonographic-pathologic correlation of 16 cases. J. Ultrasound Med. *3*:481, 1984.

Hayes, W. S., Hartman, D. S., and Sesterhenn, I.: Xanthogranulomatous pyelonephritis. Radiographics *11*:485, 1991.

Kenney, P. J.: Imaging of chronic renal infections. AJR *155*:485, 1990.

Koehler, P. R.: The roentgen diagnosis of renal inflammatory masses—special emphasis on angiographic changes. Radiology *112*:257, 1974.

Levin, D. C., Gordon, D., Kinkhabwala, M., and Becker, J. A.: Reticular neovascularity in malignant and inflammatory renal masses. Radiology *120*:61, 1976.

Malek, R. S., and Elder, J. S.: Xanthogranulomatous pyelonephritis: A critical analysis of 26 cases and of the literature. J. Urol. *119*:589, 1978.

Noyes, W. E., and Palubinskas, A.: Xanthogranulomatous pyelonephritis. J. Urol. *101*:132, 1969.

Parker, M. D., and Clark, R. L.: Evolving concepts in the diagnosis of xanthogranulomatous pyelonephritis. Urol. Radiol. *11*:7, 1989.

Rossi, P., Myers, D. H., Furey, R., and Bonfils-Roberts, E. A.: Angiography in bilateral xanthogranulomatous pyelonephritis: Case report. Radiology *90*:320, 1968.

Saeed, S. M., and Fine, G.: Xanthogranulomatous pyelonephritis. Am. J. Clin. Pathol. *39*:616, 1963.

Strasberg, Z., Jacobson, S. A., Srolovitz, H., Sedlezky, I., and Schneiderman, C.: Xanthogranulomatous pyelonephritis—radiologic considerations. J. Can. Assoc. Radiol. 21:173, 1970.

Subramanyam, B. R., Megibow, A. J., Raghavendra, B. N., and Bosniak, M. A.: Diffuse xanthogranulomatous pyelonephritis: Analysis by computed tomography and sonography. Urol. Radiol. 4:5, 1982.

Tolia, B. M., Iloreta, A., Freed, S. Z., Fruchtman, B., Bennett, B., and Newman, H. R.: Xanthogranulomatous pyelonephritis: Detailed analysis of 29 cases and a brief discussion of atypical presentations. J. Urol. 126:437, 1981.

Van Kirk, O. C., Go, R. T., and Wedel, V. J.: Sonographic features of xanthogranulomatous pyelonephritis. AJR 134:1035, 1980.

Vinik, M., Freed, T. A., Smellie, W. A. B., and Weidner, W.: Xanthogranulomatous pyelonephritis: Angiographic considerations. Radiology 92:537, 1969.

Malakoplakia

Abdou, N. I., Na Pombejara, C., Sagawa, A., Ragland, C., Stechschulte, D. J., Nilsson, U., Gourley, W., Watanabe, I., Lindsey, N. J., and Allen, M. S.: Malakoplakia: Evidence for monocyte lysosomal abnormality correctable by cholinergic agonist in vitro and in vivo. N. Engl. J. Med. 297:1413, 1977.

Cadnapaphornchai, P., Rosenberg, B. F., Taher, S., Prosnitz, E. H., and McDonald, F. D.: Renal parenchymal malakoplakia: An unusual cause of renal failure. N. Engl. J. Med. 299:1110, 1978.

Clark, R. A., Weiss, M. A., Colley, D. P., and Wyatt, G. M.: Renal malakoplakia with renal vein thrombosis. AJR 133:1170, 1979.

Cohen, M. S.: Granulomatous nephritis. Urol. Clin. North Am. 13:647, 1986.

Esparza, A. R., McKay, D. B., Cronan, J. J., and Chazan, J. A.: Renal parenchymal malakoplakia: Histologic spectrum and its relationship to megalocytic interstitial nephritis and xanthogranulomatous pyelonephritis. Am. J. Surg. Pathol. 13:225, 1989.

Gonzalez, A. C., Karcioglu, Z., Waters, B. B., and Weens, H. S.: Megalocytic interstitial nephritis: Ultrasonic and radiographic changes. Radiology 133:449, 1979.

Hartman, D. S., Davis, C. J., Jr., Lichtenstein, J.E., and Goldman, S. M.: Renal parenchymal malakoplakia. Radiology 136:33, 1980.

Kenney, P. J.: Imaging of chronic renal infections. AJR 155:485, 1990.

Lamb, G. H. R., and Ayers, A. B.: Ultrasound findings in a case of renal malakoplakia. Br. J. Radiol. 50:753, 1977.

Long, J. P. Jr., and Althausen, A. F.: Malakoplakia: A 25-year experience with a review of the literature. J. Urol. 141:1328, 1989.

Pamilo, M., and Kulatunga, A.: Renal parenchymal malakoplakia: A report of two cases: The radiological and ultrasound images. Br. J. Radiol. 57:751, 1984.

Ronald, A. R., and Simonsen, J. N.: Infections of the upper urinary tract. In Schrier, R. W., and Gottschalk, C. W. (eds.): Diseases of the Kidney. Boston, Little, Brown & Co., 1988, pp. 1065–1108.

Soberon, L. M., Zawada, E. T., Jr., Cohen, A. H., and Kaloyanides, G. J.: Renal parenchymal malakoplakia presenting as acute oliguric renal failure. Nephron 26:200, 1980.

Stanton, M. J., and Maxted, W.: Malakoplakia: A study of the literature and current concepts of pathogenesis, diagnosis and treatment. J. Urol. 125:139, 1981.

Multicystic Dysplastic Kidney Disease

Atiyeh, B., Husmann, D., and Baum, M.: Contralateral renal abnormalities in multicystic dysplastic kidney disease. J. Pediatr. 121:65, 1992.

Bartley, O., Cederbom, G., and Hegnell, B.: Multicystic renal disease in an adult. Acta Radiol. (Diagn.) 6:424, 1967.

Becker, J. A., and Robinson, T.: Congenital multicystic disease in the adult. J. Can. Assoc. Radiol. 21:165, 1970.

Bernstein, J.: The multicystic kidney and hereditary renal adysplasia. Am. J. Kidney Dis. 18:495, 1991.

Blane, C. E., Barr, M., DiPietro, M. A., Sedman, A. B., and Bloom, D. A.: Renal obstruction dysplasia: Ultrasound diagnosis and therapeutic implications. Pediatr. Radiol. 21:274, 1991.

Cooperman, L. R.: Delayed opacification in congenital multicystic dysplastic kidney, an important roentgen sign. Radiology 121:703, 1976.

Dungan, J. S., Fernandez, M. T., Abbitt, P. L., Thiagarajah, S., Howards, S. S., and Hogge, W. A.: Multicystic dysplastic kidney: Natural history of prenatally detected cases. Prenat. Diagn. 10:175, 1990.

Elkin, M.: Renal cysts and abscesses. Curr. Probl. Diagn. 5:11, 1975.

Felson, B., and Cussen, L. J.: The hydronephrotic type of unilateral congenital multicystic disease of the kidney. Semin. Roentgenol. 10:113, 1975.

Gordon, A. C., Thomas, D. F. M., Arthur, R. J., and Irving, H. C.: Multicystic dysplastic kidney: Is nephrectomy still appropriate? J. Urol. 140:1231, 1988.

Greene, L. F., Feinzaig, W., and Dahlin, D. C.: Multicystic dysplasia of the kidney: With special reference to the contralateral kidney. J. Urol. 105:482, 1971.

Griscom, N. T., Vanter, G. F., and Fellers, F. X.: Pelvoinfundibular atresia: The usual form of multicystic kidney: 44 unilateral and two bilateral cases. Semin. Roentgenol. 10:125, 1975.

Grossman, H., Rosenberg, E. R., Bowie, J. D., Ram, P., and Merten, D. F.: Sonographic diagnosis of renal cystic disease. AJR 140:81, 1983.

Hartman, D. S., and Davis, C. J.: Multicystic dysplastic kidney. In Hartman, D. S. (ed.): Renal Cystic Disease. Philadelphia, W.B. Saunders, 1989, pp. 127–142.

Hashimoto, B. E., Filly, R. A., Callen, P. W.: Multicystic dysplastic kidney in utero: Changing appearance on US. Radiology 159:107, 1986.

Kleiner, B., Filly, R. A., Mack, L., Callen, P. W.: Multicystic dysplastic kidney: Observations of contralateral disease in the fetal population. Radiology 161:27, 1986.

Kyaw, M.: The radiological diagnosis of congenital multicystic kidney. "Radiological triad." Clin. Radiol. 25:45, 1974.

Murugasu, B., Cole, B. R., Hawkins, E. P., Blanton, S. H., Conley, S. B., and Portman, R. J.: Familial renal adysplasia. Am. J. Kidney Dis. 18:490, 1991.

Osathanondh, V., and Potter, E. L: Pathogenesis of polycystic kidneys: Type 2 due to inhibition of ampullary activity. Arch. Pathol. Lab. Med. 77:474, 1964.

Pedicelli, G., Jequier, S., Bowen, A., and Boisvert, J.: Multicystic dysplastic kidneys: Spontaneous regression demonstrated with US. Radiology 160:23, 1986.

Piel, C. F.: Congenital multicystic kidney. In Gardner, K. D., and Bernstein, J. (eds.): The Cystic Kidney. Dordrecht, Kluwer Academic Publishers, 1990, pp. 393–407.

Sanders, R. C., Nussbaum, A. R., and Solez, K.: Renal dysplasia: Sonographic findings. Radiology 167:623, 1988.

Saxton, H. M., Golding, S. J., Chartler, C., and Haycock, G. D.: Diagnostic puncture in renal cystic dysplasia (multicystic kidney): Evidence on the etiology of the cysts. Br. J. Radiol. 54:555, 1981.

Spence, H. M.: Congenital unilateral multicystic kidney: An entity to be distinguished from polycystic kidney disease and other cystic disorders. J. Urol. 74:693, 1955.

Stuck, K. J., Koff, S. A., and Silver, T. M.: Ultrasonic features of multicystic dysplastic kidney: Expanded diagnostic criteria. Radiology 143:217, 1982.

Vellios, F., and Garret, R. A.: Congenital unilateral multicystic disease of the kidney: A clinical and anatomic study of seven cases. Am. J. Clin. Pathol. 35:244, 1961.

Vinocur, L., Slovis, T. L., Perimutter, A. D., Watts, F. B., Jr., and Chang, C. H.: Follow-up studies of multicystic dysplastic kidneys. Radiology 167:311, 1988.

Warshawsky, A. B., Miller, K. E., and Kaplan, G. W.: Urographic visualization of multicystic kidneys. J. Urol. 117:94, 1977.

Wood, B. P.: Renal cystic disease in infants and children. Urol. Radiol. 14:284, 1992.

12

DIAGNOSTIC SET: LARGE, UNIFOCAL, UNILATERAL

SOLID MASSES	Focal Hydronephrosis
Malignant Neoplasms	Abscess
Benign Neoplasms	Multilocular Cystic Nephroma
	Congenital Arteriovenous Malformation
FLUID-FILLED MASSES	
Simple Renal Cyst	DIFFERENTIAL DIAGNOSIS

The entities discussed in this chapter include a wide variety of pathologic lesions not usually grouped together. In the organizational format used in this text they are unified under the diagnostic set "large, unifocal, unilateral" because each usually causes enlargement of the kidney by formation of a single, focal mass. Included in this category are malignant and benign tumors, simple cyst, focal hydronephrosis, abscess, and arteriovenous malformation.

The radiologist performs two functions in regard to the unifocal renal mass. The first is *discovery* of the mass, either by excretory urography, ultrasonography, or computed tomography performed because of clinical abnormalities referable to the urinary tract or by incidental and unexpected findings noted in radiologic studies undertaken for unrelated reasons. The second, and most challenging, is *characterization of the nature* of a renal mass once it is discovered. Here, the goal of the radiologist is to separate masses that usually have little or no clinical consequence such as a simple cyst, from those that have great potential importance, such as a malignant neoplasm. Since radiologic studies do not permit specific histologic diagnosis, this goal is best achieved by classifying focal lesions as either "solid" or "fluid filled." "Solid," as used here, refers not only to completely solid tumors but also to those that contain both solid and fluid elements (i.e., complex masses). Likewise, the category, "fluid filled," includes masses that are divided into locules by solid septa. This distinction is particularly useful in directing patient management, since most solid lesions require surgery for definitive diagnosis, whereas most fluid-filled masses, being simple cysts, do not. This chapter, therefore, approaches the kidney that is enlarged by a unifocal mass according to whether the lesion is solid (including complex masses of both solid and fluid components) or fluid filled (including thick or thin-septated fluid masses)

as determined by imaging studies. Strategies for the appropriate choice of radiologic modalities—excretory urography, ultrasonography, computed tomography, magnetic resonance imaging, needle aspiration, or angiography—are discussed in Chapter 25.

There are two general patterns by which solid tumors of the kidney grow: *expansion* and *infiltration*. Each usually alters the gross morphology of the kidney in a characteristic manner that can be detected radiologically. Expansile growth occurs when neoplasia develops at an epicenter and new cells grow in all directions, pushing adjacent normal renal tissue away as the tumor increases in size. This form of growth by apposition of cells in all directions yields a tumor whose geometry is ball shaped and often surrounded by a pseudocapsule of compressed renal parenchyma that becomes fibrotic as a result of ischemia (Fig. 12–1). Infiltrative growth represents enlargement of the kidney as a result of the accumulation of abnormal cells in the interstitial spaces of the kidney. Here, the cells use the nephrons and collecting ducts as scaffolding that guides their spread diffusely throughout the kidney. The normal microscopic elements of the kidney are thus *surrounded* rather than *displaced* in this pattern of growth. The reniform shape of the enlarged kidney is thereby preserved (Fig. 12–2). Although infiltrative processes are often neoplastic, they may also be inflammatory, as discussed in the section on acute pyelonephritis in Chapter 9. Radiologically, kidneys that enlarge by virtue of infiltrative processes are bean shaped rather than ball shaped.

Some neoplasms characteristically enlarge the kidney by expansion, while others characteristically produce bean-shaped, infiltrative patterns of enlargement. These are listed in Table 12–1. Thus, the radiologic assessment of the geometry of an enlarged kidney can yield useful clues as to the underlying disease. This concept is used in this and other chap-

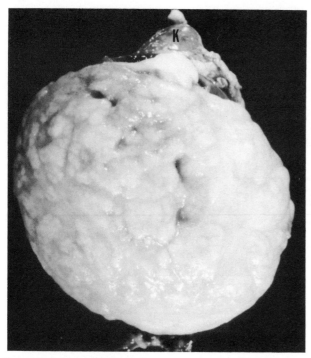

Figure 12–1. Expansile growth that creates a tumor with a ball-shaped geometry. A small amount of kidney (K) remains in the upper pole. Gross specimen, bivalved, Wilms' tumor.

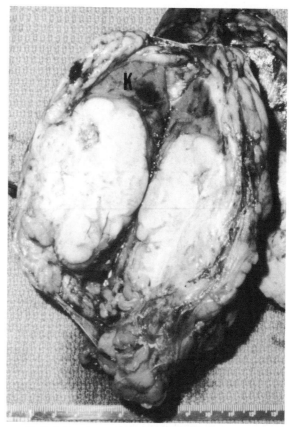

Figure 12–2. Infiltrative pattern of growth that enlarges the kidney with preservation of the reniform or bean-shaped geometry. A small amount of uninvolved kidney (K) remains in the upper pole. Gross specimen, bivalved, transitional cell carcinoma of the renal pelvis invading the kidney.

ters in attributing patterns of growth to specific diseases.

SOLID MASSES

Malignant Neoplasms

Definition

Malignant primary neoplasms of the kidney arise from epithelial cells, mature mesodermal elements, or primitive tissues. Adenocarcinoma, originating in the tubule epithelium, accounts for over 90 per cent of malignant neoplasms in the adult kidney, while Wilms' tumor (nephroblastoma) accounts for most of the primary malignant neoplasms in the kidneys of children.

Adenocarcinoma. Microscopically, adenocarcinoma may contain a variety of cell types (clear or granular cytoplasm), cell morphology (differentiated or undifferentiated), and cell arrangements (medullary, tubular, or papillary). Several cytologic and architectural features often coexist. Adenocarcinoma with a papillary architecture is thought to be associated with less aggressive biologic behavior than other forms of this tumor and thus may have a favorable prognosis. Only with extreme rarity does an adenocarcinoma contain radiologically detectable intratumoral fat.

A ball-shaped focal enlargement of the kidney rep-

Table 12–1. CHARACTERISTIC PATTERNS OF GROWTH FOR VARIOUS MALIGNANT AND BENIGN TUMORS OF THE KIDNEY*

Malignant Kidney Tumor		Benign Kidney Tumor	
Infiltration	*Expansion*	*Infiltration*	*Expansion*
Transitional cell (invasive)	Adenocarcinoma	Mesoblastic nephroma	Adenoma/oncocytoma
Lymphoma (early)	Nephroblastoma		Angiomyolipoma
Metastases†	Metastases†		Multilocular cystic nephroma
Leukemia	Mesenchymal		Juxtaglomerular cell tumor

*Infiltrative growth patterns enlarge the kidney with preservation of reniform shape, whereas expansile growth patterns create a tumor geometry that is rounded.
†Metastatic growth pattern varies according to tissue type.

resents growth of an adenocarcinoma by expansion in all directions from an epicenter at its origin in an epithelial cell of the proximal convoluted tubule. A fibrous, poorly vascularized pseudocapsule surrounds the tumor as a result of compression and ischemia of nephrons at the interface between the tumor and normal renal parenchyma. Additional pathologic features that influence the radiologic appearance of these tumors are their tendency to undergo necrosis and/or hemorrhage with secondary deposition of dystrophic calcification and the rich supply of arterial and venous channels that may develop with the cancer.

Not all adenocarcinomas are solid. Some have intermixed areas of fluid representative of hemorrhage and/or necrosis. Others, particularly those with a papillary architecture, develop *de novo* as either inherently unilocular or multilocular cysts with tumor cells lining the walls of the fluid-filled mass. This possibility must be considered in the assessment of a unilocular or multilocular fluid-filled mass, which is discussed later in this chapter. Only with extreme rarity does an adenocarcinoma arise in the wall of an otherwise benign, simple cyst.

Anatomic landmarks used to determine the stage of spread of an adenocarcinoma are the renal capsule, perirenal fat, Gerota's fascia, renal vein, inferior vena cava, and lymph nodes. Blood-borne metastases to distant organs, notably, lung, brain, bone, liver, and adrenal, are common. Two commonly used schemes of classification are tabulated in Table 12–2.

Wilms' Tumor. Wilms' tumor is derived from primitive nephrogenic blastema. The microscopic appearance of a typical case is that of a triphasic tumor composed of epithelial (glomerular and tubular), blastemal, and stromal elements. The stromal components may variably differentiate into fibroblasts, smooth or striated muscle, cartilage, osteoid, or fat. The latter accounts for the occasional radiologic detection of bone or fat in a Wilms' tumor. Wilms' tumor grows by expansion into a large ball-like mass, which frequently exhibits hemorrhage and necrosis but uncommonly contains calcium. Local venous spread and distant metastases, especially to lung and liver, are common.

Wilms' tumor may develop either as a sporadic event or in association with persistent nephrogenic blastema, a condition known as *nephroblastomatosis*. In nephroblastomatosis, microscopic foci of nephrogenic blastema, which are present as incidental findings in 1:400 autopsies of infants, undergo neoplastic or hyperplastic growth. As a result, multilobulated masses develop in one or both kidneys. Only uncommonly does nephroblastomatosis appear as a unifocal mass. However, since nephroblastomatosis is a precursor of Wilms' tumor it is discussed in this chapter rather than in those on multifocal renal masses.

Miscellaneous Malignant Tumors. Malignant renal neoplasms other than adenocarcinoma and Wilms' tumor are very uncommon. These include clear cell sarcoma and malignant rhabdoid tumor of the kidney in children and, at any age, malignant tumors of mesodermal elements, such as fibrosarcoma, myosarcoma, liposarcoma, and angioendothelioma. Chloroma, myeloblastoma, and myeloblastic sarcoma are focal masses that may develop in the kidney of patients with leukemia.

Another uncommon cause of unifocal renal enlargement is metastatic disease to the kidney. This is somewhat paradoxical, since secondary deposits in the kidney occur twice as often as primary neoplasms in autopsy series. At autopsy, however, the majority of metastases are multiple, but a few millimeters across or are seen only microscopically. Metastases usually do not grow large enough to become radiologically demonstrable because of the very brief survival period of these patients. Nevertheless, antemortem radiologic abnormalities due to a large unifocal metastatic deposit may occur in lymphoma, melanoma, carcinoma of the lung, osteogenic sarcoma, choriocarcinoma, and muscle sarcoma. With the advantage of the greater sensitivity of computed tomography over excretory urography, it is also apparent that metastases now are more often detected as bilateral and multiple masses than heretofore. Lymphoma is an exception to these generalizations regarding metastases in that it may produce large renal masses that tend to be both multiple and bilateral. These are discussed separately in Chapter 10.

Focal renal enlargement also occurs as a result of local invasion of renal parenchyma by malignant tumors arising in adjacent tissue. Transitional cell carcinoma of the pelvis, discussed in Chapter 15, is the most common example of this. Malignancy of any pararenal tissue, however, can produce the same effect.

Clinical Setting

Adenocarcinoma. Adenocarcinoma of the kidney occurs more than twice as frequently in males as in females and has a peak prevalence in the sixth decade of life. Uncommonly, adenocarcinoma is encountered in early adulthood and, rarely, in infancy and childhood. Clinical symptoms may be due to the local effect of the tumor (hematuria, pain, or palpable mass) or distant metastases (bone pain or central nervous system dysfunction). Adenocarcinoma of the kidney

Table 12–2. TWO COMMONLY USED SCHEMES FOR STAGING ADENOCARCINOMA OF THE KIDNEY

Robson	Extent of Tumor	TNM
I	Tumor confined to kidney (small) intrarenal	T1
	Tumor confined to kidney (large)	T2
II	Tumor spread to perinephric fat, but within Gerota's fascia	T3a
III	Tumor spread to renal vein	T3b
	Tumor spread to inferior vena cava	T3c
	Tumor spread to regional lymph nodes	N1–N3
IV	Tumor invasion of neighboring structures	T4
	Distant metastases	M1

is a well-known cause of constitutional or hormonal paraneoplastic syndromes, which may obscure the correct diagnosis. These include fever, erythrocytosis, hypercalcemia and constipation, anorexia, nausea, polyuria, and weight loss. Hepatic dysfunction in the absence of liver metastases also occurs and is reversible when the primary tumor is resected. Arteriovenous fistulae associated with tumor neovascularity can produce abdominal or flank bruit, high-output cardiac failure, or renal ischemia and hypertension. In a male, the sudden appearance of a varicocele, almost always left sided, signals impairment of venous drainage from the testicular vein into a renal vein occluded by a tumor. With the widespread use of computed tomography and ultrasonography, many adenocarcinomas are discovered in asymptomatic patients. Bilateral adenocarcinomas have been described in less than 2 per cent of patients. Of these, approximately one-half are bilateral at the time of initial diagnosis and the remainder develop in the contralateral kidney after initial diagnosis. Multicentricity of adenocarcinoma in the same kidney, on the other hand, occurs in as many as 9 per cent of patients. Bilaterality and multicentricity are, however, the rule when adenocarcinomas develop in patients with von Hippel-Lindau disease, in patients on dialysis with acquired cystic disease of the kidney, and in the rare cohorts of individuals with a familial form of adenocarcinoma.

Wilms' Tumor. Approximately 50 per cent of Wilms' tumors are diagnosed between the first and third years of life and 75 per cent by the fifth birthday. Wilms' tumor is uncommon in the first year of life. Those tumors that are related to heritable disorders or that are bilateral are usually diagnosed at a somewhat younger age than are those that are sporadic. The prevalence curves for adenocarcinoma and Wilms' tumor cross in the second decade of life, with Wilms' tumor rarely occurring beyond young adulthood. Several heritable and nonheritable congenital malformations are associated with Wilms' tumor, some in association with an anomaly on the short arm of chromosome 11. These include sporadic aniridia, trisomies 8 and 18, Turner's syndrome, pseudohermaphroditism with glomerulonephritis and nephrotic syndrome (Drash syndrome), other genitourinary anomalies, hemihypertrophy, Beckwith-Wiedemann syndrome, and musculoskeletal anomalies. Approximately one-third of patients with sporadic aniridia develop Wilms' tumor.

A large abdominal mass is the most common presentation for Wilms' tumor. In 5 to 10 per cent of patients, the tumor is bilateral. In these cases nephroblastomatosis is always present. Other clinical manifestations of Wilms' tumor include abdominal pain, anorexia, nausea, vomiting, fever, and gross hematuria. Venous obstruction can cause leg edema, varicocele, or the Budd-Chiari syndrome. Signs and symptoms of distant metastases are often present.

Nephroblastomatosis in its diffuse form is discovered in the newborn, infant, or child as a unilateral or bilateral abdominal mass. Small foci of persistent metanephric blastema, also part of the nephroblastomatosis complex, are asymptomatic. Nephroblasto-

matosis is a precursor of Wilms' tumor, being present in all patients with bilateral tumors and in approximately 30 per cent of those with a solitary tumor. Like Wilms' tumor, nephroblastomatosis is associated with hemihypertrophy, sporadic aniridia, pseudohermaphroditism, and Beckwith-Wiedemann syndrome. Although not malignant in and of itself, chemotherapy and radiation are used as treatment modalities in recognition of the malignant potential of nephroblastomatosis.

Miscellaneous Malignant Tumors. The miscellaneous tumors listed in the preceding section cause many of the clinical findings associated with adenocarcinoma or Wilms' tumor. Metastatic disease to the kidney is usually silent unless the lesion invades the collecting system and causes hematuria. Rarely, abdominal mass or symptoms of urinary tract infection may be the result of renal metastases. Clear cell sarcoma in childhood is frequently associated with bone metastases, while rhabdoid tumor of the kidney, also in children, has a predilection for metastatic spread to the central nervous system. Locally invasive cancer usually causes hematuria, especially when it is uroepithelial in origin.

Radiologic Findings

Excretory Urography. Most malignant neoplasms produce a ball-shaped expansion of the kidney that is seen as increased length or width or, simply, as a localized bulge (Figs. 12–3 through 12–5). A centrally

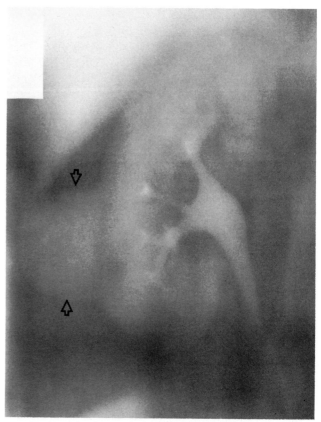

Figure 12–3. Adenocarcinoma of the kidney producing a localized bulge on the lateral contour of the kidney *(arrows)*. The interpapillary line is normal. Tomogram during excretory urography.

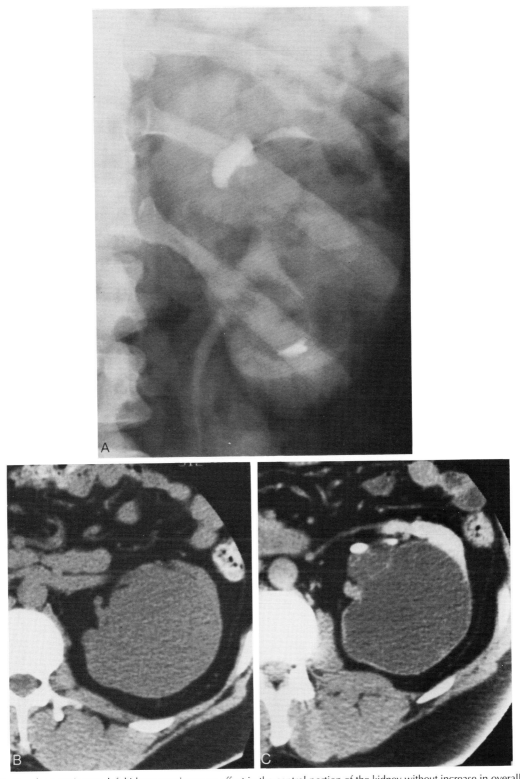

Figure 12–4. Cystic adenocarcinoma, left kidney, causing mass effect in the central portion of the kidney without increase in overall length.
   A, Excretory urogram. There is marked displacement of the infundibula and calyces and effacement of the pelvis by the tumor.
   B, Computed tomogram, unenhanced. The attenuation value of the tumor is slightly less than that of the normal kidney. *C,* Computed tomogram, contrast material enhanced. There is increased density of a thickened and slightly nodular rim of tissue on the periphery of the tumor. The bulk of the tumor enhances minimally.

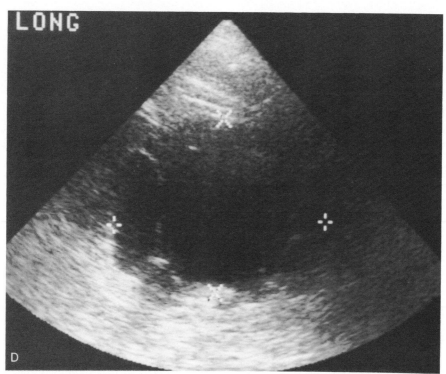

Figure 12–4 *Continued D,* Ultrasound, longitudinal section. The tumor is hypoechoic, but the far wall is poorly defined and there is no increased through-sound transmission.

located mass, however, may cause only enlargement of renal thickness, a dimension not readily measured on standard urographic projections. In this situation, both size and contour may be normal, and detection of the neoplasm will depend on infundibular, calyceal, or pelvic displacement or obliteration (Fig. 12–6). Some tumors eventually destroy the entire kidney, leaving only a large nonfunctioning mass (Fig. 12–7). Uncommonly, malignant tumors of the kidney, such as certain metastases, grow by infiltration and thereby preserve the reniform shape of the kidney even as the organ enlarges.

Tilting of the renal axis may occur if the mass grows in an exophytic manner, particularly medially. With an upper pole medial mass the axis becomes vertical, whereas a lower pole medial mass will shift the axis toward the horizontal plane. Particularly large tumors, as is often the case in Wilms' tumor and some carcinomas, may markedly displace the entire kidney in one direction or another (Fig. 12–8). Marked ventral displacement enlarges the image of the kidney on anteroposterior radiographs owing to increase in the distance of the kidney to the film.

The collecting system is frequently abnormal in the presence of a malignant neoplasm. There may be marked displacement of adjacent portions of the pelvis, infundibulum, or calyx around the tumor (see Figs. 12–4, 12–5, 12–12, and 12–17). Ureteral compression, a large dose of contrast material, or prone films are often necessary to distend the collecting structures well enough to visualize these abnormalities (see Fig. 12–6). Sometimes only minor splaying of a single ca-

lyx is present. Filling defects within the calyces, representing growth of tumor into the collecting system, are either smooth or irregular (Figs. 12–9 and 12–10). One sensitive sign of a tumor is a focal increase in the distance between the calyx (interpapillary line) and the overlying outer margin of the kidney compared with the remainder of the renal substance. This is illustrated in Figure 12–10 and schematized in Figure 4–4. Compression or invasion of a draining infundibulum by a malignant tumor can lead to focal dilatation of a group of calyces (Figs. 12–11 and 12–12). Advanced hydronephrosis of the obstructed region may develop in some patients (see Fig. 12–30).

Solid, nonnecrotic neoplasms of the kidney, regardless of the degree of vascularization, enhance during the early nephrographic phase of urography but over time do not retain their initial intensity of enhancement relative to the surrounding normal parenchyma. Enhancement reflects perfusion of the lesion with contrast material–laden blood. If perfusion of all or part of the tumor is disrupted, as occurs with hemorrhage or necrosis or in cystic neoplasms, the affected area remains relatively unenhanced throughout the urographic examination (Fig. 12–13; see also Figs. 12–5 and 12–10). The area of diminished enhancement may be small and centrally located, may be eccentric, or may involve the whole mass. The perfused, peripheral portion of a cystic or necrotic lesion is sometimes seen as a radiodense, thick wall with an irregular inner margin surrounding the relatively radiolucent center. This finding, schematized in Figure 4–4, is a feature of malignant disease.

Text continued on page 340

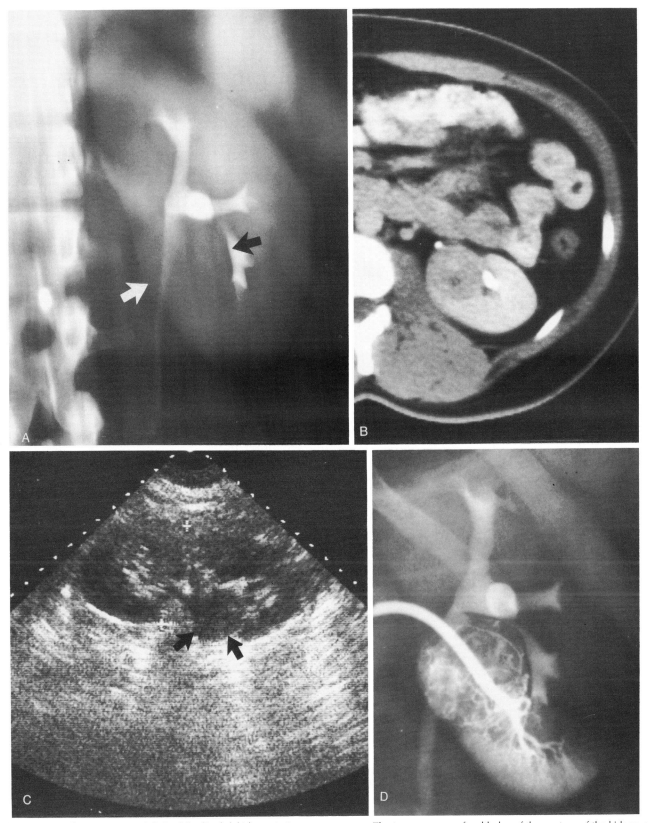

Figure 12–5. Adenocarcinoma, inferior hilar lip, left kidney. *A*, Excretory urogram. The tumor causes a focal bulge of the contour of the kidney, a slightly diminished nephrogram, as well as effacement and lateral displacement of the infundibulum and calyx of the lower pole *(arrows)*. *B*, Computed tomogram, contrast material enhanced. The small tumor, which is more easily visualized than on excretory urography, does not enhance as much as the normal renal parenchyma. A small focus of decreased central density represents hemorrhage or necrosis.

C, Ultrasonogram, coronal section. The tumor *(arrows)* is isoechoic with renal parenchyma. *D*, Selective arteriogram, accessory renal artery. There is moderate neovascularity.

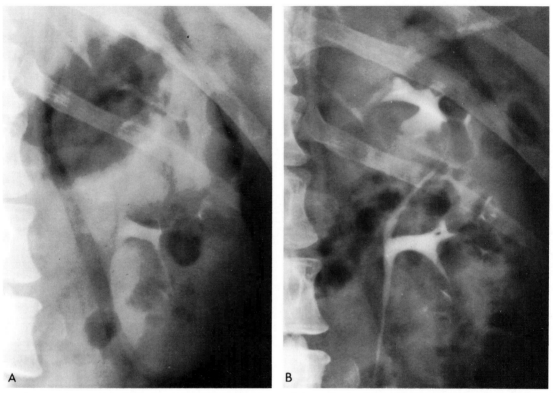

Figure 12–6. Adenocarcinoma of the kidney causing focal displacement of the collecting structures of the upper pole. *A*, Standard excretory urogram without ureteral compression. The upper pole calyces are seen faintly. *B*, Excretory urogram with effective ureteral compression results in visualization of the entire upper pole collecting system and identification of the mass lesion in the medial aspect of the upper pole.
   (Courtesy of Janet Dacie, M. B., St. Bartholomew's Hospital, London, England.)

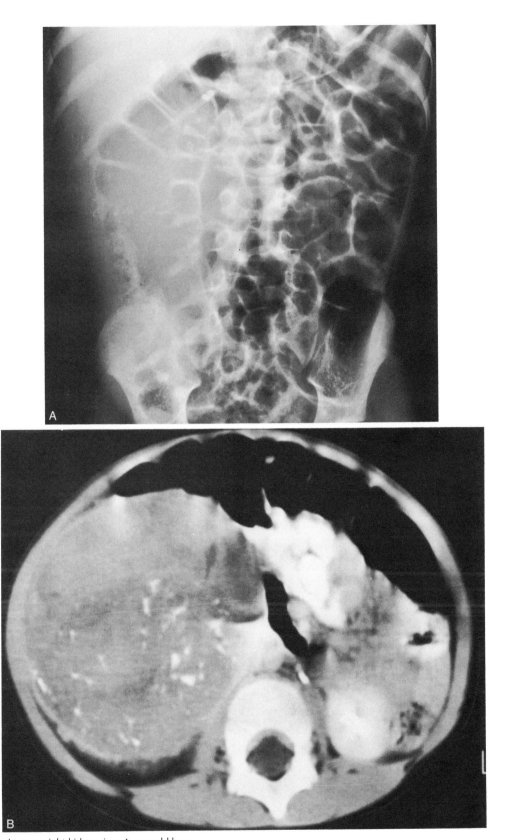

Figure 12–7. Wilms' tumor, right kidney, in a 4-year-old boy.
   A, Radiograph of abdomen. There is a large soft tissue mass filling the right mid abdomen and displacing bowel. Fine, stippled foci of calcium are visible within the tumor. *B,* Computed tomogram, contrast material enhanced. The large tumor replaces the kidney, contains numerous foci of nonperipheral dystrophic calcification, and is homogeneous.

Illustration continued on following page

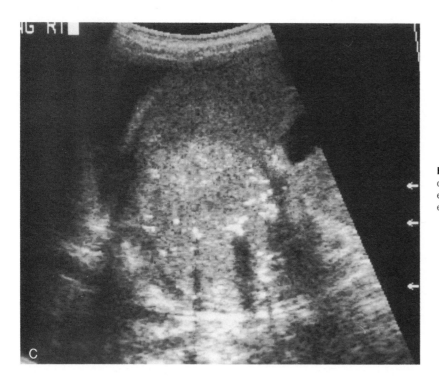

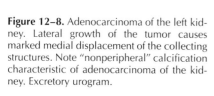

Figure 12–7 *Continued C,* Ultrasonogram, longitudinal section. The tumor is diffusely and evenly echogenic. The foci of calcification cause specular echoes and shadowing.

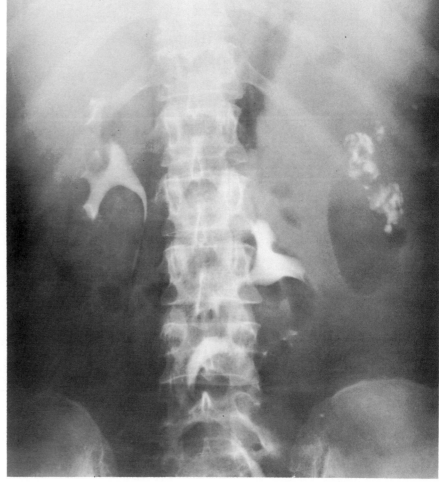

Figure 12–8. Adenocarcinoma of the left kidney. Lateral growth of the tumor causes marked medial displacement of the collecting structures. Note "nonperipheral" calcification characteristic of adenocarcinoma of the kidney. Excretory urogram.

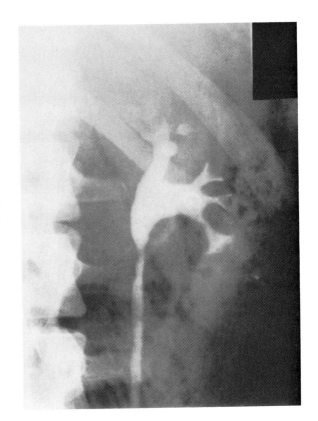

Figure 12–9. Adenocarcinoma of the kidney in a 23-year-old man seen during excretory urography as a smooth filling defect extending into the calyx of the upper pole. (Courtesy of Janet Dacie, M. B., St. Bartholomew's Hospital, London, England.)

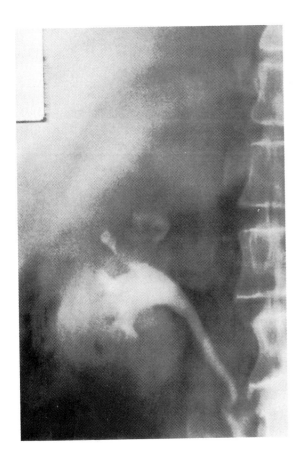

Figure 12–10. Adenocarcinoma of the kidney protruding as a smooth, lobulated filling defect into the upper collecting system. Note also the focal increase in the thickness of the upper pole caused by the tumor. (Courtesy of Professor Thomas Sherwood, M. B., University of Cambridge, Cambridge, England.)

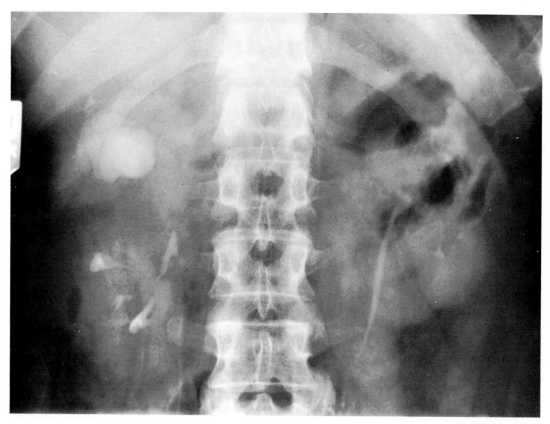

Figure 12–11. Adenocarcinoma of the right kidney causing focal dilatation of the upper pole calyces. A nephrographic defect due to the tumor replacing functioning renal tissue is apparent in the upper part of the interpolar region. Excretory urogram.

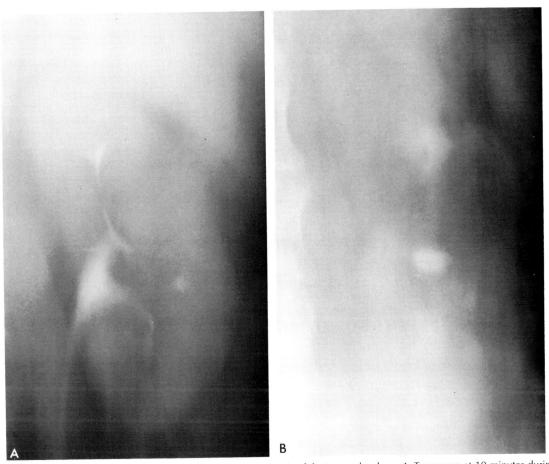

Figure 12–12. Adenocarcinoma leading to nephrographic defect as necrosis of the tumor develops. *A*, Tomogram at 10 minutes during excretory urogram. Normal nephrographic density. The tumor causes splaying of the upper interpolar collecting system.

B, Tomogram at 10 minutes during excretory urogram, 2 years after *A*. No surgical intervention followed initial urography. After a 2-year interval there is an irregular mottled nephrogram, growth of the tumor, and involvement of the collecting structures. The change in nephrographic appearance presumably represents necrosis of the tumor.

(Same case illustrated in Fig. 12–32.)

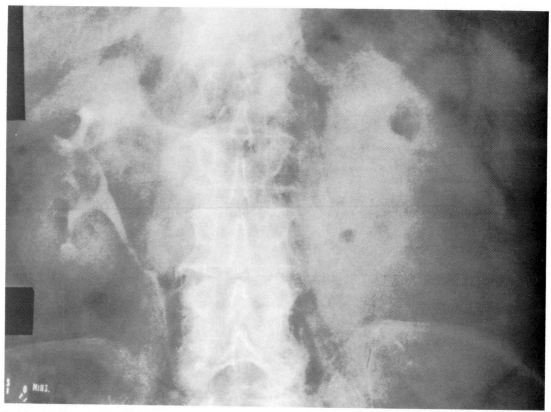

Figure 12–13. Adenocarcinoma of the left kidney with decreased enhancement, focal enlargement of the lower portion of the kidney, and a mottled nephrogram. Excretory urogram, 5-minute film.

Detecting calcium in a focal renal mass is quite useful in predicting the nature of the lesion. Based on detection by computed tomography, approximately 30 per cent of carcinomas are calcified. Only one-third of these are detected by film radiography, however. In differentiating a fluid-filled simple cyst from a solid tumor, the *location* (peripheral or nonperipheral) of calcification within the mass is a more important factor than the *pattern* of calcification (amorphous, mottled, punctate, wavy, or curvilinear). Approximately 90 per cent of all masses containing calcium in a nonperipheral location are carcinoma (see Figs. 12–7 and 12–8). Nonneoplastic conditions such as xanthogranulomatous pyelonephritis and tuberculosis as well as uncommon tumors account for the remainder. It is important to remember, however, that peripheral, curvilinear calcification, although suggestive of simple cyst, occurs in carcinoma as well (Fig. 12–14). Nonperipheral calcification occurs in approximately 5 per cent of Wilms' tumors (see Fig. 12–7).

There are other urographic findings more specifically associated with malignant masses than those already discussed. Ureteral notching in the presence of a focal renal mass is persuasive evidence of cancer (Fig. 12–15). This reflects periureteric collateral veins, which develop following invasion of the main renal vein by tumor or by propagation of thrombus from the area of the tumor. Another urographic sign that strongly suggests malignant disease is the presence of

narrow, serpiginous densities in the perirenal fat, which may be identifiable on radiographic studies (Fig. 12–16). These are dilated capsular arteries and/or veins, part of the abnormal pathways of arterial supply and venous drainage of a vascular tumor. These enlarged vessels are detectable because they are embedded in perirenal fat. Their density is enhanced during urography, but they are demonstrated best during computed tomography or angiography. Enlarged capsular veins should not be interpreted as evidence of collateral flow due to renal vein obstruction, since they may enlarge as a response to tumor hypervascularity. Although dilated capsular vessels are usually a sign of carcinoma, they may be seen in benign conditions, such as arteriovenous fistula with a high-flow state. Enlarged vessels in the perirenal fat may simulate thickened Gerota's fascia, the significance of which is discussed in Chapter 21.

In children with nephroblastomatosis, the excretory urographic findings may be normal or there may be generalized enlargement of one or both kidneys. Wilms' tumor, if present, often obscures these abnormalities, however.

Computed Tomography. Most of the characteristics of malignant tumors described in the previous section on excretory urography apply to their appearance on computed tomographic images. Because of the cross-sectional anatomic display and enhanced contrast discrimination, computed tomography has a sensitivity

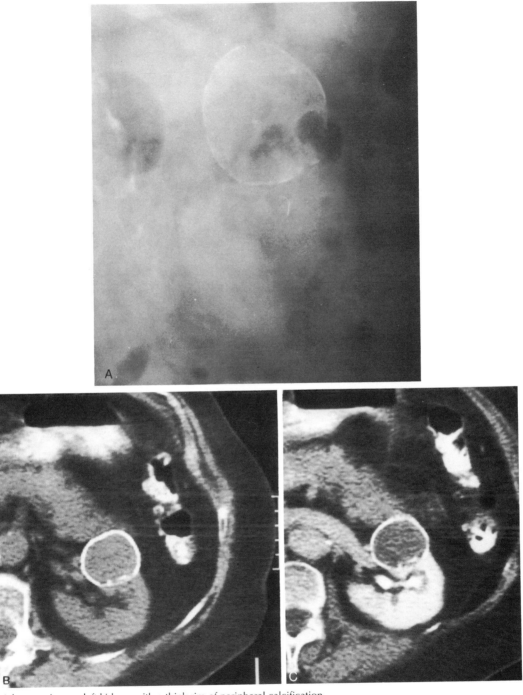

Figure 12–14. Adenocarcinoma, left kidney, with a thick rim of peripheral calcification.

A, Excretory urogram.

B, Computed tomogram without contrast material enhancement demonstrates thick rim of calcium and an attenuation value of the tumor that approximates that of the renal parenchyma.

C, Computed tomogram with contrast material demonstrates less tumor enhancement than the surrounding normal renal parenchyma.

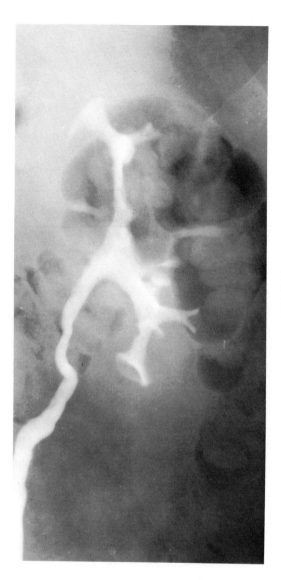

Figure 12–15. Adenocarcinoma of the kidney associated with pelvic and ureteral notching due to periureteric and peripelvic venous collaterals forming in response to renal vein obstruction by the tumor. Retrograde pyelogram. (Courtesy of Janet Dacie, M. B., St. Bartholomew's Hospital, London, England.)

of over 90 per cent compared with approximately 67 per cent for excretory urography in detecting solid mass lesions in the kidney. This advantage is particularly apparent for tumors that grow on the anterior or posterior surface of the kidney, that are deeply embedded within the parenchyma, or that are of small size (see Fig. 12–5). The attenuation value of unenhanced malignant tissue varies from slightly less than to slightly more than that of normal kidney tissue and from homogeneous to heterogeneous (Figs. 12–17 through 12–19; see also Figs. 12–4 and 12–14). Foci of decreased attenuation within the mass correspond to areas of necrosis, old hemorrhage, or cystic change. Areas of recent hemorrhage are slightly hyperdense compared with normal renal tissue. Solid malignant tumors may enhance in density to the level of surrounding normal renal parenchyma immediately after contrast material is given, but the density becomes less than that of normal tissue soon thereafter. Low-attenuation foci of old hemorrhage, necrosis, or cyst formation do not enhance. A zone of relative radiolucency surrounding a tumor that has

grown by expansion represents a fibrous pseudocapsule that has formed in response to ischemia of compressed nephrons at the interface between the neoplasm and adjacent renal parenchyma (Fig. 12–20). This finding, which has been called the "halo" sign, may also be observed by excretory urography and is encountered in benign as well as malignant masses. Tumors that have an infiltrative pattern of growth, on the other hand, cause regional enlargement without a mass circumscribed by a pseudocapsule.

Computed tomography is particularly valuable in the assessment of malignant tumors that are partially or predominantly cystic (Figs. 12–21 and 12–22; see also Figs. 12–4 and 12–14). Uncommonly, the attenuation value of the tumor contents may be equal to or only slightly higher than water and may be nonenhancing (Fig. 12–23). Usually, however, the attenuation value is sufficiently above that of water to raise the suspicion that the lesion is not an ordinary simple cyst. When a diagnosis of a cystic malignancy is suggested, additional clues derived from computed tomography are thickened walls or septations, mural

Text continued on page 349

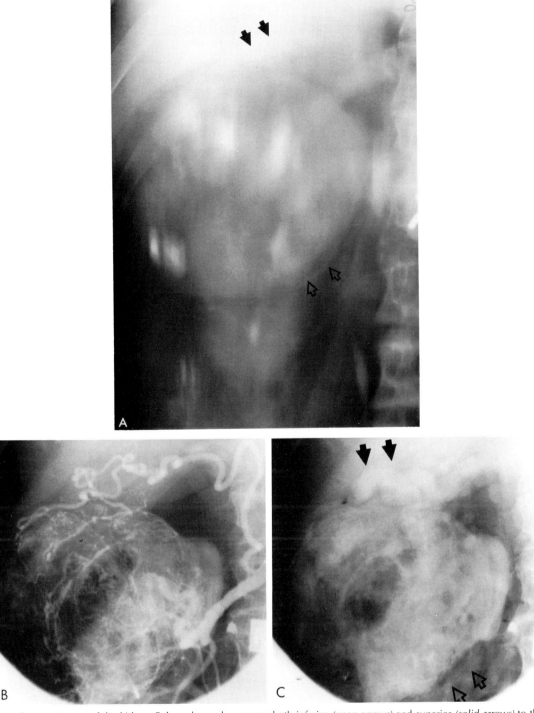

Figure 12–16. Adenocarcinoma of the kidney. Enlarged vessels are seen both inferior *(open arrows)* and superior *(solid arrows)* to the mass. The superior vessels represent parasitized adrenal arteries and veins. The inferior vessels reflect dilated renal arteries and veins.

A, Tomogram during excretory urography.

B, Arterial phase of selective renal arteriogram. The large parasitized inferior adrenal artery is seen feeding the vascular tumor.

C, Venous phase of selective renal arteriogram. Large, tortuous veins in the upper part of the tumor *(solid arrows)* drain into the inferior vena cava. Other venous structures embedded in perirenal fat drain inferior to the tumor *(open arrows)*.

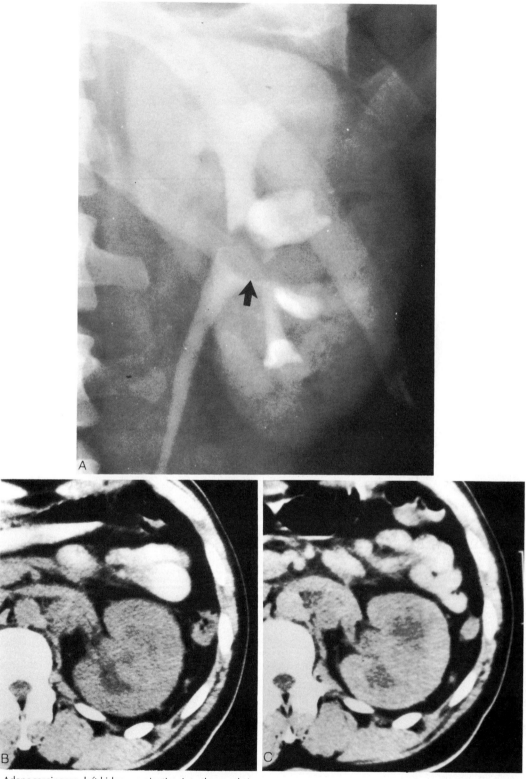

Figure 12–17. Adenocarcinoma, left kidney, projecting into the renal sinus.

A, Excretory urogram. The tumor projects into the pelvis *(arrow)* and causes partial obstruction of the calyces draining the upper and mid polar regions of the kidney. *B*, Computed tomogram, unenhanced. The tumor is isodense with renal parenchyma and partially obliterates the fat in the renal sinus. A metastatic deposit in a left para-aortic node is present.

C, Computed tomogram, contrast material enhanced. The tumor and renal tissue enhance to a similar degree.

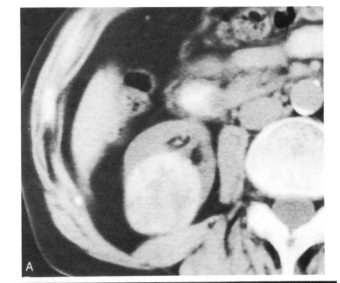

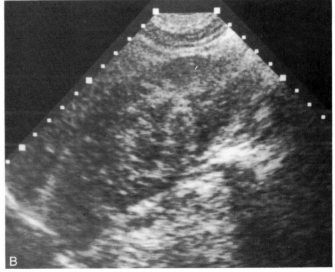

Figure 12–18. Adenocarcinoma, right kidney, with bleeding into the tumor.

A, Computed tomogram, unenhanced. The high attenuation value of the tumor represents fresh hemorrhage.

B, Ultrasonogram, longitudinal section. Most of the tumor is slightly more echogenic than the surrounding normal kidney. Some central areas of diminished echoicity are present as well.

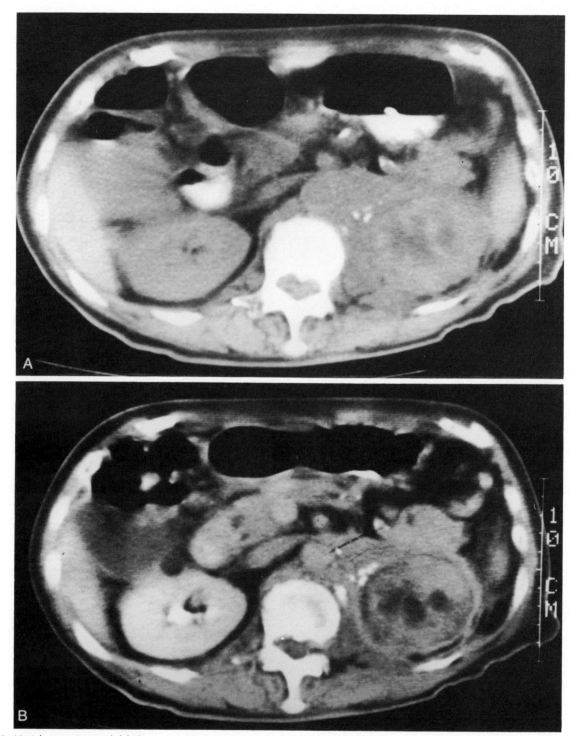

Figure 12–19. Adenocarcinoma, left kidney extending beyond the renal fascia and into regional periaortic lymph nodes.
    A, Computed tomogram, unenhanced. The tumor is composed of tissue of mixed attenuation. Low attenuation areas in the central portion of the tumor represent necrosis or old hemorrhage.
    B, Computed tomogram with contrast material enhancement better demonstrates the heterogeneous pattern of tumor enhancement.

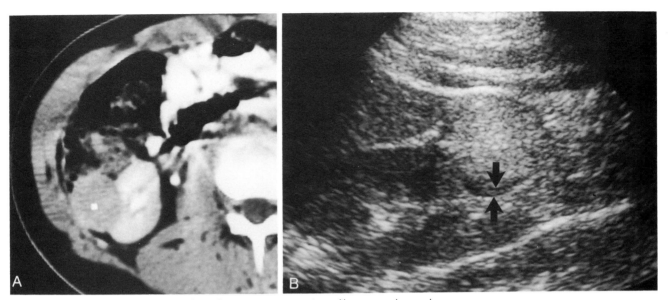

Figure 12–20. Adenocarcinoma, right kidney, demonstrating a prominent fibrous pseudocapsule.

A, Computed tomogram, contrast material enhanced. There is a faint area of relatively diminished attenuation between the tumor and the underlying renal tissue.

B, Ultrasonogram, longitudinal section. The tumor is hyperechoic relative to renal tissue. The pseudocapsule is represented by a narrow hypoechoic band at the interface between the tumor margin and adjacent kidney parenchyma *(arrows).*

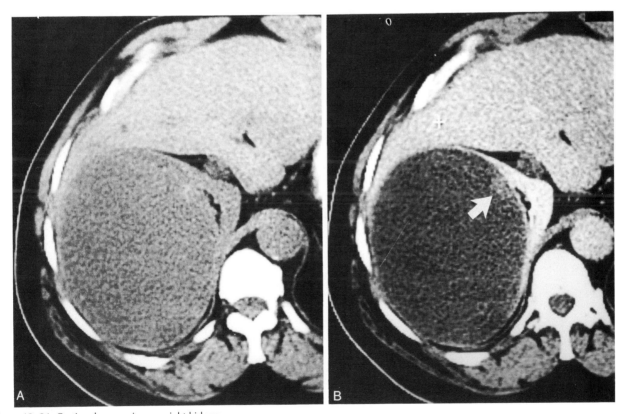

Figure 12–21. Cystic adenocarcinoma, right kidney.

A, Computed tomogram without contrast material enhancement demonstrates a tumor of homogeneous attenuation value that is less than that of renal tissue but considerable higher than that of water.

B, Computed tomogram with contrast material demonstrates enhancement of a slightly thickened wall with a mural nodule *(arrow)* becoming apparent.

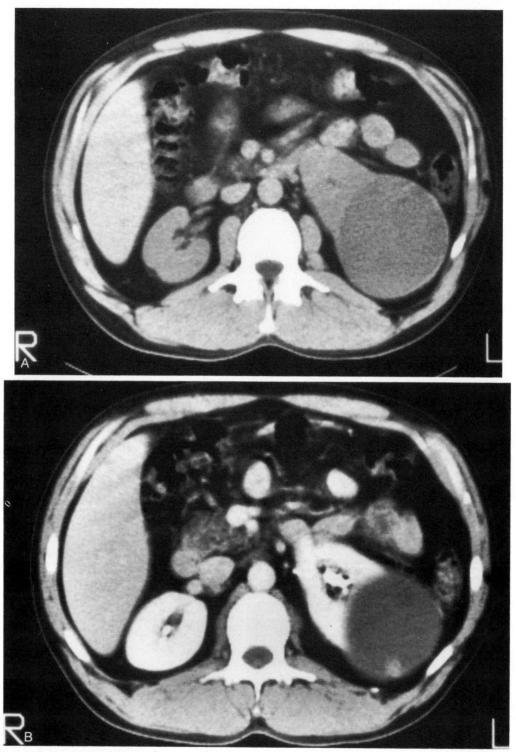

Figure 12–22. Cystic adenocarcinoma, left kidney.

   A, Computed tomogram without contrast material enhancement demonstrates an attenuation value lower than that of the renal parenchyma with a thick, slightly nodular rim.

   B, Computed tomogram with contrast material enhances the feature noted above.

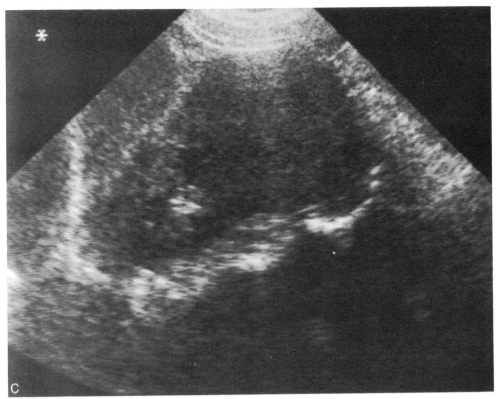

Figure 12–22 *Continued C,* Ultrasonogram, longitudinal section. Despite the "cystic" nature of the tumor, there are diffuse, low-level echoes throughout its contents.

nodules, and inhomogeneous attenuation values of the contents of the mass. Lesions other than a cystic primary or metastatic malignancy that may simulate these findings include simple cyst or pyelocalyceal diverticulum with infection or hemorrhage, abscess, hematoma, multilocular cystic nephroma, and congenital arteriovenous malformation.

The significance of the pattern and distribution of calcification in a focal mass is included in the discussion of excretory urographic findings in the preceding section. Computed tomography is the standard for detecting calcium and for characterizing its location (see Figs. 12–7 and 12–14). Calcium within a mass having an attenuation value greater than the range for water is strong evidence of malignancy, whereas a thin rim of calcification in the periphery of a mass whose contents have uniformly the attenuation value of water militates for a diagnosis of simple cyst.

Staging of malignant tumors of the kidney is best accomplished by computed tomography, particularly for detecting spread into the perirenal or pararenal spaces, extension into the renal vein or inferior vena cava, and involvement of the contralateral kidney or regional lymph nodes (Figs. 12–24 and 12–25; see also Fig. 12–19). The sensitivity of computed tomography in discovering a tumor or a thrombus in the renal vein or the inferior vena cava is similar to that of ultrasonography. However, the determination that a filling defect within these venous structures is, in fact,

a tumor rather than a clot depends on its enhancement after contrast material administration.

Computed tomography is of particular value in the initial and serial evaluation of the patient with von Hippel-Lindau disease. Multiple and bilateral cysts and adenocarcinomas of the kidneys, pheochromocytomas of the adrenal glands, and cysts of the pancreas may be present (Fig. 12–26). Similarly, computed tomography can be used for the detection of adenocarcinoma in the patient with acquired cystic disease of the kidney, as discussed in Chapter 10.

Occasionally, malignant tumors of the kidney bleed spontaneously into the subcapsular and the perirenal space. This may be the first clinical manifestation of tumor in some patients. In this situation, computed tomography readily detects the hematoma as a high-density fluid collection and usually identifies the underlying tumor, which is often small and has a cortical location.

Computed tomography is a highly reliable technique for establishing the solid or complex solid and cystic nature of a focal renal tumor and for demonstrating characteristics that suggest malignancy. There are no specific computed tomographic features that routinely permit distinction of any one particular histologic form of malignancy from another, however. Exceptions may occur, however, as in the rare demonstration of fat in a Wilms' tumor in a child. Similarly, distinction between benign and malignant tu-

Text continued on page 354

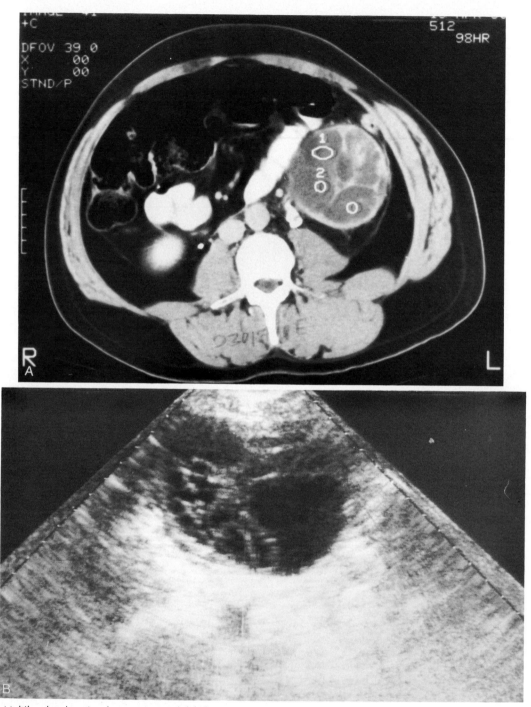

Figure 12–23. Multiloculated cystic adenocarcinoma, left kidney, containing uncomplicated fluid in the locules.

A, Computed tomogram, contrast material enhanced. The rim and septa enhance, but the attenuation value of the loculated fluid content is in the range of water (8 to 12 Hounsfield units).

B, Ultrasonogram, longitudinal section. The septa are thick, but the contents of the locules appear as uncomplicated fluid.

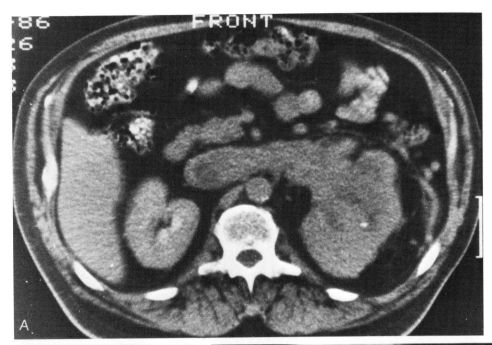

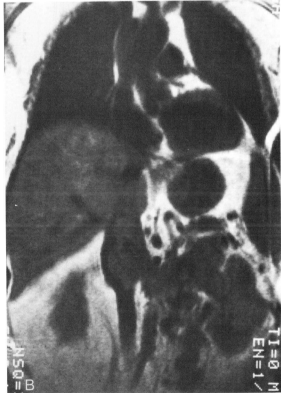

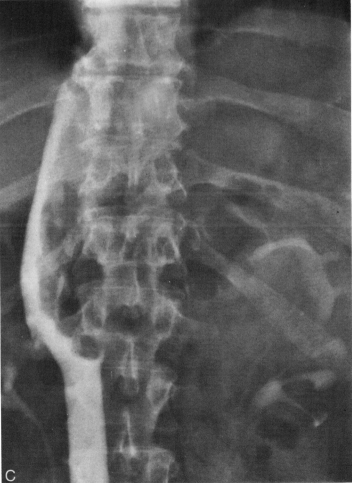

Figure 12–24. Adenocarcinoma, left kidney, with extension into renal vein and inferior vena cava.

A, Computed tomogram, contrast material enhanced. The renal vein and vena cava are enlarged and contain tumor. The same finding is demonstrated on a coronal section magnetic resonance image *(B)* and a cavogram *(C)*.

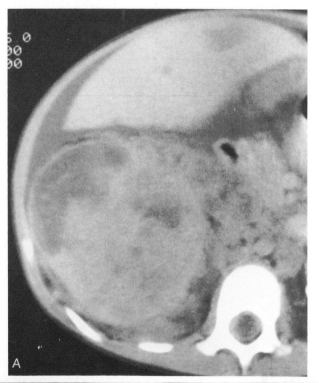

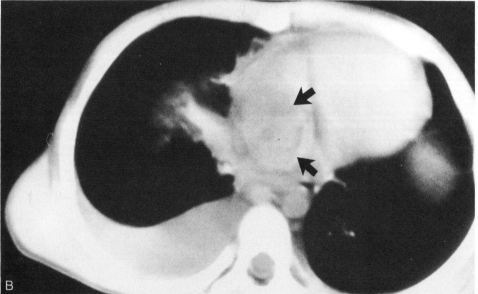

Figure 12–25. Wilms' tumor, right kidney, in a 4-year-old girl with Budd-Chiari syndrome secondary to spread of tumor to hepatic veins and the right atrium.

A, Computed tomogram with contrast material enhancement demonstrates a large tumor of mixed attenuation values with ascites.

B, Computed tomogram demonstrates tumor within the right atrium *(arrows)* as well as pleural effusion.

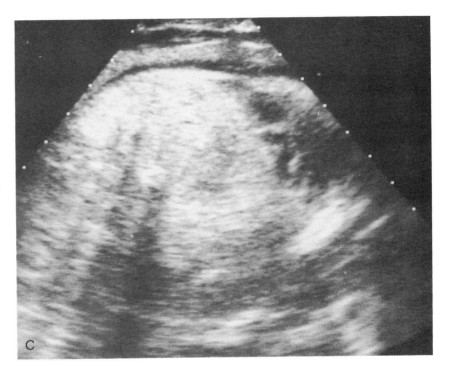

Figure 12–25 *Continued C,* Ultrasonogram, longitudinal section, demonstrates a hyperechoic pattern throughout most of the tumor.

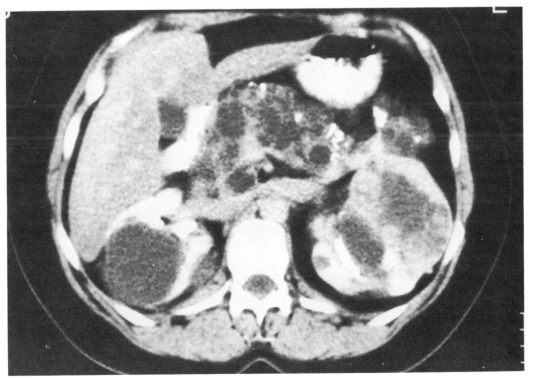

Figure 12–26. von Hippel-Lindau disease with bilateral, multiple renal adenocarcinomas and cysts as well as multiple pancreatic cysts. Computed tomogram, contrast material enhanced.

mors by computed tomographic characteristics is not feasible, except in the diagnosis of angiomyolipoma, as described in the section Benign Neoplasms, which follows.

The computed tomographic findings of nephroblastomatosis are characteristic (Fig. 12–27; see also Fig. 12–29). Multiple nodules of varying size are situated in the peripheral portions of one or both kidneys. These cause renal enlargement and create a lobulated contour. Enhancement following contrast material is absent to minimal. One or more expansile, exophytic Wilms' tumors may coexist and dominate the findings (see Fig. 12–29).

Ultrasonography. The characteristics of malignant tumors of the kidney on ultrasonography are based principally on their solid echogenic nature. The tumor margin may or may not be defined. The density of echoes produced by a solid renal mass may vary from hyperechoic to anechoic compared with renal parenchyma. Most, however, are echogenic to some degree (see Figs. 12–4, 12–5, 12–18, 12–20, 12–22, and 12–25). A solid malignant tumor that is anechoic requires distinction from a simple cyst, while one that is as echogenic as renal sinus fat simulates the appearance of angiomyolipoma.

Regardless of the echo pattern of a malignant tumor, sound transmission through a malignant tumor is impaired relative to water. As a result, malignant tumors fail to demonstrate the far wall of the tumor well and there is no acoustic enhancement beyond the lesion. Calcification within a tumor produces specular echoes and acoustic shadowing (see Fig. 12–7).

Malignant tumors that are intrinsically cystic or that have undergone cystic degeneration produce ultrasonographic images that suggest the nature of their fluid-filled components (see Figs. 12–4 and 12–23). These may vary from hypoechoic to anechoic. However, these lesions usually attenuate sound transmission more than a simple cyst does. Thus, poor far-wall enhancement and through-sound transmission in an anechoic mass militate for additional diagnostic steps, which are discussed in Chapter 25. Rarely, a cystic malignancy mimics all of the ultrasonographic features of a simple cyst.

Ultrasonography is useful in detecting renal vein enlargement, collateral venous channels in the renal hilum, and tumor or bland thrombus within the venous structures draining the kidney (Fig. 12–28). Enlargement of the renal vein may result from either occlusion or increased blood flow caused by vascular tumor. Echogenic tissue within the renal veins or inferior vena cava indicates tumor or bland thrombus in these structures.

Ultrasonography is less sensitive than computed tomography in detecting nephroblastomatosis, probably because the involved cortical tissue is sometimes isoechoic to normal renal parenchyma. Occasionally, the nephroblastomatosis nodules are hypoechoic. Ultrasonography does document well the renal enlargement and lobulated contour that are features of the nephroblastomatosis complex as well as the development of Wilms' tumor (Fig. 12–29).

Angiography. Most renal adenocarcinomas are very vascular. Common features include an enlarged renal artery, chaotically distributed intrarenal vessels of irregular size, small aneurysms, arteriovenous communications, and "lakes" of contrast material that clear slowly (Fig. 12–30). Necrosis appears as radio-

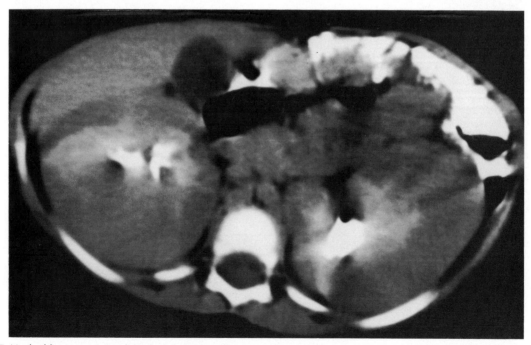

Figure 12–27. Nephroblastomatosis involving both kidneys, which are diffusely enlarged by extensive, lobulated peripheral masses that enhance minimally.

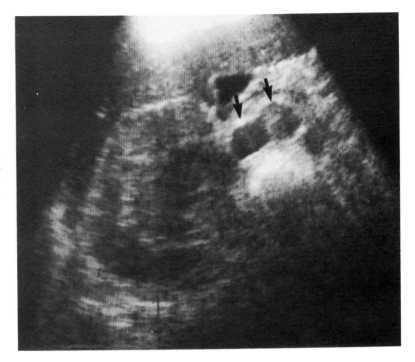

Figure 12–28. Adenocarcinoma of the right kidney extending into the renal vein and inferior vena cava *(arrows)*, both of which are enlarged and contain sound-reflecting material. Ultrasonogram, transverse section, supine.

lucent areas within the mass. The main renal vein may opacify earlier than normal owing to arteriovenous shunts. Dilated capsular veins may drain from the tumor into the main renal vein and/or into other vessels such as the intercostal, lumbar, adrenal, inferior phrenic, and gonadal veins (see Fig. 12–16). Arteries from these locations may also supply the tumor. Branches of the inferior or superior mesenteric arteries can be parasitized as tumor spreads into the mesentery.

Some adenocarcinomas are of moderate vascularity while others are hypovascular, enhance minimally during the nephrographic phase of the angiogram, and exhibit a sharp interface between tumor and adjacent normally enhanced renal parenchyma (Fig. 12–31; see also Fig. 12–5). Hypovascularity usually indicates a tumor composed of cells arranged in a papillary pattern.

Invasion of the main renal vein and inferior vena cava is common with renal adenocarcinoma and Wilms' tumor and can be established by the demonstration of a nest of arterial tumor vessels leading into the renal vein or inferior vena cava. Sometimes, linear striated capillary staining of tumor in the renal vein is seen (Fig. 12–32). Inferior vena cavography is advocated by many clinicians in the routine evaluation of patients with adenocarcinoma (see Fig. 12–24). Filling defects alone in the renal vein or inferior vena cava should not be considered conclusive evidence of venous spread of tumor, however, since propagated thrombus can produce this appearance.

Small amounts of epinephrine (5 to 10 μg) rapidly

SUMMARY OF ABNORMAL URORADIOLOGIC FINDINGS
MALIGNANT NEOPLASMS

Primary Uroradiologic Elements
    Size—large
    Contour—unifocal mass (occasional dilated capsular arteries or veins)
    Lesion distribution—unilateral
Secondary Uroradiologic Elements
    Pelvoinfundibulocalyceal system—attenuated (focal); displaced (focal); dilated (focal); replaced (focal); notched proximal ureter
    Nephrogram—replaced (focal); irregular margin; thick wall; mottled density; early density, delayed radiolucency; computed tomographic attenuation value is diminished before contrast material and enhances less than normal parenchyma
    Calcification—nonperipheral (common); peripheral (uncommon)
    Echogenicity—echogenic (common); hypoechoic (uncommon); anechoic or hyperechoic (rare); impaired through-sound transmission
    Magnetic resonance—low signal T1 (common); variable T2; enhances with contrast material

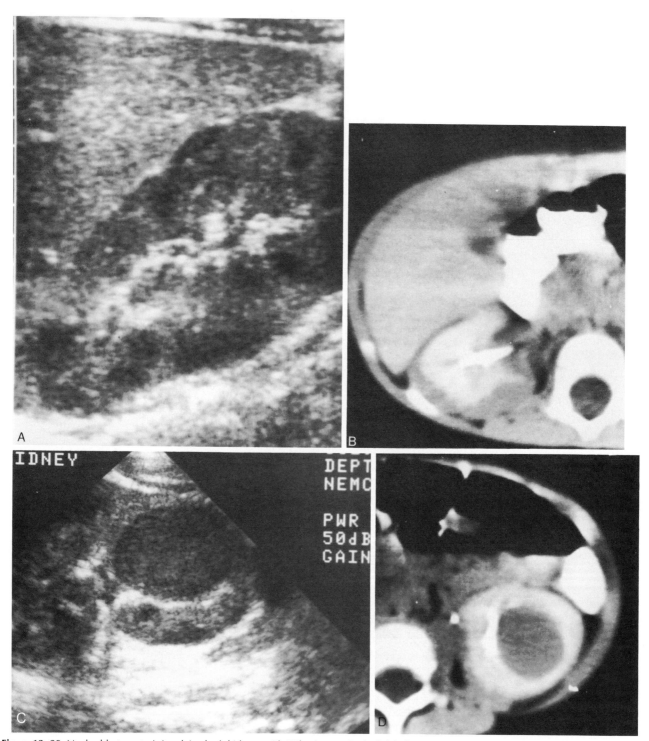

Figure 12–29. Nephroblastomatosis involving both kidneys with Wilms' tumor in the left kidney.

A, Ultrasonogram, right kidney, longitudinal section. The kidney is enlarged by the multiple, peripheral, slightly hypoechoic masses.

B, Computed tomogram with contrast material enhancement demonstrates the poorly enhancing, peripheral, lobulated tissue of nephroblastomatosis.

C, Ultrasonogram, lower pole, left kidney demonstrates expansile solid intrarenal Wilms' tumor. *D,* Computed tomogram, contrast material enhanced, lower pole of the left kidney depicts a homogeneous, poorly enhancing tumor in addition to some peripheral nephroblastomatosis.

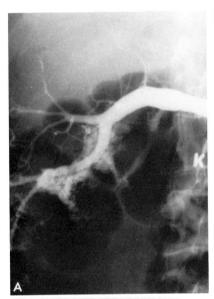

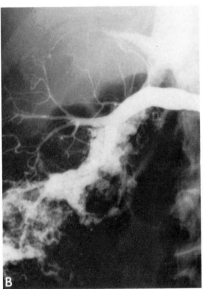

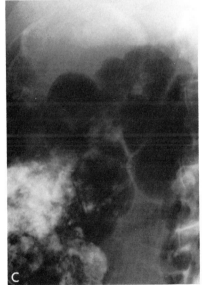

Figure 12–30. Adenocarcinoma involving the lower pole of the right kidney and causing marked hydronephrosis of the upper pole.

A and *B*, Arterial phase of selective renal arteriogram. The main renal artery is enlarged. There is rapid arteriovenous shunting into the renal veins and the inferior vena cava. The arteries to the hydronephrotic upper pole are stretched.

C, Late phase of selective renal arteriogram. "Lakes" of contrast material persist in the tumor. Thick nephrographic rims remain in the hydronephrotic upper pole.

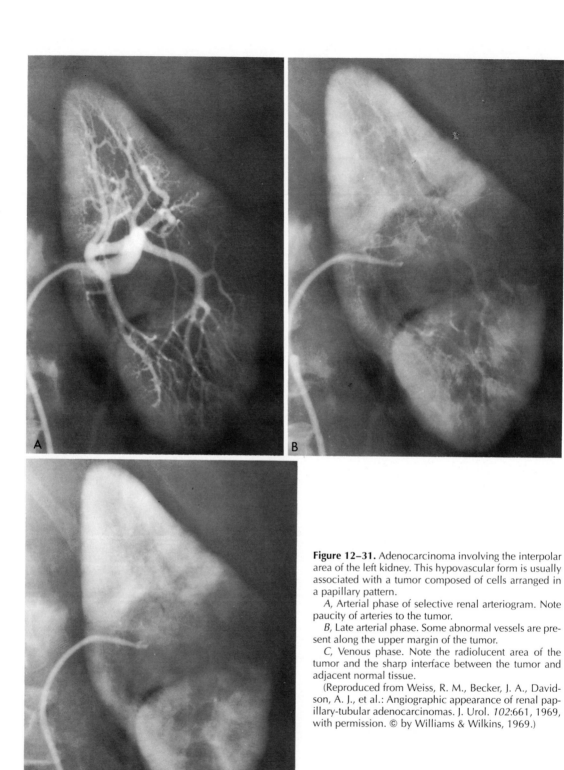

Figure 12–31. Adenocarcinoma involving the interpolar area of the left kidney. This hypovascular form is usually associated with a tumor composed of cells arranged in a papillary pattern.

A, Arterial phase of selective renal arteriogram. Note paucity of arteries to the tumor.

B, Late arterial phase. Some abnormal vessels are present along the upper margin of the tumor.

C, Venous phase. Note the radiolucent area of the tumor and the sharp interface between the tumor and adjacent normal tissue.

(Reproduced from Weiss, R. M., Becker, J. A., Davidson, A. J., et al.: Angiographic appearance of renal papillary-tubular adenocarcinomas. J. Urol. *102*:661, 1969, with permission. © by Williams & Wilkins, 1969.)

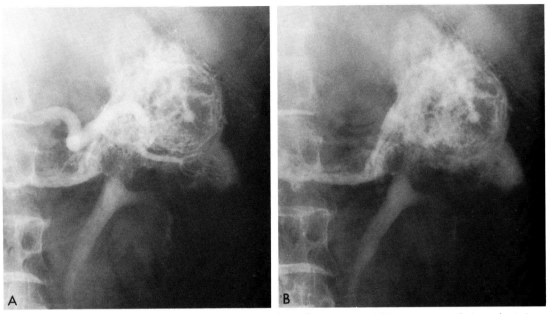

Figure 12–32. Adenocarcinoma of the kidney with invasion of the renal vein by tumor. In addition to neovascularity and arteriovenous shunts, there is linear staining of the tumor extending into the renal vein.
A, Arterial phase of selective renal arteriogram.
B, Venous phase of selective renal arteriogram.
(Same case illustrated in Fig. 12–12.)

injected into the artery of a cancer-bearing kidney causes transient contraction of normal intrarenal arteries but does not similarly affect tumor neovascularity. Contrast material injection immediately following epinephrine permits radiographic recording of this phenomenon. Failure of neovascular contraction after epinephrine is not a specific sign of cancer, however, since similar results occur in inflammatory lesions and angiomyolipoma of the kidney as well.

Wilms' tumor characteristically demonstrates moderate vascularity. The angiographic pattern of metastatic deposits in the kidney is usually similar to the vascular pattern of the primary tumor. Metastatic deposits from endocrine primary tumors, such as islet cell tumor, pheochromocytoma, and choriocarcinoma, tend to be very vascular. In general, however, angiography contributes little specific information in the diagnosis of these lesions other than confirming their solid nature by demonstrating contrast material staining during the nephrographic phase. Uroepithelial tumors that infiltrate the kidney parenchyma are also hypovascular. A fine, reticular plexus of arteries is sometimes present.

Magnetic Resonance Imaging. The information derived from magnetic resonance imaging of malignant tumors of the kidney usually duplicates that derived from computed tomography. Patterns of enhancement with gadolinium contrast material parallel those of iodinated contrast material. In selected cases, however, magnetic resonance imaging may offer special advantage for surgical planning by virtue of coronal or sagittal display of renal and retroperitoneal anatomy. This is especially applicable to situations in which the extent of venous involvement is not conclu-

sively demonstrated by computed tomography or ultrasonography.

Benign Neoplasms

Definition

Angiomyolipoma. Radiologically, the most commonly diagnosed benign kidney neoplasm is angiomyolipoma. This tumor is a hamartoma rather than a true neoplasm in that it represents excessive growth of mature fat, smooth muscle, and arteries normally present in the kidney. Hamartomas most commonly occur in tissues of ectodermal origin, such as the brain, skin, and eye. Lesions in the heart and the kidney are exceptions. A clinically apparent renal angiomyolipoma usually appears as a large tumor mass situated in one portion of the kidney. These lesions are expansile, rather than invasive, and often project into the perirenal space. At the other extreme, very small, fat-containing tumors are a common finding in the kidney at autopsy and an incidental finding on computed tomography and ultrasonography of the abdomen. These, too, are angiomyolipomas, but because of their size they cause neither symptoms nor distortion of the kidney.

Muscle and fat vary in relative amounts from one tumor to another, although most angiomyolipomas have an abundance of both tissues. Approximately 5 per cent have a fatty component that is detectable only by microscopy. Arteries found in an angiomyolipoma are characterized by an absent internal elastic membrane and a disordered adventitial cuff of smooth muscle. This is the basis for the aneurysms frequently demonstrated by arteriography. The cut surface of the tumor varies in appearance and texture, with the predominant tissue component being yellow and soft when fat is in abundance and pearl colored and firm when muscle elements are the major component. Most angiomyolipomas are very vascular. Cytologic changes of malignancy are absent.

Adenoma. An adenoma arises from tubule epithelial cells and is the benign analogue of adenocarcinoma. Adenomas usually remain small. Some pathologists classify one that has grown larger than 3 cm in diameter as adenocarcinoma, even though the cells are benign and identical in all respects to smaller lesions. Support for this practice is based on occasional cases that demonstrate a transition from benignancy to malignancy in the same lesion. Others take the position that an adenoma is benign regardless of size if all cytologic and histologic criteria for benignancy are present.

Oncocytoma. Oncocytoma, or adenoma with oncocytic features, is one type of adenoma that has received much attention in the radiologic literature. This tumor is characterized by large cells with small, uniform, round nuclei and abundant eosinophilic cytoplasm. The ultrastructural characteristic of these cells is a large number of mitochondria. Oncocytomas tend to grow to a larger size than adenomas and are usually, but not invariably, homogeneous in consistency. Calcification may occur.

Mesenchymal Tumors. Mesenchymal tissue gives rise to *juxtaglomerular cell tumor, fibroma, lipoma, myoma,* and *angioma*. The juxtaglomerular cell tumor usually distorts the contour of the kidney and always causes characteristic clinical findings, as described in the following section. Contrariwise, the other benign tumors of mesenchymal origin are usually small and do not distort either the internal architecture or the contour of the kidney. Thus, they usually escape detection during life.

A *mesoblastic nephroma* is another benign neoplasm of mesenchymal cells that is of considerable clinical importance because it is the most common solid renal mass discovered in the newborn or infant in the first few months of life. Mesoblastic nephroma is uncommonly discovered in older children and only rarely in the adult. The typical tumor is a solid, yellow-tan, unencapsulated mass that often grows large enough to replace most of the kidney parenchyma. Because the growth pattern is infiltrative, there is preservation of a reniform shape until the tumor becomes quite large. Hemorrhage and necrosis are uncommon and suggest a malignant form of this usually benign tumor.

Clinical Setting

Most angiomyolipomas are clinically silent. Discovery is usually unexpected and occurs during the investigation of the urinary tract for unrelated symptoms. Some patients present with a palpable renal mass. In others, intrarenal, subcapsular, and perirenal hemorrhage occurs and produces flank pain, hypotension, and hematuria. Angiomyolipoma is diagnosed in women more often than in men over a wide age range from young adulthood through the eighth decade. Most symptomatic angiomyolipomas occur as isolated, unifocal, unilateral kidney lesions in otherwise normal individuals. Up to 80 per cent of patients with tuberous sclerosis develop angiomyolipomas in the kidney. In these cases, involvement is usually multifocal and bilateral. Multiple, bilateral simple cysts also occur frequently in the kidneys of these patients. Other features of tuberous sclerosis include hamartomas of the face (adenoma sebaceum), fingernails, and the skin of the back as well as of the brain, eyes, bones, and heart. Epilepsy and mental retardation are frequently present. The responsible autosomal dominant gene has an incomplete expression, however, and these stigmata are not uniformly present in all patients.

Other benign tumors of the adult kidney become symptomatic when they grow large enough to cause pain or hematuria, such as with oncocytoma, or when they are metabolically active, such as with juxtaglomerular cell tumor. Here, there is an excess production of renin, causing hypertension and secondary aldosteronism, usually in young women. Severe headache and muscle weakness are noted.

Mesoblastic nephroma is usually discovered either *in utero* during an obstetric ultrasound examination or in the newborn as a large, nontender abdominal mass. Polyhydramnios is a well-recognized complication of mesoblastic nephroma developing during fetal life. This may be acute and give rise to premature labor. The size of the mass in the fetus may also cause dystocia.

Radiologic Findings

Excretory Urography. As previously mentioned, renal angiomyolipoma causes unifocal enlargement of one kidney in uncomplicated cases and bilateral, multifocal enlargement when associated with tuberous sclerosis (Fig. 12–33). One distinctive radiologic feature of this lesion is radiolucency within the mass when there is a large component of fat in the tumor (Fig. 12–34). This finding can be observed with certainty only on films obtained before administration of contrast material, since any radiolucency seen within the tumor following contrast material injection might represent necrosis or diminished perfusion in a nonhamartomatous tumor that has no fatty component. Unfortunately, fat-related radiolucency within the tumor is an infrequent radiographic observation, being reported in less than 10 per cent of patients.

Other urographic features of angiomyolipoma are the same as those of any other solid tumor, either benign or malignant, and are related to the mass effect of the lesion. These include focal collecting system attenuation and displacement or focal caliectasis due to local pressure on a draining infundibulum. Irregular obliteration of the calyces or infundibula, tumor calcification, and other signs of malignant disease, such as capsular vessels and ureteric notching, are usually not associated with benign tumors.

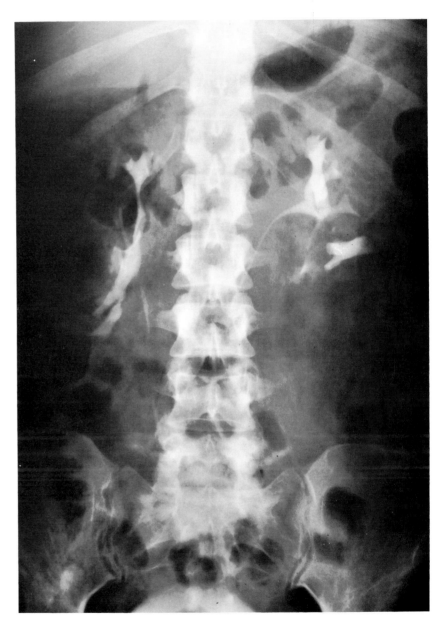

Figure 12–33. Bilateral angiomyolipomas in a patient with tuberous sclerosis. There is deformity of the pelvocalyceal system at multiple sites in both kidneys by masses that have a mottled fat radiolucency. Note also sclerotic lesions in the right iliac bone. (Courtesy of Department of Radiology, Toronto Western Hospital, Toronto, Ontario, Canada.)

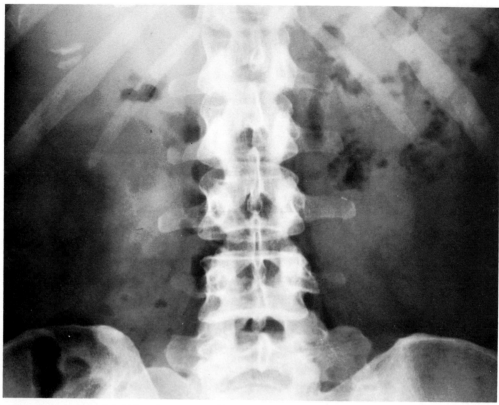

Figure 12–34. Angiomyolipoma of the right kidney in a 40-year-old woman with a palpable abdominal mass. In the right paralumbar region, there is a large, well-defined area of mottled lucency representing fat in the tumor. Preliminary film. (Courtesy of Morton Bosniak, M.D., New York University Medical Center, New York, New York.)

The urographic features of mesoblastic nephroma include a large, noncalcified mass that preserves to some extent the reniform shape of the kidney until a very large size is reached. Although the tumor may infiltrate a large portion of the kidney, excretion of contrast material is preserved to some extent. "Trapped" calyces, often seen in tumors that infiltrate rather than expand, may be present (Fig. 12–35).

Computed Tomography. Fat in a renal tumor in an adult is a finding that is virtually specific to angiomyolipoma. The demonstration of tissue with fat-equivalent negative attenuation values is the basis for the unique sensitivity of computed tomography in the detection of angiomyolipoma of the kidney (Figs. 12–36 and 12–37; see also Fig. 12–43). The fat of an angiomyolipoma is sometimes largely extrarenal and easily confused with a primary retroperitoneal tumor, such as liposarcoma. Computed tomography is valuable in this situation for detecting the nephrographic defect that indicates the true renal origin of the mass (Fig. 12–38; see also Fig. 12–43). Intermixed with the fat are muscle and blood vessels, which yield attenuation values similar to those of renal parenchyma; fresh hemorrhage, if present, is represented by higher attenuation values (Fig. 12–39). Computed tomography is also of value in documenting perinephric blood in symptomatic patients (see Fig. 12–43). If fat is not detectable in an angiomyolipoma, as is estimated to occur in 5 per cent of cases, the computed tomo-

graphic findings are those of other solid tumors, either benign or malignant (Fig. 12–40).

A benign tumor in the adult, other than angiomyolipoma, is likely to appear on computed tomography as a focal ball-shaped mass that is sharply marginated by a relatively low attenuating pseudocapsule. A smooth contour and a homogeneous internal structure are additional common features. Many of these are isodense or very slightly less dense than normal renal tissue. Contrast material enhancement is usually homogeneous and less than that of the surrounding kidney parenchyma. These features, while common to all adult benign tumors, are nonspecific. In oncocytomas, a central, clearly defined stellate area of low attenuation is sometimes present and representative of ischemic fibrosis (Fig. 12–41). This pattern overlaps the appearance of some adenocarcinomas, however, and cannot be used as a reliable indicator for the diagnosis of oncocytoma.

Mesoblastic nephroma is characteristically large and of homogeneous attenuation both before and after contrast enhancement (Fig. 12–42). Low density areas of necrosis or cyst formation are uncommon.

Ultrasonography. The fat in angiomyolipoma produces an ultrasonographic image of a mass whose echo intensity is equal to or greater than that of perirenal fat (Fig. 12–43; see also Fig. 12–36). These may be present within a large mass or appear as isolated foci of echogenicity in an otherwise normal kidney in

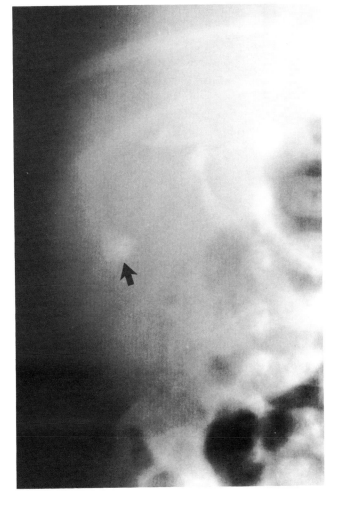

Figure 12–35. Mesoblastic nephroma involving the lower two-thirds of the right kidney. The reniform or bean shape of the kidney is preserved, and enhancement is diminished. An isolated, dilated calyx is "trapped" by the infiltrating tumor *(arrow)*.

which there is one or more tiny asymptomatic angiomyolipomas. However, this finding does not apply to all angiomyolipomas. When the fatty component is minimal, or when hemorrhage has occurred, the echo pattern has a mixed or diminished intensity. The ultrasonographic finding of a highly echogenic renal mass is not specific to angiomyolipoma, since adenocarcinoma may yield an identical image. In other respects, the ultrasonic image of an angiomyolipoma reveals a solid mass that attenuates sound and prevents both far-wall enhancement and through-sound transmission. As described previously, most of the mass may be extrarenal and give the impression of a retroperitoneal soft tissue origin rather than a renal origin.

Ultrasonography in benign tumors in the adult other than angiomyolipoma shows a solid mass composed of homogeneous tissue (see Fig. 12–41). Low-level echoes similar to those of renal tissue, a poorly defined far wall, and sound attenuation indicate only the presence of a solid mass that is indistinguishable from a malignant tumor.

Mesoblastic nephroma is usually evenly echogenic with low-level echoes (Fig. 12–44). The reniform shape of the enlarged kidney is best demonstrated by longitudinal scans, but this feature may not be appar-

ent in very large tumors. Hemorrhage, necrosis, and cyst formation are seen as focal hypoechoic areas with a larger echogenic mass. *In utero*, the tumor is readily detected in the fetal abdomen and is sometimes associated with polyhydramnios (see Fig. 12–42).

Angiography. There are no angiographic features of angiomyolipoma that permit a specific diagnosis. As might be expected from their histology, these tumors are quite vascular. Distinctive features include one dominant feeding artery with a circumferential arrangement of vessels around the tumor and multiple aneurysms of medium-sized arteries that pool contrast material (see Figs. 12–36, 12–38, and 12–40). Arteriovenous shunts are very uncommon. Any of these angiographic features may be seen in renal adenocarcinoma as well as in angiomyolipoma. Similarly, the abnormal arteries of angiomyolipoma may fail to contract following injection of epinephrine.

Oncocytoma is usually a vascular, encapsulated mass that often has a homogeneous nephrogram and occasional neovascularity. There is no characteristic arrangement of the feeding arteries that distinguishes this tumor from others that are benign or malignant. However, in common with other benign tumors, arterial encasement and venous shunting are usually absent.

Text continued on page 371

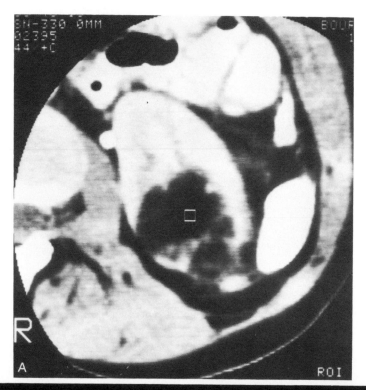

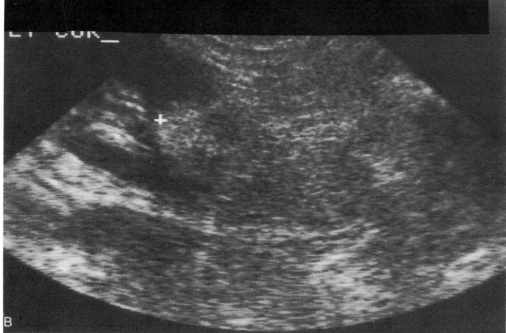

Figure 12–36. Angiomyolipoma, left kidney.

A, Computed tomogram, contrast material enhanced. The mass is composed of fat identified by negative attenuation values. The intrarenal origin of the mass is indicated by the "beak" sign.

B, Ultrasonogram, longitudinal section. The angiomyolipoma, which extends from within the lower pole of the kidney, fills the perirenal space and produces a homogeneous pattern of moderate echo intensity.

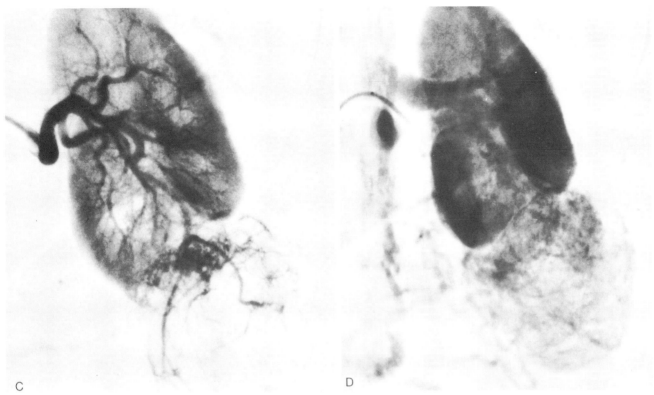

C   D

Figure 12–36 *Continued C* and *D,* Selective renal arteriogram, arterial and nephrographic phases. A single artery serves the angiomyolipoma. The vascularity is moderate, and aneurysm formation is minimal.

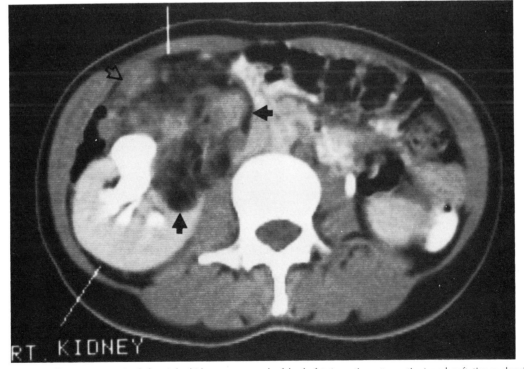

Figure 12–37. Angiomyolipoma *(arrows)* of the right kidney composed of both fat (negative attenuation) and soft tissue density. Computed tomogram, contrast material enhanced. (Courtesy of Gladys Lo, M.D., Santa Clara, California.)

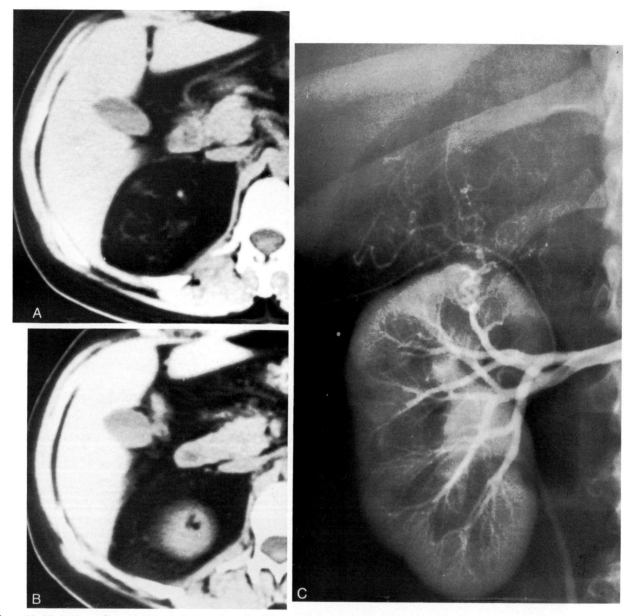

Figure 12–38. Angiomyolipoma arising in the superior pole of the right kidney. Almost all of the mass *is* extrarenal.

A, Computed tomogram with contrast material enhancement of right suprarenal area. A fat-containing tumor fills the perirenal space.

B, Computed tomogram with contrast material enhancement at level of most superior tip of the upper pole of the kidney. The nephrogram is disrupted by fatty tissue representing the site of origin of the angiomyolipoma within the renal parenchyma.

C, Selective renal arteriogram demonstrates the artery to the upper pole that supplies the angiomyolipoma.

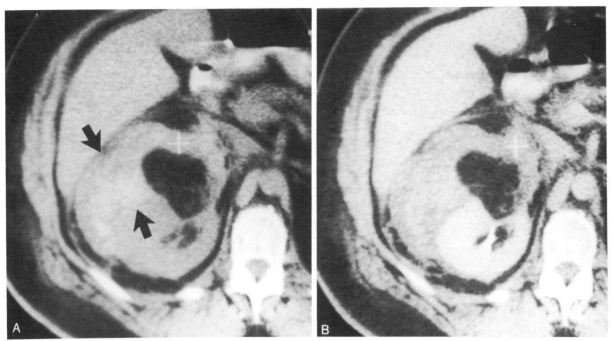

Figure 12–39. Angiomyolipoma, right kidney, with fresh hemorrhage into the adjacent perirenal space. Computed tomogram.

A, Unenhanced scan demonstrates fresh blood in the perirenal space as slightly higher attenuation tissue *(arrows)* than the renal parenchyma. The fat component of the angiomyolipoma projects into the hematoma.

B, Scan at the same level as *A* after contrast material enhancement.

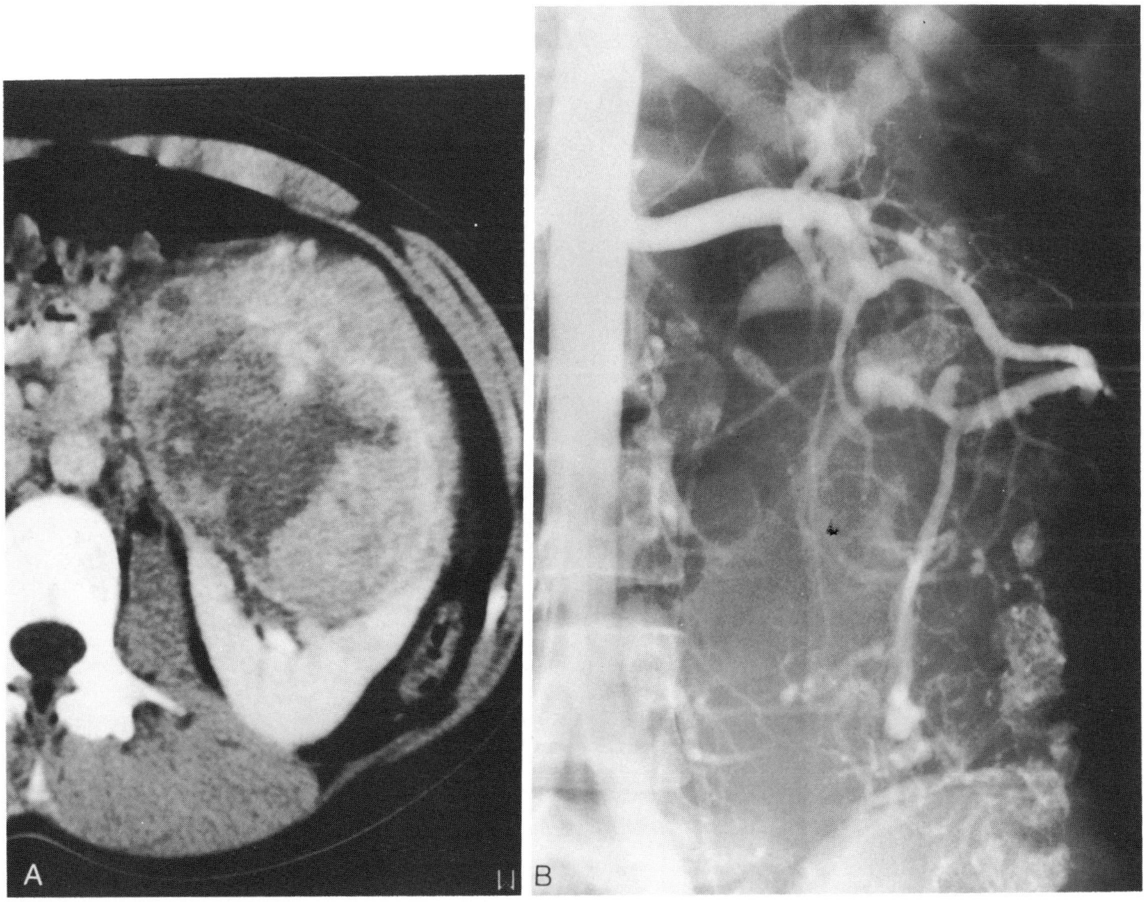

Figure 12–40. Angiomyolipoma of the left kidney with no fat detected by computed tomography.

A, Computed tomogram, contrast material enhanced. Representative section. The mass is of mixed attenuation values, but no fat was detected on contiguous thin slices throughout the lesion. The "beak" sign indicates an intrarenal origin.

B, Aortogram. A single large artery with focal aneurysms perfuses the angiomyolipoma.

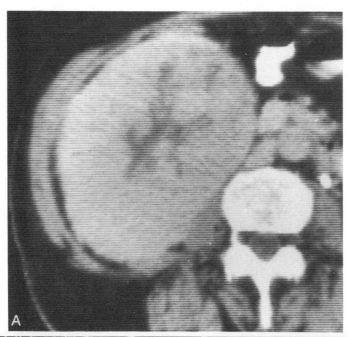

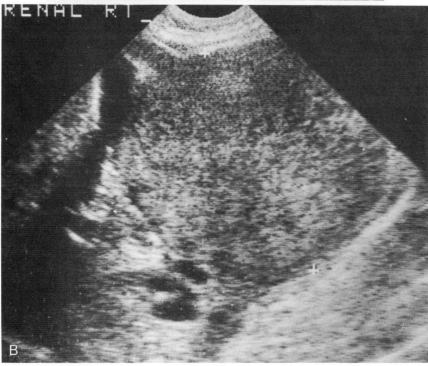

Figure 12–41. Oncocytoma, right kidney.

A, Computed tomogram, contrast material enhanced. The tumor is a ball-shaped, expansile mass of homogeneous density except for some low attenuation areas, the dominant one being central and stellate but others being peripheral and punctate. These represent ischemic and fibrotic portions of the tumor.

B, Ultrasonogram, longitudinal section. The oncocytoma produces an image of an expansile, ball-shaped mass of uniform echogenicity.

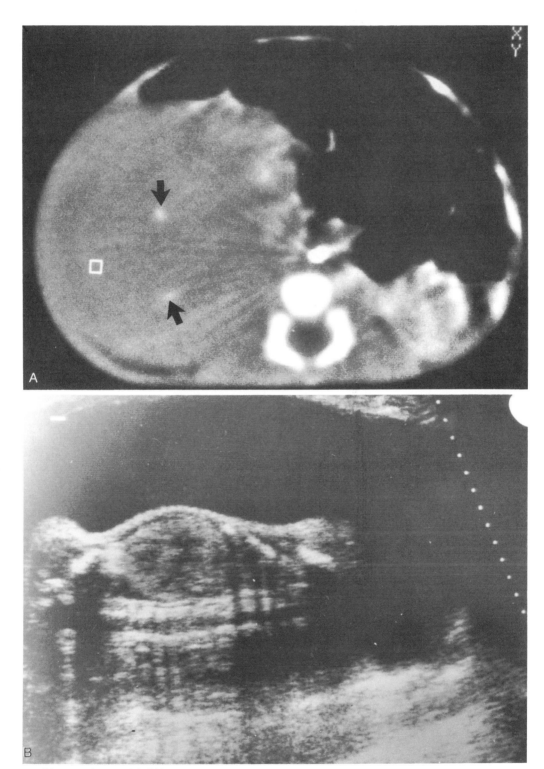

Figure 12–42. Mesoblastic nephroma, right kidney.
A, Computed tomogram, contrast material enhanced. The tumor is of homogeneous density. Two small enhanced structures *(arrows)* are seen within the mass. These represent dilated calyces "trapped" by the infiltrating neoplastic cells.
B, Prenatal ultrasonogram. A large homogeneous echogenic tumor fills the abdomen of the fetus. Polyhydramnios is present.

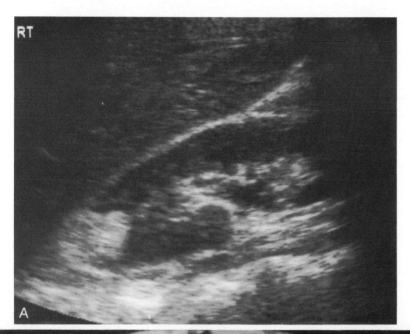

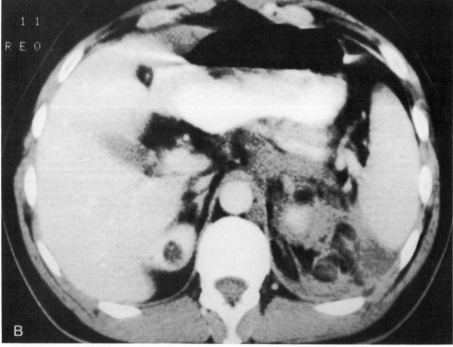

Figure 12–43. Angiomyolipoma, right kidney in a patient with tuberous sclerosis.

A, Ultrasonogram, longitudinal section. The lesion occupies the upper pole and is seen as a round, sharply marginated mass with an echogenicity equal to or slightly more than the adjacent perirenal fat.

B, Computed tomogram, contrast material enhanced. A small, fatty mass is present in the upper pole of the kidney. Perirenal blood is present in the opposite side from hemorrhage of an angiomyolipoma of the left kidney.

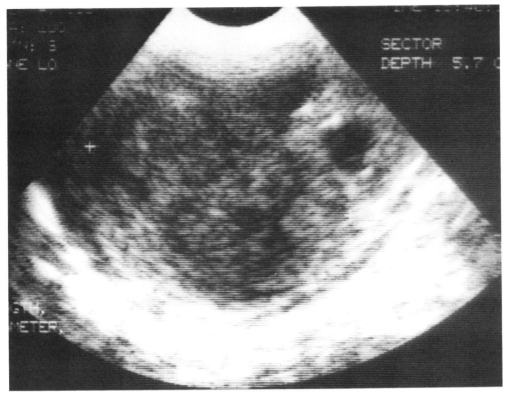

Figure 12–44. Mesoblastic nephroma, left kidney. Ultrasonogram, longitudinal section. The tumor produces a uniform pattern of echoes.

SUMMARY OF ABNORMAL URORADIOLOGIC FINDINGS
BENIGN NEOPLASMS

Preliminary Film
   Fat lucency in angiomyolipoma (uncommon)
Primary Uroradiologic Elements
   Size—large
   Contour—unifocal mass (may be multifocal with angiomyolipomas in tuberous sclerosis)
   Lesion distribution—unilateral (may be bilateral with angiomyolipomas in tuberous sclerosis)
Secondary Uroradiologic Elements
   Pelvoinfundibulocalyceal system—attenuated (focal); displaced (focal); dilated (focal)
   Nephrogram—diminished enhancement (focal); computed tomographic attenuation value is nega-
      tive (angiomyolipoma); diminished before contrast material; enhances less than normal paren-
      chyma; homogeneous (benign tumor other than angiomyolipoma)
   Echogenicity—focal hyperechoic (angiomyolipoma); echoic (benign tumor other than angiomyoli-
      poma); impaired through-sound transmission

Benign neoplasms of the kidney other than angiomyolipoma and oncocytoma are usually hypovascular. This characterization applies to juxtaglomerular cell tumor, as well. Angiography contributes little specific information in the diagnosis of these lesions other than confirming their solid nature, which is information that is more readily derived from ultrasonography or computed tomography.

FLUID-FILLED MASSES

Simple Renal Cyst

Definition

Simple parenchymal cyst is the most common unifocal mass of the kidney. With modern cross-sectional imaging, it is likely that radiologic detection approaches the true prevalence of simple cyst, which is certainly much higher than the historical estimate of 3 to 5 per cent based on autopsy studies.

The pathogenesis of renal cysts has not been conclusively established. It is clear that these are acquired lesions, however, since cysts are uncommonly present in children and increase in frequency with age. Obstruction of a renal tubule has been the generally accepted explanation, but the possibility that these develop as a result of blockage and expansion of a calyceal diverticulum has also been considered.

Simple cysts are lined with low cuboidal or flattened epithelium. The wall is composed of fibrous tissue and compressed nephrons and is only 1 to 2 mm thick in those portions that do not abut normal parenchyma. A variant form of simple fluid-filled cyst is frequently found in kidneys of patients with tuberous sclerosis, in addition to angiomyolipomas. These cysts are lined with hyperplastic columnar cells that resemble the epithelial cells of the proximal tubule. In both macroscopic and radiologic appearance, however, the cyst of tuberous sclerosis is indistinguishable from the common form of simple cyst. Multiple cysts are also associated with von Hippel-Lindau disease, neurofibromatosis, and Caroli's disease. The cysts found in von Hippel-Lindau disease are distinctive in that they are lined by hyperplastic or neoplastic cells, which may give rise to adenocarcinoma.

Simple renal cysts occur most often in the renal cortex and usually expand outward, causing a bulge on the kidney surface. When observed directly, a bluish coloration underlies the thin, glistening membrane, which is the cyst wall. This appearance explains the description of these lesions as "blue domed." Cysts vary in size and occur at single or multiple sites in one or both kidneys. The majority are reported to occur in the polar regions, particularly in the lower pole. In most cases, the cyst contains a single cavity. In some instances, thin septa divide the cyst into chambers, which may or may not communicate with each other.

The fluid within a cyst is serous, not urine, clear, and slightly yellow and has a specific gravity of 1.002 to 1.010. Small amounts of protein, urea, chlorides, and sugar are present. Lactic dehydrogenase content is considerably lower than that of serum, a finding of potential importance in the chemical evaluation of cyst aspirate. Fluid from a simple cyst should be cell free and contain little or no fat or cholesterol. If a cyst becomes infected, or if bleeding into the cyst occurs, the nature of the fluid changes accordingly. The cyst wall tends to thicken under these circumstances.

The occurrence of adenocarcinoma within the wall of a simple cyst has been the subject of a few isolated case reports. This is in contradistinction to adenocarcinoma that develops intrinsically as a cyst *de novo* or in association with von Hippel-Lindau disease, as discussed in the previous section Malignant Neoplasms. Adenocarcinoma within a cyst wall is very rare but, nevertheless, is always of concern. Much more common, on the other hand, is the coexistence of adenocarcinoma and cyst in the same kidney. This occurred in approximately 0.1 per cent of patients with carcinoma of the kidney in one large series (Emmett et al., 1963), but this figure is probably too conservative. Although the occurrence of adenocarcinoma and simple cyst in the same kidney is undoubtedly a chance relationship, these data emphasize the need for caution in ascribing a given set of urinary tract symptoms to a simple cyst discovered at urography.

The presence of several simple cysts in one or both kidneys is common. Rarely, multiple simple cysts involve only one kidney. These cases are sometimes misdiagnosed as unilateral autosomal dominant polycystic kidney disease. This diagnosis is a contradiction of terms, because by definition autosomal dominant polycystic kidney disease is always bilateral, although sometimes asymmetric. Careful recording of family history, evaluation of renal function, and search for cysts in other organs are sometimes required to differentiate multiple simple cysts in both kidneys from autosomal dominant polycystic kidney disease.

Rarely, multiple simple cysts are localized to one portion of one kidney. This cluster of cysts is not encapsulated, and there is normal renal parenchyma between the cysts on microscopic examination.

Clinical Setting

Development of simple renal cyst is very uncommon in individuals younger than age 30, but cyst formation does increase with age. Both sexes are affected equally. Most cysts grow slowly over a few years, although occasionally rapid growth can be noted. Cysts usually do not cause symptoms. If numerous or large, they may decrease renal function or produce pain. Rarely, simple cysts have caused hypertension, presumably from ischemia of compressed adjacent tissue. Cysts may rupture into the pelvocalyceal system and cause flank pain and hematuria. When this occurs, the cyst is converted into a smooth-walled cavity that communicates with the collecting system.

Radiologic Findings

Excretory Urography. Because renal cysts are usually cortical, they commonly produce focal contour expansion of the kidney outline. Calcification occurs in only 3 per cent of all cysts (Fig. 12–45). When present, it is curvilinear and thin and is deposited only along the periphery of the lesion. In one series based on film radiography (Daniel et al., 1972), 80 per cent of all kidney masses with peripheral, curvilinear calcification were simple cysts. The remaining 20 per cent were adenocarcinomas (see Fig. 12–14). These data emphasize the need for extreme caution in relying too much on a pattern of peripheral curvilinear calcification alone as a sign of benign status.

Several urographic features are characteristic of simple cyst. The nephrogram is always absent because the cyst is avascular and its fluid content, uninfluenced by glomerular filtration, does not accumulate contrast material. The interface between the cyst and the adjacent renal parenchyma is sharply defined and smooth. A 1- to 2-mm rim of tissue is opacified where the cyst protrudes beyond the confines of the kidney (Fig. 12–46). This finding, the "thin rim" sign, is due to the accumulation of contrast material in compressed nephrons and in the small vessels of the fibrous tissue portion of the capsule. The normal cortex at the margin of a slowly expanding and protruding cyst is deflected outward. This is seen in profile as an angular-shaped extension of normally dense renal tissue at the point where the cyst extends beyond the renal surface (see Fig. 12–46). This urographic finding,

the "beak" or "claw" sign, reflects slow expansion of an intrarenal mass, and it may be seen in any slow growing solid lesion, including adenocarcinoma.

When a simple cyst is completely embedded in the kidney parenchyma, the "thin rim" and "beak" signs are absent. Renal size and contour are normal. In addition, the nephrographic radiolucency of the cyst may be obscured by contrast material in parenchyma surrounding the cyst. Here, the diagnosis of simple cyst is suggested by smooth displacement of the collecting system and by tomographic definition of sharply marginated nephrographic radiolucency (Fig. 12–47).

A renal cyst causes focal displacement of adjacent portions of the pelvoinfundibulocalyceal system. The displaced, attenuated collecting structure remains smooth in contradistinction to the shagginess and obliteration that often occur when focal displacement is due to a malignant neoplasm.

Computed Tomography. A simple cyst has a homogeneous water density and a sharply demarcated margin (Fig. 12–48). The wall is either imperceptible or just barely perceptible where the cyst projects beyond the confines of the kidney. Thin septations may be identified within the cyst. Contrast material does not alter the attenuation value of the contents of a simple cyst.

Errors in the computed tomographic diagnosis of

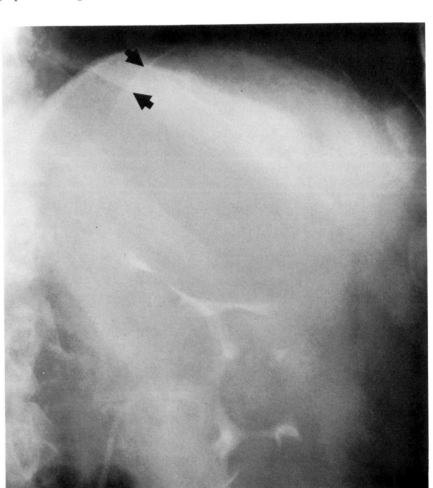

Figure 12–45. Simple cyst. Curvilinear, peripheral calcification outlines part of the cyst wall *(arrows)*. There is smooth splaying of the upper pole calyces. Excretory urogram.

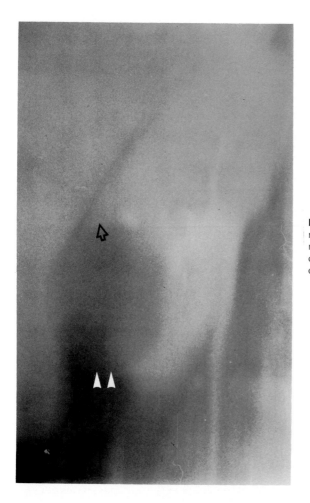

Figure 12–46. Simple cyst in the lateral portion of the lower pole. The cyst does not enhance, and there is a sharp interface between the cyst and the adjacent renal parenchyma. A "thin rim" is present along the inferior free margin of the cyst *(closed arrows)*. A "beak" sign is noted at the superior interface between the cyst and the parenchyma *(open arrow)*.

simple cyst are usually the result of partial volume averaging in very small cysts (less than 1 cm diameter) or by those that are both small and completely intrarenal. Another cause for error is the misleading impression of a thick wall that occurs when the parenchymal beak is included in the transverse cross section of the cyst (Fig. 12–49). Other sources of potential error are confusion with pyelocalyceal diverticula that have become noncommunicating, as discussed in Chapter 15.

The contents of a cyst that becomes infected or hemorrhagic produce attenuation values higher than those of water (Fig. 12–50). The density of a hemorrhagic cyst, in fact, may be the same as or greater than that of renal parenchyma on unenhanced scans (Fig. 12–51). The hyperdense cyst, therefore, may be inapparent on enhanced scans or misinterpreted as a solid mass (Fig. 12–52). Thickening of the wall of an infected or hemorrhagic cyst is also seen with computed tomography (see Fig. 12–50).

Computed tomography provides a precise display of the anatomy of a simple cyst. A conclusive computed tomographic diagnosis of simple cyst demands adherence to strict criteria. Variants such as thick mural calcification, mural nodule, thickened or irregular septation or wall, an attenuation value greater than water, and enhancement after contrast material de-

mand special considerations, which are discussed in Chapter 25.

Ultrasonography. The ultrasonographic characteristics of a simple cyst are a well-defined, smooth, anechoic mass with far-wall enhancement and increased through-sound transmission (Fig. 12–53). Each of these criteria must be fulfilled to establish a confident diagnosis by ultrasonography. Thin septa may be present (see Fig. 12–53). Small-sized cysts, cysts located in the upper pole of the left kidney, mural calcification, improper technical settings, and internal septa are factors that may degrade the ultrasound image and lead to a misdiagnosis. Infection and hemorrhage within a simple cyst usually cause internal echoes, fluid–debris level, or impaired through-sound transmission (Figs. 12–54 and 12–55; see also Fig. 12–50). The implications of these results are discussed in Chapter 25.

Magnetic Resonance. A simple cyst is of homogeneous low signal intensity on T1-weighted images and of high signal intensity on T2-weighted images. The cyst wall is smooth and sharply defined from adjacent renal parenchyma. There is no unique value intrinsic to magnetic resonance imaging in the evaluation of a cyst.

Cystography. Cyst contents can be removed by percutaneous needle aspiration and replaced with radi-

Text continued on page 382

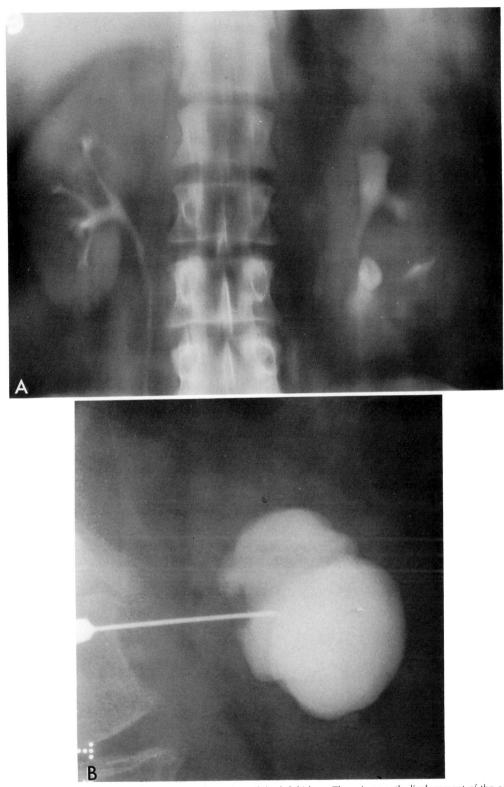

Figure 12–47. Simple cyst deeply embedded in the interpolar region of the left kidney. There is smooth displacement of the adjacent pelvis and calyces.

A, Excretory urogram. Tomogram.

B, Cystogram following needle puncture.

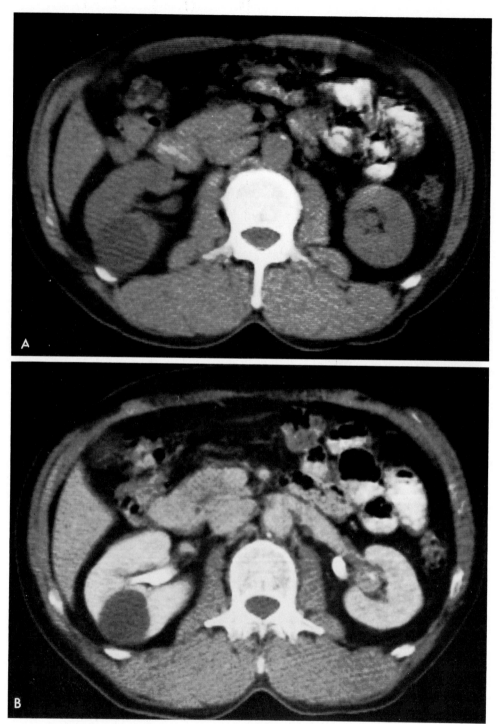

Figure 12–48. Simple cyst of the right kidney.

    A, Computed tomogram, unenhanced. The wall is smooth, and the contents have the same density as water.

    B, Computed tomogram, contrast material enhanced. The contents of the cyst do not enhance. Note the transitional cell carcinoma of the left renal pelvis.

    (Courtesy of Joy Price, M.D., Alta Bates Medical Center, Berkeley, California.)

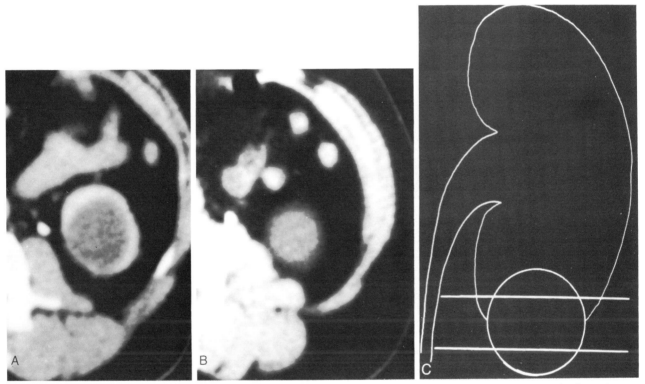

Figure 12–49. Spurious finding of a thick wall in an uncomplicated simple cyst. Computed tomograms, contrast material enhanced.
  A, The normally enhanced parenchyma surrounding the cyst simulates a thick wall.
  B, Section at a more caudal level than *A* demonstrates no visible wall surrounding the unenhanced cyst.
  C, Diagram of the level of sections *A* and *B*.

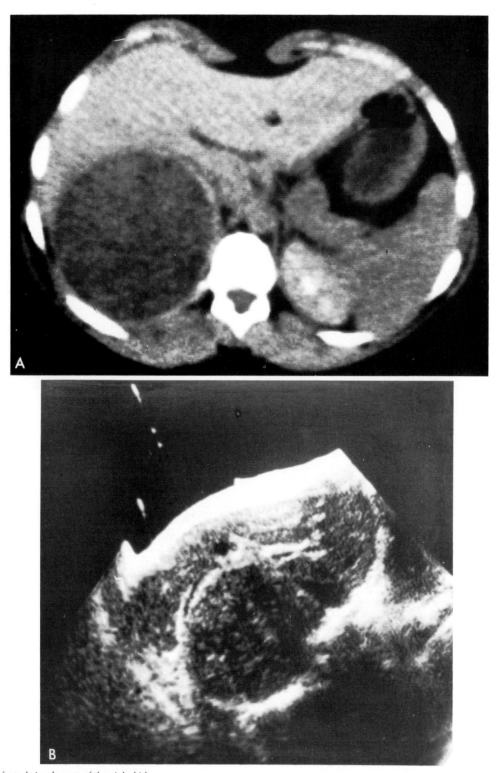

Figure 12–50. Infected simple cyst of the right kidney.
  A, Computed tomogram, contrast material enhanced. The contents of the cyst have a higher attenuation value than water and are slightly heterogeneous. Note the thickened cyst wall.
  B, Ultrasonogram, transverse section. Diffuse echogenicity is present, and there is a lack of increased through-transmission of sound. (Courtesy of César Pedrosa, M.D., and E. Ramirez, Hospital Clinico de San Carlos, Madrid, Spain.)

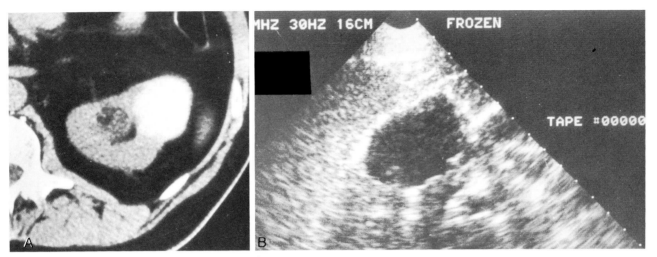

Figure 12–51. Hyperdense cyst in an asymptomatic male.
A, Computed tomogram, unenhanced. A homogeneous mass with well-defined borders is hyperdense compared with the renal parenchyma.
B, Ultrasonogram demonstrates internal echoes, a poorly defined far wall and impaired through-sound transmission.
(Kindly provided by Edward M. Meesing, M.D., and Stan L. Weiss, M.D., University of Wisconsin, Madison, Wisconsin.)

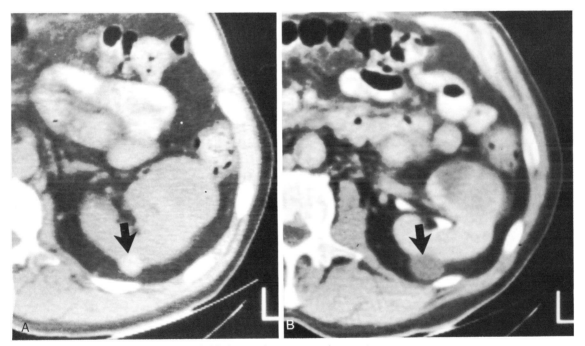

Figure 12–52. Hyperdense cyst due to hemorrhage, left kidney with coexisting adenocarcinoma.
A, Computed tomogram without contrast enhancement demonstrates a small mass *(arrow)* on the dorsal surface of the kidney.
B, Computed tomogram, contrast material enhanced. The mass *(arrow)* is hypodense relative to the renal parenchyma and simulates the appearance of a solid tumor.
(Courtesy of Steven Sussman, M.D., Durham, North Carolina.)

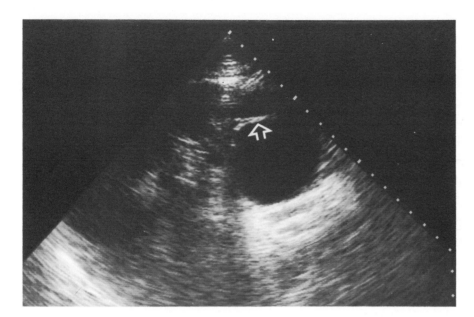

Figure 12–53. Simple cyst of the kidney demonstrating anechoicity, a well-defined far wall, and increased through-sound transmission. A thin septum is also present (*arrow*).

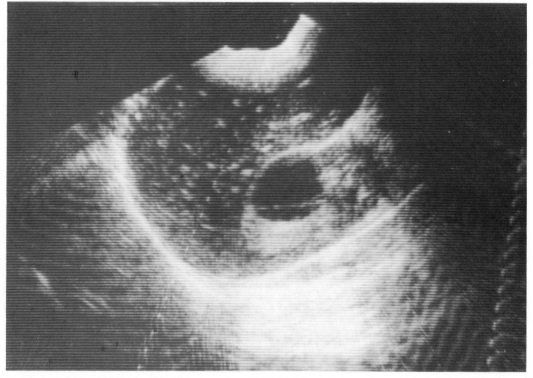

Figure 12–54. Simple cyst of the right kidney with infection, causing a fluid-debris level. Enhanced sound transmission is preserved. Ultrasonogram, longitudinal section.

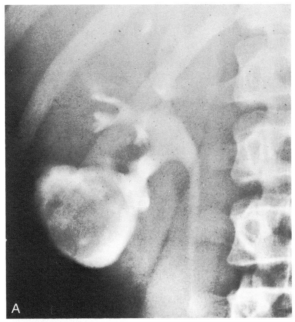

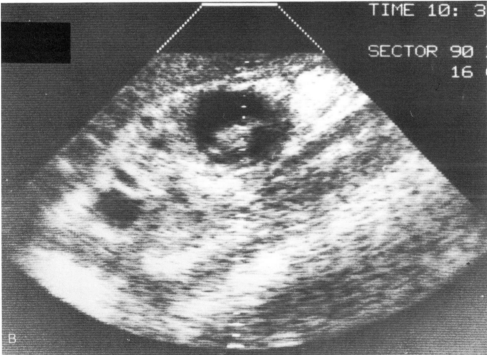

Figure 12–55. Chronic hemorrhagic cyst communicating with the pelvocalyceal system.
   A, Excretory urogram. Opacification of the cyst during the course of the study reveals a large filling defect that represented an organized blood clot.
   B, Ultrasonogram, longitudinal section. The echogenic clot within the anechoic cyst is in a dependent position.

SUMMARY OF ABNORMAL URORADIOLOGIC FINDINGS
SIMPLE RENAL CYST

Primary Uroradiologic Elements
    Size—large (when peripheral)
    Contour—unifocal mass (when peripheral)
    Lesion distribution—unilateral
Secondary Uroradiologic Elements
    Pelvoinfundibulocalyceal system—attenuated (focal); displaced (focal)
    Nephrogram—replaced (focal); smooth margin; "thin rim" sign when peripheral; "beak" sign when
       peripheral; attenuation value of water
    Calcification—uncommon; curvilinear; peripheral
    Echogenicity—anechoic; far-wall enhancement; through-sound transmission enhanced
    Cystography—smooth internal walls; clear aspirate

---

opaque contrast material or air or both (see Fig. 12–47). Complete cystography requires the study of all aspects of the cyst, either by serial computed tomographic images or by multiple radiographic projections, including horizontal beam films. All walls should be smooth and the septations thin. The aspirate from a simple cyst is clear, yellow, and free of abnormal cells. The role of cystography in the evaluation of atypical fluid-filled masses is discussed further in Chapter 25.

Angiography. Angiography demonstrates the avascular nature of simple cysts. The nephrographic defect and "beak" and "thin rim" signs are shown to better advantage than with urography because of the higher dose of contrast material administered to the kidney in a short time span. Angiography also demonstrates smooth displacement of arteries around cysts embedded deep within the kidney substance. Neovascularity, abnormal stains within the mass, early venous opacification, and pericapsular draining veins are not features of simple cysts.

The angiographic study of an infected cyst may demonstrate a hypervascular rim, neovascularity, an indistinct interface between the cyst and the adjacent renal parenchyma, or a prominent capsular artery. These findings are indistinguishable from those associated with malignant neoplasm or other forms of inflammatory disease of the kidney.

Focal Hydronephrosis

Definition

When the drainage of one portion of the kidney is obstructed, regional hydronephrosis and focal renal enlargement may develop. Overall, focal hydronephrosis is most commonly found in children with complete ureteropelvic duplication and an ectopic insertion of the ureter with or without a complicating ureterocele. In the adult, as well as in the child, obstruction may be due to a congenital cause or the result of infection, particularly tuberculosis with infundibular stenosis. Calculus and tumor obstructing an infundibulum are additional causes. Less frequent,

but still worth mentioning, is congenital ureteropelvic junction obstruction of the lower moiety of a duplicated collecting system.

Clinical Setting

Focal hydronephrosis is usually asymptomatic. Symptoms, if present, may be limited to vague abdominal or flank pain or be due to infection complicating the obstruction. A renal mass might be palpable, but this is more likely to be found in children. Focal hydronephrosis is often detected *in utero* during the course of obstetric ultrasound examination.

Radiologic Findings

Excretory Urography. Increased renal length and a localized bulge in contour are produced by focal hydronephrosis. A sharply marginated radiolucency corresponding to dilated calyces filled with nonopacified urine is seen during the nephrographic phase. This is also apparent as increased distance between the margin of the upper pole and the interpapillary line on later films. During the course of the urogram, the obstructed area will slowly opacify as contrast material passes into the dilated, urine-filled system. Detection of this transition from radiolucent to radiopaque may require filming as late as 24 to 36 hours after injection of contrast material. The wall of tissue around the dilated collecting structure is several millimeters or more in thickness and enhances in normal fashion during the urographic nephrogram. The nonobstructed calyces draining the remainder of the kidney opacify normally but may be displaced by the mass effect of the hydronephrotic segment (Fig. 12–56). Figure 4–4 illustrates these features schematically.

Pyelography. Retrograde or antegrade pyelography is sometimes valuable for precise visualization of the point of obstruction, although delayed films during urography occasionally provide the same information.

Computed Tomography. Focal hydronephrosis is seen in cross-sectional images as a smooth-walled, nonenhancing mass usually in the superior and medial part of the kidney. The homogeneous content has

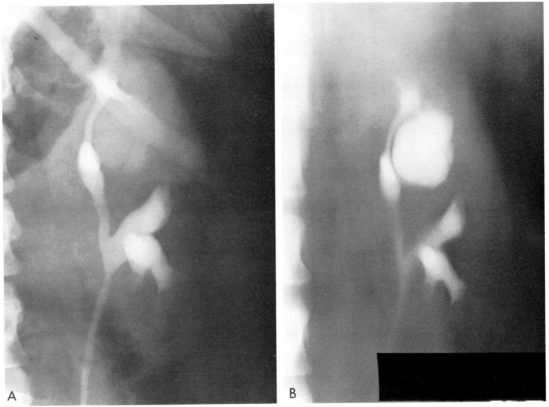

Figure 12–56. Focal hydronephrosis. Displacement of nonobstructed collecting system by an upper pole calyx dilated because of infundibular obstruction.

A, Excretory urogram, 10-minute film. There is only faint density over the dilated calyx.

B, Excretory urogram. Delayed tomogram. Late filling of the dilated calyx and the area of infundibular narrowing (possibly due to crossing vessel) are well identified.

the attenuation characteristics of water. Compressed renal tissue that comprises the wall of this mass enhances following contrast material administration (Fig. 12–57). A duplicated, obstructed ureter might also be demonstrated by computed tomography as a dilated tubular structure filled with urine having the density of water. This can usually be traced directly into the bladder, where a ureterocele is frequently present.

Ultrasonography. Ultrasound findings in focal hy-

dronephrosis are those of a thick-walled anechoic upper pole mass with an enhanced far-wall and through-sound transmission (see Fig. 12–57). Ultrasonography also identifies the dilated ureter to the point of obstruction and a ureterocele, if present.

Arteriography. Arteriography in focal hydronephrosis reveals displacement and attenuation of the arteries serving the affected portion of the kidney. None of the angiographic stigmata of neoplasm are seen with this condition.

SUMMARY OF ABNORMAL URORADIOLOGIC FINDINGS
FOCAL HYDRONEPHROSIS

Primary Uroradiologic Elements
    Size—large
    Contour—unifocal mass (usually upper pole)
    Lesion distribution—unilateral
Secondary Uroradiologic Elements
    Pelvoinfundibulocalyceal system—absent polar group (early); dilated polar group (late); displaced—
        adjacent interpolar
    Nephrogram—replaced (focal); smooth margin; thick wall; delayed opacification; attenuation value
        of water.
    Echogenicity—anechoic; far-wall enhancement; through-sound transmission enhanced

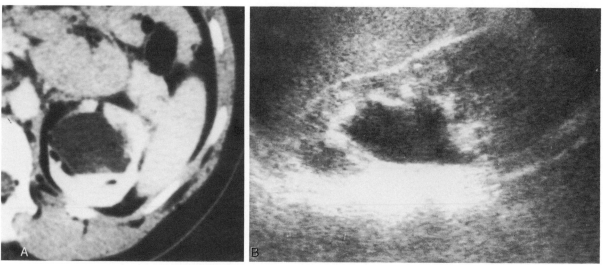

Figure 12–57. Focal hydronephrosis due to obstruction of the upper pole moiety of a completely duplicated pelvocalyceal system and ureter. Left kidney.

A, Computed tomogram, contrast material enhanced. The focal hydronephrosis appears as a water density mass with dependent layering of contrast material. The wall of the mass is compressed renal parenchyma.

B, Ultrasonogram, longitudinal section. In this projection, the dilated, fluid-filled structure has the configuration of an upper pole pelvis.

Abscess

Definition

Ascending bacterial invasion of the renal parenchyma causes a full thickness, lobar or sublobar interstitial inflammation that begins in the distribution of the medullary rays. This process, called acute tubulointerstitial nephritis, is described in detail in Chapter 9 as part of the discussion of acute pyelonephritis. If, in some individuals, the inflammatory process does not resolve spontaneously or in response to therapy in the acute phase, multiple, small foci of neutrophilic white blood cells accumulate, coalesce, and begin to form a central necrotic core. As this process progresses, a thick capsule of highly vascularized connective tissue forms around the central liquefying collection of necrotic renal parenchyma, neutrophils, and bacteria and a mature abscess is formed.

The abscess may drain through the renal capsule causing perinephritis and perinephric abscess. Sometimes cavitation and drainage into the collecting system occur.

The same process may begin with a blood-borne infection. In this circumstance, the initial tubulointerstitial infiltrate is miliary and cortical rather than a full-thickness involvement of all or part of a lobe, as is seen in ascending infections.

Clinical Setting

In the preantibiotic era, renal abscess was usually due to blood-borne metastatic seeding of *Staphylococcus aureus* from primary infection of the skin, teeth, lungs, or tonsils. Since the introduction of antibiotics, more than 80 per cent of renal and perirenal abscesses in the general population are the result of an ascending infection from the lower urinary tract. Most kidney abscesses are associated with calculous obstruction of the ureter or the pelvis. Other lesions, such as ureteropelvic junction or distal ureteral obstruction, also increase the risk for abscess. In these cases, gram-negative bacteria, particularly *Escherichia coli*, *Enterobacter aerogenes*, and *Proteus mirabilis*, predominate. Overall, males are afflicted twice as frequently as females. Immunocompromised patients are a subpopulation that is at particular risk for both blood-borne and ascending infections of the kidney leading to abscess. In this group, a variety of organisms that are not usually urinary tract pathogens may be involved.

The clinical picture may be quite nonspecific. In the acute phase, fever, chills, malaise, and signs of sepsis are present. Flank or abdominal pain may accompany a palpable renal mass. Urinalysis, including urine culture, may be normal if the infection is behind an obstructing lesion that prevents urine flow from the involved kidney. In chronic abscess, fever and leukocytosis may be minimal or absent, and localizing signs are rare. Pyuria and bacteriuria may be absent. Obviously, diagnosis on clinical grounds alone is exceedingly difficult in these patients.

Radiologic Findings

Excretory Urography. Since renal and perirenal abscesses often coexist, partial or complete obscuration of the renal outline, loss of the psoas margin, immobility of the kidney with respiration, and lumbar scoliosis concave to the side of involvement are often seen. These abnormalities may be absent if the abscess is confined solely to the kidney parenchyma. Immobility may be documented by exposing a single film during both deep inspiration and expiration.

The involved kidney is enlarged by a unifocal usually polar mass. The mass may displace or efface adjacent portions of the collecting system. A nephrographic radiolucent defect within the well-defined mass corresponds to the central collection of necrotic tissue. The wall of the mass is thick, and its inner margin is irregular (Fig. 12–58). It is not uncommon to see multiple rounded nephrographic radiolucencies representing several abscesses. Opacification of the collecting structures on the involved side is sometimes less than that seen in the contralateral kidney. Calcification is not a feature of acute or chronic renal abscess.

Computed Tomography. The appearance of a renal abscess on computed tomography varies with the evolution of the inflammatory process from early necrosis within an area of acute interstitial nephritis to an encapsulated, fluid-filled mass (Figs. 12–59 and 12–60). On unenhanced scans, the early abscess may not be discernible because it has a density equal to or slightly less than the adjacent normal parenchyma and is not circumscribed. Following contrast material administration, however, the early abscess enhances less than the remainder of the kidney and is readily identified. With time, the liquefied abscess yields attenuation values substantially below those of normal renal tissue but greater than those of water. Enhancement does not occur at this stage.

Computed tomography is highly sensitive in detect-

ing rupture of the abscess into the subcapsular and perinephric spaces (Fig. 12–61). Thickening of the renal fascia is common, especially with extension of the abscess beyond the kidney itself.

Ultrasonography. As liquefaction within the area of acute interstitial nephritis develops, there is progressive decrease of echogenicity. Eventually, the abscess becomes anechoic or demonstrates only faint internal echoes, depending on the amount of tissue debris within the cavity (see Fig. 12–61). Although the margins of the mass may be irregular, its extent is well defined by ultrasonography. At the mature, fluid-filled stage, through-sound transmission is always less than that of water but varies as a function of the amount of sound-absorbing material in the cavity of the abscess.

Angiography. As an abscess ages and a thick capsule forms, displacement of medium-sized arteries around the mass occurs. The capsule may stain intensely, and a fine, uniform set of small arteries, similar to those seen in some neoplasms, may be present. The central radiolucency of the abscess and its thick wall with irregular borders are much more apparent during angiography than during excretory urography (Fig. 12–62). With perinephritis or perinephric ab-

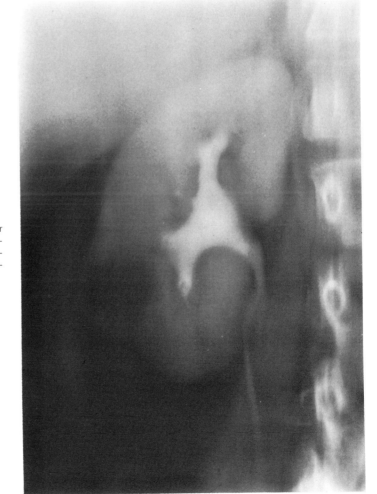

Figure 12–58. Abscess of the right kidney demonstrating contour bulge due to mass, radiolucent nephrographic defect with irregular margins, and a thick wall. Tomogram during excretory urography. (Courtesy of Robert R. Hattery, M.D., Mayo Clinic, Rochester, Minnesota.)

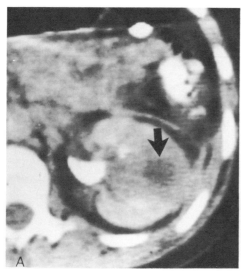

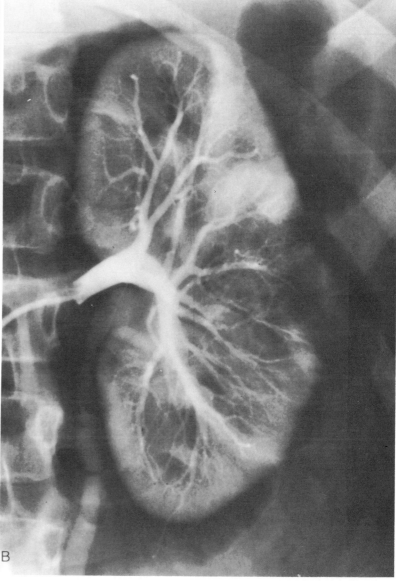

Figure 12–59. Evolving abscess, left kidney.

A, Computed tomogram, contrast material enhanced. A central low density *(arrow)* represents liquefaction within an area of tubulointerstitial nephritis seen as a well-defined larger region of diminished enhancement.

B, Selective renal arteriogram. The number of small arteries in the affected area is decreased, but the vessels are not yet displaced around the early abscess.

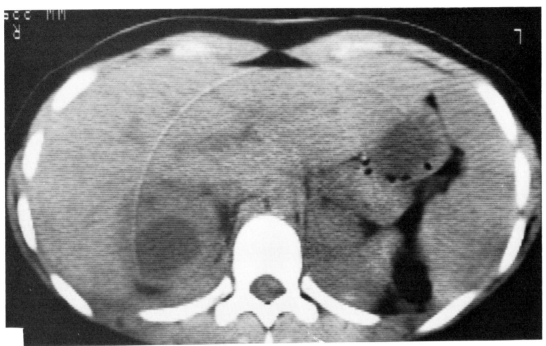

Figure 12–60. Mature (liquefied) abscess in the upper pole of the right kidney. Computed tomogram, unenhanced. The contents of the abscess have an attenuation value lower than the kidney tissue but greater than water.

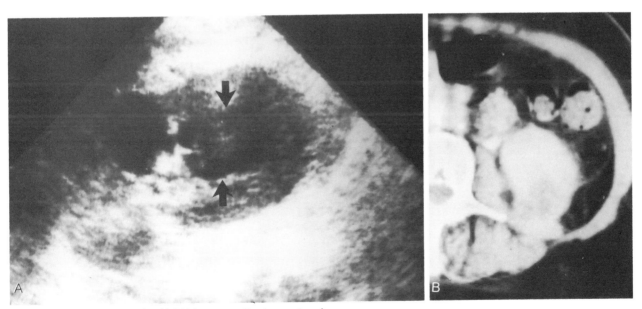

Figure 12–61. Abscess, lower pole of left kidney, extending into perirenal space.

A, Ultrasonogram, longitudinal section. The abscess *(arrows)* exhibits slight echogenicity and impaired through-sound transmission. A simple cyst is situated superior to the abscess.

B, Computed tomogram, contrast material enhanced. The abscess extends from the dorsal surface of the kidney into the perirenal space.

(Kindly provided by Sheila Sheth, M.D., and Ullrike Hamper, M.D., The Johns Hopkins University, Baltimore, Maryland.)

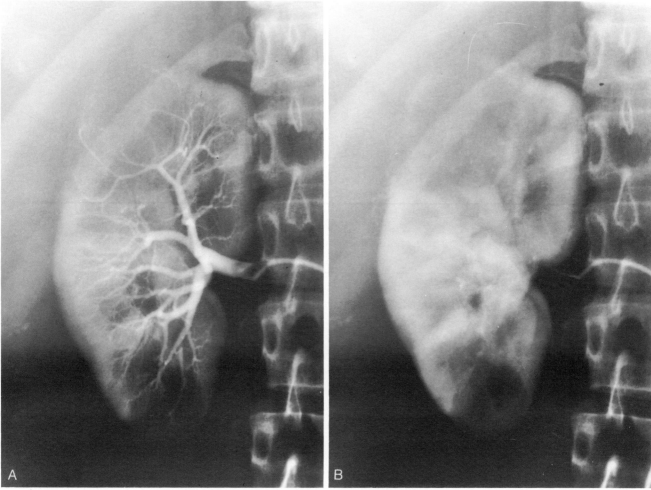

Figure 12–62. Mature abscess, upper pole of right kidney with an incidental simple cyst in the lower pole. Selective renal arteriogram.
  A, Arterial phase. Small arteries are displaced around the liquefied, encapsulated abscess.
  B, Nephrographic phase. The thick, irregular margins of the abscess are defined.

SUMMARY OF ABNORMAL URORADIOLOGIC FINDINGS
ABSCESS

Preliminary Film
  Loss of psoas margin   } when
  Scoliosis concave to involved side   perinephritis
  Immobility of kidney during respiration   } is present
Primary Uroradiologic Elements
  Size—large
  Contour—unifocal mass
  Lesion distribution—unilateral
Secondary Uroradiologic Elements
  Pelvoinfundibulocalyceal system—attenuated (focal); displaced (focal)
  Nephrogram—normal (early phase); replaced (focal)—irregular, thick wall (late phase); contrast
    material density decreased (occasional); attenuation value—normal to slightly diminished before
    contrast material administration; enhances less than normal parenchyma (early); decreased and
    nonenhancing (late)
  Echogenicity—slightly hypoechoic (early); hypoechoic to anechoic (late); variable through-sound
    transmission

scess, the capsular arteries are usually pushed outward from the kidney. None of these angiographic findings is specific to focal inflammatory disease. All of them overlap those seen in neoplastic disorders. Even early venous filling and noncontractility of feeding vessels after intra-arterial epinephrine injection have been reported.

Multilocular Cystic Nephroma

Definition

Multilocular cystic nephroma is an uncommon neoplasm composed of multiple, variably sized cysts with prominent septa. The cysts contain clear, yellow, turbid, or gelatinous fluid and do not communicate with each other. Hemorrhage is uncommon. Characteristically, although not invariably, one or more of the cysts herniate into the renal pelvis to form a nonopaque filling defect that may at times obstruct portions of the collecting system and ulcerate the uroepithelium. Multilocular cystic nephroma arises as a unifocal mass, with the remaining portion of the kidney uninvolved or compressed by the tumor.

Multilocular cystic nephroma grows by expansion and has a dense fibrous capsule. The cysts most commonly are lined by cuboidal epithelial cells that project into the cyst lumen. The stroma of the septa is usually composed of loose connective tissue with sparse cellularity, indicating the benign nature of this tumor. Rarely, however, the findings of sarcoma or Wilms' tumor are present in the septa.

Multilocular cystic nephroma is sometimes confused with multicystic dysplastic kidney. Multilocular cystic nephroma is a unifocal mass involving only a portion of an otherwise normal kidney. Multicystic dysplastic kidney, on the other hand, usually, but not invariably, involves an entire kidney. When multicystic dysplastic kidney is segmental, it lacks a fibrous capsule, a finding that is always present in multilocular cystic nephroma. Additional aspects of multicystic dysplastic kidney are discussed in Chapter 11.

Clinical Setting

Multilocular cystic nephroma has a biphasic age and sex distribution. One peak in prevalence occurs in infants and young children with a male bias, and a second peak occurs in middle-aged adults with a predominance among females. This lesion may be detected as a palpable mass, particularly in infants. Some cases present with hematuria, but many are discovered incidentally. Neither a familial incidence nor an association with congenital anomalies in other organ systems has been established.

Radiologic Findings

Excretory Urography. In multilocular cystic nephroma, the kidney is enlarged by a unifocal mass that distorts the collecting system (Fig. 12–63). Calcium may be detectable in the walls of the locules (Fig. 12–64). With careful radiographic technique, faint opacification of septa may be detectable. Otherwise, the urographic nephrogram is absent in the area of involvement. The interface between the lesion and the adjacent normally opacified renal tissue is sharply defined. Herniation of one or more cysts into the pelvis presents as a sharply defined, rounded filling defect in the opacified renal pelvis (Fig. 12–65; see also Fig. 12–63). If the prolapsed cysts are large enough or are located in a critical position, obstruction of the collecting system draining the normal portions of the kidney may occur.

Computed Tomography. Multilocular cystic nephroma is a well-marginated mass on computed tomographic images. The cysts vary greatly in size, and there may be variation in attenuation values from that of water to slightly higher (Fig. 12–66). The portion of the tumor that has prolapsed into the pelvis is readily identified (see Fig. 12–65). The thick septa that characterize this lesion enhance after contrast material is administered. Computed tomography detects calcium in the septa much more often than does standard radiography (see Fig. 12–64). The pattern of calcium deposition varies from linear to flocculent.

Ultrasonography. A sharply defined multiloculated mass with a mixture of highly echogenic septa and anechoic contents characterizes the ultrasonographic appearance of multilocular cystic nephroma (see Figs. 12–63 and 12–65). A collection of tiny cysts, each too small to be individually resolved, may be imaged as an echogenic focus. Echoes may also originate in loc-

---

SUMMARY OF ABNORMAL URORADIOLOGIC FINDINGS
MULTILOCULAR CYSTIC NEPHROMA

Primary Uroradiologic Elements
  Size—large
  Contour—unifocal mass
  Lesion distribution—unilateral
Secondary Uroradiologic Elements
  Pelvoinfundibulocalyceal system—attenuated (focal); displaced (focal); filling defects
  Nephrogram—replaced (focal); attenuation value variable above water; thick septa
  Calcification—peripheral or nonperipheral; linear to flocculent
  Echogenicity—mixed anechoic to hyperechoic; poor far-wall enhancement and through-sound
    transmission in smaller cysts
  Cystography—noncommunication between cysts

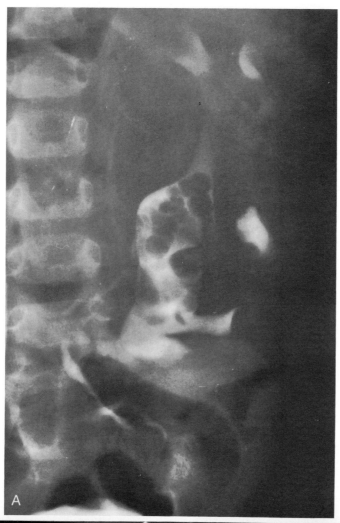

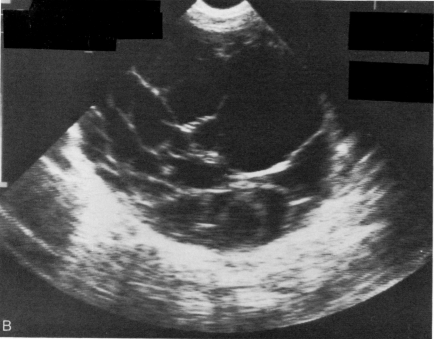

Figure 12–63. Multilocular cystic nephroma, left kidney, in a 7-year-old boy.

A, Excretory urogram. The mass distorts and displaces the central portion of the kidney. Multiple filling defects in the pelvocalyceal system represent herniated cysts.

B, Ultrasonogram, longitudinal section. The tumor is composed of numerous locules of varying size with thick septa and uncomplicated fluid.

(Kindly provided by the Department of Radiology, Alberta Children's Hospital, Calgary, Alberta, Canada.)

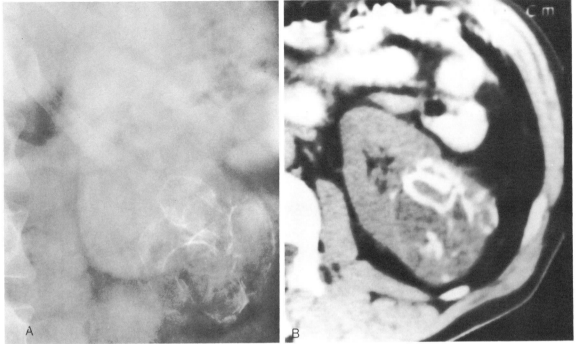

Figure 12-64. Multilocular cystic nephroma with dense calcification in the walls of involuted cysts.
A, Excretory urogram.
B, Computed tomogram, unenhanced.

ules filled with the gelatinous material found in some cysts. As a result, far-wall enhancement and increased through-sound transmission are sometimes absent. On the other hand, larger cysts with uncomplicated fluid yield characteristic findings of anechoicity, a sharply defined far wall, and increased through-sound transmission.

Cystography. Percutaneous needle aspiration of multilocular cystic nephroma yields perplexing results that are more suggestive of a solid tumor than a fluid-filled mass. The aspirate varies between fluid and gelatinous matter. The independence of each cyst cavity from the other makes it impossible to opacify the entire lesion through a needle placed in any one cyst.

Angiography. Angiography may reveal neovascularity in the form of irregular vessels coursing through the septa and around the lesion (Fig. 12-67). These are indistinguishable from neovascularity in other tumors. The septa can be seen during the angiographic nephrogram as relatively thick bands of radiodensity curving around radiolucent, fluid-filled areas.

Congenital Arteriovenous Malformation

Definition

Congenital arteriovenous malformation, also known as hemangioma, is classified as either *cirsoid* or *cavernous*. The cirsoid form is more common and is composed of multiple coiled vascular channels grouped in a cluster. This vascular mass is supplied by one or more arteries that arise at the segmental or interlobar level. Drainage of the mass is into one or more veins.

The arterial feeders and the draining veins may or may not be enlarged. The much less common cavernous form is composed of a single well-defined artery feeding into a single large chamber that is drained by a single vein. The artery and vein are often dilated. Curvilinear calcification may form in the wall of the cavernous malformation.

Congenital arteriovenous malformation is distinguished from an arteriovenous communication that results from trauma or spontaneous rupture of an aneurysm into a vein, a condition classified as *acquired arteriovenous aneurysm* or *fistula.* Here, the dominant abnormality is an arterial to venous shunt rather than a mass. This is discussed further in Chapters 26 and 27.

Clinical Setting

Congenital arteriovenous malformation occurs in all age groups. No sex predilection has been established conclusively, although a female predominance has been suggested. These malformations usually have a submucosal or mucosal relationship to the collecting system. Thus, hematuria, which may be major, is a common clinical presentation. Increased blood flow to the affected kidney is not a common feature of congenital arteriovenous malformation, unlike arteriovenous aneurysm/fistula. Thus, wide pulse pressure and high-output heart failure are absent in most cases.

Radiologic Findings

Excretory Urography. Because congenital arteriovenous malformation is usually medullary, a mass effect on the collecting system may be present (Figs. 12-68

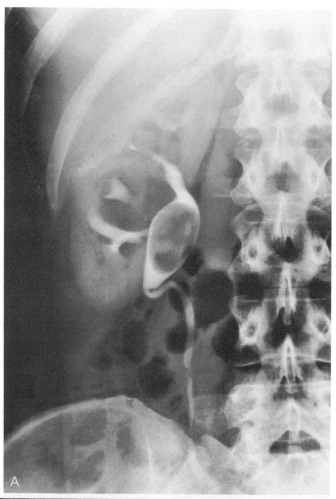

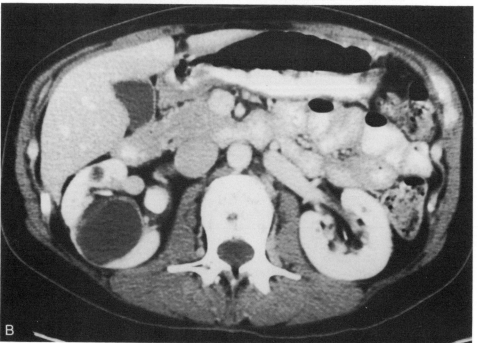

Figure 12–65. Multilocular cystic nephroma in the right kidney of a middle-aged woman. The tumor is in the central portion of the kidney. Herniation of locules produces a filling defect in the renal pelvis.

A, Excretory urogram. The mass displaces and partially obstructs infundibula and calyces.

B and *C,* Computed tomogram, contrast material enhanced. The tumor is sharply defined and composed of locules of water attenuation, some of which are herniated into the renal pelvis.

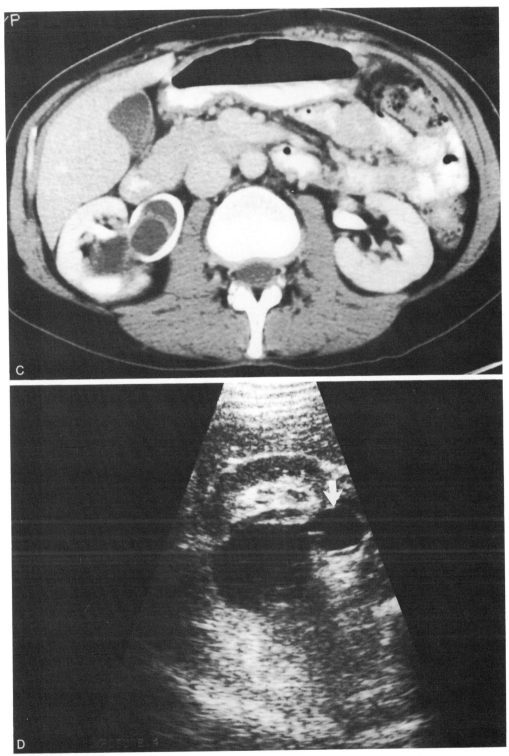

Figure 12–65 *Continued D,* Ultrasonogram, transverse section. The locules are anechoic with faint septa. The arrow indicates the locule in the pelvis.
(Kindly provided by Marge Stahl, M.D., and Wendelin Hayes, D.O., Georgetown University, Washington, D.C.)

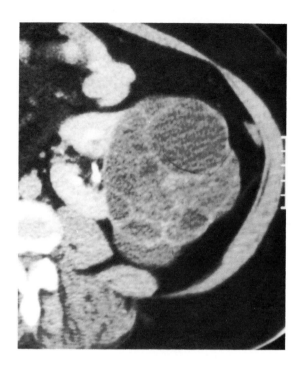

Figure 12–66. Multilocular cystic nephroma, left kidney. Computed tomogram, contrast material enhanced. The tumor is composed of multiple locules with contents of water attenuation values. The septa are prominent and enhance.

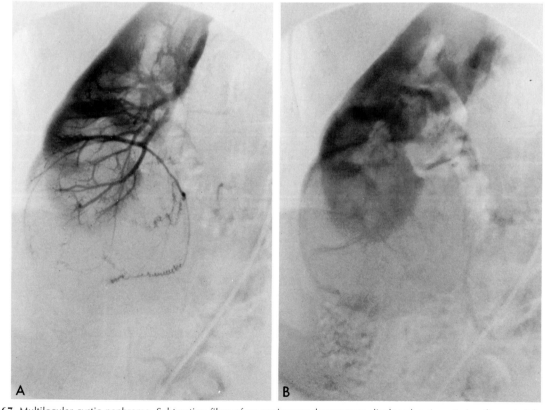

Figure 12–67. Multilocular cystic nephroma. Subtraction films of an angiogram demonstrate displaced major arteries, fine arterial supply to the septa, and the staining of the septa during the angiographic nephrogram.
   A, Arterial phase.
   B, Nephrographic phase.

and 12–69). On the other hand, the excretory urogram may be normal in a patient with a small malformation and minimal to absent bleeding. Sometimes, blood clot is the only abnormality noted. Curvilinear, peripheral calcification is sometimes present in the cavernous form of congenital arteriovenous malformation (see Fig. 12–69).

Computed Tomography. Computed tomography effectively documents the vascular nature of a congenital arteriovenous malformation by demonstrating enhancement of the entire mass with contrast material. This is best documented by a dynamic scanning technique. An enlarged feeding artery and draining vein may be identified. In other respects, the computed tomographic manifestations are the same as those noted in the preceding section Excretory Urography.

Ultrasonography. The ultrasonographic image of congenital arteriovenous malformation varies with the type. In the cirsoid form, the cluster of small vessels appears as an echoic mass, indistinguishable from a solid neoplasm (see Fig. 12–68). The cavernous form, on the other hand, yields an image of an anechoic fluid-filled mass (see Fig. 12–69). The enlarged feeding and draining vessels may also be identified. The vascular nature of an arteriovenous malformation can be established by a Doppler flow study.

Arteriography. Arteriovenous shunts with early venous opacification are not a prominent feature of congenital arteriovenous malformation and often are not

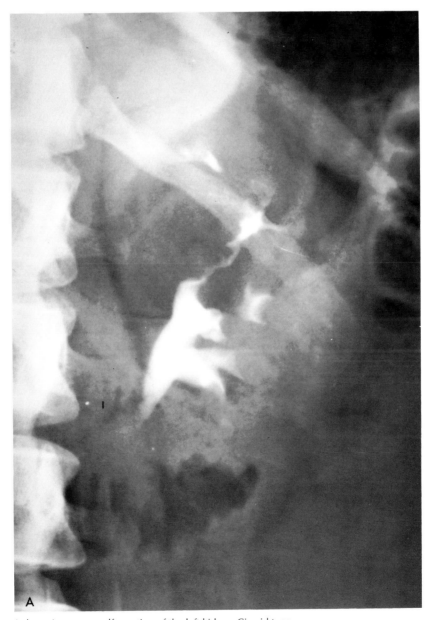

Figure 12–68. Congenital arteriovenous malformation of the left kidney. Cirsoid type.
A, Excretory urogram. A mass lesion on the medial part of the upper pole creates nodular impressions on the pelvocalyceal system.

Illustration continued on following page

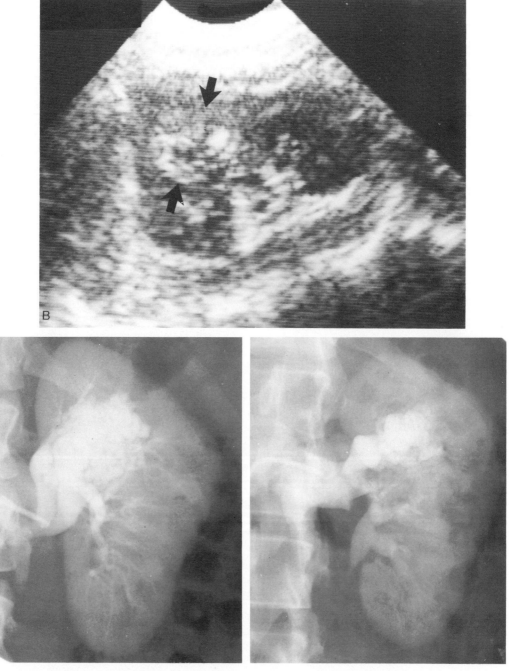

Figure 12–68 *Continued B,* Ultrasonogram, longitudinal section. The cirsoid malformation appears as an echogenic mass in the upper pole of the left kidney *(arrows).*

C, Selective left angiogram, arterial and venous phases. Note cirsoid channels.

(Courtesy of Jalil Farah, M.D., and Robert Ellwood, M.D., William Beaumont Hospital, Royal Oak, Michigan.)

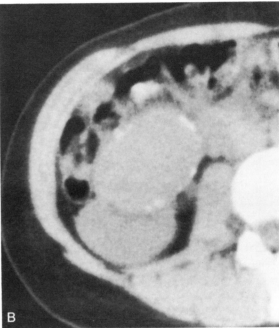

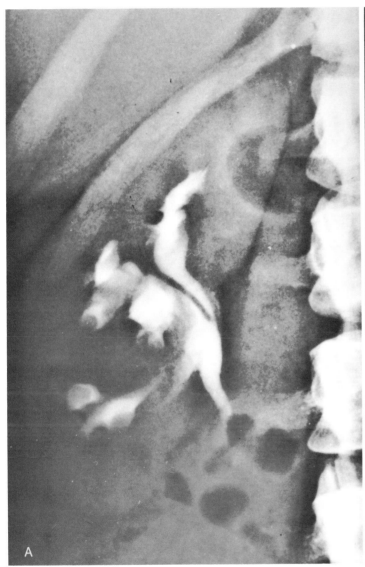

Figure 12–69. Arteriovenous malformation, right kidney. Cavernous type.

A, Excretory urogram. The malformation causes a focal displacement of the collecting system.

B, Computed tomogram, unenhanced. The malformation is of soft tissue attenuation and contains some mural calcification.

Illustration continued on following page

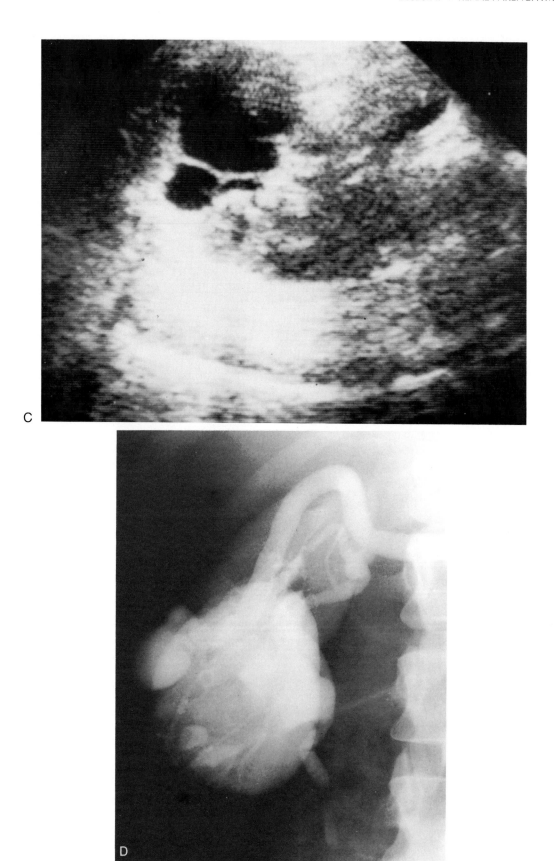

Figure 12–69 *Continued C,* Ultrasonogram, longitudinal section. The cavernous malformation has fluid characteristics and a thick septum. *D,* Selective renal arteriogram, late arterial phase. There is a single large artery supplying a large vascular chamber. Early venous filling is absent. (Courtesy of Jalil Farah, M.D., and Robert Ellwood, M.D., William Beaumont Hospital, Royal Oak, Michigan.)

**SUMMARY OF ABNORMAL URORADIOLOGIC FINDINGS
CONGENITAL ARTERIOVENOUS MALFORMATION**

Primary Uroradiologic Elements
  Size—large (may be normal)
  Contour—unifocal mass (may be normal)
  Lesion distribution—unilateral
Secondary Uroradiologic Elements
  Pelvoinfundibulocalyceal system—attenuated (focal); displaced (focal); multiple nodules
  Nephrogram—homogeneous; entire mass enhances with contrast material
  Calcification—curvilinear, peripheral
  Echogenicity—echoic mass (cirsoid); anechoic mass (cavernous)

---

present at all. The malformation, either cirsoid or cavernous, opacifies directly from the feeding artery which is usually single and enlarged. The draining vein may be single or multiple and also enlarged (see Figs. 12–68 and 12–69). A small cirsoid malformation is sometimes seen only as a poorly defined homogeneous blush during the nephrographic phase of an angiogram. In some patients, the arteriovenous malformation is too small for angiographic detection.

DIFFERENTIAL DIAGNOSIS

The differential diagnosis of unifocal masses begins with the determination of whether the lesion is solid or fluid filled. Even though certain urographic features may strongly suggest one or the other, examination of the mass by ultrasonography provides information that significantly increases diagnostic accuracy without known hazard to the patient and at relatively low cost. This technique, therefore, should be used routinely in all cases in which urographic data suggest a fluid-filled mass and in any case in which the urographic evidence for a solid tumor is equivocal. When urographic findings strongly indicate that a lesion is solid, computed tomography is often performed instead of ultrasonography. A systematic approach to the radiologic evaluation of unifocal masses is discussed in detail in Chapter 25.

Malignant tumors are usually solid and have an irregular nephrogram with mottled density and a thick pseudocapsule. Calcification, if present, is located *away* from the periphery of the mass. In cystic malignant neoplasms, the wall is thick and often contains nodules that enhance with contrast material. Additionally, the contents of a cystic neoplasm are atypical compared with the usual imaging features of uncomplicated fluid. The collecting system, in addition to being displaced, may have an irregular mucosa or may be obliterated. Serpiginous densities in perirenal fat, representing dilated vessels, and ureteral notching caused by venous collaterals are more specific signs of malignant tumor.

Angiomyolipoma produces many of the radiologic features of a malignant lesion. Fat within the tumor, whether detected as radiolucency on the preliminary film or by computed tomography, is the only finding that is virtually specific to angiomyolipoma. Fat may,

in fact, be present in Wilms' tumor, renal teratoma, or renal carcinoma, but only with extreme rarity. Although an angiomyolipoma commonly grows exophytically from the kidney into the perirenal space and may rarely extend into a renal vein, evidence of aggressive or invasive growth is absent. Other solid benign tumors have no distinctive radiologic features that permit confident differentiation from malignant tumors.

The classic urographic features of a *simple cyst* include a sharply defined radiolucent nephrographic defect, a thin wall on the outer margin of the mass, and a "beak" sign. Collecting system displacement is smooth and not obliterative, although effacement may be pronounced. Calcification, if present, is curvilinear, thin, and peripheral. A similar pattern of calcification may be present in other "benign" mass lesions, including *sclerosing lipogranuloma, renal adenoma*, and *intrarenal aneurysm*. The urographic diagnosis of cyst requires ultrasonographic or computed tomographic confirmation in most instances. Cysts that arise in the pancreas or adrenal gland can produce a concave impression on the kidney and very closely simulate the urographic appearance of a simple renal cyst. The "rim" sign is absent, however. The actual origin of a simple cyst or a cystic mass arising in the pancreas or in the adrenal gland is usually established with a high level of confidence by ultrasonography, computed tomography, or magnetic resonance imaging in the coronal or sagittal plane. A *calyceal diverticulum* may mimic a cyst on ultrasonography but can be differentiated from a cyst if contrast material enhancement demonstrates communication with the collecting system. *Renal vein varix, intrarenal aneurysm*, or *organizing hematoma* may simulate simple or complicated renal cysts on many imaging studies. The nature of a vascular lesion, however, can be confirmed using Doppler ultrasonographic techniques.

Delayed opacification of a hydronephrotic calyx and absence of an appropriate number of calyces on films early in the urographic series are hallmarks of *focal hydronephrosis*. Retrograde or antegrade pyelography usually provides a definite diagnosis.

Urography in *abscess* causing unifocal masses is nonspecific and does not alone provide a reliable basis for distinguishing this lesion from other causes of unifocal masses. Ultrasonography or computed tomography performed to document liquefaction and encapsulation leads reliably to a correct diagnosis, particularly if clinical features of infection are present.

The distinctive features of *multilocular cystic nephroma* are faintly opacified septa within an otherwise unenhancing tumor and herniation of cysts into the renal pelvis. Computed tomography is most efficacious in demonstrating these abnormalities. Unfortunately, there are rare occasions when a tumor has all of the radiologic features of a benign multilocular cystic nephroma but on pathologic examination is, in fact, a malignant variant of sarcoma, Wilms' tumor, or adenocarcinoma. This rare possibility cannot be anticipated by radiologic examination. Thus, any tumor that has the radiologic features of benign multilocular cystic nephroma must be excised to be accurately diagnosed.

When urographic and ultrasonographic evidence unequivocally indicates a simple cyst, no further investigations are needed unless the clinical findings need an explanation beyond simple cyst. Except for angiomyolipoma, definitive diagnosis of lesions that urography, ultrasonography, computed tomography, or angiography shows as solid or a mixture of fluid and solid components usually depends on pathologic examinations following surgical removal of tumor.

Bibliography

General

Hartman, D. S., Aronson, S., and Frazier, H.: Current status of imaging indeterminate renal masses. Radiol. Clin. North Am. 29:475, 1991.

Hartman, D. S.: Pediatric renal tumors. *In* Taveras, J., and Ferucci, J. (eds.): Radiology Diagnosis, Imaging, Intervention. Philadelphia, J. B. Lippincott Co., 1986, vol. 4, chapter 117, pp. 1–9.

Montie, J. E.: The incidental renal mass: Management alternatives. Urol. Clin. North Am. 18:427, 1991.

Quint, L. E., Glazer, G. M., Chenevert, T. L., Fechner, K. P., and Li, K. C.: *In vivo* and *in vitro* MR imaging of renal tumors: Histopathologic correlation and pulse sequence optimization. Radiology 169:359, 1988.

Warshauer, D. M., McCarthy, S. M., Street, L., Bookbinder, M. J., Clicleman, M. G., Richter, J., Hammers, L., Taylor, C., and Rosenfield, A. T.: Detection of renal masses: Sensitivities and specificities of excretory urography/linear tomography, US and CT. Radiology 169:363, 1988.

Malignant Neoplasms

Agnew, C. H.: Metastatic malignant melanoma of the kidney simulating primary neoplasm. AJR 80:813, 1958.

Beckwith, J. B.: Precursor lesions of Wilms' tumor: Clinical and biological implications. Med. Pediatr. Oncol. 21:158, 1993.

Bhatt, G. M., Bernardino, M. E., and Graham, S. D., Jr.: CT diagnosis of renal metastases. J. Comput. Assist. Tomogr. 7:1036, 1983.

Blath, R. A., Mancilla-Jimenez, R., and Stanley, R. J.: Clinical comparison between vascular and avascular renal cell carcinoma. J. Urol. 115:514, 1976.

Blei, C. L., Hartman, D. S., Friedman, A. C., and Davis, C. J.: Papillary renal cell carcinoma: Ultrasonic/pathologic correlation. JCU 10:429, 1982.

Boijsen, E., and Folin, J.: Angiography in the diagnosis of renal carcinoma. Radiology. 1:173, 1961.

Bosniak, M. A.: Radiographic manifestations of massive arteriovenous fistula in renal carcinoma. Radiology 85:454, 1965.

Bosniak, M. A., Stein, W., Lopez, F., Tehranian, N., and O'Connor, S.: Metastatic neoplasm to kidney. Radiology 92:989, 1969.

Brindle, M. J.: Alternative vascular channels in renal cell carcinoma. Clin. Radiol. 23:321, 1972.

Caro, G., Meisell, R., and Held, B.: Epinephrine-enhanced arteriography in renal and perirenal abscess. Radiology 92:1262, 1969.

Carter, R. J.: The pathology of renal cancer. JAMA 204:221, 1968.

Castellino, R. A.: Renal carcinoma demonstrated by post-epinephrine arteriography following normal selective arteriograms. Radiology 97:607, 1970.

Choyke, P. L., White, E. M., Zeman, R. K., Jaffe, M. H., and Clark, L. R.: Renal metastases: Clinicopathologic and radiologic correlation. Radiology 162:359, 1987.

Choyke, P. L.: MR imaging in renal cell carcinoma. Radiology 169:572, 1988.

Choyke, P. L., Filling-Katz, M. R., Shawker, T. H., Gorin, M. B., Travis, W. D., Chang, R., Seizinger, B. R., Dwyer, A. J., and Lineham, W. M.: von Hippel-Lindau Disease: Radiologic screening for visceral manifestations. Radiology 174:815, 1990.

Coleman, B. G., Arger, P. H., Mulhern, C. B., Jr., Pollack, H. M., Banner, M. P., and Arenson, R. L.: Gray-scale sonographic spectrum of hypernephromas. Radiology 137:757, 1980.

Cox, C. E., Lacy, S. S., Montgomery, W. G., and Boyce, W. H.: Renal adenocarcinoma: 28-year review. J. Urol. 104:53, 1970.

Cremin, B. J. Wilms' tumor: Ultrasound and changing concepts. Clin. Radiol. 38:465, 1987.

Cronan, J. J., Zeman, R. K., and Rosenfield, A. T.: Comparison of computerized tomography, ultrasound, and angiography in staging renal cell carcinoma. J. Urol. 127:712, 1982.

Daniel, W. W., Hartman, G. W., Witten, D. M., Farrow, G. M., and Kelalis, P. P.: Calcified renal masses: A review of ten years experience at the Mayo Clinic. Radiology 103:503, 1972.

Davidson, A. J., Hayes, W. S., Hartman, D. S., McCarthy, W. F., and Davis, C. J., Jr.: Renal oncocytoma and carcinoma: Failure of differentiation with CT. Radiology 186:693, 1993.

Davidson, A. J., and Davis, C. J.: Fat in renal adenocarcinoma: Never say never. Radiology 188:316, 1993.

Feldberg, M. A. M., and van Waes, F. G. M.: Multilocular cystic renal cell carcinoma. AJR 138:953, 1982.

Fernbach, S. K., Donaldson, J. S., Gonzalez-Crussi, F., and Sherman, J. O.: Fatty Wilms' tumor simulating teratoma: occurrence in a child with horseshoe kidney. Pediatr. Radiol. 18:424, 1988.

Fernbach, S. K., Feinstein, K. A., Donaldson, J. S., and Baum, E. S.: Nephroblastomosis: Comparison of CT with US and urography. Radiology 166:153, 1988.

Ferris, E. J., Bosniak, M. A., and O'Connor, J. F.: An angiographic sign demonstrating extension of renal carcinoma into the renal vein and vena cava. AJR 102:384, 1968.

Fishman, E. K., Hartman, D. S., Goldman, S. M., and Siegelman, S. S.: The CT appearance of Wilms' tumor. J. Comput. Assist. Tomogr. 7:659, 1983.

Forman, H. P., Middleton, W. D., Melson, G. L., and McClennan, B. L.: Hyperechoic renal cell carcinoma: Increase in detection at US. Radiology 188:431, 1993.

Genereux, G. P.: The collateral vein sign in renal neoplasm. J. Can. Assoc. Radiol. 19:46, 1968.

Glass, R. B. J., Davidson A. J., Fernbach, S. K.: Clear cell sarcoma of the kidney: CT sonographic and pathologic correlation. Radiology 180:715, 1991.

Goldstein, H. M., Kaminsky, S., Wallace, S., and Johnson, D. E.: Urographic manifestations of metastatic melanoma. AJR 121:801, 1974.

Hartman, D. S., Weatherby, E., Laskin, W. B., Brody, J. M., Corse, W., and Baluch, J. D.: Cystic renal cell carcinoma: CT findings simulating a benign hyperdense cyst: Case report. AJR 159:1235, 1992.

Hélénon, O., Chrétien, Y., Paraf, F., Melki, P., Denys, A., and Moreau, J.-F.: Renal cell carcinoma containing fat: Demonstration with CT. Radiology 188:429, 1993.

Hietala, S.-O., and Wahlqvist, L.: Metastatic tumors to the kidney: A post-mortem radiologic and clinical investigation. Acta Radiol. (Diagn.) 23:585, 1982.

Henriksson, L., and Mikaelsson, C. G.: Angiographic diagnosis of renal vein thrombosis in malignant renal tumors. Acta Radiol. (Diagn.) 14:682, 1973.

Jaffe, M. H., White, S. J., Silver, T. M., and Heidelberger, K. P.: Wilms' tumor: Ultrasonic features, pathologic correlation and diagnostic pitfalls. Radiology 140:147, 1981.

Kahn, P. C., and Wise, H. M., Jr.: The use of epinephrine in selective angiography of renal masses. J. Urol. 99:133, 1967.

Lee, K. R., Wulfsberg, E., and Kepes, J. J.: Some important radiological aspects of the kidney in Hippel-Lindau syndrome: The value of prospective study in an affected family. Radiology 122:649, 1977.

Levin, D. C., Gordon, D., Kinkhabwala, M., and Becker, J. A.: Reticular neovascularity in malignant and inflammatory renal masses. Radiology 120:61, 1976.

Levine, E., Lee, K. R., Weigel, J. W., and Farber, B.: Computed tomography in the diagnosis of renal carcinoma complicating Hippel-Lindau syndrome. Radiology 130:703, 1979.

Lokich, J. J., and Harrison, J. H.: Renal cell carcinoma: Natural history and chemotherapeutic experience. J. Urol. 114:371, 1975.

Nelson, J. A., Clark, R. E., and Palubinskas, A. J.: Osteogenic sarcoma with calcified renal metastasis. Br. J. Radiol. 44:802, 1971.

Nishitani, H., Onitsuko, H., Kauhira, K., Ono, M., Jinnouchi, Y., Ohba, T., and Matsuura, K.: Computed tomography of renal metastases. J. Comput. Assist. Tomogr. 8:727, 1984.

Palmer, J., Barry, B., Williams, R., and Briscoe, P.: Diagnosis of venous extension in renal cell carcinoma: The value of routine inferior vena cavography. Australas. Radiol. 19:265, 1975.

Pamilo, M., Suramo, I., and Päivänslao, M.: Characteristics of hypernephromas as seen with ultrasound and computed tomography. JCU 11:245, 1983.

Pollack, H. M., and Popky, G.: Spontaneous subcapsular hemorrhage: Its significance and roentgenologic diagnosis. J. Urol. 108:530, 1972.

Prati, G. F., Saggin, P., Boschiero, L., Martini, P. T., Montemezzi, S., and Muolo, A.: Small renal-cell carcinomas—clinical and imaging features. Urol. Int. 51:19, 1993.

Rafla, S.: Renal cell carcinoma: Natural history and results of treatment. Cancer 25:26, 1970.

Reiman, T. A. H., Siegel, M. J., and Shackelford, G. D.: Wilms' tumor in children: Abdominal CT and US evaluation. Radiology 160:501, 1986.

Sniderman, K. W., Krieger, J. N., Seligson, G. R., and Sos, T. A.: The radiologic and clinical aspects of calcified hypernephroma. Radiology 131:31, 1979.

Sondag, T. J., Petasnick, J. P., Patel, S. K., and Alcorn, F. S.: Hypernephromas with parasitic blood supply derived from the superior and inferior mesenteric arteries. Radiology 103:509, 1972.

Stigsson, L., Ekelund, L., and Karp, W.: Bilateral concurrent renal neoplasms: Report of eleven cases. AJR 132:37, 1977.

Strotzer, M., Lehner, K. B., and Becker, K.: Detection of fat in a renal cell carcinoma mimicking angiomyolipoma. Radiology 188:427, 1993.

Thomas, J. L., and Bernardino, M. E.: Neoplastic-induced renal vein enlargement: Sonographic detection. AJR 136:75, 1981.

Volpe, J. P., and Choyke, P. L.: The radiologic evaluation of renal metastases. Crit. Rev. Diagn. Imag. 30:219, 1990.

Wafula, J. M. C., Davies, P., and Price, H.: Acute presentation of renal tumors. Clin. Radiol. 32:585, 1981.

Weiss, R. M., Becker, J. A., Davidson, A. J., and Lytton, B.: Angiographic appearance of renal papillary-tubular adenocarcinomas. J. Urol. 102:661, 1969.

Weyman, P. J., McClennan, B. L., Stanley, R. J., Levitt, R. G., and Sagel, S. S.: Comparison of computed tomography and angiography in the evaluation of renal cell carcinoma. Radiology 137:417, 1980.

Wills, J. S., Santos, R. M., and Ashley, P. F.: Renal papillary adenocarcinoma. Clin. Radiol. 30:53, 1979.

Wong, W. S., Cochran, S. T., and Waisman, J.: The reliability of the "hypernephroma halo." AJR 137:933, 1981.

Wong, W. S., Cochran, S. T., and Boxer, R. J.: Radiographic grading system for renal cell carcinoma with clinical and pathological correlation. Radiology 144:61, 1982.

Wright, F. W.: Bilateral renal cell carcinomas. Radiology 115:543, 1975.

Yamashita, Y., Veno, S., Makita, O., Ogata, I., Hatanaka, Y., Watanabe, O., and Takahashi, M.: Hyperechoic renal tumors: Anechoic rim and intratumoral cysts in US differentiation of renal cell carcinoma from angiomyolipoma. Radiology 188:179, 1993.

Benign Neoplasms

Ambos, M. A., Bosniak, M. A., Valensi, Q. J., Madayag, M. A., and Lefleur, R. S.: Angiographic patterns in renal oncocytomas. Radiology 129:615, 1978.

Ameratunga, B.: Angiomyolipoma of the kidney. Australas. Radiol. 18:202, 1974.

Blute, M. L., Malek, R. S., and Segura, J. W.: Angiomyolipoma: Clinical metamorphosis and concepts for management. J. Urol. 139:20, 1988.

Bonavita, J. A., Pollack, H. M., and Banner, M. P.: Renal oncocytoma: Further observations and literature review. Urol. Radiol. 2:229, 1981.

Bosniak, M. A., Megibow, A. J., Hulnick, D. H., Horii, S., and Raghavendra, B. N.: CT diagnosis of renal angiomyolipoma: The importance of detecting small amounts of fat. AJR 151:497, 1988.

Bruneton, J. N., Ballanger, P., Ballanger, R., and Delorme, G.: Renal adenomas. Clin. Radiol. 30:343, 1979.

Chonko, A. M., Weiss, S. M., Stein, J. H., and Ferris, T. F.: Renal involvement in tuberous sclerosis. Am. J. Med. 56:124, 1974.

Choyke, P. L., Glenn, G. M., Walther, M. M., Zbar, B., Weiss, G. H., Alexander, R. B., Hayes, W. S., Long, J. P., Thakore, K. N., and Lineham, K. N.: The natural history of renal lesions in von Hippel-Lindau disease: A serial CT study in 28 patients. AJR 159:1229, 1992.

Compton, W. R., Lester, P. D., Kyaw, M. M., and Madsen, J.: The abdominal angiographic spectrum of tuberous sclerosis. AJR 126:807, 1976.

Cohan, R. H., Dunnick, N. R., Degesys, G. E., and Korobkin, M.: Computed tomography of renal oncocytoma. J. Comput. Assist. Tomogr. 8:284, 1984.

Conn, J. W., Bookstein, J. J., and Cohen, E. L.: Renin-secreting juxtaglomerular-cell adenoma: Preoperative clinical and angiographic diagnosis. Radiology 106:543, 1973.

Daniel, W. W., Hartman, G. W., Witten, D. W., Farrow, G. M., and Kelalis, P. P.: Calcified renal masses: A review of ten years experience at the Mayo Clinic. Radiology 103:503, 1972.

Davidson, A. J., Hayes, W. S., Hartman, D. S., McCarthy, W. F., and Davis, C. J., Jr.: Renal oncocytoma and carcinoma: Failure of differentiation with CT. Radiology 186:693, 1993.

Davidson, J. K., and Clark, D. C.: Renin-secreting juxtaglomerular-cell tumor. Br. J. Radiol. 47:594, 1974.

Davis, C. J., Sesterhan, I. A., Mostafi, F. K., and Ho, C. K.: Renal oncocytoma: Clinicopathology study of 166 patients. J. Urogen. Pathol. 1:41, 1991.

Defossez, S. M., Yoder, I. C., Papanicolaou, N., Rosen, B. R., and McGovern, F.: Nonspecific magnetic resonance appearance of renal oncocytoma: Report of three cases and review of literature. J. Urol. 145:552, 1991.

Dunnick, N. R., Hartman, D. S., Ford, K. K., Davis, C. J., Jr., and Amis, E. S., Jr.: The radiology of juxtaglomerular tumors. Radiology 147:321, 1983.

Fairchild, T. N., Dail, D. H., and Brannen, G. E.: Renal oncocytoma—bilateral, multifocal. Urology 22:355, 1983.

Feczko, P. J.: Renal hemangioma: Cause of massive hematuria. Urology 13:447, 1979.

Friedman, A. C., Hartman, D. S., Sherman, J., Lautin, E. M., and Goldman, M.: Computed tomography of abdominal fatty masses. Radiology 139:415, 1981.

Gonzalez-Crussi, F., Sotelo-Avila, C., and Kidd, J. M.: Mesenchymal renal tumors in infancy: A reappraisal. Hum. Pathol. 12:78, 1981.

Göthlin, J., and Lyrdal, F.: Haemorrhage due to renal angiomatosis. Scand. J. Urol. Nephrol. 10:170, 1976.

Hartman, D. S., Goldman, S. M., Friedman, A. C., Davis, C. J., Jr., Madewell, J. E., and Sherman, J. L.: Angiomyolipoma: Ultrasonic-pathologic correlation. Radiology 139:451, 1981.

Hartman, D. S., Lesar, M. S. C., Madewell, J. E., and Davis, C. J.: Mesoblastic nephroma: Radiologic-pathologic correlation of 20 cases. AJR 136:69, 1981.

Hartman, D. S.: Pediatric renal tumors. In Taveras, J., and Ferucci, J. (eds.): Radiology Diagnosis, Imaging, Intervention. Philadelphia, J. B. Lippincott Co., 1986, vol. 4, chapter 117, pp. 1–9.

Jander, H. P.: Renal oncocytoma: A nonentity. Radiology 130:815, 1979.

Jonutis, A. J., Davidson, A. J., and Redman, H. C.: Curvilinear calcifications in four uncommon benign renal lesions. Clin. Radiol. 24:468, 1973.

Kerr, L. A., Blute, M. L., Ryu, J. H., Swensen, S. J., and Malek, R. S.: Renal angiomyolipoma in association with pulmonary lymphangioleiomyomatosis—forme fruste of tuberous sclerosis. Urology 41:440, 1993.

Klein, M. J., and Valensi, Q. J.: Proximal tubular adenomas of kidney with so-called oncocytic features: A clinicopathologic study of 13 cases of a rarely reported neoplasm. Cancer 38:906, 1976.

Lautin, E. M, Gordon, P. M., Friedman, A. C., McCormick, J. F., Fromowitz, F. B., Goldman, M. J., Sugarman, L. A.: Radionuclide imaging and computed tomography in renal oncocytoma. Radiology 138:185, 1981.

Levine, E., and Huntrakoon, M.: Computed tomography of renal oncocytoma. AJR 141:741, 1983.

Lieber, M. M., Tomera, K. M., and Farrow, G. M.: Renal oncocytoma. J. Urol. 125:481, 1981.

Morra, M. W., and Das, S.: Renal oncocytoma—a review of histogenesis, histopathology, diagnosis, and treatment. J. Urol. 150:295, 1933.

Neisius, D., Braedel, H. U., Schridler, E., Hoene, E., and Allooss, S.: Computed tomographic and angiographic findings in renal oncocytoma. Br. J. Radiol. 61:1019, 1988.

Oesterling, J. E., Fishman, E. K., Goldman, G. M., and Marshall, F. F.: The management of renal angiomyolipoma. J. Urol. 135:1121, 1986.

Quinn, M. J., Hartman, D. S., Friedman, A. C., Sherman, J. L., Lawtin, E. M., Pyatt, R. S., Ho, C. K., Csere, R., and Fromowitz, F. B.: Renal oncocytoma: New observations. Radiology 153:49, 1984.

Raghavendra, B. N., Bosniak, M. A., and Megibow, A. J.: Small angiomyolipoma of the kidney: Sonographic-CT evaluation. AJR 141:575, 1983.

Seshanarayana, K. N., and Keats, T. E.: Angiomyolipoma of the kidney: Diagnostic roentgenographic findings. AJR 104:332, 1968.

Sherman, J. L., Hartman, D. S., Friedman, A. C., Madewell, J. E., Davis, C. J., and Goldman, S. M.: Angiomyolipoma: Computed tomographic-pathologic correlation of 17 cases. AJR 137:1221, 1981.

Tong, Y. C., Chieng, P. U., Tsai, T. C., and Lin, S. N.: Renal angiomyolipoma: Report of 24 cases. Br. J. Urol. 66:585, 1990.

Totty, W. G., McClennan, B. L., Melson, G. L., and Patel, R.: Relative value of computed tomography and ultrasonography in the assessment of renal angiomyolipoma. J. Comput. Assist. Tomogr. 5:173, 1981.

Zollikofer, C., Castanda-Zuniga, W., Nath, H. P., Velasquez, G., Formanek, A., Feinberg, S. B., and Amplatz, K.: The angiographic appearance of intrarenal leiomyoma. Radiology 136:47, 1980.

Simple Renal Cyst

Bernstein, J.: Renal cystic disease in the tuberous sclerosis complex. Pediatr. Nephrol. 7:490, 1993.

Bosniak, M. A.: The current radiological approach to renal cysts. Radiology 158:1, 1986.

Cho, K. J., Maklad, N., Curran, J., and Ting, Y. M.: Angiographic and ultrasonic findings in infected simple cysts of the kidney. AJR 127:1015, 1976.

Coleman, B. G., Arger, P. H., Mintz, M. C., Pollack, H. M., and Banner, M. P.: Hyperdense renal masses: A computed tomographic dilemma. AJR 143:291, 1984.

Daniel, W. W., Hartman, G. W., Witten, D. M., Farrow, G. M., and Kelalis, P. P.: Calcified renal masses: A review of ten years experience at the Mayo Clinic. Radiology 103:503, 1972.

Dunnick, N. R., Korobkin, M., Silverman, P. H., and Foster, W. L., Jr.: Computed tomography of high density renal cysts. J. Comput. Assist. Tomogr. 8:458, 1984.

Dunnick, N. R., Korobkin, M., and Clark, W. M.: CT demonstration of hyperdense renal carcinoma. J. Comput. Assist. Tomogr. 8:1023, 1984.

Emmett, J. L., Levine, S. R., and Woolner, L. B.: Coexistence of renal cyst and tumor: Incidence in 1007 cases. Br. J. Urol. 35:403, 1963.

Goldman, S. M., and Hartman, D. S.: The simple cyst. In Hartman, D. S. (ed.): Renal cystic disease, fascicle I. AFIP Atlas of Radiologic-Pathologic Correlation. Philadelphia, W.B. Saunders, 1989, pp. 6–37.

Hartman, D. S.: Cysts and cystic neoplasms. Urol. Radiol. 12:7, 1990.

Kleist, H., Jonsson, O., Lundstam, S., Naucler, J., Nilson, A. E., and Petterson, S.: Quantitative lipid analysis in the differential diagnosis of cystic renal lesions. Br. J. Urol. 54:441, 1982.

Ljungberg, B., Holmberg, G., Sjodin, J. G., Hietala, S. O., Stenling, R.: Renal cell carcinoma in a renal cyst: A case report and review of the literature. J. Urol. 143:797, 1990.

McHugh, K., Stringer, D. A., Hebert, D., and Babiak, C. A.: Simple renal cysts in children: Diagnosis and followup with US. Radiology 178:383, 1991.

Mitnick, J. S., Bosniak, M. A., Hilton, S., Raghavendra, B. N., Subramanyam, B. R., and Genieser, N. B.: Cystic renal disease in tuberous sclerosis. Radiology 147:85, 1983.

Moss, J. G., and Hendry, G. M. A.: The natural history of renal cysts in an infant with tuberous sclerosis: Evaluation with ultrasound. Br. J. Radiol. 61:1074, 1988.

Narla, L. D., Slovis, T. L., Watts, F. B., and Nigro, M.: The renal lesions of tuberosclerosis (cysts and angiomyolipoma): Screening with sonography and computerized tomography. Pediatr. Radiol. 18:205, 1988.

Pearlstein, A. E.: Hyperdense renal cysts. J. Comput. Assist. Tomogr. 7:1029, 1983.

Pedersen, J. F., Emamian, S. A., and Nielsen, M. B.: Simple renal cyst—relations to age and arterial blood pressure. Br. J. Radiol. 66:581, 1993.

Silverman, J. F., and Kilhenny, C.: Tumor in the wall of a simple renal cyst: Report of a case. Radiology 93:95, 1969.

Steg, A.: Renal cysts: I. Current pathogenic approach. Eur. Urol. 2:161, 1976.

Steg, A.: Renal cysts: II. Chemical and dynamic study of cystic fluid. Eur. Urol. 2:164, 1976.

Sussman, S., Cochran, S. T., Pagani, J. J., McArdle, C., Wong, W., Austin, R., Curry, N., and Kelly, K. M.: Hyperdense renal masses: A CT manifestation of hemorrhagic renal cysts. Radiology 150:207, 1984.

Weitzner, S.: Clear cell carcinoma of the free wall of a simple renal cyst. J. Urol. 106:515, 1971.

Zirinsky, K., Auh, Y. H., Rubenstein, W. A., Williams, J. J., Pasmantier, M. W., and Kazam, E.: CT of the hyperdense renal cyst: Sonographic correlation. AJR 143:151, 1984.

Focal Hydronephrosis

Cramer, B. C., Twomey, B. P., and Katz, D.: CT findings in obstructed upper moieties of duplex kidneys. J. Comput. Assist. Tomog. 7:251, 1983.

Cronan J. J., Amis, E. S., Zeman, R. K., Dorfman, G. S.: Obstruction of the upper-pole moiety in renal duplication in adults: CT evaluation. Radiology 161:17, 1986.

Koehler, P. R., and McAlister, W. H.: Nonopacified duplicated collecting systems simulating renal tumors in adults. J. Can. Assoc. Radiol. 19:4, 1968.

Mascatello, V. J., Smith, E. H., Carrera, G. F., and Teele, R. L.: Ultrasonic evaluation of the obstructed duplex kidney. AJR 129:113, 1977.

Nusbacher, N., and Bryk, D.: Hydronephrosis of the lower pole of the duplex kidney. AJR 130:967, 1978.

Winters W. D., and Lebowitz, R. L.: Importance of prenatal detection of hydronephrosis of the upper pole. AJR 155:125, 1990.

Abscess

Anderson, K. A., and McAninch, J. W.: Renal abscesses: Classification and review of 40 cases. Urology 16:333, 1980.

Combs, J. A., Crummy, A. B., and Cossman, F. P.: Angiography in renal and pararenal inflammatory lesions: The significance of early venous filling. Radiology 98:401, 1971.

Daniel, W. W., Hartman, G. W., Witten, D. M., Farrow, G. M., and

Kelalis, P. P.: Calcified renal masses: A review of ten years experience at the Mayo Clinic. Radiology 103:503, 1972.

Doolittle, K. H., and Taylor, J. H.: Renal abscess in the differential diagnosis of mass on the kidney. J. Urol. 89:649, 1963.

Elkin, M.: Renal cysts and abscesses. Curr. Prob. Diagn. Radiol. 5:36, 1975.

Evans, J. A., Meyers, M. A., and Bosniak, M. A.: Acute renal and perirenal infections. Semin. Roentgenol. 6:274, 1971.

Fair, W. R., and Higgins, M. H.: Renal abscess. J. Urol. 104:179, 1970.

Funston, M. R., Fisher, K. S., van Blerk, P. J. P., and Borte, J. H.: Acute focal bacterial nephritis or renal abscess? A sonographic diagnosis. Br. J. Urol. 54:461, 1982.

Godec, C. J., Tsai, S. H., Smith, S. J., and Cass, A. S.: Diagnostic strategy in evaluation of renal abscess. Urology 18:535, 1981.

Hoddick, W., Jeffrey, R. B., Goldberg, H. I., Federle, M. P., and Laing, F. C.: CT and sonography of severe renal and perirenal infections. AJR 140:517, 1983.

Kahn, P. C., and Wise, H. M., Jr.: Simulation of renal tumor response to epinephrine by inflammatory disease. Radiology 89:1062, 1967.

Lee, J. K. T., McClennan, B. L., Melson, G. L., and Stanley, R. J.: Acute focal bacterial nephritis: Emphasis on gray scale sonography and computed tomography. AJR 135:87, 1980.

Malgieri, J. J., Kursh, E. D., and Persky, L.: The changing clinico-pathological pattern of abscesses in or adjacent to the kidney. J. Urol. 118:230, 1977.

Salvatierra, O., Jr., Bucklew, W. B., and Morrow, J. W.: Perinephric abscess: A report of 71 cases. J. Urol. 98:296, 1967.

Multilocular Cystic Nephroma

Banner, M. P., Pollack, H. M., Chatten, J., and Witzleben, C.: Multilocular renal cysts: Radiologic-pathologic correlation. AJR 136:239, 1981.

Beckwith, J. B., and Kiviat, N. B.: Multilocular renal cysts and cystic renal tumors. AJR 136:435, 1981.

Brown, R. C., Cornell, S. H., and Culp, D. A.: Multilocular renal cysts with diffuse calcification simulating renal-cell carcinoma. Radiology 95:411, 1970.

Carlson, D. H., Carlson, D., and Simon, H.: Benign multilocular cystic nephroma. AJR 131:621, 1978.

Castiolo, O. A., Boyle, E. T., Jr., and Kramer, S. A.: Multilocular cysts of the kidney: A study of 29 patients and review of literature. Urology 37:156, 1991.

Cheng, W. S., Farrow, G. M., and Zincke, H.: The incidence of multicentricity in renal cell carcinoma. J. Urol. 146:1221, 1991.

De Campo, J. F.: Ultrasound of Wilms' tumor. Pediatr. Radiol. 16:21, 1986.

Exelby, P. R.: Wilms' tumor 1991: Clinical Evaluation and treatment. Urol. Clin. North Am. 18:589, 1991.

Felman, A. H., Hawkins, I. F., Hackett, R. L., and Talbert, J. L.: Multilocular cyst of the kidney: A case report with angiographic findings. Radiology 106:629, 1973.

Friday, R. O., Crummy, A. B., and Malek, G. H.: Multilocular renal cyst: Angiographic ultrasonic and cyst-puncture findings. Urology 3:354, 1974.

Gash, J. R., Zagoria, R. J., Dyer, R. B., and Assimos, D. G.: Imaging features of infiltrating renal lesions. Crit. Rev. Diagn. Imag. 33:4, 1992.

Grossman, H., Rosenberg, E. R., Bowie, J. D., Ram, P., and Merten, D. F.: Sonographic diagnosis of renal cystic diseases. AJR 140:81, 1983.

Hartman, D. S.: Cysts and cystic neoplasms. Urol. Radiol. 12:7, 1990.

Hohenfellner, M., Schultz-Lampel, D., Lampel, A., Steinbach, F., Cramer, B. M., and Thuroff, J. W.: Tumor in the horseshoe kidney: Clinical implications and review of embryogenesis. J. Urol. 147:1098, 1992.

Honda, H., Coffman, C. E., Berbaum, K. S., Barloon, T. J., and Masuda, K.: CT analysis of metastatic neoplasms of the kidney: Comparison with primary renal cell carcinoma. Acta Radiol. 33:39, 1992.

Javadpour, N., Dellon, A. L., and Kumpe, D. A.: Multilocular cystic disease in adults: Imitator of renal cell carcinoma. Urology 1:596, 1973.

Kallman, D. A., King, B. F., Hattery, R. R., Charboneau, J. W., Ehman, R. L., Gothman, D. A., and Blute, M. L.: Renal vein and inferior vena cava tumor thrombosis in renal cell carcinoma: CT, US, MRI and venacavography. J. Comput. Assist. Tomogr. 16:240, 1992.

Kissane, J. M., and Dehner, L. P.: Renal tumors and tumor-like lesions in pediatric patients. Pediatr. Nephrol. 6:4, 1992.

Madewell, J. E., Goldman, S. M., Davis, C. J., Jr., Hartman, D. S., Feigin, D., and Lichtenstein, J. E.: Multilocular cystic nephroma: A radiographic-pathologic correlation of 58 patients. Radiology 146:309, 1983.

Mesrobian, H.-G. J.: Wilms' tumor: Past, present, future. J. Urol. 140:231, 1988.

Parienty, R. A., Pradel, J., Imbert, M.-C., Picard, J.-D., and Savart, P.: Computed tomography of multilocular cystic nephroma. Radiology 140:135, 1981.

Powell, T., Shackman, R., and Johnson, H. D.: Multilocular cysts of the kidney. Br. J. Urol. 23:142, 1951.

Redman, J. F., and Harper, D. L.: Nephroblastoma occurring in a multilocular cystic kidney. J. Urol. 120:356, 1978.

Sisler, C. L., and Siegel, M. J.: Malignant rhabdoid tumor of the kidney: Radiologic features. Radiology 172:211, 1989.

Thijssen, A. M., Carpenter, B., Jiminez, C., and Schillinger, J.: Multilocular cyst (multilocular cystic nephroma) of the kidney: A report of 2 cases with an unusual mode of presentation. J. Urol. 142:346, 1989.

Udsom, S. V., and Melicow, M. M.: Multilocular cysts of the kidney with intrapelvic herniation of a "daughter" cyst: Report of 4 cases. J. Urol. 89:341, 1963.

Volpe, J. P., and Choyke, P. L.: The radiologic evaluation of renal metastases. Crit. Rev. Diagn. Imag. 30:219, 1990.

White, K. S., Kirks, D. R., and Bove, K. E.: Imaging of nephroblastomatosis: An overview. Radiology 182:1, 1992.

Congenital Arteriovenous Malformation

Cho, K. J., and Stanley, J. C.: Non-neoplastic congenital and acquired renal arteriovenous malformations and fistulas. Radiology 129:333, 1978.

Ekelund, L., and Göthlin, J.: Renal hemangiomas: An analysis of 13 cases diagnosed by angiography. AJR 125:788, 1975.

Honda, H., Onitsuka, H., Naitov, S., Hasoo, K., Kamoi, I., Hanada, K., Kumazoma, J., and Masuda, K.: Renal arteriovenous malformations: CT features. J. Comput. Assist. Tomogr. 15:261, 1991.

Kopchick, J. H., Bourne, N. K., Fine, S. W., Jacoshoh, H., Jacobs, S. C., and Lawson, R. K.: Congenital renal arteriovenous malformations. Urology 17:13, 1981.

Rao, A. K. R., and Kimball, W. R.: Ultrasonic appearance of an arteriovenous fistula of the kidney. JCU 6:345, 1978.

Regan, J. B., and Benson, R. C., Jr.: Congenital renal arteriovenous malformations. J. Urol. 136:1184, 1986.

Subramanyam, B. R., Lefleur, R. S., and Bosniak, M. A.: Renal arteriovenous fistulas and aneurysm: Sonographic findings. Radiology 149:261, 1983.

Takaha, M., Matsumoto, A., Ochi, K., Takeuchi, M., Takemoto, M., and Sonoda, T.: Intrarenal arteriovenous malformation. J. Urol. 124:315, 1980.

Takebayashi, S., Aida, N., and Matsui, K.: Arteriovenous malformations of the kidneys: Diagnosis and followup with color Doppler sonography in six patients. AJR 157:991, 1991.

13

PARENCHYMAL DISEASE WITH NORMAL SIZE AND CONTOUR

NEPHROCALCINOSIS

RENAL TUBERCULOSIS

DIFFERENTIAL DIAGNOSIS

In the preceding chapters the discussion has focused on diseases of the kidney that produce either abnormal kidney size or contour. However, when those diseases are excluded, there remain two important groups of abnormalities that have normal kidney size and contour. One group is characterized by generalized calcification of the renal substance, nephrocalcinosis. Primary hyperparathyroidism, the milk-alkali syndrome, hypervitaminosis D, sarcoidosis, primary and metastatic carcinoma to bone, renal tubular acidosis, medullary sponge kidney, hyperoxaluria, Bartter's syndrome, and prolonged furosemide administration in premature newborns are specific clinical entities in which kidney calcification may be radiologically detectable. A second group includes diseases in which infundibulocalyceal abnormalities are either the earliest or the only manifestations of parenchymal disease. Tuberculosis and brucellosis are included in this category.

NEPHROCALCINOSIS

Definition

When sought by careful light or electron microscopic techniques, calcium deposits are present in virtually all kidneys whether they are diseased or not. The term *nephrocalcinosis* is reserved for radiologically detectable *diffuse* calcium deposition within the renal substance and implies a metabolic or renal abnormality. Histologically, calcium is deposited in the interstitium, in tubule epithelial cells, or along basement membranes of the collecting ducts, distal convoluted tubules, or ascending limb of the loop of Henle. Concretions occur within the tubule lumina as well. In medullary cystic kidney specifically, calcium is found in communicating cystic dilatations of the distal collecting tubules. Nephrocalcinosis may be limited to the cortex or to the medulla or occur in both the cortex and the medulla. In most circumstances, however, the medulla is the only portion of the kidney parenchyma that is involved.

Deposition of calcium in the kidney occurs by either *metastatic* or *dystrophic* mechanisms or as the result of *urine stasis.*

Metastatic nephrocalcinosis usually occurs in kidneys that are morphologically normal (including normal size) but that have been subjected to metabolic disorders that promote tissue deposition of calcium, often as a result of hypercalcemia or increased tissue alkalinity. Metastatic calcification is diffuse, involves both kidneys, and is predominantly found in the medullae of the renal parenchyma.

Dystrophic calcification refers to the deposition of calcium in renal tissue that has been injured by hemorrhage, ischemia, or infarction or by suppuration or necrosis. Uncommonly, dystrophic calcification is seen as generalized, bilateral nephrocalcinosis, as in acute cortical necrosis or chronic glomerulonephritis or as a consequence of nephrotoxins. More commonly, dystrophic calcification is focal or unilateral and is not considered to fall within the definition of nephrocalcinosis. Examples include calcification in an adenocarcinoma, the wall of a simple cyst, xanthogranulomatous pyelonephritis, or tuberculosis.

Urinary stasis is the mechanism for nephrocalcinosis in medullary sponge kidney. Here, small stones form in the cystic spaces that communicate with the dilated collecting ducts.

Some diseases in which nephrocalcinosis does occur are not discussed in this chapter because in addition to radiologically detectable calcium in the renal substance, abnormalities of renal size or contour also occur. Renal papillary necrosis, acute cortical necrosis, multiple myeloma, acute tubular necrosis following

405

nephrotoxins, and chronic glomerulonephritis are examples that are covered in other chapters.

Some functional abnormalities may result from nephrocalcinosis. Much of the depression in renal function found in association with nephrocalcinosis, however, is related to an elevated serum calcium level per se. Improvement in function may occur by lowering this value even when the extent of nephrocalcinosis remains unchanged.

Clinical Setting

Conditions associated with nephrocalcinosis and normal renal size and contour can be classified as follows:

Some forms of skeletal deossification
    Primary and secondary hyperparathyroidism
    Metastatic carcinoma to bone
    Primary carcinoma

Increased intestinal absorption of calcium
    Sarcoidosis
    Milk-alkali syndrome
    Hypervitaminosis D

Miscellaneous
    Renal tubular acidosis
    Medullary sponge kidney
    Hyperoxaluria
    Bartter's syndrome
    Prolonged furosemide administration in premature newborns

The clinical aspects of each of these will be considered briefly.

Primary hyperparathyroidism is caused by an adenoma or carcinoma of a single gland or by diffuse hyperplasia of all parathyroid glands. High serum calcium and decreased serum phosphate levels are the biochemical features of this disease. Primary hyperparathyroidism has signs that are common to hypercalcemia, regardless of its cause. These include muscular weakness, myocardial failure, ulcer disease, impaired renal function, and urolithiasis. Polyuria and polydipsia reflect hypercalcemia-induced impairment of urine-concentrating ability. Normochromic, normocytic anemia, pruritus, bone pain, and tenderness may also be present in primary hyperparathyroidism.

Hypercalcemia and nephrocalcinosis occur occasionally in cases of *metastatic cancer* in which considerable bone destruction leads to a release of excessive amounts of calcium. In *primary carcinoma*, particularly of the lung or kidney, a paraneoplastic syndrome with hypercalcemia and nephrocalcinosis occurs. Inappropriate secretion of humoral factors by the tumor presumably underlies this phenomenon.

Patients with *sarcoidosis* develop hypercalcemia owing to increased intestinal sensitivity to vitamin D, which results in excessive absorption of dietary calcium. Renal disease in sarcoidosis is related principally to hypercalcemia and is not dependent on the development of nephrocalcinosis. Only rarely do sarcoid granulomas per se cause renal impairment.

Patients with the *milk-alkali syndrome* have a long history of excessive calcium ingestion, usually in the form of milk and antacids containing calcium carbonate. Positive calcium balance and alkalosis follow, although measurable hypercalcemia may be transitory. Nephrocalcinosis occurs as a result of large tubule loads of calcium and phosphate in the presence of alkaline urine and interstitial fluid.

Hypervitaminosis D results from excessive intake of this vitamin. Hypercalcemia occurs from increased absorption of calcium through the intestine, just as in sarcoidosis. Excessive vitamin D also promotes dissolution of calcium salts from bone, a second mechanism for producing hypercalcemia. These patients experience the usual symptoms of hypercalcemia and eventually develop renal failure with or without nephrocalcinosis.

Renal tubular acidosis is a form of tubule insufficiency in which there is impairment of the ability of the distal nephron to secrete hydrogen ion against a concentration gradient. As a result, the kidney is unable to excrete an acid urine (below pH 5.4) during metabolic acidosis or even under stimulus of ammonium chloride ingestion. Renal tubular acidosis associated with nephrocalcinosis and urolithiasis is known as "classic" or "distal" and takes two forms. In the *complete* form, the patient experiences states of metabolic acidosis with hyperchloremia, hypokalemia, hypercalciuria, and a high urine pH. This form may be idiopathic or may be associated with a variety of genetically transmitted, autoimmune, or toxin-induced diseases of the kidney. Nephrocalcinosis caused by other disorders may itself produce the metabolic abnormality of distal renal tubular acidosis. In the *incomplete* form of distal renal tubular acidosis, electrolytes are normal, but stone formation occurs because of an insufficient amount of citrate excreted to keep calcium soluble in the urine. Patients with distal renal tubular acidosis experience muscle weakness and paralysis and rickets and/or osteomalacia; in children, growth retardation occurs. Symptoms of stone passage are common. Azotemia may develop. Another type of renal tubular acidosis is known as the "proximal" form. Nephrocalcinosis is not a feature of this disorder.

Patients with *medullary sponge kidney* may be entirely free of urinary tract symptoms and have a normal life expectancy. When problems do occur, they are related to stone formation, urinary tract infection, and hematuria. A familial incidence has been reported rarely. Although usually seen in adults, medullary sponge kidney has been described in childhood. There is a well-established, but infrequently seen, relationship between medullary sponge kidney and congenital hemihypertrophy. Coexistence of medullary sponge kidney and primary hyperparathyroidism, reported in numerous instances, raises the possibility of a causal relationship between these two entities.

Hyperoxaluria produces nephrocalcinosis through interstitial deposition of calcium oxalate. The primary form is inherited as an autosomal recessive trait and represents enzymatic defects in the metabolic pathway of glyoxylic acid. Symptoms of calculous disease of the urinary tract occur early in childhood. Infection, hypertension, and obstructive uropathy lead to death—usually before 20 years. Acquired forms of hyperoxaluria follow ingestion of oxalate precursors, occur in association with intestinal disease (particularly regional enteritis), or are secondary to gastric bypass surgery for morbid obesity. This leads to calcium oxalate stone formation and is discussed in Chapter 14.

Bartter's syndrome is characterized by hypokalemia, metabolic alkalosis, hyperreninemia, hypoaldosteronism, and normal blood pressure. Hyperplasia of the juxtaglomerular apparatus is seen histologically. For the most part, children and adolescents are affected, although young adults have been reported with this syndrome. These abnormalities occur either sporadically or as an autosomal recessive inheritance. Individuals with Bartter's syndrome experience muscle weakness and cramps, polyuria, abdominal pain, growth failure, and mental retardation.

Furosemide-induced nephrocalcinosis occurs in low-birth-weight infants who have been treated for a prolonged period (usually 2 to 3 weeks) for congestive heart failure secondary to either patent ductus arteriosus or bronchopulmonary dysplasia. These patients develop hypercalciuria and an alkaline urine. Calcium oxalate and calcium phosphate deposition occurs both in the renal parenchyma and as stones in the pelvocalyceal system.

Radiologic Findings

Radiographic detection of calcium in the renal substance is facilitated by low kilovoltage technique and careful collimation of the x-ray beam. Films of the kidneys must be obtained before injection of contrast material, which otherwise might obscure small calcific deposits as it passes through the renal tubules. Preliminary films should be obtained in frontal and oblique projections to localize calcifications accurately within the renal substance. Tomographic cuts accomplish the same purpose. Sometimes it is difficult to determine whether a calcification is in a papilla or is lying free in the immediately adjacent calyx. This distinction can usually be resolved by careful comparison of the preliminary films with those taken after the calyces are opacified. Unless very small, the calcium deposit will usually remain faintly visible when within the papilla but become obscured when it is calyceal in location (see Fig. 13–4).

The extent of renal parenchymal calcification is highly variable (Figs. 13–1 through 13–3). In most cases of nephrocalcinosis due to deossification of the skeleton (primary hyperparathyroidism, primary or metastatic cancer, Cushing's syndrome, or adrenal corticosteroid medication) or increased absorption of calcium (sarcoidosis, milk-alkali syndrome, and hypervitaminosis D), only a few scattered punctate densities in the medullary portion of each kidney are seen. The pattern of calcium deposition in renal tubu-

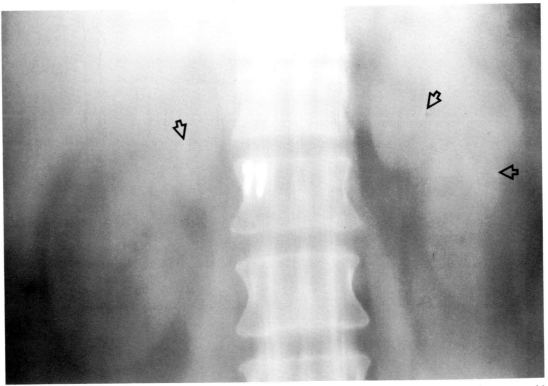

Figure 13–1. Nephrocalcinosis due to milk-alkali syndrome. Punctate densities *(arrows)* are present in both kidneys of a 61-year-old man with a 13-year history of high intake of calcium bicarbonate. Tomogram, preliminary film.

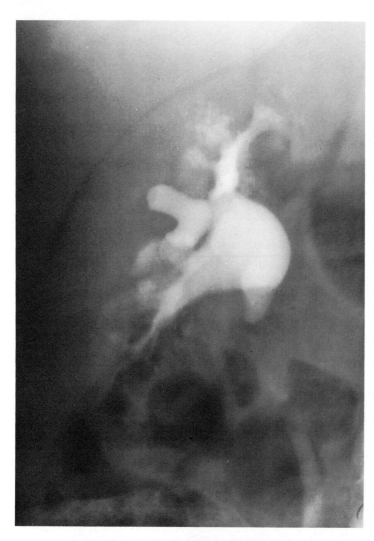

Figure 13–2. Nephrocalcinosis secondary to hypercalcemia associated with sarcoidosis. Calcifications are most apparent in the medullary portions of the upper pole. Excretory urogram. (Courtesy of Department of Diagnostic Radiology, Hammersmith Hospital, Royal Postgraduate Medical School, London, England.)

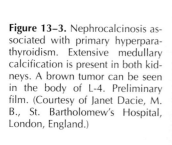

Figure 13–3. Nephrocalcinosis associated with primary hyperparathyroidism. Extensive medullary calcification is present in both kidneys. A brown tumor can be seen in the body of L-4. Preliminary film. (Courtesy of Janet Dacie, M. B., St. Bartholomew's Hospital, London, England.)

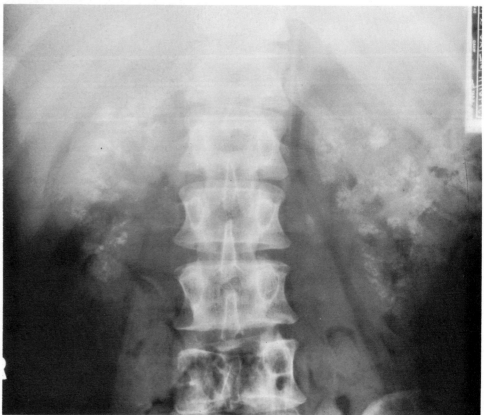

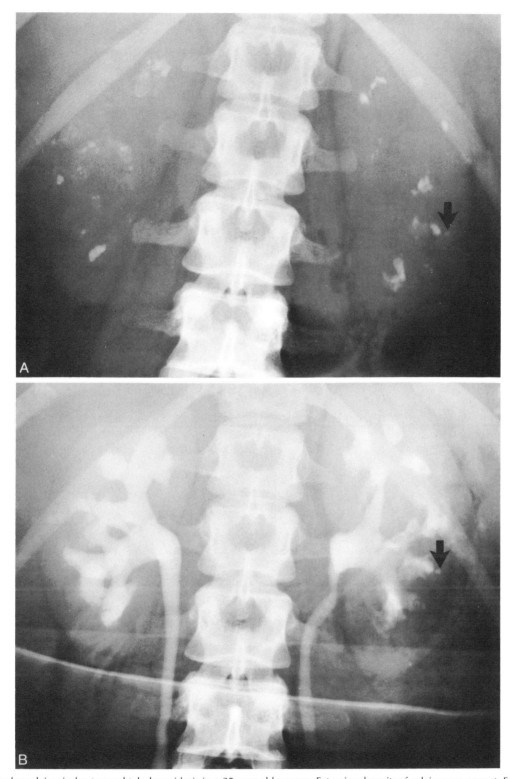

Figure 13–4. Nephrocalcinosis due to renal tubular acidosis in a 25-year-old woman. Extensive deposits of calcium are present. Evidence that the calcification is in the renal parenchyma (nephrocalcinosis) rather than in the collecting system (nephrolithiasis) is derived from the fact that individual foci can still be identified after contrast material fills the collecting system *(arrows)*.

A, Preliminary film.

B, Excretory urogram with compression. (Compare with Fig. 13–7.)

(Courtesy of the Department of Diagnostic Radiology, Hammersmith Hospital, Royal Postgraduate Medical School, London, England.) (Same patient illustrated in Fig. 14–10.)

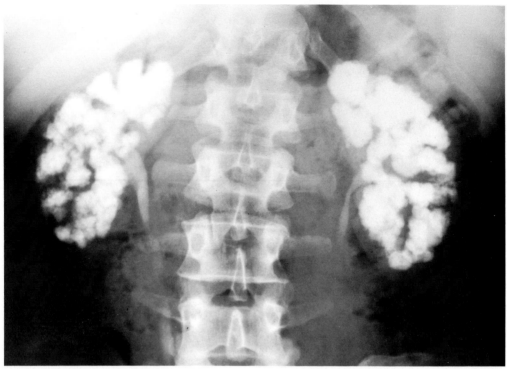

Figure 13–5. Nephrocalcinosis due to renal tubular acidosis in a 34-year-old man with skeletal deformity, first noted at age 2. Nephrocalcinosis was first detected at age 8. Dense confluent deposition of calcium in the medullae is characteristic of renal tubular acidosis. Excretory urogram. (Courtesy of Janet Dacie, M.B., St. Bartholomew's Hospital, London, England.)

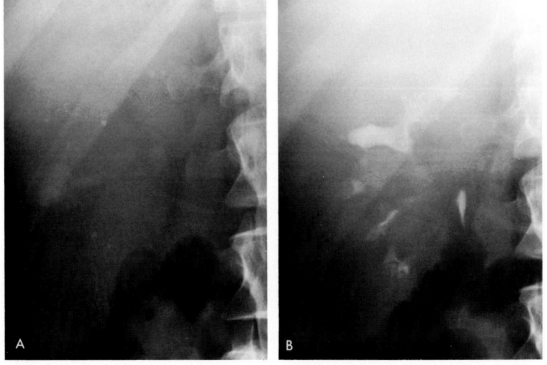

Figure 13–6. Medullary sponge kidney in a 50-year-old man. The preliminary film *(A)* demonstrates a few scattered punctate densities. During excretory urography *(B)*, additional round densities become apparent, particularly in the lower pole, as contrast material fills cystic dilatations of the collecting ducts.

lar acidosis may be similar in some cases, but more often there is very dense and extensive calcification of the medullary portions of the renal lobes (Figs. 13–4 and 13–5). This pattern is quite characteristic of renal tubular acidosis.

Medullary sponge kidney is different from other entities in this section, since a confident diagnosis can be made by detecting urographic abnormalities other than nephrocalcinosis. Because the cystic dilatations that characterize this disorder communicate with the distal collecting ducts, they fill with contrast material during urography. Therefore, those cystic spaces that do not contain stones become apparent only during urography as clusters of small, rounded opacities grouped together in the papillary tip of the renal pyramid. These vary in number from a few to many and may involve one, several, or all papillae. On the other hand, those cystic spaces that do contain stones are detected as nephrocalcinosis on the preliminary film. With contrast material enhancement, however, these baseline calcific densities become obscured as contrast material flows into the cystic spaces in which they reside and surrounds the individual calculi. This unique feature, in which baseline densities become obscured after contrast material enhancement, serves to distinguish medullary sponge kidney from other causes of nephrocalcinosis (Figs. 13–6 and 13–7; see also Fig. 13–4).

In patients with medullary sponge kidneys, many of the affected collecting ducts are ectatic rather than cystic. In these cases, numerous radiodense linear striae appear in the papillae during urography (Figs. 13–8 and 13–9). This appearance may be confused with the intense, homogeneous enhancement of the pyramids that is sometimes seen when urography is performed without ureteral compression and in the absence of ureteral obstruction. This "papillary blush" occurs in normal kidneys owing to a high dose of contrast material, normal renal function, and a state of antidiuresis induced by dehydration. Even when the papillary blush can be shown to be composed of separate, fine linear striations (the collecting tubules), it is generally held that these are normal collecting tubules that have become very dense during excretory urography. This normal, brushlike appearance is more frequently seen with low osmolality than with high osmolality contrast material. *Therefore, the diagnosis of medullary sponge kidney requires, in addition to linear striations in the papillae, the demonstration of nephrocalcinosis either by radiography or ultrasonography and/or cystic dilatations in the papillae following contrast material enhancement.*

Medullary sponge kidney has been reported with smooth enlargement of the kidneys and with congenital hemihypertrophy. In the latter circumstance, the sponge kidney may be bilateral or either ipsilateral or contralateral to the side of hypertrophy. Additionally, medullary sponge kidney may coexist with Caroli's disease and congenital hepatic fibrosis. Medullary sponge kidney has been reported in children as well as adults (see Fig. 13–9).

Unilateral medullary sponge kidney unassociated with hemihypertrophy also occurs, as does a unifocal form. However, the radiologic abnormalities of medullary sponge kidney limited to one part of a kidney may represent obstruction of papillary duct orifices by a slowly growing transitional cell carcinoma or other neoplasm (Fig. 13–10).

Nephrocalcinosis, regardless of cause, is more readily detectable by computed tomography than film radiography owing to the greater contrast resolution of the former. The search for nephrocalcinosis should include computed tomographic scanning without contrast material enhancement when standard radiographs, including tomograms, of the kidneys are normal. A ringlike pattern of medullary nephrocalcinosis has been described on computed tomograms, suggesting a predilection for crystal deposition in the corticomedullary area of the medullae.

Medullary nephrocalcinosis causes increased echogenicity in the medullae, usually sparing the cortex (Fig. 13–11). As in computed tomography, a ringlike pattern had been described on ultrasonograms as well (Fig. 13–12). Acoustic shadowing may be absent depending on the extent of crystal deposition. Increased medullary echogenicity without acoustic shadowing in nephrocalcinosis, therefore, may simulate other forms of renal parenchymal disease, as discussed in the differential diagnosis section at the end of this chapter. Ultrasonography, like computed tomography, is more sensitive than film radiography in the detection of nephrocalcinosis.

Text continued on page 417

SUMMARY OF ABNORMAL URORADIOLOGIC FINDINGS
NEPHROCALCINOSIS

Primary Uroradiologic Elements
   Size—normal (occasionally enlarged in medullary sponge kidney)
   Contour—normal
   Lesion distribution—bilateral
Secondary Uroradiologic Elements
   Papillae—linear tracts or cystic dilatation (medullary sponge kidney)
   Calcification—papilla—grouped, rounded (medullary sponge kidney); papilla and medulla—
      rounded or linear (skeletal deossification, increased calcium absorption, renal tubular acidosis,
      and hyperoxaluria); may be ringlike (computed tomography)
   Echogenicity—medullary echogenicity with or without acoustic shadowing; may be ringlike

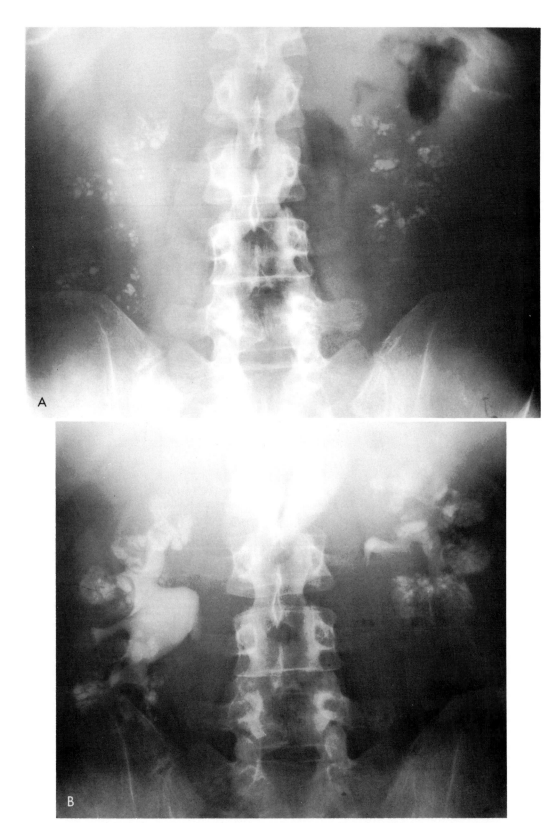

Figure 13–7. Medullary sponge kidney with advanced radiographic abnormalities in a 45-year-old woman. The preliminary film *(A)* demonstrates extensive small and large densities in the papillae. This pattern is indistinguishable from that resulting from other causes of nephrocalcinosis. The 10-minute urogram *(B)*, however, demonstrates added density accumulating in the papillae as contrast material fills those cystic spaces that do not already contain stones. At the same time, discrete foci of calcification identified on the preliminary film become obscure as contrast material flows into the cystic spaces in which they are located. These features are characteristic of medullary sponge kidney. (Compare with Fig. 13–4.)

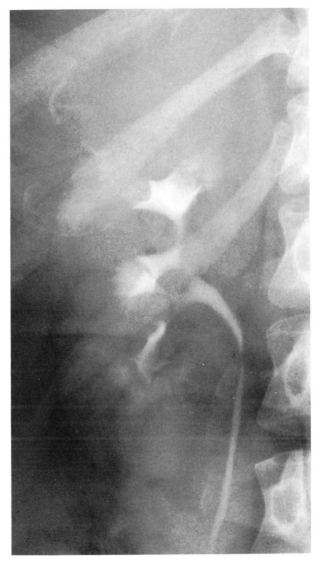

Figure 13–8. Medullary sponge kidney in a 48-year-old woman. Fine linear striations, particularly in lower pole, represent minimal changes of medullary sponge kidney. This diagnosis could not be made, however, without the cystic dilatations that were present in the papillae of the opposite kidney.

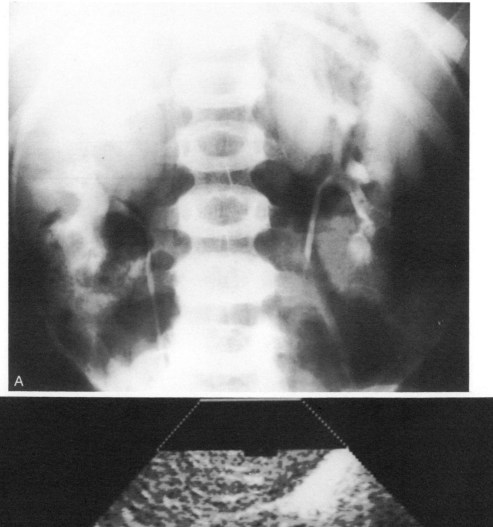

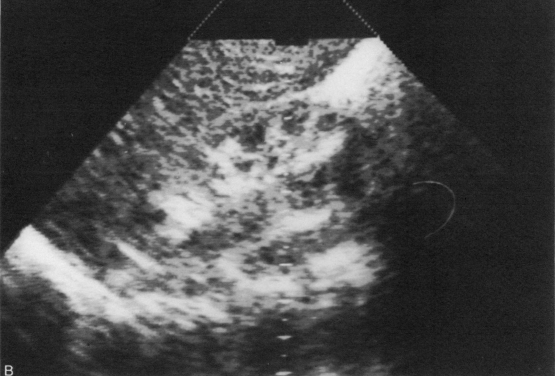

Figure 13–9. Medullary sponge kidney in a 6-year-old boy with polydipsia in whom similar findings had been present since the age of 5 months.

A, Excretory urogram. No calcification was identified on the preliminary radiograph. The collecting ducts in the papillae are distinctly ectatic. Both kidneys are enlarged.

B, Ultrasonogram, longitudinal section, right kidney. There is medullary hyperechoicity.

(Courtesy of Heidi B. Patriquin, M.D., University of Montreal, Montreal, Quebec, Canada and American Journal of Roentgenology *145*:315, 1985.)

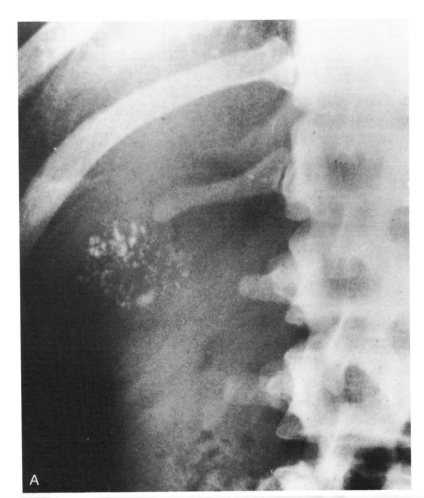

Figure 13–10. Focal medullary sponge kidney, upper pole, right kidney, at the site of a transitional cell carcinoma *(arrow)*. The preliminary film *(A)* and excretory urographic *(B)* findings are those of medullary sponge kidney. The finding of focal medullary sponge kidney requires careful evaluation of the adjacent calyx for an obstructing lesion, as illustrated in this example.

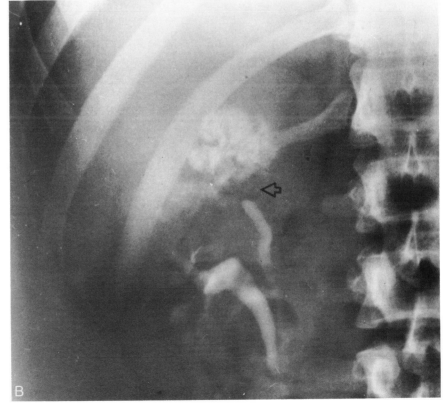

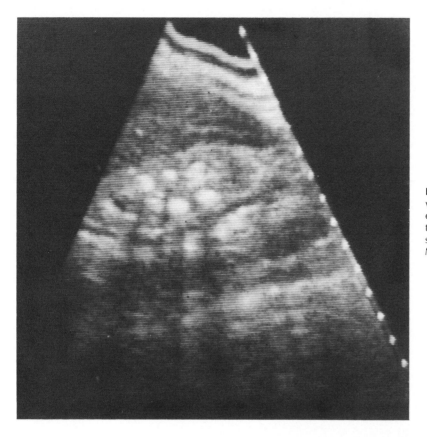

Figure 13–11. Nephrocalcinosis in a 5-year-old child with primary oxaluria. The medullae are densely echogenic, and acoustic shadowing is present. Note the sparing of the cortex. Ultrasonogram, longitudinal section of the right kidney. (Courtesy of Roy Filly, M.D., University of California, San Francisco.)

Figure 13–12. Nephrocalcinosis due to renal tubular acidosis in a 5-year-old girl with polyuria and polydipsia. Ultrasonogram, right kidney, longitudinal section. There is a ringlike pattern of hyperechoicity in the medullae. (Courtesy of the Department of Radiology and Radiologic Science, The Johns Hopkins University, Baltimore, Maryland.)

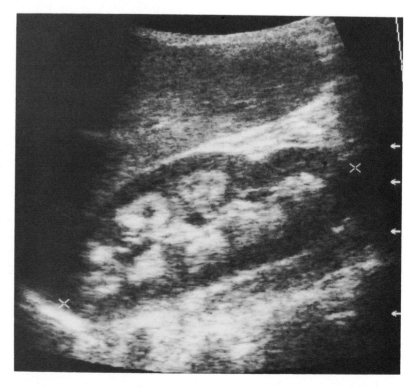

RENAL TUBERCULOSIS

Definition

Renal tuberculosis shows a wider variety of pathologic features than any other disease of the renal parenchyma. The kidney may become focally scarred or globally enlarged or may develop single or multiple masses. It may appear grossly normal or completely destroyed. Early in the disease, however, renal size and contour are normal, and the lesion first becomes radiologically detectable as minor irregularities on the surface of a papilla and its calyx. It is for this reason that renal tuberculosis is included in this chapter.

Tuberculosis of the kidney occurs as a result of metastatic seeding of *Mycobacterium tuberculosis* in the glomerular and peritubular capillary bed from a primary infection elsewhere. The organism is usually of the human, rather than bovine, type. The organisms are disseminated through the bloodstream and therefore always involve both kidneys diffusely. The subsequent course of the infection, however, is determined by the dose and virulence of the inoculum as well as by host resistance factors. Characteristically, most of the initial lesions heal, and only one or a few progress to clinically or radiologically apparent abnormalities. This happens when the bacilli erode out of their initial vascular location and spill into the tubule lumina. As a result of this migration, granulomas form along the nephron. Those occurring in the loop of Henle produce ulceration of the papillary tip. Granuloma formation, caseous necrosis, and cavitation are stages of progressive infection that cause single or multiple masses, which can ultimately destroy the entire kidney. Occasionally, these may cavitate and communicate with the collecting structure. Fibrosis and calcium deposition represent healing. The pattern of progression and healing is highly variable and produces asymmetric histologic, macroscopic, and radiologic abnormalities unique to each patient. In some cases the entire pathologic picture is limited to one or only a few papillae. As described in Chapter 15, pelvocalyceal and ureteral involvement appear as mucosal ulceration, focal or generalized dilatation, or cicatrix formation. Generalized or focal hydronephrosis follows localized scar formation in the pelvis or an infundibulum. Eventually the bladder and genital structures become involved.

Brucellosis and primary fungal infection of the kidney may produce a pathologic picture identical to that of tuberculosis.

Clinical Setting

Renal tuberculosis affects adult men more commonly than women in the general population. Reflecting on the many different pathologic manifestations, it is not surprising that the clinical picture, too, is highly variable. Most, but not all, patients have a history of tuberculosis in a site other than the kidney, usually in bone or the lungs. Infection in the primary organ may be inactive by the time renal tuberculosis becomes apparent. Therefore, a normal chest radiograph is found in about 50 per cent of patients with urinary tract tuberculosis. Only 10 to 15 per cent of patients with active genitourinary tuberculosis have active pulmonary disease at the same time. In addition to affecting the general population, tuberculosis is prevalent in immunocompromised patients, notably those with acquired immunodeficiency syndrome.

Fever, anorexia, fatigue, weakness, night sweats, and weight loss are uncommon in renal tuberculosis. Frequency is the most common urinary tract symptom. Suprapubic, groin, or flank pain; hematuria; dysuria; and complaints referable to epididymitis may be symptoms of patients with urinary tract tuberculosis. On the other hand, 10 per cent of patients are asymptomatic. Pus cells in urine that is "sterile" when cultured on standard media are the classic laboratory findings. The diagnosis is established by the demonstration of acid-fast bacilli on microscopic examination of the urine with special stains, by culture on appropriate media, or by growth of tubercle bacilli in inoculated guinea pigs.

Radiologic Findings

The single most distinctive feature of renal tuberculosis is a parenchymal cavity communicating with the collecting system. Notable also are the multiplicity of genitourinary abnormalities. Tuberculous involvement of the lumbar spine, paraspinous and psoas abscess, and calcifications in the liver, spleen, adrenal glands, and lymph nodes may coexist.

The entire genitourinary system may be radiologically normal in symptomatic renal tuberculosis. The earliest urographic abnormality is irregularity of the surface of one or more papillae or calyces at a time when renal size and contour are normal. The papilla may appear "smudged" (Fig. 13–13), or tracts of contrast material may extend into the medulla along the side of the papilla (Fig. 13–14). Papillary necrosis can become quite extensive (Figs. 13–15 and 13–16). Regardless of the degree of involvement, radiologic abnormalities are confined to a single kidney in over 70 per cent of cases.

Progressive involvement of renal parenchyma occurs in three forms, which may occur singly or in combination. First is the effect of granulomas that grow and coalesce, leading to unifocal or multifocal mass lesions. These may enlarge overall renal length, expand the thickness of the renal substance, and cause displacement of adjacent portions of the collecting system (see Fig. 13–16). Focal calcification, either circumscribed or amorphous, occurs at these sites, particularly as caseation occurs. These masses may rupture into the collecting system, leaving irregular parenchymal cavities that opacify during urography, computed tomography, or retrograde pyelography (Fig. 13–17). The second form seen in advanced renal tuberculosis is due to tissue loss and scarring, leading to surface scars over retracted papillae and dilated calyces (Fig. 13–18). Impaired excretion of contrast material may be noted in either of these two forms. A third form of renal tuberculosis is the calcified non-

Text continued on page 424

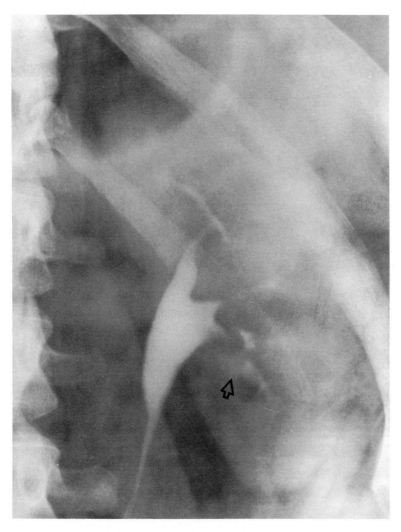

Figure 13–13. Tuberculosis. "Smudging" of contrast material along the medial side of the lower pole calyceal system *(arrow)* is a very early sign of tuberculosis. Excretory urogram.

Figure 13–14. Tuberculosis. Involvement of several papillae is manifested by collections of contrast material in a smooth cavity at one site *(open arrow)* and in irregular linear extensions in papillae at other sites *(solid arrows)*. Excretory urogram. (Courtesy of Professor Thomas Sherwood, M.B., University of Cambridge, Cambridge, England.)

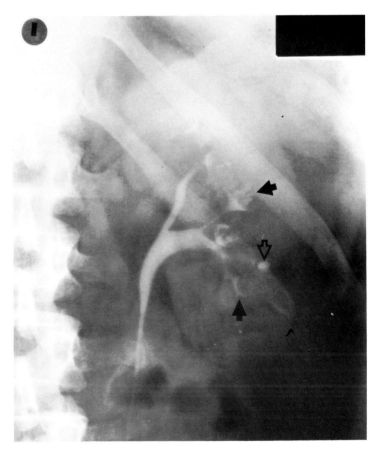

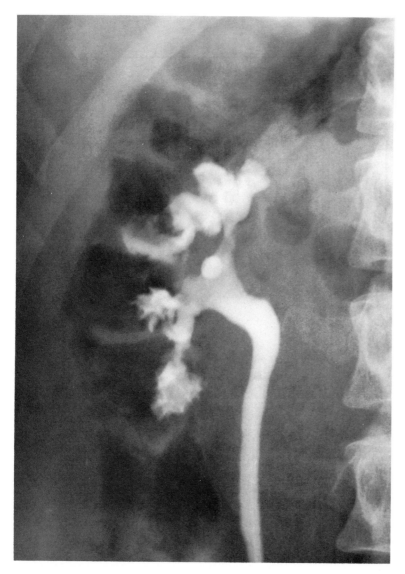

Figure 13–15. Tuberculosis causing extensive generalized papillary necrosis. Retrograde pyelogram.

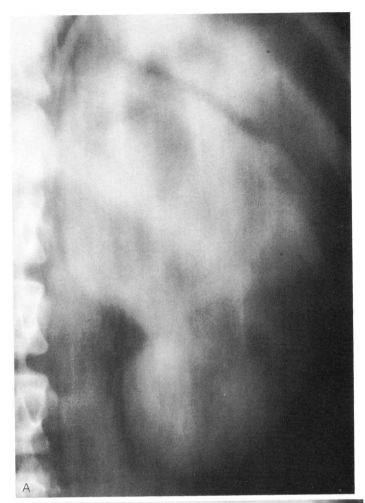

Figure 13–16. Tuberculosis affecting the dorsal portion of the left kidney. The involved area exhibits diminished enhancement and is generally enlarged with overall preservation of reniform shape. The calyces subserving the functioning ventral part of the kidney opacify but are dilated as a result of ureteral and pelvic involvement. Papillary necrosis is evident in the medullae of the ventral portion of the kidney.

   A, Excretory urogram, nephrographic phase. Tomogram.
   B, Excretory urogram, delayed film.

Illustration continued on following page

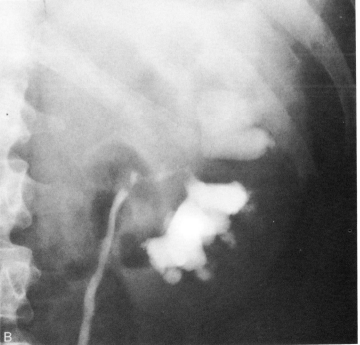

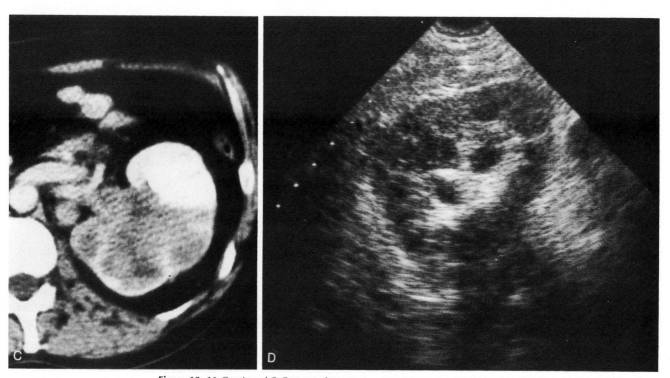

Figure 13–16 *Continued C*, Computed tomogram, contrast material enhanced.
D, Ultrasonogram, transverse section.

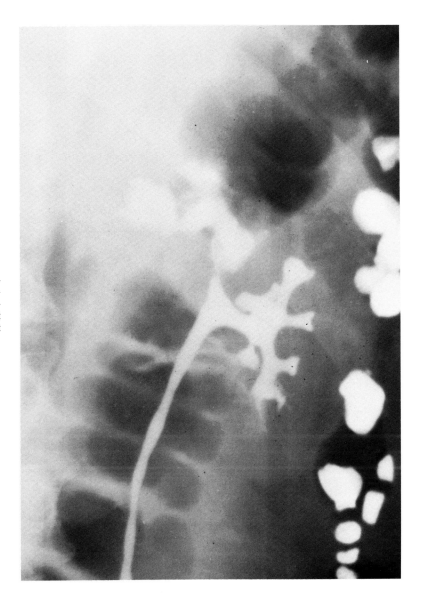

Figure 13–17. Tuberculosis. Cavitation of granulomatous masses in the upper pole has left irregular parenchymal cavities, which opacify during retrograde pyelography. Densities lateral to the kidney represent residual barium in the descending colon. (Same patient illustrated in Fig. 15–29.)

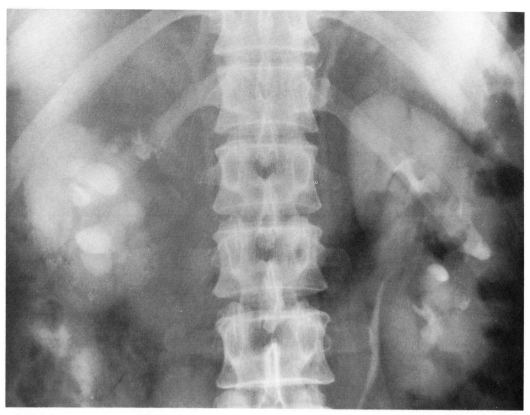

Figure 13–18. Tuberculosis causing extensive tissue loss of the right kidney. The upper pole is severely scarred and contains calcium. Papillae are not visualized, and the calyces are dilated. Mild dilatation of the interpolar and lower polar calyces of the left kidney reflect bilateral involvement. Excretory urogram.

functioning kidney representing autonephrectomy (Fig. 13–19). Calcium deposition in this stage is usually extensive, and the overall size of the destroyed tuberculous organ is often surprisingly close to normal.

In some cases the collecting system may be the only abnormal part of the kidney. The most common deformity is dilatation with an obstructing stricture. Dilatation may be limited to a single calyx whose draining infundibulum is narrowed by a scar, or it may involve the entire pelvocalyceal system (Figs. 13–20 and 13–21; see also Fig. 13–16). Occasionally, obstruction can be of such a high grade and so prolonged that severe hydronephrosis of all or part of the kidney develops (Fig. 13–22). The radiologic features of uroepithelial tuberculosis are described further in Chapters 15 and 19.

Text continued on page 429

SUMMARY OF ABNORMAL URORADIOLOGIC FINDINGS
RENAL TUBERCULOSIS

Preliminary Film
  Osseous, paraspinous changes of tuberculosis; calcification in genitourinary system, spleen, adrenals
Primary Uroradiologic Elements
  Size—normal (early); variable changes, large to small (late)
  Contour—smooth; focal/multifocal expansions, focal/multifocal scars (late)
  Lesion distribution—unilateral (20 to 30 per cent bilateral)
Secondary Uroradiologic Elements
  Papillae—irregular margin (earliest sign); retracted (late); calcified (late).
  Pelvoinfundibulocalyceal system—irregular margin (earliest sign); dilated (focal or global—most
    common sign); strictured (often infundibular); displaced (adjacent to tuberculoma); disrupted (communicating with parenchymal cavities)
  Parenchymal thickness—expanded (focal or multifocal—late); wasted (focal—late); normal (early)
  Calcification—generalized, dense (autonephrectomy); focal (circumscribed, amorphous)
  Nephrogram—contrast material density normal to diminished; replaced (focal at site of granulomas)
  Echogenicity—hyperechoic to hypoechoic masses; caliectasis; pelviectasis
  Additional features—ureter (short, straight, with reflux and multiple strictures); bladder (thick wall,
    decreased capacity); seminal vesicles and epididymides (calcified)

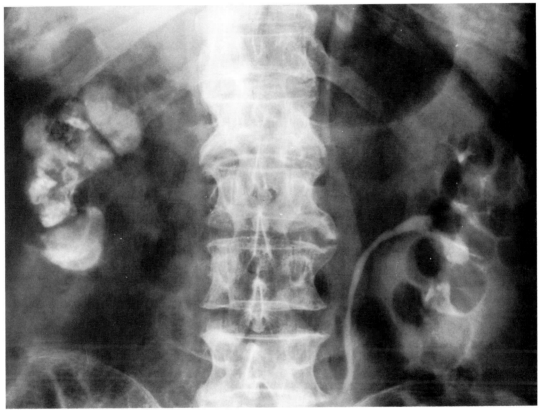

Figure 13–19. Tuberculosis resulting in right autonephrectomy. The kidney has become calcified and does not excrete contrast material. Excretory urogram.

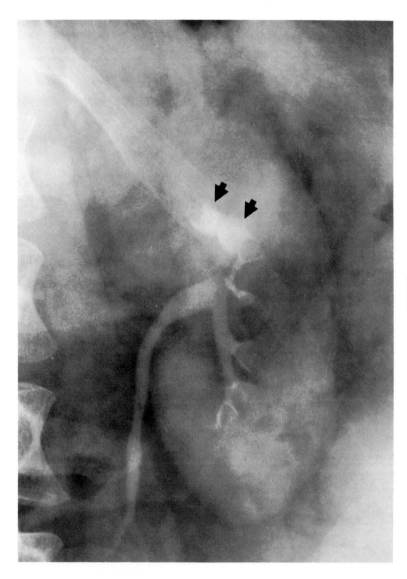

Figure 13–20. Tuberculosis causing focal caliectasis *(arrows)* due to scarring of the infundibulum draining the upper pole system. Excretory urogram.

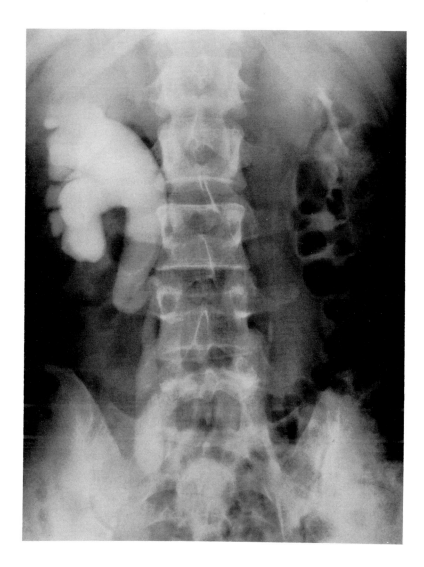

Figure 13–21. Tuberculosis. A distal right ureteral stricture has resulted in marked hydronephrosis and hydroureter. Excretory urogram.

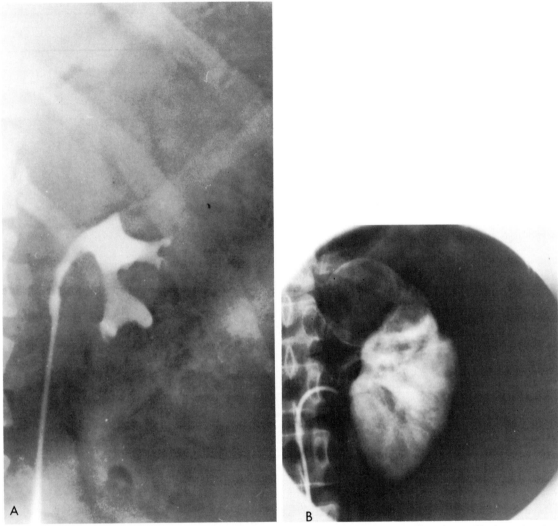

Figure 13–22. Tuberculosis. Scar formation in the infundibulum draining the left upper pole is so severe that advanced hydronephrosis of the upper pole has ensued.
A, Retrograde pyelogram. There is complete occlusion of the infundibulum to the upper pole.
B, Late phase of a selective angiogram. The thick-walled, hydronephrotic upper pole is well visualized.
(Courtesy of M. Korobkin, M.D., University of Michigan, Ann Arbor, Michigan.)

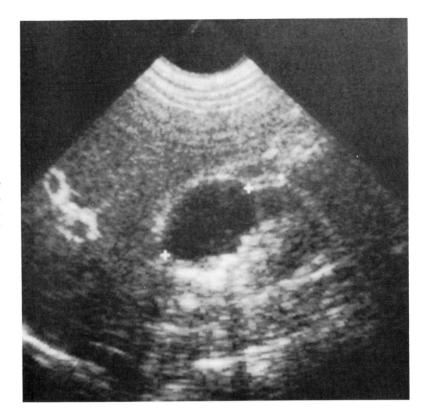

Figure 13–23. Tuberculosis. Cavitating tuberculoma of the right kidney produces an ultrasonographic image of a fluid-filled mass with low-level internal echoes. Longitudinal scan. (Courtesy of Gerald W. Friedland, M.D., Stanford University, Stanford, California.)

Detection of abnormalities in other portions of the genitourinary system is helpful in establishing the diagnosis of tuberculosis. The ureter may be shortened, dilated, and unusually straight, or it may contain multiple strictures. The bladder becomes thick walled and has a diminished capacity for urine storage as a result of tuberculous cystitis. Vesicoureteral reflux may occur. The epididymis or seminal vesicle may calcify.

The varied features of tuberculosis can be determined by computed tomography and ultrasonography, as well as by excretory urography (see Fig. 13–16). However, the latter method is more likely to detect early abnormalities of the papillae. Granulomas appear as masses that have soft tissue density on computed tomography or are echogenic on ultrasonography. Computed tomographic attenuation values decrease with caseation and liquefaction. A tuberculoma that cavitates into the pelvocalyceal system is transformed into a hypoechoic, well-defined mass (Fig. 13–23).

The angiographic features of renal tuberculosis have been described. The findings are basically those of inflammation with a tendency toward hypovascularity. There are no specific findings for tuberculosis itself. This technique should not be necessary to establish the correct diagnosis.

DIFFERENTIAL DIAGNOSIS

Nephrocalcinosis. Of all the conditions causing nephrocalcinosis in normal-sized, smooth kidneys, *medullary sponge kidney* has the most specific urographic features and should be diagnosed easily in most cases using the criteria described previously. Other causes of nephrocalcinosis have a similar pattern of calcium deposition regardless of the underlying abnormal mechanism and cannot be distinguished from each other by radiologic means. The one exception to this generalization is the pattern of very dense calcium deposition throughout the medullary portions of the renal lobe seen in *renal tubular acidosis*.

Differentiation between medullary sponge kidney, renal papillary necrosis, and tuberculosis is occasionally difficult. Unlike renal papillary necrosis and tuberculosis, destruction and sloughing of the papillae do not occur in medullary sponge kidney. Also, medullary sponge kidney calcification is rounded and clustered in cystic dilatations of collecting tubules. As contrast material flows into these cystic dilatations during urography, these baseline calcific densities are obscured while the cystic dilatations become apparent. Contrariwise, calcium deposition in both renal papillary necrosis and tuberculosis is more amorphous, involves the whole papilla, and is less uniformly patterned than in sponge kidney. Further, these baseline densities remain discrete and identifiable after contrast material enhancement. Fine linear striations in the papillae and medulla, similar to the pattern of medullary sponge kidney, may also be seen in Caroli's disease, in the juvenile form of autosomal recessive polycystic kidney disease that is characterized by severe hepatic fibrosis, portal vein hypertension, and minimal renal failure, and as a normal finding, especially when excretory urography is performed with low osmolality contrast material.

The ultrasonographic demonstration of medullary

hyperechogenicity does not necessarily indicate nephrocalcinosis. this finding is also a feature of autosomal recessive (infantile) polycystic kidney disease, autosomal dominant (adult) polycystic kidney disease presenting in infancy, and those forms of multicystic (dysplastic) kidney in which dysplasia dominates. It is also likely that in some cases of medullary sponge kidney, hyperechogenicity of the medulla occurs because of tubular ectasia alone and in the absence of nephrocalcinosis.

Tuberculosis. The early urographic abnormalities of tuberculosis may be very difficult to distinguish from other causes of renal papillary necrosis, such as analgesic abuse, sickle cell hemoglobinopathy, and diabetes mellitus (see Chapter 7). Tuberculosis, however, tends to give a smudged, ill-defined "motheaten" pattern to the papillary-calyceal area, whereas abnormal collections of contrast material in renal papillary necrosis are somewhat better defined either as linear tracts from the fornix into the medulla or as umbilicated cavities extending into the papilla. In addition, abnormalities of other forms of papillary necrosis are limited to the papillary area, while the tuberculous lesion may extend more deeply into the medulla. As these two entities progress in severity, their features diverge and differentiation becomes quite easy.

Medullary sponge kidney is similar to early renal tuberculosis in that it is limited to the papilla. However, the well-defined cystic dilatation of the distal collecting ducts, either containing calcified stones or opacifying during urography, is quite distinctive, and urographic signs of tissue destruction are absent in medullary sponge kidney.

Some cases of healed tuberculosis produce a surface scar with retraction of the underlying papilla and focal calyceal dilatation. This picture, at either a single or multiple sites, is indistinguishable from reflux nephropathy. The diagnosis of tuberculosis can be favored only if other features, such as parenchymal calcification in the scar or stricture of the collecting system or ureter, are also present.

Bibliography

Nephrocalcinosis and Medullary Sponge Kidney

Afonso, D. N., and Oliveira, A. G.: Medullary sponge kidney and congenital hemihypertrophy. Br. J. Urol. 62:187, 1988.

Al-Murrani, B., Cosgrove, D. O., Svensson, W. E., and Blaszczyk, M.: Echogenic rings—an ultrasound sign of early nephrocalcinosis. Clin. Radiol. 44:49, 1991.

Banner, M. P.: Nephrocalcinosis. In Pollack, H. M. (ed.): Clinical Urography. Philadelphia, W.B. Saunders Co., 1990, Chap. 57.

Berger, K. W., and Relman, A. S.: Renal impairment due to sarcoid infiltration of the kidney. N. Engl. J. Med. 252:44, 1955.

Bloomfield, J. A.: Large kidneys including three cases of medullary sponge kidney. J. Coll. Radiol. Australas. 7:33, 1963.

Brennan, R. P., Pearlstein, A. E., and Miller, S. A.: Computed tomography of the kidneys in a patient with methoxyflurane abuse. J. Comput. Assist. Tomogr. 12:155, 1988.

Brenner, R. J., Spring, D. B., Sebastian, A., McSherry, E. M., Genant, H. K., Palubinskas, A. J., and Morris, R. C.: Incidence of radiographically evident bone disease, nephrocalcinosis and nephrolithiasis in various types of renal tubular acidosis. N. Engl. J. Med. 307:217, 1982.

Chikos, P. M., and McDonald, G. B.: Regional enteritis complicated by nephrocalcinosis and nephrolithiasis: Case report. Radiology 121:75, 1976.

Choong, M., and Phillips, G. W. L.: Renal transitional cell carcinoma mimicking medullary sponge kidney. Br. J. Radiol. 64:275, 1991.

Conrey, W. R., and Pfister, R. C.: Radiographic findings in renal tubular acidosis: Analysis of 21 cases. Radiology 105:497, 1972.

Cumming, W. A., and Ohlsson, A.: Nephrocalcinosis in Bartter's syndrome: Demonstration by ultrasonography. Pediatr. Radiol. 14:125, 1984.

Curry, N. S., Gordon, L., Gobien, R. P., and Lott, M.: Renal medullary "rings": Possible CT manifestations of hypercalcemia. Urol. Radiol. 6:48, 1984.

Day, D. L., Scheinman, J. L., and Mahon, J.: Radiological aspects of primary hyperoxaluria. AJR 146:395, 1986.

Duncan, P. A., Sagel, I., and Farnsworth, P. B.: Medullary sponge kidney and partial Beckwith-Wiedemann syndrome: Association with congenital asymmetry. N.Y. State J. Med. 79:1222, 1979.

Eisenberg, R. L., and Pfister, R. C.: Medullary sponge kidney associated with congenital hemihypertrophy (asymmetry): A case report and survey of the literature. AJR 116:773, 1972.

Estroff, J. A., Mandell, J., and Benacerraf, B. R.: Increased renal parenchymal echogenicity in the fetus: Importance and clinical outcome. Radiology 181:135, 1991.

Falkoff, G. E., Rigsby, C. M., and Rosenfield, A. T.: Partial, combined cortical and medullary nephrocalcinosis—US and CT patterns in AIDS-associated MAI infection. Radiology 162:343, 1987.

Friedman, A., and Chesney, R. W.: Isolated renal tubular disorders. In Schrier, R. W., and Gottschalk, C. W. (eds.): Diseases of the Kidney. 4th ed. Boston, Little, Brown & Co., 1988, Chap. 21.

Gabriele, O. F.: Localized medullary cystic disease of the kidney: Sponge kidney. J. Urol. 92:253, 1964.

Garel, L., Filiatrault, D., and Robitaille, P.: Nephrocalcinosis in Bartter's syndrome. Pediatr. Nephrol. 2:315, 1988.

Gedroyc, W. M., and Saxton, H. M.: More medullary sponge variants. Clin. Radiol. 39:423, 1988.

Gilsanz, V., Fernal, W., Reid, B. S., Stanley, P., and Ramos, A.: Nephrolithiasis in premature infants. Radiology 154:107, 1985.

Ginalski, J. M., Portmann, L., and Jaeger, P.: Does medullary sponge kidney cause nephrolithiasis? AJR 155:299, 1990.

Ginalski, J. M., Schnyder, P., Portmann, L., and Jaeger, P.: Medullary sponge kidney on axial computed tomography: Comparison with excretory urography. Eur. J. Radiol. 12:104, 1991.

Ginalski, J. M., Spiegel, T., and Jaeger, P.: Use of low-osmolality contrast medium does not increase prevalence of medullary sponge kidney. Radiology 182:311, 1992.

Glazer, G. M., Callen, P. W., and Filly, R. A.: Medullary nephrocalcinosis. AJR 138:55, 1982.

Haggitt, R. C., and Pitcock, J. A.: Renal medullary calcification: A light and electron microscopic study. J. Urol. 106:342, 1971.

Harrison, A. R., and Rose, G. A.: Medullary sponge kidney. Urol. Res. 7:197, 1979.

Harrison, A. R., and Williams, J. P.: Medullary sponge kidney and congenital hemihypertrophy. Br. J. Urol. 43:552, 1971.

Hayt, D. B., Perez, L. A., Blatt, C. J., and Lee, K. L.: Direct magnification intravenous pyelography in the evaluation of medullary sponge kidney. AJR 119:701, 1973.

Hermany-Schulman, M.: Hyperechoic renal medullary pyramids in infants and children. Radiology 181:9, 1991.

Hill, G. S.: Calcium and the kidney, nephrolithiasis, and hydronephrosis. In Heptinstall, R. H. (ed.): Pathology of the Kidney. 4th ed. Boston, Little, Brown & Co., 1992, pp. 1563–1630.

Hill, S. C., Hoeg, J. M., and Avila., N. A.: Nephrocalcinosis in homozygous familial hypercholesterolemia: Ultrasound and CT findings. J. Comput. Assist. Tomogr. 15:101, 1991.

Ivemark, B. I., Lagergren, C., and Lindvall, N.: Roentgenologic diagnosis of polycystic kidney and medullary sponge kidney. Acta Radiol. (Diagn.) 10:225, 1970.

Kaiser, J. A., Mall, J. C., Salmen, B. J., and Parker, J. J.: Diagnosis of Caroli disease by computed tomography: Report of two cases. Radiology 132:661, 1979.

Kaver, I., Flanders, E. L., Kay, S., and Koontz, W. W., Jr.: Segmental medullary sponge kidney mimicking a renal mass. J. Urol. 141:1181, 1989.

Kenney, I. J., Aiken, C. G., and Lenney, W.: Furosemide-induced nephrocalcinosis in very low birth weight infants. Pediatr. Radiol. 18:323, 1988.

Kirks, D. R., and Shackelford, G. D.: Idiopathic congenital hemihypertrophy with associated ipsilateral benign nephromegaly. Radiology 115:145, 1975.

Kreel, L.: Radiological aspects of nephrocalcinosis. Clin. Radiol. 13:218, 1962.

Kuiper, J. J.: Medullary sponge kidney in three generations. N.Y. State J. Med. 71:2665, 1971.

Lalli, A. F.: Medullary sponge kidney disease. Radiology 92:92, 1969.

Lalli, A. F.: Renal parenchymal calcifications. Semin. Roentgenol. 17:101, 1982.

Longcope, W. T., and Freiman, D. G.: A study of sarcoidosis: Based on a combined investigation of 160 cases including 30 autopsies from the Johns Hopkins Hospital and Massachusetts General Hospital. Medicine 31:1, 1952.

Malek, R. S., and Kelalis, P. P.: Nephrocalcinosis in infancy and childhood. J. Urol. 114:441, 1975.

Malek, R. S.: Renal lithiasis: A practical approach. J. Urol. 118:893, 1977.

Maschio, G., Tessitore, N., D'Angelo, A., Fabris, A., Corgnati, A., Oldrizzi, L., Loschiavo, C., Lupo, A., Valvo, E., Gammaro, L., and Rugio, C.: Medullary sponge kidney and hyperparathyroidism—a puzzling association. Am. J. Nephrol. 2:77, 1982.

Morris, R. C., Yamauchi, H., Palubinskas, A. J., and Howenstine, J.: Medullary sponge kidney. Am. J. Med. 38:883, 1965.

Mortenson, J. D., Baggenstoss, A. H., Power, M. H., and Pugh, D. G.: Roentgenographic demonstration of histologically identifiable renal calcification. Radiology 62:703, 1954.

Muther, R. S., McCarron, O. A., and Bennett, W. M.: Renal manifestations of sarcoidosis. Arch. Intern Med. 141:643, 1981.

Ohlsson, L.: Normal collecting ducts—visualization at urography. Radiology 170:33, 1989.

Palubinskas, A. J.: Medullary sponge kidney. Radiology 76:911, 1961.

Palubinskas, A. J.: Renal pyramidal structure opacification in excretory urography and its relation to medullary sponge kidney. Radiology 81:963, 1963.

Parks, J. H., Coe, F. L., and Strauss, A. L.: Calcium nephrolithiasis and medullary sponge kidney in women. N. Engl. J. Med. 306:1088, 1982.

Patriquin, H. B., and O'Regan, S.: Medullary sponge kidney in childhood. AJR 145:315, 1985.

Pyrah, L. N., and Raper, F. P.: Renal calcification and calculus formation. Br. J. Urol. 27:333, 1955.

Richardson, R. E.: Nephrocalcinosis with special reference to its occurrence in renal tubular acidosis. Clin. Radiol. 13:224, 1962.

Richer, W., and Clark, M.: Sarcoidosis: A clinicopathologic review of three hundred cases, including twenty-two autopsies. Am. J. Clin. Pathol. 19:725, 1949.

Sage, M. R., Lawson, A. D., Marshall, V. R., and Ryall, R. L.: Medullary sponge kidney and urolithiasis. Clin. Radiol. 33:435, 1982.

Saxton, H. M.: Opacification of collecting ducts at urography. Radiology 170:16, 1989.

Shultz, P. K., Strife, J. L., Strife, C. F., and McDaniel, J. D.: Hyperechoic renal medullary pyramids in infants and children. Radiology 181:163, 1991.

Torres, V. E., Young, W. F., Jr., Afford, K. P., and Hattery, R. R.: Association of hypokalemia and aldosteronism and renal cysts. N. Engl. J. Med. 322:345, 1990.

Toyoda, K., Miyamoto, Y., Ida, M., Tada, S., and Utsunomiya, M.: Hyperchoic medulla of the kidneys. Radiology 173:431, 1989.

Whitehouse, R. W.: High- and low-osmolar contrast agents in urography: A comparison of the appearances with respect to pyelotubular opacification and renal length. Clin. Radiol. 37:395, 1986.

Wood, B. P.: Renal cystic disease in infants and children. Urol. Radiol. 14:284, 1992.

Yendt, E. R.: Medullary sponge kidney and nephrolithiasis. N. Engl. J. Med. 306:1106, 1982.

Tuberculosis

Bjørn-Hansen, R., and Aakhus, T.: Angiography in renal tuberculosis. Acta Radiol. (Diagn.) 11:167, 1971.

Bloom, S., Wechsler, H., and Lattimer, J. K.: Results of long term study of non-functioning tuberculous kidneys. J. Urol. 104:654, 1970.

Cremin, B. J.: Radiological imaging of urogenital tuberculosis in children with emphasis on ultrasound. Pediatr. Radiol. 17:34, 1987.

Friedenberg, R. M.: Tuberculosis of the genitourinary system. Semin. Roentgenol. 6:310, 1971.

Giustra, P. E., Watson, R. C., and Shulman, H.: Arteriographic findings in the various stages of renal tuberculosis. Radiology 100:597, 1971.

Goldman, S. M., Fishman, E. K., Hartman, D. S., Kim, Y. C., and Siegelman, S. S.: Computed tomography of renal tuberculosis and its pathological correlates. J. Comput. Assist. Tomogr. 9:771, 1985.

Kollins, S. A., Hartman, G. W., Carr, D. T., Segura, J. W., and Hattery, R. R.: Roentgenographic findings in urinary tract tuberculosis: A 10-year review. AJR 121:487, 1974.

Lattimer, J. K.: Renal tuberculosis. N. Engl. J. Med. 273:208, 1965.

Michigan, S.: Genitourinary fungal infection. J. Urol. 116:390, 1976.

Pasternack, M. S., and Rubin, R. H.: Urinary tract tuberculosis. In Schrier, R. W., and Gottschalk, C. W. (eds.): Diseases of the Kidney. 4th ed. Boston, Little, Brown & Co., 1988, pp. 993–1014.

Petereit, M. F.: Chronic renal brucellosis: A simulator of tuberculosis. Radiology 96:85, 1970.

Roylance, J., Penry, J. B., Davies, E. R., and Roberts, M.: The radiology of tuberculosis of the urinary tract. Clin. Radiol. 21:163, 1970.

Steinert, R.: Renal tuberculosis and roentgenographic examination. Acta Radiol. (Stockholm) Suppl. 53, 1943.

Wechsler, H., Westfall, M., and Lattimer, J. K.: The earliest signs and symptoms in 127 male patients with genitourinary tuberculosis. J. Urol. 83:801, 1960.

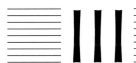

THE PELVOCALYCEAL SYSTEM AND URETER

14

INTRALUMINAL ABNORMALITIES

Abnormalities may develop within the pelvocalyceal and ureteral lumen. Such precise localization is possible when an abnormality either is completely surrounded by contrast material or moves as the patient's position is altered (Figs. 14–1 and 14–2). Localization may be difficult or impossible when the abnormality is bulky enough to prevent opacified urine from surrounding it.

Adequate distention of the pelvocalyceal system or ureter and three-dimensional reconstruction are essential measures in the accurate assessment of both extraluminal and intraluminal abnormalities of the collecting system or ureter. During excretory urography or computed tomography, distention of the pelvocalyceal system and ureter is accomplished by either contrast material–induced diuresis, abdominal compression, or both. An oral or intravenous fluid load serves the same purpose for ultrasonography. Spatial reconstruction, which is inherent in computed tomography and ultrasonography, can be achieved indirectly from radiographs by obtaining more than one projection.

UROLITHIASIS

Definition

Urolithiasis, or stone formation in the upper urinary tract, results from a complex series of incompletely understood events. This section covers stone formation and growth, the site of calculogenesis, and chemical composition.

Formation and Growth. Stones form in the kidney as crystalline aggregates with an ordered internal structure and growth pattern. Stone formation mainly occurs as a function of the level of saturation of a given ion or molecule in the urine. This, in turn, reflects either excessive renal excretion of the substance or reduced urine volume. When a substance can no longer remain in solution, precipitation and crystallization occur. In a biologic fluid, such as urine, this process is influenced significantly by pH, temperature, and urine volume as well as by the presence of stone "inhibitors."

The earliest step in calculogenesis is nucleation, which is the formation of the smallest crystal into a solid particle by the coming together of specific ions or molecules from a supersaturated state in the urine. This usually occurs on a nidus of noncrystalline organic and inorganic material. In some instances, a crystal of one type will be deposited on the surface of another type owing to similarities of crystalline lattice structure. This phenomenon, known as *epitaxy*, is of particular importance in the deposition of calcium oxalate crystals on a uric acid nucleus.

The physicochemical roles of supersaturation and pH are predominant in the formation of stones that are composed of uric acid, magnesium ammonium phosphate, and cystine. Urinary pH determines the concentration levels at which crystallization occurs. Uric acid and cystine stones form in acid urine and may be dissolved if the urine is alkalinized for a period of time. Alkaline conditions favor formation of magnesium ammonium phosphate and some mixed calcium phosphate stones.

Calcium calculogenesis is influenced significantly by stone inhibition factors and epitaxy as well as by supersaturation and pH. Normal urine contains substances that inhibit calculogenesis. Magnesium citrate and pyrophosphate are thought to inhibit growth of calcium phosphate crystals. Organic macromolecules resembling acid mucopolysaccharide probably exert a similar effect on calcium oxalate stone formation. Although the role of crystal inhibitors in stone formation has not been fully established, these substances may be deficient in patients in whom calcium stones form.

435

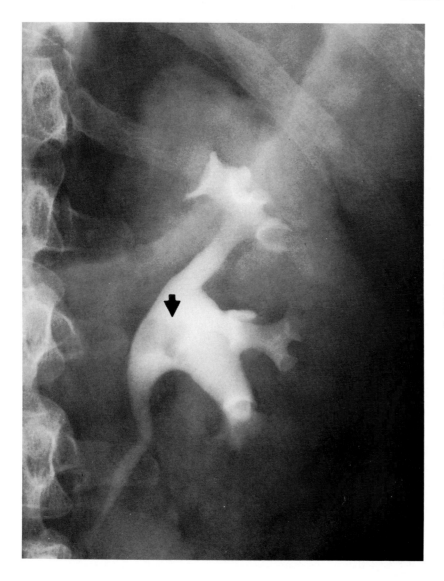

Figure 14–1. Uric acid stone in a 45-year-old patient undergoing treatment for non-Hodgkin's lymphoma. The stone *(arrow)* is completely surrounded by contrast material, establishing its intraluminal location. The stones were nonopaque on the preliminary film. Excretory urogram.

Two additional circumstances that favor stone formation and growth are urinary stasis and foreign material in the collecting system.

Site of Calculogenesis. In addition to an environment of maximal ionic or molecular concentration, stone formation requires a special sequestered site. The embryonic microcrystal must be protected against the normal flushing of the pelvocalyceal system by flowing urine. Several stone growth centers have been proposed: small, crystal-laden calyceal submucosal plaques (Randall's plaques), derived from tissue damaged by prior infection, toxic agents, or ischemia; the ostia of collecting tubules where minute crystals are impacted; forniceal lymphatics (Carr's pouches); and various sites in the nephron and the collecting duct. The concept of a protected stone growth center is supported by the deformity consistently found on the external surface of many calcium oxalate stones. This suggests attachment to a surface, perhaps the papillary tip, during nucleation and growth. After reaching a critical size, the stone is shed into the pelvocalyceal system.

Chemical Composition. Calculi are polycrystalline conglomerates that are composed of minerals (approximately 95 per cent) and organic matrix. Matrix, predominantly mucoprotein with lesser amounts of mucopolysaccharide, appears as concentric laminations, radial striations, or spherules in all stones. The role of matrix in calculogenesis is uncertain. It is possible that it is a template (nidus) for crystal growth, an inert coprecipitate of mineral crystals, or a marker of the site on the pyramid or calyx where nucleation and growth first occurred.

Approximately 90 per cent of stones found in the North American population contain calcium. Of these, about two-thirds are calcium oxalate monohydrate (crystal name = whewellite), calcium oxalate dihydrate (crystal name = wedellite), or mixed calcium phosphate. Pure calcium phosphate (crystal name = apatite) and pure or mixed calcium hydrogen phosphate (crystal name = brushite) account for less than 6 per cent of stones. The remaining calcium-containing stones are composed of magnesium ammonium phosphate (crystal name = struvite), and in most of these stones there is also either calcium phosphate or calcium oxalate.

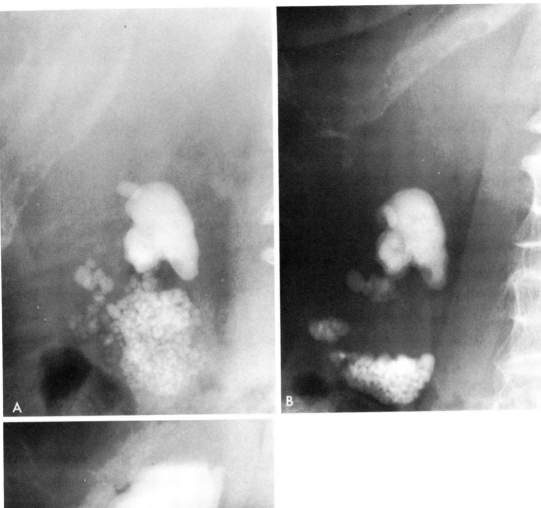

Figure 14–2. Multiple stones in a markedly dilated lower pole calyx. Staghorn calculus is at the ureteropelvic junction. The intraluminal location of the calyceal stones is established by their shifts as the patient's position is changed.

    A, Preliminary film, supine position.

    B, Preliminary film, upright position.

    C, Excretory urogram. Contrast material surrounds and obscures the stones.

Table 14–1. MINERAL COMPOSITION OF RENAL CALCULI

Crystal Name	Chemical Name	Approximate Frequency	Associated With Infection	Radiographic Opacity
Whewellite	Calcium oxalate monohydrate	34%	No	+ + +
Wedellite	Calcium oxalate dihydrate			
	Calcium oxalate plus apatite	34%	Occasionally	+ + +
Apatite, brushite, whitlockite	Calcium phosphate	6%	Occasionally	+ + +
Struvite	Magnesium ammonium phosphate	1%	Yes	– *
	Magnesium ammonium phosphate plus calcium phosphate	14%	Yes	+ +
Uric acid, urate	Uric acid, urate	7%	No	– *
Cystine	Cystine	3%	No	+
(None)	Mucoprotein/mucopolysaccharide (matrix)	Rare	Yes	– *
Xanthine	Xanthine	Very rare	No	– *

*Calculi become radiographically opaque when mixed with calcium oxalate or calcium phosphate. All calculi that are nonopaque by film radiography are opaque when imaged by computed tomography.

Approximately 10 per cent of stones are calcium-free—most of them are uric acid or cystine. Pure stones of magnesium ammonium phosphate or xanthine and matrix stones are rare, as are stones of silicates, dihydroxyadenine, and drug metabolites. A summary of the mineral composition of stones is contained in Table 14–1.

Clinical Setting

Most patients with calcium oxalate or calcium phosphate stones in industrialized countries have no identifiable underlying metabolic abnormality. The patient with *idiopathic urolithiasis* is usually male and has normal serum phosphate levels. Urinary calcium excretion is normal in up to 50 per cent of these patients. Possible factors responsible for stone formation in this group include deficiency of urine inhibitors, induction of uric acid nucleation by dietary hyperuricuria, idiopathic hyperoxaluria, or inability to acidify urine normally. The remainder of patients with idiopathic urolithiasis are hypercalciuric. Speculation on the cause of hypercalciuria has focused on increased intestinal calcium absorption ("absorptive hypercalciuria") and increased immunoreactive parathyroid hormone secretion due to a primary renal "leakage" of calcium. In the last analysis, the diagnosis of idiopathic urolithiasis rests on the exclusion of one of the known metabolic causes, which are discussed subsequently.

Stones that form in patients with *hypercalcemia* are most often calcium phosphate and only occasionally calcium oxalate. Primary hyperparathyroidism, prolonged immobilization, milk-alkali syndrome, sarcoidosis, hypervitaminosis D, neoplastic disorders, Cushing's syndrome or disease, and hyperthyroidism may all lead to hypercalcemia and stone formation. Primary hyperparathyroidism is most frequently associated with urolithiasis.

Hyperoxaluria, either primary or secondary, also causes urolithiasis. Primary hyperoxalosis is a rare autosomal recessive inherited enzyme disorder of glyoxalate metabolism. Two forms exist. Type I, the more common of the two, causes glycolic aciduria; Type II is characterized by L-glyceric aciduria. Both cause hyperoxaluria, calcium oxalate urolithiasis, and nephrocalcinosis through increased production of endogenous oxalate. Death from renal failure usually occurs before age 60 in the absence of renal dialysis.

Secondary, or acquired, hyperoxaluria occurs with conditions that cause malabsorption, rapid transit of enteric contents, and steatorrhea. These conditions include jejunoileal bypass surgery, ileal resection, and blind loop syndrome. Here, excessive intestinal fat binds intraluminal calcium ions that would normally combine with oxalate to form insoluble calcium oxalate and be eliminated in the feces. Instead, oxalate remains soluble and is absorbed in excessive amounts on reaching the colon. Hyperoxaluria and urinary tract calcium oxalate stone formation follow. These events require an intact colon.

In a nonspecific way, other chronic gastrointestinal disorders are also associated with urolithiasis, especially mixed uric acid stones. Diarrhea and operations such as ileostomy induce intestinal urate and bicarbonate loss leading to low volumes of acidic urine. Adrenocortical steroids, prolonged bed rest, and infection also predispose the patient to mixed uric acid and calcium oxalate stone. Pure uric acid stones are uncommon in these patients.

Uric acid urolithiasis is usually found in men older than age 50 without gout or any recognizable disorder of purine metabolism. Serum and urinary uric acid levels are normal. Only 25 per cent of patients with gout develop uric acid stones. Myeloproliferative disorders are associated with uric acid stones due to hyperuricemia and hyperuricuria from increased purine metabolism. Cell breakdown following chemotherapy or radiation therapy further increases the likelihood of uric acid stone formation and acute urate nephropathy.

Cystinuria is an inherited autosomal disorder of amino acid transport in the renal tubule, causing impaired reabsorption of cystine, ornithine, lysine, and arginine. The only recognized clinical consequence is cystine urolithiasis, which typically begins in the second decade of life.

Xanthinuria is a very rare, autosomal recessive inherited deficiency of xanthine oxidase resulting in increased urinary excretion of xanthine and hypoxanthine. Calculi form in approximately one-third of the affected patients.

Urinary tract infection may lead to magnesium ammonium phosphate (struvite) stones. *Proteus mirabilis* is the most common organism associated with urolithiasis, but some forms of *Pseudomonas aeruginosa*, *Klebsiella* species, *Escherichia coli*, and *Staphylococcus aureus* create conditions favorable to stone formation. These bacteria produce urease, which catalyzes the formation of ammonia from urea. Hydrolysis of ammonia produces hydroxyl (OH^-) and ammonium ions (NH_4^+), rendering the infected urine alkaline and, in turn, increasing the concentration of trivalent phosphate ion (PO_4^{3-}). A supersaturated solution of magnesium ammonium phosphate results. High urinary pH also promotes crystallization of hydroxyapatite, which is commonly incorporated in the struvite stone. Pure matrix stones have also been described with infection, but these are very rare.

Partial urinary stasis favors stone formation by causing retention of crystal aggregates and other potential niduses. Urolithiasis does not occur with complete obstruction in the absence of infection, since no precipitating solute is excreted. Stones formed as a result of partial obstruction are usually calcium phosphate, although any of the crystal systems may participate.

Any of the metabolic conditions responsible for nephrocalcinosis also favor *de novo* formation of pelvocalyceal stones. Sometimes, the stone is simply an extrusion of a concretion originally formed in the renal parenchyma as, for example, in medullary sponge kidney. Parenchymal calcification in renal tubular acidosis is particularly exuberant and also frequently leads to free stones in the collecting system.

Stone may cause acute clinical symptoms. The most dramatic is renal colic, a crescendo-decrescendo pattern of pain in the flank and lateral abdomen that often radiates into the groin, scrotum, or labia. Hematuria is usually present. Occasionally, stone disease presents as symptoms of acute or chronic urinary tract infection.

Radiologic Findings

Radiography. Detection of small opaque stones is critically dependent on proper radiographic technique. The lowest feasible kilovoltage must be used to enhance density discrimination. Careful coning of the x-ray beam enhances sharpness by reducing scattered radiation. The use of clean intensifying screens eliminates artifacts resembling stones.

Proving that a density is truly within the kidney requires either a tomogram or a constant spatial relationship between the kidney and the apparent stone in two radiographic projections. In addition to the standard frontal projection, the patient should be examined in a 30-degree posterior oblique position toward the side of suspected stone, to distinguish a kidney stone from calcification in the arteries, the lymph nodes, and the gallbladder or from opaque ingested material in the bowel (Fig. 14–3).

Tomography is an important adjunct in the evaluation of kidney stones. It can be used instead of an oblique view to clarify a suspicious shadow that is seen on an initial radiograph (Fig. 14–4). In the quest for a small stone in a patient with a strongly suggestive history, standard radiographs may be negative or suboptimal because of intestinal contents. Here, too, tomography may be of value. A range of 60 to 75 kV with a variable mAs, careful coning of the x-ray beam, and the selection of an adequate number of levels to ensure proper sampling of the kidney determine whether the use of tomography will be successful.

The radiographic appearance of a stone depends on its composition. Some stones are very dense in their entirety. Others are mixed, with a central radiodense nidus, have a homogeneous intermediate radiodensity, or are nonopaque.

The radiologic search for an opaque kidney stone must be conducted before the injection of contrast material, since radiodense calcium stones will be invisible in the midst of opaque urine (Fig. 14–5; see also Fig. 14–7). Standard radiographic technique can detect opaque stones as small as 1 mm. Mixed composition stones with a central deposit of dense calcium appear as a radiolucency that is much larger than expected on the basis of the size of the calcium density alone (Fig. 14–6). Cystine stones or struvite or uric acid calculi with small amounts of calcium have an intermediate, homogeneous density. These are slightly radiodense on preliminary films but appear radiolucent once the urine is opacified. Radiopaque ureteral stones, like kidney stones, can be detected by radiographic techniques. However, once a stone enters the ureter from the pelvocalyceal system, confirmation of its location requires opacification of the ureter since there is no longer a closely related structure such as the kidney to serve as a spatial reference (Fig. 14–7). Nonopaque stones are revealed as radiolucent filling defects only after opacification of the pelvocalyceal system or ureter and are not detectable on preliminary films (see Fig. 14–1).

A stone that is free within the collecting system is surrounded by contrast material in all projections. A small stone may be round, smooth, or jagged. Rapidly growing stones tend to branch and may fill the entire pelvocalyceal system, forming a so-called branched or staghorn calculus (Fig. 14–8). Stones may be solitary or multiple and are found anywhere in the collecting system. Stones obstruct when they impact at points of narrowing, such as an infundibulum, the ureteropel-

Text continued on page 446

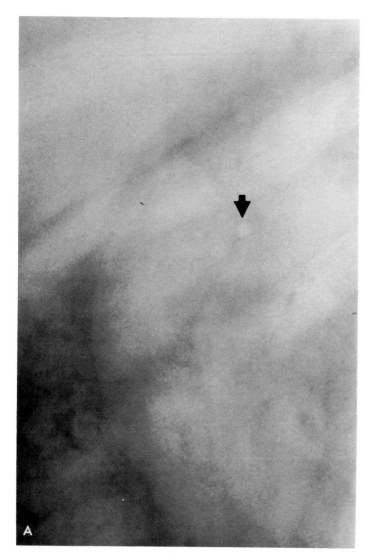

Figure 14–3. The position of this calcium oxalate stone *(arrow)* remains constant relative to the kidney on both frontal and oblique films, establishing its intrarenal location.

   A, Preliminary film, anteroposterior projection.

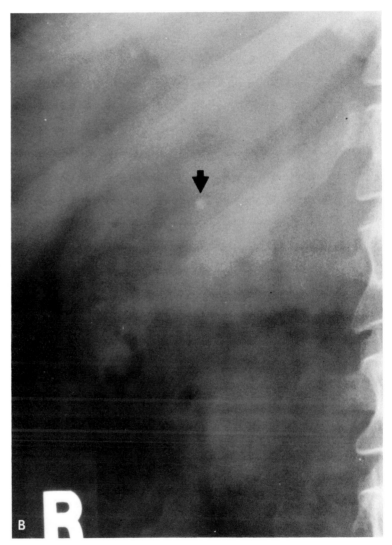

Figure 14–3 *Continued B,* Preliminary film, right posterior oblique projection. (Same patient illustrated in Fig. 14–4.)

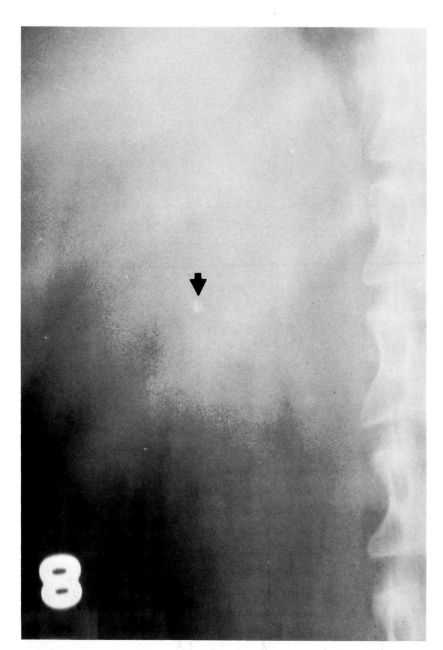

Figure 14–4. Kidney localization can be established by a tomogram demonstrating that both the stone *(arrow)* and the kidney are in focus at the same level. (Same patient illustrated in Fig. 14–3.)

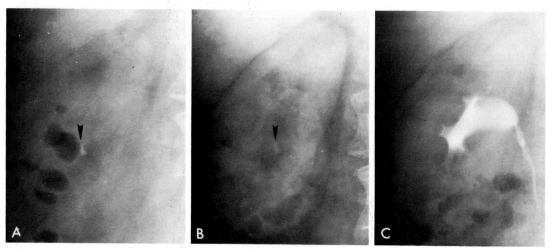

Figure 14–5. Radiopaque calculus obscured following injection of contrast material.
  A, Preliminary film. The stone *(arrow)* overlies the region of the renal pelvis.
  B, Excretory urogram, 1-minute film. The nephrogram does not affect the appearance of the stone *(arrow)*.
  C, Excretory urogram, 10-minute film. The stone is obscured by contrast material in the renal pelvis.

Figure 14–6. The size of a calculus of mixed composition is often larger than that suggested by the focal, central deposit of calcium.

A, Preliminary film. Two calculi *(arrow)* are present over the renal pelvic area. A faint band of surrounding density is suggested.

Illustration continued on following page

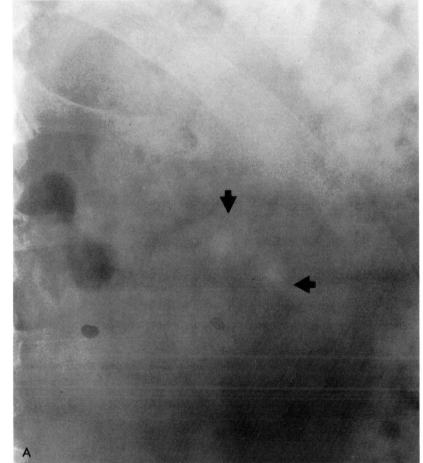

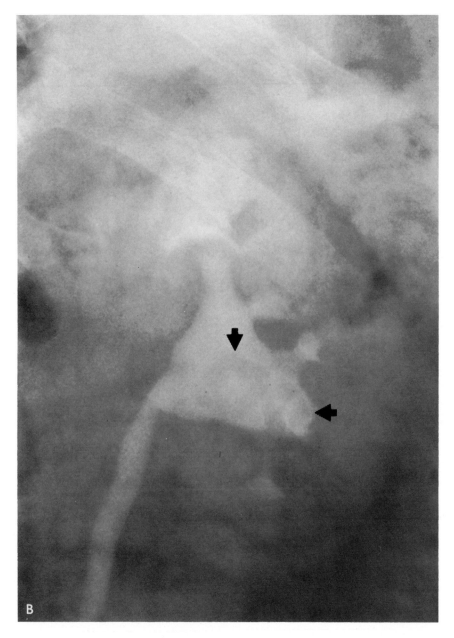

Figure 14–6 *Continued B,* Excretory urogram. Opacified urine surrounding the stones reveals a thick mantle of stone material that is radiolucent relative to opacified urine *(arrows).*

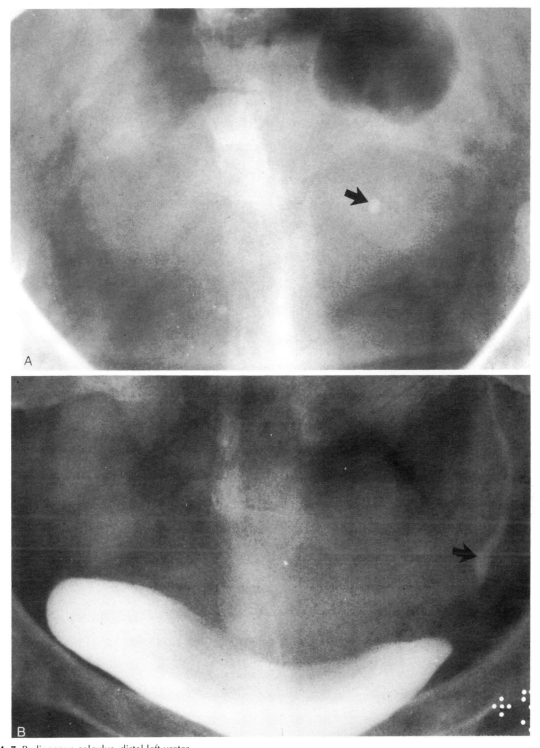

Figure 14–7. Radiopaque calculus, distal left ureter.
  A, Preliminary radiograph. The stone *(arrow)* is identified by its density, but its position relative to the urinary tract cannot be determined.
  B, Excretory urogram. Contrast material in the ureter surrounds and obscures the stone *(arrow)*, which does not obstruct the ureter.

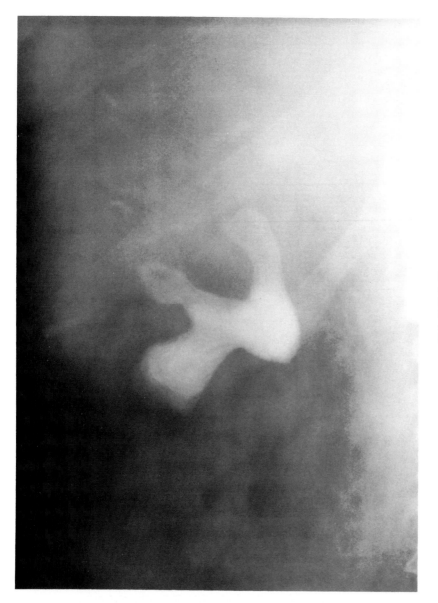

Figure 14–8. Staghorn struvite calculus with laminated pattern. Rapid growth of a stone leads to a branched shape that may fill the pelvocalyceal system. Preliminary film. (Courtesy of Joy Price, M.D., Alta Bates Medical Center, Berkeley, California.) (Same patient illustrated in Fig. 14–9.)

vic junction, the point where the ureter crosses the iliac vessels, or the insertion of the distal ureter into the bladder, causing distention proximally (Fig. 14–9; see also Fig. 14–2). When stones move, intermittent obstruction may result.

Calcium oxalate and *calcium phosphate* stones are the most opaque and typically are uniformly dense (see Fig. 14–3). These stones vary in size but only rarely reach staghorn proportions. In some metabolic disorders, pelvocalyceal calculi coexist with nephrocalcinosis (Fig. 14–10).

A pure *uric acid* stone is nonopaque on standard radiography (see Fig. 14–1). When uric acid stones are enlarged beyond 2 cm, they tend to become faintly dense, owing to impurities that have been incorporated into the lattice of the stone. Tomography is sometimes needed to demonstrate this low level of opacity. With rapid growth, a uric acid stone may form a cast of the pelvocalyceal system.

Pure *cystine* stones are homogeneous and appear as a "frosted" or "ground-glass" radiodensity intermediate between calcium and water on plain radiographs. Radiodensity, which is caused by the sulfur content of cystine, increases with size (Fig. 14–11) and laminations are absent.

The rare *xanthine* calculus is nonopaque, although as with uric acid stones, incorporation of impurities can result in faint, uniform opacity.

The radiographic density of *struvite* or *infection* stones is determined by the amount of calcium that is incorporated in the magnesium ammonium phosphate. Calcium phosphate often precipitates in layers, producing a characteristic laminated pattern of alternating bands of radiodensity and relative radiolucency. A staghorn configuration is common (see Figs. 14–8 and 14–9).

Pure matrix stone is another very rare form of nonopaque calculus, but impurities may give it a stippled appearance. Typically, matrix stones are large, branched structures, but uncommonly they are small and multiple.

Ultrasonography. Stones, regardless of their com-

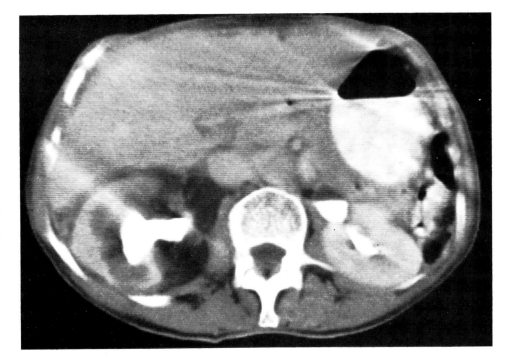

Figure 14–9. Staghorn struvite calculus impacted at the right ureteropelvic junction, causing chronic obstructive uropathy. There is diminished excretion of contrast material by the right kidney. Dilated calyces are represented by low-density areas surrounding the calculus. Computed tomogram, contrast material enhanced. (Courtesy of Joy Price, M.D., Alta Bates Medical Center, Berkeley, California.) (Same patient illustrated in Fig. 14–8.)

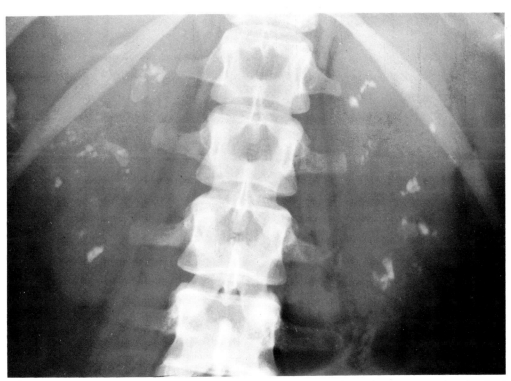

Figure 14–10. Urolithiasis in a 25-year-old woman with nephrocalcinosis due to renal tubular acidosis. Extensive deposits of calcium are present in the collecting system and renal parenchyma. Preliminary film. (Courtesy of Department of Diagnostic Radiology, Hammersmith Hospital, Royal Postgraduate Medical School, London, England.) (Same patient illustrated in Fig. 13–4.)

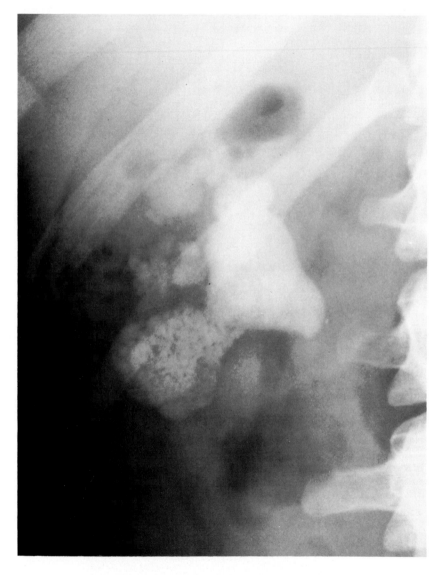

Figure 14–11. Pure cystine calculi in an 18-year-old man with elevated urinary cystine excretion and a family history of cystinuria. The radiographic density of these stones varies from faintly opaque to dense. Preliminary film. (Courtesy of Joy Price, M.D., Alta Bates Medical Center, Berkeley, California.)

position, attenuate and reflect sound. Strong echoes and a sharply marginated acoustic shadow are the ultrasonographic features that distinguish stones from other filling defects in the pelvocalyceal system and ureter (Figs. 14–12 through 14–14). Unfortunately, however, several factors may mask these features and make diagnosis by ultrasonography difficult. First, the strong echo of a stone lying centrally in a nondilated pelvis may not be discriminated from the echoes generated by the normal renal sinus. This problem can often be solved by decreasing the gain setting in a stepwise fashion until the sinus echoes disappear, leaving only the bright echo of a pelvocalyceal stone (Fig. 14–15). Second, stones produce a characteristic sharply marginated acoustic shadow with few, if any, low-level echoes only when the calculus is within the focal zone of the transducer and is comparable in size to the width of the incident ultrasound beam. Obviously, the choice of transducer is crucial in the accurate imaging of upper urinary tract stones. A third source of error occurs when a portion of the sound beam bypasses the calculus and clutters up the acoustic shadow with back-scattered echoes. The blurring of the margins of the acoustic shadow that results can be eliminated by obtaining serial ultrasonic tomographic sections. A final potential source of error is in the ultrasonographic diagnosis of matrix stones. Limited experience suggests that a matrix stone produces low-level echoes and no acoustic shadow regardless of size. In general, however, it is clear that although stones as small as 2 mm have been detected by ultrasonography under optimal conditions, the likelihood

of error varies inversely with the size of the calculus.

Gas within the pelvocalyceal system or ureter can be confused with stone, since both conditions cause bright echoes and an acoustic shadow. However, the acoustic shadow from gas is less sharply marginated than that from stone and contains high-level reverberation echoes. Lingering confusion is best resolved with the radiographic demonstration of characteristic gas radiolucency.

Computed Tomography. Computed tomography, like ultrasonography, detects urinary tract calculi and plays a major role in the differential diagnosis of nonopaque filling defects, especially in the pelvocalyceal system. Greater density discrimination accounts for the advantage of computed tomography over standard radiography. Stones that are nonopaque (uric acid) or faintly opaque (cystine) by the latter technique are visually as dense as calcium-containing stones when imaged by computed tomography (Figs. 14–16 and 14–17). However, their actual attenuation values are in a lower range than those of stone composed of calcium. Limited experience suggests that matrix stone does not have increased attenuation compared with soft tissue on computed tomography, the only apparent exception to the usual appearance of nonopaque stones on computed tomography.

Stones smaller than the thickness of the computed tomographic section can be misregistered owing to partial volume effect, obscuring the true nature of the density. A thin collimator and contiguous sections minimize this source of error.

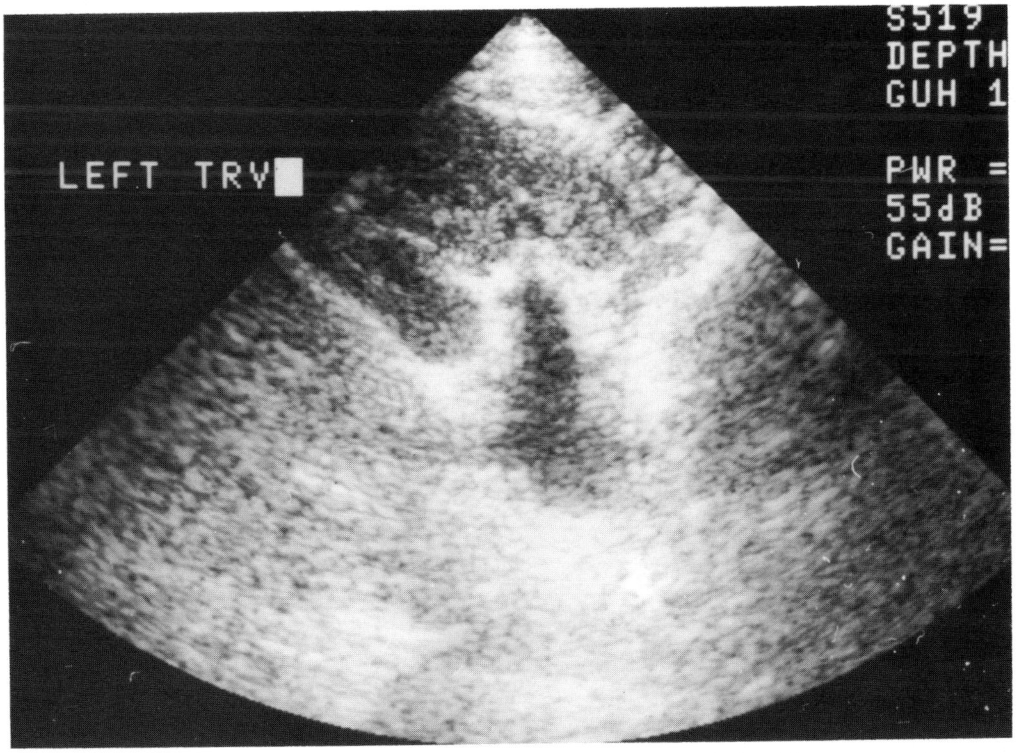

Figure 14–12. Urolithiasis producing bright echoes and a sharply marginated acoustic shadow. Ultrasonogram, transverse section.

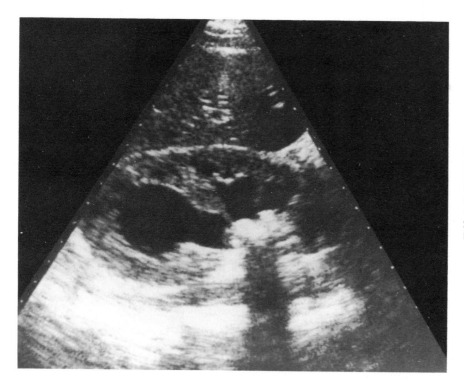

Figure 14–13. Calculus, ureteropelvic junction, left kidney, causing hydronephrosis. Ultrasonogram, transverse projection. The stone is highly echogenic and produces a sharply marginated acoustic shadow. (Kindly provided by Ulrike Hamper, M.D., and Sheila Sheth, M.D., The Johns Hopkins University, Baltimore, Maryland.)

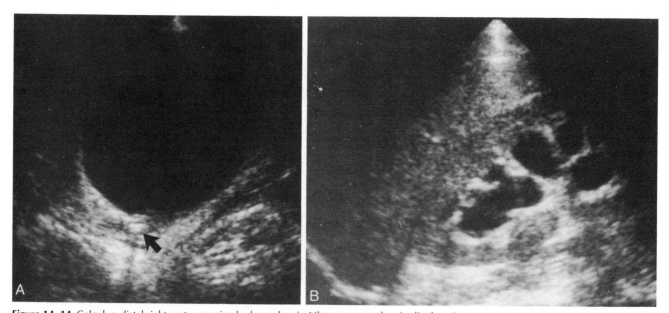

Figure 14–14. Calculus, distal right ureter, causing hydronephrosis. Ultrasonogram, longitudinal sections.
  A, Distal ureter. The small stone *(arrow)* is echogenic and produces some acoustic shadow. Because of the small size of the stone, however, the margins of the acoustic shadow are unsharp.
  B, Kidney. There is marked dilatation of the pelvocalyceal system.
  (Kindly provided by Ulrike Hamper, M.D., and Sheila Sheth, M.D., The Johns Hopkins University, Baltimore, Maryland.)

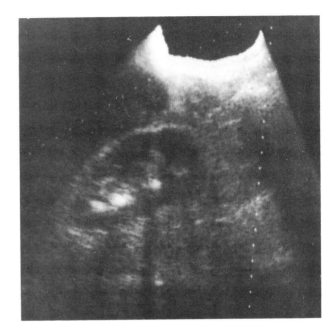

Figure 14–15. Decrease in gain setting reduces echogenicity of renal sinus fat, isolating the bright echoes of a pelvocalyceal stone. Ultrasonogram, longitudinal section.

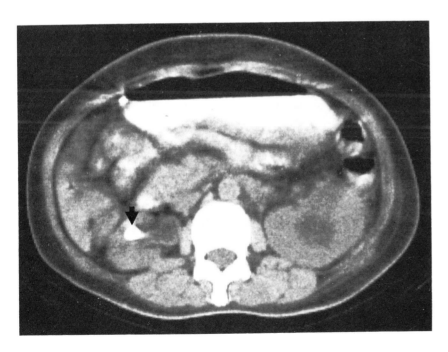

Figure 14–16. Cystine stone in the right calyx *(arrow)*. Computed tomogram, unenhanced. (Courtesy of Michael Federle, M.D., University of Pittsburgh, Pittsburgh, Pennsylvania.)

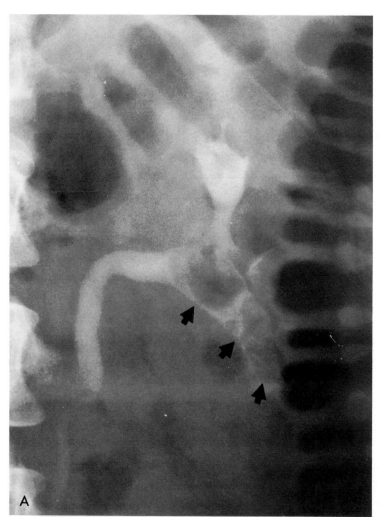

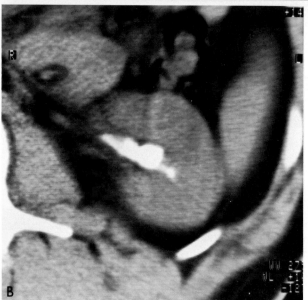

Figure 14–17. Multiple pure uric acid stones in the left pelvocalyceal system. The stones were not seen on the preliminary film and appear as nonopaque intraluminal filling defects during excretory urography. High attenuation values are noted by computed tomography.

A, Excretory urogram. Numerous nonopaque stones fill the pelvocalyceal system *(arrows).*

B, Computed tomogram without contrast material enhancement.

BLOOD CLOT

Definition

Blood clots form in the pelvocalyceal system when the volume of blood lost is large enough to cause stasis and activation of the clotting mechanism. The result is a nonopaque intraluminal mass that can obstruct the ureteropelvic junction or the ureter. Lysis occurs within 2 weeks, but rarely a fibrin mass remains, and this may eventually calcify.

Clots in the collecting system may develop simultaneously with bleeding into the renal parenchyma, the subcapsular space, the pelvocalyceal wall, or the retroperitoneal spaces. The radiologic findings of any of these may coexist.

Clinical Setting

The causes of urinary tract bleeding include trauma; tumors of the kidney parenchyma, pelvocalyceal system, or ureter; nephritis and vasculitis; arteriovenous malformation or hemangioma; rupture of an arterial aneurysm; renal venous congestion; bleeding disorders; and anticoagulant therapy. Occasionally, hematuria with clot formation is idiopathic.

The radiologist should be on guard for patients who bleed after mild trauma or during the course of anticoagulant therapy when bleeding and coagulation times are within the therapeutic range. A renal tumor, congenital anomaly, or other abnormality is sometimes discovered in this way.

Clots in the pelvocalyceal system are asymptomatic unless they obstruct the pelvocalyceal system or ureter. Other signs and symptoms reflect the event that initiated the bleeding.

Radiologic Findings

In the absence of additional bleeding, blood clots become significantly smaller or disappear within 2 weeks of formation (Fig. 14–18). This unique feature aids in the differential diagnosis of nonopaque lesions of the upper urinary tract. Otherwise, blood clots exhibit radiographic features that are common to other nonopaque intraluminal lesions. Opaque urine outlines sharp margins and may dissect between clumps of clot (Fig. 14–19). Location of the clot varies with time or with a change in the position of the patient. In major hemorrhage, the clot may form a cast of the entire pelvocalyceal system and impair urine formation by obstruction (see Fig. 14–18).

When a clot persists as a mass of fibrin, faintly opaque calcification may develop that resembles some urinary stones or calcified uroepithelial tumors (Fig.

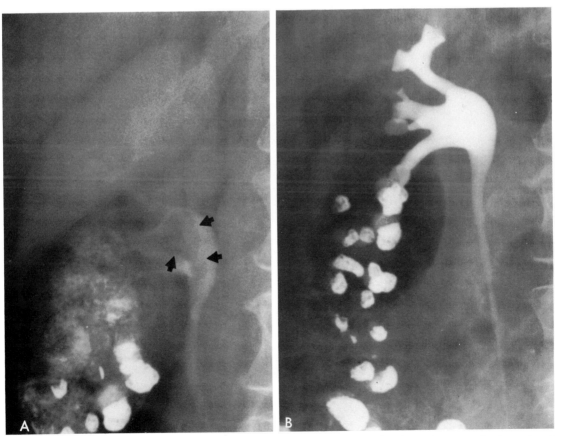

Figure 14–18. Blood clot forming a cast of the renal pelvis in an elderly woman who developed gross hematuria due to renal contusion.
  A, Excretory urogram obtained during active bleeding. Note smooth, sharply defined margin of the clot *(arrows)*.
  B, Retrograde pyelogram performed 1 week following excretory urogram. Clot has completely disappeared.

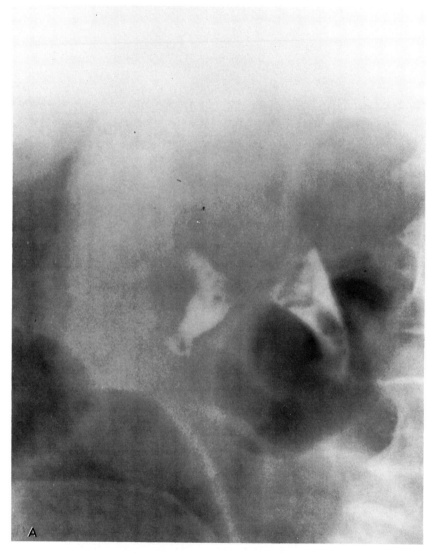

Figure 14–19. Blood clot in a 64-year-old woman with diabetes mellitus and acute bacterial nephritis. Bleeding was thought to be due to renal papillary necrosis associated with the acute bacterial nephritis.

A, Excretory urogram. Blood clots are of multiple size and shape. Note extension of opacified urine between the clumps of clot.

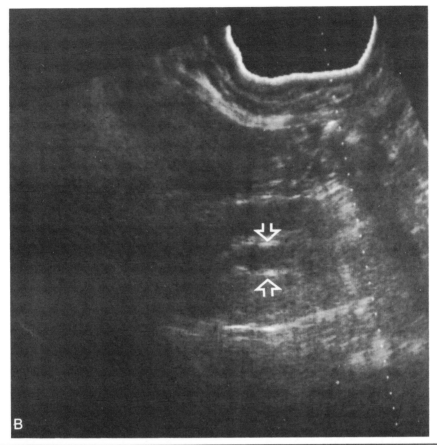

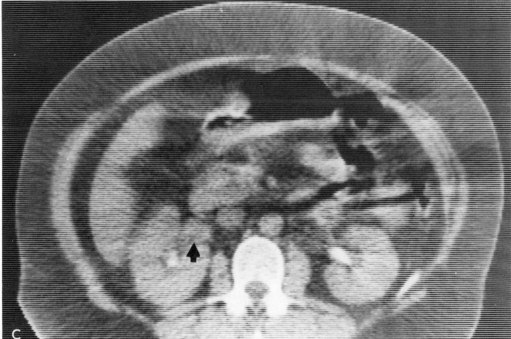

Figure 14–19 *Continued B,* Ultrasonogram, longitudinal section. A mass of low-level echoes *(arrows)* separates the high-level echoes of the central sinus complex. There is no acoustic shadowing.

C, Computed tomogram, contrast material enhanced. Clot filling the right pelvis *(arrow)* has an attenuation value equal to that of the renal parenchyma, indicating that it has not recently formed.

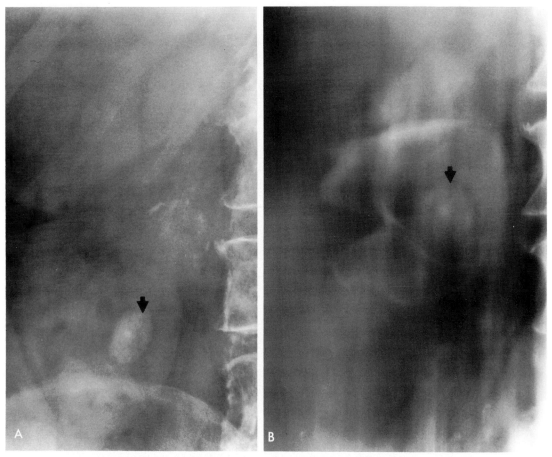

Figure 14–20. Calcified fibrinous mass developing as a residual complication of prior blood clot, pathologically confirmed.
  A, Preliminary film. Arrow identifies circumscribed area of calcification.
  B, Excretory urogram. Tomogram. A large nonopaque mass of fibrin fills the pelvocalyceal system. Focus of calcification is centrally located (arrow).

14–20). This development has been described principally in patients with calcium oxalate stones after pelvic lithotomy and may reflect a specific metabolic disorder in these patients.

The ultrasound image of clot is a mass composed of low-level echoes that separate the strong echoes of the central sinus complex (see Fig. 14–19). Unlike calculus or gas, blood clot causes neither strong echoes nor acoustic shadowing. Serial ultrasonograms are an efficient way for documenting the resolution of a clot.

The computed tomographic attenuation value of clot varies with time. When the clot is fresh, its attenuation value exceeds that of soft tissue (Fig. 14–21). Within a week, its attenuation value decreases to a level that is usually lower than that of nonenhanced renal parenchyma (see Fig. 14–19). The attenuation value of a blood clot does not increase after contrast material administration, as sometimes happens in transitional cell carcinoma. The intraluminal position of a blood clot is well defined by computed tomography if the pelvocalyceal system is distended enough to permit opacified urine to surround the mass. Neither ultrasonography nor computed tomography distinguishes blood clot from other soft tissue masses in the collecting system.

TISSUE SLOUGH

Definition

Tissue sloughed from the kidney may form free, intraluminal masses. This occurs in two forms: necrosed papilla and cholesteatoma.

When *renal papillary necrosis* evolves to the stage of frank necrosis, separation may occur between the viable and dead portions of the papilla. The slough becomes a free mass that eventually moves distally from the calyx. Calcification, if it occurs, may be present at the time of separation or develop later.

Tissue slough usually develops in patients with analgesic nephropathy and less often in cases of renal papillary necrosis due to severe urinary tract infection, obstruction, or acute bacterial nephritis. Papillary slough does not occur in S hemoglobinopathy. A complete discussion of renal papillary necrosis is found in Chapter 7.

Cholesteatoma is an unusual form of tissue slough that results from keratinizing desquamative squamous metaplasia, or epidermidalization, of the transitional cell epithelium. In this circumstance, keratin forms into either a discrete, pearly gray–whitish mass of concentric layers or an amorphous stringy collec-

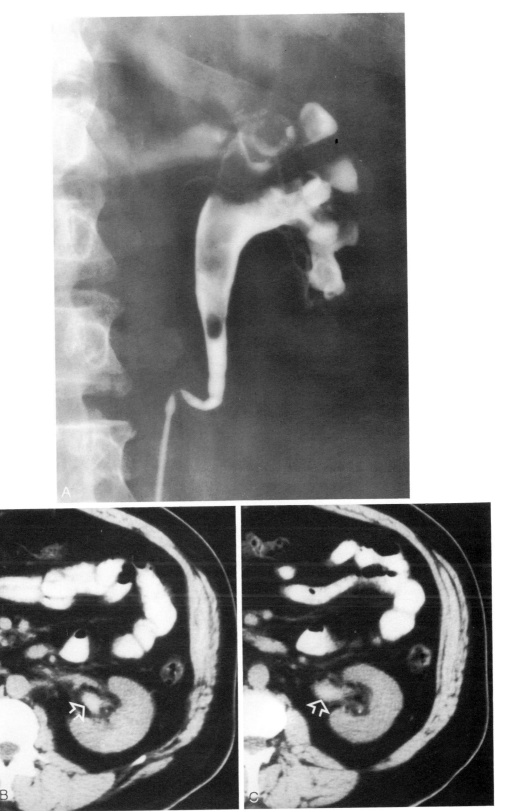

Figure 14–21. Blood clot recently formed in a 58-year-old man with gross hematuria due to an occult adenocarcinoma of the kidney.
 A, Retrograde pyelogram. The clot forms as a nonopaque filling defect in the shape of a cast of the pelvis.
 B, and *C,* Computed tomograms without contrast material enhancement in two contiguous transverse planes. The clot in the pelvis *(arrow)* is identified as tissue with an attenuation value higher than that of renal parenchyma, indicating recent formation. The carcinoma is not visualized.

tion. Either form may obstruct. Chronic inflammation from urinary tract infection or calculus disease is generally held to be the underlying cause, although this viewpoint is not without controversy (Hertle and Androulakakis, 1982). Cholesteatoma does not predispose to malignancy of the uroepithelium. The closely related, and perhaps identical, condition of leukoplakia is discussed in Chapter 15.

Clinical Setting

A papillary slough does not produce symptoms until there is obstruction of an infundibulum, the ureteropelvic junction, or the ureter. Flank pain and colic then develop. A slough may eventually pass per urethra. In other respects, the clinical setting is that of renal papillary necrosis in general, or of the specific causation, as discussed in Chapter 7.

Cholesteatoma develops in patients with chronic urinary tract infection or chronic stone disease. Hematuria and colic are often present. Occasionally, voided urine contains cornified squamous epithelium.

Radiologic Findings

A sloughed papilla appears as a triangle-shaped filling defect anywhere in the collecting system. One or more calyces will dilate, reflecting the loss of a papillary tip. Initially, the site of separation is irregular but later becomes smooth. When the urine is opacified, the slough that remains in its calyx appears as a nonopaque mass that fills the calyx except for a thin rim of surrounding opaque urine, the so-called "ring" sign (Fig. 14–22). (This finding may be seen in any of the nonopaque masses discussed in this chapter and is not specific for sloughed tissue.) A slough may migrate distally, causing dilatation proximal to a point of impaction.

Calcium is sometimes deposited along the periphery of a sloughed papilla, forming a ringlike pattern

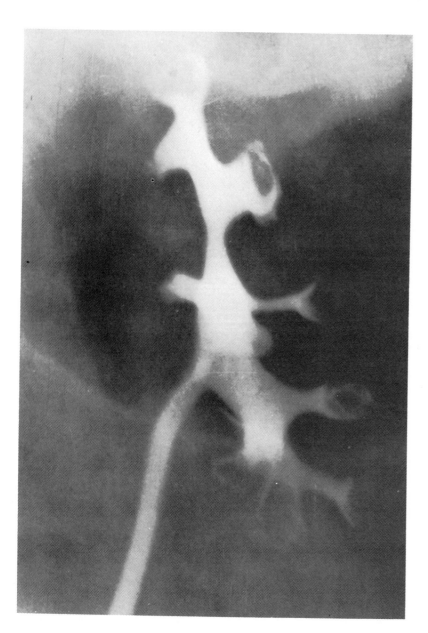

Figure 14–22. Acute renal papillary necrosis in a patient with diabetes mellitus and urinary tract infection. Papillary sloughs fill the calyces at multiple sites, leaving deformed medullae. Contrast material surrounds the sloughs, giving rise to the "ring" sign. Retrograde pyelogram. (Courtesy of the late A. J. Palubinskas, M.D., University of California, San Francisco.)

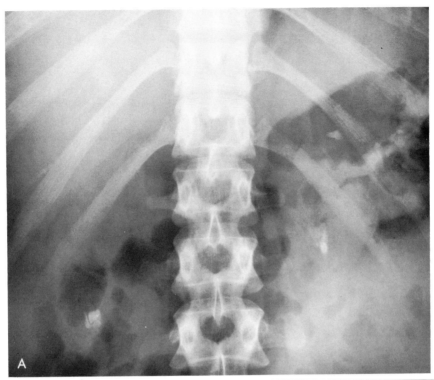

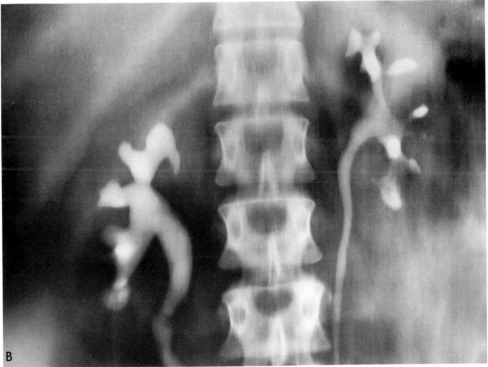

Figure 14–23. Renal papillary necrosis in 27-year-old analgesic abuser. The papillary sloughs bilaterally have calcified in a ringlike pattern. These appear as nonopaque filling defects after the urine is opacified.
  A, Preliminary film.
  B, Excretory urogram. Tomogram. Note calyceal deformities characteristic of papillary necrosis.

(Fig. 14–23). Occasionally, the whole papilla is dense, in which case the radiographic, ultrasonographic, and computed tomographic images are indistinguishable from calculus or any other calcified mass. The use of these modalities to differentiate noncalcified slough from other causes of nonopaque filling defects is discussed at the end of this chapter.

Up to one-half of the patients with cholesteatoma have urolithiasis. A cholesteatoma is usually nonopaque. Only rarely is there faint density, presumably due to microdeposits of calcium. Cholesteatoma usually presents as a rounded, intraluminal mass in the pelvocalyceal system. Contrast material extends into the concentric laminations of a cholesteatoma to produce an "onion skin" pattern of alternating density and lucency (Fig. 14–24). In amorphous forms, the filling defects are multiple and stringy, with indistinct margins. This pattern may be indistinguishable from that produced by mural lesions of the pelvocalyceal system, as discussed in Chapter 15 (Fig. 14–25). Cholesteatoma isolated in a single calyx has been reported. Computed tomography demonstrates a pel-

vocalyceal mass of relatively high attenuation value that reflects the microdeposits of calcium. Limited experience with examination of cholesteatoma by ultrasound suggests a pattern of echogenic mass without acoustic shadowing.

FUNGUS BALL
Definition

Fungus ball, or mycetoma, is a yellow-brown mass of putty-like consistency that forms from either blood-borne or ascending infection of the urinary tract by certain species of fungus. Most mycetomas are caused by *Candida albicans*. *Aspergillus* species are the second most commonly found organisms. Mycetomas have also been reported in urinary tract infection with *Cryptococcus neoformans*, *Phycomycetes* species, and *Penicillium* species. Microscopically, the ball is usually an aggregate of the mycelia (M-form) of the fungus and necrotic debris. Occasionally, the mass is composed of clumps of yeast cells (Y-form).

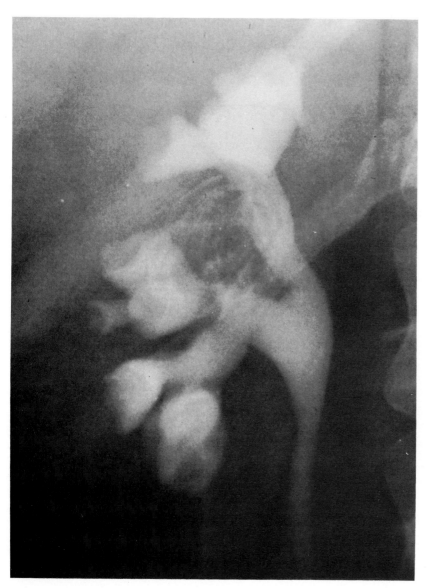

Figure 14–24. Cholesteatoma developing in a 46-year-old woman with a 2-year history of intermittent urinary tract infections. Excretory urogram reveals a 1.5-cm mass extending from the renal pelvis into the infundibulum of the upper pole. Contrast material outlines concentric laminations. (From Amberg, J. A., and Talner, L. B.: Urol. Radiol. *1*:192, 1980. Reproduced with kind permission of the authors and *Urologic Radiology*.)

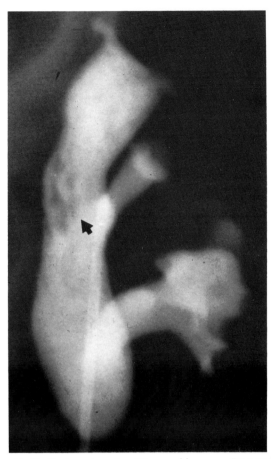

Figure 14–25. Cholesteatoma in a 72-year-old woman. Retrograde pyelogram. There is a cluster of multiple, linear, irregular lucencies with indistinct margins *(arrow).* (From Wills, J. C., Pollack, H. M., and Curtis, J. A.: AJR *136*:941, 1981. Reproduced with kind permission of the authors and *American Journal of Roentgenology.*)

Involvement of the renal parenchyma occurs in over 90 per cent of patients with blood-borne dissemination of the *Candida* species. In these cases, the fungus ball forms from mycelia shed into the pelvis from the collecting tubules and coexists with white uroepithelial plaques of thrush.

Clinical Setting

Fungal infection of the urinary tract occurs in a setting of altered host resistance. Severe debilitating disease, acquired immunodeficiency syndrome, and administration of antibiotics, adrenal corticosteroids, immunosuppressants, and antineoplastic drugs are common factors. Diabetes mellitus, drug abuse, and prolonged use of indwelling catheters are additional clinical circumstances that favor fungal infection.

The clinical findings of fungal infection of the urinary tract vary with the route of infection, the extent of renal parenchymal involvement, and the development of obstruction by the fungus ball.

Fungus ball itself may cause colic when obstruction, usually at the ureteropelvic junction, occurs. Oliguria or anuria and azotemia result from bilateral obstructing fungus balls or obstruction in a single kidney.

Other clinical findings include stranguria and funguria and passage of debris per urethra. Pneumaturia, from fermentative gases, occurs rarely.

Radiologic Findings

Fungus ball fills the renal pelvis or the ureter with a large, nonopaque mass. Multiple masses occur. Carbon dioxide, butyric acid, and lactate are fermentative gases that sometimes create a lacy radiolucent pattern within the mass. This is best noted on a preliminary film. During excretory urography or pyelography, contrast material insinuates itself into the interstices, causing a similar lacelike radiodense pattern (Fig. 14–26). A small mycetoma may move over time or with a change in the patient's position.

Hydronephrosis and impaired pelvocalyceal opacification occur when a fungus ball causes obstruction, usually at the ureteropelvic junction. Other radiologic findings that may be present with fungus ball are those due to structural damage caused by concurrent infection of the renal parenchyma (calicectasis, contour scar, papillary necrosis, and focal enlargements due to abscess) or uroepithelial thrush (mural nodules).

A fungus ball has an ultrasonographic appearance of an echogenic mass that does not cause an acoustic shadow. The computed tomographic attenuation value of a mycetoma is in the range of soft tissue. Neither ultrasonography nor computed tomography differentiates fungus ball from other intraluminal masses of soft tissue density, except when gas is detected.

FOREIGN MATERIAL
Definition

Foreign substances in the renal pelvis are derived from several sources and vary in density from radiolucent to radiopaque. These materials arrive in the pelvocalyceal system and ureter by migration through normal pathways, by passage through newly established channels, or in the case of gas-forming infection, by formation *in situ.*

A solid object placed in the bladder, either operatively or by self-insertion per urethra, may migrate through the ureter into the renal pelvis. Catheters, drains, or stents inserted into the distal ureter may do likewise, presumably as a result of reverse peristalsis induced by the foreign material. Air introduced during bladder or ureteral instrumentation and gas formed by infection and fermentation also pass retrograde into the pelvocalyceal system.

Solid objects also enter the renal pelvis directly from high-velocity wounds or by penetration from adjacent sites, as with surgically placed drains, needles, or sutures. Migration of ingested objects into the renal pelvis from the alimentary tract accounts for approximately one-fourth of renal foreign bodies in the largest reported series (Bretland and Blacklock, 1968). Penetration of the gut usually occurs at the

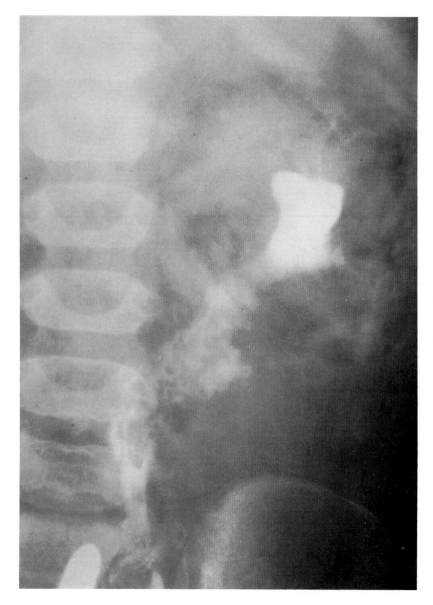

Figure 14–26. Candidiasis in the transplanted kidney of a young patient who had bilateral nephrectomies for Wilms' tumor. The pelvocalyceal system and proximal ureter are filled with an amorphous mass. Contrast material insinuates into the interstices to form a lacelike pattern. Retrograde pyelogram. (From Clark, R. E., Minagi, H., and Palubinskas, A. J.: Renal candidiasis. Radiology *101*:567, 1971. Reproduced with kind permission of the authors and *Radiology.*)

second part of the duodenum. The foreign body, often a toothpick, pin, or bone, migrates into the pelvis of the right kidney, traversing the anterior renal fascia. Much less frequently, this occurs between the fourth part of the duodenum and the left renal pelvis.

Renoalimentary fistulas *unassociated* with an ingested foreign body are due to trauma and are now rare. In the preantibiotic period, however, these fistulas developed from infection that complicated the traumatic wound. The most common form of renoalimentary fistula is renocolic, in which the renal parenchyma (not the renal pelvis) communicates with the ascending or descending colon. Rare fistulas between the kidney and the stomach, small intestine, appendix, rectum (in the case of a pelvic kidney), or lung have been recorded. Kidney cancer infrequently leads to alimentary fistulas. Even rarer is renocolic fistula due to primary carcinoma of the colon invading the kidney.

Air in the upper urinary tract is often seen with cutaneous nephrostomy, ureteroileostomy, and ureterosigmoidostomy.

Clinical Setting

The clinical features of a foreign body in the kidney vary with the initiating circumstances. A solid object within the renal pelvis, regardless of origin, is usually asymptomatic for a long period of time. Signs and symptoms, when they do arise, are those of infection or colic. Frequency, urgency, and pain are common complaints, and hematuria and pyuria are often present.

Urinary tract gas per se does not produce symptoms. The clinical findings of infection, either primary in the urinary tract or secondary to the fistula, usually dominate.

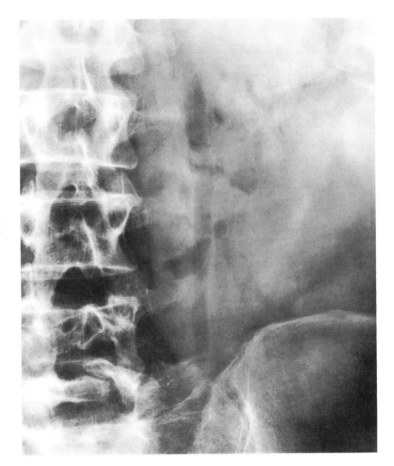

Figure 14–27. Air filling the entire left ureter through a vesicorectal fistula that formed following radical prostatectomy for carcinoma of the prostate.

Radiologic Findings

Gas in the pelvocalyceal system or ureter appears as numerous, sharply defined, round radiolucencies that change with time or with alteration of the patient's position or as complete filling of the lumen (Fig. 14–27). When a large amount of gas is present, the entire lumen is radiolucent, and its wall is sharply defined as a dense, thin line. When the patient is in an upright position, gas rises to the most cephalic portion of the collecting system (Fig. 14–28).

Solid foreign bodies have the shape and radiodensity of the material of which they are composed. Nonopaque objects may become radiopaque by encrustation with calcium crystals.

Caliectasis and pyelectasis occur if the foreign body obstructs urine flow. The radiographic signs of infection may also be associated with a foreign body.

The ultrasonographic and computed tomographic findings of foreign bodies depend on the nature of the material. Strong echoes and acoustic shadows are produced by sound reflectors such as gas or solid objects. Gas causes an acoustic shadow with poorly defined margins and high-level reverberation echoes within the shadow. Foreign material is easily detected by computed tomography, which also demonstrates abnormalities of the perirenal and pararenal spaces in cases of renoalimentary fistulas.

DIFFERENTIAL DIAGNOSIS

The abnormalities discussed in this chapter fall into two major groups: those that are radiopaque, and those that are not. The radiolucent nature of gas is a unique diagnostic feature.

The major challenge lies in distinguishing nonopaque calculus from blood clot, tissue slough, or fungus ball. Mural lesions, particularly transitional cell carcinoma, must also be considered when the location of the lesion cannot be confidently established as intraluminal by the criteria set down in the beginning of this chapter.

Ultrasonography is valuable in establishing that a nonopaque filling defect is a stone. High-level echoes and a sharply defined acoustic shadow distinguish a calculus from noncalcified tissue slough, fungus ball, blood clot, and transitional cell tumor. Acoustic shadowing due to gas must be taken into account in this assessment. Gas, of course, is easily identified by its radiographic or computed tomographic lucency.

Standard and computed tomography also aid in the assessment of a nonopaque intraluminal lesion. The diagnosis of stone is suggested by the tomographic demonstration of faint, homogeneous density in a filling defect that is nonopaque on standard films. Barely detectable calcium deposits, seen in some uroepithelial tumors, should be cautiously kept in mind, but

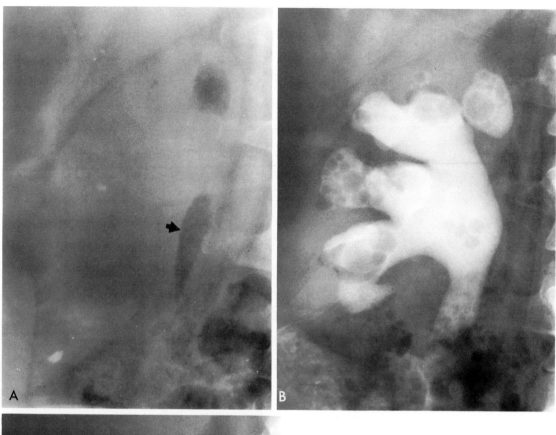

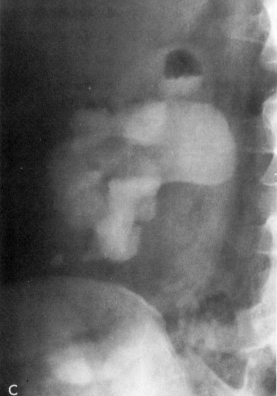

Figure 14–28. Air in the pelvocalyceal system and proximal ureter of a 60-year-old patient with cutaneous ureterostomy and urinary tract infection.

A, Preliminary film, supine position. Air fills a portion of the renal pevis *(arrow).*

B, Excretory urogram, supine position. There are numerous sharply defined lucencies within the pelvocalyceal system.

C, Excretory urogram, upright position. Gas rises to form air–fluid level.

these tumors are usually stippled rather than homogeneous. When a radiographically nonopaque filling defect is very dense by computed tomography, the diagnosis of stone is firmly established. Cholesteatoma and fresh blood clot are slightly denser than renal parenchyma, whereas most transitional cell tumors and mature blood clots will be no denser than kidney tissue.

Time-related changes in size and attenuation value are distinctive features of blood clot. Documentation requires a minimum of a few days' interval between examinations, however. In the absence of further bleeding, a clot disappears within 14 days, during which time it diminishes in computed tomographic density. Other renal abnormalities that may represent the primary cause of bleeding, papillary necrosis or tumor, for example, offer a hint as to the nature of the filling defect.

Tissue slough due to renal papillary necrosis can be recognized by the characteristic triangular shape of the shed portion of the papilla or by its location within a calyx deformed by the amputation of the papillary tip. The "ring" sign produced when the slough is surrounded by opacified urine may be mimicked by a mass of any origin that is located within the lumen of the calyx. The laminated appearance of cholesteatoma during contrast material studies suggests this diagnosis. On the other hand, when a cholesteatoma has a stringy rather than rounded mass appearance, a specific radiologic diagnosis is not possible.

A pelvic or ureteral mass with mixed soft tissue and gas densities is characteristic of a fungus ball. In the absence of gas, however, there are no radiologic features that distinguish this form of nonopaque intraluminal mass from the others discussed in this chapter.

The vast majority of radiopaque intraluminal abnormalities of the pelvocalyceal system and ureter are calculi. These are usually diagnosed accurately by their radiopaque nature, size, location, and shape. A calcified sloughed papilla is easily distinguished from stone when the calcification is deposited on the periphery of the slough. A homogeneously calcified slough, on the other hand, cannot be distinguished from a stone, except perhaps for its triangular shape or the presence of a deformed calyx. The rare, faintly calcified old blood clot is indistinguishable from a faintly calcified calculus or tumor.

Foreign bodies should be recognized by familiarity of shape, as is the case with bullets, needles, sutures, or catheters. These characteristics may become obscured by calcific encrustations, which can mask the true nature of the lesion.

Bibliography

General

Brown, R. C., Jones, M. C., Jr., Boldus, R., and Flocks, R. H.: Lesions causing radiolucent defects in the renal pelvis. AJR *119*:770, 1973.
Fein A. B., and McClennan, B.: Solitary filling defects of the ureter. Semin. Roentgenol. *21*:201, 1986.

Malek, R. S., Aguilo, J. J., and Hattery, R. R.: Radiolucent filling defects of the renal pelvis: Classification and report of unusual cases. J. Urol. *114*:508, 1975.
Parienty, R. A., Ducellier, R., Pradel, J., Lubrano, J.-M., Coquille, F., and Richard, F.: Diagnostic value of CT numbers in pelvocalyceal filling defects. Radiology *145*:743, 1982.
Pollack, H. M., Arger, P. H., Banner, M. P., Mulhern, C. B., Jr., and Coleman, B. G.: Computed tomography of renal pelvic defects. Radiology *138*:645, 1981.
Williams, B. Jr., Hartman, G. W., and Hattery, R. R.: Multiple and diffuse ureteral filling defects. Semin. Roentgenol. *21*:214, 1986.

Urolithiasis

Alter, A. J., Peterson, D. T., and Plautz, A. C., Jr.: Nonopaque calculus demonstrated by computerized tomography. J. Urol. *122*:699, 1979.
Ambos, M., and Bosniak, M. A.: Tomography of the kidney bed as an aid in differentiating renal pelvic tumor and stone. AJR *125*:331, 1975.
Banner, M. P., and Pollack, H. M.: Radiologic evaluation of urinary calculi. In Roth, R. A., and Finlayson, B. (eds.): Stones: Clinical Management of Urolithiasis. Baltimore, Williams & Wilkins, 1983, pp. 53–167.
Banner, M. P.: Calculous disease of the urinary tract. In Pollack, H. M. (ed.): Clinical Urography. Philadelphia, W.B. Saunders, 1990, pp. 1752–1925.
Boyce, W. H.: Radiology in the diagnosis and surgery of renal calculi. Radiol. Clin. North Am. *3*:89, 1965.
Brennan, R. E., Curtis, J. A., Kurtz, A. B., and Walton, J. R.: Use of tomography and ultrasound in the diagnosis of nonopaque renal calculi. JAMA *244*:594, 1980.
Brown, R. C., Loening, S. A., Ehrhardt, J. C., and Hawtrey, C. E.: Cystine calculi are radiopaque. AJR *135*:565, 1980.
Bruwer, A.: Primary renal calculi: Anderson-Carr-Randall progression? AJR *132*:751, 1979.
Carr, R. J.: A new theory on the formation of renal calculi. Br. J. Urol. *26*:105, 1954.
Clayman, R. V., and Williams, R. D.: Oxalate urolithiasis following jejuno-ileal bypass-mechanism and management. Surg. Clin. North Am. *59*:1071, 1979.
Coe, F. L., and Favus, M. J.: Nephrolithiasis. In Brenner, B. M., and Rector, F. C. (eds.): The Kidney. 4th ed. Philadelphia, W.B. Saunders, 1991, pp. 1728–1767.
Coe, F. L., Parks, J. H., and Asplin, J. R.: Medical progress: The pathogenesis and treatment of kidney stones. N. Engl. J. Med. *327*:1141, 1992.
Cook, J. H., and Lytton, B.: Intraoperative localization of renal calculi during nephrolithotomy by ultrasound scanning. J. Urol. *117*:543, 1977.
Cooke, S. A. R.: The site of calcification in the human renal papilla. Br. J. Surg. *57*:890, 1970.
Cunningham, J. J., and Cunningham M. A.: Characterization of renal stone models with gray scale echography. In vitro studies with clinical correlation. Urology *7*:315, 1976.
Drach, G. W.: Urinary lithiasis: Etiology, diagnosis and medical management. In Walsh, P. C., Retik, A. B., Stamey, T. A., and Vaughan, E. D., Jr. (eds.): Campbell's Urology. 6th ed. Philadelphia, W.B. Saunders, 1992, pp. 2085–2156.
Edell, S., and Zegel, H.: Ultrasonic evaluation of renal calculi. AJR *130*:261, 1978.
Federle, M. P., McAninch, J. W., Kaiser, J. A., Goodman, P. C., Roberts, J., and Mall, J. C.: Computed tomography of urine calculi. AJR *136*:255, 1981.
Finberg, H.: Renal ultrasound: Anatomy and technique. Semin. Ultrasound *2*:7, 1981.
Finlayson, B.: Renal lithiasis in review. Urol. Clin. North Am. *1*:181, 1974.
Gearhart, J. P., Herzberg, G. Z., and Jeffs, R. D.: Childhood urolithiasis: Experiences and advances. Pediatrics *87*:445, 1991.
Graves, F. T.: An experimental study of the anatomy of the tubules of the human kidney and its relation to calculus formation. Br. J. Urol. *54*:569, 1982.
Hillman, B. J., Drach, G. W., Tracey, P., and Gaines, J. A.: Computed tomographic analysis of renal calculi. AJR *142*:549, 1984.

Lalli, A. F.: Roentgen aspects of renal calculous disease. Urol. Clin. North Am. *1*:213, 1974.

Malek, R. S.: Urolithiasis. *In* Kelalis, P. P., Kind, L. R., and Belman, A. B. (eds.): Clinical Pediatric Urology. Philadelphia, W.B. Saunders, 1985, pp. 1093–1124.

Mall, J. C., Collins, P. A., and Lyon, E. S.: Matrix calculi. Br. J. Radiol. *48*:807, 1975.

Margolin, E. G., and Cohen, L. H.: Genitourinary calcification: An overview. Semin. Roentgenol. *17*:95, 1982.

Mulholland, S. G., Arger, P. H., Goldberg, B. B., and Pollack, H. M.: Ultrasonic differentiation of renal pelvic filling defects. J. Urol. *122*:14, 1979.

Newhouse, J. H., Prien, E. L., Amis, E. S., Jr., Dretler, S. P., and Pfister, R. C.: Computed tomographic analysis of urinary calculi. AJR *142*:545, 1984.

Pak, C. Y. C.: Etiology and treatment of urolithiasis. Am. J. Kidney Dis. *18*:624, 1991.

Patriquin, H., and Robitaille, P.: Renal calcium deposition in children: Sonographic demonstration of the Anderson-Carr progression. AJR *146*:1253, 1986.

Pollack, H. M., Arger, P. H., and Goldberg, B. B.: Ultrasonic detection of non-opaque renal calculi. Radiology *127*:233, 1978.

Prien, E. L., Sr.: The analysis of urinary calculi. Urol. Clin. North Am. *1*:229, 1974.

Prien, E. L., Sr.: The riddle of Randall's plaques J. Urol. *114*:500, 1975.

Randall, A.: Papillary pathology as a precursor of primary calculus. J. Urol. *44*:580, 1940.

Resnick, M. I., Kirsh, E. D., and Cohen, A. M.: Use of computerized tomography in the delineation of uric acid calculi. J. Urol. *131*:9, 1984.

Rosenfield, A. T., Taylor, K. J. W., Dembner, A. G., and Jacobson, P.: Ultrasound of renal sinus: New observations. AJR *133*:446, 1979.

Schlegel, J. V., Diggdon, P., and Cuellar, J.: The use of ultrasound for localizing renal calculi. J. Urol. *86*:367, 1961.

Schwartz, G., Lipschitz, S., and Becker, J. A.: Detection of renal calculi: The value of tomography. AJR:*143*, 143, 1984.

Segal, A. J., Spataro, R. F., Linke, C. A., Frank, I. N., and Rabinowitz, R.: Diagnosis of nonopaque calculi by computed tomography. Radiology *129*:447, 1978.

Sheppard, P. W., and White, F. E.: Demonstration of a matrix calculus using computed tomography. Br. J. Radiol. *60*:1028, 1987.

Singh, E. O., and Malek, R. S.: Calculus disease in the upper urinary tract. Semin. Roentgenol. *17*:113, 1982.

Smith, L. H.: Medical evaluation of urolithiasis: Etiologic aspects and diagnostic evaluation. Urol. Clin. North Am. *1*:241, 1974.

Smith, L. H.: The pathophysiology and medical treatment of urolithiasis. Semin. Nephrol. *10*:31, 1990.

Sommer, F. G., and Taylor, K. J. W.: Differentiation of acoustic shadowing due to calculi and gas collections. Radiology *135*:399, 1980.

Stafford, S. J., Jenkins, J. M., Staab, E. V., Boyce, I., and Fried, F. A.: Ultrasonic detection of renal calculi: Accuracy tested in an *in vitro* porcine kidney model. JCU *9*:359, 1981.

Stewart, H. H.: Calcifications and calculus formation in the upper urinary tract. Br. J. Urol. *27*:352, 1955.

Van Arsdalen, K. N.: Pathogenesis of renal calculi. Urol. Radiol. *6*:65, 1984.

Vermeulen, C. W., Lyon, E. S., and Ellis, J. E.: The renal papilla and calculogenesis. J. Urol. *97*:573, 1967.

Vermeulen, C. W., and Lyon, E. S.: Mechanisms of genesis and growth of calculi. Am. J. Med. *45*:684, 1968.

Wickham, J. E. A., Fry, I. K., and Wallace, D. M. A.: Computerized tomography localisation of intrarenal calculi prior to nephrolithotomy. Br. J. Urol. *52*:422, 1980.

Zwirewich, C. V., Buckley, A. R., Kidney, M. R., Sullivan, L. D., and Rowley, V. A.: Renal matrix calculus: Sonographic appearance. J. Ultrasound. Med. *9*:61, 1990.

Blood Clot

Antolak, S. J., Jr., and Mellinger, G. T.: Urologic evaluation of hematuria occurring during anticoagulant therapy. J. Urol. *101*:111, 1969.

Beck, P., and Evans, K. T.: Renal abnormalities in patient with haemophilia and Christmas disease. Clin. Radiol. *23*:349, 1972.

Navani, S., Bosniak, M. A., and Shapiro, J. H.: Varied radiographic manifestations of urinary tract bleeding. J. Urol. *100*:339, 1968.

Schaner, E. G., Balow, J. E., and Doppman, J. L.: Computed tomography in the diagnosis of subcapsular and perirenal hematoma. AJR *129*:83, 1977.

Thomas, J., Stey, A., and Aboulker, P.: Calculi on blood clots. J. Urol. (Paris) *82*:496, 1976.

Wright, F. W., Matthews, J. M., and Brock, L. G.: Complication of hemophilic disorders affecting the renal tract. Radiology *98*:571, 1971.

Tissue Slough

Amberg, J. A., and Talner, L. B.: Clinical Pathologic Conference: Cholesteatoma in a 46-year-old woman. Urol. Radiol. *1*:192, 1980.

Carsky, E. W., Prior, J. T., Moore, R., and Hamel, J.: Cholesteatoma of the kidney: Radiographic findings. Radiology *78*:796, 1962.

Eugan, J. W., Jr.: Urothelial neoplasms: Pathologic anatomy. *In* Hill, G. S. (ed.): Uropathology. New York, Churchill Livingstone, 1989, pp. 719–793.

Hare, W. S. C., and Poynter, J. D.: The radiology of renal papillary necrosis as seen in analgesic nephropathy. Clin. Radiol. *25*:423, 1974.

Hertle, L., and Androulakakis, P.: Keratinizing desquamative metaplasia of the upper urinary tract: Leukoplakia-cholesteatoma. J. Urol. *127*:631, 1982.

Osius, T. G., Harrod, C. S., and Smith, D. R.: Cholesteatoma of the renal pelvis. J. Urol. *87*:774, 1962.

Sarlis, J. N., Malakates, S. K., and Papadimitriou, D.: Cholesteatoma of renal pelvis. J. Urol. *118*:468, 1967.

Weitzner, S.: Cholesteatoma of the calix. J. Urol. *108*:365, 1972.

Fungus Ball

Biggers, R., and Edwards, J.: Anuria secondary to bilateral ureteropelvic fungus balls. Urology *15*:161, 1980.

Boldus, R. A., Brown, R. C., and Culp, D. A.: Fungus balls in renal pelvis. Radiology *102*:555, 1972.

Clark, R. E., Minagi, H., and Palubinskas, A. J.: Renal candidiasis. Radiology *101*:567, 1971.

Cohen, G. H.: Obstructive uropathy caused by ureteral candidiasis. J. Urol. *110*:285, 1973.

Comings, D. E., Turbow, B. A., and Callahan, D. H.: Obstructing *Aspergillus* cast of the renal pelvis. Arch. Intern. Med. *110*:255, 1962.

Dembner, A. G., and Pfister, R. C.: Fungal infections of the urinary tract: Demonstration by antegrade pyelography and drainage by percutaneous nephrostomy. AJR *129*:415, 1977.

Fisher, J., Mayhall, G., Duma, R., Shadomy, S., Shadomy, J., and Wathington, C.: Fungus balls of the urinary tract. South. Med. J. *72*:1281, 1979.

Gerle, R. D.: Roentgenographic features of primary renal candidiasis. AJR *119*:731, 1973.

Gilliam, J. S., and Vest, S. A.: Penicillium infection of the urinary tract. J. Urol. *65*:484, 1951.

Irby, P. B., Stoller, M. L., and McAninch, J. W.: Fungal bezoars of the upper urinary tract. J. Urol. *143*:447, 1990.

Margolin, H. N.: Fungus infection of urinary tract. Semin. Roentgenol. *6*:323, 1971.

McDonald, D. F., and Fagan, C. J.: Fungus balls in the urinary tract: Case report. AJR *114*:753, 1972.

Melchior, J., Mebust, W. K., and Valk, W. L.: Ureteral colic from a fungus ball: Unusual presentation of systemic aspergillosis. J. Urol. *108*:698, 1972.

Michigan, S.: Genitourinary fungal infection. J. Urol. *116*:390, 1976.

Stuck, K. J., Silver, T. M., Jaffe, M. H., and Bowerman, R. A.: Sonographic demonstration of renal fungus balls. Radiology *142*:473, 1981.

Warshowsky, A. B., Keiller, D., and Gittes, R. F.: Bilateral renal aspergillosis. J. Urol. *113*:8, 1975.

Foreign Material

Arthur, G. W., and Morris, D. G.: Reno-alimentary fistulae. Br. J. Surg. *53*:396, 1966.

Baird, J. M., and Spence, H. M.: Ingested foreign bodies migrating to the kidney from the gastrointestinal tract. J. Urol. *99*:675, 1968.

Bissada, N. K., Cole, A. T., and Fried, F. A.: Renoalimentary fistula: An unusual urological problem. J. Urol. *110*:273, 1973.

Bretland, M. B., and Blacklock, M. B.: Grenade fragment in the ureter. Br. J. Urol. *40*:223, 1968.

Brust, R. W., Jr., and Morgan, A. L.: Renocolic fistula secondary to carcinoma of the colon. J. Urol. *111*:439, 1974.

Eickenberg, H.-U., Amin, M., and Lich, R., Jr.: Travelling bullets in genitourinary tract. Urology *6*:224, 1975.

Frang, D.: A swallowed needle found in the kidney pelvis. J. Urol. (Paris) *71*:647, 1978.

Osmond, J. D.: Foreign bodies in the kidney. Radiology *60*:375, 1953.

Rittenberg, G. M., and Warren, E.: Air in the pelvocalyceal system: A normal finding in patients with ureteroileostomies. AJR *128*:311, 1977.

Shukri, A. M.: Reno-alimentary fistulae. Br. J. Surg. *55*:551, 1968.

Wiscott, J. W.: Hydronephrosis from shell fragment in renal pelvis. Milit. Med. *134*:1334, 1969.

15

MURAL ABNORMALITIES

Each of the dissimilar abnormalities discussed in this chapter share the same distinguishing characteristic—a primary involvement of the pelvocalyceal or ureteral wall. Except for pyelocalyceal diverticula and ureteroceles, these lesions, which are variably focal, multifocal, or diffuse, transform the normally smooth mucosa into a surface that is irregular, nodular, or sharply narrowed. In some situations, a free intraluminal component is also present but only secondary to the initiating mural event.

A mural lesion maintains a constant relationship with the pelvocalyceal wall. Opacified urine surrounds only that part of the abnormality that projects into the lumen, never completely surrounding it. Focal or multifocal mural lesions are usually sharply marginated and may form an acute angle at their site of attachment to the wall. Diffuse lesions, on the other hand, are irregular.

The radiologic criteria for mural lesions are apparent only when the pelvocalyceal system and ureter are well opacified and fully distended. This requires an adequate dose of contrast material and carefully applied abdominal compression to distend the pelvocalyceal system. Multiple projections, changes in patient position, and later re-examination are useful adjuncts. Direct opacification of the collecting system by retrograde or antegrade pyelograpy is occasionally required. Computed tomography, ultrasonography, and angiography are of secondary value in the assessment of mural lesions.

Tumors of the uroepithelium, usually transitional cell carcinoma, are the most frequently encountered mural lesions in the adult's upper urinary tract and are discussed first in this chapter. Next, congenital ureteropelvic junction obstruction is discussed. Fol-

lowing these two sections a variety of conditions, including uncommon infections, unusual responses to infection or inflammation, mural hemorrhage, longitudinal mucosal folds, and pseudodiverticulosis, are discussed. Calyceal diverticulum is an abnormality of the collecting system wall and, therefore, is discussed in this chapter even though its radiologic appearance is that of a communicating cyst rather than a mural mass. Likewise, ureterocele is included as a prolapse of the ureter into the bladder at the ureterovesical junction.

TUMORS

Definition

Approximately 8 per cent of all malignant kidney tumors have a uroepithelial origin. Transitional cell carcinoma accounts for 85 to 95 per cent of these. The remainder, for the most part, are squamous cell carcinoma. Only a very few cases of uroepithelial mucinous adenocarcinoma have been recorded. Rare, also, are primary benign and malignant tumors of the nonepithelial components of the pelvocalyceal wall and direct mural metastases.

Upper tract tumors of the uroepithelium are not evenly distributed. Transitional cell carcinoma occurs two to three times more commonly in the renal pelvis than in the ureter. Of the ureteral tumors, most occur in the distal third of that structure. There is also a well-established tendency toward multicentricity and bilaterality of transitional cell carcinomas. Bilateral upper tract metachronous and/or synchronous transitional cell carcinoma has been reported in up to 10 per cent of patients. Metachronous transitional cell carcinoma of the bladder develops in up to 40 per cent of patients with transitional cell carcinoma of the renal pelvis and in up to 55 per cent of patients with transitional cell carcinoma of the ureter.

The histologic spectrum of *transitional cell carcinoma* extends from papilloma, a thin fibrovascular core covered by normal transitional cell mucosa, to advanced cytologic and architectural features of malignancy. The gross appearance of transitional cell carcinoma varies from papillary and bulky to sessile. Some tumors are unifocal, whereas others are multiple or diffusely spread over confluent areas of the pelvocalyceal or ureteral mucosal surface.

Squamous cell carcinoma is generally thought to arise from transitional cell epithelium that has undergone squamous metaplasia in response to chronic irritation with or without infection. Many pathologists believe that these tumors are associated with leukoplakia, but others deny the idea that such association exists. Intercellular bridges and keratin pearls are specific histologic characteristics of squamous cell carcinoma. Lesions are usually single, either papillary or sessile, and highly invasive.

Mucinous adenocarcinoma is the rarest form of primary uroepithelial malignancy. This tumor, like squamous cell carcinoma, develops from metaplastic transformation of transitional cells in response to chronic inflammation. It is characterized by papillary structures with gland formation, vacuolated goblet cells, and mucin. Mucinous adenocarcinoma tends to involve broad areas of the pelvic and calyceal surface, which makes recognition more difficult than if there had been an exophytic pattern of growth.

Benign mesodermal tumors of the upper urinary tract, known as *fibroepithelial polyps,* are uncommon. Most arise in the ureter, often extending retrograde into the renal pelvis. A few originate proximal to the ureteropelvic junction. The core of these polypoid masses consists of fibrous tissue, smooth muscle, blood or lymphatic vessels, or nerve cells. The fibrous component is most often predominant. A thin layer of normal urothelium covers these polyps, which are usually elongated, thin, and occasionally divided at their tip into several fingerlike branches. The bulk of the polyp lies free in the lumen of the collecting system and is highly mobile in all directions.

Malignant nonepithelial sarcoma arising from the wall of the pelvis or calyces is extremely rare. This tumor may be derived from any of the mesenchymal components and is classified according to the predominant tissue type.

Most *metastatic tumors* involve the pelvocalyceal system or ureter by invasion from surrounding blood vessels, lymphatic channels, or lymph nodes; direct metastases occur rarely. Carcinoma of the stomach, prostate, breast, lung, cervix, and colon and melanoma account for most metastatic tumors.

Clinical Setting

Transitional cell carcinoma occurs most frequently in men and has a peak incidence in the seventh decade.

The entire uroepithelium is at risk, although the ureter is less frequently affected than the pelvocalyceal system while the upper tract as a whole is less frequently involved than the bladder. Certain epidemiologic factors increase the risk for the development of transitional cell carcinoma. These include exposure to chemicals in the dye, petroleum, rubber, and cable industries as well as in occupations such as hairdresser, leather finisher, spray painter, and textile weaver. Tobacco, coffee, artificial sweetener, tryptophan metabolites, and chronic inflammation or infection are additional risk factors. Increased prevalence of transitional cell carcinoma in patients with analgesic and Balkan nephropathy is well established. A history of transitional cell carcinoma of the bladder increases the likelihood of tumor appearing in the renal pelvis, suggesting that transitional cell carcinoma originates in unstable uroepithelium at multiple sites.

There is an eightfold increase in the risk for transitional cell carcinoma of the renal pelvis in patients with analgesic nephropathy. One or more metabolites of phenacetin are thought to be the causal agent. Unlike the population at large, among analgesic abusers, women are more frequently affected than men; a younger age group is involved; and the renal pelvis, rather than the urinary bladder, is the predominant site of tumor. The long induction time, estimated at 22 years on average, emphasizes the need for frequent and long-term surveillance of patients with analgesic nephropathy.

Squamous cell carcinoma occurs in an older age group than does transitional cell carcinoma and is generally believed to be closely associated with chronic infection and leukoplakia of the urinary tract. Calculi are present in more than half of the patients with this tumor. The prevalence in men is approximately equal to that in women. These patients follow a rapidly lethal clinical course that reflects the highly invasive behavior of squamous cell carcinoma.

Mucinous adenocarcinoma of the renal pelvis occurs only in patients with severe infection and stone disease. Branched (staghorn) calculi and hydronephrosis are frequently noted.

Malignant tumor, including the rare mural metastasis, commonly causes painless hematuria. Clots may cause intermittent obstruction and colic. Dull, persistent flank pain may also be a prominent feature. Palpable tumor is uncommon, although a hydronephrotic kidney may be felt when the tumor causes chronic obstruction.

Benign mesenchymal tumor (fibroepithelial polyp) causes hematuria and flank pain in over 50 per cent of cases. Obstruction, however, is infrequent even though the bulk of the polyp is intraluminal. These tumors occur mainly in children.

Radiologic Findings

Malignant Uroepithelial Tumors

Excretory Urography. All malignant tumors of the upper urinary tract regardless of histologic type generally have similar radiologic findings. A tumor located in the pelvocalyceal system is visualized directly by excretory urography in 60 to 70 per cent of patients. Most malignant tumors of the collecting system and ureter fulfill the criteria for a mural location, as outlined in the beginning of this chapter. However, these lesions may vary greatly in appearance. Some are single polypoid masses with a smooth, irregular, or lobular surface (Figs. 15–1 through 15–3). The same pattern may occur at multiple sites. Other lesions, particularly squamous cell carcinoma, are broad based and flat and are single or multiple (Fig. 15–4). Occasionally, there is a superficial spread over large areas, with an irregular mucosal pattern (Fig. 15–5). In some cases that arise in the pelvocalyceal system, infiltration of the renal sinus and/or parenchyma is so advanced that the kidney loses function. The intrarenal arterial branches demonstrate varying degrees of narrowing and irregularity under this circumstance (Fig. 15–6).

Contrast material trapped within the interstices of a polypoid growth causes a stippled appearance when viewed *en face* or in cross section (Fig. 15–7; see also Fig. 15–12). This pattern may suggest a malignant uroepithelial tumor in some cases but is generally not helpful in differentiating neoplastic from nonneoplastic filling defects of the pelvis. Transitional cell carcinoma may develop stippled calcific deposits that are detected infrequently by standard radiography (Fig. 15–8) but are readily seen by computed tomography. These deposits explain why the attenuation value of uroepithelial tumors is sometimes higher than that of renal parenchyma.

Indirect manifestations of a malignant tumor of the renal pelvis are nonopacification of the kidney due to hydronephrosis (Fig. 15–9; see Fig. 15–8) and a renal parenchymal mass due to infiltration of the kidney by a primary lesion in the pelvocalyceal system (Fig. 15–10). In these circumstances, diagnostic accuracy can be increased by pyelography, using either a retrograde or antegrade technique (see Figs. 15–6, 15–8, and 15–9). Either of these approaches opacifies the pelvocalyceal system better than excretory urography when renal function is compromised. Antegrade pyelogra-

Text continued on page 482

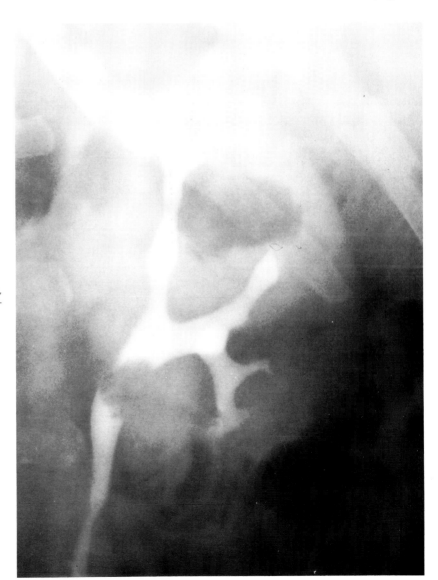

Figure 15–1. Transitional cell carcinoma. A single, lobulated, broad-based mass projects into the pelvis of the left kidney. Excretory urogram.

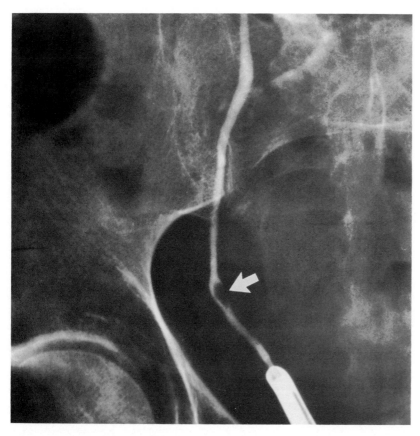

Figure 15–2. Transitional cell carcinoma, right distal ureter. Retrograde ureterogram. The tumor appears as a single, small, smooth, polypoid mass *(arrow)*.

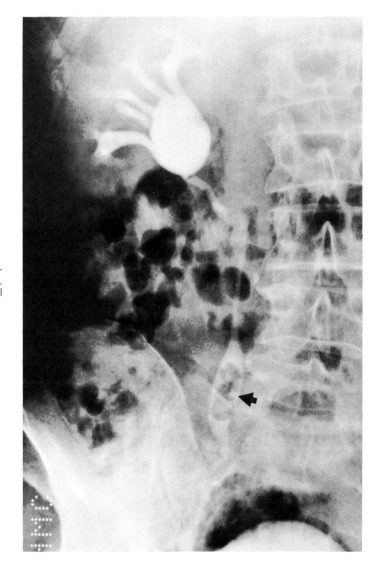

Figure 15–3. Transitional cell carcinoma, right mid ureter. Excretory urogram. The tumor *(arrow)* appears as a moderately large, lobulated, smooth mass with dilatation of the ureter just proximal and distal to the mass.

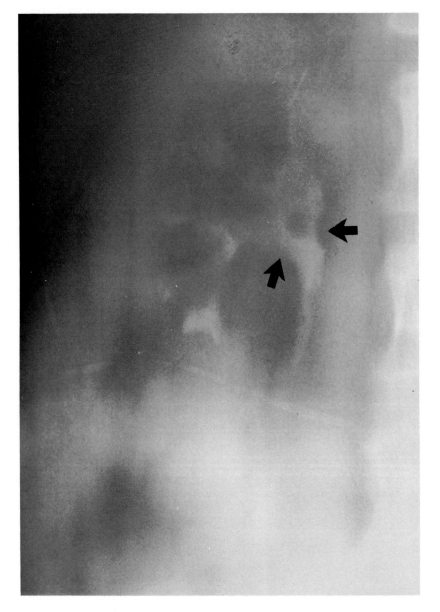

Figure 15–4. Transitional cell carcinoma. Multiple, broad-based, flat lesions *(arrows)* are present in the right renal pelvis of a 72-year-old man with gross, total hematuria. Excretory urogram.

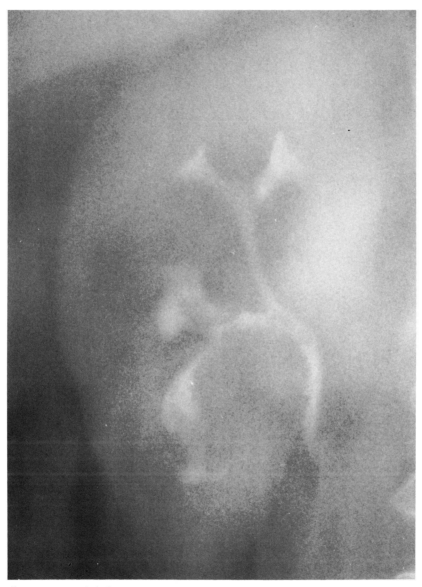

A

Figure 15–5. Transitional cell carcinoma, right kidney.

A, Excretory urogram. Superficial spread extends over a large area of the pelvocalyceal system. Caliectasis in the middle and lower poles is present. A mass effect on the inferior margin of the pelvis indicates spread of the tumor into the renal sinus fat.

Illustration continued on following page

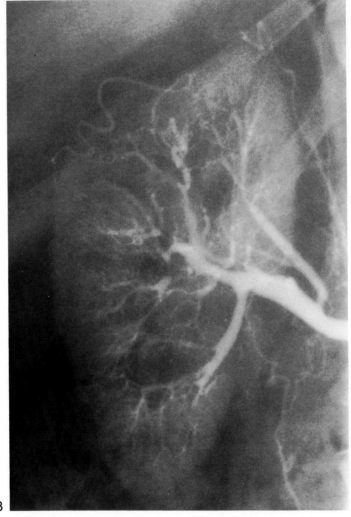

B

Figure 15–5 *Continued B,* Selective renal arteriogram, arterial phase. Encasement of the distal main renal artery and displacement of the artery to the lower pole also indicate spread of tumor into the renal sinus.

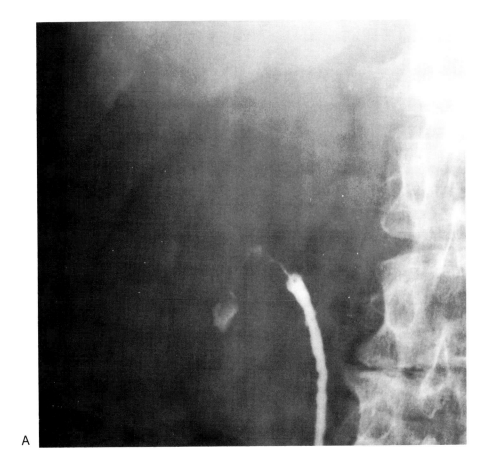

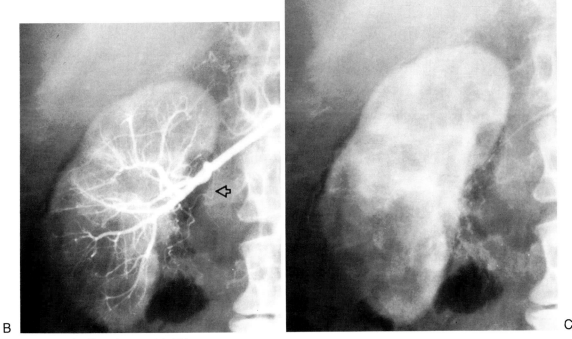

Figure 15–6. Transitional cell carcinoma, right kidney.

  A, Retrograde pyelogram. The collecting system is obliterated by infiltrating tumor.

  B and *C,* Selective renal arteriogram, arterial phase *(B)* and nephrographic phase *(C).* There is enlargement of the pelviureteric artery *(arrow),* neovascularity and tumor blush in the region of the renal pelvis, and loss of intrarenal arterial branches in the lower pole due to parenchymal invasion, which causes diminished enhancement of the lower pole nephrogram.

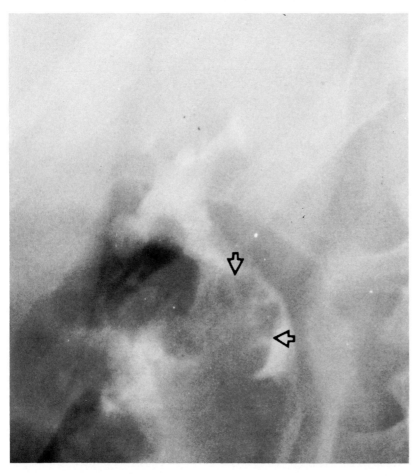

Figure 15–7. Transitional cell carcinoma. A stippled appearance is derived from contrast material that is trapped within the interstices of this polypoid growth *(arrows)*. Excretory urogram.

Figure 15–8. Transitional cell carcinoma. Stippled calcification in a bulky tumor mass, which causes obstructive uropathy.

A, Preliminary film. Fine calcific deposits *(arrows)* are present along the upper margin of the tumor.

Illustration continued on following page

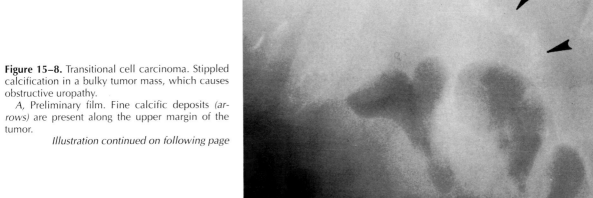

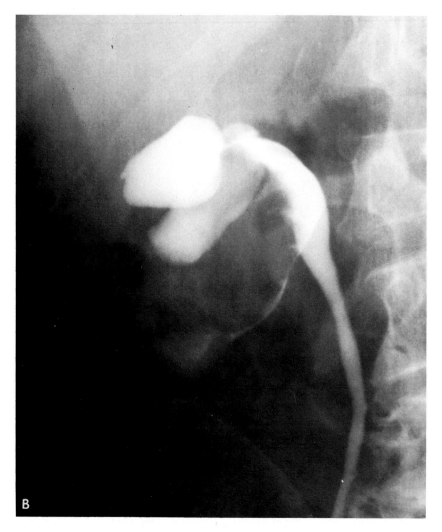

Figure 15–8 *Continued B,* Retrograde pyelogram. The tumor distorts and obstructs the pelvocalyceal system.

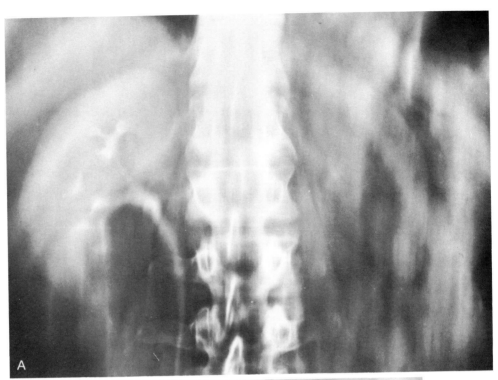

Figure 15–9. Transitional cell carcinoma, left ureter, causing loss of function of the left kidney due to hydronephrosis.

A, Excretory urogram. Tomogram. There is marked decrease in enhancement of the kidney, which is small and smooth.

B, Percutaneous antegrade pyelogram. The ureter is dilated to the point of a small nonopaque filling defect protruding into the lumen. This represents the transitional cell carcinoma.

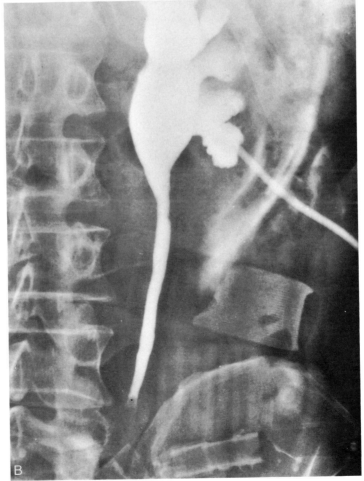

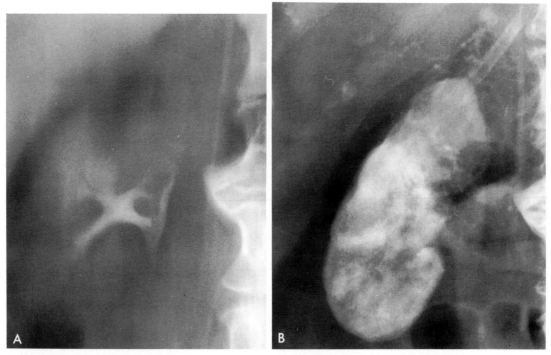

Figure 15–10. Transitional cell carcinoma arising in the pelvocalyceal system of the right kidney. Infiltration of the upper pole obliterates the vasculature and nephrons in this region, thereby diminishing the urographic and angiographic nephrograms. Note preservation of the reniform shape of the kidney despite the increase in size of the upper pole.
  A, Excretory urogram. Tomogram. Tumor also projects into the pelvis.
  B, Angiogram, nephrographic phase. There is loss of corticomedullary differentiation in addition to the decrease in the density of the upper pole nephrogram.

phy is particularly valuable when the tumor is obstructive and causes hydronephrosis. Brushing of the lesion for cytologic study can be combined with either direct approach.

A tumor located in the ureter appears as a nonopaque, irregular filling defect usually with dilatation of the ureter proximal to the mass (see Figs. 15–2 and 15–3). The ureter just distal to the tumor is also often slightly dilated. The combination of the distal margin of a nonopaque soft tissue mass invaginating into a distended segment of an opacified ureter constitutes the *chalice* or *Bergman's* sign, which can be seen on either excretory urography or pyelography (Fig. 15–11). This sign is valuable in distinguishing a nonopaque tumor from a nonopaque stone in that the latter causes spasm, rather than distention, of the segment of the ureter distal to it.

Transitional cell carcinoma located in the pelvocalyceal system sometimes infiltrates the renal parenchyma, producing a focal parenchymal mass, obliteration of the adjacent collecting system, and reduced nephrographic density in the involved region (see Fig. 15–10). These features must be distinguished from those of adenocarcinoma arising in the renal parenchyma. This can be accomplished by recognizing the preservation of the reniform shape of the enlarged kidney that is characteristic of neoplasms that infiltrate the kidney in contradistinction to the ball-shaped geometry produced by tumors that expand in all directions from an epicenter originating in the renal parenchyma. This concept is amplified in Chapter 12.

A stone that coexists with a mural lesion raises the possibility of epidermoid or mucinous adenocarcinoma. When epidermoid carcinoma develops in the presence of leukoplakia, the latter may dominate the radiologic findings and the neoplasm cannot be separately identified.

Computed Tomography. Computed tomography defines the contour and mural attachment of a uroepithelial tumor following pelvocalyceal or ureteral opacification. The soft tissue attenuation value of the tumor may increase as much as twofold after rapid intravenous injection of contrast material. The tumor appears as a mural mass projecting into the uroepithelial-lined lumen, as circumferential or eccentric thickening of the pelvic or ureteric wall, or as soft tissue infiltrating the renal sinus or periureteric fat (Figs. 15–12 through 15–14). Computed tomography offers no special advantage over excretory urography or pyelography in assessing the tumor itself. Instead, its special value is in evaluating the nature of a nonopaque filling defect in general and in staging documented uroepithelial tumors. Here, peripelvic fat obliteration, nephrographic defects, direct extension into the peripelvic or periureteric space, and lymph node enlargement provide evidence of tumor spread that may be useful in formulating therapeutic plans.

Ultrasonography. Large pelvocalyceal tumors separate the compact, dense central sinus echoes of the normal kidney and generate echoes similar in intensity to those of the renal parenchyma (see Fig. 15–13). Tumors that are too small to separate the central sinus

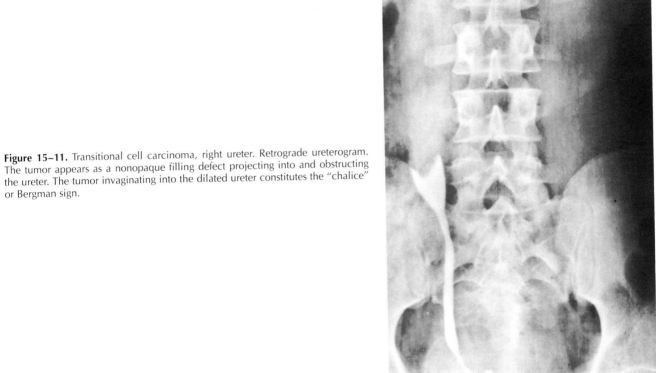

Figure 15–11. Transitional cell carcinoma, right ureter. Retrograde ureterogram. The tumor appears as a nonopaque filling defect projecting into and obstructing the ureter. The tumor invaginating into the dilated ureter constitutes the "chalice" or Bergman sign.

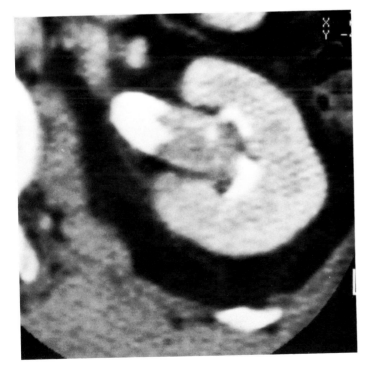

Figure 15–12. Transitional cell carcinoma. A bulky tumor fills the pelvocalyceal system of the left kidney. Differentiation between intraluminal and mural mass is not possible with a tumor of this size. Note the contrast material in the interstices of the tumor. Computed tomogram, contrast material enhanced.

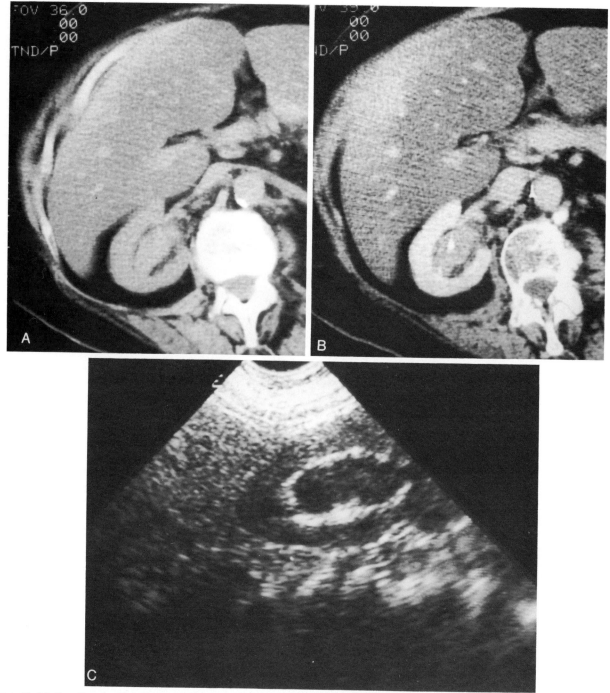

Figure 15–13. Transitional cell carcinoma, right kidney. The tumor fills the pelvocalyceal system but does not invade the sinus fat.
A, Computed tomogram, unenhanced. The carcinoma is isodense with renal parenchyma.
B, Computed tomogram, contrast material enhanced. The tumor enhances and compresses portions of the collecting system.
C, Ultrasonogram, longitudinal section. The tumor is moderately echogenic, fills the pelvis, and separates the central sinus echo complex.
(Kindly provided by Wendelin S. Hayes, D.O., Armed Forces Institute of Pathology, Washington, D.C.)

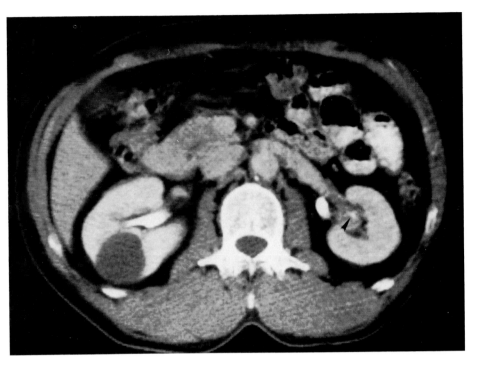

Figure 15–14. Transitional cell carcinoma in the left kidney. A small amount of intraluminal contrast material *(arrow)* is surrounded by a soft tissue mass, representing mural infiltration and extension into the renal sinus fat. The contrast material–filled structure medial to the kidney is the proximal ureter. Computed tomogram, contrast material enhanced.

echoes may not be detectable by ultrasonography. Tumors of the ureter are seen as a soft tissue mass that is often situated at the distal end of a slightly dilated ureter. Ultrasound examination does not reliably distinguish between urothelial tumor and blood clot unless the central low density pattern changes with time, which is characteristic of clot.

Ultrasonography detects infiltration of the kidney parenchyma by a tumor originating in the pelvocalyceal system. Here, the kidney size is enlarged owing to regional growth, the contour remains reniform, and the echo texture of the involved portion of the kidney is altered from that of the normal parencyhma.

Angiography. Malignant tumors of the uroepithelium are supplied by vessels of arteriolar and capillary caliber that are arranged in an irregular network. Large tumor vessels are rare. Demonstration of these poorly vascularized tumors depends on technically superior studies using selective renal artery injection of contrast material and is limited to those that arise in the pelvocalyceal system. Pharmacoangiographic and magnification techniques are sometimes useful in demonstrating otherwise inapparent tumor vessels. This bed of small arteries accounts for the contrast material enhancement of transitional cell tumors during dynamic computed tomographic scanning.

The angiographic features of malignant uroepithelial tumors include fine neovascularity, a homogeneous tumor blush, vascular encasement, and absence of arteriovenous shunts (see Fig. 15–6). Central pelvic tumors are supplied by the pelviureteric artery, which may be enlarged and/or displaced. Tumors located in the periphery of the collecting system are supplied by branches of the main renal artery. Encasement, spreading, or straightening of interlobar or arcuate arteries and a nephrographic deficit indicate parenchymal invasion (see Figs. 15–5 and 15–6). Additional angiographic abnormalities include stretching of arteries by

a dilated, obstructed pelvis and occlusion of renal artery or vein by direct tumor encasement or invasion. Parasitic blood supply develops only after invasion of the perirenal space. Angiography cannot discriminate malignant uroepithelial tumors from poorly vascularized adenocarcinoma of the kidney other than by demonstrating the morphology of infiltrative rather than expansile growth, as discussed in Chapter 12 (see Figs. 12–1 and 12–2). Similarly, the vascular patterns of malignant disease cannot reliably be distinguished from nonmalignant (inflammatory) disease.

Miscellaneous Tumors

The radiologic features of malignant, nonepithelial (mesenchymal), and metastatic tumors of the collecting system and ureter are similar to those of epithelial malignancies described in the foregoing section. Focal, blood-borne mural metastases, an uncommon event, may simulate benign conditions, such as pyelitis cystica (Fig. 15–15). Computed tomography differentiates metastases isolated to the wall from those that invade from the peripelvic or periureteric space (Fig. 15–16).

Benign mesodermal tumors (fibroepithelial polyps) of the pelvis are smooth, long, nonopaque filling defects that move freely in both antegrade and retrograde directions (Fig. 15–17). These tumors are single, bifid, or multibranched. Demonstration of the point of attachment to the pelvic wall may require multiple projections. These lesions inconstantly cause obstruction and are best identified by excretory urography.

CONGENITAL URETEROPELVIC JUNCTION OBSTRUCTION

Definition

The area where the funnel-shaped renal pelvis merges into the tubule-shaped ureter is the *ureteropelvic junc-*

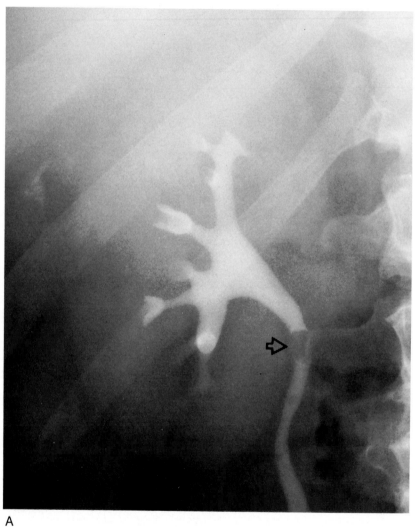

A

Figure 15–15. Mural metastases in a 59-year-old man with melanoma. There are sharply defined, oval filling defects at the right ureteropelvic junction *(arrow)* and at multiple sites in the left ureter. Some appear to be intraluminal, but all are mural. There were also blood-borne metastases to the bladder.

A, Right kidney.

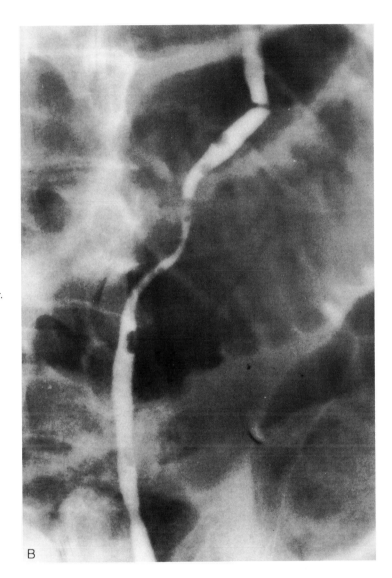

Figure 15–15 *Continued B,* Left mid ureter.

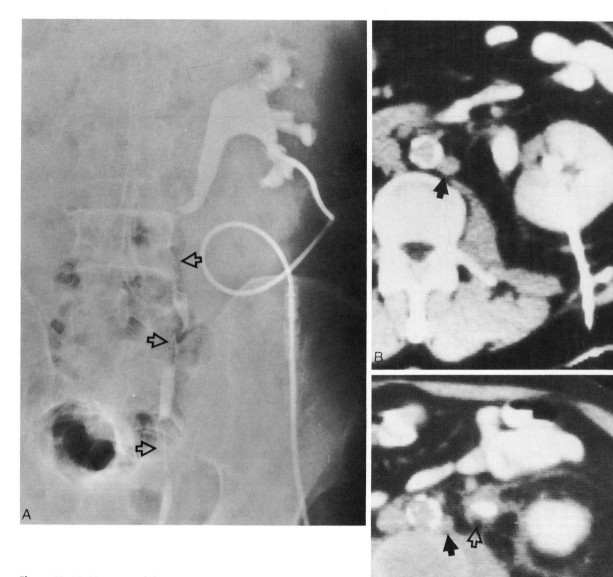

Figure 15–16. Metastases, left ureter *(open arrows)* and periaortic lymph nodes *(solid arrows)* in a man with carcinoma of the prostate.

A, Antegrade pyelogram. There are multiple segments of irregular narrowing with intervening areas of dilatation in the left ureter.

B and *C,* Computed tomograms, contrast material enhanced at the renal hilus *(B)* demonstrating an enlarged periaortic lymph node and at the level of the mid ureter *(C)* demonstrating tumor invading the ureter.

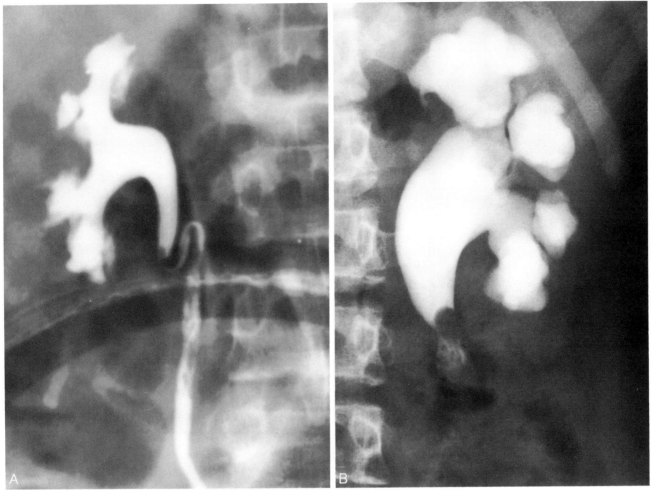

Figure 15–17. Fibroepithelial polyps, bilateral, in a child. Excretory urogram.
    A, Right kidney and proximal ureter. The polyp in the proximal ureter is a smooth, multibranched nonopaque filling defect that does not obstruct.
    B, Left kidney and proximal ureter. The polyp obstructs the ureteropelvic junction.

tion, a term embodying a general anatomic concept rather than a specific embryologic or histologic site. Congenital obstruction of this junction has been investigated extensively, but no single cause has been conclusively established. Derangement of circular and longitudinal muscle, inadequate distensibility of the ureteropelvic junctional segment due to excess inelastic collagen, and deficiency of transmitter substance at nerve endings are major theories of etiology. None of these have been validated, however. It is generally agreed that kinks, angulations, and "high insertions" of the ureter are a result, rather than a cause, of pelvic distention. Rare causes of ureteropelvic junction obstruction include crossing blood vessels, fibrous bands, ischemia, mucosal folds, aortic aneurysm, renal cyst, and eosinophilic ureteritis.

Most patients with ureteropelvic junction obstruction have no demonstrable anatomic abnormality. To explain this, Whitaker (1975) proposed a functional definition of the ureteropelvic junction as the point at which a downward moving contraction, initiated somewhere in the pelvocalyceal system, causes apposition of the ureteropelvic wall and formation of a bolus of urine. Under normal conditions, including high-flow states, efficient emptying of the pelvis follows forward propulsion of each succeeding bolus (Fig. 15–18). Whitaker theorized that congenital ureteropelvic junction obstruction occurs when the walls of the pelvis do not appose at the ureteral junction because the pelvis is not funnel shaped. The resultant failure to create a bolus impedes urine flow across the junction (Fig. 15–19). The progressive pelvic dilatation that follows incomplete drainage leads to further inefficiency of pelvic emptying. Ultimately, there is decreased glomerular filtration and progressive hypertrophy of the pelvic musculature. In extreme circumstances, hydronephrosis results.

The radiologic findings of chronic hydronephrosis are discussed in Chapter 9. Additional discussions on the forces that propel urine forward and the various causes of the dilated pelvocalyceal system are presented in Chapter 17.

Clinical Setting

Congenital ureteropelvic junction obstruction most often presents in infancy or childhood with an abdominal mass, flank or abdominal pain, failure to

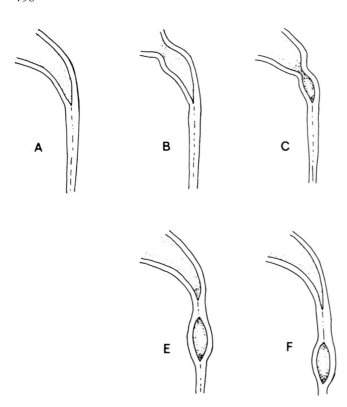

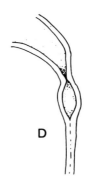

Figure 15–18. Schematic illustration of the sequence of peristalsis at the normal ureteropelvic junction.

A, Normal funnel shape of ureteropelvic junction in the resting state.

B and *C,* Peristaltic wave passes prograde through the pelvis.

D, Funnel shape of the pelvis leads to apposition of opposite walls as the peristaltic wave progresses toward the ureter.

E, A bolus forms as a result of circular contraction of muscles proximally and relaxation of muscles distally.

F, Progression of bolus occurs as longitudinally oriented force of the muscle contraction "pulls" the ureter over the bolus.

(Courtesy of R. H. Whitaker, Addenbrooke's Hospital, Cambridge, England, and Br. J. Urol. *47:*377, 1975.)

Figure 15–19. Schematic illustration of the sequence of peristalsis with congenital ureteropelvic junction obstruction.

A, The normal funnel shape of the distal pelvis either is absent in the resting state or is lost with rapid diuresis.

B, C, and *D,* A wave of contraction passes along the pelvic wall. The rounded shape precludes apposition of the walls and bolus formation.

E, Without a bolus on which to grip, the circular and longitudinal forces of muscular contraction are wasted. The junction is closed, and urine is prevented from passing through.

F, Some fluid drains through the orifice leading to the ureter because this is the weakest point in the high-pressure system.

(Courtesy of R. H. Whitaker, Addenbrooke's Hospital, Cambridge, England, and Br. J. Urol. *47:*377, 1975.)

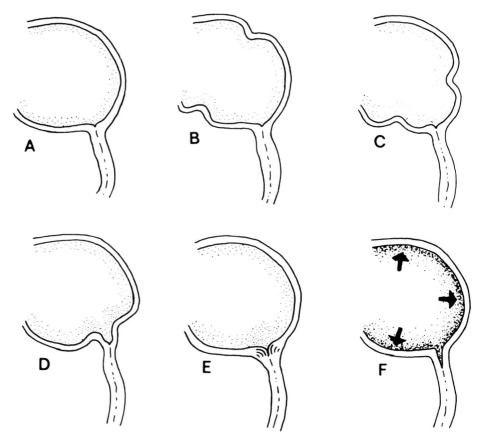

thrive, or nonspecific gastrointestinal complaints. The left kidney in males is most commonly involved. Infection, hypertension, hematuria, and stone formation are less commonly associated clinical problems. When children with congenital ureteropelvic junction obstruction sustain mild abdominal trauma, serious complications, such as hemorrhage and shock, may follow.

In adults who have congenital ureteropelvic junction obstruction, pain, hematuria, and urinary tract infection predominate. Pain is often episodic and frequently precipitated by high urine flow rates such as those produced by beer drinking.

Radiologic Findings

The classic excretory urographic findings of congenital ureteropelvic junction obstruction are a sharply defined narrowing at the junction and dilatation of the pelvocalyceal system that persists even when the patient is placed in a position that favors gravity drainage of the pelvis (Fig. 15–20). Unilateral renal enlargement, diminished parenchymal and pelvocalyceal opacification, the "rim" sign, and wasting of the kidney substance are late findings that reflect the long-term consequences of the inability of the collecting system to handle normal urine volume. These changes become most severe when the pelvis is surrounded by the renal parenchyma (intrarenal pelvis).

An extrarenal pelvis more readily dilates in response to obstruction, thereby causing less effect on parenchymal structure and function. In its most advanced form, congenital ureteropelvic junction obstruction transforms the kidney into a hydronephrotic sac.

Narrowing of the ureteropelvic junction is usually concentric (see Fig. 15–20). A sharp angulation or kink of the pelvis in relation to the proximal ureter may develop as the pelvis rotates anteriorly while it dilates (Fig. 15–21). A vessel crossing the ureteropelvic junction, usually an artery to the lower pole of the kidney, may cause a broad, tangential, sharply defined extrinsic radiolucent depression on the dilated pelvis at the junction (see Fig. 15–21). This rarely, however, is the primary cause of obstruction. In severe cases, there is no opacification of the ureter beyond the obstruction.

Antegrade and retrograde pyelography clearly demonstrate the junctional narrowing and are employed when impaired function prevents adequate opacification by excretory urography (Fig. 15–22). The ability to perform urodynamic studies during antegrade pyelography makes this approach particularly advantageous.

The angiographic, ultrasonographic, and computed tomographic abnormalities of congenital ureteropelvic junction obstruction are the same as those of chronic obstructive uropathy of any etiology. These abnormalities are discussed in Chapter 9.

The collecting system is not always dilated in con-

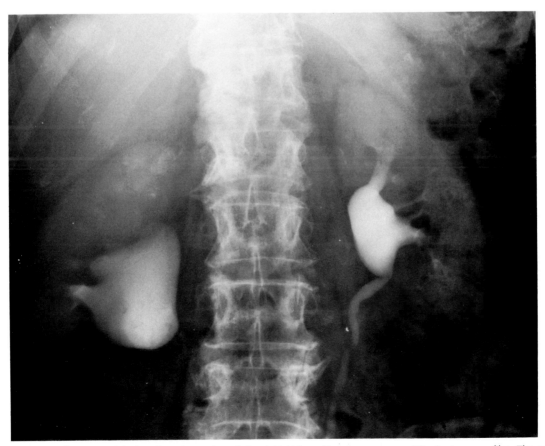

Figure 15–20. Congenital ureteropelvic junction obstruction of the right kidney. Excretory urogram, 20-minute prone film. The pelvocalyceal system is dilated and rounded. The ureter is unopacified despite the patient's prone position. (See Fig. 15–24 for the effect of a diuretic on this obstructed system.)

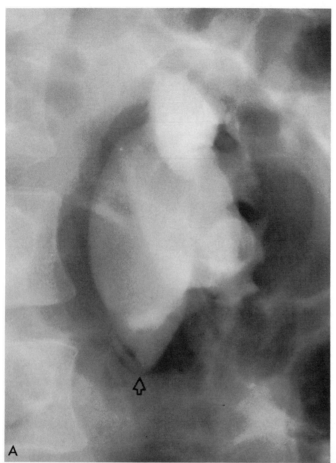

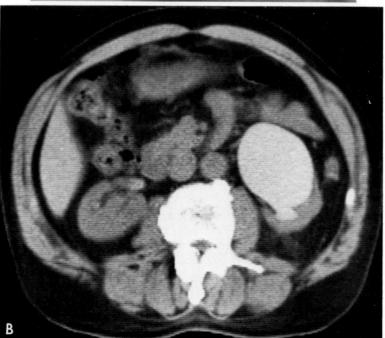

Figure 15–21. Congenital ureteropelvic junction obstruction.

A, Excretory urogram. A sharp angulation has developed as the pelvis dilates and rotates anteriorly *(arrow).* An artery running to the lower pole of the kidney and crossing this site tangentially was demonstrated by angiography.

B, Computed tomogram, contrast material enhanced. The anterior rotation of the pelvis in congenital ureteropelvic junction obstruction is well illustrated in a different patient.

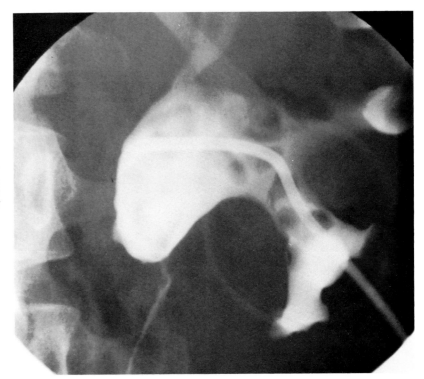

Figure 15–22. Congenital ureteropelvic junction obstruction complicated by urolithiasis, pyonephrosis, and loss of function of the left kidney. An antegrade pyelogram through the percutaneous nephrostomy opacifies the pelvocalyceal system and ureter.

genital ureteropelvic junction obstruction. Dilatation varies with both the degree of ureteropelvic dysfunction and the urine flow rate. When patients with low-grade obstruction are examined in a dehydrated state, the pelvocalyceal system may be normal or "flabby" or contain longitudinal striae representing the redundant mucosa of a usually dilated system. Long-standing obstruction leads to impaired renal function and a decrease in the amount of urine formed by the kidney. This, too, may obscure the urographic findings of obstruction (Fig. 15–23). On the other hand, a dilated pelvocalyceal system is not to be invariably equated with obstruction, an important concept that is discussed in Chapter 17.

All of the foregoing considerations underscore the need to search for congenital ureteropelvic junction obstruction under conditions of high urine flow rates. This can be accomplished easily by oral hydration or by combining a diuretic drug with either excretory urography or radionuclide renography (Fig. 15–24). One standardized protocol for diuresis urography (Whitfield, 1977) uses furosemide (40 mg), injected intravenously 20 minutes after the opacification of the urinary tract with contrast material containing 650 mg/kg of iodine. Patients should be previously hydrated. The filming sequence includes exposures at 20 minutes following contrast material administration and then again at 15 minutes after administration of the diuretic drug.

The following are evaluated in diuresis urography: (1) the size of the renal pelvis 20 minutes after the administration of contrast material alone compared with its size 15 minutes after the administration of furosemide, (2) calyceal size at the same time intervals, (3) and contrast material dilution after administration of furosemide. An increase in the area of the

renal pelvis or calyceal dilatation following the administration of the diuretic reliably predicts ureteropelvic junction obstruction, as defined by urodynamic criteria (see Chapter 17). Washout of collecting system radiopacity favors a nonobstructed system regardless of the presence of dilatation. Diuresis excretory urography provides accurate diagnostic information in approximately 85 per cent of patients with suspected congenital ureteropelvic obstruction.

Diuresis renography is performed in patients who are well hydrated in the manner described in Chapter 2. The pattern of radionuclide elimination by the kidneys is measured before and after intravenous furosemide, given at a dose of 0.5 mg/kg. Prolonged retention of the tracer after diuresis denotes obstruction. Various patterns are schematized in Figure 15–25. Specificity of diuresis renography has been reported at 88 per cent and sensitivity at 91 per cent. False-positive results occur in some dilated but nonobstructed kidneys, in azotemia, and in patients who are inadequately hydrated.

There is a small group of patients with congenital ureteropelvic junction obstruction who will not be confidently diagnosed by any of the preceding tests, including those using drug-induced diuresis. The reason for this may be the minimal nature of the functional abnormality, nondistensibility from peripelvic fibrosis caused by previous surgery, or renal functional impairment that prevents adequate excretion of either contrast material or radionuclide tracer. Here, the pressure/flow urodynamic study, originally described by Whitaker and modified by others, provides a direct measurement of pelvocalyceal pressures under controlled flow states. (See discussion in Chapter 17.) This test measures bladder pressure through a urethra-bladder catheter and renal pelvis pressure

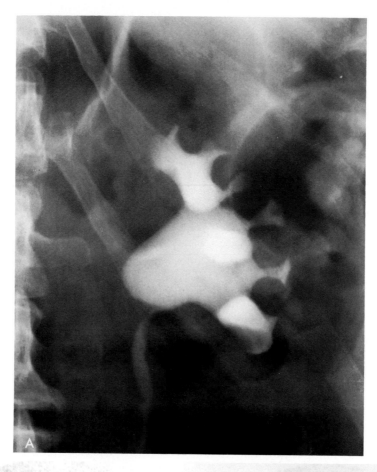

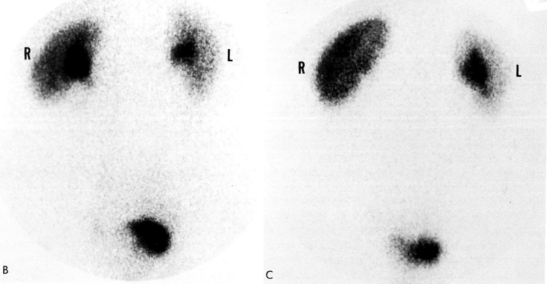

Figure 15–23. Congenital ureteropelvic obstruction causing decreased renal function. The diminished urine volume formed by the left kidney has led to normal pressure in the renal pelvis.

   A, Retrograde pyelogram, 5-minute drainage film. Although the renal pelvis is dilated, the forniceal angles are normal.

   B, 99mTc-glucoheptonate static scan, 16 minutes. Renal function on the left is 20 per cent of that on the right, but some urine is being formed, as evidenced by pelvic activity.

   C, 99mTc-glucoheptonate static scan, 3 hours. Activity in the left renal pelvis persists, while there has been loss of activity in the right renal pelvis caused by normal urine flow.

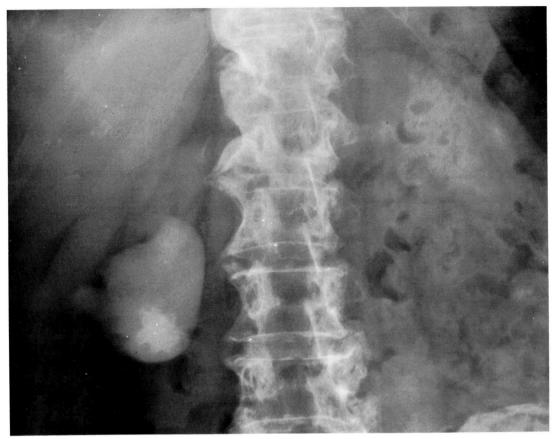

Figure 15–24. Congenital ureteropelvic obstruction of the right kidney. Excretory urogram. Film exposed 15 minutes after intravenous injection of furosemide (40 mg). The volume of the pelvis has increased, and the forniceal angles have dilated compared with the prediuretic state illustrated in Figure 15–20. The ureter remains unopacified. Note the washout of contrast material from the left kidney.

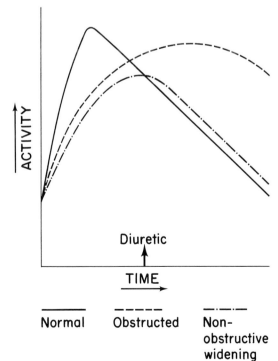

Figure 15–25. Diuresis renography. Schematized graphs of renogram activity over time in the normal, obstructed, and dilated but nonobstructed kidney. The initial slope is similar in both obstruction and nonobstructed dilatation. With injection of a diuretic drug, however, radionuclide activity decreases rapidly in nonobstructive dilatation, whereas prolonged activity is seen in obstruction.

through a catheter placed percutaneously directly into the pelvis. Proximal (pelvic) and distal (bladder) pressures are recorded at variable rates of perfusion through the percutaneous catheter. Technical details and diagnostic criteria vary from one laboratory to another (Whitaker, 1979 and 1980; Pfister and Newhouse, 1979). Pressure is measured at flow rates of up to 20 ml/min. Obstruction is generally held to exist if the pressure gradient rises above 15 cm of water under any of the conditions of the study. During the course of the Whitaker test, an antegrade pyelogram is performed. This must be correlated with pressure measurements.

Other causes of dilatation of the collecting structures in which urodynamic pressure/flow studies may be applied are discussed in Chapter 17.

INFECTION

Definition

Tuberculosis and candidiasis involve the pelvocalyceal and ureteral wall, while schistosomiasis is found in the distal ureter. Tuberculosis of the renal parenchyma is discussed in Chapter 13 and that of the bladder is presented in Chapter 19. Chapter 14 discusses fungus ball as one of the intraluminal pelvocalyceal abnormalities. A discussion of schistosomiasis of the bladder is included in Chapter 19.

Tuberculosis. The pelvocalyceal and ureteral walls are infected by bacilli that have been shed into the urine from cavitating tuberculous granulomas in the nephrons. Thickening by granulation tissue is the earliest response of the uroepithelium to *Mycobacterium tuberculosis*. In advanced cases, the muscularis and adventitia are also involved. Mucosal ulceration develops as the granulomas enlarge and coalesce, at which time the pelvic surface is diffusely irregular.

With healing, collagen and fibrous tissue replace the granulomas. As fibrosis progresses, submucosal collagen fibers are reoriented in the submucosa and cause sharply defined scars. The collecting system and ureter proximal to the cicatrix dilate as a result of increased resistance to urine flow. When healing narrows an infundibulum to the point of obliteration, the proximal calyx dilates and becomes a fluid-filled mass that is distinguishable from a cavitated parenchymal granuloma or nephrogenic cyst only by microscopic identification of the uroepithelium. As is true of all aspects of urinary tract tuberculosis, the pattern of scarring and dilatation is variable. Involvement may be at one or several sites, from an infundibulum to the distal ureter. It is rare, however, to have involvement of the distal ureter with no proximal abnormality. Destruction and retraction of the surrounding renal parenchyma cause nonobstructive dilatation of the adjacent portion of the pelvocalyceal system without distal stenoses.

Candidiasis. The upper urinary tract is infected by *Candida albicans* by either an ascending or a hematogenous route. Uroepithelial involvement, which is uncommon, is manifested by a white membrane typical of thrush, representing infiltration of the mucosa and submucosa by fungi and inflammatory cells.

Schistosomiasis (Bilharziasis). *Schistosoma haematobium* cercariae migrate to the venules of the lamina propria of the bladder and distal ureters from the portal circulation by way of hemorrhoidal and pudendal veins. Eventually, they penetrate the muscularis and submucosa of the bladder and distal ureteral wall, where ova are deposited. The cystitis and ureteritis that subsequently develop are characterized by granulomas, superficial mucosal ulcerations, and the formation of polypoid masses of granulation tissue. Eventually, fibrosis causes strictures with obstructive dilatation and calcium deposits in the dead ova.

Clinical Setting

The clinical findings of tuberculous and fungal infections of the kidney, including the uroepithelium, are discussed in Chapters 13 and 14.

Radiologic Findings

Tuberculosis. The active phase of uroepithelial tuberculosis causes marked irregularity of part or all of the collecting system and/or ureter due to both submucosal granulomas and mucosal ulceration (Fig. 15–26). Irregularity is rarely isolated, since tuberculosis usually involves a multiplicity of sites in the kidney, pelvis, and ureter.

Fibrous scars of healed tuberculosis produce sharply defined circumferential narrowings at one or several sites in the collecting system and/or ureter. These are of variable thickness and often have slightly irregular margins. The portion proximal to an obstructive narrowing dilates (Figs. 15–27 and 15–28). Fibrosis may progress during the treatment of active tuberculosis, necessitating careful serial studies during this period.

Dilatation of one or more calyces, of the entire pelvocalyceal system or of long segments of the ureter may develop without obstruction as a result of either mural fibrosis or scarring of the surrounding renal parenchyma (Figs. 15–29 and 15–30). Some patients with healed urinary tract tuberculosis develop dense calcification of the pelvocalyceal wall and ureter (Fig. 15–31).

Candidiasis. Uroepithelial thrush causes diffuse irregularity of the pelvocalyceal wall. This may occur as an isolated event or coexist with fungus ball, parenchymal damage, or both.

Schistosomiasis. Schistosomiasis usually involves the distal third of the ureters, although sometimes a more proximal infestation occurs. Asymmetry is common. Ureteral abnormalities are found in up to one-half of patients with bladder schistosomiasis. Very uncommonly, the radiologic findings of schistosomiasis are found only in the ureters.

Early manifestations are minimal dilatation, slight mucosal irregularity, and diminished peristalsis, leading to a failure to empty. With time, calcification, mural thickening and straightening, beading, and multiple segments of narrowing and dilatation develop

Text continued on page 503

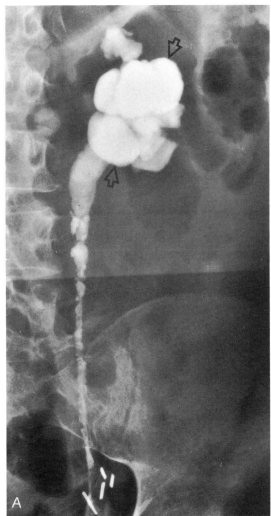

Figure 15–26. Renal and uroepithelial tuberculosis, active phase, in a 40-year-old man. There is extensive irregularity and ulceration of the entire ureter and pelvis. A large, cavitated granuloma in the kidney communicates with the collecting system.

A, Retrograde pyelogram. The opacified, cavitated granuloma *(arrows)* is superimposed on the pelvocalyceal system.

B, Computed tomogram with contrast material enhancement at the level of the kidney demonstrates the large cavity in the parenchyma.

C, Computed tomogram with contrast material enhancement at the level of the proximal ureter. The ureter *(arrow)* is thickened and enhances as a result of acute inflammation.

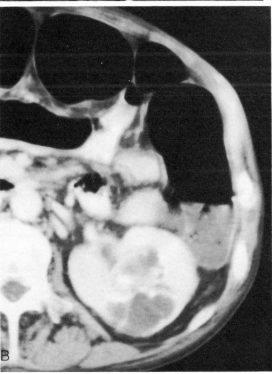

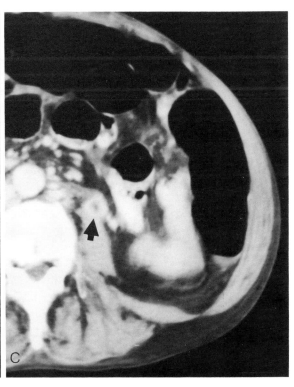

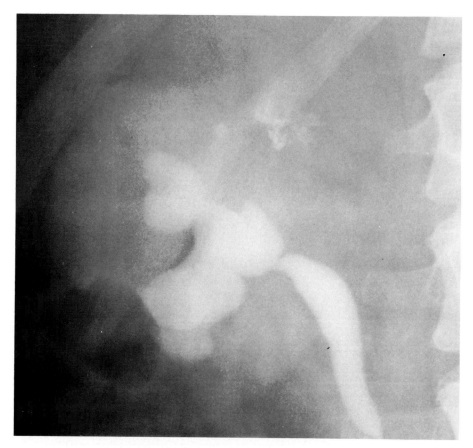

Figure 15–27. Uroepithelial tuberculosis, healed phase. There is a sharply defined circumferential narrowing, with proximal caliectasis due to obstruction. Excretory urogram.

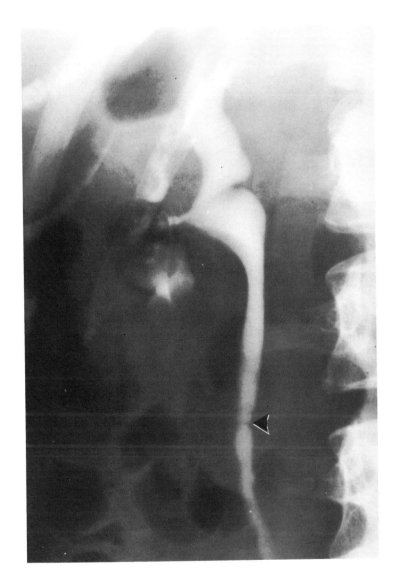

Figure 15–28. Uroepithelial tuberculosis, healed phase. Excretory urogram. A sharply circumscribed narrowing in the proximal ureter *(arrow)* does not cause obstruction. Eccentric narrowing at several sites is present distally.

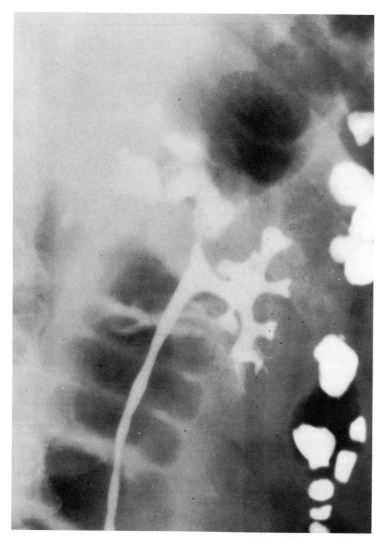

Figure 15–29. Uroepithelial tuberculosis, healed phase. Generalized dilatation of the renal pelvis and proximal ureter without obstruction is present. Also note the focal narrowing of the upper pole drainage system with a granulomatous mass in the upper pole. Retrograde pyelogram. (Same patient illustrated in Fig. 13–17.)

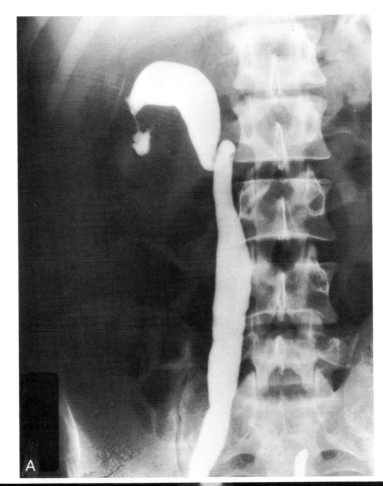

Figure 15–30. Uroepithelial tuberculosis, healed phase.

A, Retrograde pyelogram. Almost the entire ureter and pelvis are dilated. The proximal pelvis is tightly scarred.

B, Ultrasonogram, longitudinal section. There is marked caliectasis resulting from both the pelvic scar and the surrounding destroyed and retracted parenchyma.

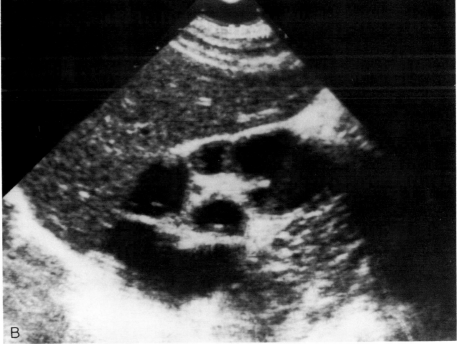

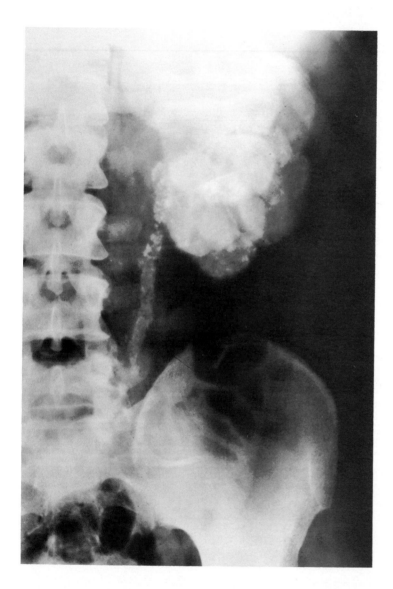

Figure 15–31. Healed tuberculosis with autonephrectomy. There is extensive calcification of the renal parenchyma, pelvis, and ureter. Abdominal radiograph.

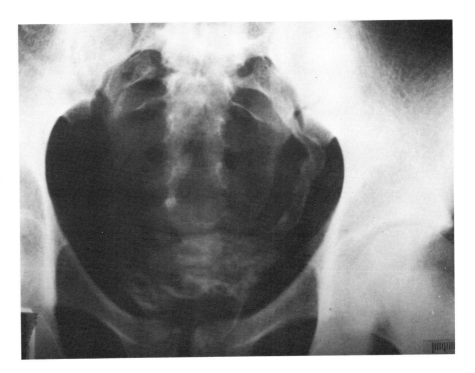

Figure 15–32. Schistosomiasis, left ureter and bladder. There is extensive, linear mural calcification. Abdominal radiograph.

(Figs. 15–32 and 15–33). In some patients there are masses of granulation tissue, known as bilharzial polyps. These are seen as solitary or multiple filling defects. Strictures may lead to hydroureter and hydronephrosis. However, hydroureter can develop from a generalized mural fibrosis and aperistalsis alone. Calcification in the wall of the ureter varies from a fine, stippled pattern to a continuous linear density. While carcinoma of the bladder uroepithelium develops more commonly in patients with schistosomiasis than in the general population, the same relationship does not hold for the ureter.

Excretory urography and voiding cystourethrography best demonstrate the abnormalities of ureteral schistosomiasis, including vesicoureteral reflux, if present. Computed tomography and ultrasonography

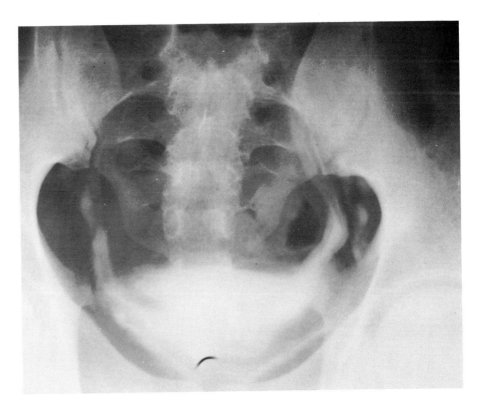

Figure 15–33. Schistosomiasis, both ureters and bladder. There is marked thickening of the ureteral and bladder walls. Vesicoureteral reflux is present. Cystogram.

best demonstrate the marked thickening of the ureteral wall that is often present.

RESPONSES TO INFECTION OR INFLAMMATION

Pyelitis and Ureteritis Cystica

Definition

Multiple small cysts in the pelvic wall are known as *pyelitis cystica* while those in the ureteral wall are referred to as *ureteritis cystica.* These form from solid buds of uroepithelium that migrate inward from the mucosal surface, become isolated in the tunica propria, and then, through metaplasia, are transformed into glandular structures that eventually fill with clear, proteinaceous fluid. Each cyst is a discrete, small mass that elevates the uroepithelium. Some grow as large as 2 cm in diameter. Spontaneous rupture sometimes occurs.

Clinical Setting

Pyelitis and ureteritis cystica develop in older patients, particularly women. The traditional viewpoint has been that the cysts form as a response to chronic infection of the urinary tract with *Escherichia coli.*

However, the fact that pyelitis cystica is found in some asymptomatic patients without a history of infection casts doubt on the validity of this premise. Clinical findings, when present, include hematuria, possibly from rupture of a cyst, and signs and symptoms of urinary tract infection.

Radiologic Findings

Pyelitis and ureteritis cystica cause persistent, unchanging filling defects in the wall of the pelvocalyceal system and the proximal ureter. These are usually discrete and widely spaced and vary in size up to 2 cm in diameter (Figs. 15–34 and 15–35). The same radiologic findings, representing mural fluid-filled blebs, may be seen as part of the Stevens-Johnson syndrome. Cysts that are small and closely grouped, an uncommon occurrence, produce a ragged appearance.

Leukoplakia

Definition

Squamous metaplasia of transitional cells with keratinization, known as *epidermidalization of the uroepithelium,* is common to both leukoplakia and cholestea-

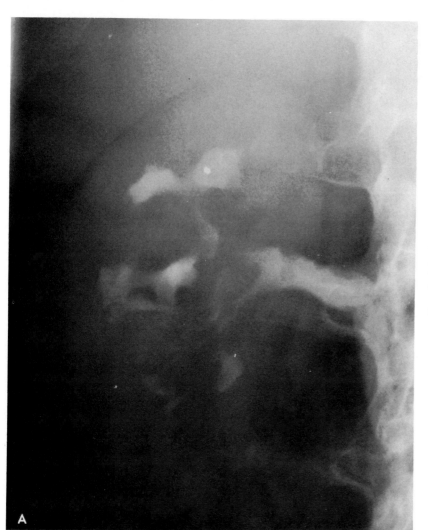

Figure 15–34. Pyelitis cystica. Multiple cysts of varying size appear as persistent, sharply marginated filling defects attached to the wall of the pelvocalyceal system in an elderly woman with chronic *E. coli* urinary tract infection.

A, Excretory urogram, right posterior oblique projection.

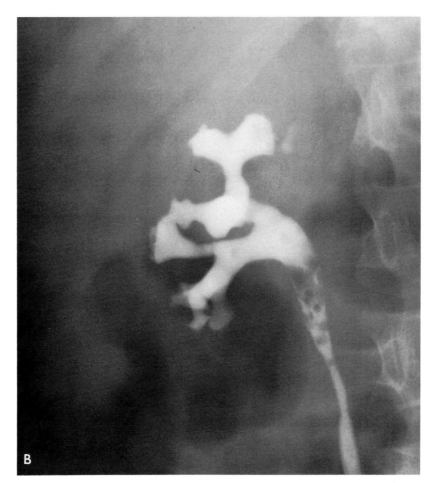

Figure 15–34 *Continued B,* Retrograde pyelogram.

toma. There is a controversy over the additional features that may characterize these two entities. The generally held view is that leukoplakia is epidermidalization plus proliferation and atypia of the basal squamous epithelial layer and that this condition is premalignant. Cholesteatoma, on the other hand, is traditionally thought of as a desquamative form of keratinizing metaplasia without malignant potential. An opposing point of view, however, proposes that leukoplakia and cholesteatoma are identical entities, characterized by metaplasia, keratinization, *and* desquamation. Proponents of this concept advocate the term *keratinizing desquamative squamous metaplasia* for both leukoplakia and cholesteatoma (Hertle and Androulakasis, 1982). Atypia and premalignant predisposition are not part of this concept. (Cholesteatoma is discussed in Chapter 14 as an intraluminal abnormality.)

Leukoplakia develops in the pelvocalyceal system and proximal ureter either as isolated patches or as a large confluent lesion. Renal calculus coexists in approximately 50 per cent of patients. Epidermoid carcinoma is said to be present in as many as 20 per cent of patients at the time that leukoplakia is diagnosed.

Clinical Setting

Leukoplakia of the upper urinary tract affects men and women equally and is most prevalent in the third to fifth decades. A history of chronic infection, often for as long as 20 years, is common. Colic and recurrent fever are frequent complaints. Passage of cornified squamous epithelium per urethra is pathognomonic of squamous metaplasia but does not distinguish leukoplakia from cholesteatoma, if such a distinction does, in fact, exist.

Radiologic Findings

Leukoplakia causes marked irregularities of the pelvocalyceal wall that are either localized (Fig. 15–36) or generalized (Fig. 15–37). The pelvocalyceal system and proximal ureter are the usual sites of involvement. Keratin that is shed into the lumen creates an irregular intraluminal mass that has a lacy pattern of contrast material within it (see Fig. 15–36). These may obstruct at the ureteropelvic junction or more distally in the ureter. As noted earlier, stone disease coexists with leukoplakia in approximately 50 per cent of affected patients.

Malakoplakia

Definition

Malakoplakia is an uncommon response to an infection of the urinary tract with *Escherichia coli.* An intracellular abnormality of macrophages, probably at the lysosomal level, is thought to prevent complete diges-

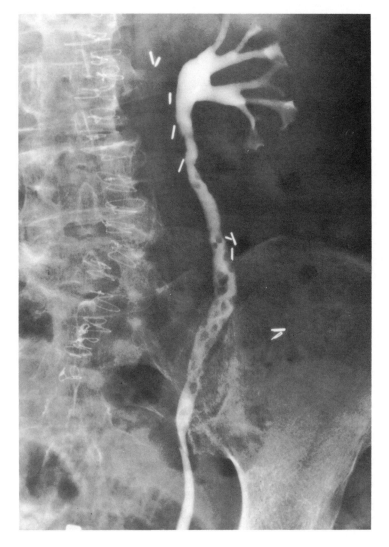

Figure 15–35. Ureteritis cystica. Multiple cysts appear as sharply marginated mural filling defects. Retrograde pyelogram. (Kindly provided by Wendelin S. Hayes, D.O., Armed Forces Institute of Radiology, Washington, D.C.)

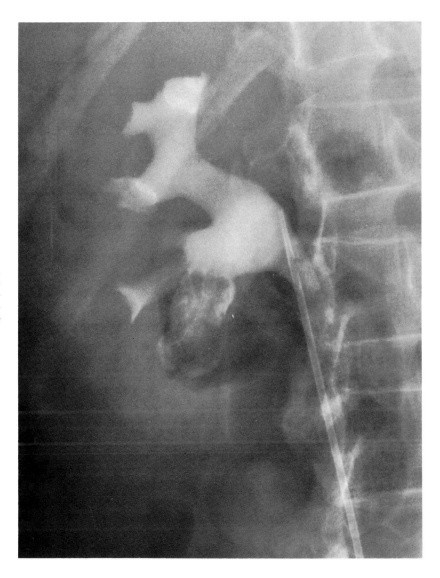

Figure 15–36. Leukoplakia. The filling defect in the collecting system of the lower pole contains a lacy pattern of contrast material, representing desquamated keratin. This presentation is indistinguishable from cholesteatoma and other intraluminal masses discussed in Chapter 14. Retrograde pyelogram.

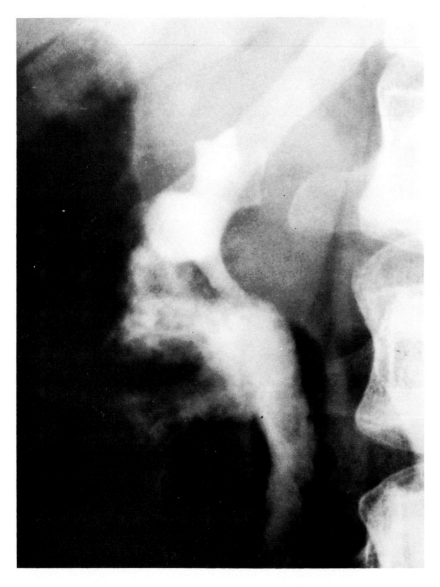

Figure 15–37. Leukoplakia. There is a generalized irregularity of the pelvocalyceal wall. Excretory urogram.

tion of phagocytosed bacteria. Submucosal granulomas dominated by large mononuclear cells with abundant cytoplasm develop. These cells contain intracytoplasmic inclusion bodies that are composed of calcium and iron-laden lysosomal material. These inclusions, known as Michaelis-Gutmann bodies, are probably bacilli in various stages of defective digestion. Michaelis-Guttman bodies may also be found in extracellular locations. The granulomas produce multiple yellow-gray or brown elevations of the mucosa.

Malakoplakia affects the bladder most frequently, but any part of the genitourinary tract, including the testes and prostate, may be involved. Renal parenchymal malakoplakia is discussed in Chapter 11 and bladder malakoplakia is discussed in Chapter 19.

Clinical Setting

Malakoplakia develops most often in women in the fifth to sixth decade in whom altered immunity is often present. Urinary tract infection with *Escherichia coli* is always present and accounts for the usual clinical findings of flank pain, dysuria, fever, hematuria,

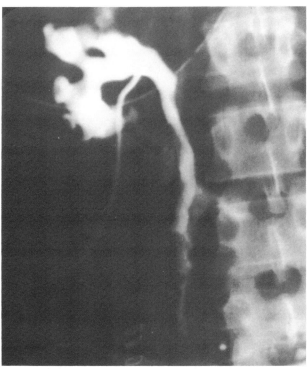

Figure 15–39. Malakoplakia involving both the pelvocalyceal system and the ureter. Multiple, irregular, mural filling defects are present throughout the ureter. Retrograde pyelogram.

proteinuria, pyuria, bacilliuria, and leukocytosis. The occurrence of obstruction and renal failure depend on the site and extent of involvement.

Radiologic Findings

Malakoplakia of the collecting system and ureter causes multiple, irregular mural filling defects and dilatation with or without obstruction (Figs. 15–38 and 15–39). Abnormalities of renal parenchymal and bladder malakoplakia usually coexist. (See Chapters 11 and 19.)

Xanthogranulomatous Pyelonephritis

The renal pelvis is scarred and contracted, and the calyces are dilated in xanthogranulomatous pyelonephritis. Pelvocalyceal system involvement invariably occurs as part of a process in which parenchymal abnormalities predominate. Xanthogranulomatous pyelonephritis is discussed in Chapter 11.

AMYLOIDOSIS
Definition

Amyloidosis of the upper urinary tract is rare and occurs as an isolated event except in children with familial Mediterranean fever. Amyloid deposits in the extrarenal part of the urinary tract are usually perivascular and limited to the submucosa. These are often calcified. The bladder is more frequently involved than the renal pelvis, the ureter, or the urethra. Most lesions are unilateral. Isolated amyloidosis, unrelated to an underlying disease, usually appears as a

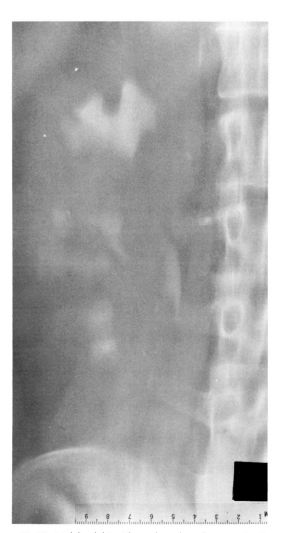

Figure 15–38. Malakoplakia. The pelvocalyceal system is distorted and irregular. Nondistensibility is present in some areas and dilatation in others. There is coexistent parenchymal involvement. Excretory urogram.

stricture with proximal dilatation. This may be found in an infundibulum of the pelvocalyceal system, at the ureteropelvic junction, or in the ureter. In systemic amyloidosis, generalized involvement causes diffuse narrowing and irregularity of the upper urinary tract, usually in association with renal amyloidosis. Amyloidosis of the kidney parenchyma is discussed in Chapter 8, and the findings of amyloidosis of the bladder are presented in Chapter 19.

Clinical Setting

Isolated amyloidosis of the upper urinary tract is either asymptomatic or associated with hematuria. Flank pain or urinary tract infection may develop in association with stricture and obstruction. In secondary amyloidosis, renal failure and the clinical manifestations of the underlying disease are likely to dominate the clinical picture.

Radiologic Findings

A linear deposit of calcium in the submucosa is sometimes seen on standard radiographs of the pelvocalyceal system. The calcium may be dense enough to create the appearance of a pelvic cast. In this situation, a thin band of relatively radiolucent mucosa separating the opacified urine from the calcified mucosa becomes apparent during excretory urography. Hydrocalyx may also result from an isolated amyloid deposit narrowing an infundibulum.

Ureteral involvement is usually limited to a single segment in which there is an elongated, irregular stricture in the distal portion of the ureter with proximal distention (Fig. 15–40). Ureteral involvement in systemic amyloidosis, most commonly seen in patients with familial Mediterranean fever, is seen as extensive narrowing and rigidity.

POLYARTERITIS NODOSA

Upper urinary tract obstruction due to ureteral stricture has been reported as a rare event in patients with polyarteritis nodosa. The underlying pathogenesis has not been elucidated.

EOSINOPHILIC URETERITIS

Ureteral stricture due to ureteral and periureteral fibrosis and eosinophilic infiltrate is another rare cause

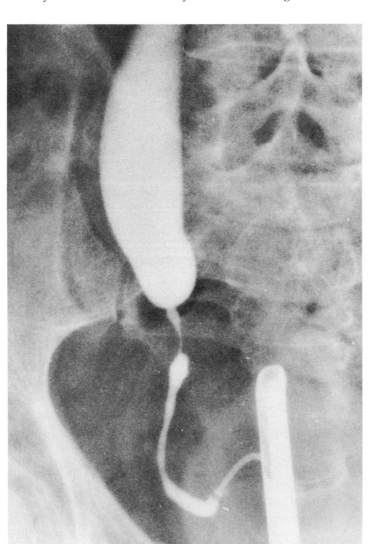

Figure 15–40. Amyloidosis, distal left ureter. Retrograde ureterogram. There is a smooth, concentric narrowing of a long segment of ureter with proximal dilatation.

of upper urinary tract obstruction. This has been described in patients with and without a history of allergy or parasite infestation. The pathologic appearance resembles that of eosinophilic cystitis. The radiologic appearance of the ureteral stricture is nonspecific.

MURAL HEMORRHAGE

Definition

There are clinical circumstances in which multiple, discrete mural pelvocalyceal or ureteral masses appear and disappear within a short time. The transient nature of these lesions strongly suggests that they are mural hematomas. However, an accurate pathologic description of this process is not available, since the conditions under which the lesions occur rarely yield tissue specimens. The clinical and radiologic features of these masses suggest multifocal sites of limited bleeding in the wall of the pelvis or ureter.

Clinical Setting

Mural hemorrhage may occur during anticoagulant therapy, as a result of blunt or penetrating abdominal trauma, in spontaneously acquired circulating anticoagulants, or as a complication of crystalluria or microurolithiasis.

Transient hematuria and flank pain are the primary clinical findings. Free blood clots, when present, are a potential cause of obstruction and renal colic.

Bleeding that develops during anticoagulant therapy, particularly when coagulation indices are within therapeutic range, may herald an underlying kidney disease, such as tumor. Radiologic studies should be carefully interpreted with this in mind.

Radiologic Findings

Mural hemorrhage produces multiple, discrete masses that project from the mucosal wall of the pelvocalyceal system or ureter (Fig. 15–41). The masses may be

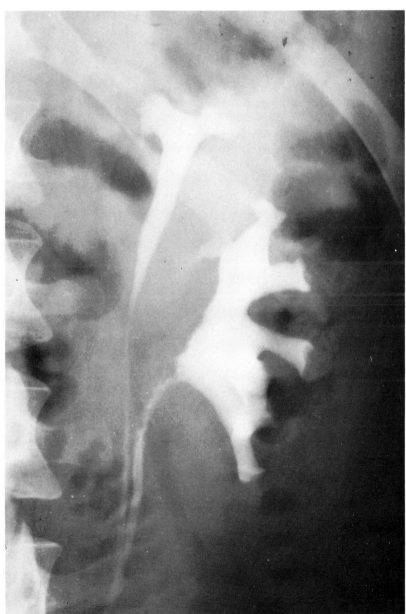

Figure 15–41. Mural hemorrhage. Multiple mural nodules are present in the pelvis of the left kidney of a 22-year-old man with penetrating trauma to the left retroperitoneum. Excretory urogram. (Courtesy of Jay A. Kaiser, M.D., and Hideyo Minagi, M.D., San Francisco General Hospital, San Francisco, California, and AJR *125*:311, 1975.)

round or oval and discrete or irregular. Coexistent intraluminal clot can cause obstruction at the uretero-pelvic junction. Computed tomography without contrast enhancement may demonstrate thickening of the uroepithelial wall and, if performed in close proximity to the acute episode of bleeding, an attenuation value of fresh blood clot. Spontaneous clearing within 2 weeks is the usual pattern.

LONGITUDINAL MUCOSAL FOLDS

Definition

The mucosa of a pelvocalyceal system that has been subjected to prolonged distention forms multiple longitudinal ridges when the system is collapsed or minimally distended. Redundant folds sometimes extend from the pelvis and upper ureter into the calycine infundibula. Neither inflammation nor edema is present. There is no support for the idea that mucosal folds are normal.

Linear radiolucent striae identical in appearance with longitudinal mucosal folds are rarely seen in renal vein thrombosis. The basis for this mural abnormality has not been established clearly, but it may be due to either edema or dilated collateral or submucosal veins.

Clinical Setting

Longitudinal mucosal folds are identified most closely with moderate to severe vesicoureteral reflux. They may also develop after relief of severe obstructive uropathy. Although this finding is usually seen in children, it is encountered in adults as well. Folds grow in prominence as the severity of reflux increases until the point at which the pelvis becomes a decompensated, dilated sac.

Longitudinal folds suggest active reflux. However, this finding can persist for years after reflux disappears or is corrected. Patients with longitudinal folds may be asymptomatic or may have findings of reflux-associated recurrent upper urinary tract infection.

Radiologic Findings

Redundant mucosal folds form fine, regular, and more or less parallel longitudinal lines of lucency within an incompletely distended pelvocalyceal system that is opacified during excretory urography, pyelography, or voiding cystourethrography with reflux (Fig. 15–42). The folds disappear when the system is distended and reappear after drainage. Radiologic evidence of reflux nephropathy may coexist.

URETERAL PSEUDODIVERTICULOSIS

Definition

Ureteral pseudodiverticulosis is an uncommon, acquired abnormality characterized by invagination of hyperplastic transitional epithelium into the lamina propria of the ureter. The underlying muscularis is sometimes effaced but remains intact. Continuity is

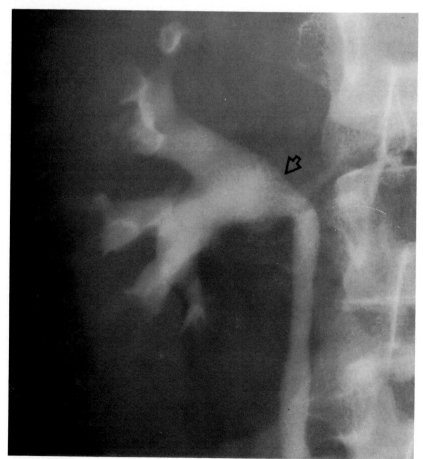

Figure 15–42. Longitudinal mucosal folds. Fine, regular linear lines of lucency (arrow) are present in the right pelvis of a young woman with documented vesicoureteral reflux. Excretory urogram.

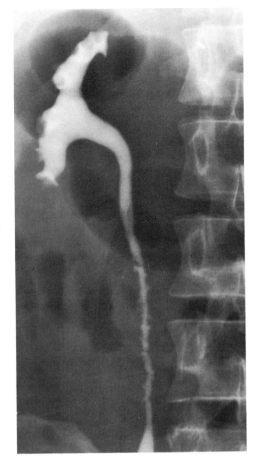

Figure 15–43. Pseudodiverticulosis, right mid ureter. Retrograde ureterogram. There are multiple, small outpouchings on both sides of the ureteral wall.

maintained between this outpouching and the ureteral lumen, thereby giving rise to the appearance of a diverticulum. Ureteritis cystica and ureteritis glandularis sometimes coexist with the pseudodiverticula.

Clinical Setting

Patients with ureteral pseudodiverticulosis are typically middle aged and older. There is frequently a history of urinary tract infection, obstruction, and/or urolithiasis. However, many are asymptomatic at the time of discovery of the pseudodiverticula. Studies of small populations of patients with this abnormality suggest the possibility of an increased prevalence of transitional cell carcinoma of the ureter or bladder and atypical urine cytology. These relationships, however, are not firmly established because of the small number of patients that have been investigated.

Radiologic Findings

Ureteral pseudodiverticulosis typically appears in the proximal and middle portions of both ureters as tiny (1 to 4 mm) outpouchings that are in continuity with the opacified ureter (Fig. 15–43). There are usually three to eight in each segment of involved ureter. Unilateral lesions are infrequent, and a solitary diverticulum is rare. The abnormality is best demonstrated by retrograde or antegrade ureteropyelography. Pseudodiverticulosis usually remains stable over time.

PYELOCALYCEAL DIVERTICULUM

Definition

Pyelocalyceal diverticula are uroepithelium-lined pouches that extend from a peripheral point of the collecting system into the adjacent renal parenchyma. Two forms have been identified on the basis of anatomic features. Type I diverticula, the more common of the two, are connected to the calyceal cup, usually at a fornix. These lesions often have a bulbous shape with a narrow connecting infundibulum of varying length. Type I diverticula occur in the polar regions, especially in the upper pole. Most measure a few millimeters in diameter. Type II diverticula develop in the interpolar region, communicate directly into the pelvis, and are usually larger and rounder than the Type I diverticula. The neck of a Type II diverticulum is short and not easily identified.

Pyelocalyceal diverticula probably have a developmental origin. The generally held opinion is that they are ureteral bud remnants that either failed to divide into fully formed calyces or were not assimilated during the process of calyceal-lobar fusion. Support for a theory of developmental origin is derived from the equal prevalence in all age groups and the frequent, although not invariable, presence of smooth muscle below the uroepithelial lining. Explanations for the genesis of pyelocalyceal diverticula as acquired abnormalities include reflux and infection, rupture of a simple renal cyst or abscess, infundibular achalasia or

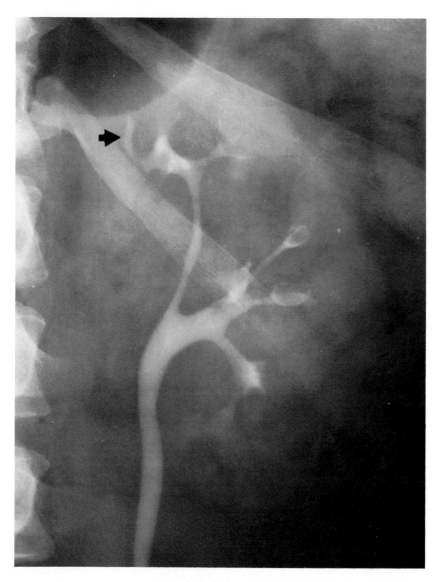

Figure 15–44. Pyelocalyceal diverticulum Type I. A single diverticulum *(arrow)* extends from a fornix of the upper pole calyx. A narrow isthmus is identifiable. Excretory urogram.

spasm, and hydrocalyx secondary to inflammatory fibrosis of an infundibulum. None of these concepts are widely supported.

Stones form in as many as 50 per cent of patients with pyelocalyceal diverticulum. These stones are either single or multiple or occur in the form of milk of calcium. The latter is a colloidal suspension of precipitated calcium salts occurring either as pure calcium phosphate, calcium carbonate, or calcium oxalate or as a mixture of any of these.

Synonyms for pelvocalyceal diverticulum are pyelogenic cyst, pericalyceal cyst, calyceal diverticulum, calyceal cyst, pyelorenal cyst, and congenital hydrocalycosis.

Clinical Setting

Pyelocalyceal diverticula are found with equal frequency at all ages and in both sexes. Most diverticula are asymptomatic and are found incidentally during excretory urography or pyelography.

Symptoms that do develop are those of infection, stone, or hemorrhage and include fever and colic. Pyuria, bacteriuria, and hematuria may develop. Some cases have been reported in which an uncomplicated diverticulum was thought to cause flank pain. Transitional cell carcinoma may arise in the uroepithelial cells that line the cavity of a pyelocalyceal diverticulum.

Radiologic Findings

Pyelocalyceal diverticula communicate with the collecting system and usually opacify during excretory urography or pyelography. However, opacification

may be delayed because of a slow exchange of urine between the two structures. For similar reasons, a diverticulum can remain opacified for a longer period of time than the freely drained portions of the pelvocalyceal system.

Type I diverticula range from 1 mm to several centimeters in diameter and are mostly found extending from a point on an upper polar calyceal cup. A narrow isthmus is frequently identified connecting the opening into the calyx with the fundus of the diverticulum. Diverticular shapes are tubular, flasklike, oval, and round (Fig. 15–44 and 15–45).

Type II diverticula occur in the interpolar region and open directly into the renal pelvis rather than into a calyx. The point of connection is often obscure (Fig. 15–46). This form of diverticula may become large enough to produce a mass effect on adjacent portions of the pelvocalyceal system and cause a defect in the nephrogram (Fig. 15–47).

Both types of diverticula appear as uncomplicated fluid-filled spaces on unenhanced computed tomographic and ultrasonographic images (see Fig. 15–45). With contrast enhancement, computed tomography demonstrates layering of contrast material in the dependent portion of the diverticulum (see Fig. 15–47).

For no apparent reason or because of occlusion of the neck from infection, edema, or scar, a diverticulum may fail to opacify during urography or pyelography. In this situation, the radiologic findings, including ultrasonographic and computed tomography, are either those of a simple cyst or a complicated cystic mass (Fig. 15–48).

A single calculus or a circumscribed collection of many small stones in the periphery of the kidney suggests a pyelocalyceal diverticulum (Fig. 15–49). These

Text continued on page 520

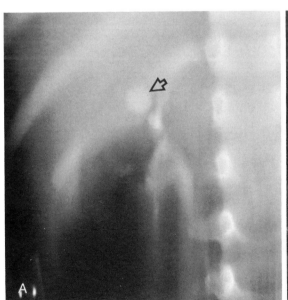 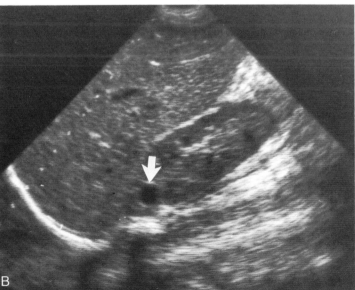

Figure 15–45. Pyelocalyceal diverticulum Type I.
A, Excretory urogram. The diverticulum *(arrow)* is round, extends from the upper pole calyx, and opacifies during contrast enhancement, indicating communication with the collecting system.
B, Ultrasonogram, longitudinal section. The diverticulum *(arrow)* appears as a fluid-filled mass that is indistinguishable from a simple nephrogenic cyst.

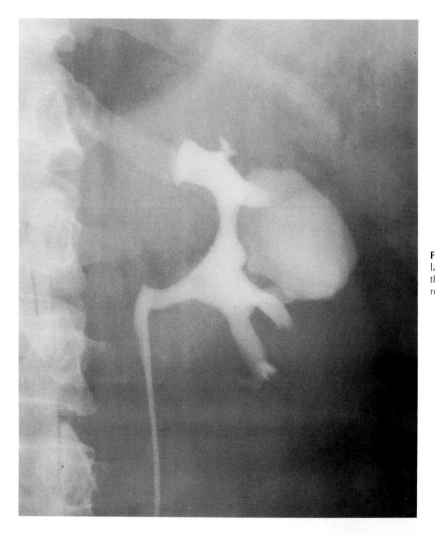

Figure 15–46. Pyelocalyceal diverticulum Type II. A large communicating fluid-filled space arises from the interpolar portion of the collecting system. Retrograde pyelogram.

Figure 15–47. Pyelocalyceal diverticulum Type II. A large communicating fluid-filled space in the interpolar region extends from the collecting system to the surface of the kidney. Computed tomogram, contrast material enhanced.

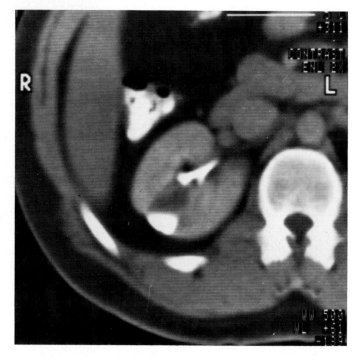

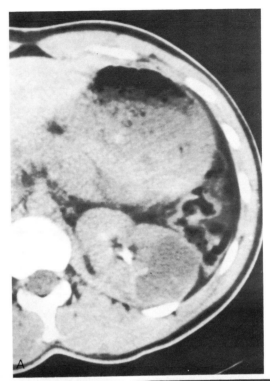

Figure 15–48. Pyelocalyceal diverticulum Type II appearing as a complicated cystic mass in a 27-year-old man.

A, Computed tomogram, contrast material enhanced. The diverticulum does not communicate, and its wall is apparently thickened as a result of expansion into the surrounding renal parenchyma.

B, Ultrasonogram, coronal section. The diverticulum *(arrow)* contains echogenic material.

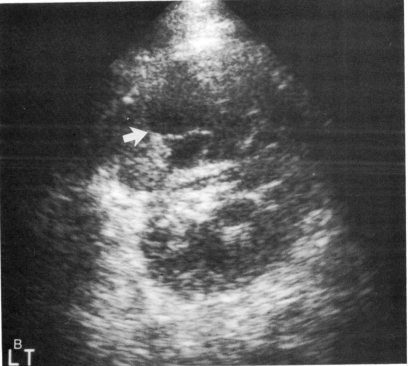

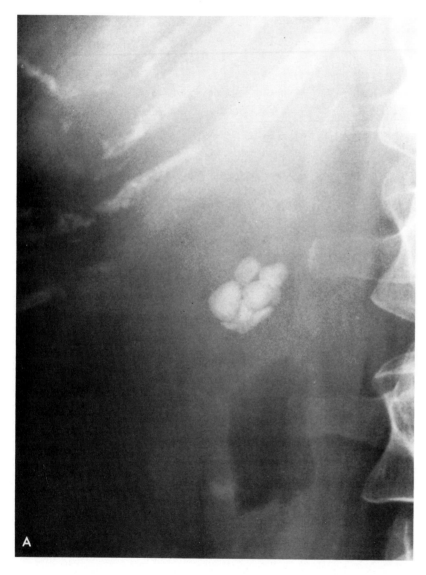

Figure 15–49. Pyelocalyceal diverticulum Type II with multiple stones.
   A, Preliminary film.

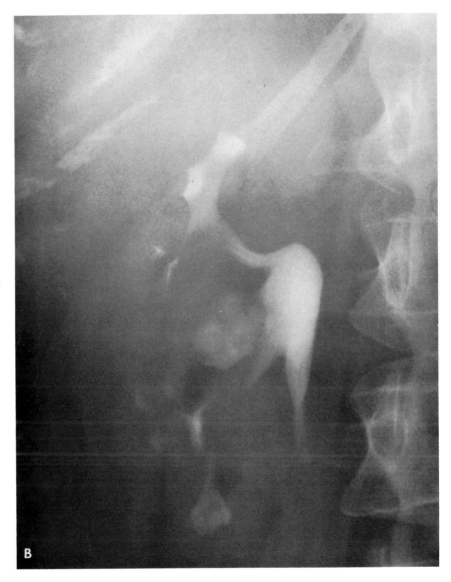

Figure 15–49 *Continued B,* Excretory urogram. Note the delayed opacification of the diverticulum.

stones may change position slightly when more than one preliminary film is available for comparison. With the patient in a prone or supine position, milk of calcium forms a round, homogeneous density that may change shape slightly with varied degrees of inspiration or alteration of the patient's position. On films exposed with a horizontal x-ray beam or on computed tomograms, the dependent portion of the milk of calcium is semilunar and there is a calcium-fluid level at the upper margin (Figs. 15–50 and 15–51). Milk of calcium is hyperechoic in the dependent portion of the diverticulum separated from the anechoic supernatant urine by a sharp linear interface (see Fig. 15–51).

The radiologic appearance of other fluid-filled lesions that communicate with the pelvocalyceal system may be identical to that of pyelocalyceal diverticula. These other lesions include a ruptured simple renal (nephrogenic) cyst and an evacuated abscess or hematoma. Mild forms of renal papillary necrosis and medullary sponge kidney can simulate a small diverticulum. These disorders are usually multiple, whereas a diverticulum almost always occurs singly. Focal cal-

iectasis (hydrocalyx) due to infundibular narrowing from tuberculous cicatrix, crossing vessel, infiltrating carcinoma, or stone may also simulate a pyelocalyceal diverticulum.

URETEROCELE

Definition

Prolapse into the bladder of the intravesicular portion of the distal ureter with an associated dilatation of the distal ureter is known as a ureterocele, a deformity that is congenital in origin. The wall of a ureterocele is composed of a thin layer of muscle and collagen interposed between the outer surface of bladder uroepithelium and the inner surface of ureteral uroepithelium.

A ureterocele may be complicated by partial or complete obstruction at its orifice or by the formation of a stone within its lumen. A ureterocele may also obstruct the other ureteral orifice(s) leading into the bladder or the bladder outlet itself. Additionally, an ectopic ureterocele may deform the ureterovesical

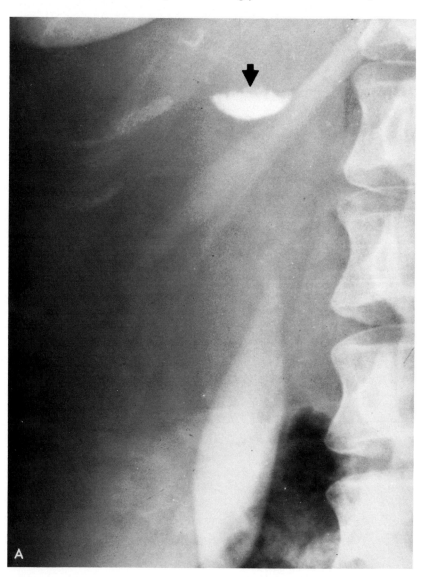

Figure 15–50. Pyelocalyceal diverticulum Type II with milk of calcium.

A, Preliminary film, upright projection obtained during oral cholecystogram. The milk of calcium forms a semilunar density with a calcium-fluid level *(arrow).*

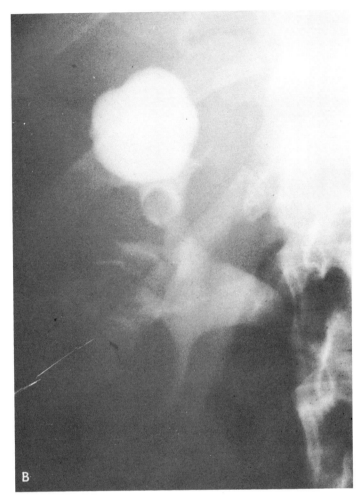

Figure 15–50 *Continued B,* Excretory urogram. Supine projection. The milk of calcium is now viewed *en face.*

junction of a normally inserted ureter and thereby cause vesicoureteral reflux.

There are several systems for classifying ureteroceles. An appropriate classification from a radiologic point of view is one that defines an "orthotopic" ureterocele as one that forms in a ureter with a normal insertion into the trigone and an "ectopic" ureterocele as one in a ureter whose insertion is ectopic. Orthotopic ureteroceles usually occur in single systems whereas ectopic ureteroceles usually occur in duplicated collecting systems.

Ureterocele is discussed in this chapter as an abnormality of the wall of the ureter. Other topics that relate to ureterocele include the embryology and anomalies of the upper urinary tract (see Chapter 3), vesicoureteral reflux (see Chapter 5), the kidney with a duplicated pelvocalyceal system (see Chapter 9), hydronephrosis and hydroureter (see Chapters 9 and 17), renal dysplasia (see Chapter 11), and focal hydrocalyx (see Chapter 12).

Clinical Setting

Orthotopic ureteroceles are usually small, unilateral, and asymptomatic. These are most often incidental findings in an adult undergoing urinary tract evaluation for an unrelated problem. A calculus may form in the ureterocele, and in some patients there may be some obstruction to urine flow with the associated risk of infection.

Ectopic ureteroceles, on the other hand, are usually large enough to cause complications that lead to their discovery in infancy or childhood. Ectopic ureteroceles that are part of a completely duplicated upper urinary tract are usually found in females and are predominantly left sided. These are very rare in individuals of African descent. A ureterocele that forms in a single ureter that is ectopically inserted usually occurs in males. Clinical problems that arise from the complications of an ectopic ureterocele include urinary tract infection, urine retention due to bladder neck obstruction, flank pain, stone formation, or an abdominal mass. Incontinence is present in females when the site of ectopic insertion is distal to the urogenital diaphragm. Prolapse of an ectopic ureterocele into the vagina may occur.

Radiologic Findings

Orthotopic ureteroceles are best defined radiologically during excretory urography. The distal ureter is minimally dilated and projects slightly into the lumen of the bladder. Opacified bladder urine surrounds the ureterocele and is separated from the dilated ureteral

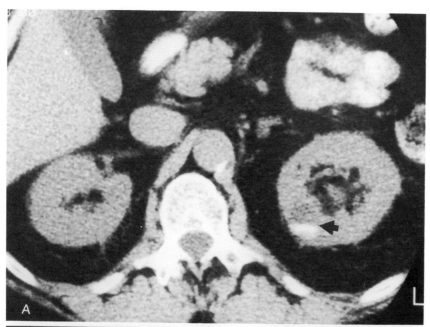

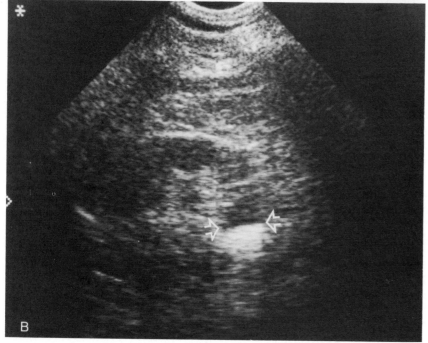

Figure 15–51. Pyelocalyceal diverticulum with milk of calcium, left kidney.

A, Computed tomogram, unenhanced. The diverticulum *(arrow)* appears as a round, low-density mass with high attenuation milk of calcium layered in its dependent portion.

B, Ultrasonogram, longitudinal projection. The supernatant fluid in the diverticulum *(arrows)* is echogenic, but much less so than the dependent milk of calcium.

(Kindly provided by Wendelin S. Hayes, D.O., Armed Forces Institute of Pathology, Washington, D.C.)

lumen by a uniformly thin line of relative radiolucency (Fig. 15–52). This represents the components of the wall of the ureterocele: the bladder and ureteral uroepithelium and the intervening muscle and collagen. This radiologic appearance, called the "cobra head" deformity, may be simulated by conditions other than ureterocele, as described in Differential Diagnosis at the end of this chapter. A calculus in the ureterocele, which may or may not obstruct, is sometimes noted (Fig. 15–53).

An ectopic ureterocele is seen on cystography as a smooth, nonopaque, intravesicular mass that is often quite large and centered toward the base of the bladder (Fig. 15–54). When defined by excretory urography or contrast material–enhanced computed tomography, the degree of enhancement of the urine within the ureterocele and its draining ureter depends on the degree of function in the related upper pole moiety. Often, opacification is absent or diminished because of hydronephrosis and/or dysplasia caused by obstruction. In this circumstance, contrast material excreted by the functioning renal units opacifies the bladder and the ureterocele appears only as a nonopaque intravesicular mass. Ultrasonography demonstrates a ureterocele as a thin, echogenic membrane in the bladder lumen in close proximity to its associated draining ureter, which is slightly to markedly dilated (Fig. 15–55). Uncomplicated fluid (urine in the bladder and distal ureter) surrounds both sides of the membrane. Dilatation of the ureter obstructed by an ectopic ureterocele is usually moderate. However, in some patients, the ureter is so dilated and tortuous that it crosses the midline and displaces both intraabdominal and retroperitoneal organs. This can be

identified by ultrasonography, computed tomography, or percutaneous ureteropyelography as a fluid-filled, elongated mass, with multiple bends in the ureter giving the appearance of septations. The dilated ureter can be traced cephalad to its associated renal unit, which is often hydronephrotic and/or dysplastic (see Fig. 15–54). Uncommonly, the draining ureter obstructed by an ectopic ureterocele is collapsed and/or diminutive owing to the absence of urine produced by its renal unit.

The size and shape of a ureterocele can change with the dynamics of voiding or alterations in bladder pressure. A ureterocele may also evert and assume the appearance of a bladder diverticulum.

DIFFERENTIAL DIAGNOSIS

The first task in evaluating an apparent mural lesion is to verify its location. Usually, small or medium-sized masses in the pelvocalyceal system readily satisfy criteria for a mural origin. A bulky, immovable, nonopaque mass that fills the collecting system or ureter, however, may be impossible to differentiate in terms of luminal or mural location. In this circumstance, differential diagnosis must be broadly based and include intraluminal abnormalities, such as nonopaque stone, blood clot, and fungus ball as well as abnormalities of mural origin. Sorting these out depends on the unique ultrasonographic or computed tomographic features of stone, the transient nature of blood clots, and the correlation of clinical and laboratory data. This is discussed in the concluding section of Chapter 14.

Malignancy of the uroepithelium is the most com-

Text continued on page 528

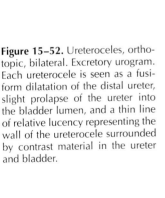

Figure 15–52. Ureteroceles, orthotopic, bilateral. Excretory urogram. Each ureterocele is seen as a fusiform dilatation of the distal ureter, slight prolapse of the ureter into the bladder lumen, and a thin line of relative lucency representing the wall of the ureterocele surrounded by contrast material in the ureter and bladder.

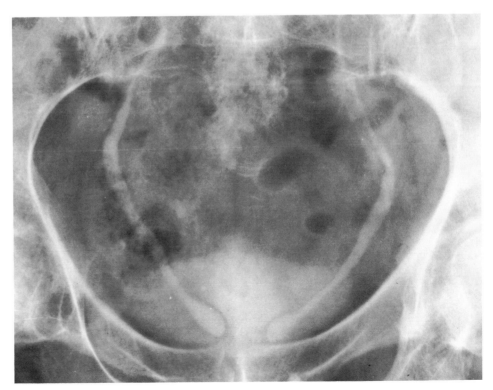

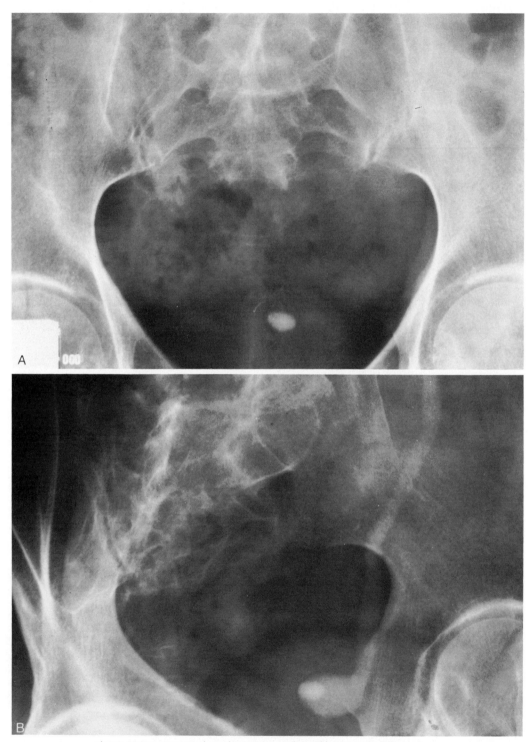

Figure 15–53. Ureterocele, orthotopic, complicated by stone and obstruction.
  A, Preliminary radiograph.
  B, Excretory urogram, left posterior oblique projection.

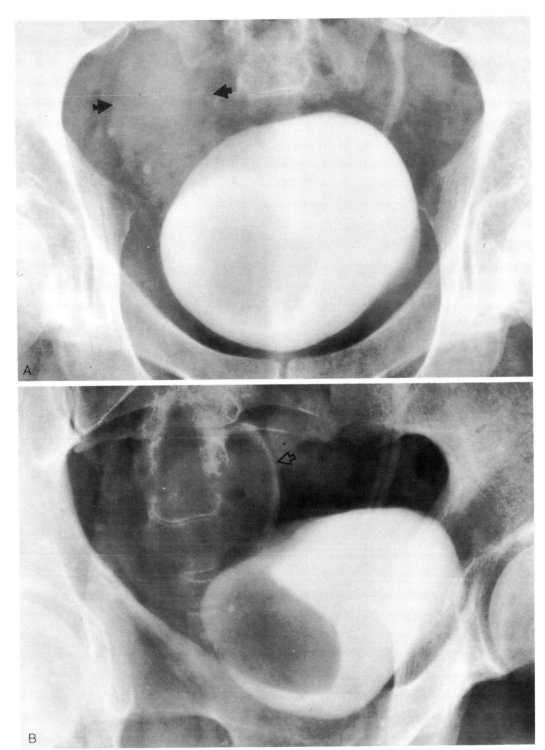

Figure 15–54. Ureterocele, ectopic, upper pole moiety of a completely duplicated right ureter and collecting system. The ureter to the upper pole is obstructed, dilated, and displaces the adjacent, nonobstructed ureter draining the lower pole moiety.

A, Excretory urogram. The large ectopic ureterocele projects into the lumen of the bladder as a smooth-walled filling defect. The dilated distal ureter is seen as a soft tissue mass *(arrows).*

B, Excretory urogram, left posterior oblique projection. The ureterocele projects into the bladder base. The ureter draining the lower pole moiety *(arrow)* is displaced by the obstructed, ectopically inserted ureter. There is complete duplication of the left ureter.

Illustration continued on following page

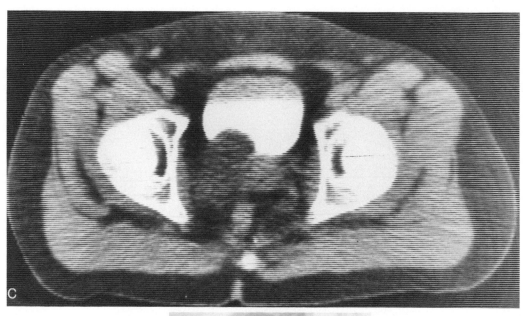

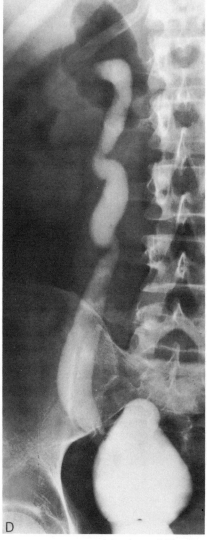

Figure 15–54 *Continued C,* Computed tomogram, contrast material enhanced. The ureterocele projects into the bladder base.
D, Antegrade pyelogram. The obstructed, dilated ureter draining the dystrophic upper pole moiety is opacified.

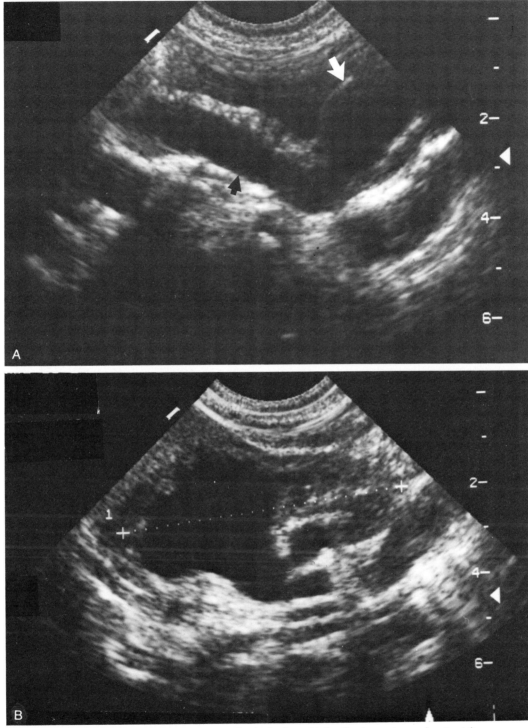

Figure 15-55. Ureterocele, ectopic, upper pole moiety of a completely duplicated left collecting system and ureter. Ultrasonograms, longitudinal projection.

A, Bladder. The dilated distal ectopic ureter *(black arrow)* enters the bladder. A thin, round, echogenic membrane *(white arrow)* represents the urine-filled ureterocele.

B, Kidney. The upper pole moiety is dilated as a result of obstruction by the ectopic ureterocele.

(Kindly provided by Steve Horii, M.D., Georgetown University, Washington, D.C.)

mon cause of an isolated focal mural mass. Uroepithelial tumors that develop in a pelvocalyceal system and invade renal tissue can be differentiated from tumors of renal parenchymal origin, such as adenocarcinoma, by an analysis of the geometry of the kidney enlargement. Tumors of uroepithelial origin preserve the reniform shape of the enlarged kidney. Most tumors of renal origin, on the other hand, grow from an epicenter and create a ball-shaped mass. This subject is discussed fully in Chapter 12. Ultimate diagnosis, of course, depends on histologic study.

Herniation of cysts from a multiocular cystic nephroma may also simulate a primary mural mass. These can be identified by their smooth surface and the coexistence of an expansile, large, multioculated, cystic tumor in adjacent renal parenchyma. Extramural abnormalities that might be confused with a lesion of mural origin include aberrant papilla, discussed in Chapter 3, and several other entities that are discussed in Chapter 16. These include tortuous blood vessels, focal fat deposits projecting from the renal sinus, endometriosis, and retroperitoneal metastases invading the ureter.

Mural masses that are multifocal, discrete, and separated from each other are due to multifocal transitional cell carcinoma, pyelitis and/or ureteritis cystica, or mural hemorrhage. The latter diagnosis is favored when there is an associated intraluminal blood clot, increased attenuation value of the lesion by computed tomography, or resolution on a repeat study performed within 2 weeks. Differentiation otherwise depends on the different clinical settings in which these entities occur.

The nature of extensive, irregular mural lesions cannot be precisely established by radiologic studies. Mural tumors of any tissue type, tuberculosis, schistosomiasis, thrush, leukoplakia, malakoplakia, xanthogranulomatous pyelonephritis, and amyloidosis may have identical appearances. Tuberculosis, however, almost always has associated renal parenchymal abnormalities, and schistosomiasis is usually limited to the distal ureter and bladder. The appearance of pseudodiverticulosis is distinctive. Otherwise, diagnosis depends on clinical and pathologic data.

Conditions that thicken the bladder mucosa and distend the distal ureter may simulate an orthotopic ureterocele. These include carcinoma of the bladder or cervix invading the ureterovesical orifice, radiation cystitis, distal ureteral calculus, or edema of the ureterovesical junction from recent passage of stone. These "pseudoureteroceles" are identified by asymmetry of the distal lumen, thickening and irregularity of the wall, the absence of intravesicular protrusion, or the coexistence of other features of the underlying abnormality.

Bibliography

General

Brennan, R. E., Curtis, J. A., Kurtz, A. B., and Dalton, J. R.: Use of tomography and ultrasound in the diagnosis of nonopaque renal calculi. JAMA 244:594, 1980.

Brown, R. C., Jones, M. C., Jr., Boldus, R., and Flocks, R. H.: Lesions causing radiolucent defects in the renal pelvis. AJR 119:770, 1973.
Fein, A. B., and McClennan, B. L.: Solitary filling defects of the ureter. Semin. Roentgenol. 21:201, 1986.
Hill, G. S.: Intrinsic and extrinsic obstruction of the urinary tract. In Hill, G. S. (ed.): Uropathology. New York, Churchill Livingstone, 1989, pp. 517–574.
Kaiser, J. A., Jacobs, R. P., and Korobkin, M.: Submucosal hemorrhage of the renal collecting system. AJR 125:311, 1975.
Malek, R. S., Aguilo, J. J., and Hattery, R. R.: Radiolucent filling defects of the renal pelvis: Classification and report of unusual cases. J. Urol. 114:508, 1975.
Pfister, R. C., and Newhouse, J. H.: Radiology of the ureter. Urology 12:15, 1978.
Pollack, H. M., Arger, P. H., Banner, M. P., Mulhern, C. B., Jr., and Coleman, B. G.: Computed tomography of renal pelvic defects. Radiology 138:645, 1981.
Smith, W. L., Weinstein, A. S., and West, J. F. Defects of renal collecting systems in patients receiving anticoagulants. Radiology 112:649, 1974.
Williamson, B. Jr., Hartman, G. W., and Hattery, R. R.: Multiple and diffuse ureteral filling defects. Semin. Roentgenol. 21:214, 1986.

Tumors

Ambos, M. A., Bosniak, M. A., Megibow, A. J., and Raghavendra, B.: Ureteral involvement by metastatic disease. Urol. Radiol. 1:105, 1979.
Apitzschi, D. E., and Meiisel, P.: Angiography of renal pelvis carcinoma. Fortschr. Geb. Roentgenstr. Nuklearmed. Erganzungsband 124:350, 1976.
Aufderheide, A. C., and Streitz, J. M.: Mucinous adenocarcinoma of the renal pelvis: Report of two cases. Cancer 33:167, 1974.
Banner, M. P., and Pollack, H. M.: Fibrous ureteral polyps. Radiology 130:73, 1979.
Baron, R. L., McClennan, B. L., Lee, J. K. T., and Lawson, T. L.: Computed tomography of transitional-cell carcinoma of the renal pelvis. Radiology 144:125, 1982.
Bergman, H., Friedenberg, R. M., and Sayegh, V.: New roentgenologic signs of carcinoma of the ureter. AJR 86:707, 1961.
Boijsen, E., and Folin, J.: Angiography in carcinoma of the renal pelvis. Acta Radiol. (Diagn.) 56:81, 1961.
Booth, C. M., Cameron, K. M., and Pugh, R. C. B.: Urothelial carcinoma of the kidney and ureter. Br. J. Urol 52:430, 1980.
Brandes, D., and Katz, R. S.: Nonepithelial tumors of the ureter and bladder. In Hill, G. S. (ed.): Uropathology. New York, Churchill Livingstone, 1989, pp. 861–872.
Burnett, K. R., Miller, J. B., and Greenbaum, E. I.: Transitional cell carcinoma: Rapid development in phenacetin abuse. AJR 134:1259, 1980.
Chew, Q. T., Nouri, M. S., and Woo, B. H.: Small renal pelvic carcinomas: Value of epinephrine magnification angiography. J. Urol. 120:243, 1978.
Colgan, J. R., III, Skaist, L., and Morrow, J. W.: Benign ureteral tumors in childhood: A case report and a plea for conservative management. J. Urol. 109:308, 1973.
Eagan, J. W.: Urothelial neoplasms: Pathologic anatomy. In Hill, G. S. (ed.): Uropathology. New York, Churchill Livingstone, 1989, pp. 719–792.
Eagan, J. W.: Urothelial neoplasms: Renal pelvis and ureter. In Hill, G. S. (ed.): Uropathology. New York, Churchill Livingstone, 1989, pp. 843–860.
Ekelund, L., and Göthlin, J.: Angiography in carcinoma of the renal pelvis and ureter. Acta Radiol. (Diagn.) 17:676, 1976.
Gaakeer, H. A., and DeRuiter, H. J.: Carcinoma of the renal pelvis following the abuse of phenacetin-containing analgesic drugs. Br. J. Urol. 51:188, 1979.
Gatewood, O. M., Goldman, S. M., Marshall, F. F., and Siegelman, S. S.: Computerized tomography in the diagnosis of transitional cell carcinoma of the kidney. J. Urol. 127:876, 1982.
Geerdsen, J.: Tumours of the renal pelvis and ureter: Symptomatology, diagnosis, treatment and prognosis. Scand. J. Urol. Nephrol. 13:287, 1979.
Gill, W. B., Lu, C. T., and Thomsen, S.: Retrograde brushing: New

technique for obtaining histologic and cytologic material from ureteral, renal pelvic and renal caliceal lesions. J. Urol. *109*:573, 1973.

Gonwa, T. A., Corbett, W. T., Schey, H. M., and Buckalew, V. M., Jr.: Analgesic-associated nephropathy and transitional cell carcinoma of the urinary tract. Ann. Intern. Med. 93:249, 1980.

Grabstald, H., Whitmore, W. F., and Melamed, M. R.: Renal pelvic tumors. JAMA *218*:845, 1971.

Grace, D. A., Taylor, W. N., Taylor, J. N., and Winter, C. C.: Carcinoma of renal pelvis: 15 year review. J. Urol. *98*:566, 1967.

Gup, A.: Benign mesodermal polyp in childhood. J. Urol. *114*:619, 1975.

Hartman, D. S., Pyatt, R. S., and Dailey, E.: Transitional cell carcinoma of the kidney with invasion into the renal vein. Urol. Radiol. *5*:83, 1983.

Hughes, F. A., III, and Davis, C. S., Jr.: Multiple benign ureteral polyps. AJR *126*:723, 1976.

Joshi, K., Jain, K., Mathur, S., and Mehrota, G. C.: Mucinous adenocarcinoma of the renal pelvis. Postgrad. Med. J. *56*:442, 1980.

Kenney, P. J., and Stanley, R. J.: Computed tomography of ureteral tumors. J. Comput. Assist. Tomogr. *11*:102, 1987.

Kinn, A. C.: Squamous cell carcinoma of the renal pelvis. Scand. J. Urol. Nephrol. *14*:77, 1980.

Lagergren, C., and Ljungqvist, A.: The arterial vasculature of renal pelvic carcinoma: An angiographic, microangiographic and histologic study. Acta Chir. Scand. *130*:321, 1965.

Leder, R. A., and Dunnick, N. R.: Transitional cell carcinoma of the pelvicalices and ureter. AJR *155*:713, 1990.

Liwnicz, B. H., Lepow, H., Schutte, H., Fernandez, R., and Caberwal, D.: Mucinous adenocarcinoma of the renal pelvis: Discussion of possible pathogenesis. J. Urol. *114*:306, 1975.

McLean, G. K., Pollack, H. M., and Banner, M. P.: The "stipple sign"—urographic harbinger of transitional cell neoplasm. Urol. Radiol. *1*:77, 1979.

Mitty, H. A., Baron, M. G., and Feller, M.: Infiltrating carcinoma of the renal pelvis: Angiographic features. Radiology *92*:994, 1969.

Murphy, D. M., Zincke, H., and Furlow, W. L.: Primary grade I transitional cell carcinoma of the renal pelvis ureter. J. Urol. *123*:629, 1980.

Narumi, Y., Sato, T., Hori, S., Kuriyama, K., Fujita, M., Kadowaki, K., Inoue, E., Maeshima, S., Fujino, Y., Saiki, S., Kuroda, M., and Kotake, T.: Squamous cell carcinoma of the uroepithelium: CT evaluation. Radiology *173*:853, 1989.

Noronha, R. F. X.: Transitional cell carcinoma of renal pelvis presenting with vascular obstruction. J. Urol. *122*:97, 1979.

Nyman, V., Oldbring, J., and Aspelin, P.: CT of carcinoma of the renal pelvis. Acta Radiol. *33*:31, 1992.

Parienty, R. A., Ducellier, R., Pradel, J., Lubrano, J.-M., Coquille, F., and Richard, F.: Diagnostic value of CT numbers in pelvocaliceal filling defects. Radiology *145*:743, 1982.

Pollack, H. M.: Long-term follow-up of the upper urinary tract for transitional cell carcinoma: How much is enough? Radiology *167*:871, 1988.

Pollen, J. J., Levine, E., and van Blerk, P. J. P.: The angiographic evaluation of renal pelvic carcinoma. Br. J. Urol. *47*:363, 1975.

Rubinstein, M. A., Walz, B. J., and Bucy, J. G.: Transitional cell carcinoma of the kidney: 25 year experience. J. Urol. *119*:595, 1978.

Segal, A. J., Spataro, R. F., Linke, C. A., Frank, I. N., and Rabinowitz, R.: Diagnosis of nonopaque calculi by computed tomography. Radiology *129*:447, 1978.

Sherwood, T.: Upper urinary tract tumours following on bladder carcinoma: Natural history of uroepithelial neoplastic disease. Br. J. Radiol. *44*:137, 1971.

Subramanyam, B. R., Raghavendra, B. N., and Madamba, M. R.: Renal transitional cell carcinoma: Sonographic and pathologic correlation. J. Clin. Ultrasound *10*:203, 1982.

Tolia, B. M., Hajdu, S. I., and Whitmore, W. F., Jr.: Leiomyosarcoma of the renal pelvis. J. Urol. *109*:974, 1973.

Toppercer, A.: Fibroepithelial tumour of the renal pelvis. Can. J. Surg. *23*:269, 1980.

Utz, D. C., and McDonald, J. R.: Squamous cell carcinoma of the kidney. J. Urol. *78*:540, 1957.

Wagle, D. C., Moore, R. H., and Murphy, G. P.: Squamous cell carcinoma of the renal pelvis. J. Urol. *111*:453, 1974.

Winalski, C. S., Lipman, J. C., and Tumeh, S. S.: Ureteral neoplasms. Radiographics *10*:271, 1990.

Youssem, D. M., Gatewood, O. M. B., Goldman, S. M., and Marshall, F. F.: Synchronous and metachronous transitional cell carcinoma of the urinary tract: Prevalence, incidence and radiographic detection. Radiology *167*:613, 1988.

Congenital Ureteropelvic Junction Obstruction

Bauer, S. B., Perlmutter, A. D., and Retik, A. B.: Anomalies of the upper urinary tract. *In* Walsh, P. C., Retik, A. B., Stamey, T. A., and Vaughan, E. D., Jr. (eds.): Campbell's Urology. 6th ed. Philadelphia, W. B. Saunders, 1992, pp. 1357–1442.

Bernstein, G. T., Mandell, J., Lebowitz, R. L., Bauer, S. B., Colodny, A. H., and Retik, A. B.: Ureteropelvic junction obstruction in the neonate. J. Urol. *140*:1216, 1988.

Chahlaoui, J., and Herba, M. J.: Ureteropelvic junction obstruction in the adult. J. Can. Assoc. Radiol. *28*:40, 1977.

Ekelund, L., Lindstedt, E., Thiesen, V., and Jönsson, M.-B.: Diuresis urography in equivocal pelvic-ureteric obstruction. Urol. Radiol. *1*:147, 1980.

English, P. J., Testa, H. J., Gosling, J. A., and Cohen, S. J.: Idiopathic hydronephrosis in childhood—a comparison between diuresis renography and upper urinary tract morphology. Br. J. Urol. *54*:603, 1982.

Friedland, G. W., Droller, M. J., and Stamey, T. A.: Obstruction of ischemic ureteropelvic junction. Urology *4*:439, 1974.

Gosling, J. A., and Dixon, J. S.: Functional obstruction of the ureter and renal pelvis: A histological and electron microscopic study. Br. J. Urol. *50*:145, 1978.

Hanna, M. K., Jeffs, R. D., Sturgess, J. M., and Barkin, M.: Ureteral structure ultrastructure: II. Congenital ureteropelvic obstruction and primary obstructive megaureter. J. Urol. *116*:725, 1976.

Hill, G. S.: Ureteropelvic junction obstruction. *In* Hill, G. S. (ed.): Uropathology. New York, Churchill Livingstone, 1989, pp. 575–598.

Jacobs, J. A., Berger, B. W., Goldman, S. M., Robbins, M. A., and Young, J. D., Jr.: Ureteropelvic obstruction in adults with previously normal pyelograms: A report of 5 cases. J. Urol. *121*:242, 1979.

Jaffee, R. B., and Middleton, A. W.: Whitaker test—differentiation of obstructive from nonobstructive uropathy. AJR *134*:9, 1980.

Johnston, J. H.: The pathogenesis of hydronephrosis in children. Br. J. Urol. *41*:724, 1969.

Johnston, J. H., Evans, J. P., Glassberg, K. I., and Shapiro, S. R.: Pelvic hydronephrosis in children: A review of 219 personal cases. J. Urol. *117*:97, 1977.

Kendall, A. R., and Karafin, L.: Intermittent hydronephrosis: Hydration pyelograpy. J. Urol. *98*:653, 1967.

Malek, R. S.: Intermittent hydronephrosis: The occult ureteropelvic obstruction. J. Urol. *130*:863, 1983.

Murnaghan, G. F.: The dynamics of the renal pelvis and ureter with reference to congenital hydronephrosis. Br. J. Urol. *30*:321, 1958.

Nixon, H. H.: Hydronephrosis in children: A clinical study of seventy-eight cases with special reference to the role of aberrant renal vessels and the results of conservative operations. Br. J. Surg. *40*:601, 1953.

Notley, R. G.: Electron microscopy of the upper ureter and pelviureteric junction. Br. J. Urol. *40*:37, 1968.

Pfister, R. C., and Newhouse, J. H.: Interventional percutaneous pyeloureteral techniques: I. Antegrade pyelography and ureteral perfusion. Radiol. Clin. North Am. *17*:341, 1979.

Powers, T. A., Grove, R. B., Bauriedel, J. K., Orr, S. C., Melton, R. E., and Bowden, R. D.: Detection of obstructed uropathy using ^{99m}technetium diethylenetriaminepentaacetic acid. J. Urol. *124*:588, 1980.

Stage, K. H., and Lewis, S.: Use of the radionuclide washout test in evaluation of suspected upper urinary obstruction. J. Urol. *125*:379, 1981.

Testa, H. J.: Nuclear medicine in diagnostic techniques. *In* O'Reilly, P. H., George, N. J. R., and Weiss, R. M. (eds.): Urology. Philadelphia, W. B. Saunders, 1990, pp. 99–117.

Wadsworth, D. E., and McClennan, B. L.: Benign causes of acquired ureteropelvic junction obstruction: A uroradiologic spectrum. Urol. Radiol. *5*:77, 1983.

Whitaker, R. H.: Some observations and theories on the wide ureter and hydronephrosis. Br. J. Urol. 47:377, 1975.

Whitaker, R. H.: The Whitaker test. Urol. Clin. North Am 6:529, 1979.

Whitaker, R. H.: Investigation of the dilated upper urinary tract. J. R. Soc. Med. 73:377, 1980.

Whitfield, H. N., Britton, K. E., Fry, I. K., Hendry, W. F., Nimmon, C. C., Travers, P., and Wickham, J. E. A.: The obstructed kidney: Correlation between renal function and urodynamic assessment. Br. J. Urol. 49:615, 1977.

Tuberculosis

Barrie, H. J., Kerr, W. K., and Gale, G. L.: The incidence and pathogenesis of tuberculous strictures of the renal pyelus. J. Urol. 98:584, 1967.

Friedenberg, R. M.: Tuberculosis of the genitourinary system. Semin. Roentgenol. 6:310, 1971.

Gow, J. G.: Genitourinary tuberculosis: A 7 year review. Br. J. Urol. 51:239, 1979.

Kollins, S. A., Hartman, G. W., Carr, D. T., Segura, J. W., and Hattery, R. R.: Roentgenographic findings in urinary tract tuberculosis: A 10 year review. AJR 121:487, 1974.

Roylance, J., Penry, J. B., Davies, E. R., and Roberts, M.: The radiology of tuberculosis of the urinary tract. Clin. Radiol. 21:163, 1970.

Candidiasis

Margolin, H. N.: Fungus infection tract. Semin. Roentgenol. 6:323, 1971.

McDonald, D. F., and Fagan, C. J.: Fungus balls in the urinary tract: Case report. AJR 114:753, 1972.

Michigan, S.: Genitourinary fungal infection. J. Urol. 116:390, 1976.

Schistosomiasis

Al-Ghorab, M. M.: Radiological manifestations of genitourinary bilharziasis. Clin. Radiol. 19:100, 1968.

Dittrich, M., and Doehring, E.: Ultrasonographical aspects of urinary schistosomiasis: Assessment of morphologic lesions in the upper and lower urinary tract. Pediatr. Radiol. 16:225, 1986.

Hugosson, C., and Olsen, P.: Early ureteric changes in Schistosoma haematobium infection. Clin. Radiol. 37:501, 1986.

Jorulf, H., and Lindstedt, E.: Urogenital schistosomiasis: CT evaluation. Radiology 157:745, 1985.

Mahmoud, A. A.: Schistosomiasis. N. Engl. J. Med. 297:1329, 1974.

Palmer, P. E. S., and Reeder, M. M.: Parasitic disease of the urinary tract. In Pollack, H. M. (ed.): Clinical Urography. Philadelphia, W. B. Saunders, 1990, pp. 999–1019.

Smith, J. H., von Lichtenberg, F., and Lehman, J. S.: Parasitic diseases of the genitourinary system. In Walsh, P. C., Retik, A. B., Stamey, T. A., Vaughan, E. D., Jr. (eds.): Campbell's Urology. 6th ed. Philadelphia, W. B. Saunders, 1992, pp. 883–927.

Umerah, B. C.: The less familiar manifestations of schistosomiasis of the urinary tract. Br. J. Radiol. 50:105, 1977.

Young, S. W., Khalid, K. H., Fariz, Z., and Mahmoud, A. H.: Urinary tract lesions of Schistosoma haematobium with detailed radiographic considerations of the bladder. Radiology 111:81, 1974.

Pyelitis Cystica

Köhler, R.: Pyelo-ureteritis cystica. Acta Radiol. (Diagn.) 4:123, 1966.

Limburg, D., and Zuidema, B. J.: Pyeloureteritis cystica. Diagn. Imaging 49:141, 1980.

Loitman, B. S., and Chiat, H.: Ureteritis cystica and pyelitis cystica. Radiology 68:345, 1957.

McNulty, M.: Pyelo-ureteritis cystica. Br. J. Radiol. 30:648, 1957.

Leukoplakia

Besmann, E. F.: Renal leukoplakia. Radiology 88:872, 1967.

Hertle, L., and Androulakasis, P.: Keratinizing desquamative squamous metaplasia of the upper urinary tract: Leukoplakia—cholesteatoma. J. Urol. 127:631, 1982.

Noyes, W. E., and Palubinskas, A. J.: Squamous metaplasia of renal pelvis. Radiology. 89:292, 1967.

Reece, R. W., and Koontz, W. W., Jr.: Leukoplakia of the urinary tract: A review. J. Urol. 114:165, 1975.

Smith, B. A., Jr., Webb, E. A., and Price, W. E.: Renal leukoplakia: Observations of behavior. J. Urol. 87:279, 1969.

Weitzner, S.: Cholesteatoma of the calix. J. Urol. 108:365, 1972.

Malakoplakia

Abdou, N. I., NaPombejara, C., Sagawa, A., Ragland, C., Stechschulte, D. J., Nilsson, U., Gourley, W., Watanabe, I., Lindsey, N. J., and Ellen, M. S.: Malakoplakia: Evidence for monocytic lysosomal abnormality correctable by cholinergic agonist in vitro and in vivo. N. Engl. J. Med. 297:1413, 1977.

Bennett, W. H.: Malacoplakia of the urinary tract: Report of three cases. J. Urol. 70:84, 1953.

Cadnaphornchai, P., Rosenberg, B. F., Taher, S., Prosnitz, E. H., and McDonald, F. D.: Renal parenchymal malakoplakia: An unusual cause of renal failure. N. Engl. J. Med. 299:1110, 1978.

Hartman, D. S., Davis, C. J., Jr., Lichtenstein, J. E., and Goldman, S. M.: Renal parenchymal malacoplakia. Radiology 136:33, 1980.

O'Dea, M. J., Malek, R. S., and Farrow, G. M.: Malacoplakia of the urinary tract: Challenges and frustrations with 10 cases. J. Urol. 118:739, 1977.

Soberon, L. M., Zawada, E. T., Jr., Cohen, A. H., and Kaloyanides, G. J.: Renal parenchymal malakoplakia presenting as acute oliguric renal failure. Nephron 26:200, 1980.

Stanton, M. J., and Maxted, W.: Malacoplakia: A study of the literature and current concepts of pathogenesis, diagnosis and treatment. J. Urol. 125:139, 1981.

Amyloidosis

Amendola, M. A.: Amyloidosis of the urinary tract. In Pollack, H. M. (ed.): Clinical Urography. Philadelphia, W. B. Saunders, 1990, pp. 2493–2500.

Chisholm, G. D., Cotter, N. B. E., and Dawson, J. M.: Primary amyloidosis of the renal pelvis. Br. Med. J. 1:736, 1967.

David, P. S., Babaria, A., March, D. E., and Goldberg, R. D. S.: Primary amyloidosis of the ureter and renal pelvis. Urol. Radiol. 9:158, 1987.

Gardner, K. D., Jr., Castellino, R. A., Kempson, R., Young, B. W., and Stamey, T. A.: Primary amyloidosis of the renal pelvis. N. Engl. J. Med. 284:1196, 1971.

Lee, K. T., and Deeths, T. M.: Localized amyloidosis of the ureter. Radiology 120:60, 1976.

Moul, J. M., and McLeod, D. C.: Bilateral organ-limited amyloidosis of the distal ureter associated with osseous metaplasia and radiographic calcifications. J. Urol. 139:807, 1988.

Pirnar, T., and Coruh, M.: Radiologic findings in renal amyloidosis of children. Pediatr. Radiol. 1:72, 1973.

Thomas, S. D., Sanders, P. W., III, and Pollack, H. M.: Primary amyloidosis of the urinary bladder and ureter: Cause of mural calcification. Urology 9:586, 1977.

Willen, R., Willen, H., Lindstedt, E., and Ekelund, L.: Localized primary amyloidosis of the ureter. Scand. J. Urol. Nephrol. 17:385, 1983.

Polyarteritis Nodosa

Hefty, T. R., Bonafede, P., and Stenzel, P.: Bilateral ureteral stricture from polyarteritis nodosa. J. Urol. 141:600, 1989.

Eosinophilic Ureteritis

Hellstrom, H. R., Davis, B. K., Shonnard, J. W., and MacPherson, T. A.: Eosinophilic pyeloureteritis: Report of a case. J. Urol. 122:833, 1979.

Uyama, T., Moriwaki, S., Aga, Y., and Yamamoto, A.: Eosinophilic ureteritis? Regional ureteritis with marked infiltration of eosinophils. Urology 18:615, 1981.

Mural Hemorrhage

Antolak, S. J., Jr., and Mellinger, C. T.: Urologic evaluation of hematuria during anticoagulant therapy. J. Urol. *101*:111, 1969.

Brannen, G. E., Wettlaufer, J. N., Stables, D. P., and Weil, R.: Intramural bleeding into a renal allograft pelvis during heparin anticoagulation. Br. J. Radiol. *52*:838, 1979.

Buntley, D. W., and McDuffie, R.: Pyeloureteral filling defects associated with anticoagulation: A case report. J. Urol. *115*:335, 1976.

Eisenberg, R. L., and Clark, R. E.: Filling defects in the renal pelvis and ureter owing to bleeding secondary to acquired circulating anticoagulants. J. Urol. *116*:662, 1976.

Higenbottam, T., Ogg, C. S., and Saxton, H. M.: Acute renal failure from the use of acetazolamide (Diamox). Postgrad. Med. J. *54*:127, 1978.

Kaiser, J. A., Jacobs, R. P., and Korobkin, M.: Submucosal hemorrhage of the renal collecting system. AJR *125*:311, 1975.

Kossol, J. M., and Patel, S. K.: Suburoepithelial hemorrhage: The value of preinfusion computed tomography. J. Comput. Assist. Tomogr. *10*:157, 1986.

Miller, V., Witten, D. M., and Shin, M. S.: Computed tomographic findings in suburothelial hemorrhage. Urol. Radiol. *4*:11, 1982.

Smith, W. L., Weinstein, A. S., and Wiot, J. F.: Defects of the renal collecting system in patients receiving anticoagulants. Radiology *113*:649, 1974.

Viamonte, M., Roen, S. A., Viamonte, M., Jr., Casal, G. L., and Rywlin, A. M.: Subepithelial hemorrhage of renal pelvis simulating neoplasm (Antopol-Goldman lesion). Urology *16*:647, 1980.

Longitudinal Mucosal Folds

Astley, R.: Striation (longitudinal mucosal folds) in the upper urinary tract: III. Urinary tract striation in children: Some experimental observations. Br. J. Radiol. *44*:452, 1971.

Cremin, B. J., and Stables, D. P.: Striation (longitudinal mucosal folds) in the upper urinary tract: II. A comparison in children and adults. Br. J. Radiol. *44*:449, 1971.

Daughtridge, T. G.: Mucosal folds in the upper urinary tract. AJR *107*:743, 1969.

Friedland, G. W., and Forsberg, L.: Striation of the renal pelvis in children. Clin. Radiol. *23*:58, 1972.

Hyde, I., and Wastie, M. L.: Striation (longitudinal mucosal folds) in the upper urinary tract: I. Striated renal pelvis and ureter in children. Br. J. Radiol. *44*:445, 1971.

Silber, I., and McAllister, W. H.: Longitudinal folds as an indirect sign of vesicoureteral reflux. J. Urol. *103*:89, 1970.

Ureteral Pseudodiverticulosis

Cochran, S. T., Waisman, J., and Barbaric, Z. L.: Radiographic and microscopic findings in multiple ureteral diverticula. Radiology *137*:631, 1980.

Wasserman, N. F., LaPointe, S., and Posalaky, I. P. Ureteral pseudodiverticulosis. Radiology *155*:561, 1985.

Wasserman, N. F., Posalaky, I. P., and Dykoski, R.: The pathology of ureteral pseudodiverticulosis. Invest. Radiol. *23*:592, 1988.

Pyelocalyceal Diverticulum

Healey, T., and Grundy, W. R.: Milk of calcium in calycine diverticula. Br. J. Radiol. *53*:845, 1980.

Middleton, A. W., Jr., and Pfister, R. C.: Stone-containing pyelocaliceal diverticulum: Embryonic, anatomic, radiologic and clinical characteristics. J. Urol. *111*:2, 1974.

Pomerantz, R. M., Kirschner, L. P., and Twigg, H. L.: Renal milk of calcium collection: Review of literature and report of case. J. Urol. *103*:18, 1970.

Rosenberg, M. A.: Milk of calcium in a renal calyceal diverticulum: Case report and review of literature. AJR *101*:714, 1967.

Siegel, M. J., and McAlister, W. H.: Calyceal diverticula in children: Unusual features and complications. Radiology *131*:79, 1979.

Spence, H. M., and Singleton, R.: Cysts and cystic disorders of the kidney: Types, diagnosis, treatment. Urol. Surv. *22*:131, 1972.

Timmons, J. W., Jr., Malek, R. S., Hattery, R. R., and de Weerd, J. H.: Caliceal diverticulum. J. Urol. *114*:6, 1975.

Williams, G., Blandy, J. P., and Tressider, G. C.: Communicating cysts and diverticula of the renal pelvis. Br. J. Urol. *41*:163, 1969.

Wulfsohn, M. A.: Pyelocaliceal diverticula. J. Urol. *123*:1, 1980.

Ureteroceles

Bauer, S. B., and Retik, A. B.: The non-obstructive ectopic ureterocele. J. Urol. *119*:804, 1978.

Bauer, S. B., Perlmutter, A. D., and Retik, A. B.: Anomalies of the upper urinary tract. *In* Walsh, P. C., Retik, A. B., Stamey, T. A., and Vaughan, E. D., Jr. (eds.): Campbell's Urology. 6th ed. Philadelphia, W. B. Saunders, 1992, pp. 1357–1442.

Mandell, J., Colodny, A. H., Lebowitz, R., Bauer, S. B., and Retik, A. B.: Ureteroceles in infants and children. J. Urol. *123*:921, 1980.

Mitty, H. A., and Schapira, H. E.: Ureterocele and pseudoureterocele: Cobra vs cancer. J. Urol. *117*:557, 1977.

Morse, F. P., III, Sears, B., and Brown, H. P.: Carcinoma of the bladder presenting as simple adult ureterocele. J. Urol. *111*:36, 1974.

Nussbaum, A. R., Dorst, J. P., Jeffs, R. D., Gearhart, J. P., and Sanders, R. C.: Ectopic ureter and ureterocele: Their varied sonographic manifestations. Radiology *159*:227, 1986.

Prewitt, L. H., Jr., and Lebowitz, R. L.: The single ectopic ureter. AJR *127*:941, 1976.

Share, J. C., and Lebowitz, R. L.: Ectopic ureterocele without ureteral and calyceal dilatation (ureterocele disproportion): Findings on urography and sonography. AJR *152*:567, 1989.

Sherwood, T., and Stevenson, J. J.: Ureteroceles in disguise. Br. J. Radiol. *42*:899, 1969.

Tanagho, E. A.: Anatomy and management of ureteroceles. J. Urol. *107*:729, 1972.

Thompson, G. J., and Kelalis, P. P.: Ureterocele: A clinical appraisal of 176 cases. J. Urol. *91*:488, 1964.

Thornbury, J. R., Silver, T. M., and Vinson, R. K.: Ureteroceles vs pseudoureteroceles in adults. Radiology *122*:81, 1977.

16

RENAL SINUS AND PERIURETERAL ABNORMALITIES

PARAPELVIC CYST

RENAL SINUS LIPOMATOSIS

VASCULAR ABNORMALITIES

SOLID TUMORS OF THE RENAL SINUS

ENDOMETRIOSIS

NEOPLASTIC AND INFLAMMATORY INFILTRATION

URETERAL DEVIATION

DIFFERENTIAL DIAGNOSIS

The abnormalities discussed in this chapter originate either in the renal sinus or in the tissue that surrounds the ureter. The renal sinus is the extension of the perinephric space into the deep recess situated on the medial border of the kidney. Contained within this space are the pelvocalyceal system, fat, and lymph nodes. Arteries, veins, lymphatic channels, and nerves of the autonomic nervous system traverse the sinus and enter or exit the kidney by penetrating the extension of the renal capsule that is invaginated into the inner recess of the sinus. The fat that fills this space surrounds the tips of the septa of Bertin and the calyces at their point of attachment to the papillae. Medially, the sinus fat is continuous with the fat of the perinephric space through which the proximal two-thirds of the ureter passes to where it pierces the caudal fusion of the anterior and posterior renal fascia at the level of the iliac crest. From this point to the ureterovesical junction the ureter is in the pelvic extraperitoneal space.

Most abnormalities of the renal sinus are focal and are best described as parapelvic, using the prefix *para* to mean "alongside" or "beside." These abnormalities cause focal displacement and smooth effacement of the pelvocalyceal system on excretory urography or pyelography and a circumscribed mass on cross-sectional tomographic techniques such as ultrasonography, computed tomography, or magnetic resonance imaging. Disorders that surround the pelvocalyceal system are described as peripelvic, using the prefix *peri* to mean "around." This distribution, which occurs mainly with renal sinus lipomatosis, causes generalized attenuation of the pelvocalyceal system.

Parapelvic cyst, renal sinus lipomatosis, vascular abnormalities, and solid tumors of the renal sinus are each discussed in the initial sections of this chapter. Some of these entities, such as pelvocalyceal impressions caused by normal blood vessels and some forms of peripelvic fat deposition, produce radiologic abnormalities but are of no clinical significance in themselves. Others cause only subtle abnormalities on excretory urography or pyelography but are readily identified by cross-sectional imaging techniques. The final sections of this chapter describe abnormalities that arise outside the ureter, but, nevertheless, are in close enough proximity to deform or displace that structure. These include endometriosis, neoplastic and inflammatory infiltration, and certain causes of deviation in the course of the ureter. Other aspects of normal and abnormal ureteral course are discussed in Chapter 3 (anatomy of the ureter), Chapter 10 (lymphoma of the renal sinus), Chapter 19 (the bladder), and Chapter 21 (the retroperitoneum).

PARAPELVIC CYST

Definition

Parapelvic cysts are spherical or ovoid, blue-gray masses that intimately attach to the renal pelvis or calyx and are filled with clear yellow fluid containing albumin, lipids, and cholesterol. Previously, these cysts, which do not communicate with the pelvocalyceal system, were thought to be mostly solitary and unilocular. Experience with computed tomography and ultrasonography, however, has shown that parapelvic cysts are often multiple or multilocular. They may fill the sinus and surround the entire collecting system, causing a pattern of effacement and stretching

533

that is usually associated with peripelvic abnormalities such as sinus lipomatosis. Rarely, a solitary cyst will insinuate itself deeply into the sinus and deform only a single calyx or infundibulum.

Parapelvic cysts are extraparenchymal lesions that probably arise from ectatic lymphatic channels. Origin in a wolffian duct remnant or as a congenital anomaly of the retroperitoneum has also been suggested. However, the microscopic appearance of the cyst wall, composed of fibrous connective tissue with collagen, lymphatic cells, and fibroblasts and a lining of flattened endothelial cells, closely resembles that of lymph vessels. This supports the concept of a lymphatic origin.

There is no consensus on the terminology for parapelvic cysts, which have also been called *pyelolymphatic, peripelvic,* or, simply, *renal sinus* or *hilar cysts.* Pyelolymphatic implies a lymphatic origin, which is only conjecture. Peripelvic is inaccurate in view of the usual parapelvic location of these cysts. Regardless of terminology, however, these cysts are uncommonly of clinical importance and are rarely subject to pathologic study.

A large parapelvic cyst may extrude from the renal sinus and cause stretching of the vascular pedicle of the kidney. Compression and displacement of a part of the pelvocalyceal system to the point of obstruction is another complication of a large cyst. Rarely, a parapelvic cyst disappears, presumably following spontaneous rupture.

Clinical Setting

Parapelvic cysts occur in all age groups. Most cysts are asymptomatic. Dull flank pain, hematuria, and the signs and symptoms of urinary tract infection, presumably secondary to obstruction, are ascribed to these lesions. If the vascular pedicle is severely stretched by a large parapelvic cyst, hyperreninemic hypertension may develop. This can be reversed by evacuation of the cyst.

Radiologic Findings

Excretory Urography. A soft tissue density in the renal sinus that causes focal displacement and smooth effacement of the adjacent portion of the pelvocalyceal system comprise the findings on excretory urography of a single parapelvic cyst (Fig. 16–1). Rarely, a halo of lucency around the mass is detected on tomograms, owing to the displacement of sinus fat. Multiple or multiloculated parapelvic cysts fill the renal sinus and cause generalized, rather than focal, effacement and stretching of the collecting system (Fig. 16–2). This pattern closely resembles that of sinus lipomatosis, except the tissue surrounding the distorted pelvocalyceal system has the radiodensity of water rather than of fat. Obstructive caliectasis may occur with either the focal or the generalized form of parapelvic cyst (see Figs. 16–1 and 16–2). The urographic nephrogram is normal, however, as would be expected of a cyst that has a sinus rather than parenchymal origin. Curvilinear calcification of the cyst wall occurs rarely.

Ultrasonography. An anechoic mass with a well-defined far wall and acoustic enhancement are the findings on ultrasound examination of parapelvic cyst (Figs. 16–3 and 16–4). These cysts are located within the normally echogenic central sinus complex, which may be either focally displaced or separated. Distinction between parapelvic cyst and hydronephrosis is dependent on the demonstration of continuity between a dilated pelvis and its branching calyces in the case of hydronephrosis (see Fig. 17–11) and the absence of branching in the case of a parapelvic cyst. Distinction on ultrasonography between a parapelvic cyst and other fluid-containing structures of the renal sinus, such as a renal artery aneurysm, a nephrogenic cyst protruding into the sinus, or a Type II pyelocalyceal diverticulum, may be impossible without the use of other diagnostic modalities including Doppler ultrasound evaluation. Interventional techniques in this region should be performed with thin-walled, 22-gauge needles to avoid serious trauma to the vascular pedicle of the kidney.

Computed Tomography. The location of a parapelvic cyst within the renal sinus is best demonstrated by computed tomography (see Figs. 16–2 through 16–4). These lesions have a homogeneous appearance with an attenuation value close to that of water. The protein content of some cysts may increase this value and make distinction from a solid tumor difficult. Some cysts are single and have a smooth outline; others are multiple, bilateral, and lobulated. Individual cysts separated by vessels and the collecting system can be identified occasionally (see Fig. 16–3). Contrast material enhancement is required to visualize the effaced pelvocalyceal system and ensure that the fluid-filled structure in the renal sinus, seen on unenhanced computed tomograms, is not a dilated pelvis (see Fig. 16–4). The attenuation value of parapelvic cysts is not changed by intravenous contrast material.

Magnetic Resonance Imaging. The magnetic resonance image of a parapelvic cyst shows a low signal mass surrounded by high signal renal sinus fat.

Angiography. Angiography demonstrates displacement and stretching of the main renal artery and its branches by a parapelvic cyst. The integrity of the renal parenchyma is best demonstrated by the angiographic nephrogram.

RENAL SINUS LIPOMATOSIS

Definition

A thin layer of loose fatty tissue in continuity with fat of the perirenal space normally envelops the other structures in the renal sinus. The amount of fat is minimal in young and lean individuals. Conversely, there is a normal increase in sinus fat with aging and obesity.

Proliferation of sinus fat also occurs abnormally in association with processes causing destruction or atrophy of renal tissue (see Fig. 21–21). In this situation,

Text continued on page 540

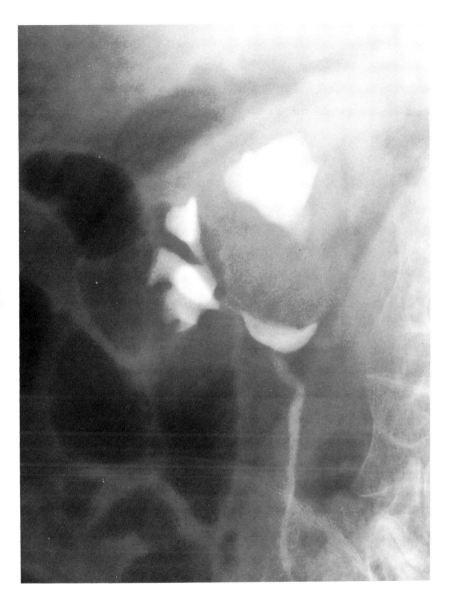

Figure 16–1. Solitary parapelvic cyst. An oval mass having the density of water focally displaces the collecting system. Effacement of the infundibula has caused caliectasis. Excretory urogram.

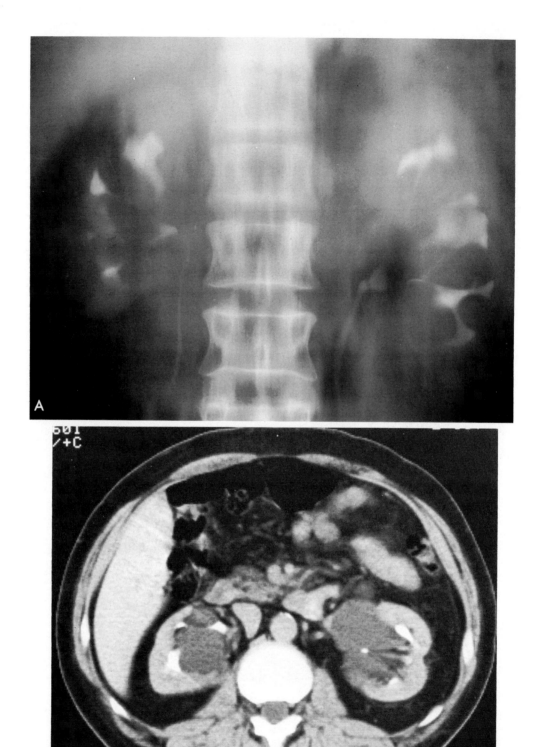

Figure 16–2. Multiple, bilateral parapelvic cysts in a 58-year-old hypertensive man. There is generalized effacement and stretching of the pelvis and infundibula of both kidneys. The tissue filling the sinuses is of water density. Caliectasis is generalized.

    A, Excretory urogram. Tomogram.

    B, Computed tomogram, contrast material enhanced. Note the smoothly marginated, homogeneous cysts.

    (Courtesy of Carol Weinstein, M.D., Good Samaritan Hospital, Portland, Oregon.)

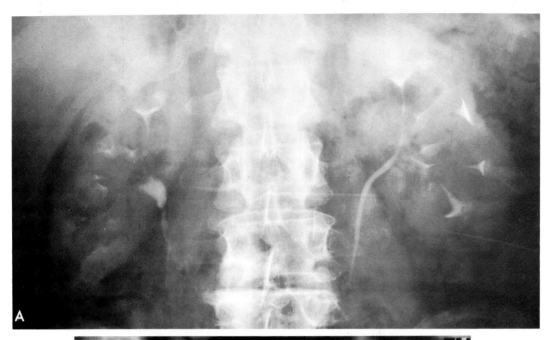

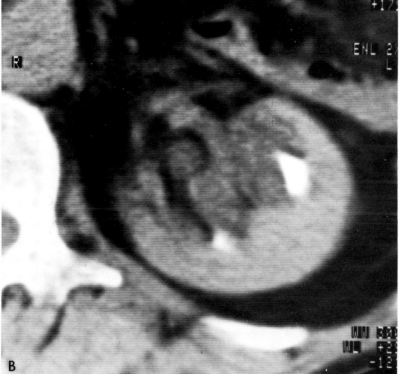

Figure 16–3. Parapelvic cysts of the left kidney and sinus lipomatosis of the right kidney.
  A, Excretory urogram. The pattern of collecting system attenuation is similar in each kidney.
  B, Computed tomogram with contrast material enhancement, taken of the upper portion of the left kidney. Individual cysts can be distinguished.

Illustration continued on following page

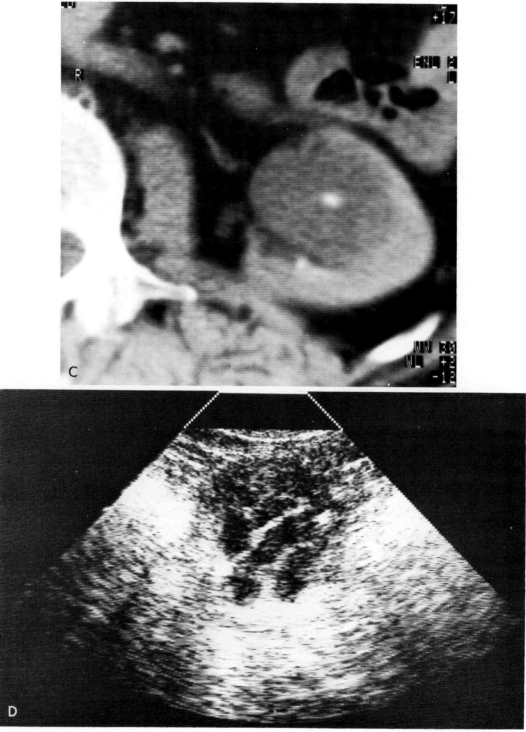

Figure 16–3 *Continued*

C, Computed tomogram with contrast material enhancement taken of the lower portion of the left kidney. Multiple cysts surround a portion of compressed collecting system.

D, Ultrasonogram. Multiple fluid-filled structures with well-defined walls and acoustic enhancement are seen. These do not communicate, in contradistinction to the findings in obstructive uropathy.

(Same patient as illustrated in Fig. 16–9.)

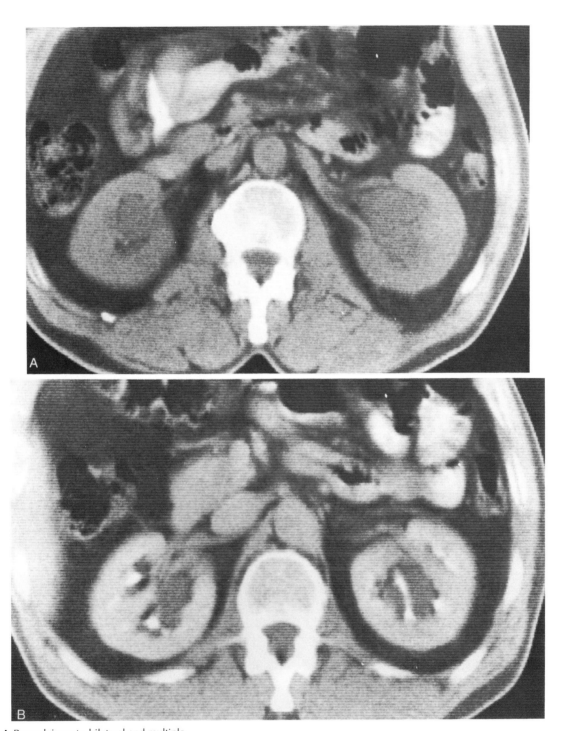

Figure 16–4. Parapelvic cysts, bilateral and multiple.
 A, Computed tomogram, unenhanced. A mass of water attenuation values fills both renal sinuses. This could represent either parapelvic cysts or hydronephrosis.
 B, Computed tomogram, contrast material enhanced. Opacification of an attenuated collecting system surrounded by the cystic masses indicates the diagnosis of parapelvic cysts.

Illustration continued on following page

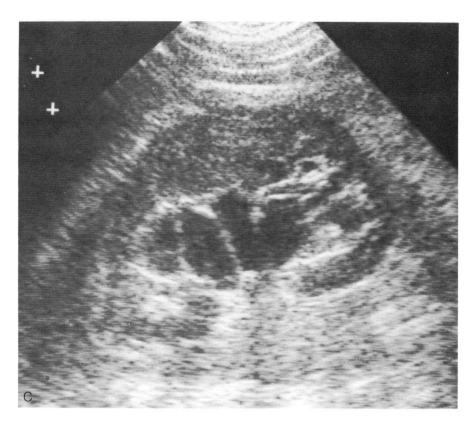

Figure 16–4 *Continued C,* Ultrasonogram, left kidney. Coronal projection. Multiple septated cystic masses fill the renal sinus. (Kindly provided by Giovanna Casola, M.D., University of California, San Diego.)

increased fat deposits preserve some of the overall kidney mass that would otherwise be reduced as renal parenchyma is lost. In rare cases, renal bulk is larger than normal and virtually the entire kidney is accounted for by greatly expanded sinus fat capped only by a very thin mantle of renal parenchyma. This extreme, which may have inflammatory cells infiltrating the proliferative sinus fat, has been referred to as "replacement lipomatosis" of the kidney.

Normal sinus fat does not affect the distensibility of the pelvocalyceal system. When fat proliferates, however, the entire collecting system becomes attenuated and loses its distensibility. Occasionally, fat collects in a single focus that deforms the adjacent pelvocalyceal system. Rarely, this projects into the wall of the pelvis and simulates a mural mass.

Synonyms for renal sinus lipomatosis are peripelvic lipomatosis, renal fibrolipomatosis (a misnomer), and, simply, peripelvic fat proliferation.

Clinical Setting

Renal sinus lipomatosis is normal in aged and obese individuals and is sometimes found in patients without known current or previous disease. By itself, fatty proliferation is asymptomatic. Clinical abnormalities that might be present reflect the primary process causing wasting, such as reflux nephropathy, atherosclerosis, or recurrent urinary tract infection.

Radiologic Findings

Normal sinus fat causes a fan-shaped, irregular radiolucency in the central part of the kidney (Fig. 16–5). Tomography is a useful adjunct when overlying gas obscures the renal sinus. A serrated interface between deep sinus fat and adjacent renal parenchyma is accentuated during the nephrographic phase of excretory urography.

Once opacified, the pelvocalyceal system appears diffusely elongated or "spider like" when the sinus fat has proliferated. The infundibula radiate from the hilus toward the parenchyma in a pattern that has been likened to the spokes of a wheel. The calyces reflect the state of the renal parenchyma and vary from normal to dilated. Renal parenchymal thickness is diminished when there is a primary underlying parenchymal disease (Fig. 16–6).

Lipomatosis is usually diffusely distributed in the renal sinus. Occasionally, fat deposits in a single focus, causing a localized deformity of the pelvis, infundibulum, or calyx. This deformity is similar in radiologic appearance to that of any other parapelvic mass except for its radiolucency (Fig. 16–7). Rarely, the focal fat deposit is small and deeply invaginates the adjacent pelvic wall, simulating a mural mass. Defining the parapelvic nature of this lesion requires a well-distended and opacified pelvocalyceal system, exposures in steep oblique projections, and, ultimately, identification of the fatty nature of the lesion by ultrasonography, computed tomography, or magnetic resonance imaging.

Sinus lipomatosis causes an echo pattern that is at least as dense as the renal parenchyma and usually denser (Figs. 16–8 and 16–9). Usually, the central sinus complex is more extensive than normal, although this finding may be obscured unless the plane of the image passes through the central axis of the sinus.

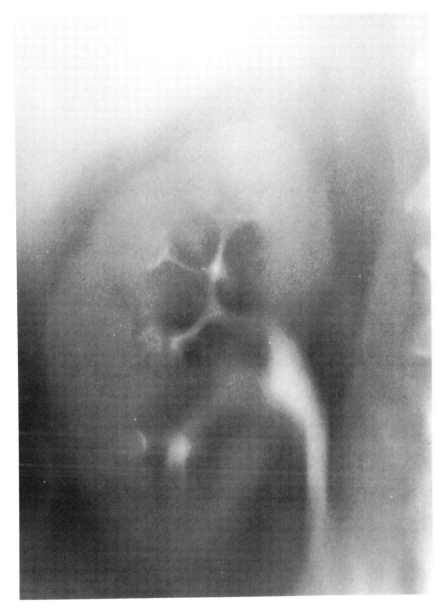

Figure 16–5. Normal renal sinus fat. The lucency in the central part of the kidney has an irregular fan shape and attenuates the pelvocalyceal system. Excretory urogram. Tomogram.

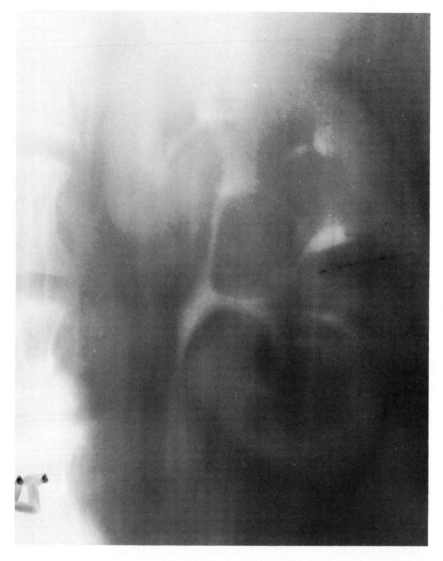

Figure 16–6. Sinus lipomatosis of the left kidney. There is diffuse elongation and attenuation of the pelvis and infundibula, mild caliectasis, and thinning of the renal parenchyma. Excretory urogram. Tomogram.

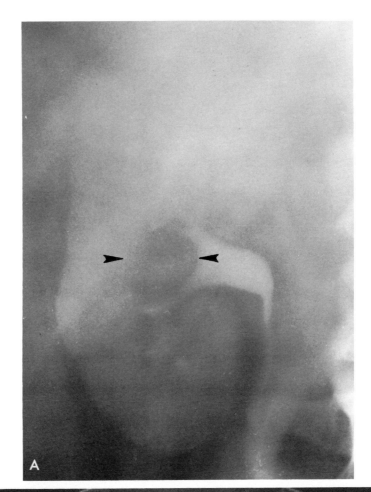

Figure 16–7. Focal sinus lipomatosis of the right kidney. The midportion of the pelvis is displaced around a radiolucent mass *(arrows)*.

A, Excretory urogram. Tomogram.

B, Computed tomogram, contrast material enhanced. The tissue at the site of pelvic distortion has the same attenuation value as perirenal fat.

(Courtesy of Joy Price, M.D., Alta Bates Medical Center, Berkeley, California.)

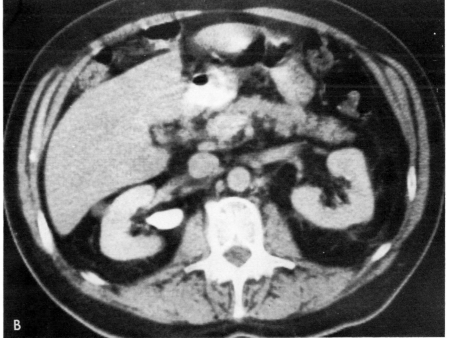

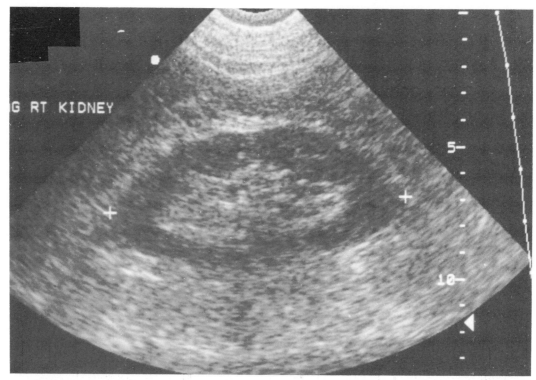

Figure 16–8. Sinus lipomatosis associated with end-stage renal failure. Ultrasonogram, longitudinal projection. There is increased prominence of the central sinus echo complex.

Computed tomography or magnetic resonance imaging unequivocally defines the fatty nature of sinus lipomatosis (see Figs. 16–7 and 16–9). Computed tomography is especially useful in examining patients with focal fat deposits that mimic other focal masses of the renal sinus.

Extensive sinus lipomatosis causes narrowing, stretching, and arching of the renal artery and its major branches. This is visualized by arteriography. The separation of arteries and the diminished number of branches are similar to what is seen with generalized parapelvic cysts.

VASCULAR ABNORMALITIES

Definition

Both arteries and veins impress on the pelvocalyceal system and ureter, either as closely apposed normal vessels or as aneurysms, collateral vessels, or varices.

Pelvocalyceal impressions by normal dorsal and ventral branches of the renal artery are common in patients with an intrarenal pelvis. Most branches cross the infundibulum to the upper pole. Other frequent sites of normal arterial impressions are the pelvis itself and the ureteropelvic junction. Normal veins passing anterior to the pelvocalyceal system produce impression in similar locations and patterns. The gonadal vein may cause a normal impression on the ureter as it follows a parallel course or, on the right side, where it crosses the ureter at approximately the level of the third lumbar vertebra.

Renal artery aneurysms are classified morphologi-

cally as either saccular or fusiform and histologically by the number of components of the arterial wall that are preserved. A "true" aneurysm is one in which intima, muscularis, and serosa are intact. The designation "false" aneurysm is used when one or more of these components are absent. An arterial aneurysm that communicates directly with dilated renal veins is described as an "arteriovenous" aneurysm or fistula.

Another useful classification of aneurysms is etiologic and includes atherosclerotic, dysplastic, post-stenotic, congenital, traumatic, and mycotic. Atherosclerosis causes true, saccular aneurysms at the origin of the main renal artery and at its major bifurcations. Atherosclerotic aneurysm of the aorta and common iliac artery also affect the course of the ureter, as discussed below. The aneurysm of arterial dysplasia is a false aneurysm or pseudoaneurysm that forms as a result of dissection. These may be large and saccular but, unlike atherosclerotic aneurysms, occur along the nonbifurcating portions of the artery. Post-stenotic aneurysms are fusiform as a result of hemodynamic forces distal to a stenosis. Arteriovenous aneurysms or fistulas are false aneurysms that follow penetrating trauma or spontaneous rupture of an atherosclerotic or mycotic aneurysm into an adjacent vein. Congenital arteriovenous malformation (hemangioma) is discussed in Chapter 12.

Extrinsic impressions on the pelvocalyceal system and ureter are also caused by collateral arteries and veins and by varices. Collateral circulation develops in response to main vessel occlusion and provides channels for renal arterial flow around a major arterial stenosis or occlusion or for venous drainage when the

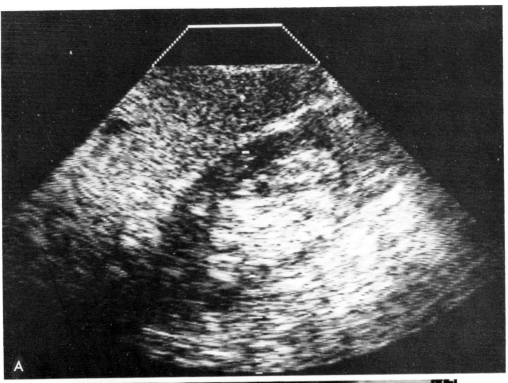

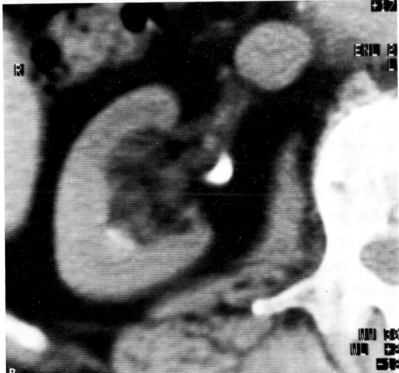

Figure 16–9. Renal sinus lipomatosis of the right kidney.

   A, Ultrasonogram, longitudinal section. The high-intensity echoes generated by the proliferated fat and other contents of the renal sinus occupy a larger than normal space.

   B, Computed tomogram, contrast material enhanced. The renal sinus contains a large volume of fat that surrounds the blood vessels. (See Fig. 16–3 for this patient's excretory urogram.)

main renal vein or inferior vena cava is occluded. Collateral pathways develop from existing vascular systems, such as the pelvic, ureteral, gonadal, adrenal, capsular, or lumbar arteries or veins as well as the ascending lumbar veins. Vascular dilatation in response to increased blood flow causes multiple impressions on the pelvocalyceal system and proximal ureter. Varices do not necessarily indicate renal vein obstruction. Any condition that increases renal blood flow, such as arteriovenous aneurysm (fistula) and vascular adenocarcinoma, may cause varices. Varices are also associated with congenital extrarenal venous malformations (left-sided or double inferior vena cava and circumaortic or retroaortic left renal vein), occlusion of the inferior vena cava, or portal vein hypertension with splenorenal shunt. Compression of the left renal vein between the aorta and the superior mesenteric artery is another cause of a renal varix that is invariably left sided. Chapters 6, 7, 21, and 26 contain additional discussions of aneurysms and collateral circulation.

Clinical Setting

Normal arteries or veins impinging on the pelvocalyceal system or ureter rarely cause symptoms. Nephralgia due to the partial obstruction, by crossing vessels, of the infundibulum that drains upper pole calyces, the so-called Fraley's syndrome, occurs rarely.

Atherosclerotic aneurysms are usually discovered in older age groups, frequently those beyond the sixth decade. Clinical abnormalities ascribed to renal artery aneurysms include flank pain, palpable mass, bruit, and hematuria. Spontaneous rupture and hyperreninemic hypertension are major complications. Aneurysms in women of child-bearing age are predisposed to spontaneous rupture during pregnancy.

Arterial dysplasia develops most frequently in women before the fifth decade. Renovascular hypertension dominates the clinical findings in these patients. Spontaneous dissection may lead to renal infarction with flank pain and hematuria. Dysplastic aneurysm per se does not cause symptoms.

The signs and symptoms of arteriovenous aneurysm (fistula) are caused by high-volume shunts. A continuous bruit in the flank or abdomen associated with a thrill is frequently present. Wide pulse pressure and diastolic hypertension may be noted. The latter is caused by the renal ischemia that follows shunting of arterial blood away from functional renal tissue. Patients with large-volume shunts are at risk for high-output congestive failure.

Renal arterial collateral circulation develops in patients with renovascular hypertension and causes no direct clinical abnormalities. Renal varices, on the other hand, cause both flank pain and hematuria, presumably from congestion of submucosal venous channels.

Right flank pain and urinary tract infection in young, parous women with dilatation of the proximal ureter has been called the "ovarian vein syndrome." These findings have been ascribed to varix or thrombosis of the right ovarian vein, which crosses the right ureter at approximately the level of the third lumbar vertebra. This syndrome, however, has not been established as a definite clinical entity.

Radiologic Findings

Normal Artery and Vein

Normal arteries produce extrinsic impressions on the pelvocalyceal system in several locations and patterns that are seen during excretory urography. The most common one is a thin linear radiolucency that crosses the superior pole infundibulum, the ureteropelvic junction, or the pelvis itself. Proximal dilatation and delayed emptying may be noted. Caliectasis due to narrowing of an infundibulum by a crossing vessel is a rare cause of nephralgia, a condition known as Fraley's syndrome. Another pattern caused by a normal artery is a concave impression on an infundibulum or the pelvis, which viewed *en face* may simulate a mural or intraluminal lesion. Steep oblique projections establish the parapelvic origin of the "filling defect" (Fig. 16–10). The arterial nature of these pelvocalyceal deformities can be established by Doppler ultrasound techniques or by arteriography and an overlay of films, but this is rarely required.

Normal renal veins cause smooth linear radiolucencies that are oriented in a horizontal or slightly oblique direction across the renal pelvis or infundibula—especially the one draining the upper pole (Figs. 16–11 and 16–12). Venous impressions are wider than those caused by arteries and change in size during the Valsalva maneuver or as the patient's position is changed. Distention of the pelvis or ureter usually effaces a venous impression but will not completely obliterate an arterial one. Steep oblique projections help to establish the parapelvic location of normal renal veins. The need for Doppler ultrasound techniques or venography is rare. The normal right gonadal vein may produce an impression on the right ureter at approximately the level of the third lumbar vertebra.

Aneurysm

Excretory Urography. Annular calcification, which occurs in more than 50 per cent of atherosclerotic renal artery aneurysms (Fig. 16–13; see also Figs. 6–1, 6–2, 6–4, and 6–6), may be confused with curvilinear calcification in kidney or gallbladder stones; lymph nodes; splenic artery aneurysms; or adrenal, parapelvic, or nephrogenic cysts. Occasionally, an aneurysm is detected as a soft tissue mass that is accentuated by surrounding sinus fat. A large renal artery aneurysm produces a concave extrinsic deformity on the adjacent portion of the pelvocalyceal system (Fig. 16–14). If viewed *en face,* this may simulate a mural mass. An aneurysm that causes renovascular ischemia may also produce notching of the pelvis by collateral arteries and other urographic features of renovascular ischemia, which are described in Chapter 6. Dysplastic or

Text continued on page 551

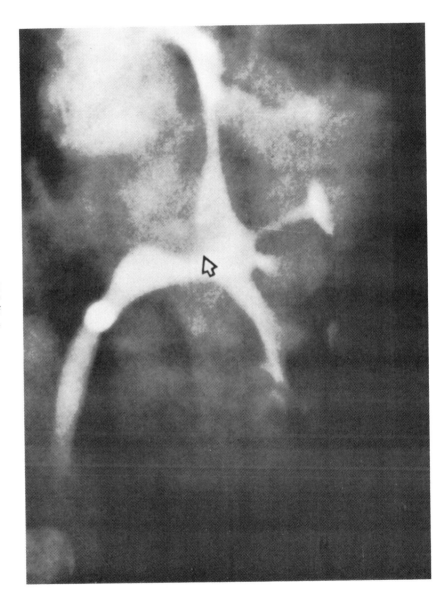

Figure 16–10. Arterial impression on the renal pelvis (arrow). A normal artery was identified by angiography. Excretory urogram. (Courtesy of Thomas A. Freed, M.D., Marin General Hospital, Greenbrae, California.)

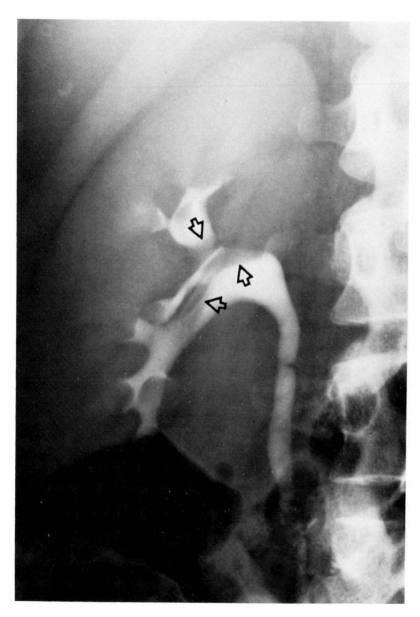

Figure 16–11. Venous impression on the renal pelvis *(arrows)*. Normal veins were identified by venography. Excretory urogram. (Courtesy of Jonathan Fish, M.D., and Daniel Kaplan, M.D., John Muir Hospital, Walnut Creek, California.)

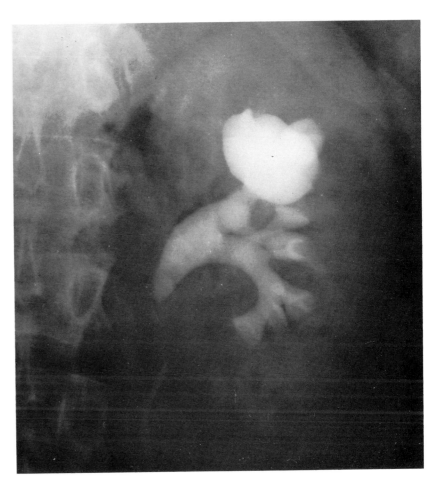

Figure 16–12. Caliectasis caused by a renal vein crossing and compressing the infundibulum of the upper pole calyx. Excretory urogram.

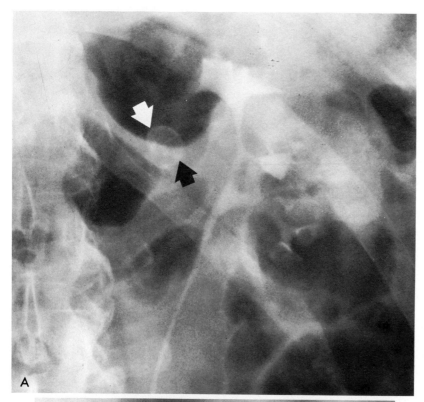

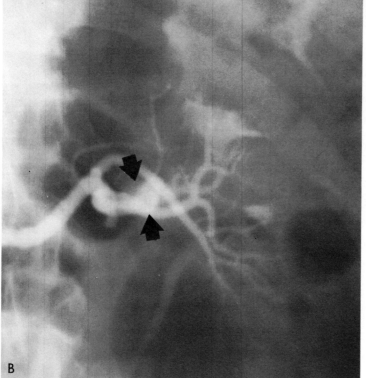

Figure 16–13. Saccular, atherosclerotic renal artery aneurysm with annular calcification *(arrows).*
  A, Excretory urogram.
  B, Renal arteriogram, arterial phase. Arrows define opacification of the aneurysmal sac.

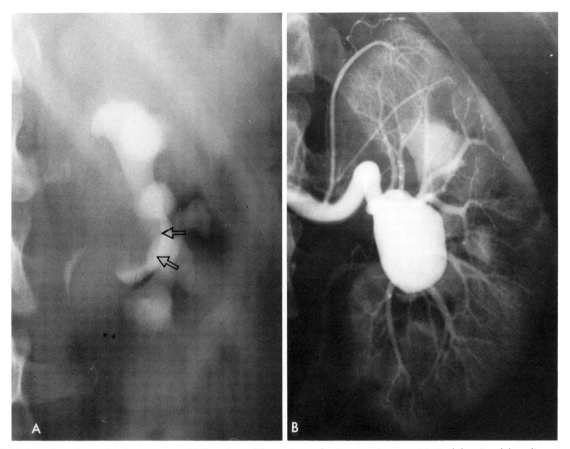

Figure 16–14. Saccular, atherosclerotic aneurysm at bifurcation of the main renal artery, causing an extrinsic deformity of the adjacent portion of the pelvis *(arrows)*.
   A, Excretory urogram.
   B, Renal arteriogram, arterial phase.

arteriovenous aneurysms of the renal artery cause urographic abnormalities that are similar to those of atherosclerosis (Fig. 16–15). Renal vein varices caused by arteriovenous aneurysm (fistula) may form a parapelvic mass as well as peripelvic and periureteral notches.

Atherosclerotic aneurysm of the aorta may cause lateral displacement of the left ureter in a manner similar to the various retroperitoneal masses that are discussed in Chapter 21. An aneurysm of the common iliac artery causes an abrupt deviation of the ureter, which passes anterior to the artery.

Angiography. Angiography is the definitive method for studying aneurysms. Atherosclerotic aneurysms are located in the proximal portion of the main renal artery or distally at bifurcations. Most are saccular (see Fig. 16–13 and 16–14). The lumen is sometimes partially filled with thrombus that obscures the true size of the aneurysm. Washout of injected contrast material from the aneurysmal sac is often delayed (Fig. 16–16). Fusiform aneurysms usually form just distal to an arterial stenosis (Fig. 16–17). Occasionally, atherosclerotic narrowing or occlusion is found in the arterial segment just distal to the aneurysm. An aortogram as well as a selective renal arteriogram is necessary to demonstrate the collateral circulation completely.

The appearance of renal arterial dysplasia varies with the histologic type. Fusiform dilatation just distal to a narrow annular radiolucent band characterizes intimal fibroplasia (Fig. 16–18). These occur in major segmental branches as well as in the main renal artery. The occurrence of multiple, small, repetitive circumarterial dilatations that protrude beyond the circumference of the normal proximal artery, the so-called string of beads, is the angiographic pattern of medial fibroplasia (Fig. 16–19). The other form of renal artery dysplasia, subadventitial fibroplasia, is associated with deformities that are not, strictly, aneurysmal in that true dilatation is absent (Fig. 16–20).

Angiography of arteriovenous aneurysms (fistulas) requires large volumes of rapidly injected contrast material because of the rapid blood flow through these lesions. Nearly immediate venous opacification is the hallmark of arteriovenous aneurysm (see Fig. 16–15). Frequently, multiple serpiginous arteriovenous channels are opacified. Large shunts cause decreased nephrographic density. These angiographic findings can be duplicated by a highly vascular adenocarcinoma.

Ultrasonography. On ultrasonography, any saccular aneurysm produces findings of a fluid-filled mass. Identification of entering and exiting vessels confirms the diagnosis of aneurysm, but such precise anatomic

Text continued on page 557

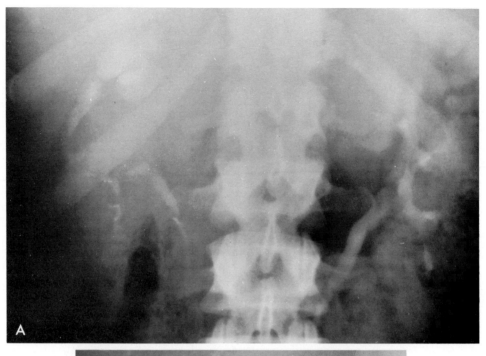

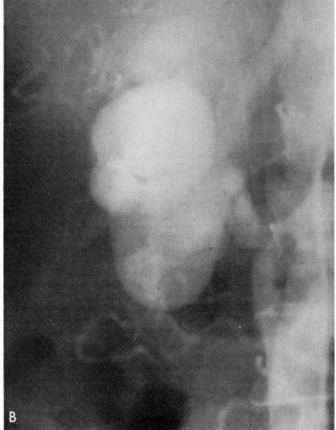

Figure 16–15. Post-traumatic arteriovenous aneurysm (fistula) following a penetrating wound of the right flank. The patient developed hypertension and a right abdominal bruit.

A, Excretory urogram. The upper pole and interpolar collecting systems are displaced and obstructed by the aneurysm.

B, Aortogram. A large arterial and venous chamber is opacified.

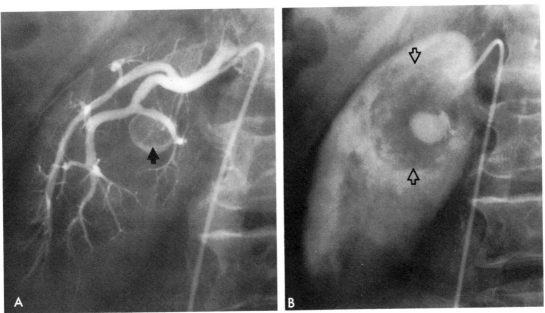

Figure 16–16. Saccular, atherosclerotic aneurysm with a thrombus partially filling the lumen *(solid arrow)*. The aneurysm had bled spontaneously and was surrounded by hematoma *(open arrows)*.
   A, Renal arteriogram, arterial phase.
   B, Renal arteriogram, nephrographic phase. There is delayed washout of contrast material from the aneurysmal sac.
(Courtesy of Joy Price, M.D., Alta Bates Medical Center, Berkeley, California.)

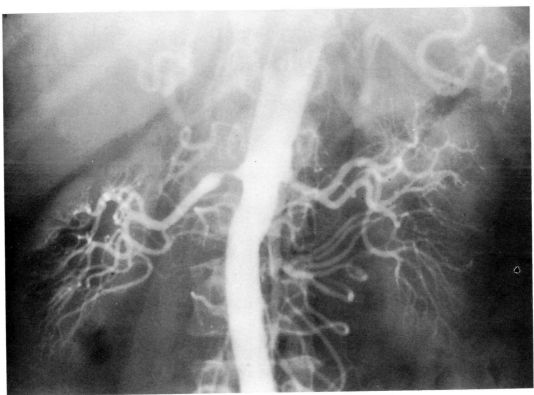

Figure 16–17. Fusiform atherosclerotic aneurysm in the right renal artery. Dilatation develops as a result of hemodynamic alterations, caused by an atherosclerotic stenosis immediately proximal to the aneurysm. Aortogram.

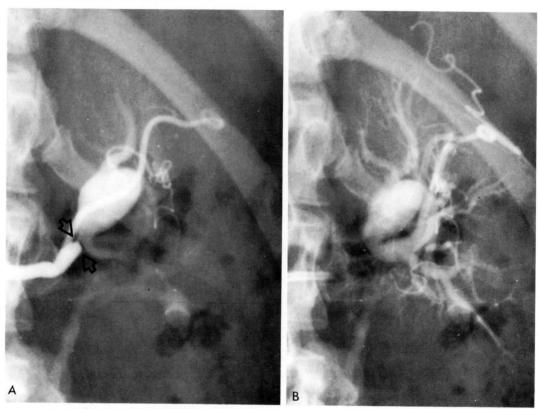

Figure 16–18. Intimal fibroplasia with post-stenotic fusiform aneurysm. This form of arterial dysplasia is characterized by a narrow annular band *(arrow).*
    A, Renal arteriogram, early phase.
    B, Renal arteriogram, late phase.
    (Courtesy of Janet Dacie, M.B., St. Bartholomew's Hospital, London, England.) (Same patient as illustrated in Figs. 6–7 and 16–21.)

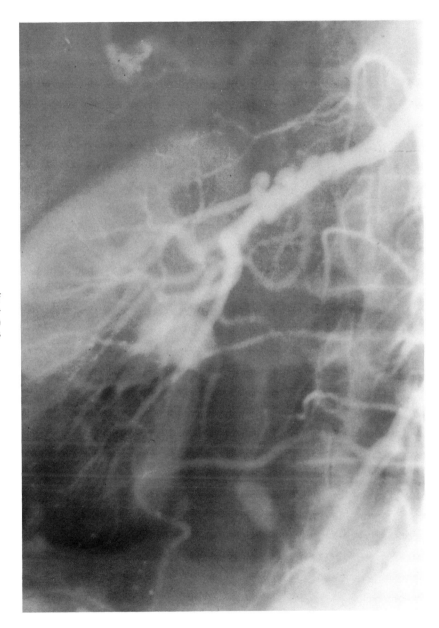

Figure 16–19. Medial fibroplasia. In this form of renal artery dysplasia there are repetitive circumarterial dilatations that protrude beyond the margin of the normal artery. Aortogram (same patient as illustrated in Fig. 26–6).

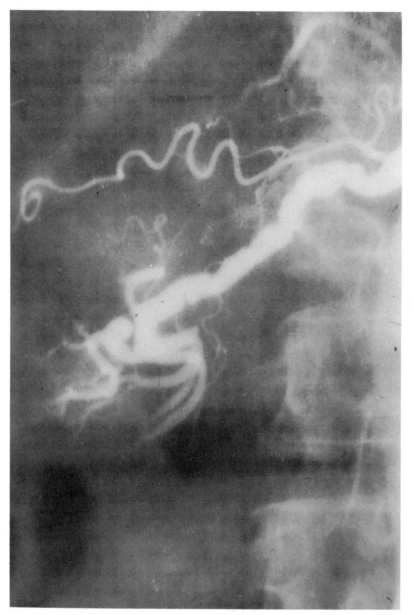

Figure 16–20. Subadventitial fibroplasia. True dilatation is absent in this type of renal artery dysplasia. Aortogram.

display is not always achieved. Flow patterns are most accurately established by Doppler techniques.

Computed Tomography and Magnetic Resonance Imaging. Computed tomography and magnetic resonance angiography are useful adjuncts in the evaluation of renal artery aneurysm. A saccular aneurysm appears as a renal sinus mass with attenuation values or signal intensity between those of water and soft tissue. The vascular nature of the mass is established by its rapid enhancement immediately following intravenous injection of a bolus of contrast material.

Collateral Circulation and Varices

Excretory Urography. Collateral arterial channels cause multiple, small, extrinsic indentations on the distended pelvocalyceal system and proximal ureter. The number and location of these indentations are determined by the site of renal artery narrowing or occlusion (Figs. 16–21 and 16–22). Notching may be limited to a single calyx or infundibulum when a segmental artery is occluded. Varices produce similar impressions on the collecting system and ureter but are usually broader or "scalloped" in comparison with the "notched" appearance of arterial collaterals

(Fig. 16–23). Additionally, varices may change in size as the patient moves from the prone to supine position or performs the Valsalva maneuver. Arterial collaterals are not subject to such variation.

Computed Tomography. Collateral arterial channels and varices are visualized as small soft tissue structures in the renal sinus or periureteral tissue. These may be confused with lymph nodes. Enhancement with contrast material, however, establishes the vascular nature of these structures.

Angiography. Arterial collaterals opacify during aortography and selective renal arteriography. Feeding vessels are enlarged and the collaterals are serpiginous; opacification is delayed (see Fig. 16–21 and 16–22). Branches of the renal artery distal to the occlusion also opacify late. Renal varices are gently undulating channels with broad lumina that opacify during the venous phase of an arteriogram (see Fig. 16–23). These are best opacified by selective venography. The techniques that facilitate venography include injection during the Valsalva maneuver, a balloon-occluding selective venous catheter, and venous injection immediately following selective renal artery injection of 6 to 8 µg of epinephrine to reduce renal blood flow and prolong venous washout time.

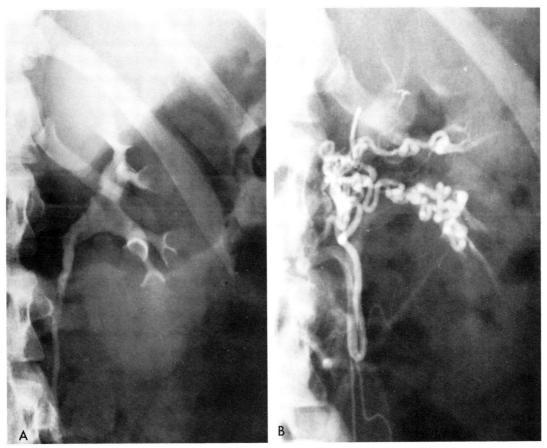

Figure 16–21. Renal arterial collaterals have caused multiple, small extrinsic indentations on the pelvis and proximal ureter of a 16-year-old girl with intimal fibroplasia of the left renal artery. (Same patient as illustrated in Figs. 6–7 and 16–18.)

A, Excretory urogram.

B, Renal arteriogram, delayed film. There are dilated, tortuous periureteric and peripelvic collaterals that correspond to the abnormalities depicted in *A*.

(Courtesy of Janet Dacie, M.B., St. Bartholomew's Hospital, London, England.)

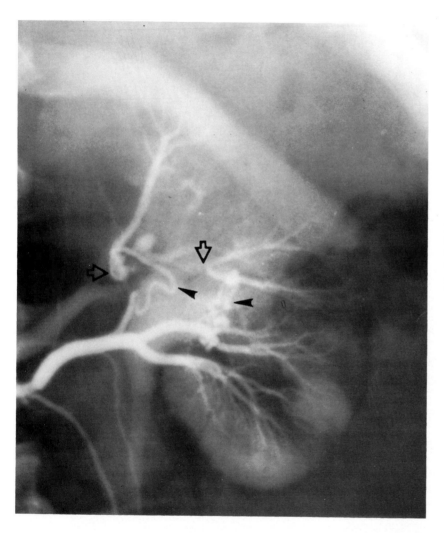

Figure 16–22. Intrarenal arterial collateral vessels *(solid arrows)* providing circulation to arcuate arteries distal to a major segmental artery occlusion *(open arrow).* This type of collateral pattern might cause notching limited to infundibula. Renal arteriogram. (Courtesy of Helen C. Redman, M.D., University of Texas at Dallas, Dallas, Texas.)

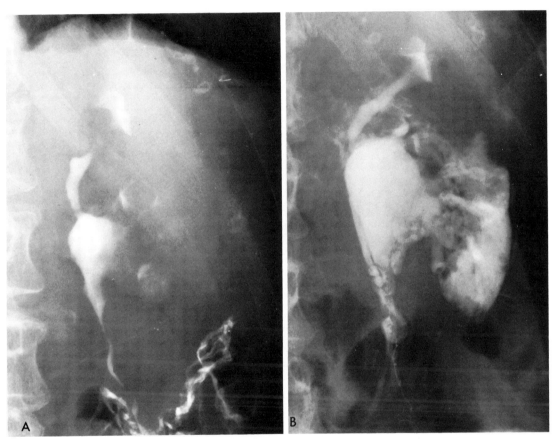

Figure 16–23. Venous collaterals. There are broad scalloped deformities of the pelvocalyceal system that correspond to dilated pelviureteric and peripelvic venous channels.

    A, Excretory urogram.

    B, Renal arteriogram, venous phase. Only a few of several renal veins have become opacified.

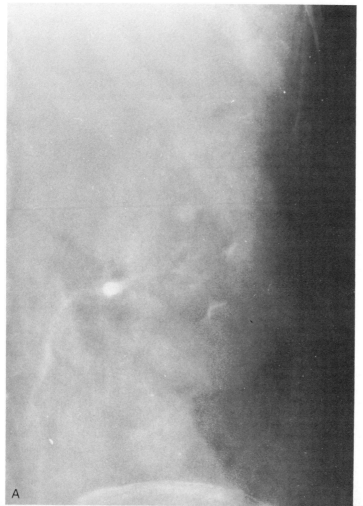

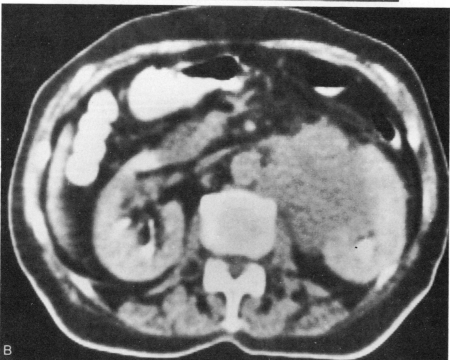

Figure 16–24. Lymphoma, retroperitoneum, in an 81-year-old woman. The lymphoma arises in the perirenal soft tissue space medial to the kidney, surrounds the pelvocalyceal system, and invades the kidney through the renal sinus.

A, Excretory urogram. The pelvis and most calyces are effaced by the infiltrating mass in the sinus.

B, Computed tomogram, contrast material enhanced. The left kidney is displaced laterally. A dilated calyx is opacified indicating obstructive uropathy.

SOLID TUMORS OF THE RENAL SINUS

Definition

Primary tumors of the renal sinus develop from any tissue within the renal sinus space. The various forms of lymphoma commonly involve sinus nodes, as discussed in Chapter 10. Fibroma, plasmacytoma, and myeloid metaplasia have also been reported in these structures. Metastases to sinus lymph nodes occur either as part of a generalized retroperitoneal process or as an isolated involvement, as with primary gonadal tumors.

Urine that leaks from the fornices of an obstructed pelvocalyceal system usually collects within the cone of the renal fascia that defines the outer limits of the perirenal space and forms a urinoma or uriniferous perirenal pseudocyst, which is discussed in Chapter 21. Uncommonly, leaked urine causes a granulomatous reaction in the renal sinus fat. A parapelvic urine granuloma containing loculated fluid is the result. These granulomas usually resolve spontaneously.

Clinical Setting

Primary renal sinus tumors may cause flank pain owing to obstructive uropathy or urinary tract infection. Symptoms of the primary underlying disease predominate in the case of renal sinus metastases.

Radiologic Findings

Soft tissue mass and focal deformity of the adjacent portion of the pelvocalyceal system are the major radiologic findings of renal sinus tumors and parapelvic urine granuloma (Fig. 16–24). A very large tumor displaces the kidney laterally and may cause anterior rotation. When renal sinus tumor is part of a diffuse infiltrating process, loss of perirenal fat, straightening, and displacement of the ureter and obliteration of the renal outline are noted.

Ultrasonography and computed tomography are particularly useful in identifying renal sinus masses (Fig. 16–25; see Fig. 16–24). Solid lesions cause echoes of varying intensity. Lymphoma, in particular, is associated with low-intensity echoes. Attenuation values on computed tomography are those of soft tissue. Following administration of intravenous contrast material, sinus masses enhance minimally, or not at all, reflecting the usual hypovascularity of retroperitoneal tumors.

A tumor that infiltrates the sinus often causes obstructive uropathy at the level of the renal pelvis. This is seen on contrast material–enhanced studies or ultrasonography as caliectasis without pelviectasis, the pelvis being prevented from distention by the surrounding infiltrative mass (see Figs. 16–24 and 16–25). The correct diagnosis of obstructive uropathy may be missed in this circumstance because of the absence of a dilated pelvis.

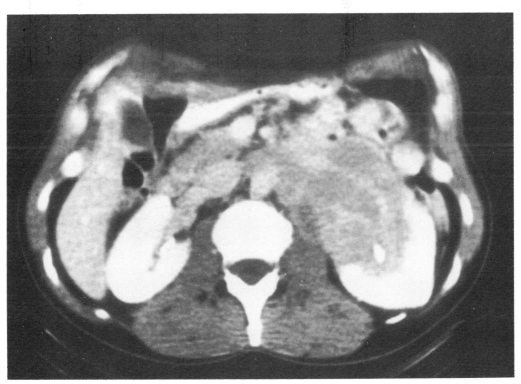

Figure 16–25. Lymphoma invading the left renal sinus in a 54-year-old man. Computed tomogram, contrast material enhanced. The kidney is displaced laterally. The tumor fills the renal sinus, causing obstructive uropathy without dilatation of the pelvis. A dilated calyx is present. The combination of caliectasis without pelviectasis is characteristic of large, infiltrating masses in the renal sinus.

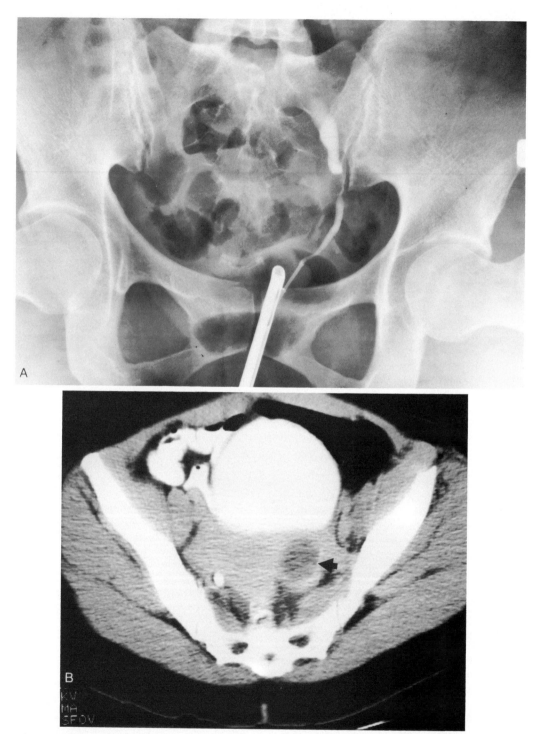

Figure 16–26. Endometriosis, left ureter.

A, Retrograde ureterogram. There is a sharply defined, smooth, concentric narrowing of a short segment of the ureter at the inferior margin of the sacroiliac joint. The proximal ureter is dilated.

B, Computed tomogram, contrast material enhanced. The endometrioma *(arrow)* is of low attenuation, representing cystic degeneration.

Illustration continued on following page

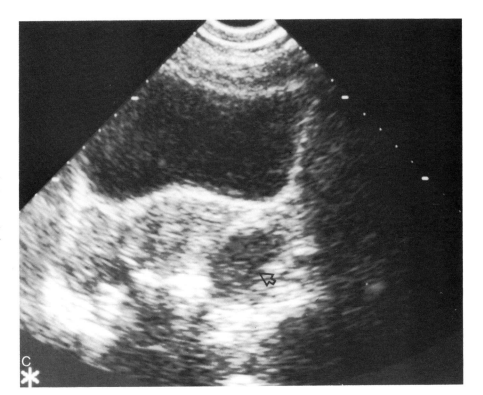

Figure 16–26 *Continued*
C, Ultrasonogram, transverse projection. The cystic endometrioma *(arrow)* is hypoechoic and contains low level echoes.
(Courtesy of Wendelin S. Hayes, D.O., Armed Forces Institute of Pathology, Washington, D.C.).

Studies of parapelvic urine granuloma with ultrasonography or computed tomography demonstrate an anechoic central component to these inflammatory soft tissue masses, which also have a corresponding area in which the attenuation value is that of water.

ENDOMETRIOSIS

Definition

Typical endometrial glands and stroma are found in ectopic locations in as many as 15 per cent of women in the child-bearing age. The mechanism for the development of endometriosis has not been clearly elucidated. Embryonic rests (müllerian duct), implantation from retrograde tubal menstruation, benign metastases, and metaplasia of coelomic epithelium have all been considered as possible explanations.

Urinary tract involvement is very uncommon and usually occurs in patients with endometriosis involving other parts of the pelvis. The bladder is far more often involved than is the ureter, as discussed in Chapter 19. The ectopic endometrium is usually extrinsic to the ureter and located in the adventitia and periureteral tissue. Less commonly, the lamina propria and muscularis are the sites of intrinsic involvement. The endometrial tissue, itself, may cause distortion of the ureter, or fibrosis may develop as a result of bleeding. Ureteral involvement is most often located at the level of the posterior attachment of the uterosacral ligament, a structure that is frequently involved in cases of pelvic endometriosis.

Clinical Setting

Ureteral endometriosis may be asymptomatic or cause flank pain, frequency, dysuria, or hematuria. Uncom-

monly, these clinical findings are related to the menstrual cycle. Although these features are usually seen only in women of child-bearing age, they may extend into the postmenopausal period.

Radiologic Findings

A smooth, tapered narrowing of a short segment of the distal one-third of the ureter is the radiologic appearance of endometriosis of the ureter (Fig. 16–26). The ureter distal to the stricture is normal. In some patients, a long segment of distal ureter is smoothly narrowed by surrounding endometrial implants (Fig. 16–27). The portion of the ureter that is involved is usually within 3 cm of the inferior margin of the sacroiliac joint, a level that corresponds to the attachment of the uterosacral ligament. Because the obstruction is often severe enough to cause hydronephrosis, visualization of the narrowed ureter may require direct retrograde or antegrade ureterography. Computed tomography or ultrasonography demonstrates the endometrial implant as a soft tissue mass usually of low attenuation or hypoechoic characteristics representing cystic degeneration (see Fig. 16–26).

NEOPLASTIC AND INFLAMMATORY INFILTRATION

The ureter may be displaced or obstructed at any level by adjacent lymph nodes that become enlarged by metastatic deposits from a distant primary neoplasm. The most common primary sites are breast, gastrointestinal tract, lung, or lymphoma. These are presented in Chapter 21 as part of a broader discussion of tumors in the retroperitoneum.

Neoplasms that originate in pelvic organs may ob-

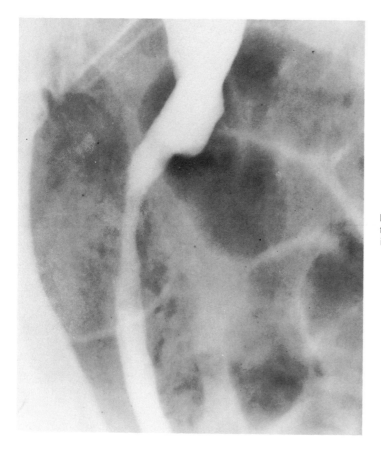

Figure 16–27. Endometriosis, distal right ureter. Retrograde ureterogram. A long segment of ureter is smoothly narrowed. There is proximal dilatation.

struct the distal ureter by direct extension to and invasion of the periureteral tissue. This complication is most often associated with carcinoma arising in the cervix, prostate, bladder, or rectosigmoid colon. A primary origin in the uterus or ovary may also grow in a similar pattern.

Ureteral deformity and obstruction may also be caused by Crohn's disease, appendicitis, diverticulitis, and pelvic inflammatory disease. Usually, the ureter is involved by direct extension of a phlegmon, abscess, or fistula. However, in some cases, periureteral fibrosis is the dominant response, and this may be remote from the primary site of inflammation. Crohn's disease of the terminal ileum and right colon and appendicitis affect the right ureter, whereas Crohn's disease of the jejunum or left colon and diverticulitis involve the left ureter. Ureteral involvement in these cases usually affects several centimeters of the ureter at the level of the pelvic brim.

Involvement of the ureter by neoplastic or inflammatory processes variably produces ureteral displacement, smooth or irregular narrowing, and/or obstruction and hydronephrosis (Fig. 16–28). Depending on the particular form and severity, these can be visualized by excretory urography or by antegrade or retrograde pyeloureterography. Computed tomography best demonstrates the periureteral component, which may be a mass that is isolated or one that is contiguous with a primary tumor or inflammatory process. Fibrosis alone causes thickening of the periureteral tissue.

URETERAL DEVIATION

The normal course of the ureter and the anomaly of retrocaval ureter are described in Chapter 3. There are numerous abnormalities extrinsic to the ureter that deviate its course. Aortic and iliac artery aneurysm are discussed earlier in this chapter. Others are described in Chapters 10 (lymphoma of the kidney), 19 (the bladder), and 21 (the retroperitoneum).

DIFFERENTIAL DIAGNOSIS

A mass in the renal sinus is usually manifested by focal displacement and effacement of the pelvocalyceal system. Unequivocal radiolucency, either on standard or tomographic films, strongly suggests the diagnosis of the focal form of renal sinus lipomatosis. Most often, the abnormality is of radiographic soft tissue density. Here, the diagnostic possibilities include parapelvic cyst, saccular aneurysm, and primary or metastatic tumor.

Ultrasonography, including Doppler evaluation, is valuable in the investigation of a parapelvic mass to establish the fluid content of a parapelvic cyst or a parapelvic urine granuloma or the vascular nature of a saccular aneurysm. In addition to flow characteristics, aneurysm is suggested when mural echoes generated by a thrombus are present. A thick wall surrounding an irregular fluid-filled cavity favors a diagnosis of urine granuloma. Focal fat deposit and solid tumor are the leading diagnostic possibilities

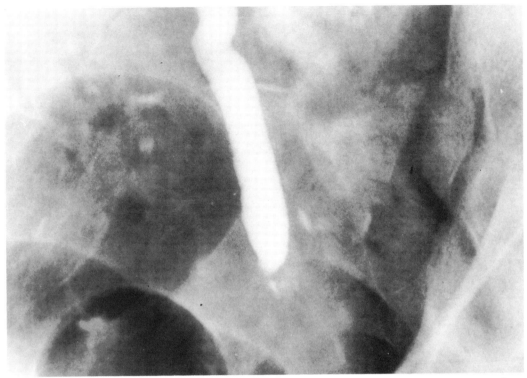

Figure 16–28. Local invasion of distal left ureter by metastatic carcinoma of the prostate. Antegrade pyelogram. There is irregular narrowing of the ureter with proximal dilatation.

when an echogenic mass without evidence of fluid is noted.

A negative computed tomographic attenuation value equal to that of perirenal fat conclusively identifies a tumorous fatty deposit. A diagnosis of saccular aneurysm is confidently established by rapid and marked enhancement of the "mass" after a bolus of intravenous contrast material is given. Angiography may still be necessary to establish the etiologic nature of the aneurysm. Computed tomography provides unequivocal evidence of the solid nature of primary and metastatic masses. Its application to the search for tumor in other parts of the retroperitoneum is basic. Finally, computed tomography may be useful in the assessment of parapelvic cyst or urine granuloma when these lesions yield equivocal findings on ultrasonographic evaluation.

Occasionally, a smooth extrinsic deformity of the collecting system develops from a process that originates in the renal parenchyma rather than in the renal sinus (Fig. 16–29). This occurs either with normal variants, such as lobar dysmorphism or a prominent hilar lip (see Chapter 3), or with true parenchymal masses, such as abscess, simple cyst, and adenocarcinoma (see Chapter 12). Normal variants usually deform infundibula or calyces, while abscess, tumor, or cyst alters the renal pelvis in addition to the peripheral collecting system. Invasion of the collecting system by malignant parenchymal tumor causes irregular pelvocalyceal deformities that simulate primary mural lesions, which are discussed in Chapter 15.

The key to differentiating extraparenchymal from parenchymal lesions that deform the pelvocalyceal system is the evaluation of the nephrogram adjacent to the mass. An intact nephrogram favors a diagnosis of a disorder that arises in the renal sinus. Disruption of the nephrogram indicates a renal parenchymal process that extends into a portion of the renal sinus. This holds true except when a malignant process of the renal sinus invades the adjacent parenchyma, a very uncommon event. The technique used to evaluate the integrity of the renal parenchyma varies with individual circumstances and might include excretory urography with tomography, radionuclide scan, computed tomography, or renal angiography (see discussion in Chapter 23).

Generalized attenuation of the pelvocalyceal system due to diffuse renal sinus lipomatosis can be reliably determined when the fatty nature of the excessive peripelvic tissue is established by characteristic findings on radiographs, tomograms, computed tomograms, ultrasonograms, or magnetic resonance imaging. These findings are absent when the collapse of the pelvocalyceal system is due to other causes, such as those discussed in Chapter 18. Generalized parapelvic cysts may deform the pelvocalyceal system in the same manner as renal sinus lipomatosis. In this situation, the fluid nature of the masses in the sinus is established by ultrasonography or computed tomography and their differentiation from hydronephrosis is established by enhancement of the attenuated pelvocalyceal system by contrast material.

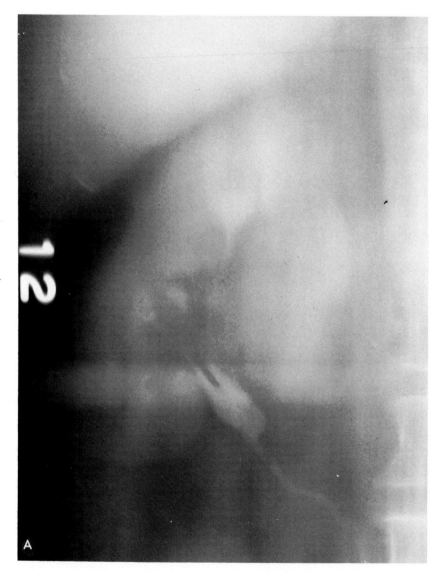

Figure 16–29. Adenocarcinoma of the right kidney presenting as a parapelvic mass. The tumor originates in the superior hilar lip and displaces the pelvocalyceal system downward.
A, Excretory urogram. Tomogram.

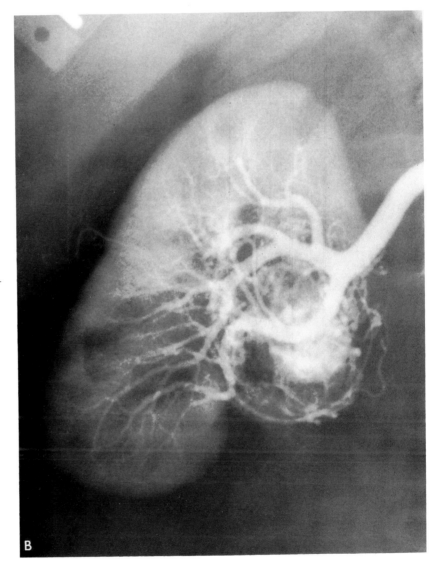

Figure 16–29 *Continued B,* Renal arteriogram, arterial phase.

Impressions on the pelvis or ureter by normal or abnormal blood vessels can be differentiated from other causes by demonstration of contrast enhancement of the arteries or veins during computed tomography or by direct visualization of the responsible vessels during angiography.

Ureteral narrowing or deformity due to the extrinsic causes discussed in this chapter are often identical in appearance to those produced by many of the mural abnormalities presented in Chapter 15. Differentiation is usually dependent on a distinctive clinical history or the demonstration of coexistent pathology such as endometriosis, Crohn's disease, diverticulitis, or the other entities that are discussed.

Bibliography

General

Fein, A. B., and McClennan, B. L.: Solitary filling defects of the ureter. Semin. Roentgenol. 21:201, 1986.

Malek, R. S., Aguilo, J. J., and Hattery, R. R.: Radiolucent filling defects of the renal pelvis: Classification and report of unusual cases. J. Urol. 114:508, 1975.

Pfister, R. C., and Newhouse, J. H.: Radiology of the ureter. Urology 12:15, 1978.

Williamson, B, Jr., Hartman, G. W., and Hattery, R. R.: Multiple and diffuse ureteral filling defects. Semin. Roentgenol. 21:214, 1986.

Parapelvic Cyst

Amis, E. S., Jr., Cronan, J. J., and Pfister, R. C.: Pseudohydronephrosis on noncontrast computed tomography. J. Comput. Assist. Tomogr, 6:511, 1982.

Amis, E. S., Jr., Cronan, J. J., and Pfister, R. C.: The spectrum of peripelvic cysts. Br. J. Urol. 55:150, 1983.

Amis, E. S., Jr., and Cronan, J. J.: The renal sinus: An imaging review and proposed nomenclature for sinus cysts. J. Urol. 139:1151, 1988.

Androvlakakis, P. A., Kirayiannis, B., and Deliveliotis, A.: The parapelvic renal cyst: A report of 8 cases with particular emphasis on diagnosis and management. Br. J. Urol. 52:342, 1980.

Bernstein, J.: The classification of renal cysts. Nephron 11:91, 1973.

Chan, J. C. M., and Kodroff, M. B.: Hypertension and hematuria secondary to parapelvic cyst. Pediatrics 65:821, 1980.

Cronan, J. J., Amis, E. S., Jr., Yoder, I. C., Kopans, D. B., Simeone, J. F., and Pfister, R. C.: Peripelvic cysts: An impostor of sonographic hydronephrosis. J. Ultrasound Med. 1:229, 1982.

Crummy, A. B., and Madsen, P. O.: Parapelvic renal cyst: The peripheral fat sign. J. Urol. 96:436, 1966.

Dana, A., Musset, D., Ody, B., Rethers, C., Lepage, T., Moreau, J.-F., and Michel, J.-R.: Abnormal renal sinus: Sonography patterns of multilocular parapelvic cysts. Urol. Radiol. 5:227, 1983.

Deliveliotis, A., and Kavadis, C.: Parapelvic cysts of the kidney: Report of seven cases. Br. J. Urol. 41:386, 1969.

Dubilier, W., Jr., and Evans, J. A.: Parapelvic cysts of the kidney. Radiology 71:409, 1958.

Hidalgo, H., Dunnick, N. R., Rosenberg, E. R., Ram, P. C., and Korbkin, M.: Parapelvic cysts: Appearance on CT and sonography. AJR 138:667, 1982.

Meier, W. L., Willscher, M. K., Novicki, D. E., and Pischinger, R. J.: Evaluation of perihilar and central renal masses using Chiba needle. J. Urol. 12:414, 1979.

Morag, B., Rubinstein, Z. J., and Solomon, A.: Computed tomography in the diagnosis of renal parapelvic cysts. J. Comput. Assist. Tomogr. 7:833, 1983.

Ralls, P. W., Esensten, M. L., Boger, D., and Halls, J. M.: Severe hydronephrosis and severe renal cystic disease: Ultrasonic differentiation. AJR 134:473, 1980.

Steel, J. F., Howe, G. E., Feeney, M. J., and Blum, J. A.: Spontaneous remission of peripelvic renal cysts. J. Urol. 114:10, 1975.

Renal Sinus Lipomatosis

Ambos, M. A., Bosniak, M. A., Gordon, R., and Madayag, M. A.: Replacement lipomatosis of the kidney. AJR 130:1087, 1978.

Case records of the Massachusetts General Hospital. Case 14-1974. N. Engl. J. Med. 290:845, 1974.

Downey, E. F., Friedman, A. C., Hartman, D. S., Pyatt, R. S., Thane, T. T., and Warnock, G. R.: Pseudocystic CT pattern of renal sinus lipomatosis. Radiology 144:840, 1982.

Fuegenburg, D., Bosniak, M., and Evans, J. A.: Renal sinus lipomatosis: Its demonstration by nephrotomography. Radiology 83:987, 1964.

Hadar, H., and Meiraz, D.: Renal sinus lipomatosis: Differentiation from space-occupying lesion with aid of computer tomography. Urology 15:86, 1980.

Honda, H., McGuire, C. W., Barloon, T. J., and Hashimoto, K.: Replacement lipomatosis of the kidney: CT features. J. Comput. Assist. Tomogr. 14:229, 1990.

Hurwitz, R. S., Benjamin, J. A., and Cooper, J. F.: Excessive proliferation of peripelvic fat of the kidney. Urology 11:448, 1978.

Scheinman, L. J., and Reibman, S. J.: Peripelvic fat simulating renal pelvic tumor. J. Urol. 123:564, 1980.

Subramanyam, B. R., Bosniak, M. A., Horii, S. C., Megibow, A. J., and Balthazar, E. J.: Replacement lipomatosis of the kidney: Diagnosis by computed tomography and sonography. Radiology 148:791, 1983.

Windholz, F.: The roentgen appearance of the central fat tissue of the kidney: Its significance in urography. Radiology 56:202, 1951.

Yeh, H.-C., Mitty, H. A., and Wolfe, B. S.: Ultrasonography of renal sinus lipomatosis. Radiology 124:799, 1977.

Vascular

Abrams, H. L., and Cornell, S. H.: Patterns of collateral flow in renal ischemia. Radiology 84:1001, 1965.

Altebarmakian, V. K., Caldamone, A. A., Dachelet, R. J., and May, A. G.: Renal artery aneurysm. Urology 13:257, 1979.

Angel, J. L., and Knuppel, R. A.: Computed tomography in diagnosis of puerperal ovarian vein thrombosis. Obstet. Gynecol. 63:61, 1984.

Baum, S., and Gillenwater, J. Y.: Renal artery impressions on the renal pelvis. J. Urol. 95:139, 1966.

Beckman, C. F., and Abrams, H. L.: Idiopathic renal vein varices: Incidence and significance. Radiology 143:649, 1982.

Beinart, C., Sniderman, K. W., Saddekni, S., Weiner, M., Vaughn, E. D., Jr., and Sos, T. A.: Left renal vein hypertension: A cause of occult hematuria. Radiology 145:647, 1982.

Boijsen, E., and Köhler, R.: Renal artery aneurysm. Acta Radiol. (Diagn.) 1:1077, 1963.

Castaneda-Zuniga, W., Zollikofer, C., Valdez-Davila, O., Nath, P. H., and Amplatz, K.: Giant aneurysms of the renal arteries: An unusual manifestation of fibromuscular dysplasia. Radiology 133:327, 1979.

Cerny, J. C., Chang, C.-Y., and Fry, W. J.: Renal artery aneurysms. Arch. Surg. 96:653, 1968.

Chait, A., Matasar, K. W., Fabian, C. E., and Mellins, H. Z.: Vascular impressions on the ureters. AJR 111:729, 1971.

Cleveland, R. H., Fellows, K. E., and Lebowitz, R. L.: Notching of the ureter and renal pelvis in children. AJR 129:837, 1977.

Derrick, F. C., Rosenblum, R. R., and Lynch, K. M., Jr.: Pathological association of the right ureter and right ovarian vein. J. Urol. 97:633, 1967.

Dykhuizen, R. F., and Roberts, J. A.: The ovarian vein syndrome. Surg. Gynecol. Obstet. 130:443, 1970.

Ekelund, L., Boijsen, E., and Lindstedt, E.: Pseudotumor of the renal pelvis caused by renal artery aneurysm. Acta Radiol. (Diagn.) 20:753, 1979.

Fishman, M. C., Pollack, H. M., Arger, P. H., and Banner, M. P.: Radiographic manifestations of spontaneous renal sinus hemorrhage. AJR 142:161, 1984.

Fraley, E. E.: Vascular obstruction of superior infundibulum causing nephralgia. N. Engl. J. Med. 275:1403, 1966.

Hayashi, M., Kume, T., and Nihira, H.: Abnormalities of renal venous system and unexplained renal hematuria. J. Urol. 124:12, 1980.

Kreel, L., and Pyle, R.: Arterial impressions on the renal pelvis. Br. J. Radiol. 35:609, 1962.

Lefleur, R. S., Ambos, M. A., and Rotheberg, M.: An unusual vascular impression on the renal pelvis. Urol. Radiol. 1:117, 1979.

Lien, H. H., and vonKrogh, J.: Varicosity of the left renal ascending lumbar communicant vein: A pitfall in CT diagnosis. Radiology 152:484, 1984.

Meng, C.-H., and Elkin, M.: Venous impression on the calyceal system. Radiology 87:878, 1966.

Mintz, M. C., Levy, D. W., Axel, L., Kressel, H. Y., et al.: Puerperal ovarian vein thrombosis: MR diagnosis. AJR 149:1273, 1987.

Painter, W. E., Di Donato, R. R., and White, R.: Renal arteriovenous aneurysm causing hydronephrosis and renal atrophy. AJR 104:306, 1968.

Pearson, J. C., Tanagho, E. A., and Palubinskas, A. J.: Non-operative diagnosis of pyelocalyceal deformity due to venous impressions. Urology 13:207, 1979.

Peterson, R. A., and Peterson, L. R.: Renal varices. J. Can. Assoc. Radiol. 31:54, 1980.

Poutasse, E. F.: Renal artery aneurysms. J. Urol. 113:443, 1975.

Rosenthal, J. T., Costello, P., and Roth, R. A.: Varicosities of renal venous system. Urology 15:427, 1980.

Slominski-Laws, M. D., Kiefer, J. H., and Vermeulen, C. W.: Arteriovenous aneurysm of the kidney. J. Urol. 75:586, 1956.

Smith, J. N., and Hinman, F., Jr.: Intrarenal arterial aneurysms. J. Urol. 97:990, 1967.

Steiner, R. M., and Wexler, L.: Renal arteriovenous fistula: Unique finding in the Marfan syndrome. J. Urol. 106:631, 1971.

Stewart, B. H., Dustan, H. P., Kiser, W. S., Meaney, T. F., Straffon, R. A., and McCormack, L. J.: Correlation of angiography and natural history in evaluation of patients with renovascular hypertension. J. Urol. 104:231, 1970.

Wendel, R. G., Crawford, E. D., and Hehman, K. N.: "Nutcracker" phenomenon: Unusual cause for renal varicosities with hematuria. J. Urol. 123:761, 1980.

Tumor of the Renal Sinus

Ambos, M. A., Bosniak, M. A., Megibow, A. J., and Raghavendra, B.: Ureteral involvement by metastatic disease. Urol. Radiol. 1:105, 1979.

Barbaric, Z. L., and Frank, I. N.: Peripelvic renal pseudocyst due to obstruction. AJR 129:1097, 1977.

Friedman, A. C., Hartman, D. S., Sherman, J., Lautin, E. M., and Goldman, M.: Computed tomography of abdominal fatty masses. Radiology 139:415, 1981.

Grossman, I. W., and Kopilnick, M. D.: Peripelvic renal fibroma: Radiographical, pathological and ultrastructural study of a unique lesion. J. Urol. 105:174, 1971.

Olivares, R. L., Jr., McDaniel, E. C., McCallum, D. C., and Mackenzie, J. R.: Peripelvic urine granuloma simulating a renal neoplasm. J. Urol. 107:693, 1972.

Redlin, L., Francis, R. S., and Orlando, M. M.: Renal abnormalities in agnogenic myeloid metaplasia. Radiology 12:605, 1976.

Rubin, B. E.: Computed tomography in the evaluation of renal lymphoma. J. Comput. Assist. Tomogr. 3:759, 1979.

Silver, T. M., Thornbury, J. R., and Teears, R. J.: Renal peripelvic plasmacytoma: Unusual radiographic findings. AJR 128:313, 1977.

Endometriosis

Bennington, J. L., and Beckwith, J. B.: Tumors of the Kidney, Renal Pelvis, and Ureter. AFIP Atlas of Tumor Pathology, second series, fascicle 12. Washington, D.C., Armed Forces Institute of Pathology, 1975.

Hill, G. S.: Uropathology. New York, Churchill Livingstone, 1989.

Kane, C., and Drovin, P.: Obstructive uropathy associated with endometriosis. Am. J. Obstet. Gynecol. 151:207, 1985.

Langmade, C. F.: Pelvic endometriosis and ureteral obstruction. Am. J. Obstet. Gynecol. 122:463, 1975.

Laube, D. W., Calderwood, G. S., and Benda, J. A.: Endometriosis causing ureteral obstruction. Obstet. Gynecol. 65:695, 1985.

Lucero, S. P., Wise, H. A., Kirsh, G., Devoe, K., Hess, M. L., Kandawalla, N. C., and Drago, J. R.: Ureteric obstruction secondary to endometriosis. Br. J. Urol. 61:201, 1988.

Older, R. A.: Endometriosis of the genitourinary tract. In Pollack, H. M. (ed.): Clinical Urography. Philadelphia, W.B. Saunders, 1990, pp. 2485–2492.

Olive, D. L., and Schwartz, L. B.: Endometriosis. N. Engl. J. Med. 328:1759, 1993.

Pollack, H. M., and Wills, J. J.: Radiographic features of ureteral endometriosis. AJR 131:627, 1978.

Reddy, A. N., and Evans, A. T.: Endometriosis of the ureters. J. Urol. 111:474, 1974.

Shook, T. E., and Nyberg, L. M.: Endometriosis of the urinary tract. Urology 31:1, 1988.

Stiehm, W. D., Becker, J. A., and Weiss, R. M.: Ureteral endometriosis. Radiology 102:563, 1972.

Neoplastic and Inflammatory Infiltration

Abrams, H. L., Spiro, R., and Goldstein, N.: Metastases in carcinoma: Analysis of 1000 autopsied cases. Cancer 3:74, 1950.

Cohen, W. M., Freed, S. Z., and Hasson, J.: Metastatic cancer of the ureter: A review of the literature and case presentations. J. Urol. 112:188, 1974.

Demos, T. C., and Moncada, R.: Inflammatory gastrointestinal disease presenting as genitourinary disease. Urology 13:115, 1979.

Gelister, J. S. K., Falzon, M., Crawford, R., Chapple, C. R., and Hendry, W. F.: Urinary tract metastasis from renal carcinoma. Br. J. Urol. 69:250, 1992.

Geller, S. A., Lin, C.-S.: Ureteral obstruction from metastatic breast carcinoma. Arch Pathol 99:476, 1975.

Miller, W. A., and Spear, J. L.: Periureteral and ureteral metastases from carcinoma of the cervix. Radiology 107:533, 1973.

Recloux, P., Weiser, M., Piccart, M., and Sculier, J. P.: Ureteral obstruction in patients with breast cancer. Cancer 61:1904, 1988.

Richie, J. P., Withers, G., and Ehrlich, R. M.: Ureteral obstruction secondary to metastatic tumors. Surg. Gynecol. Obstet. 148:355, 1979.

Shield, D. E., Lytton, B., Weiss, R. M., Schiff, M., Jr.: Urologic complications of inflammatory bowel disease. J. Urol. 115:701, 1976.

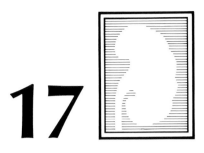

17

THE DILATED PELVOCALYCEAL SYSTEM

The uroradiologic tradition that equated dilatation of the urinary tract with obstruction has been in question ever since voiding cystourethrography first demonstrated that dilatation of nonobstructed upper tracts occurred solely as a consequence of vesicoureteral reflux. Now, the concept of nonobstructive dilatation of the renal collecting system and ureter is firmly established and multiple causes have been identified. Thus, proper analysis of a dilated upper urinary tract requires consideration of both obstructive and nonobstructive factors.

In the first section of this chapter the discussion is about the forces that propel urine from the calyces to the bladder. These forces are fundamental to an understanding of dilatation of the upper urinary tract, regardless of cause. Next, the variable pathophysiologic expressions of urinary tract obstruction and their radiologic analogues are described as a function of a continuum of time extending from acute to chronic. This discussion also takes into account those cases in which obstruction is intermediate, intermittent, or equivocal. The numerous specific causes of obstruction (e.g., congenital, neoplastic, inflammatory), presented in other chapters, are not enumerated. The concluding section of this chapter is a discussion of nonobstructive dilatation, particularly the specific conditions that are associated with this finding.

DYNAMICS OF URINE PROPULSION

The upper urinary tract is normally a low pressure system that contains a small volume of urine. *Peristalsis* is the principal force that propels urine forward. *Nephronic pressure* and *gravity* also contribute to the transport of urine through this system. It is useful to consider each of these factors when trying to understand the various circumstances of pelvocalyceal and ureteral dilatation.

Nephronic Pressure

Nephronic pressure is the hydrodynamic force imparted to tubule fluid by glomerular filtration and by the secretion and reabsorption of water and solutes by tubule cells. Each of these factors influences upper tract dilatation by their effect on the pressure and the volume of formed urine. For example, urine formation in acute extrarenal obstruction persists because the balance between continued perfusion of the glomerular capillaries and uninterrupted reabsorption of water by the distal tubules favors ongoing glomerular filtration, although at a reduced rate. The continued formation of urine in the presence of outflow obstruction, however, leads to slight dilatation of the upper tract to the point of the obstruction and invariable blunting with occasional rupture of the calyceal fornices, reflecting both volume and pressure increases. In diabetes insipidus, on the other hand, dilatation occurs without an obstructing lesion because nephrons produce a larger than normal volume of urine as a result of their inability to reabsorb water at the distal tubule and collecting duct level.

Peristalsis

Peristalsis originates in the proximal portion of the pelvocalyceal system, presumably at a pacemaker site in specially adapted calyceal muscle. The stimulus for contraction is thought to be passive stretching of the calyceal wall by urine. The electrical excitation that stimulates the contractile wave spreads from one smooth muscle cell to another through very close anatomic contacts called nexuses. Nerves play no role in the propagation of peristalsis. Muscle contraction first becomes visible in the renal pelvis and continues distally as a coordinated wave. The frequency of peristaltic contractions increases as the volume of urine increases. At very high urine flow rates, peristalsis ceases, and urine flows in a continuous column into the bladder, propelled by nephronic pressure and when the patient is upright, by gravity.

The concepts of Whitaker (1975) provide a comprehensive basis for understanding normal and abnormal peristalsis. The contraction wave that moves down the renal pelvis does not propel urine forward until it reaches a point at which the pelvis becomes funnel shaped, a configuration that permits apposition of its walls. The ureteropelvic junction is the site at which apposition first occurs. It is Whitaker's contention that apposition of the walls is essential for bolus formation and that bolus formation, in turn, is a prerequisite for peristalsis. Propulsion of urine from the ureteropelvic junction forward is the result of the resolution of the forces of contraction of the spirally arranged ureteric muscle into circular and longitudinal vectors in relation to the bolus. Effective peristalsis requires obliteration of the lumen of the ureter at the top of the bolus by a strong circular contraction, by relaxation ahead of the bolus, and by a longitudinally directed muscle contraction that has the effect of pulling the ureter

over the bolus. This sequence is illustrated in Figures 17-1 and 17-2.

A variety of disorders of peristalsis cause dilatation of the renal pelvis and ureter. These include abnormality in the shape of the ureteropelvic junction (discussed in Chapter 15), congenital or acquired deficiencies of the wall of the pelvis and ureter, and functional incoordination between the longitudinal and circular forces of muscular contraction, discussed in the concluding section of this chapter.

Gravity

The upright position favors forward flow of urine by adding the effect of gravity to that of nephron pressure and peristalsis. Under low to moderate flow conditions, peristalsis is very effective, and the relative contribution of gravity is minimal. This is not the case, however, when a high urine flow rate converts the pelvis and ureter into a wide column of continuously moving urine. Here, the contribution of peristalsis is negligible compared with that of nephronic pressure and gravity.

The role of gravity in emptying the collecting system is assessed by radiologic examination in the upright or prone position. This is an important step in evaluating the dilated pelvis and ureter. Emptying of a dilated system by placing a patient upright for a few minutes is evidence against obstruction. However, caution is required in interpretation of findings because in some cases of partial obstruction, gravity contributes the extra force needed to empty the con-

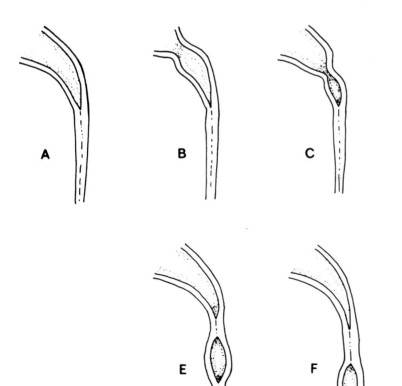

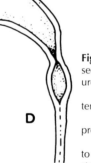

Figure 17–1. Schematic illustration of sequence of peristalsis at the normal ureteropelvic junction.

A, Normal funnel shape of the ureteropelvic junction at rest.

B and *C,* Peristaltic wave passes prograde through the pelvis.

D, Funnel shape of the pelvis leads to apposition of opposite walls as peristaltic wave progresses toward the ureter.

E, A bolus forms as a result of circular contraction of muscles proximally and relaxation of muscles distally.

F, Progression of bolus occurs as the longitudinally oriented force of muscle contraction "pulls" the ureter over the bolus.

(Courtesy of R. H. Whitaker, Addenbrooke's Hospital, Cambridge, England, and the Br. J. Urol. *47*:377, 1975.)

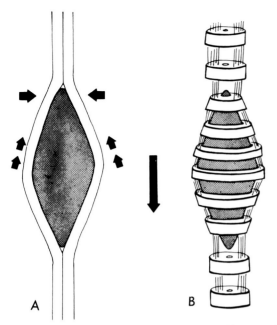

Figure 17–2. Schematic illustration of the resolution of forces and the ureteral muscle action in normal ureteral peristalsis.

A, Resolution of forces into circular and longitudinal sectors in relation to the bolus.

B, Representation of muscle contraction and relaxation in relation to the bolus.

(Courtesy of R. H. Whitaker, Addenbrooke's Hospital, Cambridge, England, and the Br. J. Urol. *47:*377, 1975.)

tents of a proximally dilated system across a narrowed segment. On the other hand, dilatation proximal to a narrowing that persists in the upright position is evidence for obstruction.

OBSTRUCTIVE UROPATHY

Whitaker defines urinary tract obstruction as a "narrowing such that the proximal pressure must be raised to transmit the usual flow through it" (1975). This implies that neither *dilatation nor increased pelvic pressure is invariably present in obstruction,* although some degree of dilatation is usually present. According to this definition, the diagnosis of obstruction requires the measurement of hydrostatic pressure proximal and distal to a demonstrable narrowing at known urine flow rates. The pressure/flow technique of Whitaker, described in Chapter 15, is the invasive method by which these parameters can be studied directly. However, the goal for assessing the dilated upper urinary tract is to use the various imaging modalities that indirectly measure these elements, allowing the radiologist to avoid, whenever possible, the need for invasive techniques.

In obstruction, the degree of collecting system dilatation and of damage to the structure and function of the kidney is determined by both the chronicity and the severity of the offending lesion. Acute obstruction creates a constellation of abnormalities quite distinct from those created by chronic obstruction (Fig. 17–3). Radiologic patterns in intermittent obstruction differ from those seen with unrelenting lesions. Each of these are considered in the following sections.

Acute Obstruction

Driven by hemodynamic pressure from perfusion of glomerular capillaries, urine production continues in acute obstruction, although at a greatly reduced rate. Hydrostatic pressure proximal to the obstruction rises as newly formed urine moves into the obstructed system. Urine formation eventually would cease if it were not for factors that partially compensate for the increasing pressure. These include continued water reabsorption by the distal tubules and collecting ducts and leakage of urine into veins, lymphatics, and the renal sinus through ruptured calyceal fornices. Some urine may also pass between tubule cells and into the interstitial space of the kidney. The passage of urine around the obstructing lesion is yet another compensating factor. The net effect of these changes is a balanced state in which urine formation continues, although at a reduced rate.

The foregoing considerations indicate that the major impact of acute obstruction on the kidney is functional, rather than structural. Blunting of the forniceal angles is the most reliable and consistent anatomic representation of increased hydrostatic pressure in the pelvocalyceal system, and forniceal rupture is the extreme consequence of elevated urine pressure. Dilata-

Figure 17–3. Schematic illustration of the differences in pelvocalyceal dilatation, renal function (pelvic pressure), and structural kidney damage between acute and chronic obstruction. In acute obstruction there is minimal dilatation, marked increase in pelvic pressure, and no structural damage. Chronic obstruction is characterized by marked dilatation and normal pelvic pressures as nephron damage permanently slows the rate of urine formation. Numbers refer to intrapelvic pressure in centimeters of water.

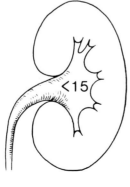

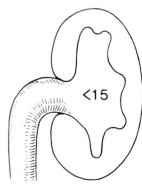

NORMAL   ACUTE
                             OBSTRUCTION   CHRONIC
                                                      OBSTRUCTION

tion of the upper urinary tract to the point of obstruction is always minimal to moderate (Fig. 17–4). Except for forniceal rupture, structural damage to the kidney does not occur in acute obstruction. The delayed appearance of contrast material during urography or of radioactivity during radionuclide studies with a filtered agent reflects a decrease in glomerular filtration rate caused by elevated tubule pressure. Nevertheless, glomerular filtration does continue and a gradual increase over time in nephrographic radiodensity or radioactivity occurs in these respective studies. As contrast material or tracer slowly passes prograde through the tubule lumina and collecting ducts, the minimally dilated collecting system and ureter proximal to the obstruction are visualized. Leakage of urine through ruptured fornices is shown by contrast material in renal sinus tissue or, more rarely, in the medullary interstitium, renal veins, or lymphatics. This is classified, respectively, as *pyelosinus, pyelointerstitial, pyelovenous,* or *pyelolymphatic backflow.* The dense nephrogram and dilated collecting structures persist over time and are not influenced by gravity when the patient is examined in the upright position. The upright position, however, is useful in moving contrast material distally to visualize the point of obstruction.

The functional defects of acute obstruction are most pronounced in patients whose pelvocalyceal systems are "intrarenal" and thus not readily distensible (Fig. 17–5). In comparison, "extrarenal" systems dilate more and have a less severe functional defect. Of all the radiologic features of acute obstruction (these are presented in Chapter 9), blunting of the calyceal fornices, forniceal rupture, and failure of a dilated system to drain under the influence of gravity are most specific.

Ultrasonography is highly sensitive in detecting moderate to marked dilatation of the collecting system. This degree of dilatation, however, is not a usual feature of acute obstruction. Therefore, there is always a significant possibility of a false-negative result when ultrasonography, even when combined with an abdominal radiograph to detect opaque calculus, is used to diagnose acute obstruction in patients with acute colic and hematuria. Likewise, it is impossible to distinguish by ultrasonography mild dilatation due to obstruction from a normal extrarenal pelvis. Under ordinary circumstances, excretory urography is the preferred technique for investigating possible acute obstruction of the urinary tract.

Chronic Obstruction

The elevated hydrostatic pressure of acute unrelieved obstruction eventually causes moderate to marked dilatation of the collecting system and ureter to the level of obstruction, wasting of the renal parenchyma, and reduction in renal blood flow. These features of chronic obstruction evolve over time and represent both structural and functional changes. As nephrons atrophy and renal blood flow diminishes, the amount of urine formed progressively diminishes to equal the amount that can leave the system. Thus, the pelvocalyceal system eventually converts from an initial high pressure, minimally dilated acutely obstructed structure to a passively dilated, low pressure chronically obstructed sac, with a slow exchange of urine (see Fig. 17–3).

Chronic obstruction is usually associated with mild and nonspecific symptoms or is asymptomatic. Causes of chronic obstruction include ureteropelvic junction obstruction; urolithiasis; ureteral stricture; periureteral fibrosis; primary, metastatic, and retroperitoneal tumors; congenital anomalies; and a wide variety of bladder and bladder outlet abnormalities, as discussed in other chapters.

The extent of renal damage caused by a chronic obstructive lesion is determined by both duration and degree of obstruction. In extreme cases, the kidney is transformed into a functionless, fluid-filled, flank mass composed of a thin rim of severely atrophied parenchyma and is minimally perfused by stretched, branchless arteries (Fig. 17–6). In this instance, a flank mass is detectable by abdominal radiography alone and by excretory urography. The fluid-filled nature of the mass is established by either ultrasonography or computed tomography. Pyelography can demonstrate the site of obstruction. When performed by the antegrade route, pressure in the hydronephrotic kidney, usually less than 10 cm of water, can be measured.

Abnormalities less severe than the preceding extreme example are more common. Even with moderate to marked dilatation, the pelvis can usually be distinguished from the calyces. The renal parenchyma is variably thinned. The density of the nephrogram is diminished because of the decreased clearance of contrast material by compromised nephrons. An increasingly dense nephrogram is not seen in chronic obstruction, reflecting the normal hydrostatic pressure of urine in the collecting system. Early in the course of the excretory urogram, thin bands of slightly radiodense parenchyma, the "rim" sign, surround the dilated, not yet opacified calyces, producing a "negative pyelogram" (Figs. 17–7 and 17–8). In some patients with chronic obstruction, a thin curvilinear area of enhancement develops during the course of urography at the interface between the inner medulla and the adjacent dilated calyces. This "calyceal crescent" sign represents concentrated contrast material in distal collecting ducts whose orientation has been distorted by calyceal dilatation (Fig. 17–9). Collecting system opacification is delayed. In less severe circumstances, only moderate dilatation of the collecting system and wasting of the renal parenchyma are noted (Fig. 17–10). In some patients, obstruction is partial and nonprogressive. In these cases, dilatation of the collecting system may disappear and the radiologic findings of obstruction can be evoked only by a challenge to the kidney to increase urine production by using a diuretic agent, as discussed below and in Chapter 15.

Slow uptake and prolonged activity in the radioisotope renogram are the hallmarks of moderate chronic obstructive uropathy, but these can also be seen in dilated nonobstructed systems. Renography, includ-

Text continued on page 583

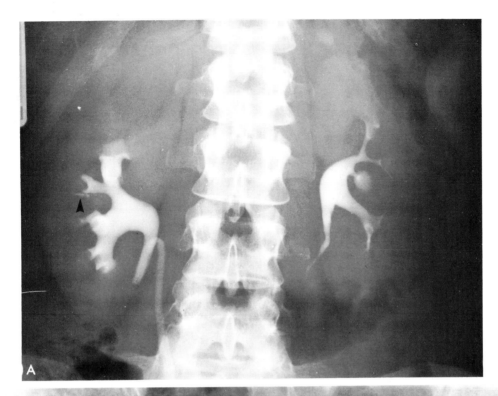

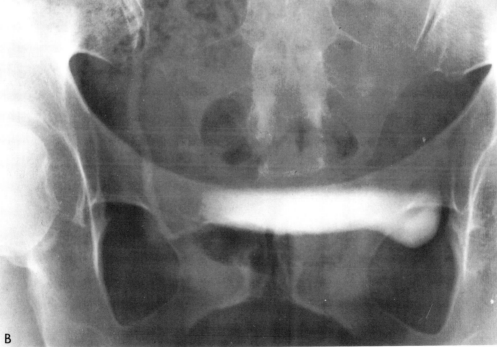

Figure 17–4. Acute obstructive uropathy due to stone in the distal right ureter. There is minimal enlargement of the pelvocalyceal system. Dilatation of the forniceal angles and leakage of contrast material into the sinus *(arrowhead)* through a ruptured fornix reflect elevated hydrostatic pressure in the pelvis of the kidney. Despite the added force of gravity when the patient is upright, the system does not drain.

A, Excretory urogram, 20-minute film.

B, Upright, postvoid film of the bladder. (Same patient illustrated in Fig. 9–15.)

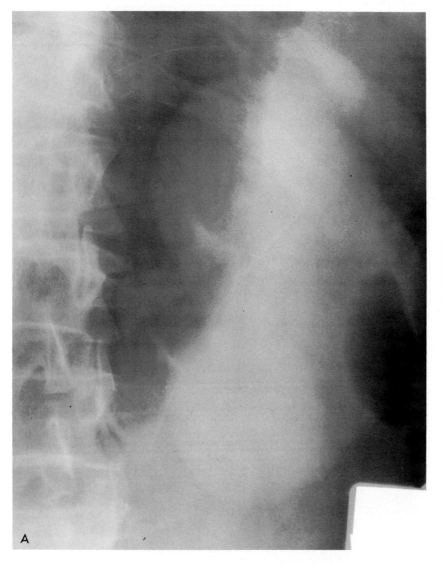

Figure 17–5. Acute obstructive uropathy of the left kidney due to stone. The "intrarenal" location of the pelvis causes pronounced transitory functional effects, seen as an increasingly dense nephrogram and a marked delay in pelvocalyceal opacification.

A, Excretory urogram, 10-minute film.

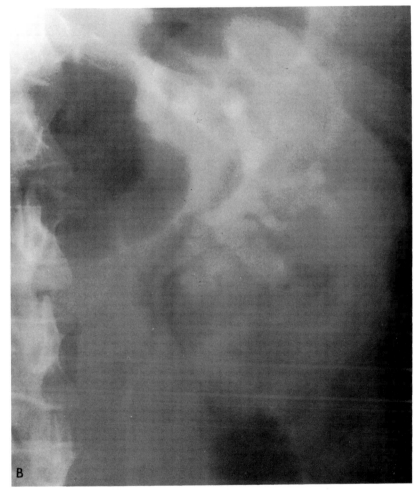

Figure 17–5 *Continued B,* Excretory urogram, 1-hour film. There has been spontaneous passage of a stone into the bladder.

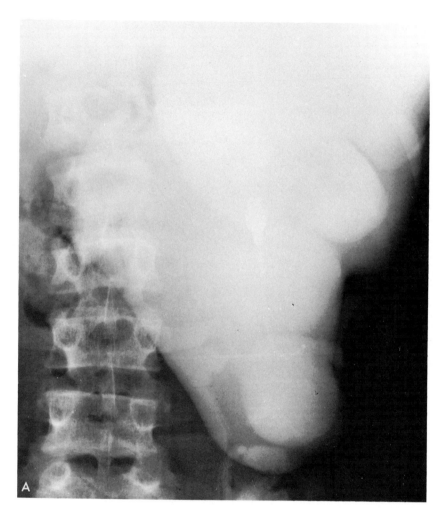

Figure 17–6. Chronic obstructive uropathy due to ureteropelvic junction obstruction in a 16-year-old boy with congenital unilateral kidney and renal failure. In this extreme example, the kidney has become a large, urine-filled sac with minimal perfusion by stretched, branchless arteries.

A, Antegrade pyelogram.

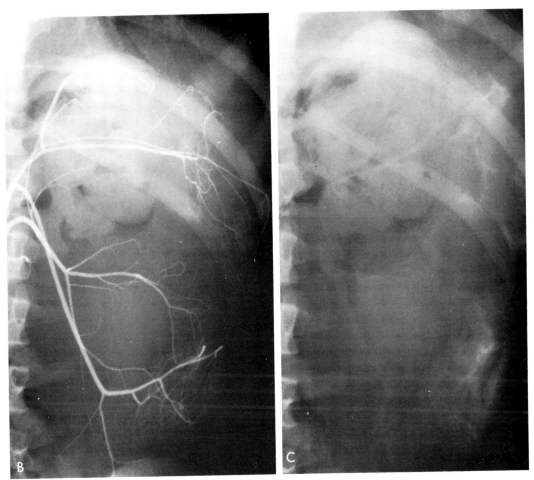

Figure 17–6 *Continued B,* Renal arteriogram, arterial phase.
C, Renal arteriogram, late phase. Thin bands of compressed renal tissue, the "rim" sign, are opacified.

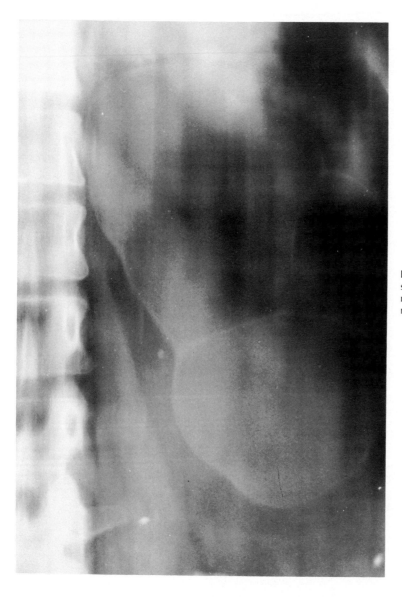

Figure 17–7. Chronic obstructive uropathy causing a "rim" sign. Excretory urogram. There is nephrographic enhancement of strikingly thin renal parenchyma representing residua of atrophied cortex and medulla.

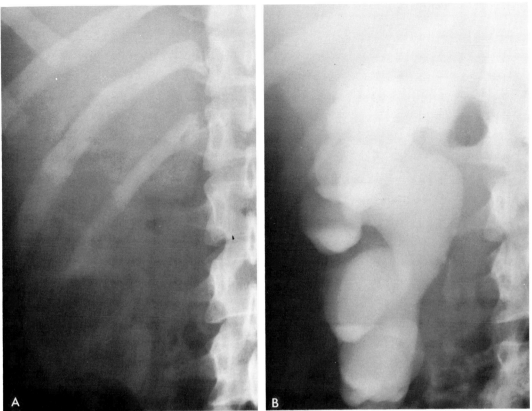

Figure 17–8. Chronic obstructive uropathy in a 27-year-old woman with long-standing ureteropelvic junction obstruction.

A, Excretory urogram. Early film demonstrates the nephrogram of compressed parenchyma surrounding the nonopacified calyces, the "negative pyelogram."

B, Excretory urogram. The previously radiolucent dilated calyces are opacified on a delayed upright film.

(Same patient illustrated in Fig. 9–20.)

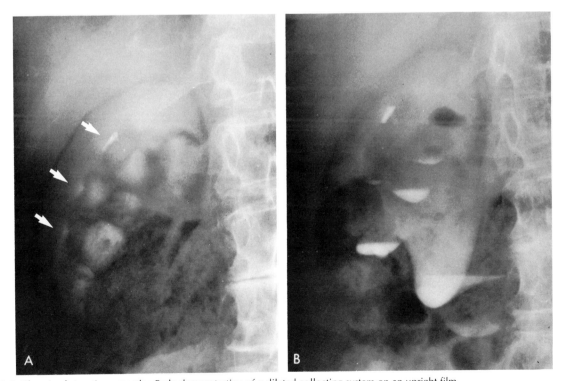

Figure 17–9. Chronic obstructive uropathy. Early demonstration of a dilated collecting system on an upright film.

A, Excretory urogram, supine film. Narrow, semilunar bands of contrast material *(arrows)* called "calyceal crescents" are present at the interface between renal parenchyma and the faintly opacified dilated calyces.

B, Excretory urogram, upright film. Layering of contrast material facilitates visualization of the dilated calyces.

581

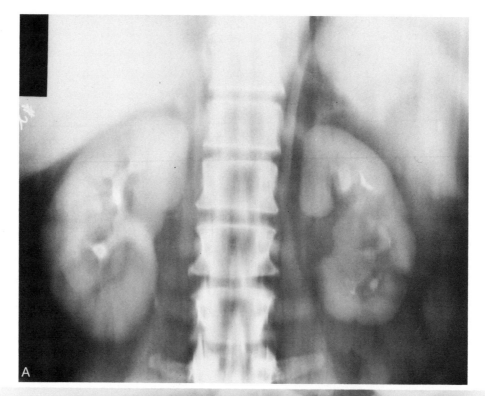

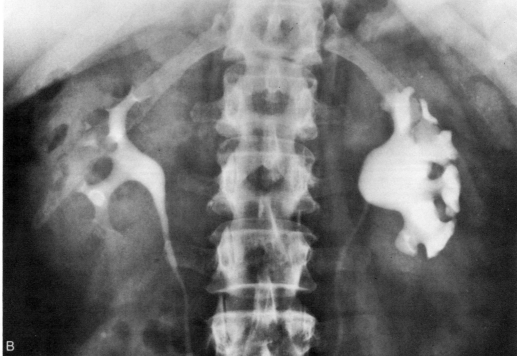

Figure 17–10. Chronic obstructive uropathy of the left kidney, intermediate grade. There is moderate parenchymal thinning and collecting system dilatation, but the time–density pattern of the nephrogram is normal, indicating a stable state.
  A, Excretory urogram, 3-minute tomogram.
  B, Excretory urogram, 10-minute film.

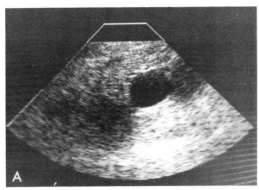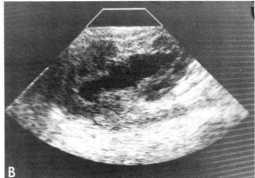

Figure 17–11. Chronic obstructive uropathy. Ultrasonogram. The dilated oval pelvis, seen on a medial longitudinal section (A), communicates with the intrarenal portion of the pelvocalyceal system, seen on a more lateral longitudinal section (B).

ing diuresis renography, is discussed below and in Chapter 2.

Screening for chronic obstructive uropathy is most efficaciously performed with ultrasonography, using the criteria described in Chapter 9 (Fig. 17–11). When combined with a radiograph of the abdomen to exclude a false-negative result caused by staghorn calculus, the sensitivity of ultrasonography in detecting a dilated collecting system approaches 100 per cent (Table 17–1). Other, very uncommon sources of false-negative results are acute renal failure superimposed on chronic obstruction and neoplastic, inflammatory, or desmoplastic processes in the renal sinus and periureteral tissue that prevent dilatation of the obstructed collecting system and ureter. All dilated systems are not due to obstruction, however. Therefore, false-positive tests occur and account for a specificity of approximately 75 per cent. These results, however, are to be expected in a screening test and do not detract from the value of ultrasonography as the primary technique for the diagnosis of chronic obstruction. The causes of nonobstructive dilatation of the collecting system that account for false-positive results are discussed in the last section of this chapter.

Computed tomography is also a very accurate technique for the detection of dilatation of the collecting system. Contrast material enhancement is sometimes

needed to establish that the dilated fluid-filled structure is in fact the pelvocalyceal system rather than a noncommunicating parapelvic cyst (Fig. 17–12; see also Fig. 16–4). Additionally, computed tomography is more likely than ultrasonography to image the obstructing lesion. Often, though, computed tomography will only identify dilatation and not provide the information needed to separate obstructive from nonobstructive causes. The ultimate identification of a lesion responsible for the obstruction often requires retrograde or antegrade pyelography (see Fig. 17–6). Additional features of chronic obstructive uropathy are discussed in Chapter 9.

Intermediate, Intermittent, and Equivocal Forms of Obstruction

Diagnosis of acute and chronic obstruction is straightforward in most patients when excretory urography and ultrasonography are used, with occasional assistance from radionuclide renography, computed tomography, or pyelography. There is a group of patients in whom these standard studies produce normal or equivocal results, yet in whom there is convincing clinical evidence for obstruction. Most of these patients have functional obstructions at the ureteropelvic junction, as discussed in Chapter 15. In patients who experience obstruction intermittently, correct diagnosis requires examination during symptomatic periods, so-called acute urography. Other patients have obstructive lesions of intermediate severity that are occult except when studied during a condition of diuresis that challenges the ability of the collecting system and the ureter to accommodate large urine flow rates. Equivocal findings of obstruction may also be encountered in patients whose dilatation is due to nonobstructive causes or in patients whose collecting systems are not distensible because of prior surgery and peripelvic fibrosis.

To evaluate any of these possibilities, standard tests must be modified to evoke evidence of obstruction. *Diuresis urography* and *diuresis renography* assess the ability of the upper tract to transport urine under conditions of high flow rates. Respectively, these techniques evaluate dilatation and emptying of the upper

Table 17–1. DECISION MATRIX FOR DETECTION OF CHRONIC OBSTRUCTIVE UROPATHY BY ULTRASOUND*

		Chronic Obstructive Uropathy	
		+	−
Dilated Collecting System	+	True Positive 0.98 (Sensitivity)	False Positive 0.25
	−	False Negative 0.02	True Negative 0.75 (Specificity)

*Overall accuracy is 0.97. False-negative results can be reduced by combining the ultrasonogram with an abdominal radiograph. (From Ellenbogen, P. H., et al.: Sensitivity of gray scale ultrasound in detecting urinary tract obstruction. AJR 130:731, 1978.)

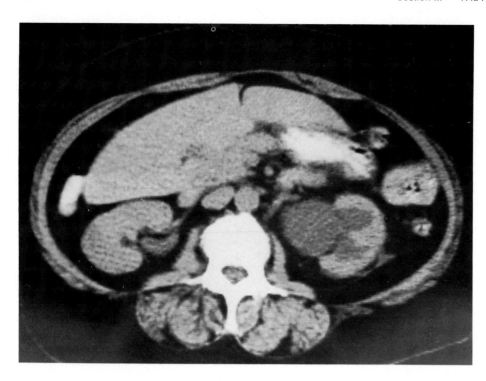

Figure 17–12. Chronic obstructive uropathy of the left kidney. The attenuation value of the dilated pelvocalyceal system is that of water. Note the wasting of the renal parenchyma, which is a feature of chronic obstruction. Computed tomogram, nonenhanced. (Same patient illustrated in Fig. 9–23.)

urinary tract and the shape of the renogram curve before and after a diuresis provoked by intravenous furosemide. These tests help separate patients whose obstruction is mild or intermittent from those whose dilated pelvis is not due to obstruction at all (Fig. 17–13). When these tests fail to resolve the question of obstruction, a pressure/flow urodynamic study permits direct measurement of pressure in the renal pelvis and bladder under conditions of controlled flow, as discussed in Chapter 15.

In patients with obstruction, the goal is to select for surgery those who have periods of continuous or intermittent high pelvic pressure under conditions of usual urine flow rates, since this is the circumstance that eventually causes deterioration of renal function.

NONOBSTRUCTIVE DILATATION

Vesicoureteral Reflux

Persistent reflux of large volumes of urine through the vesicoureteral junction may dilate the ureter and pelvocalyceal system. Reflux is often found in infants or children and most commonly results from an abnormally short segment of terminal ureter traversing the bladder wall, commonly with a more obtuse angle of insertion than is normally present in nonrefluxing ureters. Usually, this mural segment of the distal ureter lengthens and its angle of insertion becomes more acute as the child grows. Reflux then disappears spontaneously and without consequence. There are some children, however, in whom this does not occur. In them, reflux may be massive and persistent, causing the collecting system and the ureter to dilate and the kidney to suffer global atrophy as a result of a "water-hammer" effect on the parenchyma (Fig. 17–14). This

is termed *reflux atrophy* and is discussed in Chapter 6 as one cause of the unilateral, small, smooth kidney. Reflux atrophy is distinct from another complication of major vesicoureteral reflux, the focal scarring of reflux nephropathy (chronic atrophic pyelonephritis). (See discussion in Chapter 5.) Either of these reflux-induced structural alterations of the kidney persist into adulthood as permanent damage, although both originate in infancy or early childhood.

Vesicoureteral reflux is not always caused by a short, obtusely angled, mural segment of distal ureter. A bladder diverticulum located adjacent to the ureteral orifice may become large enough to transform a nonrefluxing orifice into one that allows vesicoureteral reflux. This sometimes occurs in infants and children as a result of a congenital deficiency of muscle in the posterolateral wall of the bladder where the ureters insert. Known as a *Hutch diverticulum* this deformity may actually incorporate the ureteral orifice into the diverticulum itself. Reflux may also occur in patients with bladder outlet obstruction, such as posterior urethral valves in male children, or in dysmorphic conditions, such as prune-belly syndrome. At any age, reflux can develop *de novo* as a consequence of neurologic disorders of the bladder.

One potentially misleading appearance associated with massive vesicoureteral reflux in children is the coexistence of a large capacity, thin-walled bladder and marked upper urinary tract dilatation. This combination has been termed *megacystis-megaureter syndrome* but is actually nothing more than the effect of large volumes of refluxed urine refilling the bladder after voiding and maintaining its distended state.

Pelvocalyceal dilatation due to recurrent overdistention by refluxed urine is usually persistent. The appearance on excretory urography or ultrasonog-

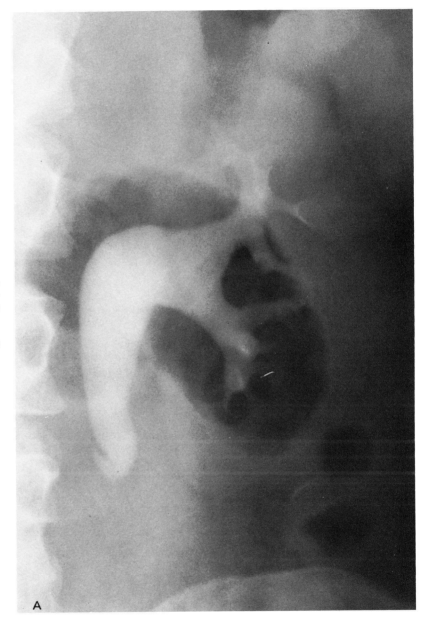

Figure 17–13. Negative diuresis urogram. The appearance of the pelvocalyceal system simulates obstruction at the ureteropelvic junction, although the normal forniceal angles suggest otherwise.

A, Excretory urogram, 20-minute film.

Illustration continued on following page

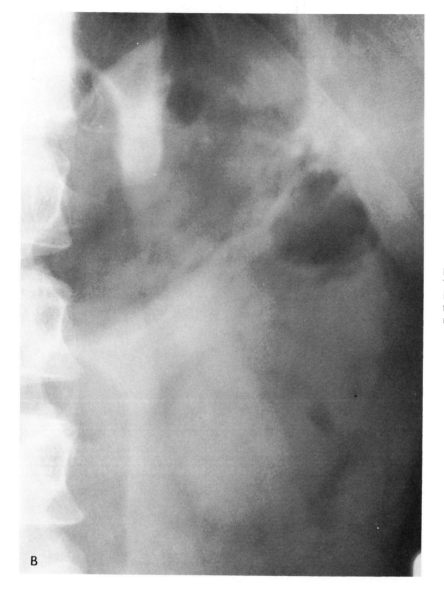

Figure 17–13 *Continued B,* Excretory urogram. This film was taken 15 minutes after intravenous injection of 40 mg of furosemide. Washout of contrast material from the collecting structures eliminates obstruction as a cause of dilatation.

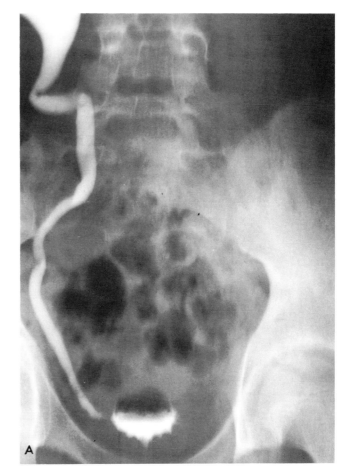

Figure 17–14. Vesicoureteral reflux into the right pelvocalyceal system of an 11-year-old girl with recurrent urinary tract infection. This reflux has led to dilatation of the pelvocalyceal system and global parenchymal atrophy.

A, Voiding cystourethrogram.

B, Excretory urogram. Note the longitudinal mucosal folds in the right pelvis due to incomplete distention of the collecting system.

(Same patient illustrated in Fig. 5–7.)

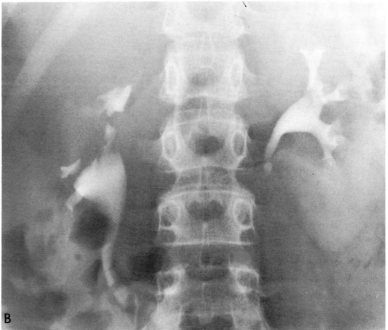

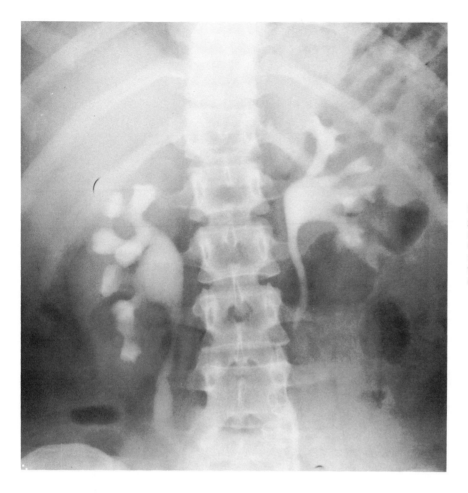

Figure 17–15. Pelvocalyceal dilatation and global parenchymal wasting in the right kidney of a 26-year-old woman without prior urologic history. In the absence of concurrent reflux and a pertinent history, it is impossible to determine a responsible cause. Excretory urogram.

raphy is indistinguishable from pelvocalyceal dilatation due to other causes discussed in this chapter. In some patients, the dilatation of the collecting system may not be apparent when the patient is examined in an antidiuretic state. Instead, the collecting system appears redundant or flaccid or longitudinal folds are noted, as discussed in Chapter 15 (see Fig. 17–14). The dilated nature of the collecting system in these cases becomes apparent only when the examination is repeated with diuresis.

Although reflux as a cause of dilatation of the pelvocalyceal system and ureter is sometimes demonstrable by voiding cystourethrography in the adult, dilatation may be the residual effect of prior, spontaneously corrected reflux, in which case voiding cystourethrography fails to identify the etiology (Fig. 17–15). In this circumstance, vesicoureteral reflux cannot be distinguished from other nonobstructive causes of dilatation.

Infection

Dilatation of the pelvocalyceal system and ureter sometimes occurs with acute pyelonephritis (Fig. 17–16). Presumably, this results from inhibition of the muscular activity of the ureter and the pelvis by pathogens, possibly through release of endotoxin. Appropriate antibiotic therapy quickly reverses this effect. Other abnormalities seen by urography or ultrasonography during the early phase of acute pyelonephritis are described in Chapter 9.

High Flow States

Diabetes insipidus, osmotic diuresis, and unilateral kidney are all examples of high flow states. *Diabetes insipidus* occurs when the kidney is unable to maximally concentrate urine. Normally, vasopressin produced by the hypothalamus-hypophysis acts on distal tubules and collecting ducts to increase water reabsorption and thereby concentrate the urine. Either deficient hypothalamic-hypophyseal production of vasopressin or insensitivity of the renal tubules to normal amounts of endogenous vasopressin causes diabetes insipidus.

Hypothalamic diabetes insipidus develops when vasopressin production is reduced by more than 90 per cent. This usually occurs following pituitary destruction by tumor (usually craniopharyngioma), by surgery, or as a complication of meningitis or head trauma. Rarely, hypothalamic diabetes insipidus is present on a hereditary basis. Hypothalamic diabetes insipidus is characterized by the ability of the kidney to concentrate urine in response to exogenous vasopressin and its inability to do so with water deprivation alone.

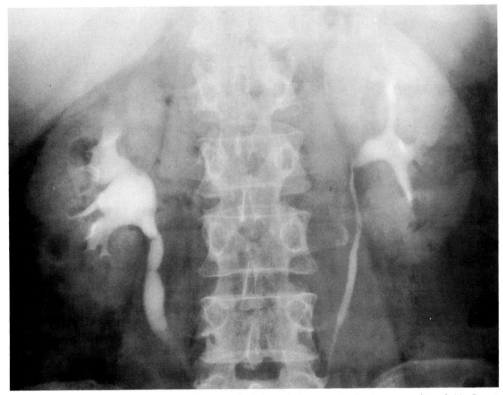

Figure 17–16. Dilatation of the pelvocalyceal system of the right kidney during an episode of acute pyelonephritis. Excretory urogram.

Another form of diabetes insipidus is due to compulsive intake of large amounts of water, a condition known as *psychogenic water intoxication*. In this condition, excessive fluid intake inhibits normal hypothalamic-hypophyseal production of vasopressin. Increased concentration of urine following water deprivation characterizes this form of diabetes insipidus.

Primary nephrogenic diabetes insipidus occurs when distal tubules and collecting ducts are unable to respond to either endogenous or exogenous vasopressin. This is a rare sex-linked recessive genetic disorder found mainly in infants and young males.

As part of a major renal disorder, the kidney may become incapable of maximally concentrating urine. *Secondary nephrogenic diabetes insipidus* develops in association with drug toxicity, analgesic nephropathy, sickle cell anemia, hypokalemia or hypercalcemia from any cause, chronic uremic nephropathy, postobstructive nephropathy, reflux nephropathy (chronic atrophic pyelonephritis), amyloidosis, and sarcoidosis. No specific tubule lesion that accounts for polyuria in these conditions has been identified.

Patients with diabetes insipidus complain of polyuria, polydipsia, and constipation and excrete hypotonic urine. Excessive water excretion may cause severe dehydration, which in infants or children can lead to convulsions and death.

The pelvocalyceal systems, ureters, and bladder are dilated in all forms of diabetes insipidus as the volume of urine formed overwhelms the peristaltic capacity of the ureter (Fig. 17–17). Overdistention even-

tually leads to loss of ureteral muscle tone. The ureter then becomes a passive conduit between the kidney and the bladder, and urine is propelled only by nephronic pressure and gravity. Marked distention of the bladder may contribute further to upper tract distention by obstructing the ureterovesical junction. Global wasting of the kidney, including effacement of the papillae, occurs as increased hydrostatic pressure causes renal parenchymal atrophy. Collecting system dilatation and renal wasting are readily visualized by excretory urography, ultrasonography, and computed tomography.

Moderate dilatation of the calyces, pelvis, and ureter is also seen during osmotic diuresis from any cause and in the single kidney that has undergone compensatory hypertrophy (Fig. 17–18).

Congenital Megacalyces

Uniform dilatation of the calyces due to underdevelopment of the papillae constitutes congenital megacalyces. The medullary tip is of a semilunar shape that caps, rather than projects as a cone into the calyx. The calyces are polygonal and have a mosaic or faceted appearance.

The pathogenesis of congenital megacalyces has not been established. Suggested possibilities are faulty ureteral bud division, primary hypoplasia of glomeruli in the juxtamedullary cortex, functional infundibular achalasia due to maldevelopment of smooth muscle fibers of the pelvocalyceal junction, and transient collecting system obstruction *in utero*, caused by

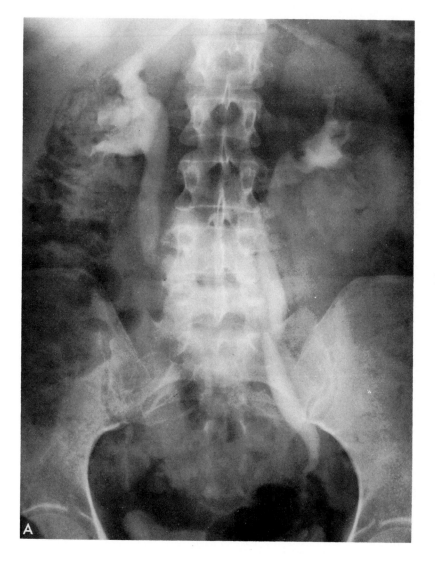

Figure 17–17. Bilateral pelvocalyceal and ureteral dilatation due to diabetes insipidus. Drainage occurs when the patient is in the upright position.
  A, Excretory urogram. Patient is supine.

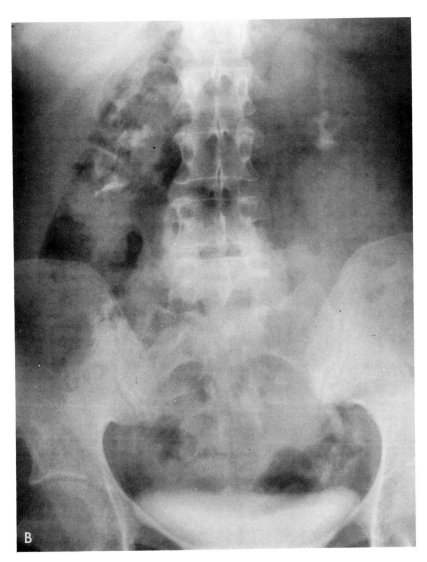

Figure 17–17 *Continued B,* Excretory urogram. Patient is upright.

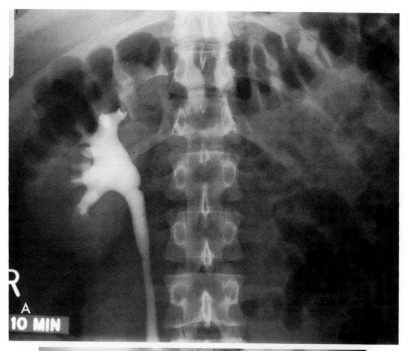

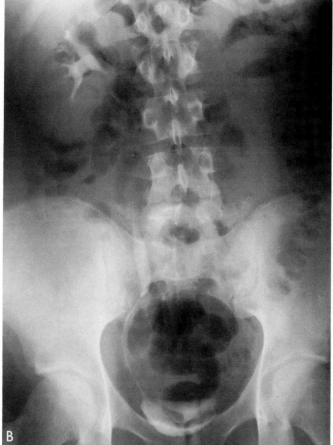

Figure 17–18. Pelvocalyceal and ureteral dilatation due to a high flow state in a patient with congenital absence of one kidney. Drainage occurs when the patient is in the upright position.

A, Excretory urogram. Patient is supine.

B, Excretory urogram. Patient is upright.

involuting folds in the proximal portion of the fetal ureter.

The diagnosis of congenital megacalyces should be considered only in patients whose characteristic calyceal deformities exist without prior or concurrent obstruction. Vesicoureteral reflux must also be excluded. Stasis of urine in the enlarged calyces predisposes the patient to infection and stone formation, which are the major clinical abnormalities in these patients.

Renal function, as measured by creatinine clearance or serum creatinine, is normal in patients with congenital megacalyces. This is an important feature in differentiating this abnormality from postobstructive atrophy. Some data suggest a moderate defect in concentrating ability of kidneys with congenital megacalyces (Talner and Gittes, 1974).

Congenital megacalyces is usually unilateral. Contrast material appears at the same time in the affected and the normal kidney during excretory urography, but maximum opacification of the pelvocalyceal system is delayed in the abnormal kidney because of the dilution effect of the large volume of urine in its collecting system. The renal pelvis and infundibula are often capacious but otherwise normal (Fig. 17–19). Other features of congenital megacalyces on excretory urography are normal to increased number of calyces, normal to increased length of kidney, and decreased thickness of renal parenchyma due to both expanded calyceal volume and thinning of the medulla. The papillary tips are either absent or very shallow. Congenital megacalyces is not progressive. The occasional finding of a dilated ureter has been cited as evidence for obstruction as a pathogenetic factor.

Stones and infection complicate the urographic appearance of congenital megacalyces and preclude confident distinction from other entities, especially postobstructive atrophy.

Ultrasonography and computed tomography demonstrate dilatation of the calyces and reduction in thickness of the renal parenchyma. Neither of these techniques, however, is useful in distinguishing congenital megacalyces from other nonobstructive causes of a dilated collecting system.

Renal arteries visualized during angiography are normal except for slight displacement by large calyces. The angiographic nephrogram demonstrates that the reduction of parenchymal thickness in congenital megacalyces is due only to a medullary deformity, since the cortex retains its normal thickness of 0.5 to 0.8 mm. The normal thickness of the cortex can also be demonstrated by magnetic resonance imaging.

Quantitative renal radionuclide studies with either ^{99m}Tc-DTPA or ^{99m}Tc-DMSA demonstrate normal glomerular function in the kidney with congenital megacalyces and distinguish these kidneys from those whose similar structural deformity is accompanied by a permanent loss of nephrons. Examples of the latter include postobstructive atrophy or pressure atrophy from vesicoureteral reflux. Radionuclide renograms with tracers that measure excretion (^{131}I -iodohippurate sodium or ^{99m}Tc-DTPA) show marked prolongation of the excretory phase in the congenital megacalyces

kidney. This result, simulating obstruction, is due to the gradual mixing of isotope with the large volume of urine in the dilated calyces (see Fig. 17–19). The diuresis renogram will exclude obstruction in this situation. These aspects of radionuclide imaging are discussed further in Chapter 2.

Postobstructive Atrophy

The renal changes following relief of urinary tract obstruction include generalized papillary atrophy, global thinning of the parenchyma, and generalized dilatation of the pelvocalyceal system. Some of the dilatation, particularly that involving the calyces, is due to atrophy of surrounding tissue. Altered smooth muscle morphology may also contribute to postobstructive pelvocalyceal dilatation.

Persistent collecting system dilatation after surgical correction of obstruction raises the possibility of ineffective surgery. Diuresis studies (urography or renography) or pressure/flow measurement usually resolve this question.

Pelvocalyceal dilatation in postobstructive atrophy produces abnormalities on urography, ultrasonography, and computed tomography that are identical to nonobstructive dilatation caused by other forms of parenchymal atrophy or maldevelopment (see Fig. 17–15). Impaired function of the postobstructive kidney is detectable by radionuclide techniques and is a basis for distinction from congenital megacalyces. (A discussion of other aspects of postobstructive atrophy appears in Chapter 6.)

Pregnancy

As a result of pregnancy, the collecting systems and ureters dilate, and peristaltic activity diminishes. Microscopically, there is hypertrophy of ureteropelvic smooth muscle and hyperplasia of connective tissue. These changes affect about 90 per cent of women during the course of pregnancy, appearing as early as the end of the first trimester and becoming maximal in the third trimester. Dilatation of the ureter extends only to the level of the pelvic brim; distal to this point the caliber is normal. Dilatation during pregnancy far more often involves the right collecting system and ureter than the left. Only one-third of patients demonstrate any left-sided changes at all, and even less often does left-sided dilatation predominate. Most changes arising from pregnancy resolve within a few weeks after delivery. Persistent dilatation after parturition is usually caused by urinary tract infection acquired during pregnancy.

The cause of upper tract dilatation during pregnancy has been debated extensively but never precisely defined. The muscle-relaxing effects of progesterone-like hormones and partial mechanical obstruction are two likely contributing factors. Suggested causes of obstruction include thickening of muscle and connective tissue in the distal segment of the ureter, compression by a dilated ovarian vein, compression by iliac vessels, and pressure from the

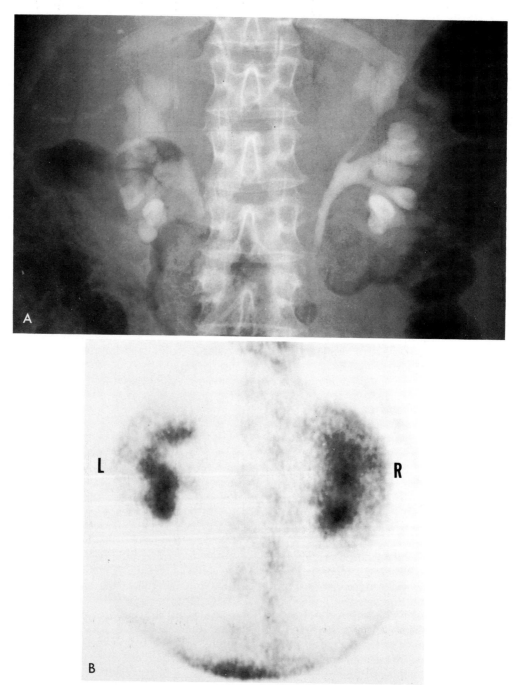

Figure 17–19. Congenital bilateral megacalyces (presumed diagnosis) in a 57-year-old woman with a normal urologic history and normal renal function. The excretory urogram was performed because a radionuclide bone scan suggested bilateral obstruction.

   A, Excretory urogram. Dilatation of calyces, polycalycosis, and flattened papillae are present.

   B, Radionuclide bone scan, delayed image. Activity has persisted in the dilated collecting systems, simulating obstruction.

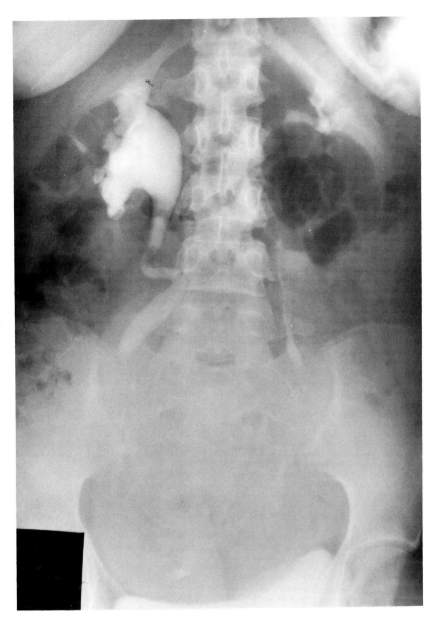

Figure 17–20. Dilatation of the right collecting system associated with pregnancy. Dilatation of the right ureter usually extends to the pelvic brim. Excretory urogram.

gravid uterus, which rotates to the right as it enlarges. Hypertrophy of Waldeyer's sheath, a connective tissue envelope around the distal ureter, might cause dilatation either by direct compression or by preventing hormonally induced relaxation of the distal ureter. None of these considerations alone explains the predominant involvement of the right side, the absence of distal ureteral dilatation, and the appearance of these changes early in pregnancy before the uterus is large enough to produce pressure on the ureter. It is likely that the cause is multifactorial.

The dilated collecting system and ureter associated with sluggish peristalsis predisposes the patient to urinary tract infection. Otherwise, this condition is without consequence.

Excretory urography, which is rarely required during pregnancy, demonstrates generalized dilatation that is usually limited to the right side of the pelvocalyceal system and ureter to the pelvic brim and a

normal caliber of the distal ureter (Fig. 17–20). Ultrasonography also detects the dilatation and is an efficacious method for establishing pregnancy as a cause.

Prune-Belly Syndrome

Congenital absence or deficiency of abdominal musculature, cryptorchidism, and dystrophic urinary tract abnormalities constitute the major findings of the prune-belly syndrome. This condition, which occurs predominantly in males, is also known as the *Eagle-Barrett* or *triad syndrome.*

Urinary tract abnormalities in prune-belly syndrome are dominated by marked dilatation, elongation, and tortuosity of the ureters. Obstruction of the ureter or of the lower urinary tract is only rarely present. Ureteral dilatation is most marked distally, and vesicoureteral reflux is usually present. Diminished to absent peristalsis reflects a patchy absence of

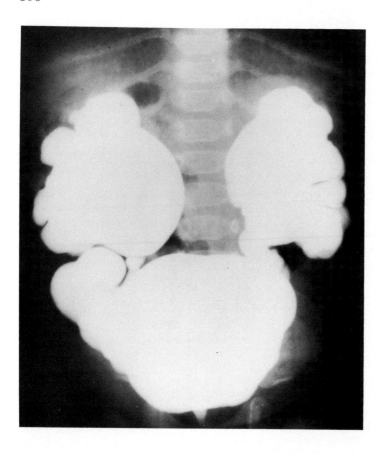

Figure 17–21. Prune-belly syndrome in a newborn with renal failure. Cystogram. There is marked dilatation of the bladder and the upper urinary tracts with renal parenchymal wasting.

ureteral muscle interspersed with abnormal amounts of fibrous and collagenous tissue. Similar histologic findings are present in the bladder, which is usually dilated, but not trabeculated. A urachal cyst or diverticulum often coexists. The prostatic urethra is dilated and elongated, the prostate is hypoplastic, and the verumontanum is absent to small. (See Chapter 19 for further discussion of the bladder in prune-belly syndrome.) The kidneys variably demonstrate pelvocalyceal dilatation, parenchymal dysplasia, small size, and diminished function. In some cases, the kidneys are normal.

The clinical consequences of prune-belly syndrome vary from death *in utero* or in the neonatal period with Potter's syndrome to minimal symptoms and an extended life span. Renal failure and urosepsis are the principal complications of those who survive with moderate to severe expression of this disorder.

Excretory urography, ultrasonography, and voiding cystourethrography demonstrate the previously described abnormalities of the urinary tract in patients with prune-belly syndrome (Fig. 17–21). In some cases, the question of a coexistent obstructing lesion must be resolved with the pressure/flow study of Whitaker.

Primary Megaureter

The term *primary megaureter* is used here to describe a ureter that has a normally tapered distal segment but is otherwise dilated over a varying length, from a few

centimeters immediately proximal to the distal tapered end to and including the pelvocalyceal system. In extreme examples, renal atrophy accompanies hydronephrosis and hydroureter. Excluded from this definition are dilatation of the ureter due to vesicoureteral reflux and the other causes of nonobstructed dilatation discussed in the preceding sections as well as ureters obstructed by demonstrable mechanical obstruction.

The nature of primary megaureter has not been fully elaborated. The tapered distal segment is normal in caliber, freely allows passage of a retrograde catheter, but is aperistaltic. This is the segment that is thought to be abnormal. The more proximal dilated segment, on the other hand, exhibits normal or increased peristalsis and the bolus of urine within this segment is often incompletely propelled into the bladder. These abnormalities are generally considered secondary to the defect of the distal aperistaltic segment. Despite these observations, no consistent, specific histologic abnormality has been identified either in the tapered distal or the more proximal dilated segments. These findings, however, point to a functional impairment of peristalsis in the distal ureter, perhaps because of disordered arrangement of muscle.

Inclusion of primary megaureter in this section on nonobstructed dilatation of the ureter is arbitrary and based on the absence of a mechanical obstructing lesion. A valid argument could be made to classify this entity as a functional obstruction in the same manner as most cases of ureteropelvic junction obstruction. Indeed, moderate to severe primary megaureter meets Whitaker's criteria for obstruction, as discussed earlier in this chapter.

As a congenital abnormality, primary megaureter is found in all ages, although severe instances usually come to medical attention in infancy and childhood. A tendency toward predominance in males and left-sided involvement has been reported. Bilaterality has been noted in up to 50 per cent of patients and other anomalies in up to 40 per cent of cases. These include ipsilateral ureteropelvic junction obstruction, contralateral agenesis, contralateral or ipsilateral vesicoureteral reflux, contralateral ureteral ectopia or duplication, and ipsilateral megacalyces, among others.

Severity of primary megureter varies from minimal and inconsequential to severe functional obstruction with hydroureter, hydronephrosis, and impaired kidney function. Clinical findings, when present, include pain, hematuria, abdominal mass, or the signs and symptoms of urinary tract infection.

Primary megaureter is best studied by excretory urography. In mild cases, there is a 2- to 3-cm fusiform dilatation of the distal ureter just proximal to a tapered extravesical distal segment of up to 4 cm in length. With increased severity, the ureter dilates more proximally to include the pelvocalyceal system (Fig. 17–22). In extreme cases, there is wasting of the renal parenchyma and evidence of impaired excretion of contrast material (Fig. 17–23). Characteristically, the ureters lack tortuosity despite considerable dilatation. Fluoroscopy during excretory urography or real-time ultrasonography permit visualization of peristalsis, which, depending on severity, may be normal, increased, or diminished. Ineffective emptying and a to and fro movement of the urine in the dilated portion of the ureter is a frequent finding. Patients with advanced degrees of primary megaureter demonstrate obstructive patterns in diuresis urography or renography and in pressure/flow urodynamic studies.

DIFFERENTIAL DIAGNOSIS

Separating intermediate, intermittent, and equivocal forms of obstruction from the various nonobstructive causes of dilatation is the first challenge in evaluating

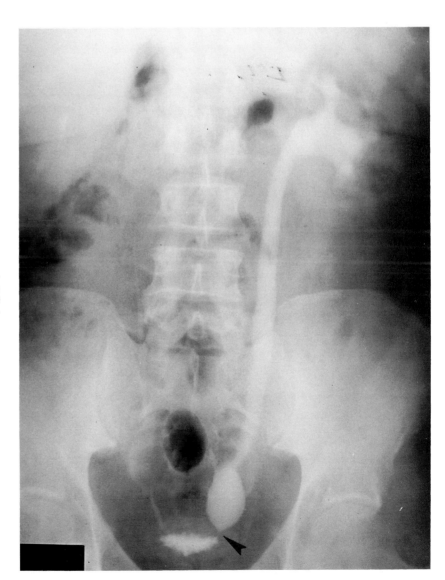

Figure 17–22. Primary megaureter with dilatation that includes the pelvocalyceal system as well as the ureter. Note fusiform narrowing of the most distal portion of the left ureter *(arrow)*. Excretory urogram, postvoid film.

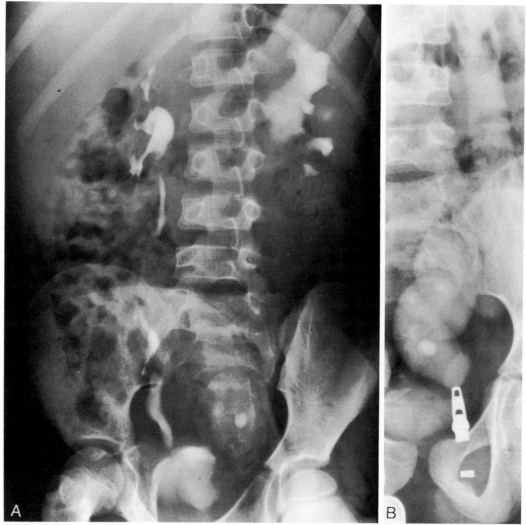

Figure 17–23. Primary megaureter causing marked dilatation of the left ureter and pelvis as well as wasting of the renal parenchyma. A nonobstructing stone is present in the pelvic portion of the ureter.

A, Excretory urogram, right posterior oblique projection. The left pelvis is dilated and the renal parenchyma wasted. A stone is seen overlying the coccyx. The bladder is deformed and effaced by the adjacent dilated, but unopacified, distal ureter.

B, Delayed film. The markedly dilated ureter with a dense stone is well visualized.

(Courtesy of Wendelin S. Hayes, D.O., Armed Forces Institute of Pathology, Washington, D.C.)

patients whose radiologic findings do not clearly point to obstruction. Diuresis urography and diuresis renography meet this challenge in most instances by demonstrating either further distention or prolonged retention of radioactivity in those who are obstructed or the rapid washout of contrast material or radionuclide in those who are not. The use of urodynamic pressure/flow studies is required only when the diuresis studies yield inconclusive results.

Once obstruction is eliminated as a cause of upper tract dilatation, vesicoureteral reflux must be considered. Voiding cystourethrography, using either radiographic or radionuclide techniques, accomplishes this with a high degree of accuracy but only when reflux is concurrent. Unfortunately, this is not the rule in adults whose renal damage occurred during infancy or childhood from reflux that has long since been resolved. Unless identified by relevant historical data, often not available in this frequently asymptomatic condition, these patients will be indistinguishable from those with other causes of nonobstructive collecting system dilatation.

Nonobstructive and nonreflux dilatation of the pelvocalyceal system and ureter is sometimes accompanied by wasting of the renal parenchyma in patients with prior reflux, in the various forms of high flow states, in postobstructive atrophy, in prune-belly syndrome, and in primary megaureter. In each of these, atrophy is accompanied by impaired function of the affected kidney, as measured by radionuclide techniques. Dilatation of the collecting system and decreased parenchymal thickness are also features of congenital magacalyces, but in this circumstance radionuclide studies of the affected kidney demonstrate normal function.

If nonobstructive dilatation occurs unaccompanied by thinning of the renal parenchyma, identification of a specific cause will be solely dependent on correlation with clinical data, if available. Radiologic criteria alone are insufficient.

Finally, in the evaluation of patients with a dilated upper urinary tract, awareness should be maintained of the occasional coexistence of two independent abnormalities, the radiologic findings of which may overlap. Combinations of ureteropelvic and ureterovesical junction obstruction, congenital megacalyces and primary megaureter, and primary megaureter and vesicoureteral reflux have been documented in a few instances. Also, it is important to exclude the effect of elevated bladder pressure as a cause of a dilated ureter. This may be seen not only in patients with bladder outflow obstruction but also in patients with voluntary infrequent voiding or, simply, filled bladders.

Bibliography

General

Bernstein, G. T., Mandell, J., Lebowitz, R. L., Bauer, S. B., Colodny, A. H., and Retik, A. B.: Ureteropelvic junction obstruction in the neonate. J. Urol. *140* (part 2):1216, 1988.
Brown, T., Mandell, J., and Lebowitz, R. L.: Neonatal hydronephrosis in the era of sonography. AJR *148*:959, 1987.

Clark, W. R., and Malek, R. S.: Ureteropelvic junction obstruction: I. Observations on the classic type in adults. J. Urol. *138*:276, 1987.
Curry, N. S., Gobien, R. P., and Schabel, S. I.: Minimal-dilatation obstructive nephropathy. Radiology *143*:531, 1982.
Dixon, J. S., and Gosling, J. A.: An evaluation of idiopathic hydronephrosis using light and electron microscopy. Ann. R. Coll. Surg. Engl. *62*:216, 1980.
Editorial: The dilated upper urinary tract. Br. Med. J. *1*:1382, 1979.
Fernbach, S. K.: The dilated urinary tract in children. Urol. Radiol. *14*:34, 1992.
Friedland, G. W.: Miscellaneous congenital anomalies of the genitourinary tract. *In* Pollack, H. M. (ed.): Clinical Urography. Philadelphia, W.B. Saunders, 1990, pp. 771–787.
Gillenwater, J. Y.: The pathophysiology of urinary obstruction. *In* Walsh, P. C., Retik, A. B., Stamey, T. A., and Vaughan, E. D., Jr., (eds.): Campbell's Urology. 6th ed. Philadelphia, W.B. Saunders, 1992, pp. 497–532.
Gosling, J. A., and Dixon, J. S.: Functional obstruction of the ureter and renal pelvis: A histological and electron microscopic study. Br. J. Urol. *50*:145, 1978.
Hill, G. S.: Basic Physiology and Morphology of Hydronephrosis, *In* Hill, G. S. (ed.): Uropathology. New York, Churchill Livingstone, 1989, pp. 467–515.
Hill, G. S.: Intrinsic and extrinsic obstruction of the urinary tract. *In* Hill, G. S. (ed.): Uropathology. New York, Churchill Livingstone, 1989, pp. 467–515 and 517–574.
Hill, G. S.: Ureteropelvic junction obstruction. *In* Hill, G. S. (ed.): Uropathology. New York, Churchill Livingstone, 1989, pp. 575–598.
Hoffer, F. A., and Lebowitz, R. L.: Intermittent hydronephrosis: A unique feature of ureteropelvic junction obstruction caused by a crossing renal vessel. Radiology *156*:655, 1985.
Koff, S. A.: Problematic ureteropelvic junction obstruction. J. Urol. *138*:390, 1987.
McGrath, M. A., Estroff, J., and Lebowitz, R. L.: The coexistence of obstruction at the ureteropelvic and ureterovesical junction. AJR *149*:403, 1987.
Newhouse, J. H., Amis, E. S., Jr., and Pfister, R. C.: Urinary obstruction: Pitfalls in the use of delayed contrast material washout for diagnosis. Radiology *151*:319, 1984.
O'Reilly, P. H., Lupton, E. W., Testa, H. J., Shields, R. A., Carrol, R. N. P., and Edwards, E. C.: The dilated, non-obstructed renal pelvis. Br. J. Urol. *53*:205, 1981.
O'Reilly, P. H.: Role of modern radiological investigations in obstructive uropathy. Br. Med. J. *284*:1847, 1982.
Platt, J. F., Rubin, J. M., Ellis, J. H., and DiPietro, M. A.: Duplex Doppler US of the kidney: Differentiation of obstructive from nonobstructive dilatation. Radiology *171*:515, 1989.
Sherwood, T.: The dilated upper urinary tract. Radiol. Clin. North Am. *17*:333, 1979.
Shopfner, C. E.: Ureteropelvic junction obstruction. AJR *98*:148, 1966.
Shopfner, C. E.: Nonobstructive hydronephrosis and hydroureter. AJR *98*:172, 1966.
Talner, L. B.: Urinary obstruction. *In* Pollack, H. M. (ed.): Clinical Urography. Philadelphia, W. B. Saunders, 1990, pp. 1535–1628.
Talner, L. B.: Specific causes of obstruction. *In* Pollack, H. M. (ed.): Clinical Urography. Philadelphia, W.B. Saunders, 1990, pp. 1629–1751.
Weiss, R. M.: Physiology and pharmacology of the renal pelvis and ureter. *In* Walsh, P. C., Retik, A. B., Stamey, T. A., and Vaughan, E. D., Jr. (eds.): Campbell's Urology. 6th ed. Philadelphia, W. B. Saunders, 1992, pp. 111–141.
Whitaker, R. H.: Some observations and theories on the wide ureter and hydronephrosis. Br. J. Urol. *47*:377, 1975.
Whitaker, R. H.: Pathophysiology of ureteric obstruction. *In* Williams, D. I., and Chisholm, G. D. (eds.): Scientific Foundation of Urology, Volume II. Urogenital Tract: Oncology and the Urologic Armamentarium. London, William Heinemann, 1976, pp. 18–22.
Whitaker, R. H., and Johnson, J. H.: A simple classification of wide ureters. Br. J. Urol. *47*:781, 1976.
Whitaker, R. H.: Investigation of the dilated upper urinary tract. J. R. Soc. Med. *73*:377, 1980.
Whitfield, H. N., Britton, K. E., Fry, I. K., Hendry, W. F., Nimmon,

C. C., Travers, P., and Wickham, J. E. A.: The obstructed kidney: Correlation between renal function and urodynamic assessment. Br. J. Urol. *49*:615, 1977.

Techniques

Britton, K. E., Whitfield, H. N., Nimmon, C. C., Hendry, W. F., and Wickham, J. E. A.: Obstructive nephropathy: successful evaluation with radionuclides. Lancet *1*:905, 1979.

Choyke, P. L.: The urogram: Are rumors of its death premature? Radiology *184*:33, 1992.

Ekelund, L., Lindstedt, E., Thiesen, V., and Jönsson, M.-B.: Diuresis urography in equivocal pelvic-ureteric obstruction. Urol. Radiol. *1*:147, 1980.

Ellenbogen, P. H., Scheible, F. W., Talner, L. B., and Leopold, G. R.: Sensitivity of gray scale ultrasound in detecting urinary tract obstruction. AJR *130*:731, 1978.

Haddad, M. C., Sharif, H. S., Shahed, M. S., Mutaiery, M. A., Samihan, A. M., Sammak, B. M., Southcombe, L. A., and Crawford, A. D.: Renal colic: Diagnosis and outcome. Radiology *184*:83, 1992.

Jaffe, R. B., and Middleton, A. W.: Whitaker test: Differentiation of obstructive from nonobstructive uropathy. AJR *134*:9, 1980.

Koff, S. A., Thrall, J. H., and Keyes, J. W., Jr.: Diuretic radionuclide urography: Non-invasive method for evaluating nephroureteral dilatation. J. Urol. *122*:451, 1979.

Lupton, E. W., O'Reilly, P. H., Testa, H. J., Gosling, J. A., and Dixon, J. S.: Diuresis renography in idiopathic hydronephrosis. Ann. R. Coll. Surg. Engl. *62*:216, 1980.

Nilson, A. E., Avrell, M., Bratt, C. G., and Nilsson, S.: Diuretic urography in the assessment of obstruction of the pelviureteric junction. Acta Radiol. (Diagn.) *21*:499, 1980.

O'Reilly, P. H.: Current status of diuretic renography. In Freeman, L. M., and Weismann, H. S. (eds.): Nuclear Medicine Annual. New York, Raven Press, 1987, pp. 173–192.

O'Reilly, P. H.: Investigation of obstructive uropathy. In O'Reilly, P. H., George, N. J. R., Weiss, R. M. (eds.): Diagnostic Techniques in Urology. Philadelphia, W.B. Saunders, 1990, pp. 401–425.

Pfister, R. C., and Newhouse, J. H.: Interventional pyeloureteral techniques: I. Antegrade pyelography and ureteral perfusion. Radiol. Clin. North Am. *17*:341, 1979.

Powers, T. A., Grove, R. B., Bauriedel, J. K., Orr, S. C., Melton, R. E., and Bowden, R. D.: Detection of obstructive uropathy using 99mtechnetium diethylenetriaminepentaacetic acid. J. Urol. *124*:588, 1980.

Sanders, R. C., and Hartman, D. S.: The sonographic destruction between multicystic kidney and hydronephrosis. Radiology *151*:621, 1984.

Scola, F. H., Cronan, J. J., and Schepps, B.: Grade I hydronephrosis: Pulsed Doppler US evaluation. Radiology *171*:519, 1989.

Stage, K. H., and Lewis, S.: Use of the radionuclide washout test in evaluation of suspected upper urinary tract obstruction. J. Urol. *125*:379, 1981.

Whitfield, H. N., Britton, K. E., Hendry, W. F., and Wickham, J. E. A.: Furosemide intravenous urography in the diagnosis of pelviureteric junction obstruction. Br. J. Urol. *51*:445, 1979.

Whitfield, H. N., Harrison, N. W., Sherwood, T., and Williams, D. I.: Upper urinary tract obstruction: Pressure/flow studies in children. Br. J. Urol. *48*:427, 1976.

Whitaker, R. H.: Methods of assessing obstruction in dilated ureters. Br. J. Urol. *45*:15, 1973.

Whitaker, R. H.: The Whitaker test. Urol. Clin. North Am. *6*:529, 1979.

Whitaker, R. H.: Perfusion Pressure Flow Studies. In O'Reilly, P. H., George, N. J. R., and Weiss, R. M. (eds.): Diagnostic Techniques in Urology. Philadelphia, W.B. Saunders, 1990, pp. 135–142.

Nonobstructive Dilatation

Bailey, R. R., and Rolleston, G. L.: Kidney length and ureteric dilatation in the puerperium. J. Obstet. Gynaecol. Br. Common. *78*:55, 1971.

Blickman, J. G., and Lebowitz, R. L.: The coexistence of primary megaureter and reflux. AJR *143*:1053, 1984.

Burbige, K. A., Lebowitz, R. L., Colodny, A. H., Bauer, S. B., and

Retik, A. B.: The megacystic-megaureter syndrome. J. Urol. *131*:113, 1984.

Burbige, K. A., Amodio, J., Berdon, W. E., Hensle, T. W., Blanc, W., and Lattimer, J. K.: Prune-belly syndrome. J. Urol. *137*:86, 1987.

Garcia, C. J., Taylor, K. J. W., and Weiss, R. M.: Congenital megacalyces: Ultrasound appearance. J. Ultrasound Med. *6*:163, 1987.

Greskovich, F. J., III, and Nyberg, L. M.: The prune-belly syndrome: A review of its etiology, defects, treatment and prognosis. J. Urol. *140*:707, 1988.

Guyer, P. B., and Delaney, D. J.: Over-distensibility of the female upper urinary tract. Clin. Radiol. *25*:367, 1974.

Hamilton, S., and Fitzpatrick, J. M.: Primary non-obstructive megaureter in adults. Clin. Radiol. *38*:181, 1987.

Hanna, M. K., and Wyatt, J. K.: Primary obstructive megaureter in adults. J. Urol. *113*:328, 1975.

Harrison, R. B., Ramchandani, P., and Allen, J. T.: Psychogenic polydipsia—unusual cause for hydronephrosis. AJR *133*:327, 1979.

Hellström, M., Jodal, V., Märild, S., and Wettergren, B.: Ureteral dilatation in children with febrile urinary tract infection or bacteruria. AJR *148*:483, 1987.

Johnston, J. H.: Megacalicosis: A burnt-out obstruction? J. Urol. *110*:344, 1973.

Kass, E. J., Silver, T. M., Konnak, J. W., Thornbury, J. R., and Wolfman, M. G.: The urographic findings in acute pyelonephritis: Non-obstructive hydronephrosis. J. Urol. *116*:544, 1976.

King, L. R.: Megaloureter: Definition, diagnosis and management. J. Urol. *123*:222, 1980.

King, L. R.: Vesicoureteral reflux, megaureter and ureteral reimplantation. In Walsh, P. C., Retik, A. B., Stamey, T. A., and Vaughan, E. D., Jr. (eds.): Campbell's Urology. 6th ed. Philadelphia, W.B. Saunders, 1992, pp. 1689–1742.

Kleeman, F. J.: Unilateral megacalicosis. J. Urol. *110*:378, 1973.

Manson, A. D., Yalowitz, P. A., Randall, R. V., and Greene, L. F.: Dilatation of the urinary tract associated with pituitary and nephrogenic diabetes insipidus. J. Urol. *103*:327, 1970.

Marchant, D. J.: Effects of pregnancy and progestational agents on the urinary tract. Am. J. Obstet. Gynecol. *112*:487, 1972.

Mark, L. K., and Möel, M.: Primary megaloureter. Radiology *93*:345, 1969.

McLoughlin, A. P., III, Pfister, R. C., Leadbetter, W. F., Salzstein, S. L., and Kessler, W. D.: The pathophysiology of primary megaloureter. J. Urol. *109*:805, 1973.

Miller, S. S., and Winston, M. C.: Nephrogenic diabetes insipidus. Radiology *87*:893, 1966.

O'Reilly, P. H., Lawson, R. S., Shields, R. A., Testa, H. J., Carroll, R. N. P., and Charlton-Edwards, E.: The dilated, nonobstructed renal pelvis. Br. J. Urol. *53*:205, 1981.

Paltiel, H. J., and Lebowitz, R. L.: Neonatal hydronephrosis due to primary vesicoureter reflux: Trends in diagnosis and treatment. Radiology *170*:787, 1989.

Pfister, R. C., and Hendren, W. H.: Primary megaureter in children and adults: Clinical and pathophysiologic features of 150 ureters. Urology *12*:160, 1978.

Pfister, R. C., McLaughlin, A. P., III, and Leadbetter, W. F.: Radiological evaluation of primary megaureter. Radiology *99*:503, 1971.

Schulman, A., and Herlinger, H.: Urinary tract dilatation in pregnancy. Br. J. Radiol. *48*:638, 1975.

Shapiro, S. R., Woerner, S., Adelman, R. D., and Palmer, J. M.: Diabetes insipidus and hydronephrosis. J. Urol. *119*:715, 1979.

Spiro, F. I., and Fry, I. K.: Ureteric dilatation in non-pregnant women. Proc. R. Soc. Med. *63*:462, 1970.

Talner, L. B., and Gittes, R. F.: Megacalyces. Clin Radiol. *23*:355, 1972.

Talner, L. B., and Gittes, R. F.: Megacalyces: Further observations and differentiation from obstructive renal disease. AJR *121*:473, 1974.

Vargas, B., and Lebowitz, R. L.: The coexistence of congenital megacalyces and primary megaureter. AJR *147*:313, 1986.

Waltzer, W. C.: The urinary tract in pregnancy. J. Urol. *125*:271, 1981.

Weber, A. L., Pfister, R. C., James, A. E., Jr., and Hendren, W. H.: Megaureter in infants and children: Roentgenologic, clinical and surgical aspects. AJR *112*:170, 1971.

Whitaker, R. H., and Flower, C. D. R.: Megacalices—how broad a spectrum? Br. J. Urol. *53*:1, 1981.

Willi, U. V., and Lebowitz, R. L.: The so-called megaureter-megacystis syndrome. AJR *133*:409, 1979.

18

THE EFFACED PELVOCALYCEAL SYSTEM AND URETER

EXTRINSIC COMPRESSION
   Global Enlargement of Renal Parenchyma
   Masses or Masslike Abnormalities of the
   Renal Sinus
	SPASM/INFLAMMATION
	
	INFILTRATION
	
	OLIGURIA

The abnormalities discussed in this chapter have in common the feature of a collapsed pelvocalyceal system and/or ureter. Four broad categories account for this appearance: *extrinsic compression* by diseases of the renal parenchyma or renal sinus, *spasm/inflammation* or *infiltration* of the upper urinary tract, and *oliguric states*, in which the volume of urine formed is insufficient to distend the collecting system.

Specific entities in these categories are discussed in other chapters. In this chapter they are brought together only in summary form because generalized effacement of the collecting system is sometimes the predominant finding and the point of departure in radiologic diagnosis. Table 18–1 is a list of the various causes of effacement.

EXTRINSIC COMPRESSION

Global Enlargement of Renal Parenchyma

Generalized enlargement of the renal parenchyma often causes indistensibility of the collecting system. Excessive renal bulk occurs with cellular infiltration or proliferation, with deposition of abnormal proteins, or with the accumulation of interstitial edema or blood. These processes often reduce urine volume, which also contributes to the collapse of the pelvocalyceal system and ureter.

Bilateral renal enlargement by cellular infiltration or proliferation occurs with proliferative or necrotizing disorders of glomeruli. Neoplastic infiltrations are associated with leukemia, lymphoma, or mesoblastic nephroma; and inflammatory cell infiltration causes bilateral nephromegaly in acute interstitial nephritis. Amyloidosis and multiple myeloma are examples of renal enlargement due to deposition of abnormal pro-

teins. Acute tubular necrosis and acute cortical necrosis have a similar effect as a result of abnormal fluid accumulation within the renal parenchyma. Intratubular and interstitial depositions of uric acid crystals cause large smooth kidneys in acute urate nephropa-

Table 18–1. CAUSES OF EFFACEMENT OF THE PELVOCALYCEAL SYSTEM AND/OR URETER

Extrinsic Compression
  Global Enlargement of Renal Parenchyma—Bilateral
    Proliferative or necrotizing disorders of glomeruli
    Amyloidosis
    Multiple myeloma
    Neoplastic infiltrates (leukemia, lymphoma, mesoblastic
      nephroma)
    Acute tubular necrosis
    Acute cortical necrosis
    Acute interstitial nephritis
    Acute urate nephropathy
  Global Enlargement of Renal Parenchyma—Unilateral
    Renal vein thrombosis
    Acute arterial infarction
    Acute bacterial nephritis
  Renal Sinus Masses or Masslike Abnormalities
    Renal sinus lipomatosis
    Parapelvic cyst
    Hemorrhage
    Renal sinus neoplasm, especially lymphoma
Spasm/Inflammation
  Infection
    Acute pyelonephritis
    Acute bacterial nephritis
    Acute tuberculosis and candidiasis
  Hematuria
Infiltration
  Malignant uroepithelial tumors
Oliguria
  Antidiuretic state
  Renal ischemia
  Oliguric renal failure

thy. Each of these processes affects both kidneys uniformly, and both are discussed in Chapter 8.

Unilateral renal enlargement with effacement of the collecting system may follow renal vein thrombosis or acute arterial infarction with swelling of the interstices of the kidney by blood and congested intrarenal capillaries and veins. Engorgement may be so severe and urine production so limited that retrograde pyelography is needed to opacify the collapsed collecting system. Generalized effacement of the pelvocalyceal system is also found in acute bacterial nephritis. Effacement in this circumstance is caused by acute inflammatory cell infiltrate, reduced urine flow, and spasm of the collecting system. Chapter 9 discusses in detail causes of unilateral renal enlargement that might be associated with an effaced collecting system.

Masses or Masslike Abnormalities of the Renal Sinus

Renal sinus lipomatosis characteristically elongates and attenuates the pelvis and infundibula. This condition, which is usually bilateral, is associated with aging and obesity or as a response to pathologic loss of renal parenchyma. The surrounding renal parenchyma is sometimes wasted. Excessive fat deposition in the renal sinus is most readily detected by computed tomography or ultrasonography.

Some parapelvic cysts insinuate themselves around the pelvis and infundibula and cause a urographic appearance similar to that of renal sinus lipomatosis. Distinction between these two disorders can be made reliably by ultrasonography, computed tomography, or magnetic resonance imaging. Renal sinus lipomatosis and parapelvic cyst are discussed in Chapter 16.

Spontaneous hemorrhage into the renal sinus has been described in patients on anticoagulant therapy. This self-limiting process causes attenuation of the pelvocalyceal system, impaired excretion of contrast material, and, occasionally, caliectasis. Blood in the sinus produces an initially high-density mass that disappears within a few weeks.

A neoplasm in the renal sinus, either primary or metastatic, may surround the pelvocalyceal system and proximal ureter. Similarly, more distal portions of the ureter may be surrounded by tumor in the perirenal space. As a result, the predominant radiologic finding may be a lack of distensibility of these structures. Lymphoma invading the kidney by a transsinus route, as described in Chapter 10, characteristically causes such an abnormality. Other entities that produce similar findings in the ureter are discussed in Chapters 16 and 21.

SPASM/INFLAMMATION

One manifestation of acute pyelonephritis is generalized effacement of the pelvocalyceal system. The precise mechanism for this is unclear. Spasm of the smooth muscles of the collecting system wall is the likely explanation, although swelling of the kidney may play a role as well. Paradoxically, some patients with acute pyelonephritis have a dilated pelvocalyceal system and ureter as a result of paralysis of the smooth muscle by bacterial endotoxins.

Effacement of the pelvis and calyces is always present in acute bacterial nephritis in which oliguria, parenchymal swelling, and spasm contribute to this effect. Acute infection is discussed in Chapter 9.

Uroepithelial tuberculosis and candidiasis cause submucosal granulomas, mucosal ulcerations, and, eventually, fibrosis and mural thickening. These conditions render the collecting system and ureter nondistensible. They are discussed in Chapter 15.

Upper urinary tract bleeding, whether from the kidney or directly from uroepithelial structures, can cause effacement of the collecting system, presumably as a result of irritation of pelvocalyceal smooth muscle. This reverts to normal as bleeding ceases.

INFILTRATION

Malignant uroepithelial tumors, most commonly transitional cell carcinoma, may grow either superficially or infiltrate deeply over a large area of the pelvocalyceal system or ureter. Either of these patterns may cause generalized effacement of the upper tract in association with a nodular mucosal pattern, which is discussed in Chapter 15.

OLIGURIA

The pelvocalyceal system and ureter are collapsed in the oliguric kidney, just as they are distended by a large volume of urine in high flow states, such as diabetes insipidus. Collapse is readily reversed by a fluid load when oliguria is due to the antidiuretic effect of water deprivation. However, no such easy reversal occurs when oliguria reflects primary renal vascular or parenchymal disease. In these situations, effacement of the pelvocalyceal system is one radiologic abnormality among many that reflect the underlying disorder. For example, a collapsed upper urinary tract due to oliguria caused by severe renal artery stenosis will be a unilateral phenomenon, accompanied by those other radiologic signs of ischemia that are discussed in Chapter 6. On the other hand, oliguria caused by acute renal failure will be associated with bilaterally enlarged smooth kidneys, which are discussed in Chapter 8.

Bibliography

Global Enlargement—Bilateral

See Bibliography for Chapter 8.

Global Enlargement—Unilateral

See Bibliography for Chapter 9.

Renal Sinus and Periureteral Masses or Masslike Abnormalities

See Bibliography for Chapter 16.

Spasm/Inflammation

See Bibliographies for Chapter 9 (Acute Pyelonephritis and Acute Bacterial Nephritis); Chapter 15 (Acute Tuberculosis, Candidiasis, and Xanthogranulomatous Pyelonephritis); and Chapter 11 (Xanthogranulomatous Pyelonephritis).

Infiltration

See Bibliography for Chapter 15.

Oliguria

See Bibliographies for Chapter 6 (Renal Ischemia) and Chapter 8 (Acute Renal Failure).

IV

THE LOWER URINARY TRACT

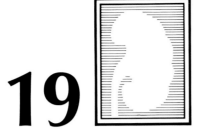

WENDELIN S. HAYES

19

THE URINARY BLADDER

ANATOMY

The urinary bladder is a distensible, muscular pouch that serves as a reservoir for urine. Thus, the contour and size of the bladder varies with the degree of filling. The bladder is predominately a pelvic organ, lying behind the pubic symphysis when empty and rising above the symphysis and high in the pelvis when full. The superior surface of the bladder, called the *dome*, is covered by peritoneum. The space between the anterior bladder wall and the posterior aspect of the symphysis pubis is known as the anterior perivesical space, or the *space of Retzius.* In the female, the uterus and vagina are posterior and inferior to the bladder while the fallopian tubes and ovaries are lateral and superior. In the male, the rectum is posterior, the seminal vesicles and ampulla of the vas deferens posteroinferior, and the prostate inferior to the bladder.

Transitional epithelium forms a bladder lining that is seven to eight cells thick from the basement membrane to the lumen. The muscular wall consists of a complex arrangement of interlacing smooth muscle bundles distinct from the lamina propria that supports the bladder mucosa. The muscle bundles, longi-

tudinal or circular, freely cross each other with no definite orientation except around the bladder neck, where three distinct layers can be identified.

The most inferior portion of the urinary bladder is the bladder neck, which leads to the urethra. The pubocervical or puboprostatic ligaments support the urethrovesical junction. The internal sphincter is at the bladder neck.

The bladder is a very vascular structure with arterial blood supply from the superior, middle, and inferior vesical arteries, which are branches of the hypogastric artery, and from smaller branches of the obturator and inferior gluteal arteries. Branches of the uterine and vaginal arteries supply the bladder base in the female.

A rich plexus of veins surrounds the bladder, terminating in the hypogastric veins. The vesicovenous plexus also communicates with the hemorrhoidal veins, which drain into the intervertebral venous plexus.

The ureters enter the bladder at the posterior portion of the trigone. At the posterior aspect of the trigone there is a muscular ridge lying between the ureteral orifices, the *interureteric ridge.* The trigone is triangular, with its apex anterior and its base at the interureteral ridge.

EMBRYOLOGY AND ANOMALIES

Agenesis

Agenesis of the bladder represents persistence of the cloaca due to failure of the urorectal septum to form and partition the cloaca into an anterior bladder and a posterior rectum. Agenesis of the bladder is a rare anomaly that has been reported predominantly in females. Associated renal and genital anomalies include bilateral renal agenesis, dysplastic kidney, hydronephrosis, solitary kidney, and absence of the prostate and seminal vesicles. Complications include recurrent urinary tract infections, incontinence, and renal failure.

Duplication and Septation

Complete duplication of the urinary bladder and related anomalies are extremely rare. Two bladders lie side by side, separated by a peritoneal fold. Each bladder wall consists of the normal mucosal and muscular layers, and each has a ureter from the ipsilateral kidney. Each bladder has a separate urethra. Duplication of the bladder is often associated with duplication of the genital and distal gastrointestinal tracts, of the external genitalia, and, less commonly, of the lower spine. Congenital anomalies of the kidney and ureters may coexist.

Duplication of the bladder may be partial or incomplete with communication at the inferior portion of both bladders. In this circumstance, drainage is through a common urethra. Fewer associated anomalies are seen with incomplete than with complete bladder duplication. The radiologic appearance of a partially duplicated bladder has been described as "valentine" shaped.

Another anomaly of bladder compartmentalization is division of a single bladder into two portions by a septum in the sagittal or coronal plane. The complete septum results in a ureter draining into the closed portion, resulting in a dysplastic or nonfunctional kidney. Excretory urography demonstrates one functioning kidney with an associated hemibladder.

Exstrophy/Epispadias

Exstrophy of the bladder and epispadias occur as a spectrum of defects in the formation of the anterior abdominal wall caused by varying degrees of failure of midline fusion of the mesodermal tissue below the umbilicus. Exstrophy is the most common anomaly of the bladder. Males are affected more often than females by a ratio of 2:1. In its most severe manifestation, the rectus abdominus muscle is widely separated and the bladder lies open and everted on the anterior abdominal wall. The bladder mucosa is continuous with the skin. The exposed transitional cell mucosa often undergoes metaplasia, creating an increased risk for adenocarcinoma of the bladder. With an associated epispadias, the urethral mucosa covers the dorsum of a short penis and the urethra opens on the dorsal surface of the penis. In the female, the urethra is short, the labia are widely separated, and the clitoris is cleaved. The upper urinary tract is usually normal.

A radiograph of the pelvis in the exstrophy/epispadias anomaly demonstrates diastasis of the pubic symphysis (Fig. 19–1). On excretory urography there is a wide lateral curve of the pelvic portion of the distal ureters, which then turn medially and slightly upward and pass through the bladder wall in a perpendicular direction. The most distal portion of the ureters is slightly dilated. The remainder of the upper tracts is usually normal.

Prune-Belly Syndrome

Prune-belly syndrome (Eagle-Barrett syndrome, triad syndrome) is a rare congenital syndrome, usually affecting males, in which there is deficiency or hypoplasia of abdominal muscles, undescended testicles, and anomalies of the urinary tract. The syndrome is usually readily recognized at birth because of the characteristic thin, wrinkled abdominal wall that is the result of absent abdominal musculature. Detection may occur later in life in patients with mild manifestations. The major prognostic factor in patients with prune-belly syndrome is related to the severity of the urinary tract abnormalities.

The bladder is frequently very large with a wall of variable thickness. Bladder musculature is replaced by collagen. The bladder is often elongated, without trabeculation, and attached to the umbilicus, where a patent urachus, urachal diverticulum, or cyst may be apparent.

The appearance of the ureter in prune-belly syndrome is discussed in Chapter 17.

THE URACHUS

Anomalies

The urachus develops from the superior portion of the urogenital sinus and connects the dome of the bladder to the allantoic duct during fetal life. Before birth, the urachus obliterates and becomes a vestigial structure known as the *medial umbilical ligament.* In the absence of complete obliteration, the urachus persists in one of four types of congenital anomalies: *patent urachus, urachal cyst, urachal sinus,* or *urachal diverticulum* (Fig. 19–2).

Patent urachus represents the failure of the entire course of the urachus to close, resulting in an open channel between the bladder and the umbilicus. A patent urachus is usually diagnosed in the newborn when urine is noted leaking from the umbilicus.

A urachal cyst forms when both the umbilical and the vesical ends of the urachal lumen close, but an intervening portion remains patent and fluid filled. This generally occurs in that part of the urachus that is closest to the bladder. Urachal cysts usually remain obscure until complicated by infection or, more rarely, tumor. The clinical findings that result, such as mid-

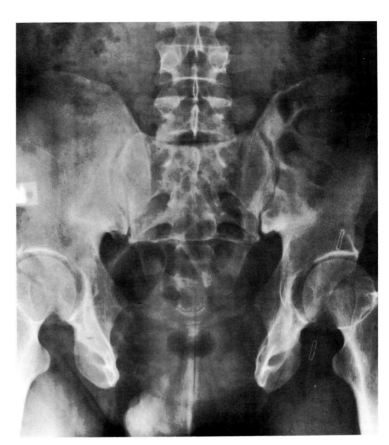

Figure 19–1. Bladder exstrophy. The radiograph of the pelvis reveals diastasis of the symphysis pubis.

abdominal or suprapubic pain, fever, dysuria, or a palpable mass with associated urinary tract symptoms often mimic a variety of acute abdominal or pelvic inflammatory processes. Rarely, spontaneous drainage of a urachal cyst through the umbilicus occurs.

Urachal sinus is a blind-ending dilatation of the urachus at the umbilical end, whereas urachal diverticulum is a similar deformity that communicates with the anterosuperior aspect of the bladder as a result of failure of closure of the urachus at the bladder. A urachal diverticulum sometimes occurs in boys with urethral obstruction and may also be associated with prune-belly syndrome without outlet obstruction.

A patent urachus is directly demonstrated by retrograde injection of contrast material into its orifice at the umbilicus. This anomaly may also be identified during a voiding cystourethrogram in the lateral projection or by ultrasonography as a fluid-filled tubular structure extending from the bladder to the umbilicus (Fig. 19–3). Urethral atresia or posterior urethral valve with bladder outlet obstruction coexists with patent urachus in up to 30 per cent of cases. Here, voiding cystourethrography demonstrates these additional, complicating features. A urachal diverticulum is identified as a urine-filled anterosuperior extension from the bladder dome by cystography, voiding cystourethrography, ultrasonography, computed tomography, or magnetic resonance imaging. The latter three modalities may be used to identify an uncomplicated urachal cyst or sinus as a collection of simple fluid localized in the midline of the anterior abdominal wall between the umbilicus and the pubis and often contiguous with the bladder dome. Needle aspiration and contrast material instillation may also be used. A urachal cyst complicated by infection or neoplasm demonstrates additional features of fluid with mixed echogenicity, higher than water attenuation values, or soft tissue components and thickening of the urachal wall. Radiologic evaluation with computed tomography, ultrasonography, or needle aspiration allows for a definitive diagnosis (Figs. 19–4 and 19–5).

Malignant Tumors

The urachus is lined by transitional cell epithelium, which uncommonly undergoes metaplasia and malignant transformation into mucinous adenocarcinoma. Nonmucinous adenocarcinoma, squamous cell carcinoma, transitional cell carcinoma, and sarcoma of the urachus are rarer than mucinous adenocarcinoma. Urachal neoplasms are situated at the vesicourachal junction at the dome of the bladder and, at the time of diagnosis, are often quite large. Local spread of tumor, which has commonly occurred by the time of diagnosis, is into the anterior abdominal wall, the bladder, the space of Retzius, and the peritoneum. Distant spread is into regional lymph nodes and beyond.

Urachal adenocarcinoma is most prevalent between the fifth and eight decades of life and affects males more often than females by a ratio of approximately 3:1. Because the site of origin of urachal carcinoma is

Text continued on page 614

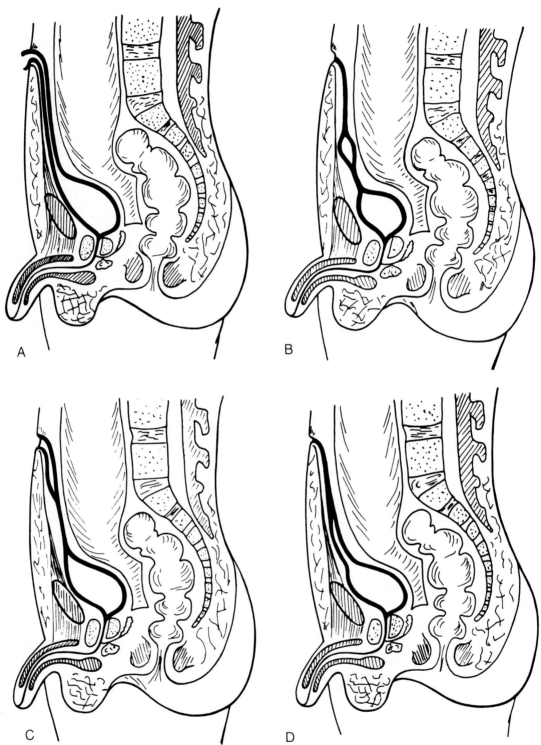

Figure 19–2. Congenital urachal anomalies.
  A, Patent urachus.
  B, Urachal cyst.
  C, Urachal sinus.
  D, Urachal diverticulum.
  (From Schnyder, A., and Candardjis, G.: Vesicourachal diverticulum: CT diagnosis in two adults. AJR *137*:1063–1065, 1981. Reproduced with kind permission of the authors and *American Journal of Roentgenology.*)

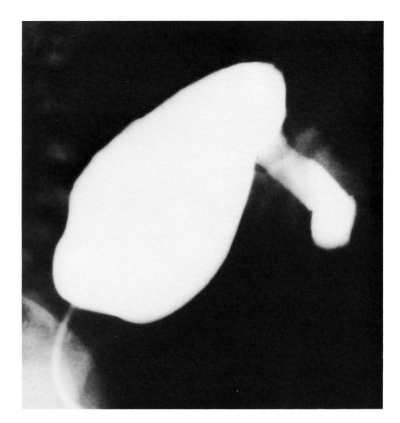

Figure 19–3. Patent urachus. A voiding cystourethrogram demonstrates contrast material in a patent urachus, which extends through the umbilicus into the umbilical stump ending in a blind pouch.

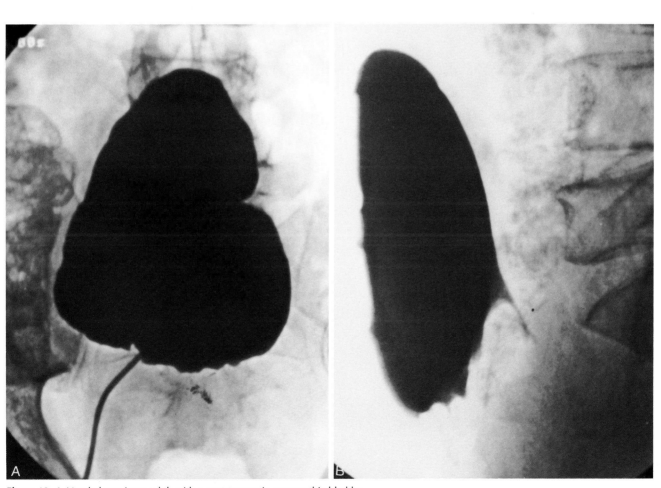

Figure 19–4. Urachal cyst in an adult with a post-traumatic neuropathic bladder.
A and *B,* Frontal and lateral radiographs. Opacification of a urachal cyst following percutaneous puncture reveals a predominantly smooth wall cyst. There is no communication to the bladder.

Illustration continued on following page

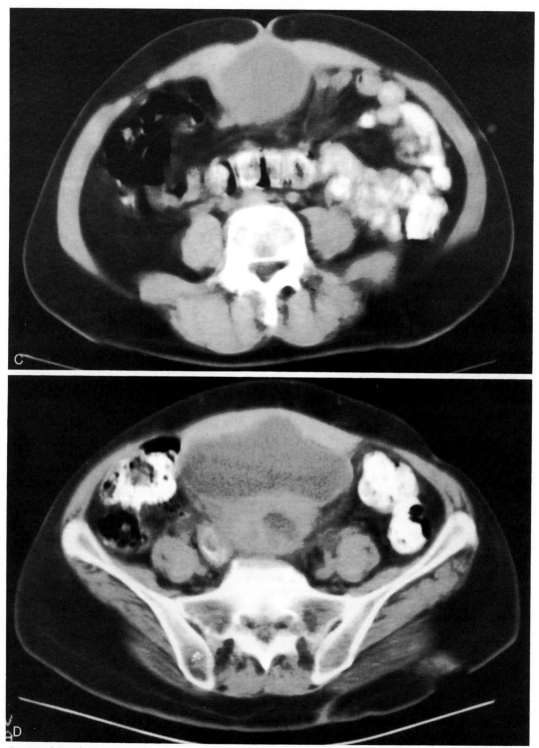

Figure 19–4. *Continued C* and *D,* Computed tomograms without contrast material enhancement at the level of the umbilicus *(C)* and pelvis *(D)* demonstrate the extent of the cyst.

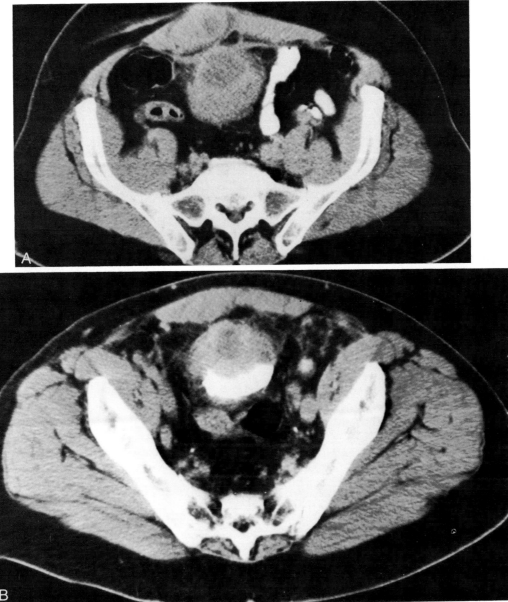

Figure 19–5. Infected urachal cyst in an adult with persistent lower abdominal pain. Computed tomograms with contrast material enhancement demonstrate an irregular mass of variable attenuation values that extended from level of the umbilicus to the dome of the bladder.
A, Upper section demonstrates involvement of the rectus abdominis muscle.
B, Section at the level of dome of the opacified bladder.

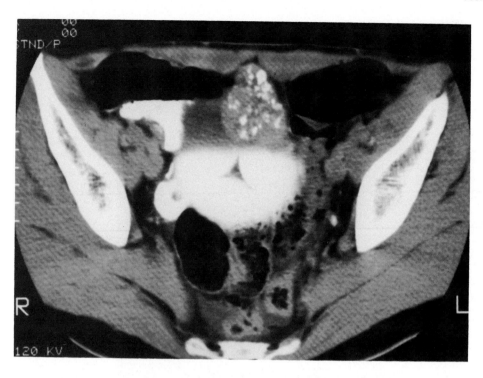

Figure 19–6. Urachal adenocarcinoma. Computed tomogram with contrast material enhancement. There is a calcified, soft tissue midline mass in the anterior aspect of the bladder dome.

not one that leads to early clinical findings and because of the lack of fascial barriers in the area, spread is extensive and the prognosis for urachal carcinoma is poor.

Hematuria is the most common symptom of urachal carcinoma, but this often occurs only after significant tumor growth. Less commonly, patients present with dysuria, frequency, abdominal pain, or a lower abdominal or suprapubic mass. Gross or microscopic mucus is present in the urine in as many as 25 per cent of patients.

An abdominal radiograph may show a supravesical soft tissue mass with calcification. Urachal adenocarcinoma is best defined radiologically by ultrasonography or computed tomography as a soft tissue mass in the anterosuperior portion of the bladder. Hemorrhage or necrosis may be seen as hypoechoic or low attenuation areas within the tumor. Dystrophic calcification is often present within the mass, which is characteristically located in the midline and often involves the anterior abdominal wall and adjacent bladder wall (Fig. 19–6). Intravesical growth, as seen by either computed tomography or ultrasonography, represents advanced disease.

DIVERTICULUM

Most bladder diverticula are acquired in association with long-standing bladder outlet obstruction, including those due to neuropathic disorders of the bladder. Most commonly, diverticula are encountered in older men with benign prostatic enlargement, prostatitis, or carcinoma of the prostate. Other causes include urethral stricture and, in infants, congenital urethral valve or stricture. In females, bladder diverticula may develop in outlet obstruction owing to urethral carcinoma or diverticulum.

A congenital bladder diverticulum, on the other hand, is uncommon and develops as a result of herniation of bladder mucosa through the detrusor muscle of the bladder, usually at a location slightly above and lateral to a ureteral orifice. This so-called *Hutch diverticulum* may vary from small to quite large and cause either obstruction of or vesicoureteral reflux into the ipsilateral ureter. In male infants, bladder diverticula must be distinguished from protrusions of the urinary bladder bilaterally into the inguinal rings anteriorly. These outpouchings, known as "bladder ears," are transient and usually disappear with aging.

An acquired bladder diverticulum begins as a small outpouching of mucosa that evaginates between hypertrophied detrusor muscle bundles but does not extend beyond the outer margin of the bladder wall. This structure is called a *cellule* (Fig. 19–7). Only when the cellule protrudes beyond the outer margin of the bladder wall is it referred to as a diverticulum. Most acquired diverticula develop in the base of the bladder, often just anterolateral to a ureteral orifice. Diverticula can vary in size and become much larger than the bladder. They may be single or multiple. Large diverticula may cause ureteral deviation or obstruction, vesicoureteral reflux, urinary tract infection, or calculi (Fig. 19–8). Some diverticula grow large enough to deform the bladder and cause urinary retention (Fig. 19–9). Diverticula are lined by uroepithelium and, therefore, may be the site of carcinoma of the bladder. Because a diverticulum lacks a layer of muscle, carcinoma arising in a diverticulum is likely to spread faster than one that arises in the bladder lumen.

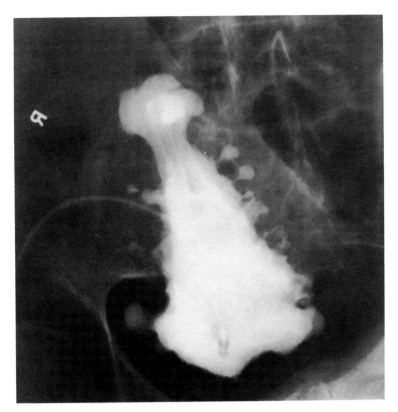

Figure 19–7. Cellule. There are multiple outpouchings between hypertrophic detrusor muscle bundles. Cystogram.

Bladder diverticula are best studied radiologically by cystography, voiding cystourethrography, ultrasonography, computed tomography, or excretory urography. Their appearance varies with location, size, effect on adjacent structures, and the presence of complicating stone or tumor. A large diverticulum originating near the ureterovesical junction may deviate the ipsilateral ureter medially. A diverticulum may also displace the bladder, giving rise to the same appearance as a soft tissue mass originating in the extravesical retroperitoneum. A wide-neck diverticulum fills and empties readily with the bladder. If the neck of the diverticulum is narrow, poor emptying may lead to urine stasis, chronic infection, and stone formation. Radiographs obtained after voiding are valuable in this regard. Ultrasonography is a particularly effective modality for the evaluation of a bladder diverticulum, which appears as a fluid-filled outpouching of the bladder that communicates to the lumen. Calculi within a diverticulum are echogenic and produce an acoustic shadow. Tumor within the diverticulum produces a filling defect on excretory urography or computed tomography or a soft tissue mass within the diverticulum on ultrasonograpy (Fig. 19–10).

INTRALUMINAL FILLING DEFECTS

Bladder calculi occur most often in adults as a result of urine stasis due to bladder neck obstruction or neuropathic bladder dysfunction combined with urinary tract infection. Urine stasis may also occur in bladder diverticulum. Long-term bladder instrumentation or

other foreign bodies are additional conditions that promote calculus formation. *Proteus mirabilis* is the organism most commonly associated with bladder infection and stone formation.

Patients with bladder calculi may be asymptomatic, and the stones discovered only as an incidental finding during radiologic or cystoscopic evaluation. Symptoms, when present, include pain and difficulty in urination, sometimes due to intermittent obstruction of the bladder neck by the calculus. Microscopic hematuria is frequently present because of associated irritation of the bladder mucosa.

Bladder calculi vary in density on radiographs from densely opaque to nonopaque. They may be solitary or multiple and vary in size and shape. The composition of the calculi will determine whether they appear homogeneous or laminated (Fig. 19–11). With contrast material in the bladder, the calculi may be obscured. Most, however, are seen as filling defects within the contrast material–filled bladder. Mobility of the stones can be demonstrated on oblique or erect projections. On ultrasonography, bladder calculi of all types are identified as echogenic structures within the fluid-filled bladder with associated acoustic shadowing. Mobility of the stones can be easily demonstrated with real-time ultrasonography. Calculi that are not opaque on radiographs are well demonstrated on unenhanced computed tomography because their attenuation values are high enough to appear dense.

Other etiologies that must be considered in the diagnosis of intraluminal bladder filling defects include fungus ball, foreign material, blood clot, and sloughed papilla. These are usually distinguished by the clinical

Text continued on page 620

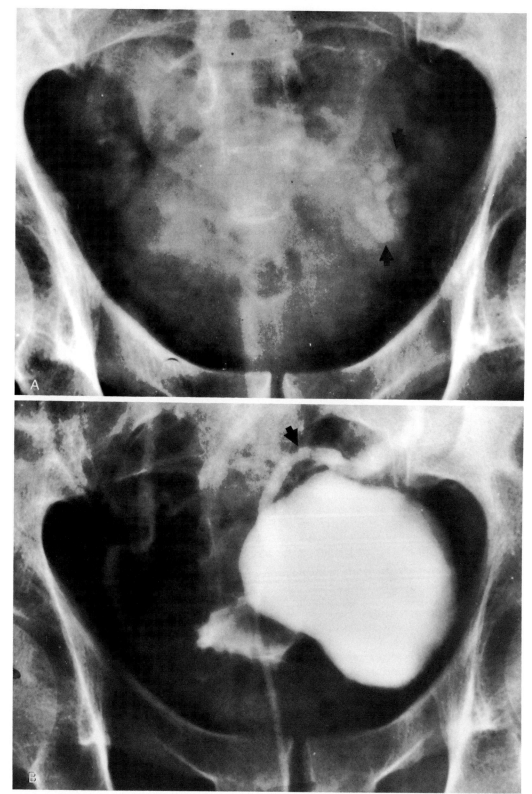

Figure 19–8. Bladder diverticulum containing multiple calculi.

A, Radiograph of pelvis demonstrates left-sided multiple densities *(arrows).*

B, Excretory urogram, postvoid film, demonstrates opacification of a large bladder diverticulum. The calculi are obscured by the contrast material. Note medial deviation of the ipsilateral ureter by the diverticulum *(arrow).*

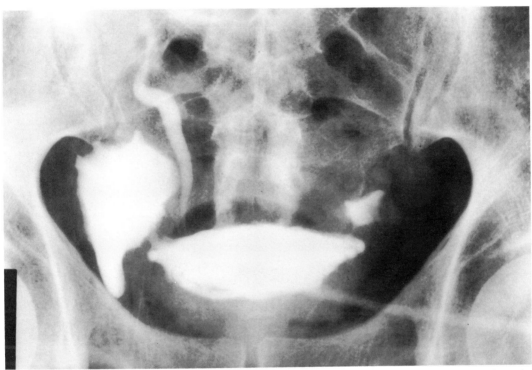

Figure 19–9. Bladder diverticula. A cystogram demonstrates a large right-sided diverticulum and a small left-sided diverticulum. The narrow neck leading through the bladder wall is visualized in both. Reflux of contrast material into the right ureter is present.

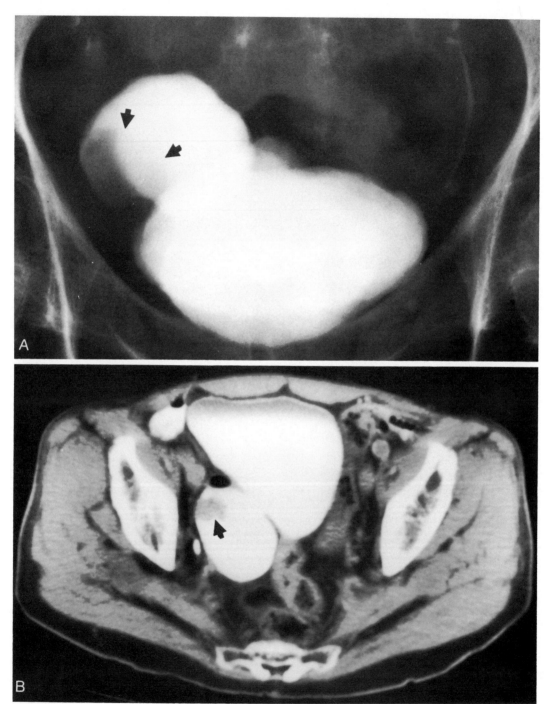

Figure 19–10. Carcinoma within a bladder diverticulum.
   A, Excretory urogram demonstrates an intraluminal filling defect *(arrows)* within a right-sided bladder diverticulum.
   B, Computed tomogram with contrast material enhancement reveals irregular mural-based mass *(arrow)* protruding into the lumen of the bladder diverticulum.

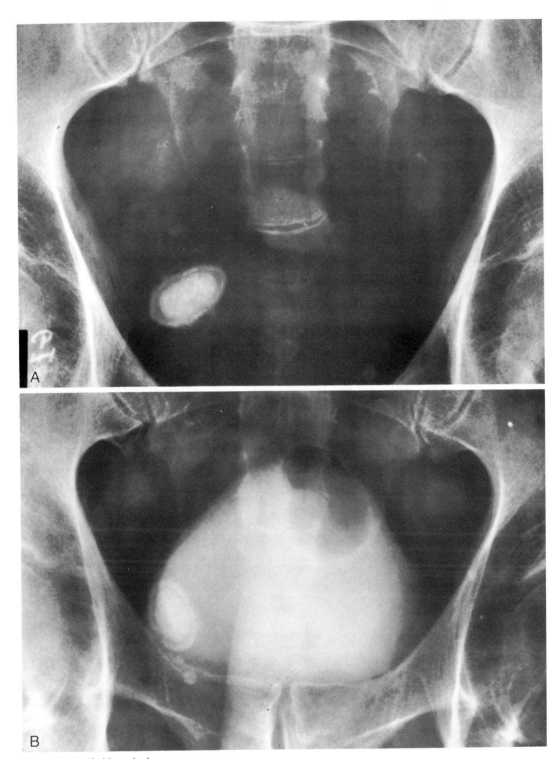

Figure 19–11. Bladder calculus.
A, Radiograph of the pelvis demonstrates a laminated bladder calculus.
B, Excretory urogram, right lateral decubitus view. The calculus has moved with the change in position of the patient.

setting in which they occur or exhibit other characteristics, as discussed subsequently and in Chapter 14.

INFECTION
Acute Cystitis

Acute cystitis due to bacterial infection is most commonly the result of invasion of the bladder through the urethra by coliform bacteria that have colonized the perineum. The short length of the female urethra contributes to the striking predilection of acute cystitis for females compared with males. *Escherichia coli* is the most common organism causing acute cystitis. Other pathogens include *Klebsiella* species, *Enterobacter* species, *Proteus mirabilis*, *Pseudomonas aeruginosa*, *Staphylococcus* species, *Streptococcus faecalis*, *Serratia* species, and *Candida albicans*.

Dysuria, urinary frequency and urgency, and gross hematuria are the most common clinical features of acute cystitis. However, patients may be asymptomatic. Pyuria and bacteriuria are the dominant laboratory findings.

The acutely infected bladder is often normal in appearance radiologically. Cystography is usually not performed in patients with acute symptoms because of the risk of inducing bacteremia. Mucosal inflammation and edema may cause thickened bladder mucosa with a cobblestone appearance. Bladder irritability may lead to reduced bladder capacity.

Emphysematous Cystitis

Acute bacterial cystitis in patients with diabetes mellitus may sometimes be associated with the formation of both intraluminal and intramural bladder gas, a condition known as emphysematous cystitis. *Escherichia coli* is the most common pathogen.

Other organisms that may cause gas-forming bladder infection are *Aerobacter aerogenes*, *Staphylococcus aureus*, *Streptococcus* species, *Proteus* species, *Nocardia* species, and *Candida albicans*. The gas in emphysematous cystitis is carbon dioxide, which is produced by bacterial fermentation of urine glucose within the bladder wall.

Most patients with emphysematous cystitis are elderly and have a history of long-standing or poorly controlled diabetes mellitus. In addition to the symptoms of cystitis described in the previous section, pneumaturia may be present. Unlike emphysematous pyelonephritis, described in Chapter 9, emphysematous cystitis is not life threatening and usually responds to appropriate antimicrobial therapy and control of the patient's diabetes mellitus.

Standard radiographs of the lower abdomen demonstrate gas within the bladder wall as a mottled or streaky radiolucency. Associated gas is often present in the bladder lumen, and this changes location with change in the position of the patient. An excretory urogram confirms the location of the mural gas (Fig. 19–12). The bladder wall may appear thickened and irregular as a reflection of inflammation and edema.

Occasionally, gas extends into the ureters or perivesical soft tissue. Intraluminal gas due to infection must be differentiated from that due to vesicovaginal or vesicoenteric fistula or recent surgical or diagnostic instrumentation (Fig. 19–13).

Tuberculosis

Tuberculosis of the bladder results from a descending infection from the upper urinary tract and, therefore, usually coexists with renal or ureteral abnormalities as well. Initially, the ureteral orifice becomes edematous and ulcerated. Ureteral obstruction may follow. The inflammatory process may progress to involve any portion of the bladder, resulting in multiple mural irregularities. Eventually, fibrosis of the bladder wall causes asymmetry and contraction of the bladder. If fibrosis involves the ureteral orifice, either stricture or a rigid, dilated ureteral orifice with vesicoureteral reflux develops. The reader is referred to Chapter 13 for a discussion of tuberculosis of the kidney and to Chapter 15 for a discussion of tuberculosis of the pelvocalyceal system and ureter.

Schistosomiasis

Schistosomiasis (bilharziasis) is a parasitic infection prevalent in Eastern Africa, the Middle East, and Southwest Asia. Of the three types of *Schistosoma* species that occur in endemic areas, it is *Schistosoma haematobium* that affects the urinary tract, particularly the bladder. The cercariae penetrate the skin of humans and migrate to the venules of the lamina propria of the bladder and distal ureters by way of the portal circulation and the hemorrhoidal and pudendal veins. Eventually, they penetrate the muscularis and submucosa of the bladder and distal ureters, where ova are deposited. The cystitis and ureteritis that subsequently develop are characterized by granulomas, superficial mucosal ulcerations, and the formation of polypoid masses of granulation tissue. Fibrosis and calcium deposition in dead ova eventually develop.

Patients with bladder schistosomiasis develop hematuria, dysuria, and frequency. A fibrotic bladder with reduced capacity is a late complication. Additionally, bladder schistosomiasis carries an increased risk for carcinoma of the bladder, particularly squamous cell carcinoma.

The radiologic features of bladder schistosomiasis vary with the duration of the infestation. Initially, the bladder mucosa demonstrates a prominent and irregular pattern representing nonspecific acute inflammation, edema, and granulomas in the submucosa. As a late manifestation, calcification forms in patterns that vary from focal to linear deposits with a distribution that in some patients is limited to segments while in others involves the entire bladder (Fig. 19–14). With repeat schistosomal and secondary infections the bladder becomes contracted. Bladder carcinoma that develops as a complication of schistosomiasis produces the additional feature of a soft tissue mass that

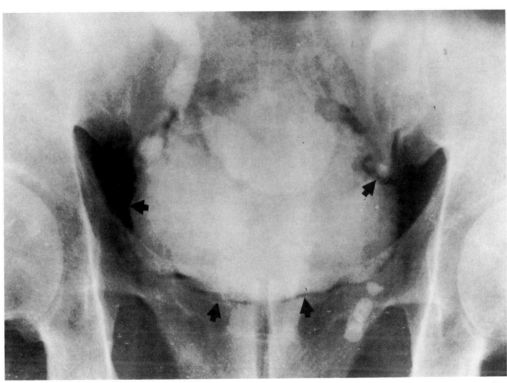

Figure 19–12. Emphysematous cystitis in a patient with diabetes mellitus. Linear radiolucencies *(arrows)* represent gas within the wall of the bladder. Excretory urogram.

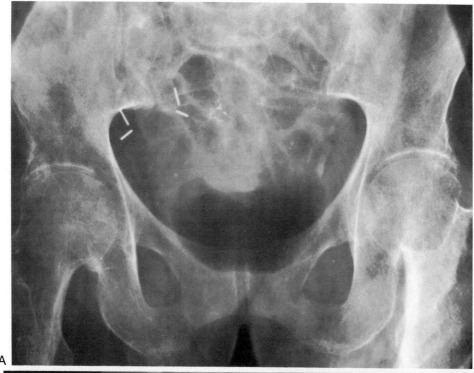

A

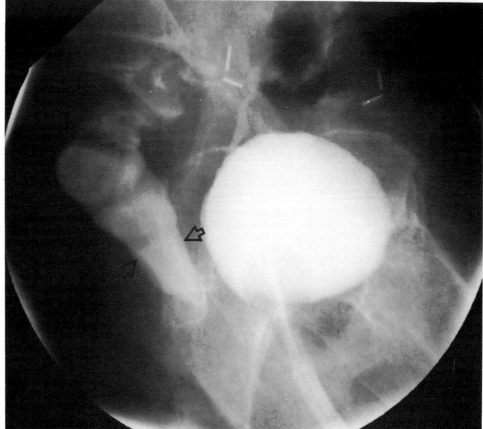

B

Figure 19–13. Intraluminal bladder gas secondary to a vesicoenteric fistula.
    A, Radiograph of the pelvis demonstrates gas lucency within the bladder.
    B, Cystogram. The rectosigmoid colon *(arrows)* opacifies with contrast material introduced into the bladder.

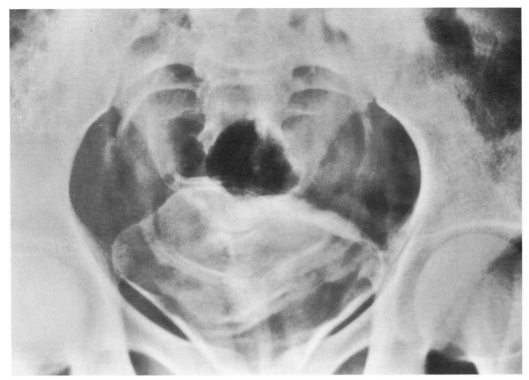

Figure 19–14. Schistosomiasis. There is dense calcification of the bladder wall. Radiograph of pelvis.

may create asymmetry or discontinuity in the pattern of mural calcification.

Schistosomiasis of the ureter is discussed in Chapter 15.

Candidiasis

Fungal infections of the bladder are almost always due to *Candida* species, especially *Candida albicans.* Risk factors for fungal cystitis include immunocompromised states, debilitation, diabetes mellitus, long-term antibiotic or corticosteroid therapy, prematurity, and extended bladder catheterization. The bladder mucosa is diffusely thickened by acute inflammation, and patients develop urgency, frequency, dysuria, and suprapubic pain. Hematuria is present.

Radiologically, a nonspecific pattern of bladder wall thickening and irregularity is seen. A fungus ball, if present, appears as a nonopaque, irregular filling defect within the bladder lumen. This may contain gas (Fig. 19–15). In some patients, multiple small fungus balls are present rather than one large ball.

Candidiasis of the upper urinary tract is discussed in Chapters 14 and 15.

Malakoplakia

Malakoplakia is an uncommon granulomatous response to an infection of the urinary tract, predominantly with *Escherichia coli.* An intracellular abnormality of macrophages, probably at the lysosomal level, is thought to prevent complete digestion of phagocytosed bacteria. Submucosal granulomas dominated by large mononuclear cells with abundant cytoplasm de-

velop. Intracellular and extracellular inclusion bodies composed of calcium and iron-ladened lysosomal material are present. These inclusions, known as Michaelis-Gutmann bodies, are probably bacilli in various stages of defective digestion. The granulomas produce multiple yellow-gray or brown elevations of the mucosa.

Malakoplakia affects any part of the genitourinary tract, including the testes and prostate, but the bladder is involved most frequently. Malakoplakia of the kidney is discussed in Chapter 11 and that of the pelvis and ureter in Chapter 15.

Malakoplakia affects females most often, predominantly in the fifth to sixth decades of life. Symptoms are generally those of urinary tract infection and bladder irritability. Hematuria is commonly present.

The radiologic appearance of malakoplakia of the bladder is that of single or multiple mural filling defects, especially in the trigone or bladder base (Fig. 19–16). Radiologic differentiation from neoplasm is not possible.

INFLAMMATION
Radiation Cystitis

Cystitis sometimes develops as a result of external or intracavitary radiation therapy for primary urothelial neoplasms or other pelvic malignancies. This is usually mild. In some patients, however, a severe cystitis occurs either in an *acute* or a *delayed* form.

In acute radiation cystitis, edema, hyperemia, petechiae, and ulceration of the bladder wall develop. Clinically, symptoms of bladder inflammation, such

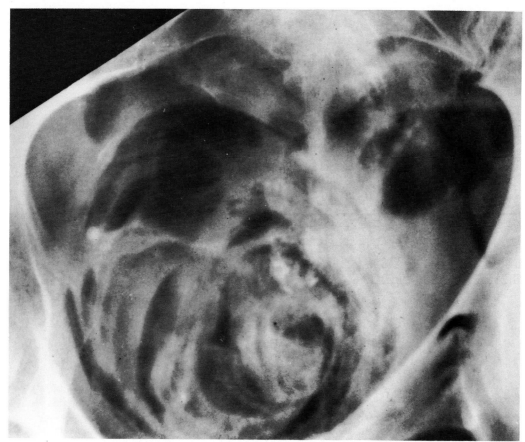

Figure 19–15. Fungus ball in bladder due to candidiasis. Radiograph of the pelvis demonstrates a laminated, gas-containing filling defect within the bladder.

as frequency and dysuria as well as hematuria, become manifest. Radiologic studies, if abnormal, demonstrate prominence and irregularity of bladder mucosa, bladder irritability, and increased contractility. These findings, however, are not specific for radiation.

Delayed radiation cystitis develops up to 4 years following therapy, depending on dose and host susceptibility. Here, the pathologic findings are interstitial fibrosis, obliterative endarteritis, and telangiectasia of the bladder mucosa. Severe hematuria may be a complicating factor. The radiologic findings in delayed radiation cystitis are dominated by extensive fibrosis causing reduced bladder capacity, a thickened bladder wall, and, in some cases, upper tract obstruction (Fig. 19–17). Calcification is rare.

Cyclophosphamide Cystitis

Cyclophosphamide, used as an antineoplastic or immunosuppressive agent, produces metabolites that are cytotoxic to uroepithelium. The bladder is especially susceptible, presumably reflecting an exposure time that is more prolonged than that in the upper urinary tract. Cystitis occurs in as many as 40 per cent of patients receiving cyclophosphamide, which is also considered a risk factor for carcinoma of the bladder.

In acute cyclophosphamide cystitis, the bladder mucosa becomes edematous and hyperemic. Ulceration and hemorrhage may ensue. Radiologic findings

at this stage include bladder wall thickening and irregularity with intraluminal filling defects due to blood clots. Acute cyclophosphamide cystitis may evolve into a chronic form characterized by bladder fibrosis, and, in some patients, persistent bladder hemorrhage. Radiologically, this stage is seen as a contracted, low capacity bladder (Fig. 19–18).

Eosinophilic Cystitis

Eosinophilic cystitis is a rare inflammatory condition of unknown etiology that occurs in both children and adults. A predilection for patients with asthma, allergies, parasite infestation, eosinophilic gastroenteritis, and bladder trauma has been reported.

The bladder mucosa exhibits erythema, edema, thickening, and ulceration in eosinophilic cystitis. Histologically, the lamina propria is infiltrated with eosinophils, lymphocytes, plasma cells, mast cells, and histiocytes. The clinical findings of irritative bladder symptoms and hematuria and the radiologic findings of a thickened, irregular bladder wall are nonspecific.

Eosinophilic ureteritis is discussed in Chapter 15.

Interstitial Cystitis

Interstitial cystitis is a syndrome of unknown etiology that is characterized by chronic, severe suprapubic pain, urinary frequency, urgency, dysuria, nocturia,

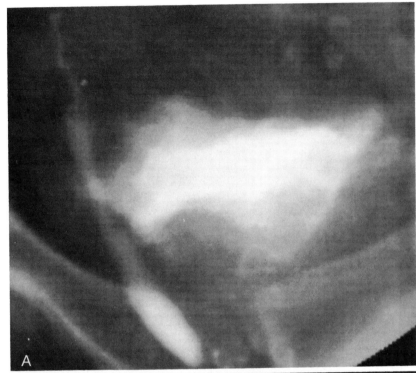

Figure 19–16. Malakoplakia, bladder.
A, Excretory urogram. Extensive, irregular filling defects are seen throughout the bladder wall.
B, Computed tomogram demonstrates diffuse thickening of the bladder.

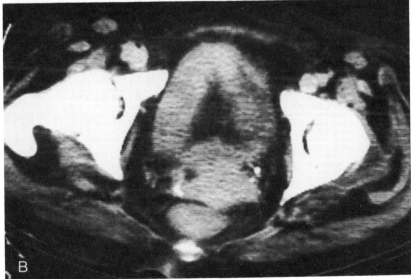

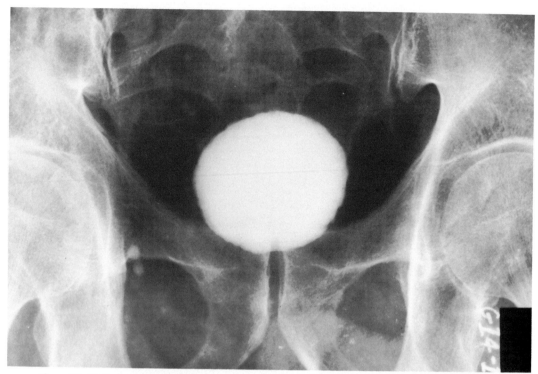

Figure 19–17. Radiation cystitis. The bladder wall is slightly irregular and contracted. Excretory urogram.

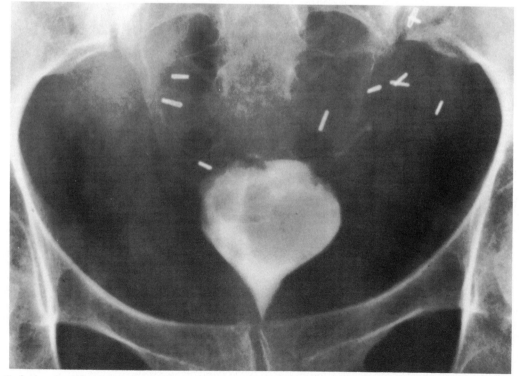

Figure 19–18. Cyclophosphamide cystitis. The bladder is contracted and deformed by fibrosis. Filling defects within the bladder represent blood clots. Excretory urogram.

reduced bladder capacity, and the absence of urinary tract infection. Females between the ages of 50 and 60 years are most frequently affected. The bladder mucosa is characterized by foci of pinpoint petechial hemorrhage, known as glomerulations. Splitting or cracking of the urothelium tends to occur with bladder distention. Linear ulcers, known as *Hunner's ulcers*, may be seen. Microscopically, there is a pancystitis with mast cell infiltration of detrusor muscle bundles. Radiologic examination reveals a small contracted bladder with a smooth or irregular wall.

PROLIFERATIVE AND INFILTRATING DISORDERS

Cystitis Glandularis and Cystitis Cystica

Cystitis cystica and cystitis glandularis are part of a continuum of metaplastic changes that begin in solid buds of uroepithelium, known as *Brunn's nests*, that project into the lamina propria, where they become isolated. Mucinous metaplasia of cells at the center of Brunn's nests leads to the formation of cysts that may markedly dilate, creating a condition known as *cystitis cystica*. Frank gland formation may follow the discharge of the mucinous secretions at the mucosal surface. This condition is known as *cystitis glandularis.*

The traditional view has been that cystitis glandularis and cystitis cystica are associated with chronic infection or irritation of the bladder. However, the fact that these same changes may be found in the bladders of asymptomatic patients without such a history raises the possibility that they may be a normal uro-

epithelial variant. Likewise, the possibility that cystitis cystica and cystitis glandularis are precursor lesions for carcinoma of the bladder has been suggested but not clearly established, except in the presence of exstrophy of the bladder.

Cystitis cystica and cystitis glandularis appear as multiple, discrete, small masses that elevate the uroepithelium. Some may be as large as 2 cm in diameter, while others may become confluent, giving rise to a cobblestone pattern. These abnormalities are most often seen at the bladder trigone and base.

Cystitis glandularis and cystitis cystica are most often encountered clinically in women and children with chronic urinary tract infections. The same findings also occur in association with pelvic lipomatosis and bladder exstrophy (Fig. 19–19).

Sharply defined, small projections from the wall of the bladder characterize the radiologic appearance of cystitis cystica and cystitis glandularis. These may be single or multiple and, when numerous, resemble a cobblestone pattern. Sometimes the lesions are irregular or lobulated, an appearance that may be difficult to differentiate from bladder carcinoma (Fig. 19–20).

Ureteritis cystica and pyelitis cystica are similar conditions occurring in the upper urinary tract. These are discussed in Chapter 15.

Endometriosis

Involvement of the urinary tract by endometrial implants occurs in less than 2 per cent of patients with endometriosis. When this does occur, the bladder is

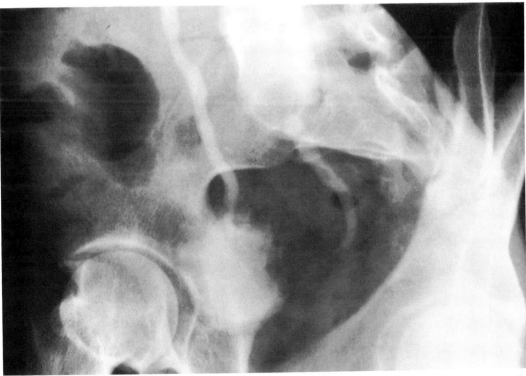

Figure 19–19. Pelvic lipomatosis and cystitis glandularis in a 34-year-old black man. The bladder is small, is displaced by surrounding fat, and has multiple mucosal irregularities. There is slight obstruction at the right ureterovesical junction.

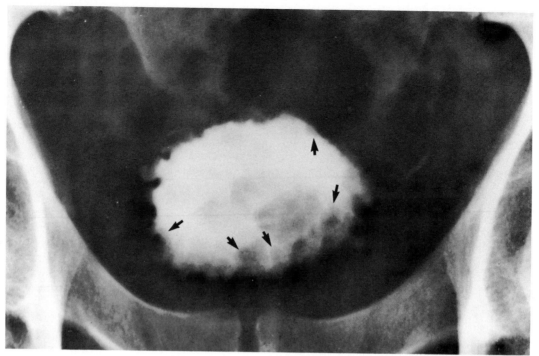

Figure 19–20. Cystitis cystica and cystitis glandularis. There are multiple filling defects *(arrows)* throughout the bladder wall giving rise to a cobblestone appearance. Excretory urogram.

far more frequently affected than are the ureters or the kidneys. Urinary tract endometriosis is most commonly seen in patients between 30 and 35 years of age, although bladder endometriosis has been reported in postmenopausal women on hormonal therapy and, rarely, in men receiving hormonal therapy for prostate carcinoma.

Endometriosis that involves the bladder wall appears as blue-black nodules that protrude into the bladder lumen. Implants may also be present on the serosal surface of the bladder. These cause cramping pain, dysuria, frequency, hematuria, and, in some cases, a palpable mass. These findings, including the cystoscopic appearance of the bladder mucosa, may be cyclic in relation to menstruation. Endometrial implants that are limited to the serosal surface of the bladder may be asymptomatic.

Endometrial deposits in the wall of the bladder are seen radiologically as mural filling defects that are indistinguishable from other abnormalities that arise in the bladder wall, including carcinoma. These are best detected radiologically by cystography or ultrasonography. Serosal implants are often not visualized by radiologic methods.

Endometriosis of the ureter is discussed in Chapter 16.

Amyloidosis

Amyloidosis of the urinary bladder is usually primary and isolated, rather than part of a generalized disorder. Bladder amyloid appears as a submucosal nodule that often has an overlying mucosal ulceration. In some cases, the pattern is irregular or cobblestoned.

The lateral aspects of the bladder, rather than the trigone, are usually involved. Amyloid deposits at the ureteral orifice lead to progressive dilatation of the upper urinary tract. Globular deposits of pale eosinophilic material in the submucosa and in arteries and veins are seen microscopically.

Amyloidosis of the bladder is most prevalent in adults between the fifth and seventh decades of life. Gross, painless hematuria, which is sometimes life threatening, is the presenting symptom in the majority of patients.

Radiologically, amyloidosis appears as an irregular, mural mass that is indistinguishable from other lesions of mural origin, including carcinoma. Linear or nodular deposits of calcium in the lamina propria may be present. When these are present, cystography demonstrates a thin radiolucent line of mucosa separating the calcium deposits from the contrast material in the bladder cavity.

Amyloidosis of the kidney is discussed in Chapter 8 and that of the ureter in Chapter 15.

NEOPLASMS

Benign Tumors

Benign tumors of the bladder are rare and, with the exception of nephrogenic adenoma, almost always nonepithelial. These include leiomyoma, hemangioma, paraganglioma, and neurofibroma. Lymphangioma, fibrous histiocytoma, fibroma, fibromyxoma, osteoma, fibroepithelial polyp, and granular cell tumor have also been reported in isolated instances.

Most benign bladder tumors are submucosal and

do not erode the overlying mucosa. As a result, hematuria is uncommon and symptoms reflect the size and location of the tumor particularly if obstruction of the ureter or bladder outlet is present. There are no radiologic findings that permit the specific diagnosis of a benign bladder tumor.

Nephrogenic adenoma has been classified as a benign neoplasm by some, while others view this lesion as a metaplastic uroepithelial response to chronic inflammation associated with bladder calculi, chronic indwelling catheter, prior surgery, or trauma. Histologically, a nephrogenic adenoma is composed of papillary fronds and tubules that are usually covered by transitional epithelium. These produce a polypoid or papillary lesion that in gross appearance may be mistaken for carcinoma.

Nephrogenic adenoma is encountered most frequently in young adults, and males are affected more commonly than females. Unlike most benign tumors, the clinical setting for nephrogenic adenoma includes signs and symptoms of chronic irritation or infection, including dysuria, urgency, frequency, and microscopic hematuria.

On radiologic investigation, nephrogenic adenoma appears as a single tumor or as multiple mural masses that have no distinguishing features from other benign or malignant tumors (Fig. 19–21).

Leiomyoma is the most common benign bladder tumor and is of mesenchymal origin. Females are three times more frequently affected than are males. Leiomyoma is usually located in the trigone. Most leiomyomas are well encapsulated and submucosal and project into the bladder lumen. Some extend from their submucosal origin into the perivesical soft tissue, while others may have both an intravesical and an extravesical component. Occasionally, a leiomyoma is pedunculated.

A leiomyoma that projects into the bladder lumen appears as a sharply circumscribed filling defect on contrast material–enhanced radiologic studies, such as cystography, excretory urography, or computed tomography (Fig. 19–22). Similar characteristics are identified with those modalities, such as ultrasonography or magnetic resonance imaging, that differentiate soft tissue from bladder urine without the use of contrast material. A leiomyoma that has an extravesical pattern of growth is identified as a soft tissue mass in the perivesical region causing extrinsic deformity of the bladder.

Hemangioma of the bladder is uncommon. Coexisting cutaneous hemangiomas of the thigh, lower abdomen, and perineum occur in as many as 30 per cent of cases. Individuals with the Klippel-Trenaunay syndrome have associated hemangioma of the bladder in up to 6 per cent of cases. These hemangiomas, therefore, may be diagnosed within a specific clinical context. Most bladder hemangiomas are of the cavernous rather than the cirsoid type and are quite variable in size, number, and location within the bladder. Hemangioma is usually detected in the first 2 decades of life as a result of hematuria, which may be severe. With the use of standard radiography or computed tomography, hemangioma cannot be differentiated from other bladder tumors unless phleboliths are present within the soft tissue bladder wall mass (Fig. 19–23). The vascular nature of the mass, which is ap-

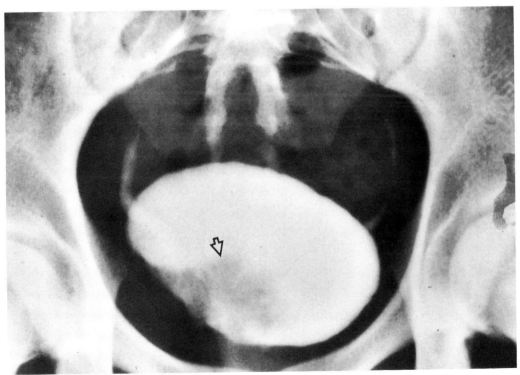

Figure 19–21. Nephrogenic adenoma. There is an irregular filling defect *(arrow)* on the right side of the bladder. Excretory urogram.

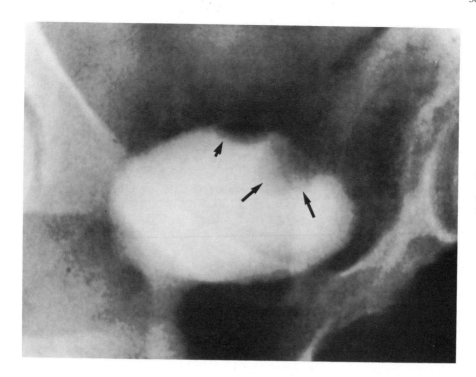

Figure 19–22. Leiomyoma. A filling defect *(arrows)* with smooth margins is present on the left side of the bladder. The lucency in the dome *(short arrow)* is air. Cystogram.

parent by cystoscopy, can be identified by contrast material–enhanced computed tomography as well as selective angiography of the internal iliac artery.

Paraganglioma is a rare bladder tumor of neurogenic origin that accounts for less than 1 per cent of all extra-adrenal paragangliomas. Paraganglioma in the bladder produces a mural soft tissue mass of similar gross morphology to other forms of benign and malignant tumors. The trigone is the most common location, followed by the dome and the lateral walls of the bladder. A bladder paraganglioma that is metabolically active creates the setting for a unique clinical presentation in which hypertension, palpitation, headache, blurred vision, diaphoresis, anxiety, and syncope are variably exacerbated during urination. Hematuria is frequently present.

Paraganglioma of the bladder appears on radiologic studies as an intramural mass that is indistinguishable from other tumor types (Fig. 19–24). Distinctive features that are often present are a high signal intensity on T2-weighted magnetic resonance images, tumor uptake using the radionuclide metaiodobenzylguanidine, and, less distinctively, neovascularity and tumor stain demonstrated by angiography. With magnetic resonance imaging, moderately T2-weighted sequences delineate the lesion from urine. These and other aspects of adrenal and extra-adrenal paraganglioma are discussed in Chapters 21 and 22.

Neurofibromatosis rarely involves the urinary tract. When this occurs, the bladder is the most likely site. The neurofibromas are soft tissue masses that may be intravesical or extravesical. In some patients the bladder lumen is lobulated or irregular as a result of diffuse infiltration. This limits bladder capacity as well. The diagnosis of neurofibroma of the bladder is dependent on the radiologic demonstration of these ab-

normalities in a patient with the cutaneous manifestations of neurofibromatosis.

Malignant Tumors

Uroepithelial Carcinoma

Carcinoma of the bladder epithelium is the most common malignancy of the urinary tract. Transitional cell carcinoma accounts for approximately 90 per cent of all bladder malignancies. Less frequent histologic types are squamous cell carcinoma (5 per cent) and adenocarcinoma (2 per cent). Nonepithelial malignancies account for the remainder.

Transitional cell carcinoma of the bladder is closely associated with a number of risk factors. These include environmental exposure to the aniline dye metabolites, benzidine and napthylamine, and to a variety of aromatic amines. Pelvic radiation, tobacco smoking, and cyclophosphamide therapy are additional risk factors. Patients with chronic uroepithelial irritation and inflammation associated with, for example, chronic bladder instrumentation, chronic urinary tract infection, calculi, and schistosomiasis are at particular risk for squamous cell carcinoma. The very uncommon adenocarcinoma of the bladder is usually seen in urachal anomalies and in patients with bladder exstrophy, and possibly in conditions associated with metaplasia of the transitional cell epithelium.

The prevalence of carcinoma of the bladder reaches a peak in the seventh decade of life. Males are affected more often than females by a ratio of 3:1. Hematuria is the most common clinical finding and may occur even in the absence of irritative symptoms, such as dysuria, urgency, or suprapubic pain. The trigone and lateral and posterior walls of the bladder are the most common location for transitional cell carcinoma.

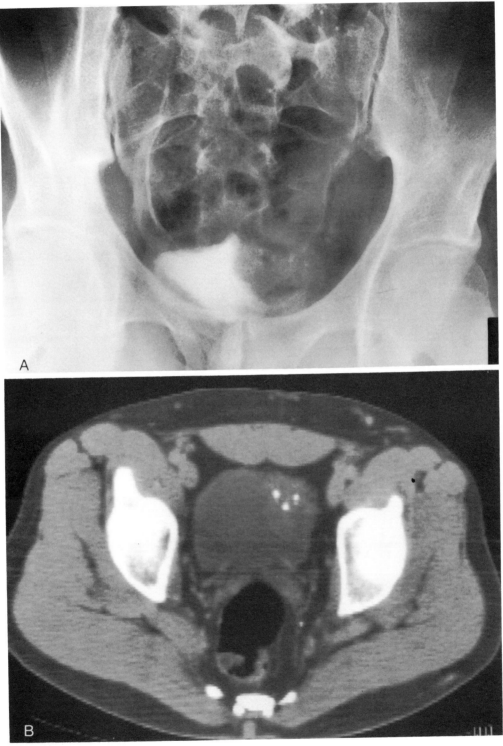

Figure 19–23. Hemangioma.
  A, Excretory urogram. There is a large mass attached to the wall of the bladder. Faint, punctate densities within the mass represent phleboliths.
  B, Computed tomogram without contrast enhancement demonstrates the mural mass and phleboliths protruding into the urine-filled bladder lumen.

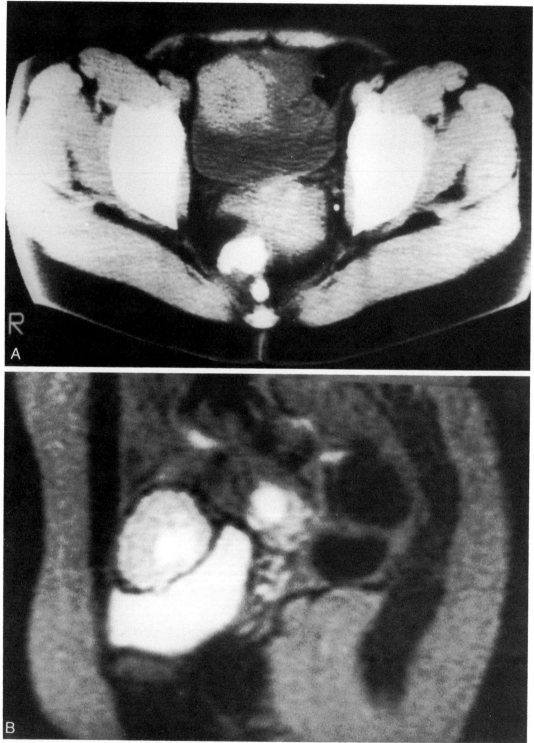

Figure 19–24. Paraganglioma.
   A, Computed tomogram, unenhanced. There is a round mass in the dome of the bladder.
   B, Magnetic resonance image, T2-weighted, sagittal plane. The mass in the dome of the bladder has a high signal intensity.

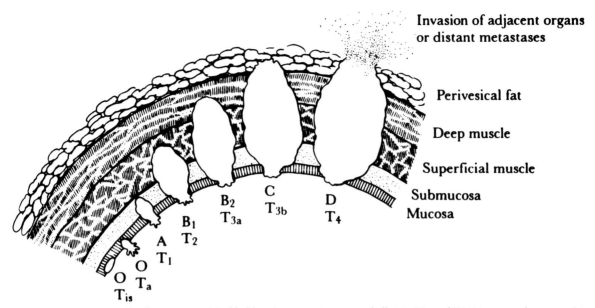

Figure 19–25. Staging of transitional cell carcinoma of the bladder. The Jewett-Strong-Marshall (A,B,C,D) and TNM (tumor-node-metastasis) systems are illustrated. (Reprinted with permission from Amis, E. S., Jr., and Newhouse, J. H.: Essentials of Uroradiology. Boston: Little, Brown & Company, 1991.)

Any histologic type of epithelial bladder malignancy can be staged according to the established systems of classifications. The two schemes used for staging of a uroepithelial malignancy are the Jewett-Strong-Marshall and the American Joint Committee TNM systems (Fig. 19–25). Most transitional cell carcinomas are superficial at the time of diagnosis, that is, Stage O or A of Jewett-Strong-Marshall or Tis, Ta, or T1 in the TNM system. In general, squamous cell carcinoma is more infiltrative and aggressive than transitional cell carcinoma. In addition to local invasion and regional lymph node involvement, distant hematogenous metastases should be sought, especially in the lung, liver, and skeleton.

The diagnosis of bladder malignancy is based on biopsy during cystocopy. Histologic features, such as cellular differentiation, cell type, grading, and depth of involvement as well as multiplicity of lesions and tumor stage, determine therapy.

Commonly, radiologic studies are normal in patients with bladder malignancy. When detectable, the malignancy appears as an irregularity distorting the wall or projecting into the lumen of the contrast material–filled bladder. When cystography or excretory

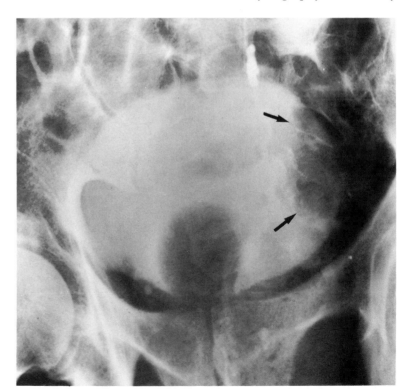

Figure 19–26. Transitional cell carcinoma. There is a large filling defect *(arrows)* on the left. A Foley balloon catheter is in place.

urography is performed, carefully collimated oblique and postvoid films are often necessary for confirmation of a suspected abnormality (Figs. 19–26 and 19–27). Rarely, calcification in an area of tumor necrosis or cystic degeneration is detected on standard radiographs of the bladder. A uroepithelial malignancy near a ureteral orifice may cause a slight dilatation of the intramural portion of the distal ureter, giving rise to an appearance that simulates a ureterocele. This "pseudoureterocele" can be differentiated from a true ureterocele by the fact that the dilated segment in the latter condition prolapses into the bladder lumen, whereas the dilated segment in a pseudoureterocele remains within the bladder wall. Retrograde ureteropyelography is the most efficacious technique for assessing the upper urinary tracts for synchronous, multicentric tumors and for evaluation of ureteral obstruction, which is associated with both bladder muscularis invasion and lymph node metastases. Bladder diverticula should be carefully evaluated as the possible site of malignancy (see Fig. 19–10).

Transabdominal ultrasonography of the distended bladder demonstrates a malignant tumor as a soft tissue structure protruding into the urine-filled bladder lumen. Infiltration of bladder wall may produce a pattern of echogenicity that is distinct from the normal echogenic appearance of the muscle in some patients (Fig. 19–28). The degree of penetration through the bladder muscle, however, cannot be accurately assessed with ultrasonography. Similarly, ultrasonography is not a reliable technique for evaluating spread of a bladder malignancy into either the perivesical soft tissue or regional lymph nodes.

Computed tomography with contrast material in the bladder demonstrates findings similar to those described earlier for excretory urography and cystography (Fig. 19–29). In addition, computed tomography is able to suggest macroscopic tumor spread to the perivesical tissue, the pelvic sidewalls, and the pelvic and para-aortic lymph nodes. However, overstaging by computed tomography may occur in patients with abnormal perivesical tissue density caused by radiation therapy, transurethral biopsy, or partial cystectomy. Computed tomographic guided biopsy of enlarged lymph nodes can be performed to determine metastatic involvement.

Magnetic resonance imaging of bladder malignancy visualizes the primary tumor in a manner similar to the previously described techniques (Fig. 19–30). Additional advantage can be gained with magnetic resonance imaging by virtue of its ability to display the anatomy of the region in both coronal and sagittal projections. This may be of particular value for lesions that are situated in the bladder base or the bladder dome and for evaluating involvement of the seminal vesicles and prostate. Magnetic resonance imaging also distinguishes superficial and deep muscle invasion of the bladder.

Rhabdomyosarcoma

Rhabdomyosarcoma is the most common soft tissue sarcoma of childhood. As many as 20 per cent of these tumors occur in the genitourinary system, usually in the bladder and less often in the prostate, vagina, testicle, pelvic floor, perineum, and retroperitoneum. Rhabdomyosarcomas that arise in the genitourinary system are usually of the histologic and cytologic subclassification of *embryonal*. *Sarcoma botryoides* is another subclassification characterized by the gross appearance of a grapelike polypoid tumor, usually in hollow viscera such as the bladder or vagina. Males are more often affected than are females by a ratio of 2:1, and most of these tumors develop before 5 years of age.

Embryonal rhabdomyosarcoma usually originates in the submucosa of the posterior wall of the bladder, in the region of the trigone and bladder neck. Tumor growth is usually intraluminal as a polypoid mass with glistening, mucoid, pale gray surfaces. This is the characteristic pattern for sarcoma botryoides. Symptoms of bladder outlet obstruction, a palpable lower abdominal mass, and hematuria are the usual clinical findings.

Radiologic findings in embryonal rhabdomyosarcoma that are growing in the botryoides pattern are those of a lobulated soft tissue mass in the base of the bladder. These are apparent as multiple, nodular filling defects on studies using contrast material in the bladder or as echogenic soft tissue of similar description within the urine-filled bladder by ultrasonography (Fig. 19–31). The tumor may fill the bladder lumen, obstruct the bladder outlet, or invade the perivesical soft tissue.

Lymphoma

Lymphomatous involvement of the bladder is more common in non-Hodgkin's lymphoma than in Hodgkin's disease and usually occurs in disseminated disease. The radiologic findings are those of any other mural neoplasm that causes irregularity, thickening, and nodularity of the bladder wall (Fig. 19–32). Involvement of other sites coexist.

Primary lymphoma of the bladder is rare, accounting for less than 1 per cent of tumors of the bladder. Primary lymphoma appears as a lobulated, submucosal mass that is radiologically indistinguishable from transitional cell carcinoma.

EXTRAVESICAL LESIONS

Crohn's Disease

Genitourinary complications occur in as many as one-fourth of patients with Crohn's disease. Bladder involvement results from direct extension from an adjacent loop of involved bowel, which becomes fixed to the peritoneal surface of the bladder. The bladder wall thickens, and the mucosa becomes prominent. An enterovesical fistula may follow. Although this is most commonly seen on the right side in patients with terminal ileal or ileocolic disease, the same process may also occur on the left side as a result of involvement of the sigmoid colon.

Bladder involvement usually occurs in a setting of

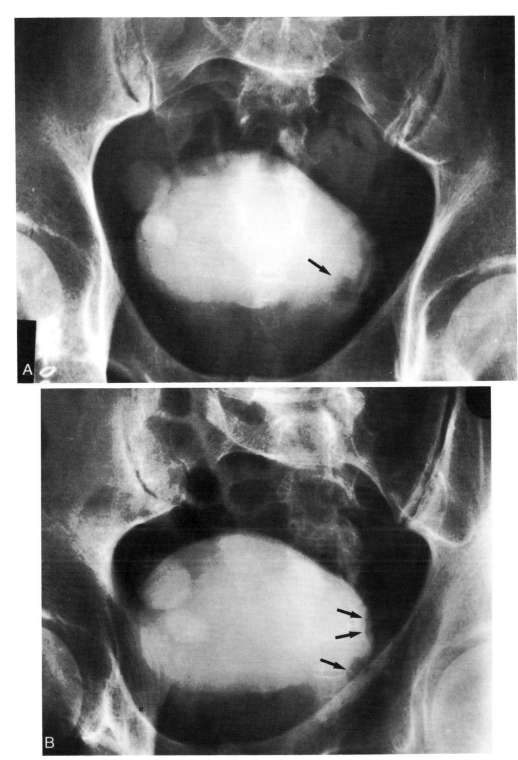

Figure 19–27. Transitional cell carcinoma, small multiple foci. Excretory urogram.
 A, An anteroposterior radiograph demonstrates a small filling defect *(arrow)* on the left side of the bladder with associated irregularity of the wall.
 B, A shallow oblique projection demonstrates multiple irregular lesions *(arrows).*

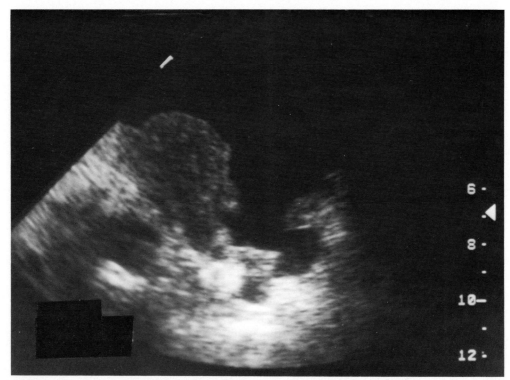

Figure 19–28. Transitional cell carcinoma. Ultrasonogram, transverse projection. There is an irregular, echoic mass projecting into the urine-filled lumen. (Kindly provided by Ulrike Hamper, M.D., and Sheila Sheth, M.D., The Johns Hopkins University, Baltimore, Maryland.)

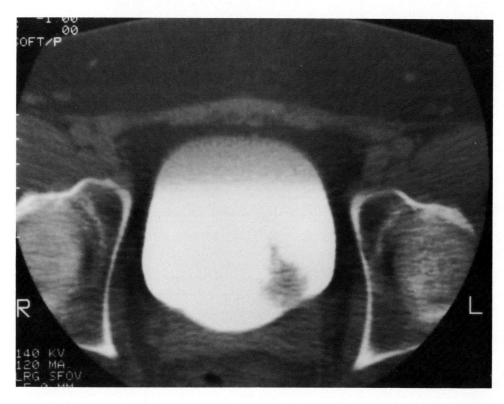

Figure 19–29. Transitional cell carcinoma. Computed tomogram, contrast material enhanced. An irregular mural-based mass protrudes into the bladder lumen. (Kindly provided by Peter L. Choyke, M.D., National Institutes of Health, Bethesda, Maryland.)

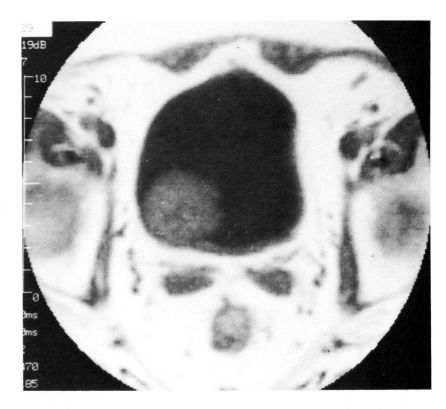

Figure 19–30. Transitional cell carcinoma. Magnetic resonance image, T1-weighted, axial section. The tumor is seen as a rounded, soft tissue mass protruding into the bladder lumen. (Kindly provided by Peter L. Choyke, M.D., National Institutes of Health, Bethesda, Maryland.)

a long-standing history of Crohn's disease. Symptoms are those of lower urinary tract inflammation and/or infection and, if a fistula is present, pneumaturia. However, in some patients, these may constitute the initial clinical findings.

Radiologic studies using enteric and urinary tract opacification demonstrate fixation of involved bowel to the peritoneal surface of the bladder with an associated inflammatory mass. The bladder, itself, may be tethered to the inflammatory mass with mural thickening and mucosal irregularity (Fig. 19–33). An enterovesical fistula is demonstrable either through contrast material moving from bowel to bladder or in the reverse direction. These abnormalities are best demonstrated by barium small bowel studies, excretory urography, cystography, or computed tomography.

Diverticulitis of the sigmoid colon and appendiceal abscess are additional inflammatory conditions of the bowel that may affect the bladder in a manner similar to that of Crohn's disease.

Pelvic Lipomatosis

Proliferation of mature fat in the extraperitoneal space of the pelvis occurs as an idiopathic process. Limited demographic studies of this poorly understood abnormality suggest a predominance in black males of all ages. Symptoms, when present, reflect bladder inflammation or obstruction of the bladder outlet or rectum. Symptoms may also be quite nonspecific.

Symmetric, circumferential external compression, elongation and elevation of the bladder and the rectosigmoid, and medial deviation of the distal ureters are the major consequences of pelvic lipomatosis. The

iliac veins and the caudal portion of the inferior vena cava may be similarly narrowed. In the inflammatory form of pelvic lipomatosis, cystitis, including cystitis glandularis and cystica, may also be noted. In severe cases, this may be associated with ureteral obstruction and obstructive uropathy.

Fat proliferation is recognizable on standard radiographs as increased lucency of perivesical soft tissue and as an increased amount of tissue with computed tomographic or magnetic resonance imaging characteristics of normal fat. The deformities of the bladder, rectosigmoid, and ureters described previously are best demonstrated radiologically by cystography, excretory urography, barium enema, or CT (Fig. 19–34). Ultrasonography demonstrates the abnormal bladder contour as well as the surrounding echogenic fat without evidence of a definite mass.

Miscellaneous Conditions

Extrinsic compression of the bladder and medial deviation of the distal ureter are also caused by iliopsoas muscle hypertrophy, a narrow bony pelvis, lymphadenopathy, pelvic hematoma, lymphocele, iliac artery aneursym, iliac vein varices, and neoplasms arising in perivesical tissue including the spine and bony pelvis (Fig. 19–35). These may be symmetric and bilateral or eccentric and focal. Many of these conditions have a distinctive clinical setting with associated characteristic radiologic findings that permit an accurate diagnosis.

Carcinoma of the sigmoid colon may involve the bladder wall, and, in some circumstances, produce a colovesical fistula.

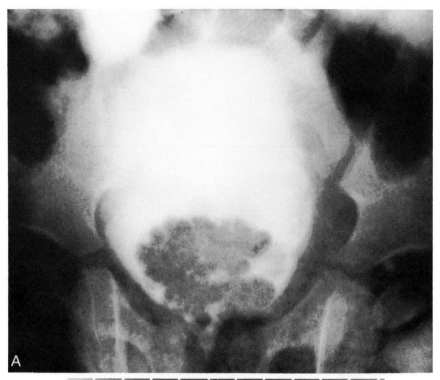

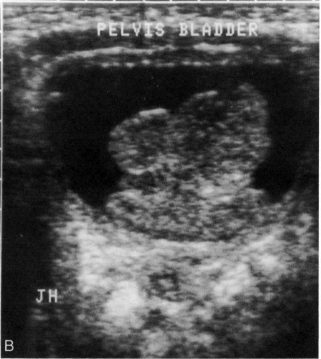

Figure 19–31. Rhabdomyosarcoma, bladder, in a 15-month-old female infant.

A, Ultrasonogram demonstrates a lobulated soft tissue mass within the bladder.

B, Excretory urogram. The mass is composed of multiple, grapelike lobules.

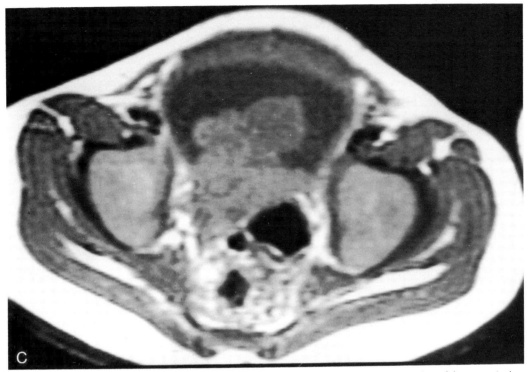

Figure 19–31. *Continued C,* Magnetic resonance image, T1-weighted, axial projection. Posterior extension of the tumor is demonstrated.

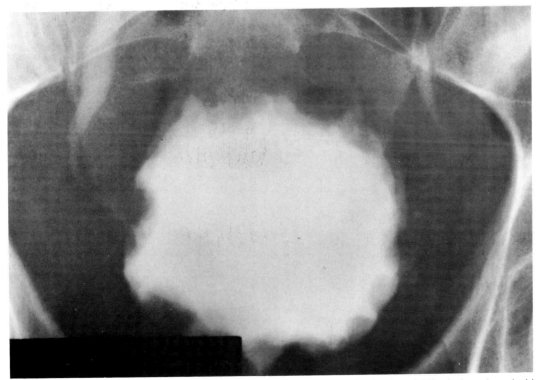

Figure 19–32. Lymphoma. An excretory urogram demonstrates multiple mural nodules distributed diffusely throughout the bladder.

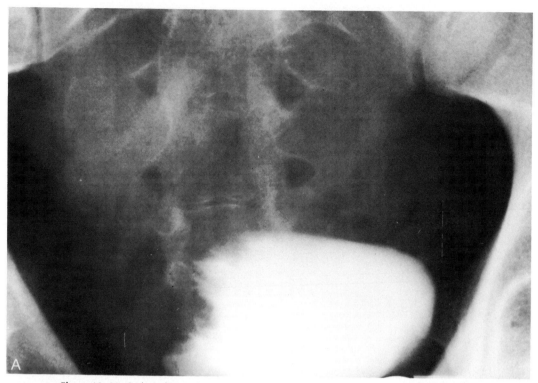

Figure 19–33. Crohn's disease in a young male with dysuria.
A, Excretory urogram. The right side of the bladder has a tethered or spiculated appearance.

TRAUMA

Bladder injury results from penetrating, blunt, or iatrogenic trauma. Approximately 10 per cent of patients with pelvic fracture have an associated bladder injury.

Sandler and colleagues (1986) have classified bladder injury into five types:

Type 1   Bladder contusion
Type 2   Intraperitoneal rupture
Type 3   Interstitial bladder rupture
Type 4   Extraperitoneal rupture
      a. Simple
      b. Complex
Type 5   Combined bladder injury

Bladder contusion (Type 1) results from an incomplete or nonperforating tear of the bladder mucosa. This is the most common type of bladder injury and is often present in patients with a pelvic hematoma. The diagnosis of bladder contusion is one of exclusion of other types of injury in the traumatized patient with hematuria. The cystogram is normal.

Intraperitoneal bladder rupture (Type 2) occurs at the dome of the bladder. This follows a sudden rise in intravesical pressure, as might occur with blunt abdominal trauma, especially in the presence of a distended bladder. Individuals involved in an automobile accident while wearing a lap-type seat belt are at particular risk for intraperitoneal bladder rupture. Children, whose distended bladder typically protrudes into the peritoneal space, are also more likely to experience this type of bladder injury. Radiologic demonstration of a Type 2 bladder injury depends on the demonstration of contrast material entering the peritoneal cavity from the bladder. The contrast material surrounds loops of bowel and intraperitoneal viscera and fills the paracolic gutters (Fig. 19–36).

Interstitial (Type 3) bladder injury is rare and characterized by incomplete perforation of the serosa with an intact mucosa. There is an irregularity of the bladder wall demonstrated by cystography but no extravesical leakage of contrast material.

Extraperitoneal rupture (Type 4) of the bladder due to blunt trauma is almost always associated with a spicule of bone from a fracture of the anterior pelvic arch lacerating the bladder base. In some cases the bladder tear occurs at a site that is remote from the pelvic fracture, suggesting a compression and bursting mechanism rather than a direct laceration. Contrast material leakage in a *simple* Type 4 injury is limited to the pelvic extraperitoneal space, while a *complex* Type 4 injury is characterized by spread of contrast material beyond this space and into the scrotum, the retroperitoneum, thigh, penis, or anterior abdominal wall (Figs. 19–37 and 19–38). Severe complex Type 4 injury may be confused with a Type 2 (intraperitoneal) bladder rupture.

Retrograde cystography should be used to evaluate a suspected bladder injury, but only after an associated urethral injury is first excluded by a retrograde urethrogram, as described in Chapter 20. Following a preliminary radiograph, dilute (approximately 25 per cent) contrast material is instilled slowly into the bladder using gravity drip. The study should be per-

Text continued on page 646

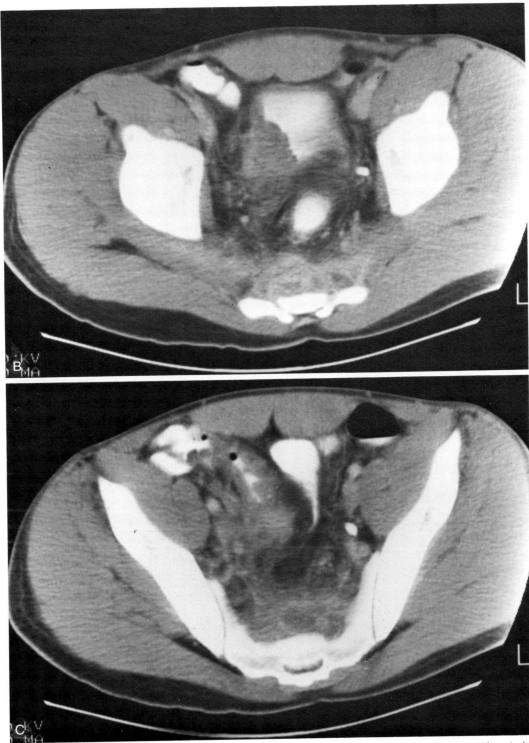

Figure 19–33 *Continued B,* Computed tomogram with contrast material enhancement at the level of the bladder base. There is thickening of the right lateral wall of the bladder, strands of soft tissue density in the perivesical fat, and increased presacral soft tissue.

C, Computed tomogram with contrast material enhancement at the level of the bladder dome. The thickened terminal ileum deforms the right side of the bladder.

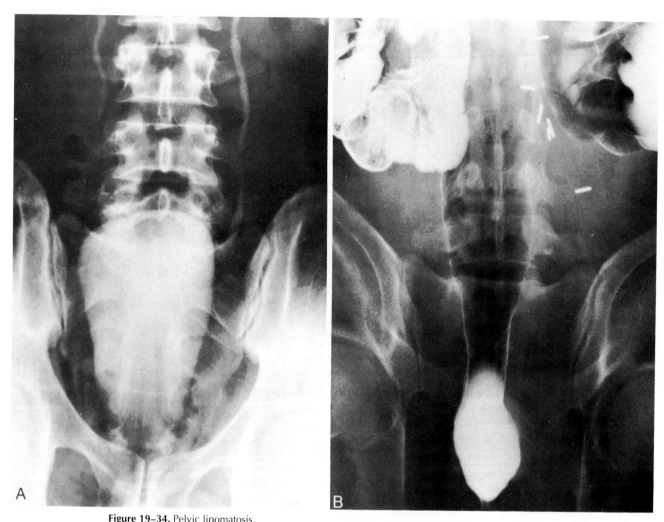

Figure 19–34. Pelvic lipomatosis.
A, Excretory urogram demonstrates symmetric compression of the bladder.
B, Barium enema. There is extrinsic compression and straightening of the rectum and rectosigmoid.

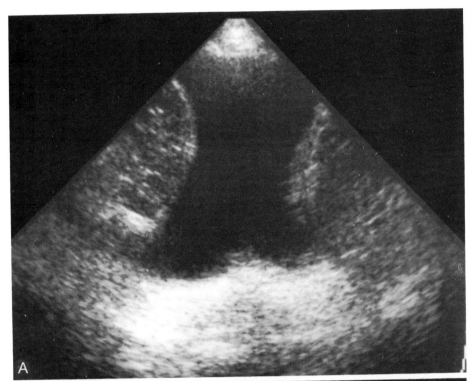

Figure 19–35. Lymphoma, retroperitoneal lymph nodes, causing bilateral and symmetric extrinsic compression of the bladder.

A, Ultrasonogram, transverse projection.

B, Computed tomogram, contrast material enhanced.

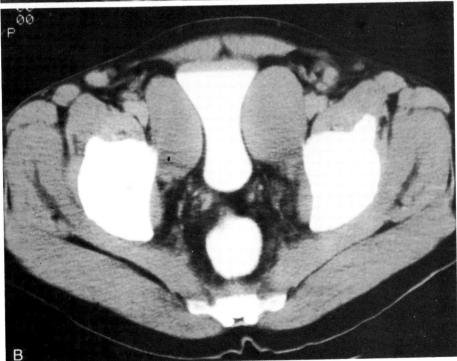

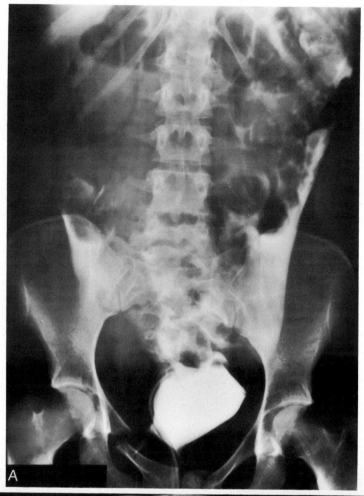

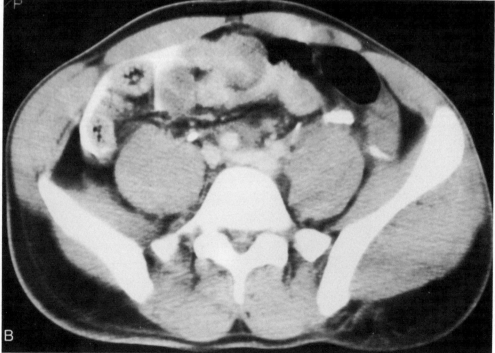

Figure 19–36. Bladder rupture, intraperitoneal, in two patients.
   A, A cystogram demonstrates contrast material outlining loops of small and large bowel.
   B, Computed tomogram, contrast material enhanced. Contrast material surrounds loops of bowel.

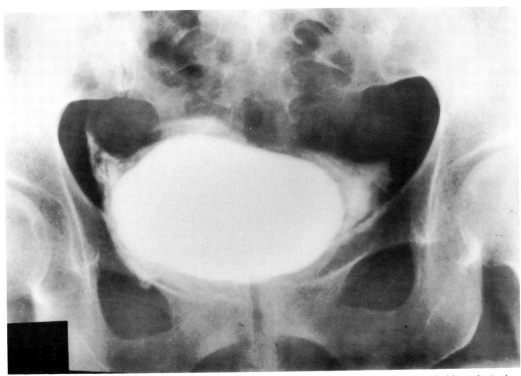

Figure 19–37. Bladder rupture, *simple* extraperitoneal. Cystogram. The leakage of contrast material from the bladder is limited to the perivesical extraperitoneal space of the pelvis.

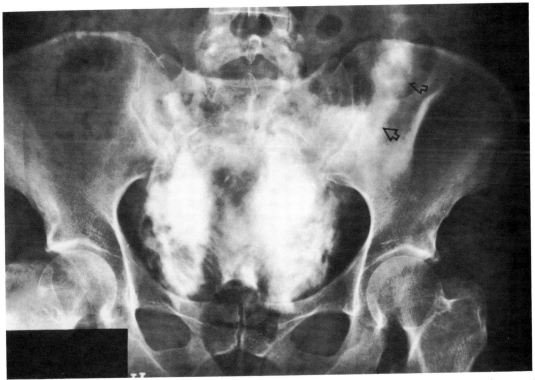

Figure 19–38. Bladder rupture, *complex* extraperitoneal. Cystogram. Contrast material has dissected from the perivesical extraperitoneal space superiorly into the pararenal compartment of the retroperitoneum *(arrows)*.

formed under fluoroscopic control, if possible. Otherwise, an initial radiograph obtained after instillation of approximately 100 ml of contrast material and serial radiographs thereafter are required to monitor the course of the examination. The earliest images, obtained either by fluoroscopy or radiography, must be carefully evaluated for leakage of contrast material outside the bladder lumen. If this is not detected, additional contrast material up to a volume of between 300 and 400 ml is given. Oblique projections assist in the detection of a small amount of extravesical contrast material, but these may be difficult to obtain in the setting of acute trauma. A radiograph after draining the bladder is essential at the completion of the study to detect those cases in which the leakage of contrast material outside the bladder is seen only at this point in the examination.

Bibliography

Anatomy

Tanagho, E. A.: Anatomy of the lower urinary tract. In Walsh, P. C., Retik, A. B., Stamey, T. A., and Vaughan, E. D., Jr. (eds): Campbell's Urology. 6th ed. Philadelphia, W.B. Saunders, 1992, pp. 40–69.

Embryology and Anomalies

Abrahamson, J.: Double bladder and related anomalies: Clinical and embryological aspects and a case report. Br. J. Urol. 33:195, 1961.

Dunetz, G. N., and Bauer, S. B.: Complete duplication of bladder and urethra. Urology 15:179, 1985.

Gearhart, J. P., and Jeffs, R. D.: Exstrophy of the bladder, epispadias, and other bladder anomalies. In Walsh, P. C., Retik, A. B., Stamey, T. A., Vaughan, E. D., Jr., (eds.): Campbell's Urology. 6th ed. Philadelphia, W.B. Saunders, 1992, pp. 1772–1821.

Hill, G. S.: Anomalies of the bladder and urethra. In Hill, G. S. (ed.): Uropathology. New York, Churchill Livingstone, 1989, pp. 235–278.

Kapoor, R., and Saha, M. M.: Complete duplication of the bladder, urethra and external genitalia in a neonate: A case report. J. Urol. 137:1243, 1987.

Metoki, R., Orikasa, S., Ohta, S., and Kanetoh, H.: A case of bladder agenesis. J. Urol. 136:662, 1986.

Richman, T. S., and Taylor, K. J. W.: Sonographic demonstration of bladder duplication. AJR 139:604, 1982.

Satter, E. J., and Mossman, H. W.: A case report of double bladder and double urethra in the female child. J. Urol. 79:274, 1958.

Tortora, F. L. Jr., Lucey, D. T., Fried, F. A., and Mandell, J.: Absence of the bladder. J. Urol. 129:1235, 1983.

White, P., and Lebowitz, R. L.: Exstrophy of the bladder. Radiol. Clin. North Am. 15:93, 1977.

The Urachus

Avni, E. F., Matos, C., Diard, F., and Schulman, C. C.: Midline omphalovesical anomalies in children: Contribution of ultrasound imaging. Urol. Radiol. 10:189, 1988.

Bauer, S. B., and Retik, A. B. Urachal anomalies and related umbilical discorders. Urol. Clin. North Am. 5:195, 1978.

Berman, S. M., Tolia, B. M., Laor, E., Reid, R. E., Schweizerhof, S. P., Freed, S. Z.: Urachal remnants in adults. Urology 31:17, 1988.

Brick, S. H., Friedman, A. C., Pollack, H. M., Fishman, E. K., Radecki, P. D., Siegelbaum, M. H., Mitchell, D. G., Lev-Toaff, A. S., Caroline, D. F.: Urachal carcinoma: CT findings. Radiology 169:377, 1988.

Goldman, I. L., Caldamone, A. A., Gauderer, M., Hampel, N., Wesselhoeft, C. W., and Elder, J. S.: Infected urachal cysts: A review of 10 cases. J. Urol. 140:375, 1988.

Grogono, J. L., and Shepheard, B. G. F.: Carcinoma of the urachus. Br. J. Urol. 41:222, 1969.

Narumi, Y., Sato, T., Kuriyama, K., Fujita, M., Saiki, S., Kuroda, M., Miki, T., and Kotake, T.: Vesical dome tumors: Significance of extravesical extension on CT. Radiology 169:383, 1988.

Schnyder, P. A., and Candardjis, G.: Vesicourachal diverticulum. CT diagnosis in two adults. AJR 137:1063, 1981.

Sheldon, C. A., Clayman, R. V., Gonzalez, R., Williams, R. D., and Fraley, E. E.: Malignant urachal lesions. J. Urol. 131:1, 1984.

Spataro, R. F., Davis, R. S., McLachlan, M. S. F., Linke, C. A., and Barbaric, Z. L. Urachal abnormalities in the adult. Radiology 149:659, 1983.

Stanfield, N. J., and Shearer, R. J. Prostatism, obstructive uropathy and uraemia associated with a urachal cyst. Br. J. Urol. 53:482, 1981.

Thomas, A. J., Pollack, M. S., and Libshitz, H. I. Urachal carcinoma: Evaluation with computed tomography. Urol. Radiol. 8:194, 1986.

Williams, B. D., and Fisk, J. D.: Sonographic diagnosis of giant urachal cyst in the adult. AJR 136:417, 1981.

Diverticulum

Hill, G. S.: Lower urinary tract obstruction. In Hill, G. S. (ed.): Uropathology. New York, Churchill Livingstone, 1989, pp. 599–622.

Jarow, J. P., and Brendler, C. B.: Urinary retention caused by a large bladder diverticulum: A simple method of diverticectomy. J. Urol. 139:1260, 1988.

Schiff, M. Jr., and Lytton, B.: Congenital diverticulum of the bladder. J. Urol. 104:111, 1970.

Taylor, W. N., Alton, D., Toguri, A., Churchill, B. M., and Schillinger, J. F.: Bladder diverticula causing posterior urethral obstruction in children. J. Urol. 122:415, 1979.

Intraluminal Filling Defects

Amendola, M. A., Sonda, L. P., Diokno, A. C., and Vidyasagar, M.: Bladder calculi complicating intermittent clean catheterization. AJR 141:751, 1983.

Lebowitz, R. L., and Vargas, B.: Stones in the urinary bladder in children and young adults. AJR 148:491, 1987.

Infection

Bailey, H.: Cystitis emphysematosa: 19 cases with intraluminal and interstitial collections of gas. AJR 86:850, 1961.

Bartkowski, D. P., and Lanesky, J. R.: Emphysematous prostatitis and cystitis secondary to Candida albicans. J. Urol. 139:1063, 1988.

Harold, D. L., Koff, S. A., and Kass, E. J.: Candida albicans "fungus ball" in bladder. Urology 9:662, 1977.

Jorulf, H., and Lindstedt, E.: Urogenital schistosomiasis: CT evaluation. Radiology 157:745, 1985.

McDonald, D. F., and Fagan, C. J. Fungus balls in the urinary bladder. Am. J. Roentgenol. Radium Ther. Nucl. Med. 114:753, 1972.

Olmo, J. M. C., Carcamo, P., Deiriarte, E. G., Jimenez, F., Martinezpineiro, L., and Martinezpineiro, J. A.: Genitourinary malakoplakia. Br. J. Urol. 72:6, 1993.

Pollack, H. M., Bauner, M. P., Martinez, L. O., and Hodson, C. J.: Diagnostic considerations in urinary bladder wall calcification. AJR 136:791, 1981.

Rohner, T. J., and Tuliszewski, R. M. Fungal cystitis: Awareness, diagnosis and treatment. J. Urol. 124:142, 1980.

Tomaszewski, J. E.: Cystitis. In Hill, G. S. (ed.): Uropathology. New York, Churchill Livingstone, 1989, pp. 431–454.

Inflammation

Aron, B. S., and Schlesinger, A.: Complications of radiation therapy: The genitourinary tract. Semin. Roentogenol. 9:65, 1974.

Ehrlich, R. M., Freedman, A., Goldsobel, A. B., and Stiehm, E. R.: The use of sodium 2-mercaptoethane sulfonate to prevent cyclophosphamide cystitis. J. Urol. 131:960, 1984.

Gillenwater, J. Y., and Wein, A. J.: Summary of the National Institute of Arthritis, Diabetes, Digestive and Kidney Diseases workshop on interstitial cystitis, National Institutes of Health, Bethesda, Maryland, August 28–29, 1987. J. Urol. *140*:203, 1988.

Hellstrom, H. R., Davis, B. K., and Shonnard, J. W.: Eosinophilic cystitis: A study of 16 cases. Am. J. Clin. Pathol. *72*:777, 1979.

Holm-Bentzen, M., and Lose, G.: Pathology and pathogenesis of interstitial cystitis. Urology *29*:8, 1987.

Kessler, W. O., Clark, P. L., and Kaplan, G. W.: Eosinophilic cystitis. Urology *6*:499, 1975.

Klein, F. A., and Smith, M. J. V.: Urinary complications of cyclophosphamide therapy: Etiology, prevention, and management. South. Med. J. *76*:1413, 1983.

Larsen, S., Thompson, S. A., Hald, T., Barnard, R. J., Gilpin, C. J., Dixon, J. S., and Gosling, J. A.: Mast cells in interstitial cystitis. Br. J. Urol. *54*:283, 1982.

Maatman, T. J., Novick, A. C., Montague, D. K., Levin, H. S.: Radiation-induced cystitis following intracavitary irradiation for superficial bladder cancer. J. Urol. *130*:338, 1983.

Messing, E. M.: The diagnosis of interstitial cystitis. Urology *29*:4, 1987.

Messing, E. M., and Stamey, T. A.: Interstitial cystitis. Urology *12*:381, 1978.

Mitas, J. A., II, and Thompson, T.: Ureteral involvement complicating eosinophilic cystitis. Urology *26*:67, 1985.

Nkposong, E. O., and Attah, E. B.: Eosinophilic cystitis. Eur. Urol. *4*:274, 1978.

Palubinskas, A. J.: Eosinophilic cystitis: Case report of eosinophilic infiltration of the urinary bladder. Radiology *75*:589, 1960.

Philips, F. S., Sternberg, S. S., Cronin, A. P., and Vidal, P. M.: Cyclophosphamide and urinary bladder toxicity. Cancer Res *21*:1577, 1961.

Renert, W. A., Berdon, W. E., and Baker, D. H.: Hemorrhagic cystitis and vesicoureteral reflux secondary to cytotoxic therapy for childhood malignancies. AJR *117*:664, 1973.

Sircus, S. I., Sant, G. R., and Ucci, A. A.: Bladder detrusor endometriosis mimicking interstitial cystitis. Urology *32*:339, 1988.

Stanton, M. J., and Maxted, W.: Malacoplakia: A study of the literature and current concepts of pathogenesis, diagnosis and treatment. J. Urol. *125*:139, 1981.

Sutphin, M., and Middleton, A. W., Jr.: Eosinophilic cystitis in children: A self-limited process. J. Urol. *132*:117, 1984.

Tomaszewski, J. E.: Cystitis. *In* Hill, G. S. (ed.): Uropathology. New York, Churchill Livingstone, 1989, pp. 431–454.

Watson, N. A., and Notley, R. G.: Urological complications of cyclophosphamide. Br. J. Urol. *45*:606, 1973.

Proliferative and Infiltrating Disorders

Abramovici, I., Chiatt, S., and Nussenson, M.: Massive hematuria and perforation in a case of amyloidosis of the bladder: Case report and review of the literature. J. Urol. *118*:964, 1977.

Amendola, M. A.: Amyloidosis of the urinary tract. *In* Pollack, H. M. (ed.): Clinical Urography. Philadelphia, W.B. Saunders, 1990, pp. 2493–2500.

Davies, G., and Castro, J. E.: Cystitis glandularis. Urology *10*:128, 1977.

Edwards, P. D., Hurm, R. A., and Jaeschke, W. H.: Conversion of cystitis glandularis to adenocarcinoma. J. Urol. *108*:568, 1972.

Malek, R. S., Greene, L. F., and Farrow, G. M.: Amyloidosis of the urinary bladder. Br. J. Urol. *43*:189, 1971.

Missen, G. A. K., and Tribe, C. R.: Catastrophic haemorrhage from the bladder due to unrecognized secondary amyloidosis. Br. J. Urol. *42*:43, 1970.

Older, R. A.: Endometriosis of the genitourinary tract. *In* Pollack, H. M. (ed.): Clinical Urography. Philadelphia, W.B. Saunders, 1990, pp. 2486–2492.

Sarma, K. P.: Cystitis cystica (cystosis) with bladder cancer. J. Urol. *120*:169, 1978.

Shook, T. E., and Nyberg, L. M.: Endometriosis of the urinary tract. Urology *31*:1, 1988.

Susmano, D., Rubenstein, A. B., Dakin, A. R., and Lloyd, F. A.: Cystitis glandularis and adenocarcinoma of the bladder. J. Urol. *105*:671, 1971.

Thomas, S. D., Sanders, P. W., III, and Pollack, H. M.: Primary amyloidosis of the urinary bladder and ureter: Cause of mural calcification. Urology *9*:586, 1977.

Tomaszewski, J. E.: Cystitis. *In* Hill, G. S., (ed.): Uropathology. New York, Churchill Livingstone, 1989, pp. 431–454.

Neoplasms

Abenoza, P., Manivel, C., and Fraley, E. E.: Primary adenocarcinoma of urinary bladder: Clinicopathologic study of 16 cases. Urology *29*:9, 1987.

Albert, N. E.: Leiomyoma of the bladder: Preoperative diagnosis by ultrasound. Urology *17*:486, 1981.

Amendola, M. A., Glazer, G. M., Grossman, H. B., Aisen, A. M., and Francis, I. R.: Staging of bladder carcinoma: MRI-CT-Surgical correlation. AJR *146*:1179, 1986.

Amis, E. S., Jr., and Newhouse, J. H.: Essentials of Uroradiology. Boston, Little, Brown & Co., 1991, p. 300.

Azouz, E. M.: Hematuria, rectal bleeding and pelvic phleboliths in children with the Klippel-Trenaunay syndrome. Pediatr. Radiol. *13*:82, 1983.

Baker, M. E., Silverman, P. M., and Korobkin, M.: Computed tomography of prostatic and bladder rhabdomyosarcomas. J. Comput. Assist. Tomogr. *9*:780, 1985.

Belis, J. A., Post, G. J., Rochman, S. C., and Milam, D. F.: Genitourinary leiomyomas. Urology *13*:424, 1979.

Bessette, P. L., Abell, M. R., and Herwig, K. R.: A clinicopathologic study of squamous cell carcinoma of the bladder. J. Urol. *112*:66, 1974.

Binkovitz, L. A., Hattery, R. R., and LeRoy, A. J.: Primary lymphoma of the bladder. Urol. Radiol. *9*:231, 1988.

Bhagavan, B. S., Tiamson, E. M., Wenk, R. E., Berger, B. W., Hamamoto, G., and Eggleston, J. C.: Nephrogenic adenoma of the urinary bladder and urethra. Hum. Pathol. *12*:907, 1981.

Blute, M. L., Engen, D. E., Travis, W. D., and Kvols, L. K.: Primary signet ring cell adenocarcinoma of the bladder. J. Urol. *141*:17, 1989.

Bornstein, I., Charboneau, J. W., and Hartman, G. W.: Leiomyoma of the bladder: Sonographic and urographic findings. J. Ultrasound Med. *5*:407, 1986.

Brenner, D. W., and Schellhammer, P. F.: Upper tract urothelial malignancy after cyclophosphamide therapy: A case report and literature review. J. Urol. *137*:1226, 1987.

Bryan, P. J., Butler, H. E., LiPuma, J. P., Resnick, M. I., and Kursh, E. D.: CT and MR imaging in staging bladder neoplasms. J. Comput. Assist. Tomogr. *11*:96, 1987.

Buy, J. N., Moss, A. A., Guinet, C., Ghossain, M. A., Malbec, L., Arrive, L., and Vadrot, D.: MR staging of bladder carcinoma: Correlation with pathologic findings. Radiology *169*:695, 1988.

Caceres, J., Mata, J. M., Lucaya, J., Palmer, J., and Donoso, L.: Hemangioma of the bladder. Radiographics *11*:161, 1991.

Carlson, D. H., and Wilkinson, R. H.: Neurofibromatosis of the bladder in children. Radiology *105*:401, 1972.

Charnsangavej, C.: Lymphoma of the genitourinary tract. Radiol. Clin. North Am. *28*:865, 1990.

Das, S., and Amar, A. D.: Vesical diverticulum associated with bladder carcinoma: Therapeutic implications. J. Urol. *136*:1013, 1986.

Das, S., Bulusu, N. V., and Lowe, P.: Primary vesical pheochromocytoma. Urology *21*:20, 1983.

Deniz, E., Shimkus, G. J., and Weller, C. G.: Pelvic neurofibromatosis: Localized von Recklinghausen's disease of the bladder. J. Urol. *96*:906, 1966.

Dershaw, D. D., and Scher, H. I.: Sonography in evaluation of carcinoma of bladder. Urology *29*:454, 1987.

Eagan, J. W., Jr.: Urothelial neoplasms: Urinary bladder. *In* Hill, G. S. (ed.): Uropathology. New York, Churchill Livingstone, 1989, pp. 793–842.

Eagan, J. W., Jr.: Nonepithelial tumors of the ureters and bladder. *In* Hill, G. S. (ed.): Uropathology. New York, Churchill Livingstone, 1989, pp. 861–872.

Fisher, M. R., Hricak, H., and Tanagho, E. A.: Urinary bladder MR imaging. Radiology *157*:471, 1985.

Gonzalez, J. A., Watts, J. C., and Alderson, T. P.: Nephrogenic adenoma of the bladder: Report of 10 cases. J. Urol. *139*:45, 1988.

Hatch, T. R., and Barry, J. M.: The valve of excretory urography in staging bladder cancer. J. Urol. *135*:49, 1986.

Hays, D. M., Raney, R. B., Jr., Lawrence, W., Soule, E. H., Gehan, E.

A., and Tefft, M.: Bladder and prostatic tumors in the Intergroup Rhabdomyosarcoma Study (IRS-I). Cancer 50:1472, 1982.

Hillman, B. J., Silvert, M., Cook, G., Stanisic, T., Bjelland, J., Claypool, H. R., Haber, K., and Mellins, H. Z.: Recognition of bladder tumors by excretory urography. Radiology 138:319, 1981.

Hockley, N. M., Bihrle, R., Bennett, R. M., III, and Curry, J. M.: Congenital genitournary hemangiomas in a patient with the Klippel-Trenaunay syndrome: Management with the neodymium: YAG laser. J. Urol. 141:940, 1989.

Husband, J. E. S., Olliff, J. F. C., Williams, M. P., Heron, C. W., and Cherryman, G. R.: Bladder cancer: Staging with CT and MR imaging. Radiology 173:435, 1989.

Illescas, F. F., Baker, M. E., and Weinerth, J. L.: Bladder leiomyoma: Advantages of sonography over computed tomography. Urol. Radiol. 8:216, 1986.

Jacobo, E., Loening, S., Schmidt, J. D., and Culp, D. A.: Primary adenocarcinoma of the bladder: A retrospective study of 20 patients. J. Urol. 117:54, 1977.

Jacobs, M. A., Bavendam, T., and Leach, G. E.: Bladder leiomyoma. Urology 34:56, 1989.

Klein, T. W., and Kaplan, G. W.: Klippel-Trenaunay syndrome associated with urinary tract hemangiomas. J. Urol. 114:596, 1975.

Leestma, J. E., and Price, E. B.: Paraganglioma of the urinary bladder. Cancer 28:1063, 1971.

Lowe, F. C., Goldman, S. M., and Oesterling, J. E.: Computerized tomography in evaluation of transitional cell carcinoma in bladder diverticula. Urology 34:390, 1989.

Lower, G. M., Jr.: Concepts in causality: Chemically induced human urinary bladder cancer. Cancer 49:1056, 1982.

Maurer, H. M.: Rhabdomyosarcoma. Pediatr. Ann. 8:35, 1979.

Miyake, O., Namiki, M., Sonoda, T., and Kitamura, H.: Secondary involvement of genitourinary organs in malignant lymphoma. Urol. Int. 42:360, 1987.

Rholl, K. S., Lee, J. K. T., Heiken, J. P., Ling, D., and Glazer, H. S.: Primary bladder carcinoma: Evaluation with MR imaging. Radiology 163:117, 1987.

Shapiro, E., and Strother, D.: Pediatric genitourinary rhabdomyosarcoma. J. Urol. 148:1761, 1992.

Silverberg, E., and Lubera, J. A.: Cancer statistics, 1988. Cancer 83:5, 1988.

Stilmant, M. M., and Siroky, M. B.: Nephrogenic adenoma associated with intravesical bacillus Calmette-Guérin treatment: A report of 2 cases. J. Urol. 135:359, 1986.

Thornbury, J. R., Silver, T. M., and Vinson, R. K.: Ureteroceles vs. pseudoureteroceles in adults. Radiology 122:81, 1977.

Vargas, A. D., and Mendez, R.: Leiomyoma of bladder. Urology 21:308, 1983.

Wallace, D. M., Chisholm, G. D., and Hendry, W. F.: T.N.M. classification for urological tumours (U.I.C.C.)—1974. Br. J. Urol. 47:1, 1975.

Warshawsky, R., Bow, S. N., Waldbaum, R. S., and Cintron, J.: Bladder pheochromocytoma with MR correlation. J. Comput. Assist. Tomogr. 13:714, 1989.

Wenz, W., Sommerkamp, H., and Dinkel, E.: Leiomyoma of bladder. Urol. Radiol. 8:114, 1986.

Whitmore, W. F., Jr.: Bladder cancer: An overview. CA 38:213, 1988.

Yousem, D. M., Gatewood, O. M. B., Goldman, S. M., and Marshall, F. F.: Synchronous and metachronous transitional cell carcinoma of the urinary tract: Prevalence, incidence, and radiographic detection. Radiology 167:613, 1988.

Zimmerman, K., Amis, E. S., Jr., and Newhouse, J. H.: Nephrogenic adenoma of the bladder: Urographic spectrum. Urol. Radiol. 11:123, 1989.

Zingas, A. P., Kling, G. A., Crotte, E., Shumaker, E., and Vazquez, P. M.: Computed tomography of nephrogenic adenoma of the urinary bladder. J. Comput. Assist. Tomogr. 10:979, 1986.

Extravesical Lesions

Banner, M. P.: Genitourinary complications of inflammatory bowel disease. Radiol. Clin. North Am. 25:199, 1987.

Carpenter, A. A.: Pelvic lipomatosis: Successful surgical treatment. J. Urol. 110:397, 1973.

Chang, S. F.: Pear-shaped bladder caused by large iliopsoas muscles. Radiology 128:349, 1978.

Enzinger, F. M., and Weiss, S. W.: Soft Tissue Tumors. St. Louis, C. V. Mosby Co., 1983, pp. 233–234.

Heyns, C. F.: Pelvic lipomatosis: A review of its diagnosis and management. J. Urol. 146:267, 1991.

Hill, G. S.: Intrinsic and extrinsic obstruction of the urinary tract. In Hill, G. S. (ed.): Uropathology. New York, Churchill Livingstone, 1989, pp. 235–278 and 517–574.

Merine, D., Fishman, E. K., Kuhlman, J. E., Jones, B., Bayless, T. M., and Siegelman, S.: Bladder involvement in Crohn disease: Role of CT in detection and evaluation. J. Comput. Assist. Tomogr. 13:90, 1989.

Resnick, M. I., and Kursh, E. D.: Extrinsic obstruction of the ureter. In Walsh, P. C., Retik, A. B., Stamey, T. A., and Vaughan, E. D., Jr. (eds.): Campbell's Urology. 6th ed. Philadelphia, W.B. Saunders, 1992, pp. 533–570.

Wechsler, R. J., and Brennan, R. E.: Teardrop bladder: Additional considerations. Radiology 144:281, 1982.

Trauma

Carroll, P. R., and McAninch, J. W.: Major bladder trauma: The accuracy of cystography. J. Urol. 130:887, 1983.

Carroll, P. R., and McAninch, J. W.: Major bladder trauma: Mechanisms of injury and a unified method of diagnosis and repair. J. Urol. 132:254, 1984.

Cass, A. S., and Luxenberg, M.: Features of 164 bladder ruptures. J. Urol. 138:743, 1987.

Corriere, J. N., Jr., and Harris, J. D.: The management of urologic injuries in blunt pelvic trauma. Radiol. Clin. North Am. 19:187, 1981.

Corriere, J. N., Jr., and Sandler, C. M.: Mechanisms of injury, patterns of extravasation and management of extraperitoneal bladder rupture due to blunt trauma. J. Urol. 139:43, 1988.

Palmer, J. K., Benson, G. S., and Corriere, J. N., Jr.: Diagnosis and initial management of urological injuries associated with 200 consecutive pelvic fractures. J. Urol. 130:712, 1983.

Sandler, C. M., Hall, J. T., Rodriguez, M. B., and Corriere, J. N., Jr.: Bladder injury in blunt pelvic trauma. Radiology 158:633, 1986.

Sandler, C. M., Phillips, J. M., Harris, J. D., and Toombs, B. D.: Radiology of the bladder and urethra in blunt pelvic trauma. Radiol. Clin. North Am. 19:195, 1981.

Sigler, L. J., Addonizio, J. C., Fernandez, R., and Schutte, H.: Incidence and treatment of bladder perforation following bladder biopsy. Urology 26:10, 1985.

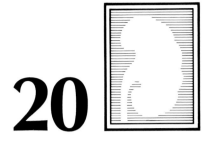

WENDELIN S. HAYES

20

THE URETHRA

This chapter describes the normal anatomy, anomalies, and acquired diseases of the urethra. The focus of this chapter is on the male urethra, which is far more complex in all respects than the female urethra. Material on the female urethra is included in each section, where appropriate.

ANATOMY

The male urethra is divided into two parts delineated by the inferior aspect of the urogenital diaphragm. The *posterior urethra* extends from the bladder neck distally to the inferior urogenital diaphragm, while the *anterior urethra* extends distally from the same landmark to the penile meatus. Figure 20–1 illustrates the anatomic landmarks of the urethra.

The posterior urethra is divided into *prostatic* and *membranous* segments. The prostatic portion extends from the bladder neck to the proximal margin of the urogenital diaphragm and is surrounded by the prostate gland. It is lined by transitional epithelium. A mound of smooth muscle along its posterior wall forms a prominent landmark, the *verumontanum* (Fig. 20–2). On either side of the verumontanum are the openings of the ejaculatory ducts. The orifice of the prostatic *utricle,* a vestige of the müllerian duct, is located in the midline of the proximal verumontanum. The membranous urethra is approximately 1 cm in length, traverses the urogenital diaphragm, and has a lining of stratified columnar epithelial cells (Fig. 20–3).

The anterior urethra is divided into the *bulbous* and the *penile* or *pendulous* segments. The bulbous urethra extends from the inferior margin of the urogenital diaphragm distally to the penoscrotal junction inferiorly. The proximal one-half of the bulbous urethra is dilated and has a symmetric cone shape at its proximal end when distended (Fig. 20–4). The penile urethra extends from the penoscrotal junction to the external meatus distally. The *fossa navicularis* is the slightly dilated, 1- to 1.5-cm segment of the penile urethra that narrows just proximal to the meatus. The mucosa of the entire anterior urethra is stratified columnar epithelium except at the meatus, which is lined by stratified squamous epithelium.

There are numerous mucus-producing glands, known as the *paraurethral glands of Littré,* along the anterior urethra. These glands are most numerous in the bulbous urethra. An additional set of glands, *Cowper's glands,* are situated within the urogenital diaphragm and drain through two long ducts into the bulbous urethra.

The urethra in adult females is approximately 4 cm in length and 6 mm in diameter (Fig. 20–5). This structure courses obliquely from the bladder neck to the urethral orifice.

ANOMALIES

Posterior Urethral Valve

Type I posterior urethral valve is an anomaly of wolffian duct origin that results from malposition, thickening, and fusion of the *plicae colliculi* of the urethral

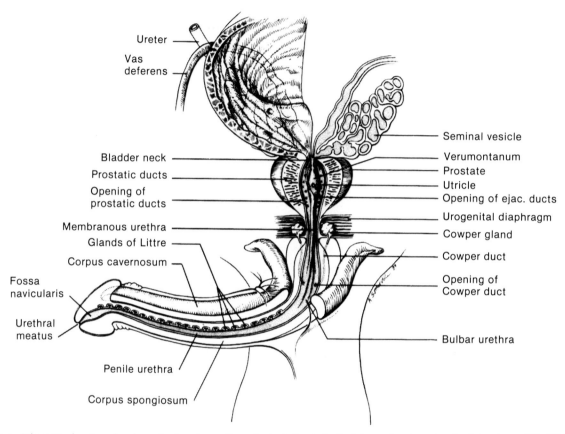

Figure 20–1. Schematic drawing of male urethral anatomy. (From Amis, E. S., et al.: Radiology of male periurethral structures. AJR *151*:321–324, 1988. Reproduced with kind permission of the authors and *American Journal of Roentgenology.*)

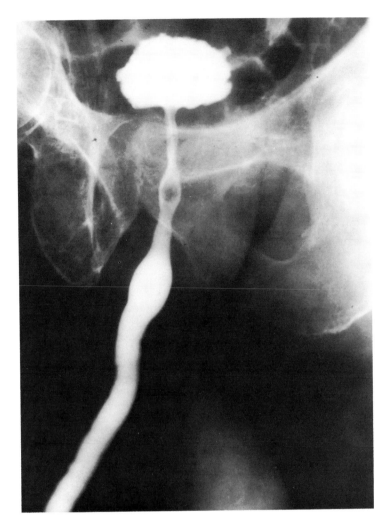

Figure 20–2. Normal male urethra. The verumontanum is seen as an oval filling defect in the prostatic urethra. Voiding cystourethrogram. (Kindly provided by Stanford M. Goldman, M.D., The Johns Hopkins University, Baltimore, Maryland.)

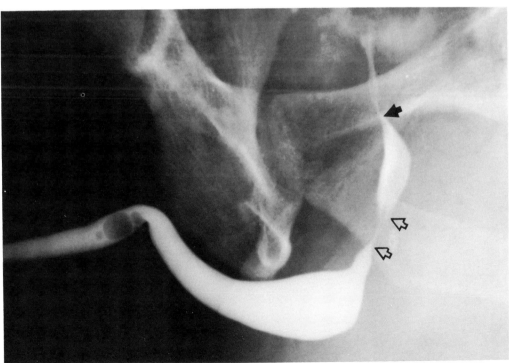

Figure 20–3. Normal male urethra. The prostatic urethra extends from the bladder neck *(solid arrow)* to the membranous urethra, which traverses the urogenital diaphragm *(open arrows)*. Several air bubbles are just distal to the penoscrotal junction. Retrograde urethrogram. (Kindly provided by William H. Bush, Jr., M.D., University of Washington, Seattle.)

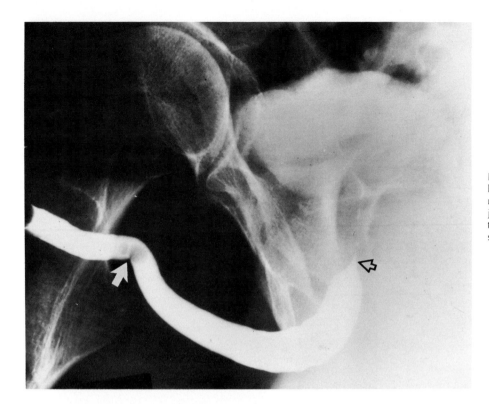

Figure 20–4. Normal male urethra. The bulbous urethra *(arrows)* extends from the membranous urethra to the penoscrotal junction. Retrograde urethrogram. (Courtesy of William H. Bush, Jr., M.D., University of Washington, Seattle.)

crest. The urethral crest is a musculomembranous structure that extends inferiorly from the verumontanum and divides into two or four plicae colliculi. These pass inferiorly, encircle the urethra, and terminate on the anterior aspect of the membranous urethra. Type I posterior urethral valve occurs when the wolffian duct originates more anterior than normal.

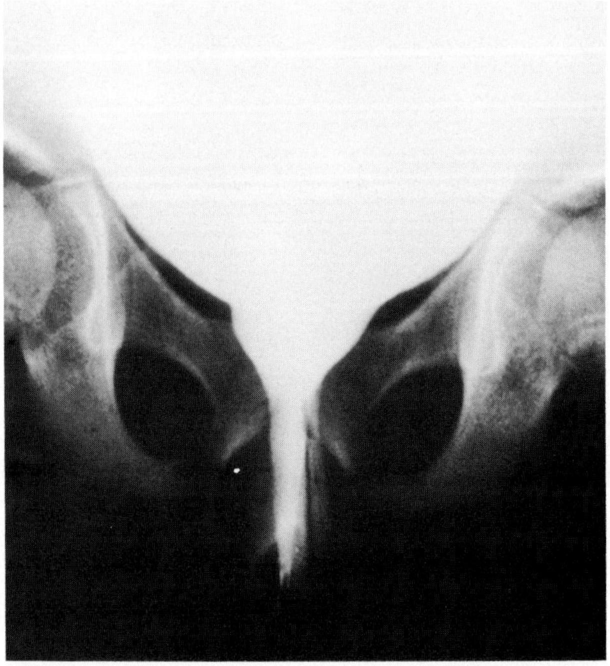

Figure 20–5. Normal female urethra. Voiding cystourethrogram. (Courtesy of William H. Bush, Jr., M.D., University of Washington, Seattle.)

In this situation the plicae colliculi form a thick, fused, valvelike cusp.

Type II posterior urethral valve has been classically described as a mucosal fold that extends from above the verumontanum toward the bladder base. It is likely that a Type II posterior urethral valve is, in fact, a manifestation of bladder neck obstruction, rather than a true posterior urethral anomaly.

Type III posterior urethral valve is a disklike membrane with a central orifice. This is transversely oriented across the urethral lumen and is not related to the verumontanum.

Type I posterior urethral valve produces a variable degree of obstruction, which may become manifest from the fetal period into adulthood. Older children and adults are more likely to have voiding disturbances or urinary tract infection, while those patients who are diagnosed *in utero*, in infancy, or early childhood are more likely to have clinical findings of urinary tract obstruction. An obvious abnormality of the urinary stream is not necessarily present when partial obstruction is compensated for by muscular hypertrophy of the bladder. In some children, clinical findings are obscure and include failure to thrive and recurrent vomiting. Patients with severe hydroureter, hydronephrosis, and obstructive nephropathy are likely to also have renal dysplasia and renal failure. This combination in the fetus leads to diminished urine output and oligohydramnios, as well as the other components of Potter's syndrome, including a high mortality rate in the perinatal period.

Radiologic findings in the patient with a posterior urethral valve vary with the age at which it is discovered. In the fetus with severe obstruction, ultrasonography demonstrates renal dysplasia, dilated renal pelves, tortuous and dilated ureters, bladder distention and oligohydramnios. Occasionally, dilatation of the posterior urethra is identified. The same urinary tract findings are noted after birth along with a small thorax and radiographic evidence of pulmonary hypoplasia. Ultrasonography at any age may also identify bladder wall thickening and trabeculation and a dilated posterior urethra (Fig. 20–6). Perirenal fluid collections and ascites are sometimes noted.

Voiding cystourethrography demonstrates dilatation and elongation of the posterior urethra (Fig. 20–7). A linear radiolucent band representing the valve may be seen (Fig. 20–8). The verumontanum is often enlarged. The bladder neck commonly hypertrophies and, thus, appears narrow in relationship to the dilated posterior urethra. Unilateral or bilateral vesicoureteral reflux is present in as many as 50 per cent of patients whose posterior urethral valve is discovered within the first year of life. If a cystogram is performed, retrograde passage of a urethral catheter is typically unimpeded by a Type I valve but may be difficult with a Type III valve. Bladder hypertrophy, trabeculation, sacculation, and diverticula are also demonstrated by cystography.

Diverticulum of the Anterior Urethra and Anterior Urethral Valve

A diverticulum of the anterior urethra develops on the ventral surface of the penile urethra, either as a result of incomplete development of the corpus spongiosum focally or incomplete fusion of a segment of the urethral plate. The diverticulum is usually oval, and its distal lip is thin and valvelike. It is this thin, anterior lip that has been called an anterior urethral valve.

The diverticulum fills during voiding, thereby narrowing and obstructing the true urethra. Incomplete bladder emptying and bladder infections are complications. Dribbling at the end of urination may also be present.

During voiding cystourethrography, the typical saccular diverticulum of the anterior urethra fills with contrast material and appears as an oval-shaped structure on the ventral aspect of the anterior urethra (Fig. 20–9). With distention of the diverticulum, partial or complete outflow obstruction occurs.

Megalourethra

Megalourethra is a rare anomaly that results from abnormal development of the corpus spongiosum and, less frequently, the corpus cavernosum. Congenital dilatation of the penile urethra without obstruction results. This anomaly may coexist with other urinary tract anomalies, including prune-belly syndrome, renal dysplasia, megaureter, megacystis, and bladder diverticulum, as well as vesicoureteral reflux. Both the phallus and the urethra are enlarged in megalourethra. Since sepsis may follow instrumentation

of the urethra, radiologic investigation of this disorder is best conducted by antegrade voiding techniques rather than retrograde urethrography.

Congenital Meatal Stenosis

Congenital meatal stenosis is a pinpoint narrowing of the urethral orifice frequently seen to some degree in patients with hypospadias. This condition is rare. Acquired meatal stenosis is more common than congenital stenosis and usually results from meatitis complicating circumcision.

Voiding cystourethrography in a patient with meatal stenosis demonstrates dilatation of the urethra proximal to a narrowed meatal orifice. Radiologic evaluation of meatal stenosis, however, is usually not required.

Hypospadias/Epispadias

Hypospadias is a condition in which the urethral meatus opens onto the ventral surface of the penis at a point proximal to the tip of the glans. In epispadias, in contradistinction, the urethral orifice is located on the dorsal aspect of the penis. Epispadias is usually seen in association with the various forms of exstrophy, which are discussed in Chapter 19. Epispadias in the female is associated with a short, patulous urethra, widely separated labia, and a bifid clitoris.

In either hypospadias or epispadias, voiding cystourethrography demonstrates a foreshortened urethra.

Urethral Duplication

Urethral duplication usually occurs either as complete or incomplete anomalies. *Complete* duplication takes several forms: two separate structures originate from the bladder and persist with separate external drainage; a common urethra originates from the bladder and duplicates distally; or a duplicated origin unites distally into a single external orifice. In *incomplete* duplication, an accessory urethra that does not communicate with either the bladder or the main urethra opens on the dorsal or ventral surface of the penis. Uncommonly, an accessory urethra arises from the main urethra and ends blindly in the periurethral tissue. In most cases, both the primary urethra and the accessory urethra are in the sagittal plane. The ventrally positioned urethra is usually the more functional one and also the urethra that is more easily catheterized regardless of its meatal position. Urethral duplication also occurs as a component of partial or complete caudal duplication anomalies, which include bladder duplication.

Specific clinical symptoms vary with the type of duplication. Patients with patent urethral duplication are either asymptomatic or exhibit a double urinary stream. Incontinence, infection, and dysuria are present occasionally.

A voiding cystourethrogram and a retrograde ure-

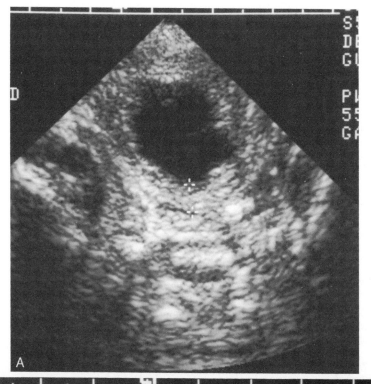

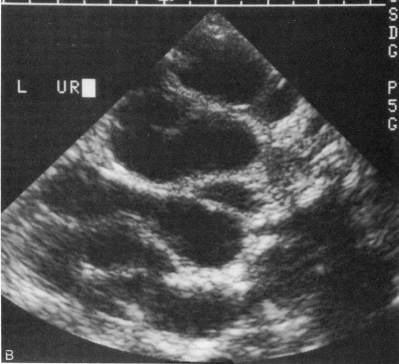

Figure 20–6. Posterior urethral valve in a newborn. Ultrasonograms.

A, Bladder, transverse section. The bladder wall *(cursors)* is thickened.

B, Left ureter, transverse section. The ureter is dilated and tortuous.

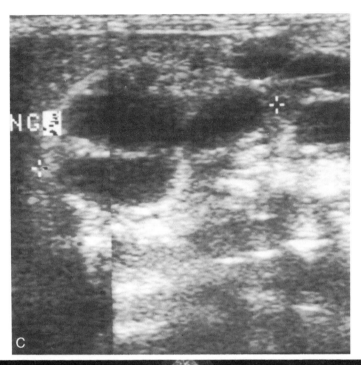

Figure 20–6. *Continued C,* Right kidney, longitudinal section.
D, Left kidney, longitudinal section. Hydronephrosis is present.

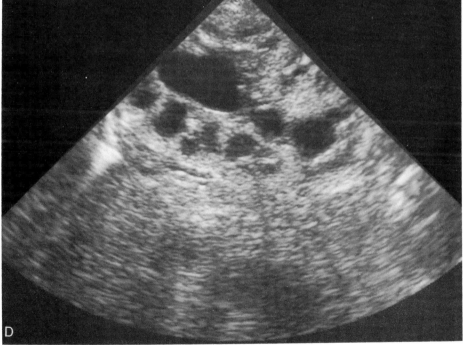

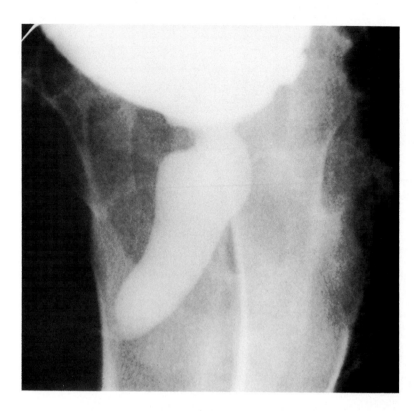

Figure 20–7. Posterior urethral valve in a newborn. Voiding cystourethrogram. There is dilatation and elongation of the posterior urethra with an abrupt change in caliber at the site of the valve as well as a prominent indentation on the posterior aspect of the bladder neck.

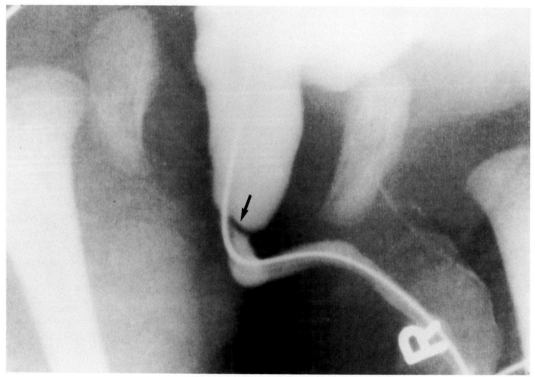

Figure 20–8. Posterior urethral valve in a newborn. Voiding cystourethrogram. The posterior urethra is dilated proximal to the sharply defined valve *(arrow)*.

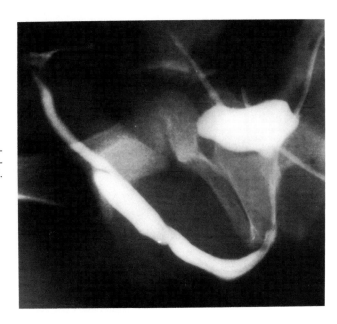

Figure 20–9. Congenital diverticulum of the urethra. Voiding cystoure-throgram. The saccular diverticulum is an elongated, oval-shaped structure on the ventral aspect of the anterior urethra. (Courtesy of Stanford M. Goldman, M.D., The Johns Hopkins University, Baltimore, Maryland.)

throgram, which may require two catheters in some patients, demonstrate the two urethral channels.

Congenital Urethral Stricture

A true congenital urethral stricture is one that is limited to a localized narrowing at the junction of the posterior and anterior urethra. Segmental urethral stenosis or complete atresia is rarely seen, often in association with severe cases of prune-belly syndrome.

INFECTION
Gonorrhea

Infection of the urethra by *Neisseria gonorrhoeae* most commonly involves the glands of Littré in the bulbous urethra and frequently leads to stricture formation in this part of the urethra. However, any portion of the urethra may be involved. The bacteria provoke an inflammatory response in the urethral submucosa that is characterized by cell necrosis and granulation tissue. A periurethral abscess may form in the glands of Littré and eventually drain into the urethra, forming a pseudodiverticulum. If the abscess extends into the perineum, fistulas between the urethra and the skin create a so-called "watering pot" perineum.

The clinical hallmarks of acute gonococcal urethritis are a purulent urethral discharge and dysuria. Acute symptoms may resolve without antibiotic therapy. In the absence of effective therapy for the acute infection, the organism may persist in the glands of Littré, causing a thin urethral discharge and favoring the development of fibrosis and stricture. Obstructive voiding symptoms may occur months to years after the initial gonococcal infection.

Radiologic evaluation by retrograde urethrography in gonococcal urethritis is usually limited to circumstances in which there are complications of the acute infection. A periurethral abscess that has drained into

the urethra is seen as a diverticulum-like collection of contrast material that communicates with the urethra. Fistulas between the urethra and the skin, the "watering pot" perineum, are also opacified during retrograde urethrography (Fig. 20–10). Postgonococcal strictures are often irregular in appearance, are several centimeters in length, and most often involve the bulbous urethra (Fig. 20–11). There is often associated filling of the glands of Littré as well as Cowper's duct and gland. In some patients the stricture may be quite localized (Fig. 20–12). Stricture formation in the most proximal part of the bulbous urethra leads to a loss of the normal cone shape of this segment. When the urethra is examined by voiding cystourethrography, reflux of contrast material into dilated prostatic ducts may be noted (Fig. 20–13). This represents increased hydrostatic pressure proximal to a stricture.

Tuberculosis

Tuberculosis of the urethra results from a descending infection from the upper urinary tract or is secondary to tuberculosis of the prostate. Although the prostate is involved in up to 70 per cent of cases of genital tuberculosis, the urethra is rarely affected. When the urethra is involved, the bulbous and membranous segments are the most common sites. Periurethral and prostatic caseating granulomas as well as fistulas between the urethra and the perineum are frequently present. The latter complication causes the same "watering pot" appearance as that described in gonorrhea.

Tuberculosis of the kidney is discussed in Chapter 13, that of the pelvis and ureter in Chapter 15, and that of the bladder in Chapter 19.

Schistosomiasis

Urethritis secondary to *Schistosomiasis haematobium* occurs in association with bladder involvement. Fistulas

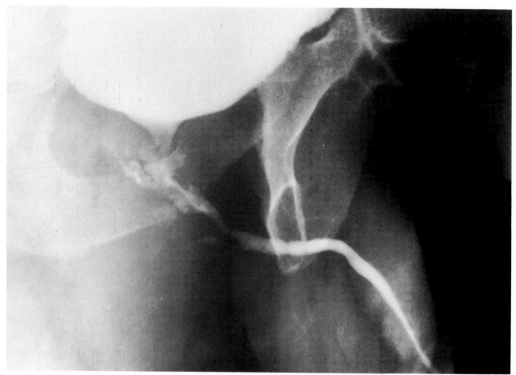

Figure 20–10. Gonorrheal urethritis complicated by fistulas and sinuses. Retrograde urethrogram. There is irregular narrowing of the bulbar urethra with multiple sinuses.

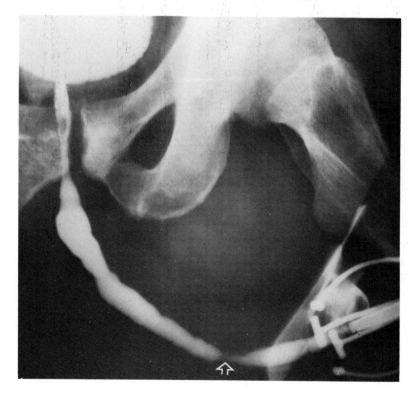

Figure 20–11. Gonorrheal urethritis with late stricture. Retrograde urethrogram. There is diffuse urethral narrowing. The glands of Littré are faintly opacified in the most narrowed segment *(arrow).*

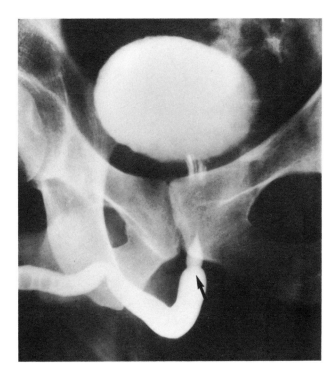

Figure 20–12. Gonorrheal urethritis with late stricture. Retrograde urethrogram. There is a localized stricture *(arrow)* in the bulbous urethra.

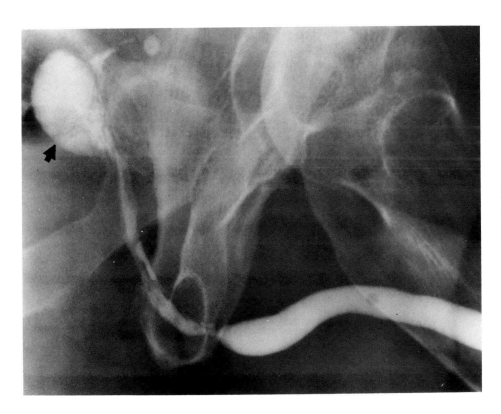

Figure 20–13. Gonorrheal urethritis and stricture. Retrograde urethrogram. There is a long stricture of the proximal portion of the bulbous urethra and reflux of contrast material into the prostate *(arrow)*.

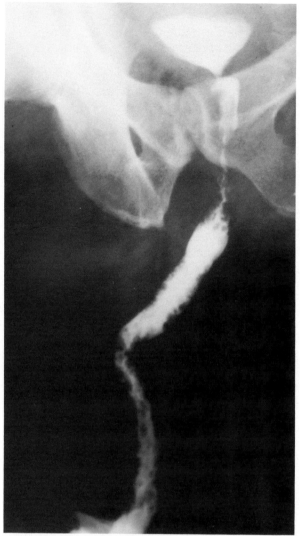

Figure 20–14. Condylomata acuminata. Retrograde urethrogram. There are multiple filling defects throughout the entire urethra. (From Pollack, H.M., et al.: Urethrographic manifestations of venereal warts (condyloma acuminata). Radiology *126*:643–646, 1978. Reproduced with kind permission of the authors and *Radiology*.)

that develop involve the bulbar urethra, the scrotum, and the perineum. Long strictures of the penile urethra also occur. Schistosomiasis of the prostate often coexists.

Schistosomiasis of the ureter is discussed in Chapter 15 and that of the bladder in Chapter 19.

Condylomata Acuminata

Condylomata acuminata is a viral infection that is manifested by formation of verrucae on the skin of the genital, perineal, and perianal regions. Intraurethral extension occurs in as many as 5 per cent of patients and is clinically suspected with the appearance of meatal condylomata, or when urethral discharge or irritative voiding symptoms develop in patients with genital verrucae. Involvement of the bladder may also occur.

With urethrography, multiple nonobstructive filling defects are present, at times involving the entire urethra. These range from 1.0 to 10.0 mm (Fig. 20–14).

NEOPLASMS

Benign Tumors

Fibrous urethral polyps arise in the prostatic urethra in the region of the verumontanum. They are pedunculated and composed of a loose, fibrous, connective tissue core covered by transitional cell epithelium.

Urethral polyps are a rare cause of bladder outlet obstruction in boys. Most cases are diagnosed in boys between 3 and 10 years of age. The polyp may prolapse from the urethra into the bladder, causing intermittent obstruction and hematuria.

Both retrograde and voiding cystourethrography demonstrate the mobility of these polyps, which appear as oval filling defects in the posterior urethra that prolapse into the membranous or bulbous urethra during voiding (Figs. 20–15 and 20–16). Without voiding, a filling defect may be detected at the bladder base on any study that uses contrast material to fill the bladder. Ultrasonographically, a fibrous polyp appears as an echogenic polypoid mass in the bladder base.

Miscellaneous benign tumors that rarely occur in the urethra include *hemangioma, leiomyoma, and benign prostatic epithelial polyp.*

Malignant Tumors

Malignant tumors of the urethra are rare. Most are *squamous cell carcinomas* that arise in the bulbomem-

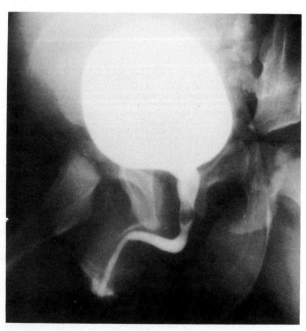

Figure 20–15. Congenital urethral polyp. Voiding cystourethrogram. The polyp appears as a round filling defect in the posterior urethra. (Courtesy of William H. Bush, Jr., M.D., University of Washington, Seattle.)

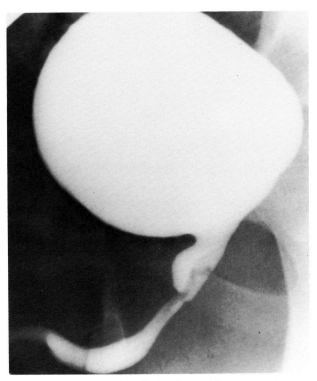

Figure 20–16. Congenital urethral polyp. Voiding cystourethrogram. The polyp appears as an elongated structure in the posterior urethra. (Courtesy of Stanford M. Goldman, M.D., The Johns Hopkins University, Baltimore, Maryland.)

branous urethra. *Transitional cell carcinoma,* usually involving the prostatic urethra, and *adenocarcinoma,* originating in either Cowper's glands or the glands of Littré, are far less common than squamous cell carcinoma. Predisposing factors for squamous cell carcinoma of the urethra include chronic irritation, gonococcal urethritis, urethral trauma, and stricture.

A malignant tumor of the male urethra has a peak prevalence between 50 and 70 years of age. Clinical manifestations include obstructive symptoms, palpable mass, or a periurethral abscess or fistula. Lesions of the proximal urethra are often more advanced at the time of diagnosis than are those of the distal urethra and, therefore, have a worse prognosis. Additionally, tumors of the proximal urethra tend to infiltrate the perineum, scrotum, prostate, and bladder.

Urethral carcinoma appears on retrograde urethrography as a narrow and often long, irregular stricture (Figs. 20–17 and 20–18). Less commonly, the carcinoma produces a filling defect within the urethral lumen. A change in the appearance of a pre-existing stricture or recurrent stricture after urethroplasty raises the suspicion of urethral carcinoma.

Squamous cell carcinoma is the most commonly occurring malignant tumor of the female urethra, as is true in the male. The distal third of the urethra is the most frequent site for squamous cell carcinoma, while transitional cell carcinoma or adenocarcinoma usually involves the proximal urethra. Females with malignant urethral tumors usually exhibit a bleeding mass.

Sarcoma arising in the mesenchymal supporting tissue of the urethra is extremely rare. Histologic types include rhabdomyosarcoma, leiomyosarcoma, malignant fibrous histiocytoma, and myxosarcoma. Also rare is *primary or metastatic melanoma* of the urethra. Other *metastases* may occur from primary malignancies arising in the prostate, colon, rectum, bladder, kidney, ureter, and testes. The penis is usually also involved.

TRAUMA

The urethra may be injured by blunt, penetrating, or iatrogenic causes. Injury of the male urethra is classi-

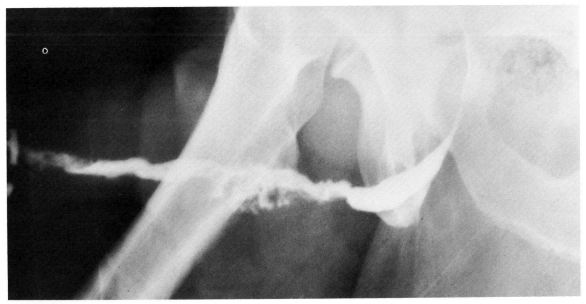

Figure 20–17. Squamous cell carcinoma, anterior urethra. Retrograde urethrogram. The tumor produces an irregular narrowing of a long segment of the anterior urethra.

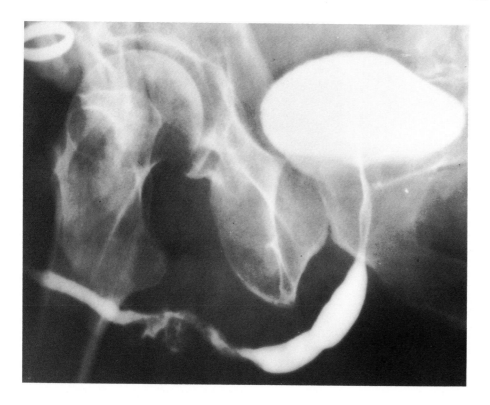

Figure 20–18. Squamous cell carcinoma, anterior urethra. Retrograde urethrogram. There is a mass in the distal urethra associated with a long, irregular stricture.

fied either as a posterior urethral injury, which is typically associated with pelvic fracture, or as an anterior urethral injury, which is usually not associated with pelvic fracture. Posterior urethral and bladder injuries sometimes coexist.

Urethral injury in the female is an extremely rare event because of its short length and lack of ligamentous fixation to adjacent structures.

Posterior Urethral Injury

A posterior urethral injury occurs in as many as 10 per cent of males with pelvic fracture. The urethra is subject to a shearing force when a pelvic fracture disrupts the urogenital diaphragm and the puboprostatic ligaments, resulting in displacement of the prostate gland.

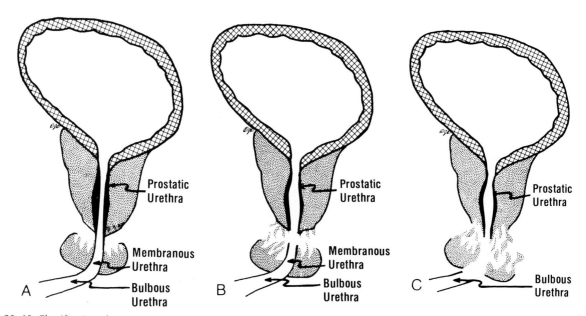

Figure 20–19. Classification of posterior urethral injuries. Schematic drawing.
  A, Type I.
  B, Type II.
  C, Type III.
  (From Sandler, C.M., et al.: Posterior urethral injuries after pelvic fracture. AJR *137*:1233–1237, 1981. Reproduced with kind permission of the authors and *American Journal of Roentgenology.*)

The radiologic classification of posterior urethral injury is based on the following definitions, which are illustrated in Figure 20–19:

Type I. The posterior urethra is intact but stretched and elongated. The prostate is displaced proximally owing to the disruption of the moorings of the prostate. Resultant hematoma elevates the bladder high in the pelvis. No contrast material is present in the periurethral tissue.

Type II. Disruption of the urethra occurs above the urogenital diaphragm at the junction of the posterior and membranous urethra. Contrast material is present in the extraperitoneal space of the pelvis above the urogenital diaphragm.

Type III. The membranous urethra is disrupted with extension of the injury to the proximal bulbous urethra and/or disruption of the urogenital diaphragm. Contrast material extends into the soft tissue both above and below the urogenital diaphragm. Depending on the degree of disruption of the urogenital diaphragm, contrast material may also be seen in the perineum (Fig. 20–20).

Type III posterior urethral injury occurs most frequently. Both Type II and Type III urethral tears may be partial or complete. During urethrography, partial filling of the bladder suggests a partial tear.

The classic clinical findings in posterior urethral injury include blood at the urethral meatus, inability to void spontaneously, and a palpable bladder. Digital rectal examination of the prostate gland may reveal superior displacement of the prostate. The absence of these findings, however, does not preclude a urethral injury.

Radiologic examination of the urethra in the setting of acute trauma must be performed with retrograde instillation of contrast material at the meatus or fossa navicularis, preferably under fluoroscopic control. Any attempt to catheterize the urethra beyond the fossa navicularis carries the risk of false passage of the catheter, conversion of a partial to a complete tear, contamination of a hematoma, or hemorrhage in the prostate. Abnormal radiologic findings in the urethra correspond to the preceding descriptions for the classification of urethral injury. Associated abnormalities relating to the bladder or pelvis as well as findings of other abdominal trauma may be present. Some of these are discussed in Chapters 19 and 27.

The radiologic evaluation for the late complications of urethral trauma include assessment of integrity of the urethral lumen, false passages, bladder incontinence, and stricture formation. Stricture may form after either partial or complete urethral tear (Fig. 20–21).

Combined Urethral and Bladder Injury

Bladder injury is present in as many as 20 per cent of males with posterior urethral injury. Bladder involvement may be demonstrated at the time of retrograde urethrography, if the urethral injury is incomplete and some bladder opacification occurs. An attempt should not be made to completely distend the bladder with contrast material during retrograde urethrography once a posterior urethral injury is detected. Rather, the examination of the bladder should be performed after a suprapubic catheter is in place.

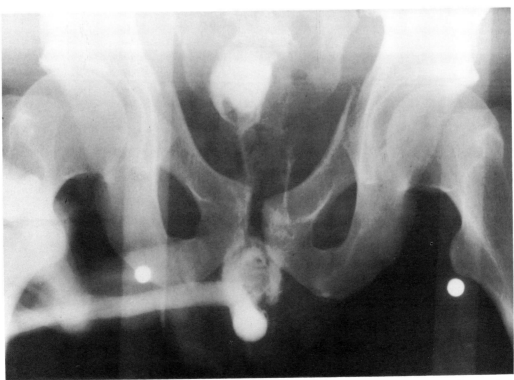

Figure 20–20. Posterior urethral injury, Type III. Retrograde urethrogram. There is contrast material in perineal and perivesical soft tissue.

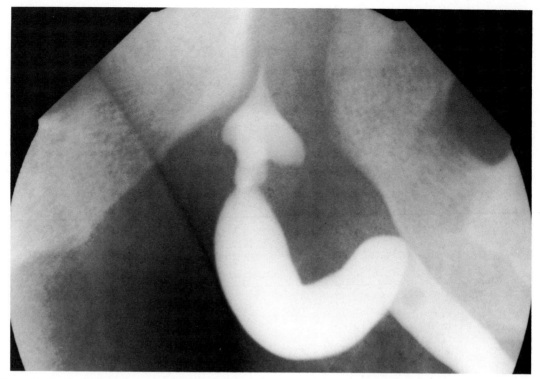

Figure 20–21. Urethral stricture, post-traumatic. Retrograde urethrogram demonstrates a proximal bulbar urethral stricture.

Anterior Urethral Injury

Injury of the anterior urethra results from a direct blow to the perineum or a straddle injury involving the bulbous urethra. Straddle injuries most often occur as a result of falling astride a parallel bar, the frame of a bicycle, or the top of a fence rail or steel beam. The force of a straddle injury compresses the bulbous urethra against the inferior pubis, resulting in contusion or partial or complete urethral tear. The corpus spongiosum may also be affected. Typically, there is no associated pelvic fracture. Anterior urethral trauma is less common than is trauma to the posterior urethra.

Retrograde urethrography should be performed as described previously for suspected posterior urethral injuries. Contusion of the anterior urethra gives rise to the same clinical features as more serious injuries of the anterior urethra, but the radiologic appearance of the urethra is normal. Partial or complete urethral rupture is demonstrated with a more severe straddle injury. If Buck's fascia is torn, contrast material may extend into the scrotum, perineum, or anterior abdominal wall. A stricture may form as a long-term complication of straddle injury. These occur generally in the proximal bulbous urethra and are usually short, measuring 0.5 cm or less.

Penetrating Urethral Injury

Penetrating wounds of the perineum or buttocks may involve either the anterior or the posterior urethra. The anterior urethra is more commonly involved. Ex-

amination of the patient with suspected penetrating injury of the urethra should follow the previously described guidelines for retrograde urethrography.

Iatrogenic Anterior Urethral Injury

Urethral injury from surgical instrumentation, long-term transurethral bladder catheterization, abdominoperineal resection, or radiation may cause a stricture to form over time. Stricture related to a long-term transurethral bladder catheter follows pressure necrosis and is most likely to occur at the penoscrotal junction or the bulbomembranous segment.

MISCELLANEOUS

Diverticulum of the Female Urethra

A diverticulum of the female urethra is most likely the result of dilatation of periurethral glands, although maternal birth trauma has also been considered as a cause. An uncomplicated diverticulum may cause dribbling after voiding. If the diverticulum becomes infected, the clinical findings are those of purulent discharge, dyspareunia, and a palpable mass. Stones, which may form within the diverticulum, are detectable on radiographs of the region (Fig. 20–22). Radiologic demonstration of a female urethral diverticulum may occur during a voiding cystogram, on a postvoiding film of the region, or following retrograde opacification of the urethra through an occluding catheter.

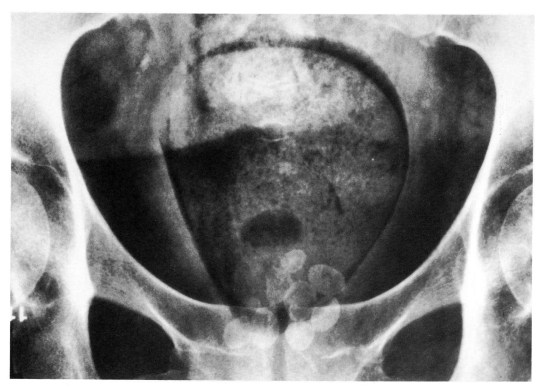

Figure 20–22. Diverticulum in a female urethra complicated by multiple calculi.

Figure 20–23. Syringocele. Retrograde urethrogram. The smooth filling defect in the bulbous urethra *(solid arrow)* results from dilatation of the terminal portion of one of Cowper's ducts. The syringocele itself does not fill with contrast material. There is faint visualization of the contralateral Cowper's duct *(open arrow)*. Only a portion of the prostatic urethra is visualized on this study.

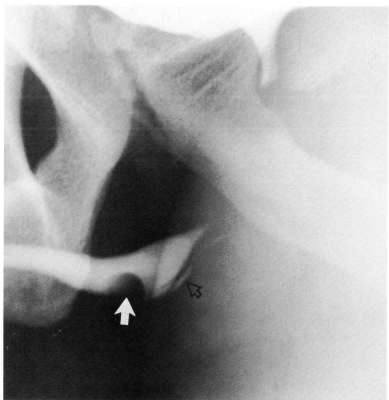

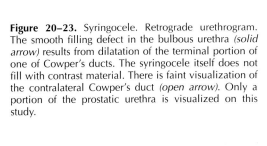

Cowper's Duct Cyst

Cowper's glands are paired structures located on either side of the membranous urethra within the urogenital diaphragm. Their ducts enter the proximal bulbar urethra. Cowper's glands function as accessory male sex organs that contribute to semen coagulation and urethral lubrication.

Abnormalities of Cowper's duct are uncommon. Syringoceles or cystic dilations occur most commonly in infants and young children secondary to narrowing of the duct orifice. Clinical findings include recurrent urinary tract infection or irritative and obstructive voiding symptoms. Rarely, Cowper's duct cyst appears as a perineal mass.

The dilated duct is seen radiologically as a filling defect on the ventral surface of the bulbar urethra (Fig. 20–23). Reflux of contrast material into a patulous or perforated syringocele opacifies the dilated duct.

Bibliography

Anatomy

Amis, E. S., Jr., Newhouse, J. H., and Cronan, J. J.: Radiology of male periurethral structures. AJR 151:321, 1988.
McCallum, R. W.: The adult male urethra: Normal anatomy, pathology and method of urethrography. Radiol. Clin. North Am. 17:227, 1979.
Tanagho, E. A.: Anatomy of the lower urinary tract. In Walsh, P. C., Retik, A. B., Stamey, T. A., and Vaughan, E. D., Jr. (eds.): Campbell's Urology. 6th ed. Philadelphia, W.B. Saunders, 1992, pp. 40–69.

Anomalies

Appel, R. A., Kaplan, G. W., Brock, W. A., and Streit, D.: Megalourethra. J. Urol. 135:747, 1986.
Cremin, B. J.: A review of the ultrasonic appearances of posterior urethral valve and ureteroceles. Pediatr. Radiol. 16:357, 1986.
Das, S., and Brosman, S. A.: Duplication of the male urethra. J. Urol. 117:452, 1977.
Duckett, J. W.: Hypospadias. In Walsh, P. C., Retik, A. B., Stamey, T. A., and Vaughan, E. D., Jr. (eds.): Campbell's Urology. 6th ed. Philadelphia, W.B. Saunders, 1992, pp. 1903–1919.
Effmann, E. L., Lebowitz, R. L., and Colodny, A. H.: Duplication of the urethra. Radiology 119:179, 1976.
Gonzales, E. T., Jr.: Posterior urethral valves and other urethral anomalies. In Walsh, P. C., Retik, A. B., Stamey, T. A., and Vaughan, E. D., Jr. (eds.): Campbell's Urology. 6th ed. Philadelphia, W. B. Saunders, 1992, pp. 1872–1892.
Hulbert, W. C., and Duckett, J.: Current views on posterior urethral valves. Pediatr. Ann. 17:31, 1988.
Hill, G. S.: Anomalies of the bladder and urethra. In Hill, G. S. (ed.): Uropathology. New York, Churchill Livingstone, 1989, pp. 235–277.
Kirks, D. R., and Grossman, H.: Congenital saccular anterior urethral diverticulum. Radiology 140:367, 1981.
Macpherson, R. I., Leithiser, R. E., Gordon, L., and Turner, W. R.: Posterior urethral valves: An update and review. Radiographics 6:753, 1986.
Mahony, B. S., Callen, P. W., and Filly, R. A.: Fetal urethral obstruction: US evaluation. Radiology 157:221, 1985.
Mininberg, D. T., and Genvert, H. P.: Posterior urethral valves: Role of temporary and permanent urinary diversion. Urology 33:205, 1989.
Nakayama, D. K., Harrison, M. R., and de Lorimer, A. A.: Prognosis of posterior urethral valves presenting at birth. J. Pediatr. Surg. 21:43, 1986.
Psihramis, K. E., Colodny, A. H., Lebowitz, R. L., Retik, A. B., and

Bauer, S. B.: Complete patent duplication of the urethra. J. Urol. 136:63, 1986.
Saltzman, B., Mininberg, D. T., and Muecke, E. C.: Epispadias: Contending with continence. Urology 16:256, 1985.
Sant, G. R., and Kaleli, A.: Cowper's syringocele causing incontinence in an adult. J. Urol. 133:279, 1985.
Scherz, H. C., Kaplan, G. W., and Packer, M. G.: Anterior urethral valves in the fossa navicularis in children. J. Urol. 138:1211, 1987.
Shrom, S. H., Cromie, W. J., and Duckett, J. W.: Megalourethra. Urology 17:152, 1981.
Young, H. H., Frontz, W. A., and Baldwin, J. C.: Congenital obstruction of the posterior urethra. J. Urol. 3:289, 1919.

Infection

Bissada, N. K., Cole, A. T., and Fried, F. A.: Extensive condylomas acuminata of the entire male urethra and the bladder. J. Urol. 112:201, 1974.
Harrison, W. O.: Gonococcal urethritis. Urol. Clin. North Am. 11:45, 1984.
McCallum, R. W.: The adult male urethra: Normal anatomy, pathology and method of urethrography. Radiol. Clin. North Am. 17:227, 1979.
Osegbe, D. N., and Amaku, E. O.: Gonococcal strictures in young patients. Urology 18:37, 1981.
Osoba, A. O., and Alausa, O.: Gonococcal urethral stricture and watering-can perineum. Br. J. Vener. Dis. 52:387, 1976.
Pollack, H. M., DeBenedictis, T. J., Marmar, J. L., and Praiss, D. E.: Urethrographic manifestations of venereal warts (condyloma acuminata). Radiology 126:643, 1978.
Sawczuk, I., Badillo, F., and Olsson, C. A.: Condylomata acuminata: Diagnosis and follow-up by retrograde urethrography. Urol. Radiol. 5:273, 1983.
Singh, M., and Blandy, J. P.: The pathology of urethral stricture. J. Urol. 115:673, 1976.
Symes, J. M., and Blandy, J. P.: Tuberculosis of the male urethra. Br. J. Urol. 45:432, 1973.
Tomaszewski, J. E.: Urethritis. In Hill, G. S. (ed.): Uropathology. New York, Churchill Livingstone, 1989, pp. 455–466.
Wein, A. J., and Benson, G. S.: Treatment of urethral condyloma acuminatum with 5-fluorouracil cream. Urology 9:413, 1977.

Neoplasms

Bagley, F. H., and Davidson, A. I.: Congenital urethral polyp in a child. Br. J. Urol. 48:278, 1976.
Bolduan, J. P., and Farah, R. N.: Primary urethral neoplasms: Review of 30 cases. J. Urol. 125:198, 1981.
Caro, P. A., Rosenberg, H. K., and Snyder, H. M., III: Congenital urethral polyp. AJR 147:1041, 1986.
Craig, J. R., and Hart, W. R.: Benign polyps with prostatic-type epithelium of the urethra. Am. J. Clin. Pathol. 63:343, 1975.
Grabstald, H.: Tumors of the urethra in men and women. Cancer 32:1236, 1973.
Hopkins, S. C., Nag, S. K., and Soloway, M. S.: Primary carcinoma of male urethra. Urology 23:128, 1984.
Kaplan, G. W., Bulkley, G. J., and Grayhack, J. T.: Carcinoma of the male urethra. J. Urol. 98:365, 1967.
Katz, R. S.: Tumors and tumorlike conditions of the male urethra. In Hill, G. S. (ed.): Uropathology. New York, Churchill Livingstone, 1989, pp. 1369–1380.
Kimche, D., and Lask, D.: Congenital polyp of the prostatic urethra. J. Urol. 127:134, 1982.
Levine, R. L.: Urethral cancer. Cancer 45:1965, 1980.
Zulian, R. A. S., Brito, R. R., and Borges, H. J.: Transurethral resection of pedunculated congenital polyps of the posterior urethra. Br. J. Urol. 54:45, 1982.

Trauma

Barbagli, G., Selli, C., Stomaci, N., Rose, A. D., Trippitelli, A., and Lenzi, R.: Urethral trauma: Radiological aspects and treatment options. J. Trauma 27:256, 1987.

Coffield, K. S., and Weems, W. L.: Experience with management of posterior urethral injury associated with pelvic fractures. J. Urol. *117*:722, 1977.

Colapinto, V., and McCallum, R. W.: Injury to the male posterior urethra in fractured pelvis: A new classification. J. Urol. *118*:575, 1977.

Corriere, J. N., Jr., and Harris, J. D.: The management of urologic injuries in blunt pelvic trauma. Radiol. Clin. North Am. *19*:187, 1981.

Morehouse, D. D., and Mackinnon, K. J.: Management of prostato-membranous urethral disruption: 13-year experience. J. Urol. *123*:173, 1980.

Lentz, H. C., Mebust, W. K., Foret, J. D., and Melchior, J.: Urethral strictures following transurethral prostatectomy: Review of 2,223 resections. J. Urol. *117*:194, 1977.

Palmer, J. K., Benson, G. S., and Corriere, J. N., Jr.: Diagnosis and initial management of urological injuries associated with 200 consecutive pelvic fractures. J. Urol. *130*:712, 1983.

Perry, M. O., and Husmann, D. A.: Urethral injuries in female subjects following pelvic fractures. J. Urol. *147*:139, 1992.

Peters, P. C., and Sagalowsky, A. I.: Genitourinary trauma. *In* Walsh, P. C., Retik, A. B., Stamey, T. A., and Vaughan, E. D., Jr. (eds.): Campbell's Urology. 6th ed. Philadelphia, W. B. Saunders, 1992, pp. 2571–2594.

Pierce, J. M., Jr.: Disruptions of the anterior urethra. Urol. Clin. North Am. *16*: 329, 1989.

Sandler, C. M., and Corriere, J. N., Jr.: Urethrography in the diagnosis of acute urethral injuries. Urol. Clin. North Am. *16*:283, 1989.

Sandler, C. M., Harris, J. H., Jr., Corriere, J. N., Jr., and Toombs, B. D.: Posterior urethral injuries after pelvic fracture. AJR *137*:1233, 1981.

Sandler, C. M., Phillips, J. M., Harris, J. D., and Toombs, B. D.: Radiology of the bladder and urethra in blunt pelvic trauma. Radiol. Clin. North Am. *19*:195, 1981.

Miscellaneous

Gonzales, E. T., Jr.: Posterior urethral valves and other urethral anomalies. *In* Walsh, P. C., Retik, A. B., Stamey, and T. A., Vaughan, E. D., Jr. (eds.): Campbell's Urology. 6th ed. Philadelphia, W.B. Saunders, 1992, pp. 1886–1888.

Maizels, M., Stephens, F. D., King, L. R., and Firlit, C. F.: Cowper's syringocele: A classification of dilatations of Cowper's gland duct based upon clinical characteristics of 8 boys. J. Urol. *129*:111, 1983.

Raz, S., Little, N. A., and Juma, S.: Female urology. *In* Walsh, P. C., Retik, A. B., Stamey, T. A., and Vaughan, E. D., Jr. (eds.): Campbell's Urology. 6th ed. Philadelphia, W.B. Saunders, 1992, pp. 2813–2816.

Redman, J. F., and Rountree, G. A.: Pronounced dilatation of Cowper's gland duct manifest as a perineal mass: A recommendation for management. J. Urol. *139*:87, 1988.

Yaffe, D., and Zissin, R.: Cowper's gland duct: Radiographic findings. Urol. Radiol. *13*:123, 1991.

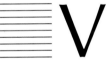

V
THE
RETROPERITONEUM
AND ADRENAL

21

THE RETROPERITONEUM

The advent of computed tomography, ultrasonography, and magnetic resonance imaging, has opened a new era for the anatomic study of the retroperitoneum. The spatial and density resolution and cross-sectional anatomic display of computed tomography, augmented by the intrinsic contrast provided by abundant fat usually found in the retroperitoneum, combine to yield images of exquisite accuracy and clinical usefulness. The same attributes apply to images generated by magnetic resonance. Ultrasonography, although effective in defining fluid collections and solid tumors whose echo pattern is distinctive from the normally echogenic retroperitoneal fat, is not as efficacious in evaluating retroperitoneal disorders.

This chapter first presents the anatomy of the retroperitoneum and then describes the various pathologic processes that affect each of the three compartments that constitute the retroperitoneum. This is followed by a discussion of primary retroperitoneal neoplasms, retroperitoneal lymphadenopathy, retroperitoneal fibrosis, and pseudotumors of the retroperitoneum. Excluded from consideration are the solid organs other than the kidney that are contained within the retroperitoneum.

ANATOMY

The retroperitoneum is a large space bounded anteriorly by the posterior parietal peritoneum and posteriorly by the transversalis fascia (Figs. 21–1 through 21–5). The diaphragm marks the cephalic limits; and the level of the pelvic brim marks the approximate caudal extent of this area.

Each side of the retroperitoneum is divided into three compartments by two separate layers of medium to dense collagenous connective tissue fascia,

mainly orientated in a coronal plane, one anterior and the other posterior to the kidney and adrenal gland. The *anterior renal fascia* (Gerota's fascia) is a thin layer of connective tissue that is sometimes difficult to distinguish, whereas the *posterior renal fascia* (Zuckerkandl's fascia) is slightly thicker and consistently identifiable. A normal fascial thickness of up to 3 mm has been reported, although most fasciae measure approximately 1 mm (Fig. 21–6). These two sheaths, which together constitute the *renal fascia*, blend together laterally to form a single membrane, the *lateroconal fascia*. This structure extends posterolateral to the ascending or descending colon, where it fuses with the parietal peritoneum. Superiorly, both layers of renal fasciae blend with the diaphragmatic fascia to form the cephalic limit of the retroperitoneum. Inferiorly, the caudal extent is marked by the fusion of anterior and posterior leaves with the iliac fascia and the periureteric connective tissue at the level of the iliac crest. The medial extent of the anterior renal fascia blends into the connective tissue and fat that surrounds the great vessels behind the pancreas and duodenum. The posterior renal fascia fuses along its medial margin with the fascia of the psoas and the quadratus lumborum muscles. These medial relationships effectively close one perirenal space from direct communication with the other side.

The *renal capsule* is a firm, smooth sheet of fibrous tissue with a thin layer of smooth muscle that invests the kidney. The capsule adheres to the underlying parenchyma through fine connective tissue processes and bridging blood vessels that allow easy stripping of the capsule away from the normal kidney. With disease, the capsule thickens and becomes more adherent. The subcapsular area is a potential space where fluid can collect.

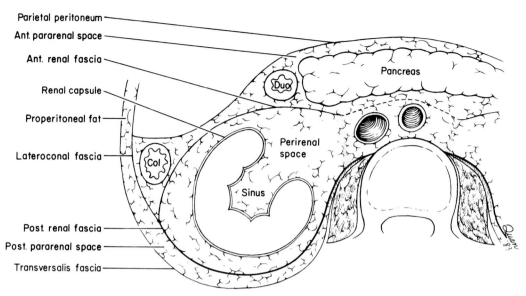

Figure 21–1. Diagram of the cross-sectional anatomy of the right retroperitoneum at the level of the renal sinus.

The *perirenal space,* encompassed by the anterior and posterior renal fasciae, contains the kidney and adrenal gland. Abundant fat fills this space, particularly posterior and inferior to the lower pole of the kidney. This fat acts as natural contrast material and accounts for the visualization of the renal outline and the upper one-half of the psoas muscle on standard radiographs (Fig. 21–7). The superior and inferior capsular arteries that originate variably from the main renal artery, its proximal major branches, and the inferior adrenal artery course through the perirenal fat in proximity to the kidney and supply blood to both the capsule and the perirenal fat. The middle capsular artery is a *recur-*

rent artery extending from the superior or inferior artery or arises directly from an arcuate branch of the renal artery that perforates the cortex and extends into the perirenal fat. Capsular veins parallel the arteries but have an extensive potential collateral network. The renal sinus is a continuation of the perirenal space where it invaginates into the hilum of the kidney. The contents of the sinus (pelvocalyceal system, proximal ureter, and neurovascular and lymphatic structures) are thus contents of the perirenal space. (These are discussed separately in Chapter 16.) The perinephric fat is traversed by fibrils that extend from the renal capsule to the renal fascia. These bridging septa are

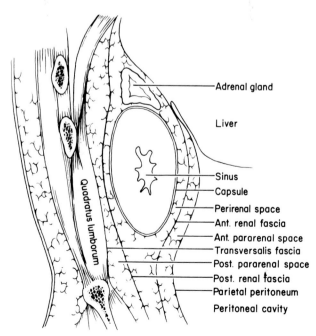

Figure 21–2. Diagram of the parasagittal anatomy of the right retroperitoneum at the level of the renal sinus.

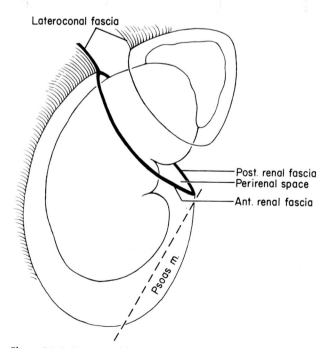

Figure 21–3. Diagram of the right renal fascia in a frontal projection.

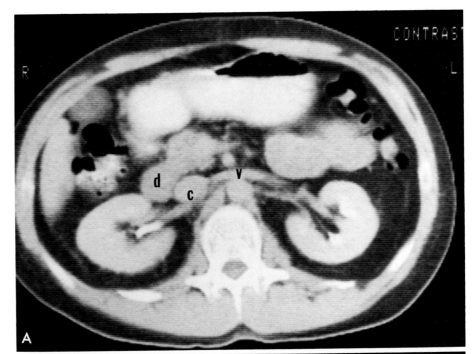

Figure 21–4. Anatomy of the retroperitoneum. Computed tomogram, contrast material enhanced.

A, Section at the level of the renal sinus. The left renal vein (v) passes anterior to the renal artery and crosses the midline between the aorta and the superior mesenteric artery before entering the inferior vena cava (c). The various compartments and structures can be identified using Figure 21–1. Note the relationship of the descending duodenum (d) to the right kidney.

B, Section at the level of the lower poles. Note the relationship of the ascending and descending colon and the descending duodenum (d) to the kidneys and perirenal spaces.

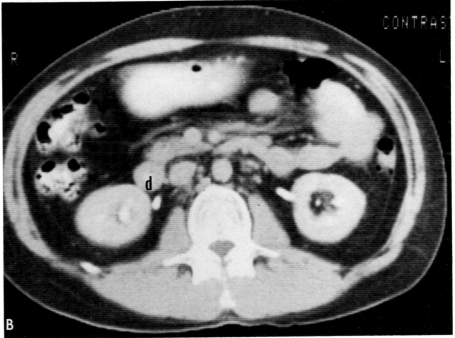

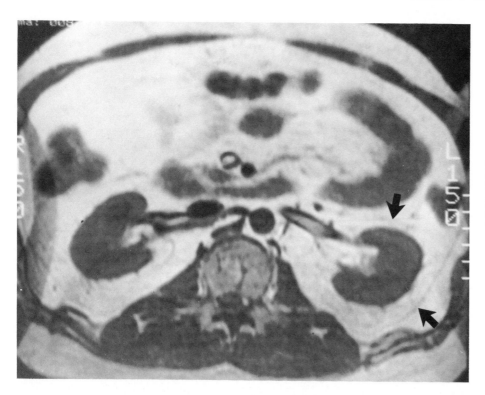

Figure 21–5. Anatomy of the retroperitoneum. Magnetic resonance, T1-weighted image. Fat in the perirenal and pararenal space and the renal sinuses is represented by high intensity signal. The fascia around the left kidney is well visualized *(arrows)*.

easily visualized when they become thickened by fluid or other disease processes (Fig. 21–8). In addition to connecting the renal capsule and fascia, some of these septations connect the anterior and posterior leaves of the renal fascia, while others arise from the capsule and are more or less parallel to the surface of the kidney. The posterior renorenal septum is an important structure that runs from the anterolateral to the posteromedial aspect of the renal capsule.

The *anterior pararenal space* is limited anteriorly by the posterior parietal peritoneum and posteriorly by

the anterior renal fascia. The pancreas; the descending, transverse, and ascending duodenum; the ascending and descending colon; and the splenic, hepatic, and proximal superior mesenteric arteries are contained within this space. Unlike the two perirenal spaces, the anterior pararenal space communicates across the midline. Fat deposition in this space is usually sparse. The anterior and posterior pararenal spaces potentially communicate along their inferior margin.

The *posterior pararenal space* is bounded by the trans-

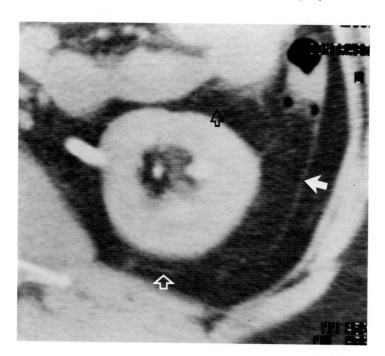

Figure 21–6. Normal renal fascia. Computed tomogram, contrast material enhanced. *Open arrow*, renal fascia; *solid arrow*, lateroconal fascia.

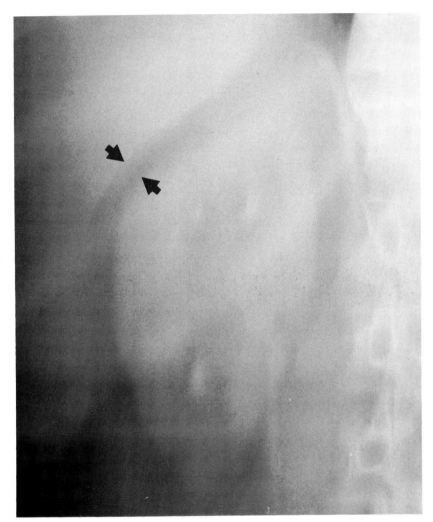

Figure 21–7. Normal perirenal space filled with fat *(arrows)*. Excretory urogram. Tomogram.

versalis fascia. The medial extent of this space is limited by the fusion of the posterior renal fascia with the fasciae of the psoas and quadratus lumborum muscles. Nevertheless, there is a potential communication with the prevertebral retrocrural space, which, in turn, leads to the mediastinum. Laterally, the fat of the posterior pararenal space continues as the properitoneal "flank stripe." The fat of this space outlines the lower one-half of the psoas muscle. The posterior pararenal space contains no organs.

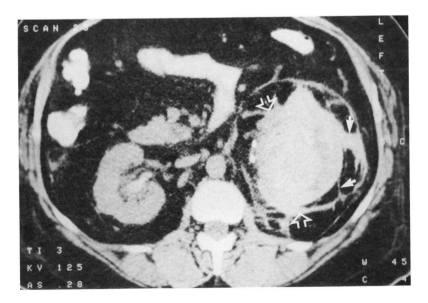

Figure 21–8. Prominent bridging septa. Computed tomogram, unenhanced. Extracorporeal shock wave lithotripsy was complicated by perirenal hemorrhage. Blood surrounds the kidney *(open arrows)* and is contained by bridging septa *(solid arrows)* that are parallel to the renal capsule. Perpendicular septa extending to the renal fascia are thickened.

ABNORMALITIES OF THE RETROPERITONEAL SPACES

Renal Fasciae

The renal fasciae, even when abnormal, are visualized infrequently during excretory urography and then almost always with tomography. During computed tomography, on the other hand, the fasciae are seen in most normal individuals. Edema, hyperemia, or fibrosis thicken the fasciae in a variety of conditions, including nephrolithiasis, upper urinary tract infection, carcinoma, lymphoma, subcapsular hematoma, renal infarction, and prior renal surgery (Figs. 21–9 and 21–10). Nonrenal causes of fascial thickening include leaking abdominal aneurysm, infection of the perinephric space, acute or chronic pancreatitis, retroperitoneal tumor, pancreatic carcinoma, peritonitis, ascites due to cirrhosis, retroperitoneal fibrosis, and radiation therapy.

Linear bands of density within the perirenal fat oriented roughly parallel to the renal outline are sometimes seen during excretory urography, especially with tomography, in the presence of highly vascular renal carcinoma (Fig. 21–11). These linear or serpiginous densities, caused by capsular arteries and veins that have enlarged in response to the high volume of blood flow to and from the tumor, might be confused with thickened renal fascia. Computed tomography, especially with dynamic techniques, clearly identifies the vascular nature of these structures.

Perirenal Space

Fluid. Abnormalities that arise either within the kidney or within structures of the adjacent retroperitoneal spaces may cause fluid to accumulate in the perirenal space. The most common fluid accumulations are blood, pus, and urine.

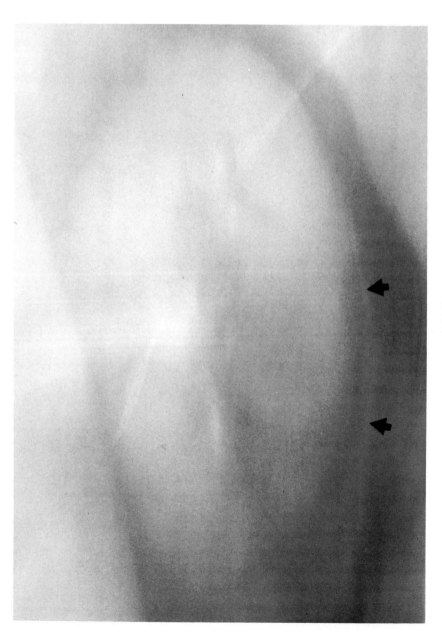

Figure 21–9. Thickened renal fascia *(arrows)* in a 70-year-old man with chronic urinary tract infection. Excretory urogram.

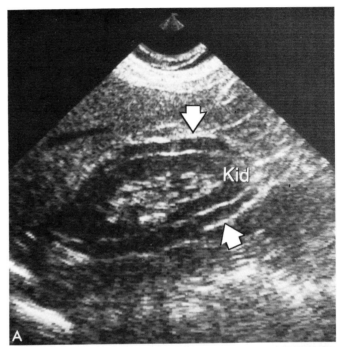

Figure 21–10. Thickened renal fascia.

A, Ultrasonogram, longitudinal section, supine. Right kidney (Kid). The renal fascia is identified by arrows.

B, Computed tomogram. Arrows identify thickened fasciae.

(Courtesy of Department of Radiology, Vancouver General Hospital, Vancouver, British Columbia, Canada.)

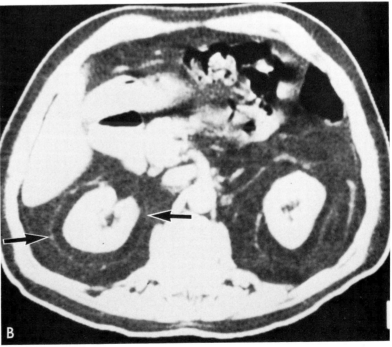

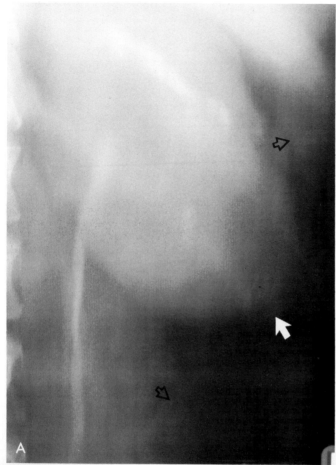

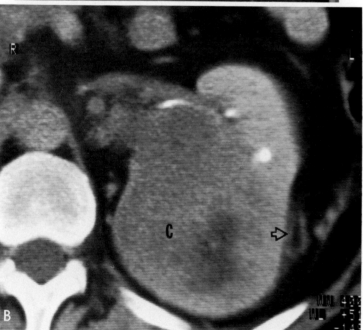

Figure 21–11. Enlarged blood vessels *(arrows)* simulating thickened renal fascia. These vessels have enlarged in response to increased blood flow to a very vascular renal carcinoma (C).

A, Excretory urogram. Tomogram.

B, Computed tomogram, contrast material enhanced.

Fluid that collects slowly and in small to moderate amounts usually localizes in the posterior and inferior aspects of the perirenal space, behind and below the lower pole of the kidney (Figs. 21–12 and 21–13). Acute distention of the perirenal space by a large amount of fluid transforms the normal inferomedial orientation of this space into a vertical axis, obliterates the outline of the kidney and upper one-half of the psoas muscle, and displaces the kidney in an anterior, medial, and superior direction. When the volume of fluid is extensive, anterior displacement of the descending duodenum and/or lateral displacement of the retroperitoneal part of the ascending or descending colon may occur depending on the location of the fluid. Occasionally a large perirenal collection of fluid causes a concave deformity of the renal contour similar to that seen with a subcapsular fluid collection (Fig. 21–14).

A *perirenal hematoma* may result from trauma; leaking aneurysm; renal, adrenal, or other retroperitoneal tumors; vasculitis; bleeding diathesis; or renal infarct. Fresh blood typically has a homogeneous attenuation value of 50 to 80 Hounsfield units. Five to 15 days after hemorrhage, clumps of high attenuation material are usually intermingled with surrounding water-density fluid (Fig. 21–15). Nontraumatic perirenal he-morrhage is often termed *spontaneous*. Carcinoma and angiomyolipoma of the kidney are each the cause of approximately 30 per cent of cases of spontaneous perirenal hematoma. For patients with a spontaneous perirenal hematoma in whom a mass is not detected on initial computed tomography, serial repeat examinations should be obtained until the hematoma has completely resolved.

Pus from suppurative processes, either in the kidney or in the pararenal spaces, may extend into the perirenal space (see Fig. 21–14). In pancreatitis, this is facilitated by the release of digestive enzymes, which, at a minimum, increase the density of perirenal fat owing to edema.

Urine may leak into the perirenal space as a result of an acute or subacute outflow obstruction, as occurs with ureteral obstruction or penetrating or blunt trauma (Fig. 21–16). In acute obstruction due to stone, urine enters the perirenal space through rupture of a calyceal fornix that is distended by increased hydrostatic pressure in the pelvocalyceal system. When patients are studied with excretory urography, the contrast material–induced osmotic diuresis adds to the already elevated pressure of urine in the renal pelvis. Thus, the likelihood of forniceal rupture and urine leakage increases with the amount of contrast material

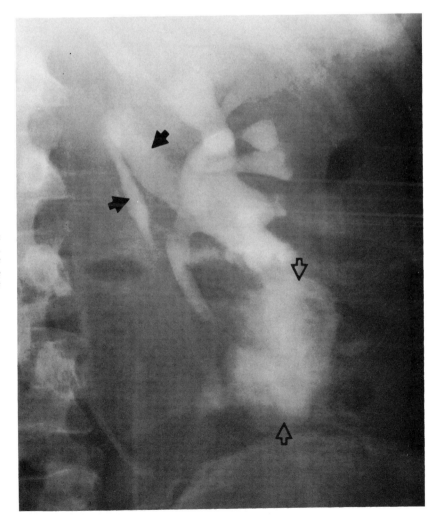

Figure 21–12. Perirenal leakage of urine due to subacute obstruction 7 days after pyelolithotomy. Opacified urine has collected medial to the kidney *(solid arrows)* and posterior and inferior to the lower pole of the kidney *(open arrows)*. Excretory urogram.

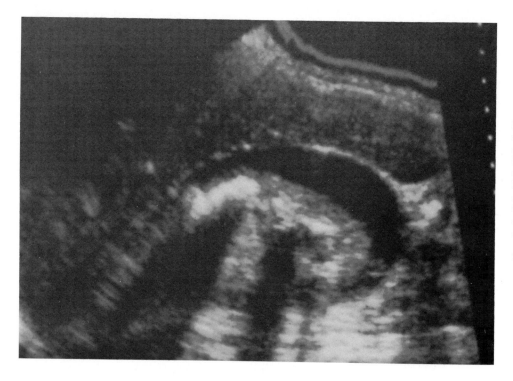

Figure 21–13. Large perirenal fluid collection of urine in a patient with chronic obstruction of the right kidney due to urolithiasis. The localization of the urine is atypical in being mainly anterior. Note the acoustic shadows caused by urolithiasis and the thickened renal fascia. Ultrasonogram, longitudinal axis, supine. (Courtesy of Hedvig Hricak, M.D., University of California, San Francisco.)

given. Rupture may also occur from a previously dilated calyx and progress directly through the renal parenchyma and into the subcapsular and perirenal spaces. This situation is likely to occur when preexisting disease has thinned the parenchyma. Acute leakage of urine into the perirenal space due to trauma occurs at any point where the pelvocalyceal system or proximal ureter is disrupted.

Urine that slowly leaks into the perirenal space over a long period of time creates a unique condition known as *urinoma*. This urine collection has also been termed a *uriniferous perirenal pseudocyst, pseudohydronephrosis, hydrocele renalis, perirenal cyst, perinephric cyst,* and *pararenal pseudocyst.* Here, an encapsulated extrapelvocalyceal collection of urine forms from urine leakage through a rent in the collecting system or the proximal ureter when chronic ureteral obstruction is present. Accidental or surgical trauma, congenital obstruction in children, ureteral tumor, stone, blood clot, and periureteric fibrosis are among the usual causes of the obstruction. As urine leaks into the perirenal space, normal fat is transformed into a

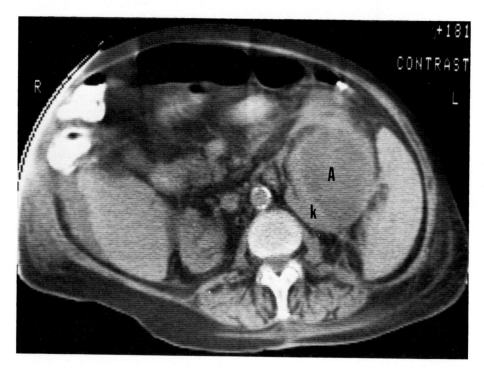

Figure 21–14. Left perinephric abscess in an elderly woman with chronic renal failure. Computed tomogram, unenhanced. The abscess (A) has a lower attenuation value than the kidney and is surrounded by a thick capsule. Both kidneys are small, and the left kidney (k) is deformed by pressure from the perinephric abscess.

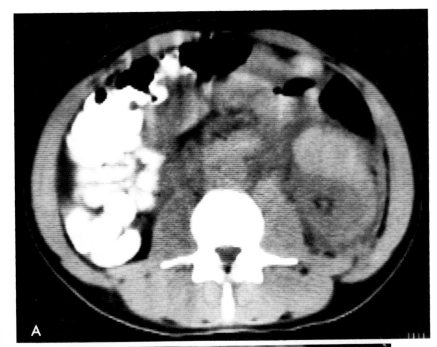

Figure 21–15. Acute perirenal hematoma in a 38-year-old man with left abdominal pain. Idiopathic.

A, Computed tomogram, initial examination. Fresh blood fills the left perirenal space and has a higher attenuation value than the renal parenchyma.

B, Computed tomogram, initial examination. After contrast material is administered, the kidney becomes isodense with the freshly clotted blood.

Illustration continued on following page

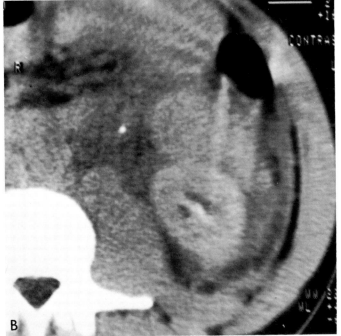

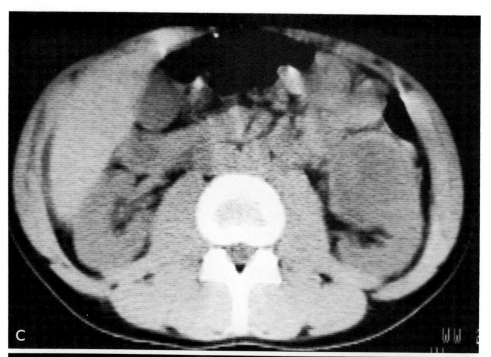

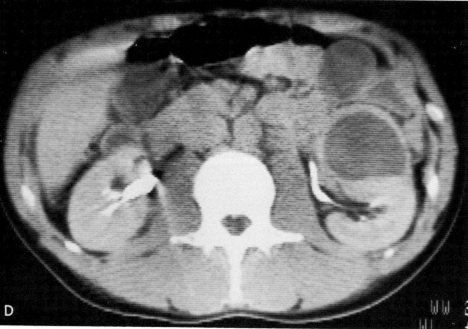

Figure 21–15 *Continued C,* Computed tomogram, 6 weeks after initial examination. The blood clot has decreased in attenuation value and is now slightly less dense than renal parenchyma before administration of contrast material.

D, Computed tomogram, 6 weeks after initial examination. The blood clot does not enhance. A thick capsule has formed.

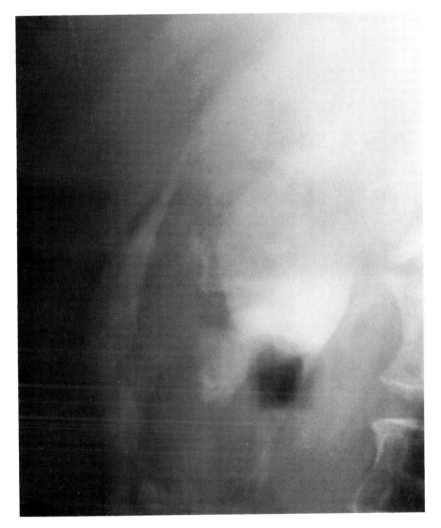

Figure 21–16. Perirenal urine collection following subacute obstruction of the right proximal ureter by a metastasis from a colon tumor in a 71-year-old man. Opacified urine can be detected in the perirenal space and the renal sinus. Excretory urogram.

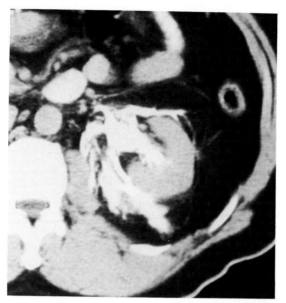

Figure 21–17. Urinoma complicating acute obstruction. Computed tomogram, contrast material enhanced. Contrast material fills the renal sinus and perirenal space.

dense, reddish fibrous mass that is covered by distended veins. The wall of the pseudocyst contains fatty or fibrous debris, blood clot, and crystals of urine salts. The mature pseudocyst is the end result of this process of lipolysis and fibroblastic round cell stimulation. A false capsule forms within 2 weeks and matures in approximately 6 weeks.

Clinical manifestations of urinoma are a palpable flank mass and vague abdominal distress or tenderness. There is little, if any, fever. The mass appears slowly after the initiating event, often with a latent period of 4 or more months.

Urinoma has a radiologic appearance of a soft tissue mass whose axis usually, but not always, approximates the cone of renal fascia (see Fig. 21–3). Large lesions displace the kidney superiorly and deviate the lower pole laterally. The proximal ureter is sometimes displaced medially, occasionally to an extreme degree. Perirenal fat remote from the pseudocyst remains uninvolved so that both the upper psoas margin and the contour of the superior half of the kidney are preserved. Additionally, radiologic and ultrasonographic findings of chronic obstruction are present. Active extravasation is sometimes seen following injection of contrast material (Fig. 21–17). The fluid nature of the urinoma can be accurately defined by ultrasonography, computed tomography, or magnetic resonance imaging. Debris or blood may produce low-level echoes or raise the computed tomographic attenuation values.

Tumor. Tumor involvement of the perirenal space usually occurs by direct extension from the kidney or the pararenal spaces, although rarely primary tumors arise directly from perirenal fat (see Fig. 21–29). Primary tumors arising in the perirenal space are discussed in the following section. Whereas fluid in the perirenal space usually has a homogeneous density and is smoothly marginated, as seen by cross-sec-

tional imaging methods, malignant tumors are often inhomogeneous and have irregular margins and attenuation values that are greater than the patient's normal fat. Contrast material enhancement often occurs in solid perirenal tumors.

Caution should be exercised in assessing invasiveness of a tumor by computed tomography or magnetic resonance imaging. A bulky tumor may intimately contact an adjacent space or organ without actual invasion. Contiguity of structures, therefore, should not by itself be used as evidence for invasion in the staging of tumors.

Gas. Gas may extend into the perirenal space from a gas-forming renal infection, from penetrating trauma, by extension from the pararenal space, or by spread from the extraperitoneal portion of the true pelvis (Figs. 21–18 and 21–19). Pancreatic inflammation, perforated duodenum, and diverticulitis are the usual causes of perirenal gas that originates in the anterior pararenal space (Fig. 21–20).

Fat. Peripelvic fat, including that of the renal sinus, as well as pararenal fat may become diffusely increased in obesity, in pelvic lipomatosis, and in association with aging. Severe renal parenchymal atrophy may be associated with massive fat deposition in the renal sinus and perinephric space. This phenomenon is known as *replacement lipomatosis* and is usually associated with long-standing renal inflammatory disease (Fig. 21–21).

Abnormal Vessels. Renal venous collaterals enlarge in renal vein thrombosis and are seen by computed tomography as a network of fine, linear densities in the perirenal fat that may be difficult to distinguish from fibrous septa (Fig. 21–22). A multitude of pathways exist and include the following veins: renoazygous, gastrorenal, adrenolumbar, inferior phrenic, adrenorenal, splenorenal, renolumbar, gonadal, and ureteral. These veins pass through perirenal fat and provide systemic or portal drainage from the kidney by way of subcapsular and perforating renal veins.

Engorged renal arteries and veins that form in the perirenal fat in association with hypervascular renal carcinoma were previously discussed (see Fig. 21–11). These must be differentiated from thickened renal fascia and collateral veins.

Subcapsular Space

Traditionally, it has been held that distinction between a subcapsular and perirenal fluid collection was easily made on computed tomography. Fluid was considered subcapsular in location when it was immediately contiguous with a portion of the renal parenchyma and flattened its normal convex border. Typically, fat was present between the fluid collection and Gerota's fascia, which was preserved. In contrast, a fluid collection was diagnosed as perinephric when it surrounded a major portion of the kidney, was contiguous with and obliterated the renal fascia, replaced the normal perinephric fat, and typically did not flatten or distort the renal contour.

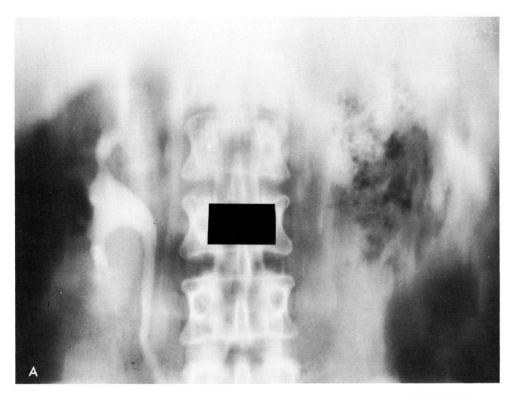

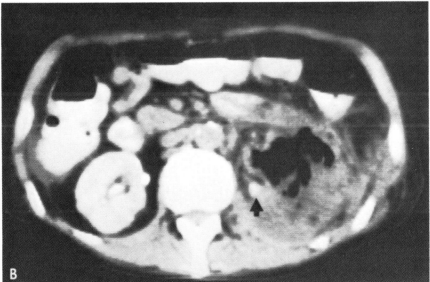

Figure 21–18. Gas-forming infection of the left perirenal space, presumably arising in the kidney.

A, Excretory urogram. Tomogram. Multiple radiolucent collections are present on the left side, and there is obliteration of the left psoas and kidney margins. The left pelvocalyceal system is faintly opacified.

B, Computed tomogram, contrast material enhanced. Gas and fluid fill the inferior portion of the left perirenal space. Note the opacified ureter partially surrounded by gas *(arrow).*

(Courtesy of Joshua Becker, M.D., State University of New York, Downstate Medical Center, Brooklyn.)

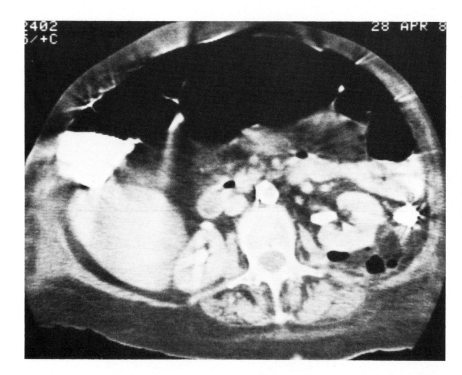

Figure 21–19. Extension of gas-forming diverticular abscess into the left perirenal space. Computed tomogram, contrast material enhanced. (Courtesy of Stuart London, M.D., Oakland, California.)

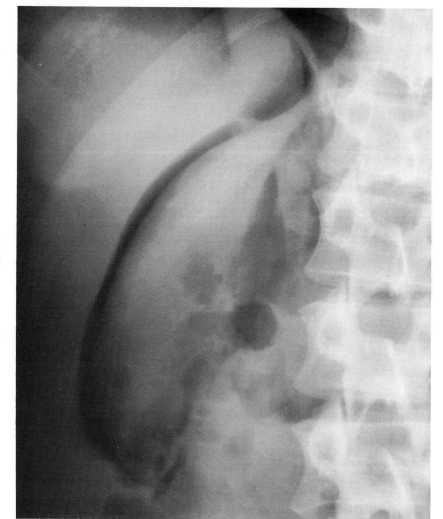

Figure 21–20. Gas in the right perirenal space due to perforation of descending duodenum. (Courtesy of Hedvig Hricak, M.D., University of California, San Francisco.)

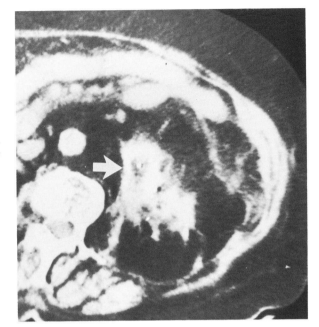

Figure 21–21. Replacement lipomatosis. Computed tomogram, contrast material enhanced. The left kidney *(arrow)* is distorted by severe inflammatory disease. There has been a compensatory increase in the perirenal fat.

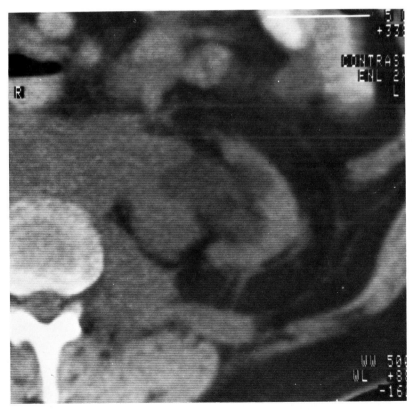

Figure 21–22. Renal venous collaterals in a patient with occlusion of the left renal vein secondary to metastatic deposits in the left renal sinus and around the aorta and inferior vena cava. Fine linear densities in the perirenal fat represent venous collaterals. These may be difficult to distinguish from fibrous septa. Computed tomogram, contrast material enhanced.

Careful anatomic studies of the perinephric space, however, have revised these concepts by demonstrating that the perinephric space is not one compartment but is subdivided by bridging septa and by the reno-renal septum. Perirenal fluid collections localized by these septa are indistinguishable from subcapsular fluid collections. Differentiation in most cases is not important from a management point of view.

The most common subcapsular/localized perinephric fluid collection is blood. Although there are many nonneoplastic causes such as trauma, vasculitis, bleeding diathesis, renal infarction, or intrinsic renal disease (Fig. 21–23), carcinoma or angiomyolipoma of the kidney must always be considered as the cause, especially in a nontraumatic or spontaneous setting. Pus is less likely to accumulate in the subcapsular space or localized perinephric space as the proteolytic enzymes often enable direct extension through the capsule, septa, and even the renal fascia into the paranephric spaces. Occasionally, a subcapsular/localized perinephric hematoma becomes secondarily infected, resulting in a thick-walled localized inflammatory mass. Most frequently, subcapsular/localized perinephric fluid collections are identified following trauma. Management is usually conservative, and in most cases they resolve spontaneously. Less commonly, however, the hematoma does not resolve and becomes chronic. Renovascular (ischemic) hypertension may follow, a phenomenon known as "Page" kidney. Biconvex, lentiform calcification is characteristic of chronic subcapsular or loculated perinephric hemorrhage (Fig. 21–24).

Anterior Pararenal Space

Pancreatitis is the most common cause of a fluid collection in the anterior pararenal space. Large fluid collections in the anterior pararenal space extend toward the peritoneal cavity, displacing the small intestine ventrally and the ascending or descending colon laterally (Fig. 21–25). The properitoneal "flank stripe," renal outline, perirenal fat, and psoas margins are maintained. Proteolytic enzymes disrupt the small septal fibers that connect the lateral conal fascia to the anterior renal fascia. Fluid dissects between the two major layers of the posterior renal fascia, producing a characteristic wedge-shaped appearance of the retrorenal fluid. Typically the fat within the posterior pararenal space is compressed but preserved (Fig. 21–26).

Posterior Pararenal Space

Abnormalities of the posterior pararenal space develop through the spread of disease from the anterior pararenal space, the retrocrural space, extraperitoneal pelvic structures, the perirenal space, or adjacent organs. Spontaneous hemorrhage, extension of osteomyelitis of the spine, and lymphatic extension of tumor from the pelvis or lower extremities are several examples. Primary tumors of posterior pararenal fat and connective tissue occur as well.

Abnormalities that extend into the posterior pararenal space obliterate the lower one-half of the psoas muscle and the properitoneal flank stripe. The kidney may be displaced in an anterior and superior direction (Fig. 21–27). Fluid collections have an inferomedial axis similar to that of the inferior cone of the perirenal fascia.

PRIMARY RETROPERITONEAL TUMORS

The term *primary retroperitoneal tumor* is reserved for a neoplasm that originates within the soft tissue between the parietal peritoneum and transversalis fascia but does not arise from a retroperitoneal organ such as the kidney or adrenal. Most primary retroperitoneal neoplasms arise from mesenchyme, neurogenic tissue, or embryonic rests, as summarized in Table 21–1. Using this definition, and by including lymph nodes as a retroperitoneal organ, lymphoma is not considered a primary retroperitoneal tumor. Lymphangioma, although best considered a developmental malformation and not a true neoplasm, is an important retroperitoneal mass that can be confused with primary retroperitoneal tumors.

Table 21–1. DIFFERENTIAL FEATURES OF THE MOST COMMON PRIMARY RETROPERITONEAL TUMORS

Tumor	Features
MESENCHYMAL NEOPLASMS	
Liposarcoma	Fatty component on computed tomography or magnetic resonance imaging
Leiomyosarcoma	Nonfatty; conspicuous necrosis; intravascular component
Malignant fibrous histiocytoma	Nonfatty; less necrotic than leiomyosarcoma; no vascular invasion
NEUROGENIC NEOPLASMS	
Nerve sheath tumors	History of neurofibromatosis; dumbbell growth through neural foramen; bone erosion
Neuroblastoma	Occurs in children; paraspinal; elevated vanillylmandelic acid levels; 80% calcify
Ganglioneuroma	Young adults; paraspinal location; bone erosion
Paraganglioma	Hypertension; elevated vanillylmandelic acid levels; paraspinal; very bright on T2-weighted magnetic resonance imaging; positive MIBG scan
NEOPLASMS DERIVED FROM EMBRYONIC RESTS	
Teratoma	Children and young adults; calcification (clumps or shards); cystic component; fat (sebum or adipose tissue); dermoid plug
Germ cell malignancies (e.g., yolk sac tumor)	Children or young adults; elevated tumor tissue markers
Extrarenal Wilms' tumor	Children; very rare; arise along urogenital ridge between kidney and gonad
DEVELOPMENTAL MALFORMATION	
Lymphangioma	Elongated shape; uniloculated or multiloculated cystic mass, crosses multiple spaces

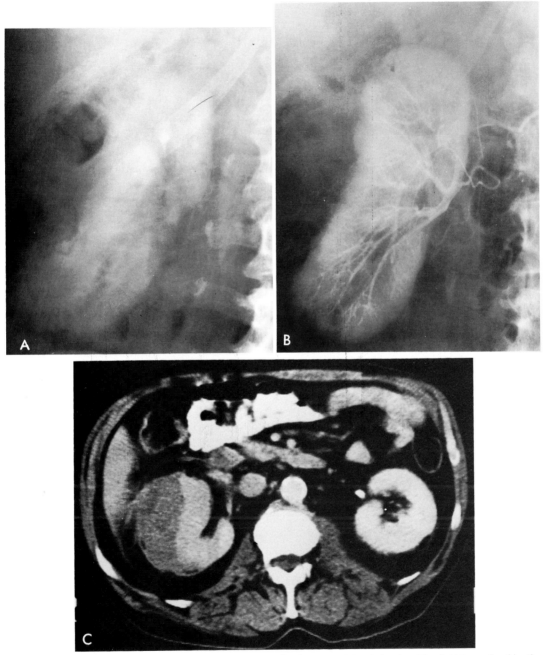

Figure 21–23. Subcapsular hematoma forming in the left kidney as a result of an acute lobar infarction. The fluid is confined by the capsule and causes a broad concave deformity of the underlying renal parenchyma.

A, Excretory urogram.
B, Selective arteriogram, late arterial phase.
C, Computed tomogram, contrast material enhanced.
(Courtesy of Stuart London, M.D., Oakland, California.)

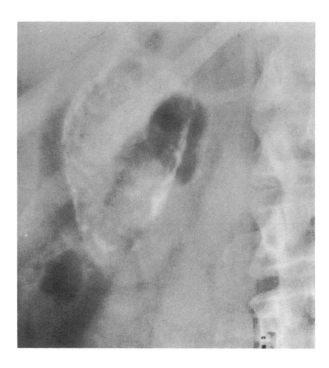

Figure 21–24. Chronic, calcified subcapsular/localized perinephric hemorrhage. Plain abdominal film. There is a biconvex, lentiform calcification overlying the lateral margin of the right kidney.

To establish the diagnosis of a primary retroperitoneal tumor radiologically and pathologically, it is necessary to demonstrate that the mass is truly retroperitoneal in location, yet one that does not originate from a retroperitoneal organ. This can be quite difficult or impossible when the tumor is very large or there has been invasion into adjacent viscera. Of principal importance for surgical planning, however, is establishing the extent of involvement and the relationship of the tumor to normal structures.

Because of the obscure nature of symptoms produced by retroperitoneal tumors, initial radiologic investigation often includes abdominal radiography and contrast studies of the gastrointestinal tract or urinary tract. These typically demonstrate a soft tissue mass and displacement of organs without intrinsic involvement (Fig. 21–28). Calcification, often present, is rarely specific enough to be useful in refining diagnostic choices. Formed bone suggests teratoma, or very rarely, mesenchymoma. Fat, seen as a radiolucency on radiographs, occurs in liposarcoma, lipoma, or teratoma. However, fat-containing renal angiomyolipoma or adrenal myelolipoma may sometimes simulate the same findings as a fatty primary retroperitoneal tumor.

By using barium studies or excretory urography it may be difficult, if not impossible, to define the intraperitoneal or retroperitoneal location of a large abdominal mass. Since the kidney and ureter are retroperitoneal, however, displacement of these structures is often a sensitive sign of retroperitoneal pathology (see Fig. 21–28). Once a retroperitoneal tumor is suspected, computed tomography or magnetic resonance imaging should be used (see Fig. 21–28). These imaging modalities can determine the likely site of origin and describe the gross morphology. In some cases a specific histologic diagnosis can be confidently pre-

dicted on the basis of radiologic features, as in liposarcoma or teratoma.

Unlike computed tomography, magnetic resonance imaging provides images in the coronal and sagittal planes that are sometimes advantageous in defining the relationship of a retroperitoneal tumor to the kidney or adrenal gland and in assessing the patency of the large vessels of the abdomen (Fig. 21–29). Regarding staging, however, it is important to realize that demonstration of contiguity between a tumor and an adjacent organ, such as the liver, kidney, or bowel, does not necessarily signify invasion. Invasion is most reliably demonstrated radiologically by the angiographic demonstration of neovascularity derived from the principal arterial supply to the organ in question. Ultrasonography and radionuclide techniques are of limited use in the evaluation of most retroperitoneal tumors except for specific situations such as the metaiodobenzylguanidine (MIBG) radionuclide scan for suspected paraganglioma. This is discussed in Chapters 2 and 22.

Mesenchymal

Liposarcoma is the most common primary retroperitoneal malignancy of mesenchymal origin. Most occur between the fourth and sixth decades of life. Women are slightly more commonly affected than are men. Liposarcoma is a malignancy of undifferentiated mesenchymal cells from its inception rather than a malignant transformation of previously normal retroperitoneal fat. Like other retroperitoneal tumors, symptoms caused by liposarcoma are insidious and the tumor is usually quite large before it is detected. Computed tomographic and magnetic resonance images correlate closely with the histologic findings. Well-differentiated tumors contain fat that has imaging charac-

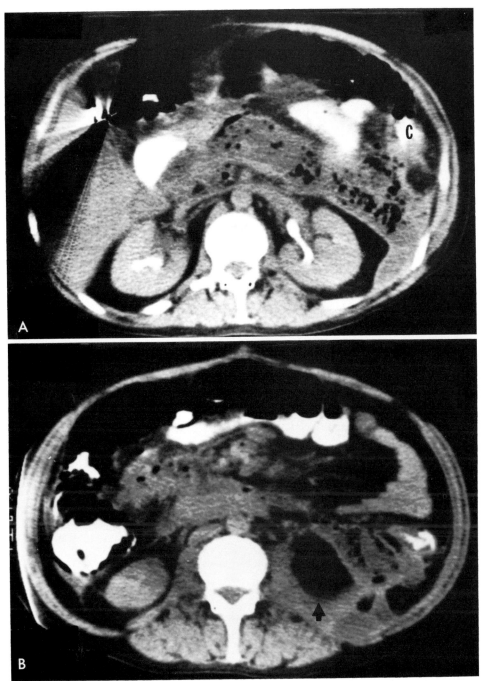

Figure 21–25. Abscess in the anterior pararenal space due to acute pancreatitis. The abscess, which also contains gas, points toward the peritoneal cavity and displaces the descending colon (C) anteriorly and laterally. Note preservation of the integrity of the renal fascia and the perirenal space.

A, Computed tomogram with contrast material enhancement at the level of the renal sinus.

B, Computed tomogram at the level of the inferior cone of the renal fascia. Note the extension of the abscess into the posterior pararenal space *(arrow)* and preservation of the perirenal space within the cone of the renal fascia.

(Courtesy of Philip M. Weinerman, M.D., Ohio State University, Columbus, Ohio.)

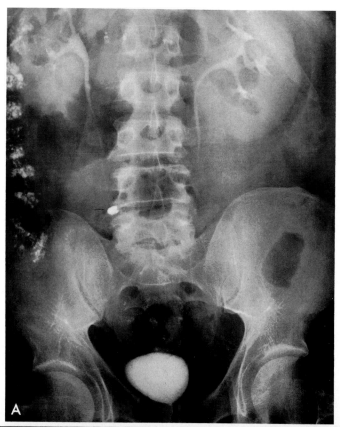

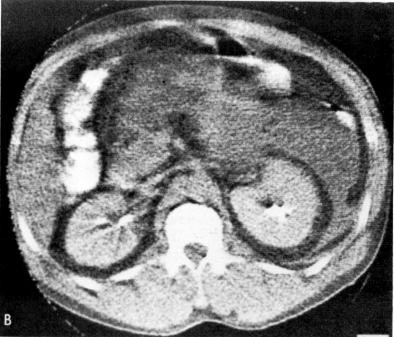

Figure 21–26. Acute pancreatitis causing inflammatory changes limited to the anterior pararenal space. Preservation of the normal perirenal fat causes a radiolucent "halo" around the left kidney.

A, Excretory urogram.

B, Computed tomogram, contrast material enhanced.

(From Susman, N., Hammerman, A. M., and Cohen, E.: The renal halo sign in pancreatitis. Radiology *142:*323, 1982. With kind permission of the authors and *Radiology.*)

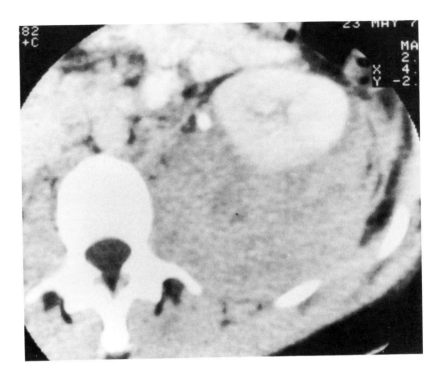

Figure 21–27. Posterior paranephric and perinephric hemorrhage following renal biopsy. Computed tomogram, contrast material enhanced. The hematoma, which is less dense than the enhanced kidney, displaces the kidney anteriorly and obliterates both the psoas muscles and the posterior renal fascia.

teristics indistinguishable from normal retroperitoneal or subcutaneous fat (Fig. 21–30; see also Fig. 21–28). Poorly differentiated pleomorphic, round cell, or myxoid liposarcomas often have little to no radiologically detectable fat and, therefore, are impossible to differentiate from other forms of retroperitoneal tumors that are not fat bearing (Fig. 21–31; see also Fig. 21–29). Eighty to 90 per cent of retroperitoneal liposarcomas have sufficient fat for detection by radiologic techniques. Complete surgical removal of retroperitoneal liposarcoma is often difficult owing to its infiltrating margins. Recurrence and/or distant metastases are common.

Leiomyosarcoma is the second most common primary retroperitoneal tumor derived from mesenchyme. It is thought to arise from smooth muscle within the retroperitoneum, including the wall of the inferior vena cava. Two-thirds to three-fourths of these tumors occur in women, usually in the fifth or sixth decade of life. Three dominant growth patterns for leiomyosarcoma have been identified: completely extravascular (62 per cent), completely intravascular within the lumen of the inferior vena cava (5 per cent), and a pattern of combined extraluminal and intraluminal growth (33 per cent) (Hartman et al, 1992). Extravascular tumors usually present as mass, pain, and weight loss. Tumors with an intraluminal vena caval component may present with Budd-Chiari syndrome, nephrotic syndrome, or lower extremity edema depending on the extent and location of the tumor thrombus. Necrosis is a conspicuous, pathologic feature of retroperitoneal leiomyosarcoma and is seen radiologically as attenuation values and signal intensities intermediate between soft tissue and uncomplicated fluid. A leiomyosarcoma that does not have a vascular component is seen radiologically as a usually necrotic mass that displaces retroperitoneal organs (Fig. 21–32). This appearance is similar to many other primary, non–fat-containing tumors of the retroperitoneum. Radiologic studies are suggestive of leiomyosarcoma when a solid tumor has both extravascular and intravascular components or is completely intravascular and expands the lumen of the inferior vena cava (Fig. 21–33).

Malignant fibrous histiocytoma is the third most common mesenchymal primary retroperitoneal malignancy. These are most commonly detected during the sixth decade of life. Males are slightly more frequently affected than are females. Presenting complaints and physical findings are nonspecific and include pain, fever, mass, and weight loss. Radiologic studies usually demonstrate a noncalcified mass displacing adjacent retroperitoneal organs. On computed tomography and magnetic resonance images, malignant fibrous histiocytoma does not contain fat and tends to demonstrate less evidence of necrosis than does the typical leiomyosarcoma. Most malignant fibrous histiocytomas are moderately vascular or hypervascular (Fig. 21–34). Unlike retroperitoneal leiomyosarcoma, malignant fibrous histiocytoma does not involve the inferior vena cava.

Miscellaneous tumors of mesenchymal origin are less common than liposarcoma, leiomyosarcoma, and malignant fibrous histiocytoma. These include malignancies of cartilage, bone, mesothelial tissue, and blood vessels. There are no distinctive radiologic features associated with any of these tumors.

Neurogenic

Nerve sheath tumors, such as neurilemmoma (schwannoma) or neurofibroma, may present either as a soli-

Text continued on page 698

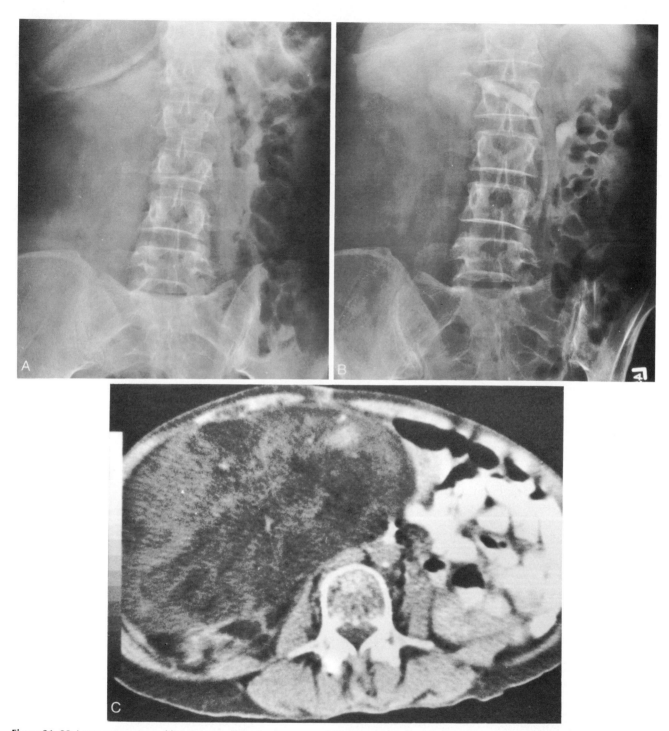

Figure 21–28. Large retroperitoneal liposarcoma. There is a large noncalcified fatty mass that displaces the right kidney but is separate from it. The ascending colon is displaced across the midline. The mass is more lucent than adjacent soft tissue on the abdominal radiograph and has fatty regions clearly demonstrable with computed tomography.

A, Abdominal radiograph.

B, Excretory urogram.

C, Computed tomogram, contrast material enhanced.

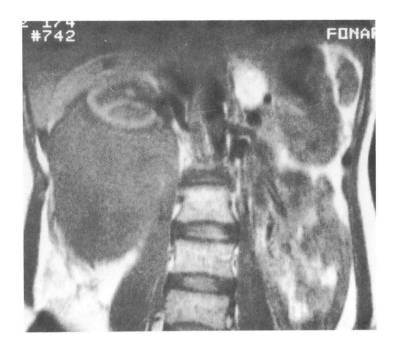

Figure 21–29. Perinephric liposarcoma. T1-weighted coronal magnetic resonance image. A large mass fills the right perinephric space. The kidney is displaced but is otherwise normal. The tumor does not contain detectable fat.

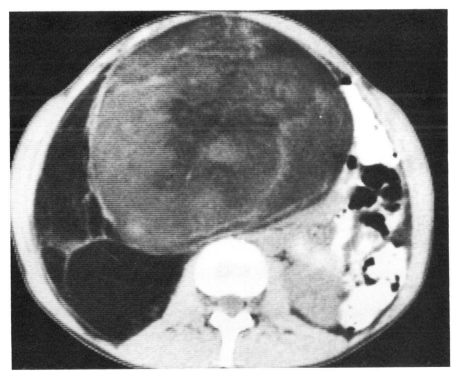

Figure 21–30. Liposarcoma. Computed tomogram. A large tumor displaces the aorta and bowel. The tissue in the lateral part of the tumor is well-differentiated fat and is identical in attenuation values to normal retroperitoneal or subcutaneous fat. The medial portion of the tumor is of higher density and represents areas of hemorrhage or poorly differentiated tumor.

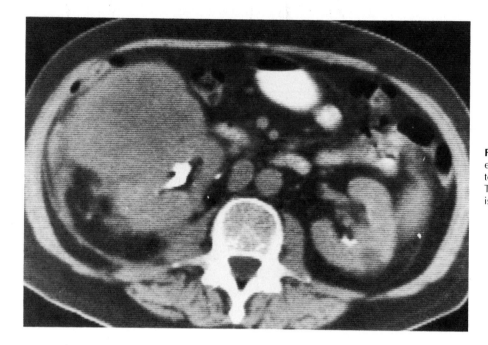

Figure 21–31. Liposarcoma, poorly differentiated, invading the kidney. Computed tomogram, contrast material enhanced. The tumor contains no detectable fat and is inseparable from the kidney.

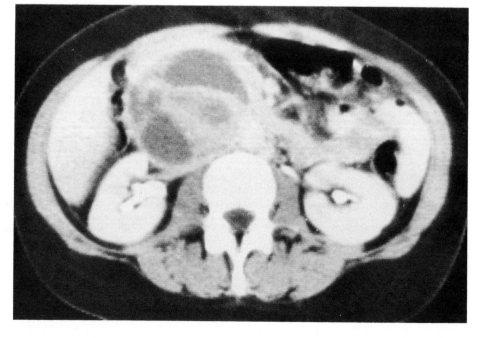

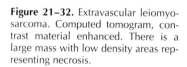

Figure 21–32. Extravascular leiomyosarcoma. Computed tomogram, contrast material enhanced. There is a large mass with low density areas representing necrosis.

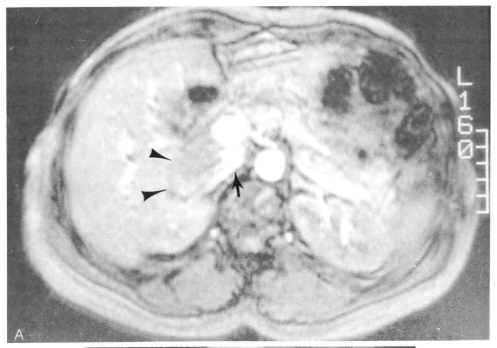

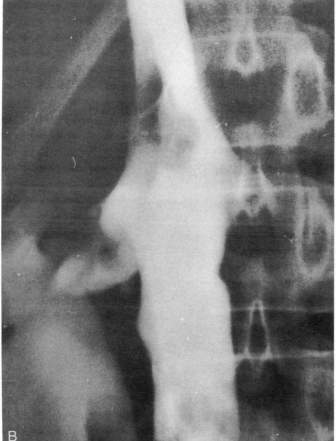

Figure 21–33. Leiomyosarcoma with extravascular and intravascular components. An extraluminal mass *(arrowheads)* indents the inferior vena cava *(arrow)*. The intraluminal component is conspicuous on the cavogram. This combination of findings is very suggestive of leiomyosarcoma.

    A, Magnetic resonance image, gradient-echo.

    B, Cavogram.

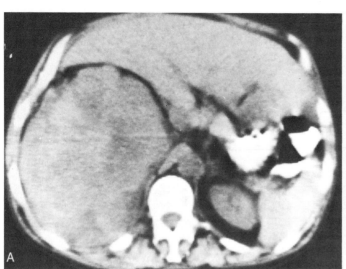
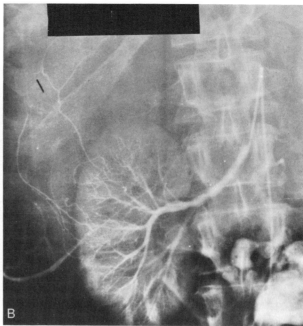

Figure 21–34. Malignant fibrous histiocytoma. There is a large hypovascular mass displacing the right kidney inferiorly. Necrosis is not a prominent feature.
A, Computed tomogram, unenhanced.
B, Selective arteriogram.

tary retroperitoneal mass or, in the case of neurofibroma, as a complication of neurofibromatosis. These tumors are usually encountered in patients who are younger than those with mesenchymal tumors. Both males and females are equally affected. Nerve sheath tumors occur along the course of peripheral or sympathetic nerves. They may be benign or malignant. Small tumors are usually well defined and sharply circumscribed (Fig. 21–35). Large tumors often demonstrate necrosis. Although computed tomography and magnetic resonance imaging define, localize, and determine tumor extent, they do not permit differentiation between benign and malignant nerve sheath tumors. The radionuclide gallium, on the other hand, may be useful in this regard, since uptake occurs in malignant but not in benign neural neoplasms.

A diagnosis of nerve sheath tumor may be suggested by clinical or radiologic manifestations of neurofibromatosis, a bilobed dumbbell-shaped mass with one component extending into a neural foramen, or a well-defined mass associated with adjacent smooth erosion of the spine or the undersurface of a rib.

Neuroblastoma, ganglioneuroblastoma, and *ganglioneuroma* are derived from sympathetic ganglion cells. Although most originate within the adrenal medulla, these tumors may arise anywhere along the chain of sympathetic ganglia. Extra-adrenal forms of these tumors, therefore, are paraspinal or presacral-retrorectal in location. Neuroblastoma is the malignant tumor of sympathetic ganglion cells, while ganglioneuroma is the benign form. Ganglioneuroblastoma contains both differentiated and undifferentiated elements, and its biologic behavior is variable. In the newborn, neuro-

blastoma may rarely differentiate into a less aggressive ganglioneuroblastoma or benign ganglioneuroma.

The clinical and radiologic features of the extra-adrenal sympathoblast-derived tumors are similar to those that arise in the adrenal gland, as discussed in Chapter 22. These include presentation in childhood for neuroblastoma and ganglioneuroblastoma and in young adults for ganglioneuroma, abnormally high levels of urinary vanillylmandelic acid (especially with neuroblastoma and ganglioneuroblastoma), origin in a paraspinal or presacral-retrorectal location, punctate tumoral calcification, and invasion of the spinal canal (Fig. 21–36).

Paraganglioma, like the neuroblastoma line of tumors, usually arises within the adrenal medulla, where they are termed *pheochromocytoma.* They may, however, arise from paraganglionic cells located anywhere along the chain of sympathetic ganglia. Approximately 10 per cent of all paragangliomas are extra-adrenal. Males are affected more frequently than are females. Most patients are diagnosed between the ages of 30 and 45 years. Most paragangliomas are hormonally active and cause clinical findings related to excess secretion of catecholamine. These include headache, sweating, palpitations, and hypertension. Approximately 10 per cent of paragangliomas are multiple and separate. Rarely, a continuous chain of paragangliomas occurs in a paraspinal location, a condition known as *paragangliomatosis.*

The most common location of extra-adrenal, retroperitoneal paraganglioma is between the origin of the inferior mesenteric artery and the aortic bifurcation, a

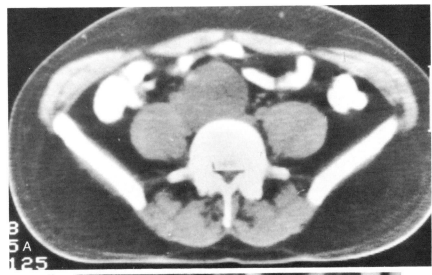

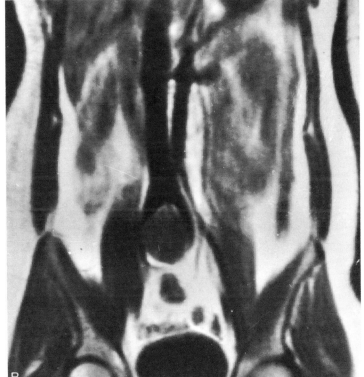

Figure 21–35. Nerve sheath tumor. There is a well-defined soft tissue mass near the bifurcation of the aorta and inferior vena cava.

A, Computed tomogram.

B, Magnetic resonance image, T1-weighted, coronal section.

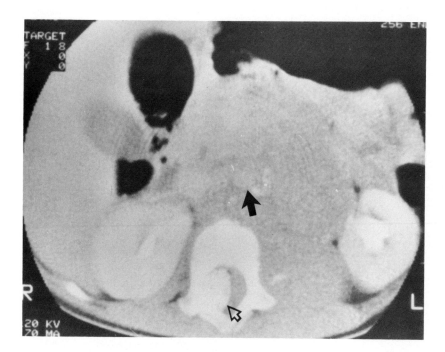

Figure 21–36. Neuroblastoma. Computed tomogram after intrathecal and intravenous contrast material administration. A large calcified mass displaces and partially obstructs the left kidney. The aorta *(solid arrow)* is displaced ventrally. The tumor has invaded the spinal canal and displaces the thecal sac *(open arrow)* to the right.

region known as the organ of Zuckerkandl (Fig. 21–37). The second most common site of occurrence is the renal hilum (Fig. 21–38). The least frequently involved location is suprarenal and extra-adrenal. Ten to 15 per cent of extra-adrenal paragangliomas are malignant. Although malignant paragangliomas are larger than benign paragangliomas, distinction between benign and malignant cannot be achieved radiologically unless metastases are identified.

Computed tomography typically demonstrates a well-defined para-aortic mass. Tumors less than 7 cm are usually homogeneous and sharply marginated. Larger tumors frequently demonstrate irregular margins and heterogeneous density. Most paragangliomas are very bright on T2-weighted magnetic resonance images. Radionuclide studies with MIBG demonstrate increased activity in the tumor. This technique is especially useful for identifying multiple tumors or metastases, as described in Chapter 2. Imaging features of paraganglioma are similar to adrenal pheochromocytoma and are discussed in Chapter 22 (see Fig. 22–18).

Clinical and radiologic features that support a diagnosis of paraganglioma include abnormally high levels of serum catecholamine (75 to 90 per cent of cases), a history of a previously resected paraganglioma, a para-aortic location, bright signal on T2-weighted magnetic resonance images, and a positive MIBG radionuclide scan.

Embryonic Remnants

Teratoma is the most common primary retroperitoneal tumor arising from an embryonic rest. Females are more commonly involved than males by a ratio of 3:1. Age distribution is bimodal, with a peak in the first 6 months of life and a second peak in early adulthood. Most retroperitoneal teratomas are mature and dis-

place rather than invade adjacent organs. Complete excision of a mature teratoma is curative since they neither metastasize nor recur.

The radiologic findings of retroperitoneal teratoma are illustrated in Figure 21–39. Ninety percent of retroperitoneal teratomas calcify, usually in a pattern of congealed clumps or linear shards. Unlike ovarian teratomas, formed teeth are very uncommon in primary retroperitoneal teratomas. Seventy-five per cent of retroperitoneal teratomas have a cystic component. A characteristic feature of a cystic teratoma is an eccentric protrusion of either solid or solid and cystic tissue into the cyst. This protrusion, known as a *dermoid plug* or *Rokitansky body*, is detected in less than 50 per cent of cases. Fat is detected by radiologic techniques in 60 per cent of cases, usually in the form of adipose tissue or, far less commonly, as sebum. Sebum is fat that is liquid at body temperature and is recognized on computed tomography as a fat–fluid level composed of a negative attenuation value supernatant material and a dependent fluid collection with an attenuation value of water. A fat-containing retroperitoneal tumor in childhood is most likely a teratoma, although a benign lipoma will produce similar features.

Primary retroperitoneal tumors other than teratoma that are derived from embryonic tissue include *germ cell tumors* (Fig. 21–40) and *extrarenal Wilms' tumor.* Primary retroperitoneal germ cell tumors are rare. Most are thought to be metastases from an occult primary in the testicle. Similar to primary germ cell tumors of the testicle, tumor tissue markers, such as alpha-fetoprotein and human chorionic growth hormone, may be elevated in primary germ cell tumors of the retroperitoneum. Extrarenal Wilms' tumor is extremely rare and is thought to originate from the metanephric blastema of the embryonic urogenital ridge. Most, therefore, arise near the midline and between the kidney and the ovary or testicle.

Text continued on page 707

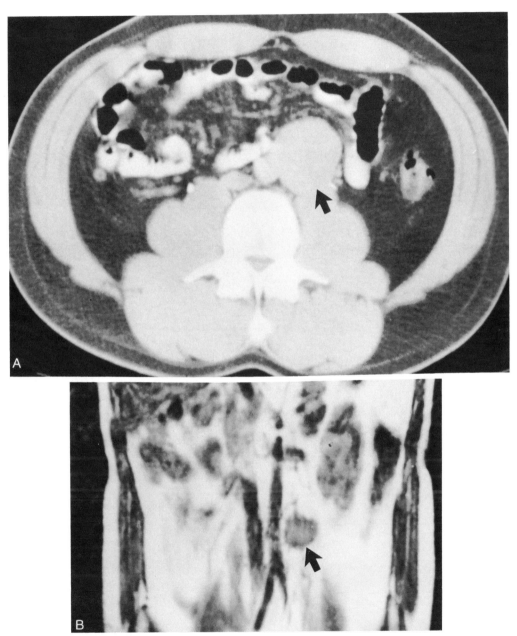

Figure 21–37. Paraganglioma located in the organ of Zuckerkandl. There is a well-defined mass *(arrow)* near the aortic bifurcation.
  A, Computed tomogram, contrast material enhanced.
  B, Magnetic resonance image, T1-weighted, coronal section.

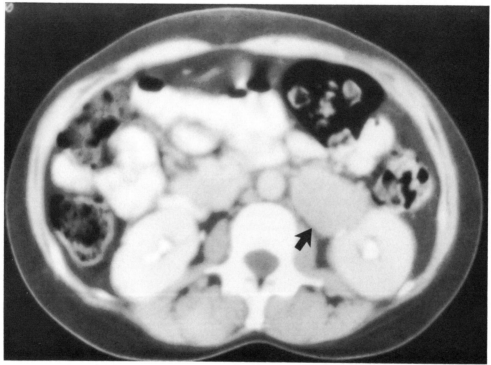

Figure 21–38. Paraganglioma, left renal hilum. Computed tomogram, contrast material enhanced. There is a well-defined extrarenal mass *(arrow)* adjacent to the left renal hilum.

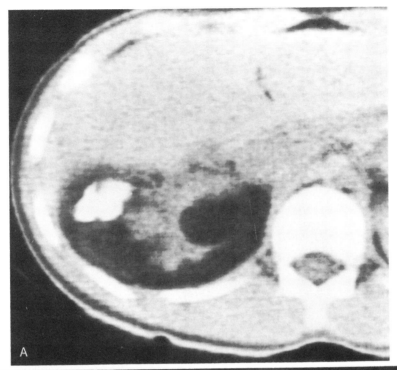

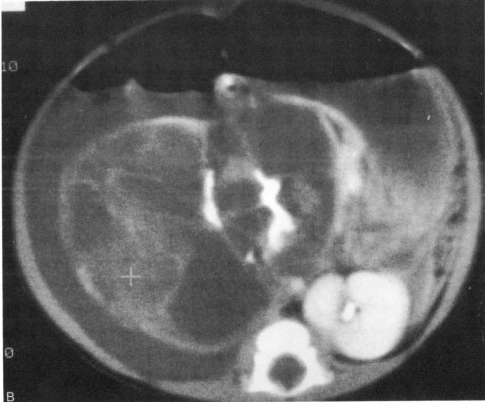

Figure 21–39. Teratoma, retroperitoneum. Characteristic radiologic features are illustrated in four different cases.
 A, Computed tomogram, contrast material enhanced. Congealed calcification and adipose tissue.
 B, Computed tomogram, contrast material enhanced. Linear shards of calcification and prominent cysts.

Illustration continued on following page

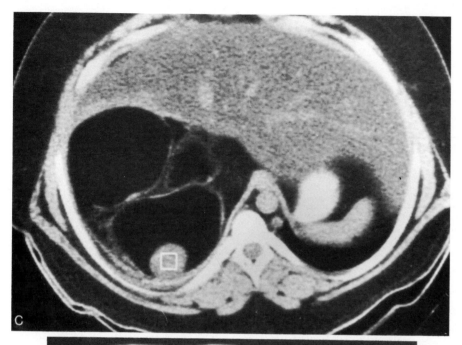

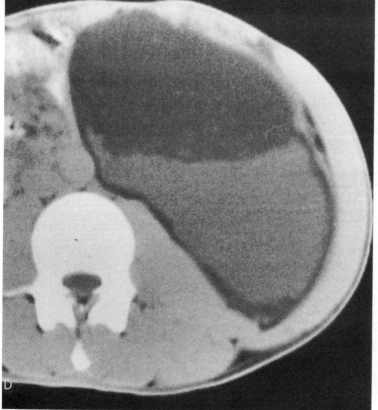

Figure 21–39. *Continued C,* Computed tomogram, contrast material enhanced. Multiple cysts with dermoid plug or Rokitansky body *(cursor).*

D, Computed tomogram, unenhanced. Fat–fluid level representative of sebum.

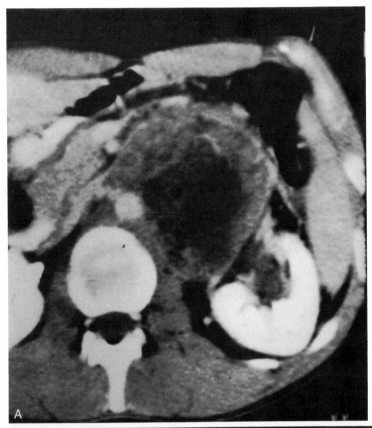

Figure 21–40. Endodermal sinus tumor originating in the retroperitoneum. The cystic and necrotic tumor displaces adjacent structures.

A, Computed tomogram, contrast material enhanced.

B, Ultrasonogram, longitudinal section.

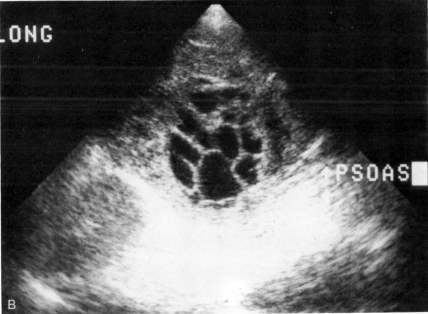

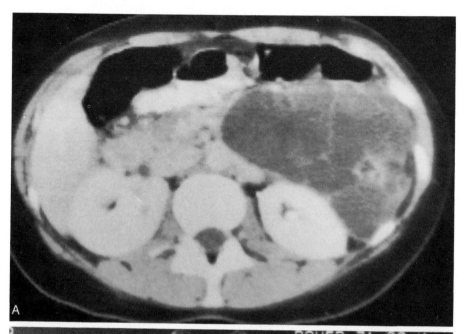

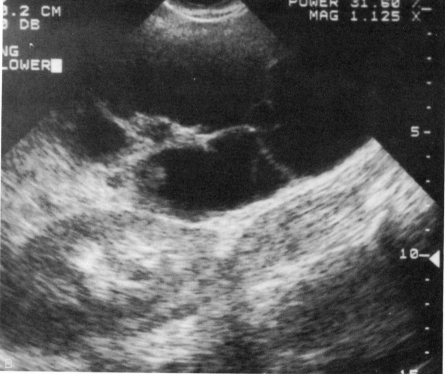

Figure 21–41. Lymphangioma, retroperitoneum. The mass is composed of multiple locules separated by thin septa and containing uncomplicated fluid.

A, Computed tomogram, contrast material enhanced.

B, Ultrasonogram, coronal section.

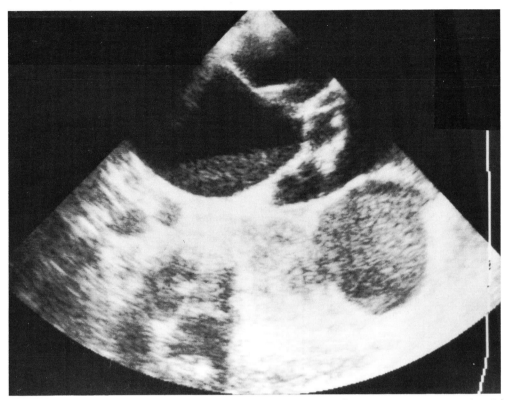

Figure 21–42. Lymphangioma, retroperitoneum, complicated by hemorrhage or infection. Ultrasonogram, transverse section. Echogenic debris in cysts is shown, some of which is layered in dependent portions of locules.

Developmental Malformation

Lymphangioma is a developmental malformation in which lymphangiectasia follows the failure of developing lymphatic tissue to establish normal communication with the remainder of the lymphatic system. Although not a true neoplasm, it must be considered in the diagnosis of retroperitoneal masses. In lymphangioma, abnormal lymphatic channels dilate to form a unilocular or multilocular cystic mass. Lymphangioma is usually discovered early in life, but it may occur in adulthood as well. There is no sex predilection. The most common clinical findings include pain, abdominal distention, fever, fatigue, weight loss, and hematuria.

The most characteristic radiologic features of lymphangioma include a unilocular or multilocular cystic elongated mass that crosses more than one compartment of the retroperitoneum (Fig. 21–41). The ultrasonographic and computed tomographic characteristics of the cyst contents are usually those of uncomplicated fluid. Some solid elements may be present as a result of infection or hemorrhage (Fig. 21–42). Calcification and chyle are uncommon.

RETROPERITONEAL LYMPHADENOPATHY

Retroperitoneal lymph nodes may be para-aortic, paracaval, interaortocaval, renal hilar, and suprahilar. Lymph nodes are recognized as abnormal when they are enlarged, are increased in number, or exhibit an internal architecture.

Computed tomography is the best technique for detecting enlarged retroperitoneal lymph nodes. Structures that must be differentiated from adenopathy include bowel loops, left-sided inferior vena cava, retroaortic or circumaortic left renal vein, dilated normal veins, the diaphragmatic crus, retroperitoneal hemorrhage (especially due to aneurysm), and retroperitoneal fibrosis. Accurate assessment requires complete opacification of the small bowel with dilute oral contrast material to distinguish loops of intestine. Intravenous contrast material may be required to identify vascular structures. Scans should be obtained in suspended expiration with 10-mm collimation.

Normal lymph nodes are between 3 and 10 mm in diameter and are round or oval soft tissue density structures in the para-aortic and paracaval areas. Isolated nodes that measure 10 to 15 mm in diameter are suspicious for abnormality. Lymph nodes that exceed 15 mm in cross-sectional diameter are definitely abnormal. It is useful to remember that between the aorta and the left psoas muscle there is normally no extranodal structure larger than 5 mm in diameter. Loss of the normal lateral contour of the aorta strongly suggests para-aortic adenopathy.

Abnormal lymph nodes may be solitary or multiple and may occur in clusters or conglomerate masses (Fig. 21–43). In patients with known lymphoproliferative disease, clusters of more than the usual number of normal-sized lymph nodes are usually abnormal. The attenuation value of abnormal lymph nodes varies from that associated with tissue necrosis to normal

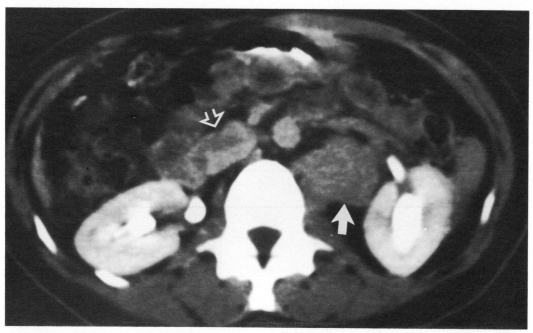

Figure 21–43. Retroperitoneal adenopathy due to Castleman's disease. Computed tomogram, contrast material enhanced. A conglomeration of lymph nodes *(solid arrow)* displaces and obstructs the left kidney. Paracaval lymphadenopathy is also present *(open arrow)* but is difficult to distinguish from intestinal loops because of insufficient oral contrast material.

tissue density (Fig. 21–44). These may be homogeneous or heterogeneous. Very negative attenuation values are seen in *lipoplastic lymphadenopathy* or fatty replacement of lymph nodes. Attenuation values of up to approximately 120 Hounsfield units have been described in patients with Hodgkin's disease or with metastases from primary carcinoma of the breast or ovary. Calcification of lymph nodes may occur following chemotherapy or in patients with retroperitoneal lymph node metastases from a primary testicular tumor.

Lymphadenopathy may be recognized as a small number of enlarged nodes, a conglomerate group of contiguous nodes, or a large confluent homogeneous mass in which individual nodes are no longer identifiable (Fig. 21–45; see also Fig. 21–43). It is impossible to differentiate benign and malignant causes for node enlargement by computed tomography alone. Likewise, computed tomography cannot depict focal architectural change in either normal-sized or consistently enlarged nodes. Thus, a negative examination does not exclude lymph node pathology.

Magnetic resonance imaging may provide useful complementary information when computed tomography is inconclusive (Fig. 21–46). Abnormal lymph nodes usually exhibit low or intermediate signal intensity on T1-weighted or proton-density images. On T2-weighted images, abnormal lymph nodes have a high signal and may resemble fat. Magnetic resonance may differentiate abnormal lymph nodes with high signal intensity from blood vessels in which the flow void phenomenon produces a low signal intensity. Likewise, magnetic resonance may differentiate tumor-bearing nodes from fibrosis following chemotherapy or radiation therapy by virtue of the fact that

fibrosis usually produces a low signal intensity on T2-weighted images compared with the typical high signal intensity of tumor.

Lymphangiography is more sensitive at detecting architectural abnormalities in normal-sized lymph nodes than is computed tomography. Therefore, lymphangiography is useful when computed tomography is equivocal or negative.

RETROPERITONEAL FIBROSIS

Retroperitoneal fibrosis results from the proliferation of fibrous tissue in a midline and para-aortic distribution. Most cases of retroperitoneal fibrosis are idiopathic, a condition known as *Ormond's disease*. There are, however, a number of specific etiologies, including *aortic hemorrhage, aortitis,* and, possibly, isolated *aortic atherosclerosis. Retroperitoneal malignancy,* especially metastases, may also produce this abnormality by provoking a desmoplastic response to tumor cells. Sclerosing Hodgkin's disease, in particular, has been associated with this occurrence. Other conditions that may be associated with retroperitoneal fibrosis are *methysergide toxicity, inflammatory bowel disease, extravasation of blood or urine* into the retroperitoneum, *prior surgery* or *radiation* to the region, and *collagen vascular disease.* The latter may also occur with Reidel's thyroiditis and sclerosing mediastinitis.

Idiopathic retroperitoneal fibrosis most commonly occurs in patients between 40 and 60 years of age. Males are more commonly affected than are females by a ratio of 2:1. Pathologically, the fibrotic mass is predominantly sagittal and parasagittal, typically extending from below the level of the kidneys to the bifurcation of the great vessels. The fibrotic tissue may

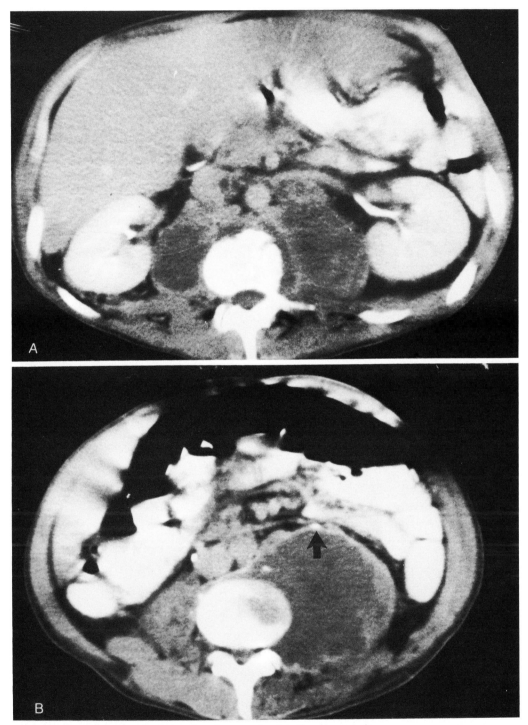

Figure 21–44. Lymphoma associated with necrotic lymph nodes extending into the psoas muscles.

A, Computed tomogram, contrast material enhanced. The mass lateral to the aorta is a necrotic left para-aortic lymph node. Lymph nodes are also present behind the aorta and between the aorta and the inferior vena cava. Enlarged nodes surround and distort the inferior vena cava. Both psoas muscles are involved.

B, Computed tomogram with contrast material enhancement caudal to *A.* The ureter *(arrow)* is displaced anteriorly by an enlarged psoas muscle infiltrated by tumor.

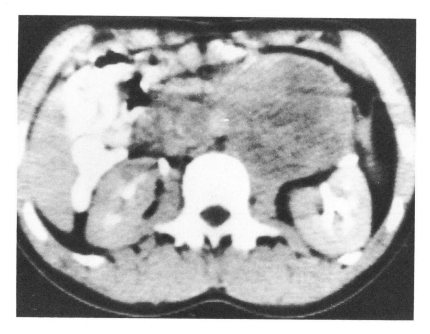

Figure 21–45. Lymphadenopathy presenting as a confluent retroperitoneal mass. Computed tomogram, contrast material enhanced. Individual lymph nodes have congealed into a single large mass. The aorta is displaced ventrally. A smaller confluent mass is present to the right of the aorta.

involve the inferior vena cava, aorta, ureters, and occasionally the iliac and renal veins in a symmetric or asymmetric distribution. Microscopically idiopathic retroperitoneal fibrosis is characterized by collagen, fibroblasts, and inflammatory cells when it is at a mature stage of development. Considerable vascularity is present initially. The presence of neoplastic cells excludes the diagnosis of idiopathic retroperitoneal fibrosis and confirms that the fibrotic process is a desmoplastic response to malignancy.

The clinical and laboratory findings of idiopathic retroperitoneal fibrosis are nonspecific and include fever, back pain, and elevated erythrocyte sedimentation rate. Less common signs and symptoms include lower extremity swelling due to venous occlusion, oliguria or anuria caused by ureteral obstruction, and constipation due to rectal involvement.

Excretory urography typically demonstrates bilateral hydronephrosis, which may be asymmetric and sometimes even unilateral. Rarely, the ureters and kidneys are uninvolved. Retrograde studies demonstrate a smooth tapering of the ureters that is most pronounced at the pelvic brim (Fig. 21–47). The ureteral narrowing may vary from focal to involvement of a long segment. Despite the ureteral narrowing and obstructive uropathy, there is no impediment to the retrograde passage of a ureteral catheter. Ureteral encasement by retroperitoneal fibrosis is usually not associated with medial displacement, although a slight degree of medial deviation sometimes occurs.

Computed tomography typically demonstrates a homogeneous soft tissue mass that extends from the infrarenal para-aortic region to the bifurcation of the aorta and encases the aorta, inferior vena cava, and ureters. Ureteral involvement with subsequent proximal ureteral dilatation and hydronephrosis may be asymmetric or unilateral. The aorta is typically not displaced ventrally (see Fig. 21–47). Contrast enhancement varies with the age of the process. In its earliest

stages of development, enhancement occurs as a manifestation of increased vascularity associated with active inflammation. Later, the dense organized fibrous tissue has less vascularity and, correspondingly, does not enhance.

It has been suggested that magnetic resonance imaging might permit distinction between benign or nonneoplastic retroperitoneal fibrosis and malignant retroperitoneal fibrosis. In nonmalignant retroperitoneal fibrosis, a low or intermediate signal intensity on T1- and T2-weighted images has been reported in contrast to a higher signal intensity on T2-weighted images in most malignancies. Magnetic resonance imaging also demonstrates the effect of the fibrotic mass on flowing blood in the aorta and inferior vena cava.

Ultrasonography demonstrates retroperitoneal fibrosis as a poorly marginated, periaortic mass that is typically echo free or hypoechoic. Associated hydronephrosis is easily evaluated by ultrasonography as well. Body habitus, bowel gas, and adjacent bony structures may degrade the ultrasonographic imaging of retroperitoneal fibrosis.

Venacavography is not necessary for the evaluation of most cases of retroperitoneal fibrosis. In particular problems, cavography may be used to demonstrate displacement, extrinsic compression, or complete obstruction of the inferior vena cava.

Atypical manifestations of retroperitoneal fibrosis include ventral displacement of the aorta (Fig. 21–48), disease confined to the pelvis, involvement of the perirenal space, displacement of the retroperitoneal bowel, and vascular occlusion. Very rarely, computed tomography is normal.

PSEUDOTUMORS OF THE RETROPERITONEUM

Left para-aortic pseudotumors can be a source of error in interpreting transverse cross sections of the retro-

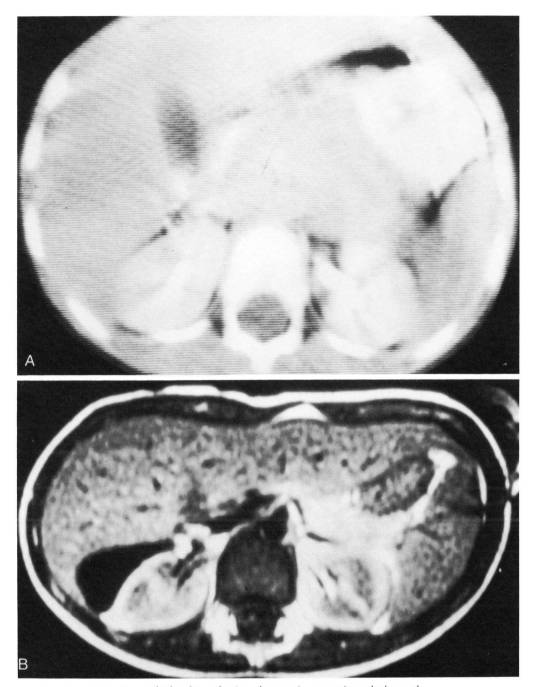

Figure 21–46. Magnetic resonance imaging applied to the evaluation of uncertain retroperitoneal adenopathy.

A, Computed tomogram, contrast material enhanced. There is a soft tissue mass between the spine and stomach that was thought to represent retroperitoneal lymphadenopathy.

B, Magnetic resonance image at the same level as *A.* There is no adenopathy. The retroperitoneal spaces are normal.

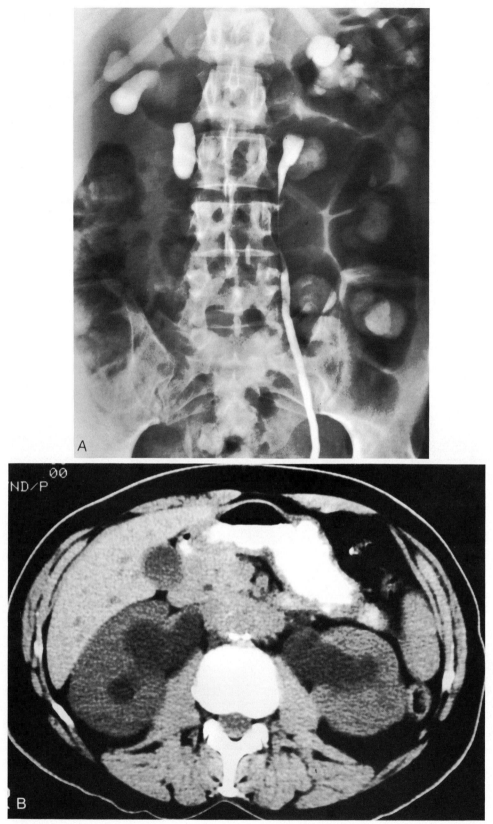

Figure 21–47. Retroperitoneal fibrosis.

A, Retrograde pyelogram. The fibrotic mass encases the left ureter, resulting in a long, smooth stricture and hydronephrosis. Similar findings were present involving the right ureter.

B, Computed tomogram, unenhanced. The attenuation value of the fibrotic mass is similar to that of the psoas muscles. The fibrotic mass surrounds the partially calcified aorta and the inferior vena cava. Note that the aorta maintains its normal position just ventral to the spine.

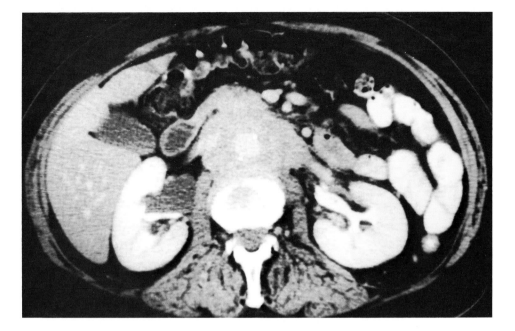

Figure 21–48. Retroperitoneal fibrosis. Computed tomogram, contrast material enhanced. Unilateral hydronephrosis and the ventral displacement of the aorta from the spine are unusual manifestations of retroperitoneal fibrosis. Confident radiologic differentiation from lymphoma is impossible.

peritoneum. These are caused by normal or variant vascular or intestinal structures, such as a duplicated inferior vena cava, a normal splenic artery or vein, an enlarged azygos vein from congenital or acquired processes, a circumaortic or retroaortic left renal vein, an enlarged left gonadal vein, loops of small bowel, displaced organs as a result of prior surgery, an extrarenal pelvis, and duplicated ureters. Oral and intravenous contrast material administration, particularly using dynamic techniques, is valuable in ruling out pseudotumors that cause potential interpretative errors.

Bibliography

Retroperitoneal Anatomy and Spaces

Dodds, W. J., Darweesh, R. M. A., Lawson, T. L., Stewart, E. T., Foley, W. D., Kishk, S. M. A., and Hollwarth, M.: The retroperitoneal spaces revisited. AJR *157*:1155, 1986.

Feuerstein, I. M., Zeman, R. K., Jaffe, M. H., Clark, L. R., and David, C. L.: Perirenal cobwebs: The expanding CT differential diagnosis. J. Comput. Assist. Tomogr. *8*:1128, 1984.

Honda, H., McGuire, C. W., Barloon, T. J., and Harshimoto, K.: Replacement lipomatosis of the kidney: CT features. J. Comput. Assist. Tomogr. *14*:229, 1990.

Kneeland, J. B., Auh, Y. H., Rubenstein, W. A., Zirinsky, K., Morrison, H., Whalen, J. P., and Kazam, E.: Perirenal spaces: CT evidence for communication across the midline. Radiology *164*:657, 1987.

Kochkodan, E. J., and Haggar, A. M.: Visualization of the renal fascia: A normal finding in urography. AJR *140*:1243, 1983.

Korobkin, M., Silverman, P. M., Quint, L. E., and Francis I. R.: CT of the extraperitoneal space: Normal anatomy and fluid collections. AJR *159*:933, 1992.

Kunin, M.: Bridging septa of the perinephric space: Anatomic, pathologic and diagnostic considerations. Radiology *158*:361, 1986.

Love, L., Meyers, M. A., Churchill, R. J., Reynes, C. J., et al.: Computed tomography of the extraperitoneal space. AJR *136*:781, 1981.

Marincek, B., Young, S. W., and Castellino, R. A.: A CT scanning approach to the evaluation of left paraaortic pseudotumors. J. Comput. Assist. Tomogr. *5*:723, 1981.

Meyers, M. A., Whalen, J. P., Peelle, K., and Berne, A. S.: Radiologic features of extraperitoneal effusions. Radiology *104*:249, 1972.

Meyers, M. A., Whalen, J. P., and Evans, J. A.: Diagnosis of perirenal and subcapsular masses: Anatomic-radiologic correlation. AJR *121*:523, 1974.

Meyers, M. A.: The reno-alimentary relationships: Anatomic-roentgen study of their clinical significance. AJR *123*:386, 1975.

Meyers, M. A.: Uriniferous perirenal pseudocyst: New observations. Radiology *117*:539, 1975.

Mitchell, G. A. G.: Renal fascia. Br. J. Surg. *37*:257, 1950.

Parienty, R. A., Pradel, J., Picard, J.-D. Ducellier, R., et al.: Visibility and thickening of the renal fascia on computed tomographs. Radiology *139*:119, 1981.

Raptopoulos, V., Kleinman, P. K., Marks, S. Jr., Snyder, M., and Silverman, P. M.: Renal fascial pathway: Posterior extension of pancreatic effusions with in the anterior pararenal space. Radiology *158*:367, 1986.

Rubenstein, W. A., and Whalen, J. P.: Extraperitoneal spaces. AJR *157*:1162, 1986.

Somogyi, J., Cohen, W. N., Omer, M. M., and Makhuli, Z.: Communication of right and left perirenal spaces demonstrated by computed tomography. J. Comput. Assist. Tomogr. *3*:270, 1979.

Susman, N., Hammerman, A. M., and Cohen, E.: The renal halo sign in pancreatitis. Radiology *142*:323, 1982.

Thomas, A. M. K., and Carr, D. H.: Visibility of the renal fascia at intravenous urography. Clin. Radiol. *35*:177, 1984.

Thornbury, J. R.: Perirenal anatomy: Normal and abnormal. Radiol. Clin. North Am. *17*:321, 1979.

Winfield, A. C., Gerlock, A. J., Jr., and Shaff, M. I.: Perirenal cobwebs: A CT sign of renal vein thrombosis. J. Comput. Assist. Tomogr. *5*:705, 1981.

Retroperitoneal Tumors

Davidson, A. J., and Hartman, D. S.: Imaging strategies for neoplasms of the kidney, adrenal gland and retroperitoneum. CA *37*:151, 1987.

Davidson, A. J., Hartman, D. S., and Goldman, S. M.: Mature teratoma of the retroperitoneum: Radiologic, pathologic, and clinical correlation. Radiology *172*:421, 1989.

Enzinger, R. M., and Weiss, S. W.: Soft Tissue Tumors. St. Louis, C.V. Mosby, 1983.

Hartman, D. S., Hayes, W. S., Choyke, P. L., and Tibbetts, G. P.: Leiomyosarcoma of the retroperitoneum and inferior vena cava: Radiologic-pathologic correlation. Radiographics *12*:1203, 1992.

Hayes, W. S., Davidson, A. J., Grimley, P. M., and Hartman, D. S.:

Extraadrenal retroperitoneal paraganglioma: Clinical, pathologic, and CT findings. Presented before the Society of Uroradiology, Naples, Florida, 1989.

Lee, J. K. T.: Magnetic resonance imaging of the retroperitoneum. Urol. Radiol. *10*:48, 1988.

Levine, E., Huntarakoon, M., and Wetzel, L. H.: Malignant nerve-sheath neoplasms in neurofibromatosis: Distinction from benign tumors by using imaging techniques. AJR *149*:1059, 1987.

Retroperitoneal Lymphadenopathy

Einstein, D. M.: Abdominal lymphadenopathy: Spectrum of CT findings. Radiographics *11*:457, 1991.

Hartman, D. S.: Retroperitoneal tumors and lymphadenopathy. Urol. Radiol. *12*:132, 1990.

Lien, H. H., et al.: Normal and anomalous structures simulating retroperitoneal lymphadenopathy at computed tomography. Acta Radiol. *29*:385, 1988.

Sagel, S. S., and Lee, J. K. T.: Retroperitoneal lymphadenopathy. *In* Taveras, J. E. Ferrucci, J. T.: (eds.): Radiology: Diagnosis—Imaging—Intervention. Philadelphia, J.B. Lippincott, 1988.

Retroperitoneal Fibrosis

Amis, E. S.: Retroperitoneal fibrosis. AJR *157*:321, 1991.

Arrive, L., Hricak, H., Tavares, N. J., and Miller, T. R.: Malignant versus nonmalignant retroperitoneal fibrosis: Differentiation with MR imaging. Radiology *172*:139, 1989.

Mulligan, S. A., Holley, H. C., Koehler, R. E., Koslin, D. B., Rubin, E., Berland, L. L., and Kenney, P. J.: CT and MR imaging in the evaluation of retroperitoneal fibrosis. J. Comput. Assist. Tomogr. *13*:277, 1989.

Rominger, M. G., and Kenney, P. J.: Perirenal involvement by retroperitoneal fibrosis: The usefulness of MRI to establish diagnosis. Urol. Radiol. *13*:173, 1992.

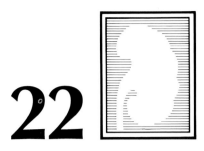

22

THE ADRENAL

NORMAL ANATOMY

The adrenal glands are located within the perinephric space and are completely surrounded by perirenal fat. Each gland weighs approximately 4 gm, 90 per cent of which is cortex and only 10 per cent medulla. The two portions of the adrenal, each of different embryologic origin, are autonomous with respect to hormone production and pathologic states.

The adrenal cortex is derived from mesoderm and is involved in the synthesis of mineralocorticoids, glucocorticoids, androgens, and estrogens. Cortical neoplasms include adenoma and carcinoma, both of which may hyperfunction. Cortical hyperplasia usually results from excessive stimulation of adrenocorticotropic hormone (ACTH) but may be primary.

The adrenal medulla is derived from neural crest ectoderm and is involved in the synthesis of epinephrine and norepinephrine. Medullary tumors include neuroblastoma, ganglioneuroblastoma, ganglioneuroma, and pheochromocytoma.

The right adrenal gland is suprarenal in location and at a more cephalic position than the left adrenal gland (Fig. 22–1). It is usually detected on axial images at the level just superior to the upper pole of the right kidney and dorsal to the inferior vena cava. Right adrenal masses are truly suprarenal, and large masses often displace the right kidney inferiorly. The medial limb of the right gland is more conspicuous than the lateral (horizontal) limb. The limbs of the normal adrenal gland are usually thinner than the adjacent diaphragmatic crura, although the medial

limb of the right gland normally can be as thick as 5 mm.

The normal left adrenal is slightly more caudal relative to the kidney than is the right gland (see Fig. 22–1). It is usually detected on axial sections obtained at the same level as the upper pole of the left kidney. Left adrenal masses often compress the ventral surface of the kidney, but unlike right adrenal masses usually do not displace the kidney inferiorly. On axial sections the left adrenal has the appearance of an inverted V or Y.

The splenic vein is another useful landmark to identify the left adrenal gland and to determine the origin of retroperitoneal masses. The left adrenal gland is positioned between the left kidney and the splenic vein. Adrenal masses classically arise dorsal to the splenic vein, whereas pancreatic masses originate ventral to the splenic vein (see Fig. 22–15). Normal adrenal glands vary in size and shape but are always straight or concave. Glands that are round or convex are abnormal and signify either enlargement or a mass.

There are several conditions that may simulate an adrenal mass. On the left side, a "pseudotumor" may be due to fluid-filled gastric fundus or gastric diverticulum, accessory spleen, tortuous splenic vein, inferior phrenic vein, exophytic upper pole renal mass, pancreatic mass, or diaphragmatic crura. On the right side, interposition of colon between liver and kidney, a fluid-filled duodenum, a caudal lobe of the liver, or an exophytic upper pole renal mass may be confused with an adrenal mass. Most of these misleading ap-

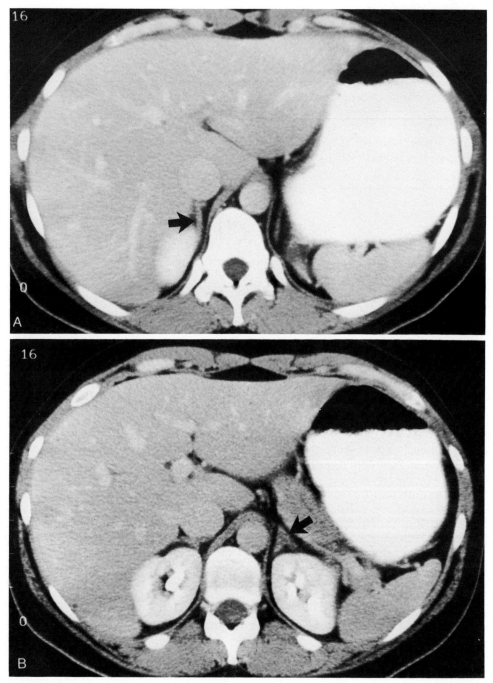

Figure 22–1. Normal adrenal glands. Computed tomograms, contrast material enhanced.
   A, The medial limb of the right adrenal gland *(arrow)* is dorsal to the inferior vena cava and ventral to the upper pole of the kidney.
   B, The left adrenal gland *(arrow)* has an inverted V appearance.

pearances can be distinguished by a carefully performed bolus, contrast material–enhanced, dynamic computed tomogram with an adequate amount of oral contrast material or by magnetic resonance imaging in several planes.

IMAGING MODALITIES

Although there are many imaging modalities to evaluate the adrenal glands, no single technique is perfect for all clinical problems. In most cases, multiple modalities are utilized. It is imperative to correlate all images with biochemical results and clinical findings.

Computed tomography is the procedure of choice for resolving most clinical problems relating to the adrenal gland. The spatial resolution of computed tomography is unsurpassed when contiguous, thin 3- to 5-mm sections are obtained. Spiral computed tomography avoids misregistration artifacts, thereby improving accuracy. Although providing excellent morphologic information, computed tomography does not provide functional data. In many cases computed tomography is unable to differentiate a nonhyperfunctioning adenoma from metastases to the adrenal, which is one of the most commonly encountered problems in adrenal imaging.

Although the spatial resolution of magnetic resonance imaging is slightly inferior to that of computed tomography, it may be very helpful in selected cases. Coronal or sagittal images may confirm the adrenal gland origin of a mass while axial images are equivocal. The flow void phenomenon seen with magnetic resonance imaging allows excellent evaluation of vascular patency, especially when other modalities are indeterminate. Contrast resolution of magnetic resonance imaging is superior to that of computed tomography. Pheochromocytoma has a characteristic high signal on T2-weighted images. Likewise, differentiation of metastases from nonhyperfunctioning adenoma is possible in many cases.

Radionuclide imaging of the adrenal is most useful when functional information is required. There are two main pharmaceuticals that have potential for general use. Metaiodobenzylguanidine (MIBG) is an analogue of norepinephrine and is useful in detecting functioning medullary tumors. NP-59 (beta-iodomethyl-19-norcholesterol) depicts glucocorticoid, mineralocorticoid, and androgen secretion. Both are labeled with iodine 131 or iodine 123.

MIBG is especially useful in detecting extra-adrenal paraganglioma, multiple paragangliomas, metastatic or recurrent paraganglioma, and neuroblastoma. MIBG is, however, costly and time consuming, taking up to 3 days to complete a study.

NP-59 is not commonly used because of its lack of general availability. Since it accumulates in areas of cortical hormone synthesis, its primary application is in the evaluation of incidentally detected adrenal masses with normal adrenal function. The term *nonfunctioning* adenoma is a misnomer. Those greater than 2 cm in diameter usually demonstrate some ac-

cumulation of NP-59. Thus, they are better considered non*hyper*functioning adenomas. In contrast, absence of discernable NP-59 uptake in an adrenal mass greater than 2 cm in diameter indicates a hypofunctioning or destructive lesion, such as metastases. Disadvantages of NP-59 include a 5- to 7-day interval between injection of the radiopharmaceutical and the imaging study and a relatively high radiation dose to the adrenal gland.

Radionuclide evaluation of the adrenal gland is discussed further in Chapter 2.

Adrenal venous sampling, although somewhat technically difficult, provides functional information by obtaining blood samples for metabolic assay. This is especially useful when morphologic data are equivocal or contradictory with clinical or laboratory data. Venous sampling is most widely used in differentiating adenoma from hyperplasia in patients with hyperaldosteronism. In these cases the adenoma is often small and difficult to image. Bilateral samples are required, and, ideally, these should be collected simultaneously. Sampling before and after the administration of ACTH also provides useful information. With this technique, a ratio of aldosterone to cortisol should be calculated before and after ACTH stimulation to correct for varying dilution of adrenal vein blood in each sample.

An adenoma demonstrates elevated levels of aldosterone in the ipsilateral vein with a positive response to stimulation with ACTH. The contralateral gland produces suppressed levels of aldosterone and does not respond to ACTH. Hyperplasia, on the other hand, demonstrates elevated aldosterone levels from both adrenal veins, with further increase following ACTH.

Inferior vena cavography may be required to detect the intraluminal component of an adrenal malignancy, such as carcinoma or pheochromocytoma. This technique may be especially useful in those cases in which magnetic resonance imaging, ultrasonography, or computed tomography are equivocal.

Adrenal arteriography is rarely required. It is potentially dangerous in patients with pheochromocytoma and rarely diagnostic for a specific histologic diagnosis. Computed tomography and magnetic resonance imaging almost always provide the morphologic information required for surgical planning.

APPROACH TO ADRENAL IMAGING

Adrenal imaging can be conveniently divided into two main categories: the radiologic evaluation of abnormal adrenal function and the evaluation of abnormal adrenal morphology with normal adrenal function (nonhyperfunctioning adrenal masses). Abnormal adrenal function can be further subdivided into hyperfunction, either cortical or medullary, or adrenal insufficiency (Addison's disease).

In patients with abnormal adrenal function, the primary task of the radiologist is to detect and characterize the adrenal pathology and pathophysiology. For example, in a patient with known hypercortisolism, it is the radiologist's objective to determine whether the cause is hyperplasia, adenoma, or carcinoma.

When confronted with abnormal adrenal morphology and apparent normal adrenal function, it is essential to confirm by laboratory studies that the adrenal glands are truly not hyperfunctioning. In many cases cortical or medullary hormones will be mildly elevated, thus allowing a specific diagnosis. These so-called nonfunctional masses are usually encountered as incidental findings while imaging other clinical problems. Although there are many causes for a non-hyperfunctioning adrenal mass, differential features are often present that will enable a specific diagnosis.

ABNORMAL ADRENAL FUNCTION

Cushing's Syndrome (Hypercortisolism)

Cushing's syndrome (hypercortisolism) is the result of excessive glucocorticoid production. Clinical features include truncal obesity, "buffalo hump," "moon" face, hirsutism, and muscle atrophy. Hypertension is common. The diagnosis of Cushing's syndrome is established by finding elevated levels of free cortisol in a 24-hour urine collection.

Once the diagnosis has been established, determination of the etiology is important, as outlined in Table 22–1. Excluding exogenous sources, in adults 70 to 85 per cent of cases are due to ACTH-producing pituitary adenoma causing bilateral hyperplasia. Ten to 20 per cent of cases result from an adrenal adenoma, and 5 to 10 per cent are caused by adrenal carcinoma. In children, Cushing's syndrome is usually caused by carcinoma.

Most cases of adrenal hyperplasia result from excessive ACTH production by a pituitary adenoma, which is known as Cushing's *disease*. In 10 to 15 per cent of cases, however, excessive ACTH is produced ectopically (e.g., oat cell carcinoma, bronchial carcinoid, pheochromocytoma). Rare etiologies of adrenal hyperplasia include hypothalamic tumors and primary pigmented nodular adrenal disease.

· Patients with Cushing's syndrome should be initially evaluated with computed tomography of the

---

Table 22–1. CAUSES OF CUSHING'S SYNDROME

Exogenous adrenal steroids
Adrenal hyperplasia (70%–85%)
  Pituitary adenoma (Cushing's disease)
  Ectopic adrenocorticotropic hormone
    Oat cell carcinoma
    Bronchial carcinoid
    Pheochromocytoma
    Islet cell tumor
    Medullary thyroid carcinoma
    Thymic carcinoid
    Ovarian tumor
  Hypothalamus (rare)
  Primary pigmented nodular
    adrenal disease (rare)
Adrenal adenoma (10%–20%)
Adrenal carcinoma (5%–10%)

---

adrenal glands. Adrenal imaging in these patients is facilitated by the abundant retroperitoneal fat that is usually present. Hyperplasia is suggested when one of four patterns is present: bilateral adrenal enlargement, normal glands, multiple small nodules, or a multinodular gland with a dominant nodule. Diffuse bilateral enlargement is the most common pattern. It is recognized as enlargement of the entire gland without a focal mass (Fig. 22–2). The limbs are thicker and sometimes longer than normal. If both adrenals are enlarged, the diagnosis of hyperplasia can be made confidently since bilateral adenomas are extremely rare.

Hyperplastic adrenal glands frequently appear normal or only slightly enlarged on computed tomography (Fig. 22–3). A normal computed tomographic study never excludes the diagnosis of adrenal hyperplasia, which can be established on the basis of biochemical studies demonstrating hypercortisolism alone.

Uncommonly, adrenal hyperplasia is multinodular. The nodules are almost always less than 3 cm in diameter and frequently less than 1 cm in diameter. In most cases there is enlargement of the gland between individual nodules.

Rarely, a multinodular gland may have a single dominant nodule that may be mistaken for an adenoma (Fig. 22–4). If ipsilateral adrenalectomy were performed in this circumstance, Cushing's syndrome would persist postoperatively owing to the occult contralateral hyperplasia. In these cases it is especially important to not overlook subtle signs of hyperplasia, such as other, smaller nodules or slight adrenal enlargement.

Careful evaluation of the computed tomographic pattern of hyperplasia may be useful in determining its pathophysiology. In classic pituitary-dependent Cushing's disease caused by an ACTH-producing pituitary tumor, approximately one-half of the adrenal glands appear normal and one-half are mildly enlarged. Marked enlargement, that is, a right medial limb that is larger than 10 mm in thickness, is not seen in classic pituitary-dependent Cushing's disease and usually signifies ectopic ACTH production (Fig. 22–5).

Petrosal venous sampling is more accurate than computed tomography in determining the pathogenesis of the adrenal hyperplasia. Bilateral simultaneous sampling of the inferior petrosal sinuses is extremely sensitive, specific, and accurate for diagnosing Cushing's disease and distinguishing that entity from ectopic ACTH sources. Lack of a gradient indicates an ectopic source for ACTH production.

Ten to 20 per cent of cases of Cushing's syndrome are caused by an adrenal adenoma. A functioning adenoma that causes hypercortisolism is usually easily detected on computed tomography since it is usually larger than 2 cm in diameter and is surrounded by abundant retroperitoneal fat (Fig. 22–6). Most adenomas have a smooth, round or oval contour that is well delineated. The contralateral adrenal gland is usually smaller than normal because of ACTH

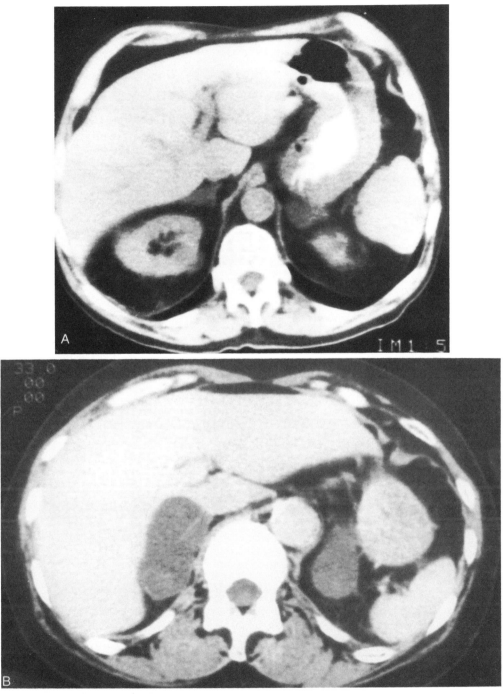

Figure 22–2. Hyperplasia, adrenal, in two patients.
A, Computed tomogram, contrast material enhanced. Both adrenal glands are mildly enlarged.
B, Computed tomogram, contrast material enhanced. There is marked enlargement of both glands, which are lobular with convex contours.

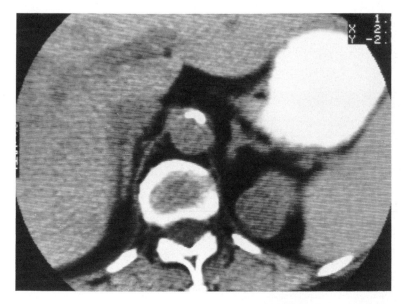

Figure 22–3. Hyperplasia with minimal enlargement. Computed tomogram without contrast material. Both glands maintain their normal shape, but the limbs are thicker than the adjacent diaphragmatic crura.

Figure 22–4. Macronodular hyperplasia with a dominant nodule.

A and *B,* Computed tomograms without contrast material at two contiguous levels. There is a small right adrenal mass *(solid arrow)* that could be confused with an adenoma. Careful evaluation of the left gland, however, demonstrates two additional nodules *(open arrows).* In a patient with adrenal hyperfunction, these findings are most consistent with macronodular hyperplasia.

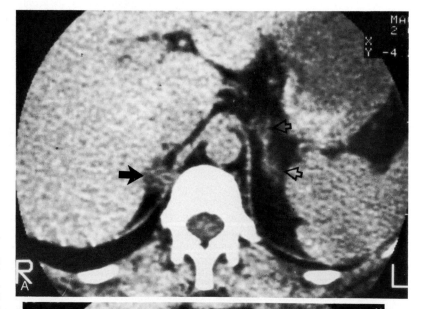

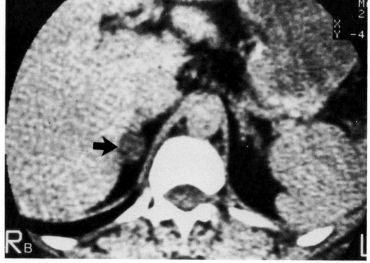

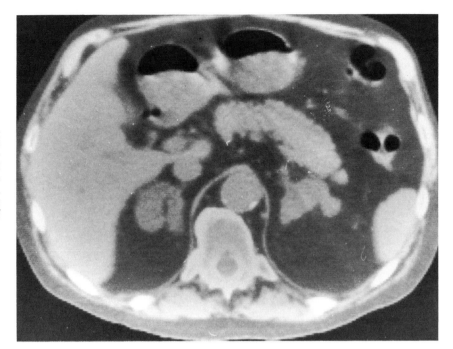

Figure 22–5. Hyperplasia, adrenal, due to ectopic adrenocorticotropic hormone produced by a small cell carcinoma of the lung. Computed tomogram, unenhanced. The increased amount of retroperitoneal fat facilitates evaluation of the massively enlarged adrenal glands. Enlargement to this degree usually results from an ectopic rather than a pituitary source of adrenocorticotropic hormone.

suppression by the functioning adenoma. Computed tomographic features that differentiate adenoma from carcinoma include smooth contour, sharp margination, a size less than 5 cm in diameter, and absence of hemorrhage or necrosis. Approximately 15 per cent of adenomas calcify, but this feature is not helpful in differentiating adenoma from carcinoma.

Although two-thirds of adrenal cortical carcinomas demonstrate some degree of biochemical hyperfunction, only 5 to 10 per cent of adult cases of Cushing's syndrome are caused by carcinoma. In contrast, most childhood cases of Cushing's syndrome are caused by carcinoma. Adrenal cortical carcinoma is suspected when any of the following computed tomography findings are present: a mass greater than 5 cm in diameter, necrosis, hemorrhage, inhomogeneous enhancement (Fig. 22–7), venous extension into an adrenal or renal vein or into the inferior vena cava (Fig. 22–8), distant metastases (especially lung, lymph nodes, liver), or invasion into adjacent viscera. Thirty to 40 per cent of carcinomas calcify. As mentioned previously, calcification by itself does not distinguish benign from malignant disease.

Magnetic resonance imaging is usually not necessary in most cases of Cushing's syndrome but may be useful in selected circumstances (Fig. 22–9). Adrenal carcinoma is typically hypointense compared with liver on T1-weighted images and hyperintense compared with liver on T2-weighted images. The coronal or sagittal images may help define adrenal from renal origin if axial computed tomography is equivocal. Magnetic resonance imaging is also useful for documenting the extent of venous invasion and may be helpful in differentiating tumor thrombus from non-tumor venous thrombus when gadolinium-enhanced scans are performed.

Hyperaldosteronism

Primary hyperaldosteronism is the result of elevated aldosterone production by the adrenal cortex with subsequent hypertension, hypokalemia, and suppression of plasma renin activity. Approximately 80 per cent of cases of primary hyperaldosteronism have a unilateral cortical adenoma, a condition known as *Conn's syndrome*. Most of the remaining cases have bilateral micronodular or macronodular hyperplasia. It is very rare to have an adrenal carcinoma that produces only aldosterone. Differentiation is extremely important since an adenoma is treated surgically while patients with hyperplasia are treated medically. Surgical resection of adenoma usually results in improvement or cure of hypertension and electrolyte disturbances, whereas surgical intervention in hyperplasia usually does not result in prolonged improvement of these abnormalities.

Computed tomography in patients with hyperaldosteronism is less often diagnostic than in patients with Cushing's syndrome because in the former the tumor is usually smaller and there is no increase in periadrenal retroperitoneal fat compared with the latter. The average aldosterone-producing adenoma measures only 1.7 cm in diameter, with a range of 0.5 to 3.5 cm (Fig. 22–10). Overlapping sections of 1.5- to 3.0-mm thickness, therefore, are recommended. Because of increased cytoplasmic lipid in aldosterone-producing adenoma, the computed tomographic attenuation values in patients with primary aldosteronism are usually lower than in patients with Cushing's syndrome. Occasionally, the attenuation value is similar to water and an adenoma mimics a small adrenal cyst.

Patients with clinical findings that support the di-

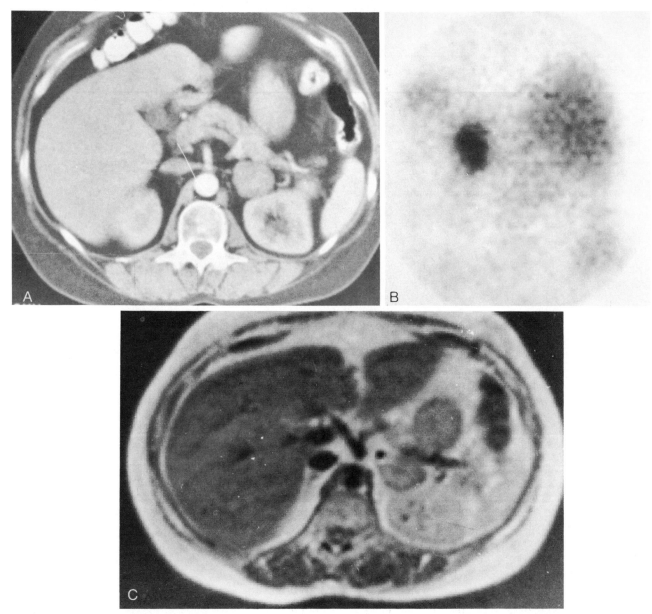

Figure 22–6. Adrenal adenoma.
  A, Computed tomogram, contrast material enhanced. There is a well-defined 3.5-cm mass between the pancreas and the left kidney.
  B, NP-59 radionuclide scan, posterior view. The mass accumulates NP-59.
  C, Magnetic resonance image, T2 weighted. The mass has a signal that is slightly brighter than that of liver. Compare with the signal intensity of metastases illustrated in Figure 22–21*B.*

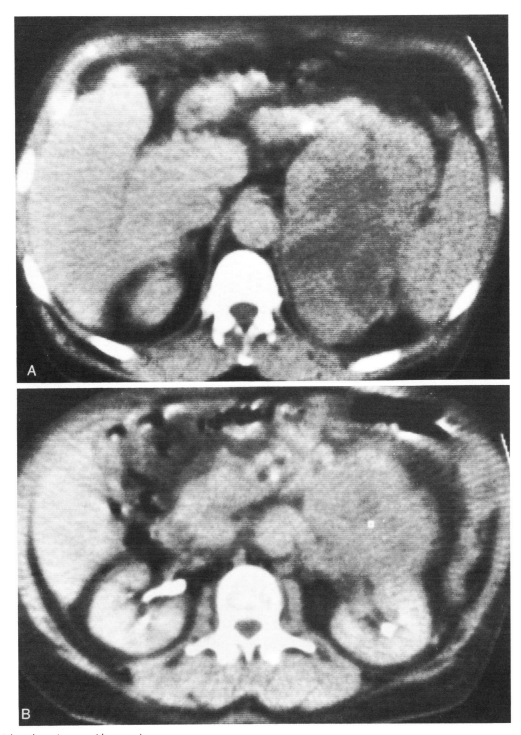

Figure 22–7. Adrenal carcinoma with necrosis.
 A and *B*, Computed tomograms with contrast material enhancement at two levels. There is a large left adrenal tumor adjacent to, but separate from, the kidney. Necrotic zones are conspicuous. Radiologic differentiation from other large adrenal masses is possible only if cortical hormone levels are elevated.

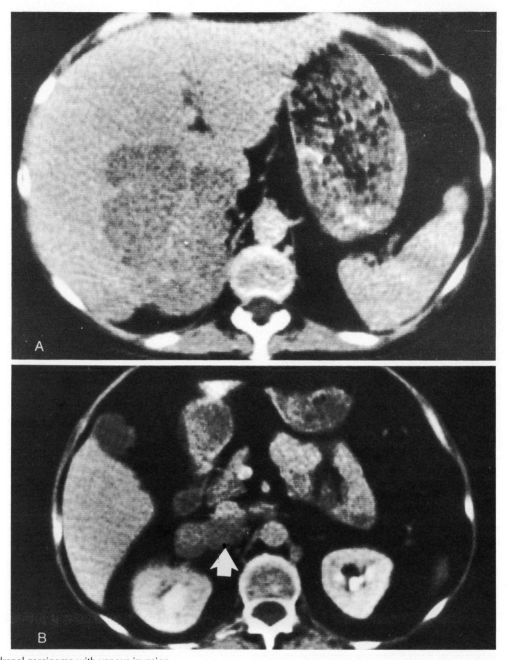

Figure 22–8. Adrenal carcinoma with venous invasion.
    A, Computed tomogram, contrast material enhanced. There is a large lobulated right-sided mass that cannot be separated from the liver.
    B, Computed tomogram, contrast material enhanced caudal to *A.* The mass *(arrow)* is separate from the kidney but displaces the inferior vena cava ventrally.

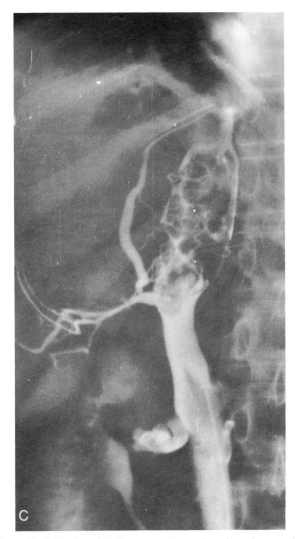

Figure 22–8 *Continued C,* Cavogram. Tumor thrombus obstructs the inferior vena cava. Carcinoma is the most common adrenal tumor with venous invasion.

agnosis of an adenoma and who also have an obvious unilateral nodule and a normal contralateral gland on computed tomography do not require venous sampling. Utilizing thin-section computed tomography, two-thirds of patients with hyperplasia have small micronodules while one-third have normal-appearing adrenal glands. In cases with multiple bilateral nodules, computed tomography cannot reliably permit distinction between hyperplasia and adenoma. Occasionally it is difficult to decide if a nodule less than 2 cm in diameter seen on computed tomography represents an adenoma or a single nodule in hyperplastic glands (Fig. 22–11). Therefore, all patients with bilateral nodules or equivocal findings on computed tomography require venous sampling, as do patients with bilaterally normal glands.

Virilization

Virilization refers to the appearance of adult masculine characteristics in prepubertal males or in females of any age. It is often called the *adrenogenital syndrome* and can be caused by congenital adrenal cortical hyperplasia or neoplasia. Most cases are seen in children.

Congenital adrenal hyperplasia is caused by an enzymatic deficiency (usually 21-hydroxylase) in the biosynthetic pathway of adrenal steroids. This results in ineffective adrenal steroid production with overproduction and accumulation of cortisol precursors. Some of these produce androgenic effects and hyperplasia of the adrenal cortex. Overproduction of androgens causes masculinization owing to inhibition of differentiation of the embryonic genital tract along female lines. In 30 per cent of cases, mineralocorticoid production is also impaired, leading to hyponatremia, hyperkalemia, hypoglycemia, and hypotension. The hyperplastic adrenal glands are usually larger than normal while maintaining a normal shape.

Adrenal adenoma or carcinoma may also produce virilization. However, this occurs in the neonatal period with extreme rarity, which helps in their differentiation from congenital adrenal hyperplasia. With a virilizing adrenal tumor, size is not as reliable a criterion in differentiating adenoma from carcinoma as it is in Cushing's syndrome. In children, some benign adenomas are larger than 5 cm in diameter. In adults, the majority of adrenal virilizing tumors are malignant.

Feminization

Feminization from adrenal hyperfunction is very rare. It usually occurs in adult males who present with gynecomastia, testicular atrophy, feminizing hair changes, and loss of libido. In the adult, feminization is almost always due to carcinoma whereas in children it is more likely caused by an adenoma.

Mixed Endocrine Syndrome

Mixed endocrine syndrome refers to any combination of hypercortisolism, hyperaldosteronism, virilization or feminization syndromes. These are usually associated with adrenal cortical carcinoma. Cushing's syndrome caused by adrenal adenoma or hyperplasia may be associated with increased levels of sex hormones and/or their precursors, but actual clinical signs of virilization or feminization with Cushing's syndrome are usually seen only in adrenal carcinoma.

Neuroblastoma/Ganglioneuroblastoma

Neuroblastoma is a highly malignant neoplasm that arises most commonly in the adrenal medulla but may also originate in any sympathetic ganglia in an extra-adrenal location. Neuroblastoma is the most common solid, extracranial tumor in infants and children and the second most common intra-abdominal tumor in children after Wilms' tumor. Ninety percent of neuroblastomas become manifest within the first 8

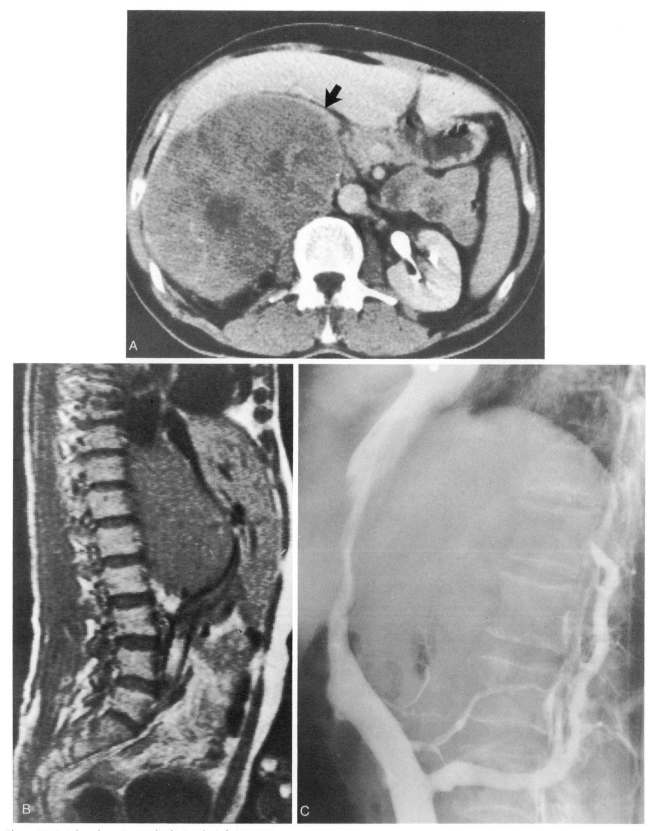

Figure 22–9. Adrenal carcinoma displacing the inferior vena cava.

A, Computed tomogram, contrast material enhanced. A large inhomogeneous mass displaces the inferior vena cava ventrally *(arrow)*. It is impossible to be certain whether tumor has extended into the inferior vena cava.

B, Magnetic resonance image, T1-weighted, sagittal section. The inferior vena cava is displaced but patent.

C, Cavogram. The inferior vena cava is narrowed but is free of tumor thrombus. Posterior collateral veins are prominent.

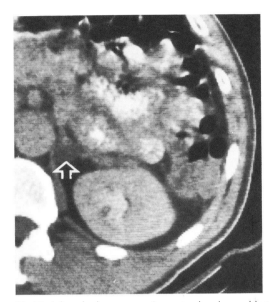

Figure 22–10. Adrenal adenoma causing secondary hyperaldosteronism (Conn's syndrome). Computed tomogram, contrast material enhanced. There is a small, well-defined mass *(arrow)* arising in the left adrenal. Characteristically mineralocorticoid-secreting adrenal adenomas have abundant tumor lipid with a resultant attenuation value near that of water.

years of life, while 50 per cent of patients are younger than 2 years of age when diagnosed. Both sexes are equally affected.

About one-half of patients with neuroblastoma present with a palpable mass, often with accompanying pain and fever. In 90 per cent of patients, there is an elevated level of vanillylmandelic acid that is the basis of the diagnosis. If there is intraspinal extension of tumor, then pain, paraplegia, limb weakness, urinary retention, constipation, or loss of bladder and bowel control become manifest. Neuroblastoma may be associated with spontaneous chaotic eye movements, particularly when voluntary eye movement is attempted, a condition known as opsoclonus-myoclonus. Watery diarrhea with hypokalemic achlorhydria due to a vasoactive polypeptide is present in approximately 10 per cent of patients with neuroblastoma.

Staging is extremely important in patient management and prognosis. A tumor confined to the adrenal gland is Stage I, while one that extends in continuity with the adrenal gland but remains on one side of the body is Stage II. Stage III is a localized tumor that crosses the midline, while Stage IV involves distant metastases. In Stage IV-S (special) metastases are confined to skin, bone marrow, or liver.

Pathologically, neuroblastoma is a solid, poorly defined tumor with conspicuous areas of hemorrhage and necrosis. Large tumors frequently engulf the aorta and other retroperitoneal structures. The kidneys and ureters are usually displaced laterally. Direct invasion into liver, kidney, pancreas, or the spinal canal is common. Rarely, neuroblastoma is cystic as a result of extensive hemorrhage and necrosis.

Ganglioneuroblastoma is a composite tumor that contains both mature ganglion cells and primitive neuroblastemal elements and is, in fact, a differentiating or maturing neuroblastoma. As such, a ganglioneuroblastoma has a better prognosis than a neuroblastoma. It is impossible to differentiate the two tumors radiologically.

Surgical excision remains the most successful means of therapy for neuroblastoma and ganglioneuroblastoma. The role of the radiologist is to determine extent of tumor, and, if possible, resectability. Regardless of size, tumors that invade major vessels, such as aorta, celiac plexus, or superior mesenteric artery, are not resectable. Tumors that cross the midline but do not come into contact with large vessels or are adherent to only one side of vessel may be resectable. Intraspinal extension is treated by decompressive laminectomy and debulking of tumor.

The ultrasonographic appearance of most abdominal neuroblastomas is that of a tumor of variable echogenicity with irregular hyperechoic areas intermixed with less echogenic areas. These correspond to foci of hemorrhage, necrosis, and microcalcification. Ultrasonography is usually able to demonstrate that the mass is extrarenal, thus establishing neuroblastoma rather than Wilms' tumor as the most likely diagnosis.

Computed tomography typically demonstrates a calcified, inhomogeneous solid mass with areas of hemorrhage and necrosis. Enhancement is usually inhomogeneous. Computed tomography nicely demonstrates the relation of the tumor to adjacent organs and blood vessels. Intrathecal contrast material facilitates detection of spinal extension, which can also be seen by magnetic resonance imaging without myelography. Neuroblastoma arising from the adrenal is similar in appearance to extra-adrenal neuroblastoma (see Fig. 21–36).

Magnetic resonance imaging is sometimes helpful in evaluating the extent of a tumor for planning either radiation or surgical therapy, as well as for monitoring tumor size as a follow-up (Fig. 22–12). Magnetic resonance imaging does require sedation in very young patients but obviates the need for intrathecal injection of contrast material. On T1-weighted images metastases in the medullary cavities of bones can also be imaged as low signal foci relative to higher signal in bone marrow.

On any imaging modality, a cystic neuroblastoma may be difficult to distinguish from adrenal hemorrhage, as discussed subsequently in this chapter. Differential features favoring neuroblastoma include elevated vanillylmandelic acid, discovery beyond the neonatal period, failure to regress over time, and the presence of a solid component (Fig. 22–13).

Neuroblastoma that develops in infants younger than 1 year of age is less aggressive and associated with a better prognosis than neuroblastoma that arises in older children. In neonatal neuroblastoma, therefore, a neuroblastoma may mature into a well-differentiated, benign neoplasm (i.e., a ganglioneuroma). This, however, is extremely rare.

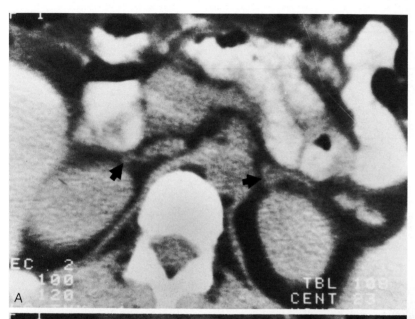

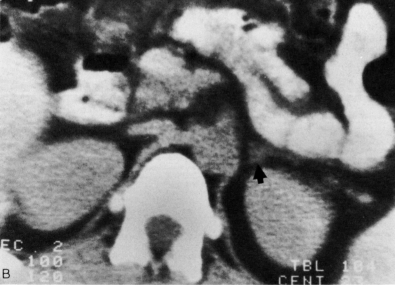

Figure 22–11. Adrenal hyperplasia, bilateral, causing hyperaldosteronism.

A and *B,* Computed tomograms, contrast material enhanced, consecutive 4-mm thick sections. There is a small nodular mass in each adrenal gland *(arrows).* Venous sampling demonstrated elevated levels of mineralocorticoids in each gland.

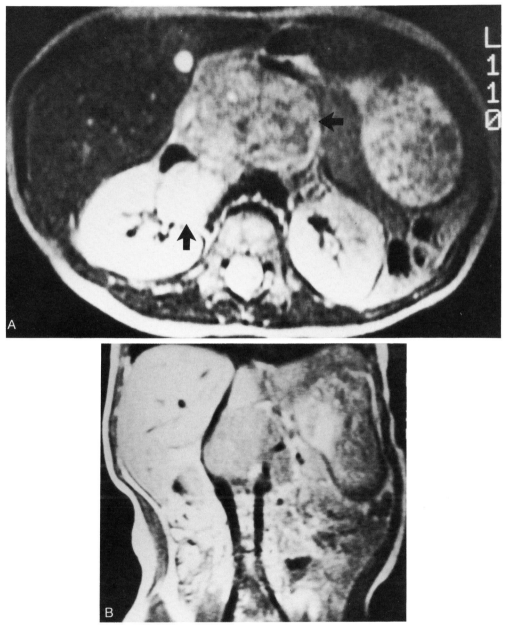

Figure 22–12. Neuroblastoma, Stage 3 (crosses midline). There is a lobulated heterogeneous mass with two discrete components. One is medial to the right kidney, and the other is ventral to the aorta *(arrows)*. The inferior vena cava is displaced laterally and ventrally and is separated from the aorta, which is patent and in normal position.

A, Magnetic resonance image, axial section.

B, Magnetic resonance image, coronal section.

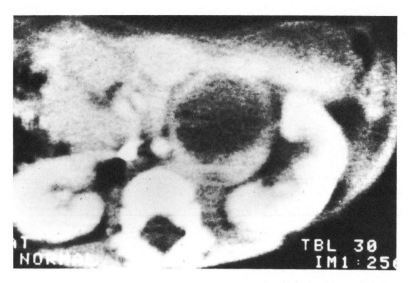

Figure 22–13. Neuroblastoma, cystic, in a 4-month-old infant with an abdominal mass. Computed tomogram, contrast material enhanced. There is a thick-walled, cystic adrenal mass displacing and distorting the left kidney.

Ganglioneuroma

Ganglioneuroma is a benign neoplasm that is composed of ganglion cells, a variable number of Schwann cells, and collagen. Ganglioneuroma occurs at all ages; most are asymptomatic. Adrenal ganglioneuroma is rarely associated with hypertension despite the fact that levels of urinary catecholamines and their metabolites are often elevated. *Verner-Morrison syndrome* consists of watery diarrhea, hypochlorhydria, and alkalosis due to secretion of a vasoactive intestinal polypeptide by a ganglioneuroma.

Ganglioneuromas are usually oval or spherical and sharply marginated. Calcification may be present. Large amounts of hemorrhage and necrosis are un-common. Most tumors are uniformly solid. Radiologic features of ganglioneuroma are nonspecific (Fig. 22–14). The diagnosis of ganglioneuroma can be suggested in a nonhypertensive patient with an adrenal mass and an elevated level of catecholamine and catecholamine metabolites or with Verner-Morrison syndrome.

Pheochromocytoma

Pheochromocytoma is a neoplasm of the adrenal medulla composed of paraganglionic cells that contain catecholamines. The term *pheochromocytoma* should be restricted to tumors that arise within the adrenal

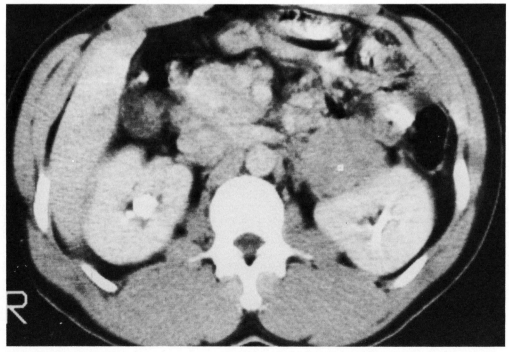

Figure 22–14. Ganglioneuroma. Computed tomogram, contrast material enhanced. A well-defined 5-cm homogeneous adrenal mass compresses the left kidney.

gland. The same tumor arising in the sympathetic chain outside the adrenal gland should be referred to as a paraganglioma rather than an extra-adrenal pheochromocytoma. These are discussed in Chapter 21.

Excess catecholamine production causes labile or sustained hypertension combined with episodes of perspiration, palpitations, and anxiety. The 24-hour urine vanillylmandelic acid level is elevated in over 90 per cent of patients. The presence of free norepinephrine in a 24-hour urine specimen is the most sensitive indicator of functioning paraganglioma. Plasma catecholamine measurement is less accurate than assays of urine because secretion by a paraganglioma is often intermittent and because intravenous sampling may cause a stress-related increase in plasma catecholamine levels.

Pheochromocytoma has been associated with *multiple endocrine neoplasia 2 syndrome, multiple endocrine neoplasia 3 syndrome, tuberous sclerosis, von Hippel-Lindau disease, neurofibromatosis, and Carney's syndrome.* Fifty percent of patients with multiple endocrine neoplasia syndrome are asymptomatic.

The mean diameter of a pheochromocytoma is 6 cm, although in association with the multiple endocrine neoplasia syndromes the tumor is often smaller and difficult to image. The term *medullary hyperplasia* has been applied to hyperfunctioning nodules less than 1 cm in diameter. Hemorrhage and necrosis are common in large pheochromocytomas. Indeed, the tumor may become cystic as a result of extensive hemorrhage. About 10 per cent of pheochromocytomas calcify and 10 per cent are associated with extra-adrenal paragangliomas or are bilateral.

Approximately 10 per cent of pheochromocytomas are malignant. However, both the radiologic and histologic diagnosis of malignancy is dependent on the presence of metastases rather than an inherent, distinctive set of features. Frequent sites of metastases include bone, lymph nodes, lung, and liver. Extension or direct invasion into the inferior vena cava is not common. Recurrence of metastases 3 to 5 years after resection of a primary malignant pheochromocytoma tumor may occur.

The optimal strategy for the radiologic evaluation of a patient with suspected pheochromocytoma is controversial. Computed tomography has a high sensitivity (more than 90 per cent) in the detection of functioning pheochromocytoma. Contrast material is rarely required. Glucagon is contraindicated because it may provoke a hypertensive crisis. A small tumor is usually homogeneous, while a large tumor often contains areas of diminished attenuation reflecting necrosis (Fig. 22–15). Those with extensive hemorrhage may be confused radiologically with an adrenal cyst (Fig. 22–16). As stated earlier, bilateral pheochromocytomas are present in about 10 per cent of cases (Fig. 22–17).

There are, however, several important limitations of computed tomography. It is impossible to differentiate pheochromocytoma from other types of adrenal tumors by computed tomography alone. Clip artifacts often make evaluation for recurrence following surgery difficult. Computed tomography appears to be less reliable than magnetic resonance imaging and radionuclide studies for very small nodules (medullary hyperplasia), for extra-adrenal tumors, and for metastatic disease. Despite these limitations, computed tomography is the preferred technique for initial evaluation of a patient with clinical evidence of a catecholamine-producing tumor.

Magnetic resonance imaging is another excellent technique to evaluate a patient with suspected pheochromocytoma. Magnetic resonance imaging is particularly useful in detecting extra-adrenal paragangliomas, especially those arising in the wall of the bladder and paracardiac region, in evaluating the postoperative patient, in patients with hypertension and only

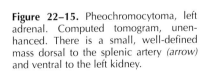

Figure 22–15. Pheochromocytoma, left adrenal. Computed tomogram, unenhanced. There is a small, well-defined mass dorsal to the splenic artery *(arrow)* and ventral to the left kidney.

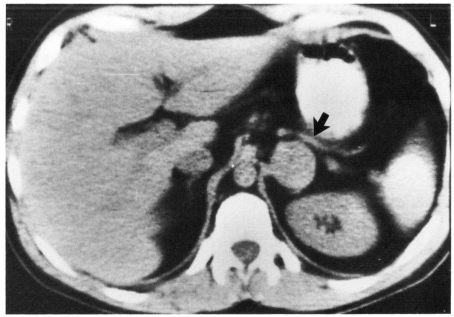

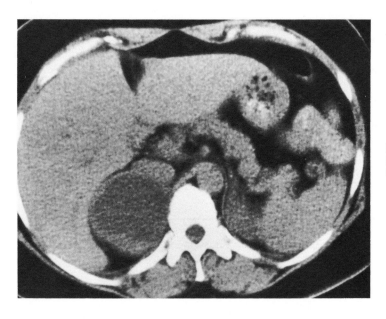

Figure 22–16. Pheochromocytoma, cystic, right adrenal. Computed tomogram, unenhanced. There is a 6-cm thick-walled cystic adrenal mass dorsal to the inferior vena cava.

mildly elevated catecholamine levels, and in patients at increased risk for developing paraganglioma (e.g., von Hippel-Lindau syndrome).

On T1-weighted images, a pheochromocytoma has a signal intensity that is lower than or equivalent to that of liver, kidney, or muscle, while on T2-weighted images, the signal intensity is very high (see Fig. 22–17A). A pheochromocytoma exhibits inhomogeneous enhancement after injection of gadolinium. These signal characteristics readily support the diagnosis of pheochromocytoma in the appropriate clinical setting.

MIBG is a norepinephrine analogue that may be useful as a radionuclide agent when other imaging modalities are equivocal because it accumulates at sites of norepinephrine synthesis. It is especially helpful in detecting medullary hyperplasia, recurrence, metastases, or extra-adrenal paragangliomas (see Fig. 22–17B). MIBG has the advantage of imaging the entire body with one dose of the radionuclide. Disadvantages of MIBG include limited availability, relatively poor spatial resolution, and the length of the procedure (1 to 3 days). The specificity of an MIBG scan is not 100 per cent. Other tumors, such as neuroblastoma, carcinoid, medullary carcinoma, choriocarcinoma, and atypical schwannoma can also accumulate the radionuclide, although in a clinical setting

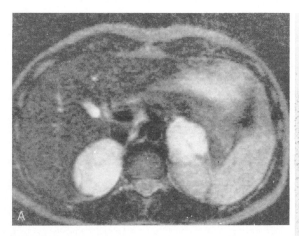

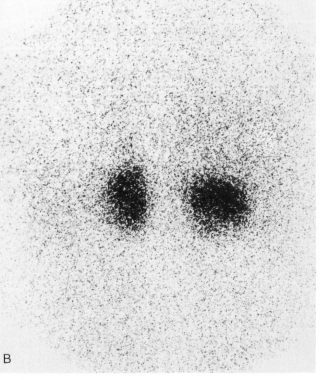

Figure 22–17. Pheochromocytoma, bilateral.
  A, Magnetic resonance image, T2 weighted. Both tumors have a very bright signal.
  B, MIBG scan. There is uptake of radionuclide by both tumors.

different from that of pheochromocytoma. This technique is also discussed in Chapter 2.

Addison's Disease

Addison's disease (adrenal insufficiency) results from reduced secretion of adrenal steroid hormones to a level below that required for endocrine homeostasis. Advanced cases are usually readily apparent clinically. Recognition of early disease, however, is often difficult. The most common symptoms of adrenal insufficiency are slowly progressive fatigability, weakness, anorexia, weight loss, cutaneous and mucosal pigmentation, hypotension, and, occasionally, hypoglycemia. These features are nonspecific and easily confused with other, more common, chronic illnesses. Occasionally, sudden, massive adrenal destruction due to sepsis or adrenal hemorrhage causes acute adrenal insufficiency that presents as fulminating shock.

Although there are many causes of Addison's disease, as enumerated in Table 22–2, two radiologic patterns dominate. The most common pattern is that of adrenal atrophy with diminutive glands (Fig. 22–18). In these cases glandular atrophy is idiopathic and presumed to be due to autoimmune destruction. These patients are often cachectic and not efficaciously examined by computed tomography because of absent retroperitoneal fat and the small size of both adrenal glands. The other major pattern seen in Addison's disease is that of bilateral adrenal enlargement with preservation of the adrenal shape (Fig. 22–19). This occurs when the adrenal gland is replaced by inflammatory or neoplastic cells, abnormal metabolites, or hemorrhage.

Table 22–2. CAUSES OF ADRENAL INSUFFICIENCY

Idiopathic atrophy (autoimmune)
Replacement diseases
    Tuberculosis
    Histoplasmosis
    Blastomycosis
    Amyloidosis
    Hemorrhage
    Metastatic disease
    Lymphoma

ABNORMAL ADRENAL MORPHOLOGY WITH NORMAL FUNCTION

The most common causes of an adrenal mass with normal adrenal function are a nonhyperfunctioning adenoma, metastatic disease, cyst, hemorrhage, myelolipoma, and granulomatous disease. Rare causes of a nonfunctioning mass include mesenchymal tumor (e.g., leiomyosarcoma), primary melanoma, and hemangioma. Rare causes of bilateral adrenal enlargement include extramedullary hematopoiesis and Wolman's disease. Additionally, the functional adrenal masses previously discussed must also be considered since occasionally they are nonfunctional, as for example, the 10 per cent of pheochromocytomas that do not hyperfunction.

Metastases

The adrenal gland is the fourth most common site for metastatic disease, surpassed only by lung, liver, and bone. At autopsy about one-fourth of patients with epithelial malignancy have metastases to the adrenal.

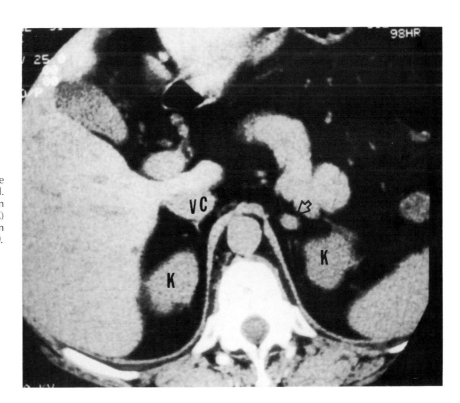

Figure 22–18. Addison's disease, destructive pattern. Computed tomogram, unenhanced. The adrenal glands are barely visible as thin linear densities between the right kidney (K) and the inferior vena cava (VC) and between the left kidney (K) and the splenic vein *(arrow).*

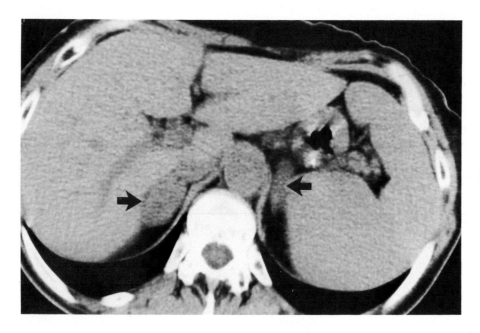

Figure 22–19. Addison's disease, replacement pattern, in a patient with histoplasmosis. Computed tomogram, unenhanced. Both glands *(arrows)* are enlarged with convex margins.

The most common primary neoplasms that metastasize to the adrenal are carcinoma of lung, breast, thyroid, or colon, lymphoma, and melanoma.

In most patients metastases to the adrenal gland are not apparent clinically. A large tumor or one that is complicated by hemorrhage may cause flank pain or a palpable mass. Even with complete replacement of both glands, adrenal insufficiency is uncommon. Steroids used as part of a chemotherapeutic regimen may mask Addison's disease.

There are five pathologic and radiologic patterns of metastases to the adrenal gland: small (less than 5 cm in diameter) mass, large (more than 5 cm in diameter) mass, multiple masses, diffuse adrenal enlargement, and normal-appearing glands. The computed tomographic findings, however, cannot distinguish metastases from other entities that affect the adrenal gland.

Typically the small (less than 5 cm) mass is homogeneous but may have mixed density (Fig. 22–20). Rarely, increased attenuation values caused by hemorrhage or calcification is present. It is impossible to distinguish a metastasis from a nonhyperfunctioning adenoma on the basis of computed tomographic appearance alone. Magnetic resonance imaging and NP-59 radionuclide scan may be helpful in this differentiation. Metastases to the adrenal gland are typically isointense with liver on T1-weighted images and brighter than liver on T2-weighted images (Fig. 22–21). As previously noted, adenoma typically has a signal intensity similar to liver on both T1- and T2-weighted images (see Fig. 22–6). Using liver signal intensity as a reference, however, may be misleading when the liver is affected by pathologic processes such as iron deposition, hepatitis, or fatty infiltration.

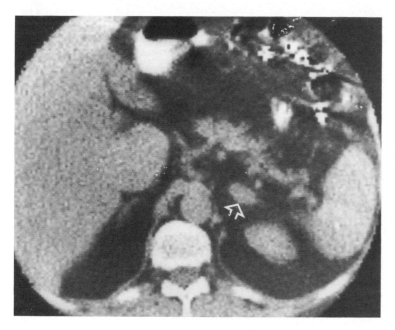

Figure 22–20. Metastases producing a small mass in left adrenal. Computed tomogram, contrast material enhanced. The metastasis *(arrow)* was from a small cell carcinoma of the lung.

Figure 22–21. Metastases to both adrenal glands from renal cell carcinoma. There are masses in both adrenal glands *(arrowheads)*, as well as a mass in the liver *(arrows)*. On the T2-weighted image *(B)* the signal intensity of the metastases is greater than the uninvolved liver. Compare with the signal intensity of an adenoma illustrated in Figure 22–6C.

A, T1-weighted magnetic resonance image.

B, T2-weighted magnetic resonance image at the same level.

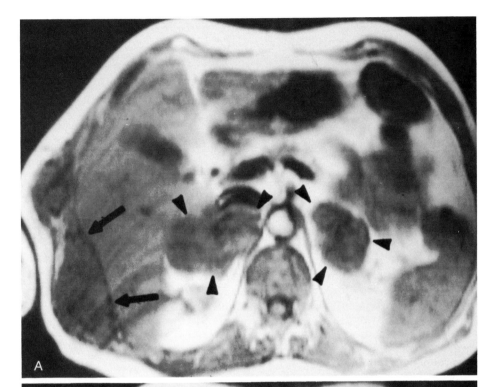

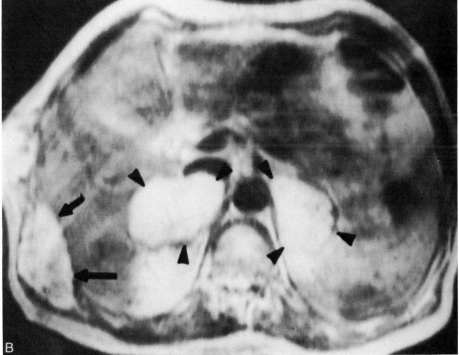

Because adenomas generally contain small amounts of fat, while metastases do not, fat suppression techniques may be helpful in some cases. If the mass decreases in signal intensity on fat suppression, it is likely benign. Otherwise, it is likely malignant (Mitchell et al., 1992). Calculated T2-weighted values have also been used; values less than 60 msec imply benign disease, while those greater than 65 msec imply malignant disease. Enhancement characteristics on dynamic, enhanced magnetic resonance images have also been reported to be helpful. A combination of the above techniques may prove optimal in avoiding biopsy. An adrenal metastasis of any size does not accumulate NP-59, whereas a nonhyperfunctioning adenoma greater than 2 cm in diameter does accumulate radionuclide.

An adrenal metastasis larger than 5 cm in diameter is less of a diagnostic problem than is a small metastatic nodule in that it is usually associated with advanced disease and a known primary site (Fig. 22–22). Large metastases are often inhomogeneous owing to hemorrhage or necrosis. Occasionally, hemorrhage extends into the perinephric space (Fig. 22–23).

Multiple adrenal masses or bilateral adrenal enlargement signifying diffuse infiltration are additional manifestations of metastatic disease to the adrenal gland (Figs. 22–24 and 22–25). When the metastases are small, the intervening gland is normal in size. With both patterns there is frequently other evidence of abdominal metastases, such as adenopathy or liver metastases. Calcification, most likely the result of prior hemorrhage and/or necrosis, may occur in approximately 16 per cent of cases with these patterns.

The radiologic identification of a normal adrenal gland does not exclude microscopic metastatic disease. In one series of patients with small cell lung carcinoma, biopsy of adrenal glands that appeared normal on computed tomography were found to contain malignant cells in 17 per cent of patients (Pagani, 1983).

Lymphoma

Adrenal gland involvement is found in up to 25 per cent of patients with lymphoma at autopsy. Non-Hodgkin's lymphoma is more likely to involve the adrenal than is Hodgkin's disease. The most common pattern is diffuse enlargement with oval, round, or triangular-shaped glands (see Fig. 22–24). Bilateral involvement occurs in 50 per cent of cases and is frequently accompanied by retroperitoneal lymphadenopathy. Necrosis is uncommon in the absence of prior chemotherapy or radiation therapy. Primary lymphoma of the adrenal gland is extremely rare.

Cyst

An adrenal cyst is an uncommon, fluid-filled, nonneoplastic mass that is usually detected as an incidental finding in a patient with no other evidence of adrenal disease. A large cyst may cause pain. Although the exact etiology in many cases is uncertain, the majority are believed to be pseudocysts that have evolved from prior adrenal hemorrhage, as discussed in the section that follows. A typical adrenal cyst has a fluid-filled center surrounded by a thin wall that does not enhance. This radiologic appearance is similar to a renal cyst, except that up to 15 per cent of adrenal cysts develop peripheral calcification (Fig. 22–26). However, a cystic neoplasm, such as a pheochromocytoma, or rarely an adrenal abscess may produce a similar appearance (see Fig. 22–16).

Hemorrhage

Hemorrhage is the most common cause of an adrenal mass in the neonatal period. This usually occurs in

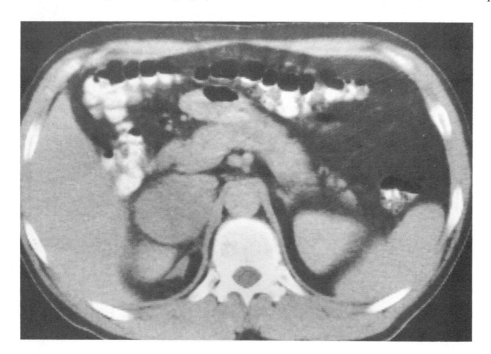

Figure 22–22. Metastases producing a large mass in the right adrenal. Computed tomogram, contrast material enhanced. A melanoma had been excised several years previously.

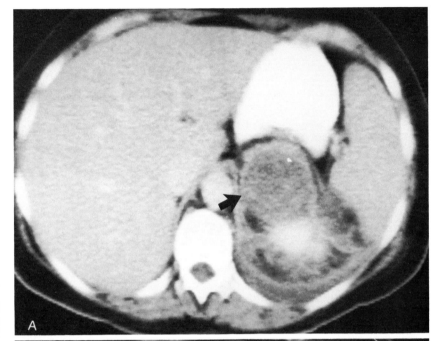

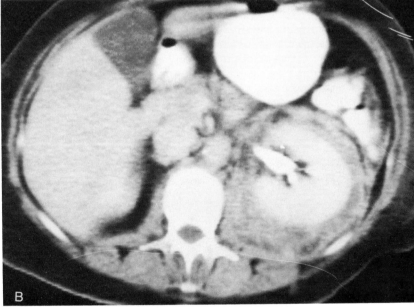

Figure 22–23. Metastasis to the adrenal complicated by perinephric hemorrhage.

A, Computed tomogram with contrast material enhancement through the upper pole of the left kidney. There is a large inhomogeneous adrenal mass *(arrow)* that is separate from the kidney.

B, Computed tomogram with contrast material enhancement caudal to *A*. There is blood in the perinephric space.

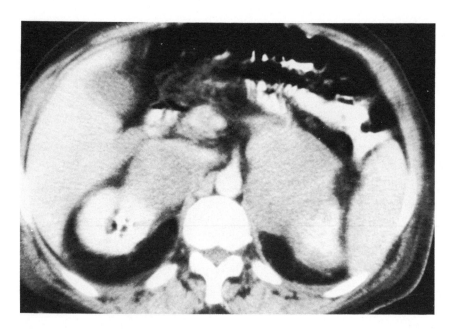

Figure 22–24. Metastases, bilateral, secondary to lymphoma. Computed tomogram, contrast material enhanced. Large masses replace both adrenal glands.

association with birth trauma, hypoxia, renal vein thrombosis, sepsis, coagulopathy, or macrosomia related to maternal diabetes mellitus. The clinical triad of mass, blood loss anemia, and prolonged jaundice is characteristic for neonatal adrenal hemorrhage. In hemorrhage due to birth trauma, the right gland is more frequently involved than the left, possibly because the right adrenal gland is compressed between the spine and the liver. Although 10 per cent of cases of adrenal hemorrhage are bilateral, adrenal insufficiency is very uncommon.

In the adult, adrenal hemorrhage may result from severe stress, burns, sepsis, hypertension, renal vein thrombosis, liver transplantation affecting the right adrenal, underlying adrenal disease (especially tumors), anticoagulation therapy, and trauma. *Waterhouse-Friedrichson syndrome* was originally described as bilateral adrenal hemorrhage complicating meningococcal septicemia. Recently, this definition has been

expanded to include bilateral adrenal hemorrhage as a complication of any cause of sepsis. Bilateral adrenal hemorrhage in the adult may cause acute adrenal insufficiency and death if not recognized and treated with adrenal corticosteroids. The diagnosis is frequently delayed, however, because clinical findings are often nonspecific.

The ultrasonographic appearance of adrenal hemorrhage varies with the acuteness of the process. Acute hemorrhage often appears as a round or oval suprarenal mass that is slightly hyperechoic relative to liver. Occasionally the echo pattern suggests a solid mass. With time, the lesion becomes more hypoechoic and cystlike. An organizing hematoma decreases in size, becomes multiloculated and, typically, resolves or calcifies over time (Figs. 22–27 and 22–28). If a suspected hematoma does not resolve, regress, or calcify, or if the patient becomes febrile or demonstrates an elevated urinary vanillylmandelic acid value, alternative

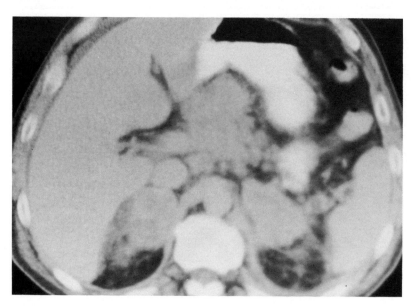

Figure 22–25. Metastases, bilateral. Computed tomogram, unenhanced. There is an ill-defined, inhomogeneous right adrenal mass. The left gland is large and has convex margins and a triangular shape. Extensive celiac adenopathy dorsal to the stomach and stranding in the perinephric fat are additional evidence of disseminated disease.

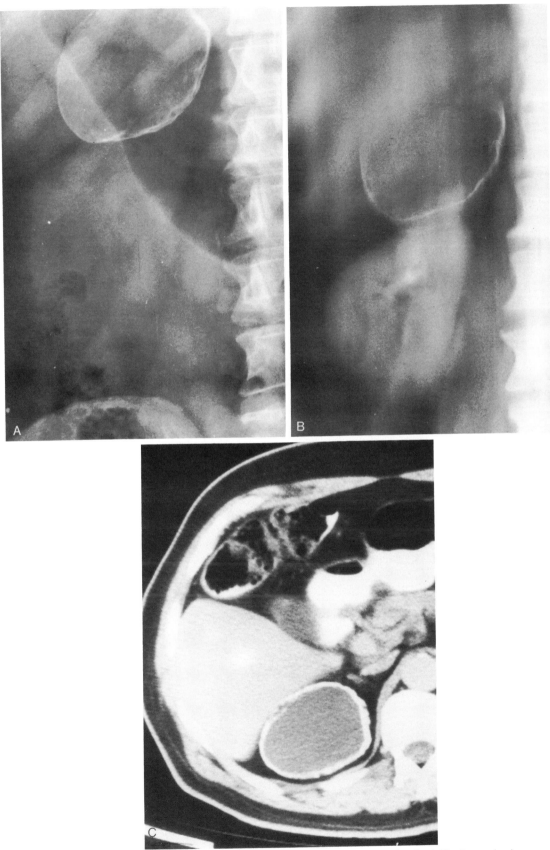

Figure 22–26. Cyst, calcified, right adrenal. There is a well-defined, suprarenal mass with peripheral calcification and a homogeneous water density center.

A, Abdominal radiograph.

B, Excretory urogram, tomogram.

C, Computed tomogram, contrast material enhanced.

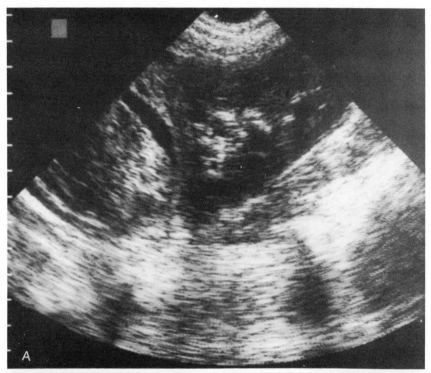

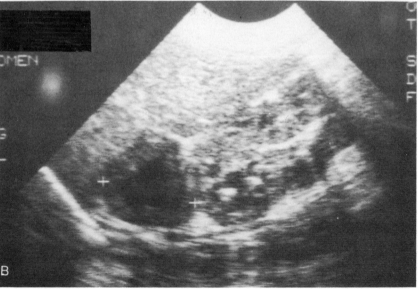

Figure 22–27. Hemorrhage, adrenal in three patients with different ultrasonographic patterns.
 A, Solid-appearing hemorrhage.
 B, Cystic hemorrhage with a thick wall and internal echoes.

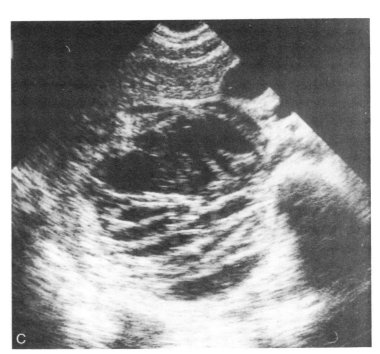

Figure 22–27. *Continued C,* Multiloculated, organizing hemorrhage.

diagnoses must be considered. These would include adrenal abscess complicating adrenal hemorrhage or a rare neonatal adrenal neoplasm, such as a congenital neuroblastoma.

The computed tomographic findings of adrenal hemorrhage vary with the age of the lesion and whether it is masslike or infiltrative. Initially, a hematoma exhibits increased attenuation values in the range of 50 to 90 Hounsfield units. This appears hyperdense relative to unenhanced renal parenchyma. Hemorrhage in the form of a mass is usually inhomogeneous and may be associated with a perinephric component (Fig. 22–29). This appearance may be identical to an adrenal tumor that has bled. When hemorrhage is infiltra-

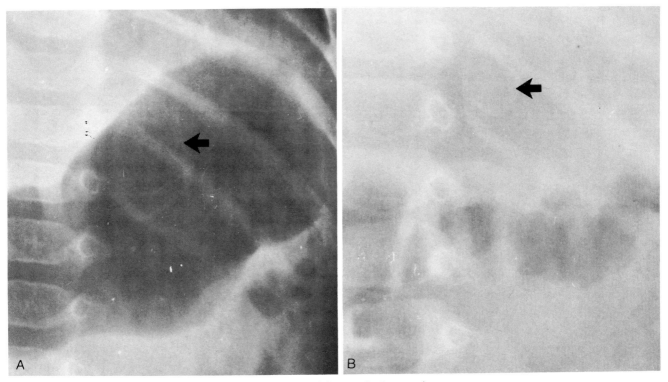

Figure 22–28. Hemorrhage, left adrenal, with calcification and decrease in size over time.
A, Abdominal radiograph at 1 month of age. A mass with peripheral calcification *(arrow)* overlies the 11th and 12th posterior ribs.
B, Abdominal radiograph. Ten months later the calcified mass *(arrow)* has diminished in size.

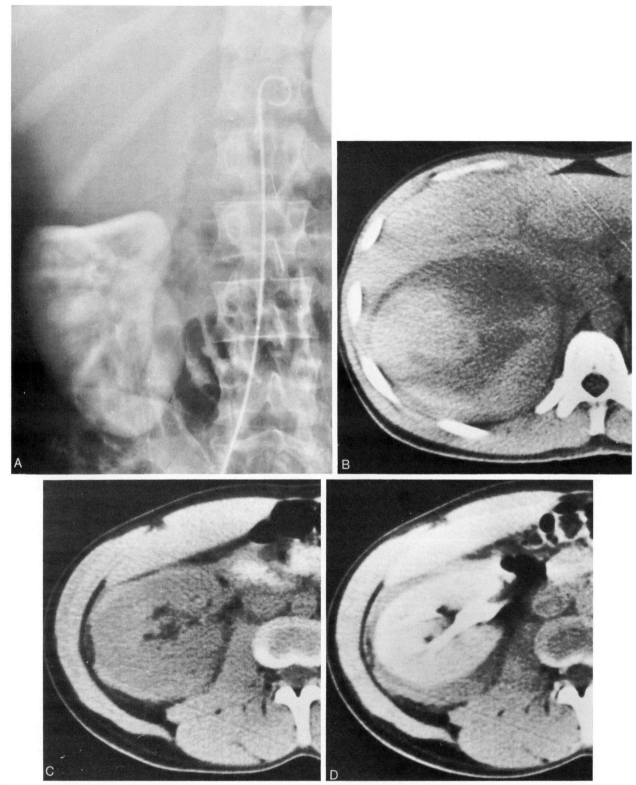

Figure 22–29. Hemorrhage, right adrenal, presenting as a large mass with extension of blood into perinephric space.

A, Aortogram, nephrographic phase. There is inferior displacement of the right kidney by a large, extrarenal mass.

B, Computed tomogram without contrast material enhancement through the mass demonstrates mixed densities. The high density area corresponds to fresh hemorrhage.

C, Computed tomogram without contrast material enhancement at the level of the right renal pelvis. The high density blood in the perinephric space forms a thin rim around the unenhanced kidney.

D, Computed tomogram, contrast material enhanced at the same level as *C* confirms the nonenhancing perinephric hemorrhage.

tive rather than masslike, the adrenal gland is enlarged with convex thickening of the limbs (Fig. 22–30). This appearance may simulate one of the infiltrative diseases listed in Table 22–7. However, high attenuation values are characteristic for hemorrhage.

As the hematoma organizes, the attenuation values decrease and the lesion becomes cystic (Fig. 22–31). The wall of the cystic hematoma is initially thick and irregular but eventually becomes thin and frequently calcifies. At this stage, differentiation between an adrenal cyst and a mature cystic hematoma becomes impossible. Indeed, many apparent adrenal cysts are likely the result of an organized adrenal hemorrhage.

The appearance of adrenal hemorrhage with magnetic resonance imaging varies with the evolution of hemoglobin breakdown. Immediately after a hematoma is formed, it appears relatively hypointense on T1-weighted images and hyperintense on T2-weighted images. Over time, T1-weighted images may reveal the formation of a relatively bright ring that progresses inward toward the center of the lesion. The periphery, which may contain hemosiderin laden macrophages, may produce a thin dark rim on both T1- and T2-weighted images in subacute or chronic hematoma (Fig. 22–32). Although fat and hemorrhage are both bright on T1-weighted images, distinction can usually be made on T2-weighted images since fat will not appear brighter than normal fat elsewhere in the body, whereas hemorrhage often does. This, in addition to the ringlike pattern, is highly suggestive of hemorrhage.

Myelolipoma

Myelolipoma is an uncommon, benign, metabolically inactive tumor composed of adipose and myeloid tissue. It is usually detected as an incidental finding in adults undergoing an examination for unrelated clinical indications. Autopsy series have shown a prevalence of less than 0.2 per cent and an equal sex distribution. Almost all adrenal myelolipomas originate in the adrenal cortex and are often 10 cm in diameter or larger. Rarely, myelolipoma occurs in an extra-adrenal retroperitoneal location. All myelolipomas contain fat as adipose tissue and myeloid elements in proportions that vary considerably. However, most have sufficient fat to permit detection by computed tomography or magnetic resonance imaging.

Symptoms produced by a myelolipoma relate to the size of the tumor. Spontaneous bleeding can cause acute flank pain or even hypovolemic shock and is more likely to occur in tumors that are composed of myeloid tissue.

The radiologic appearance of myelolipoma depends on the relative amount of fat and of myeloid tissue and whether there has been hemorrhage. In most lesions, the fatty component is predominant and recognizable as radiolucency on abdominal radiographs, as a hyperechoic mass on ultrasonograms, as a mass with negative attenuation values on computed tomograms, or as bright signal intensity mass on T1-

weighted magnetic resonance images (Fig. 22–33). Distinction between fat and hemorrhage may be difficult on T1-weighted images since both appear bright. T2-weighted images usually enable differentiation in that fat does not appear brighter than normal fat elsewhere in the body, whereas hemorrhage often does. Fat suppression techniques may be extremely helpful in differentiating fat from hemorrhage.

The finding of a fat-containing, well-marginated tumor in the region of the adrenal gland strongly suggests the diagnosis of myelolipoma. Rarely, a metastasis or other aggressive lesion may engulf normal retroperitoneal fat as it spreads and may simulate the appearance of fat-containing tumor. Calcification is often present, especially in myelolipomas that have bled.

A myelolipoma that is composed primarily of myeloid tissue may be hypoechoic on ultrasonography and have characteristics of red marrow on other imaging studies. In the absence of radiologically detectable fat, a confident radiologic diagnosis of myelolipoma is not possible (Fig. 22–34). Biopsy may be very helpful in cases with equivocal findings of fat. In cases complicated by infarction or hematoma, the margins of the tumor may become irregular owing to blood dissecting into the retroperitoneal fat. Here, findings of acute, subacute, or chronic bleeding become superimposed on the tumor.

Granulomatous Disease

Infections that produce granulomatous reaction in the adrenal glands (usually tuberculosis or histoplasmosis) typically cause bilateral enlargement. Adrenal destruction with Addison's disease occurs in the absence of appropriate treatment. Historically, tuberculosis was the most common cause of Addison's disease.

Adrenal glands enlarged by granulomatous disease have rounded contours and resemble inflated balloons. Extension beyond the adrenal is very unusual. On computed tomography, enlarged glands usually contain lucent areas that represent necrosis. The contour may be smooth or lobular (see Fig. 22–19). With treatment, the glands often decrease in size and may become normal in appearance. Calcification may be stippled or solid when it occurs. Occasionally, a dense zone of calcification without evidence of a normal adrenal remnant is the only manifestation of healed granulomatous disease.

Uncommonly, granulomatous disease of the adrenal gland forms a mass, such as a tuberculoma. Such an appearance is impossible to differentiate from the nonfunctioning masses discussed earlier.

Rare Adrenal Masses

Rare adrenal tumors include mesenchymal tumors, such as *leiomyosarcoma, primary melanoma*, and *hemangioma*. These usually present as a large adrenal mass with normal adrenal function. Although the presence of phleboliths and contrast material pooling on angi-

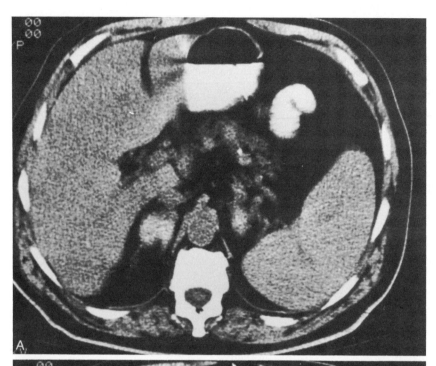

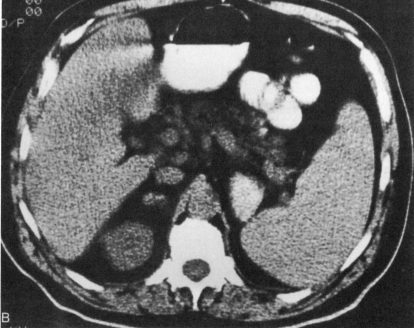

Figure 22–30. Hemorrhage, bilateral adrenal, in a 60-year-old man with sepsis.

A and *B,* Computed tomogram without contrast material enhancement at two adjacent levels. Both adrenals are enlarged and their attenuation is greater than that of liver, a finding seen with acute hemorrhage.

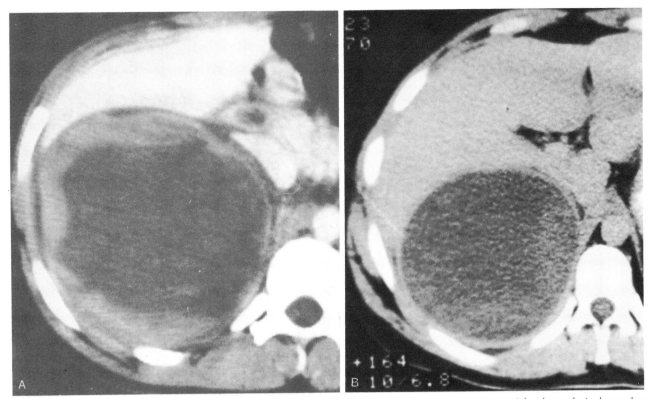

Figure 22–31. Hemorrhage, organizing in right adrenal in two patients. Computed tomogram, contrast material enhanced. As hemorrhage organizes, its attenuation value approaches that of water. The wall may be thick and irregular *(A)* or thin and smooth *(B)*. In the latter case, differentiation from an adrenal cyst is extremely difficult. (Compare with Fig. 22–26.)

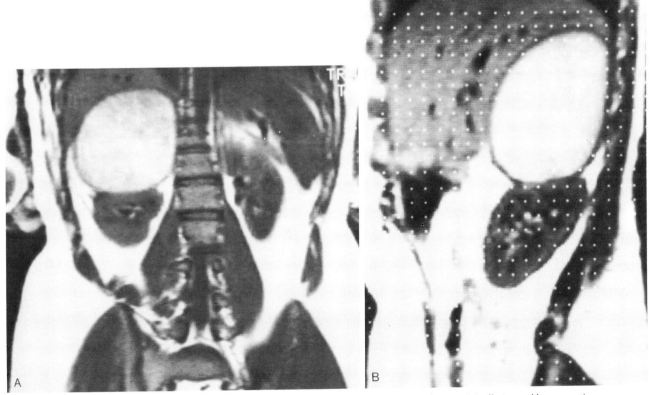

Figure 22–32. Hemorrhage, right adrenal. Magnetic resonance images. Adrenal hemorrhage is characteristically imaged by magnetic resonance as a well-defined, mildly heterogeneous mass with a signal that is slightly less intense than adjacent retroperitoneal fat. Differentiation from myelolipoma is difficult when utilizing T1-weighted images. (Compare with Fig. 22–33*B*.)

A, T1-weighted image, coronal section.

B, T1-weighted image, sagittal section.

745

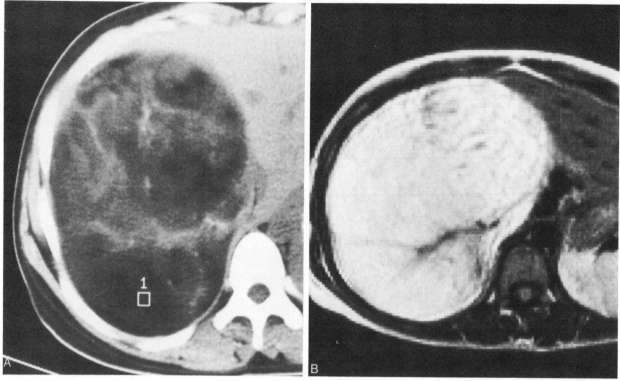

Figure 22–33. Myelolipoma, right adrenal. Fatty areas within the tumor are similar to normal subcutaneous fat. The higher density strands on computed tomography and the low signal areas on the magnetic resonance scan correspond to areas of hemorrhage or myeloid tissue.
  A, Computed tomogram, unenhanced.
  B, Magnetic resonance image, T1 weighted.

ography has been reported as characteristic for hemangioma, an accurate diagnosis is rarely made prospectively. Likewise, a specific radiologic diagnosis is rarely possible in cases of mesenchymal adrenal tumors.

Extramedullary hematopoiesis is a rare cause of adrenal enlargement. It may be seen in diseases associated with decreased red blood cell production by bone marrow. Adrenal enlargement in extramedullary hematopoiesis may, in part, result from hemorrhage that sometimes is a complicating factor.

Wolman's disease (familial xanthomatosis) is a rare metabolic disease that involves the adrenal glands. A disturbance in fat metabolism results in an abnormal

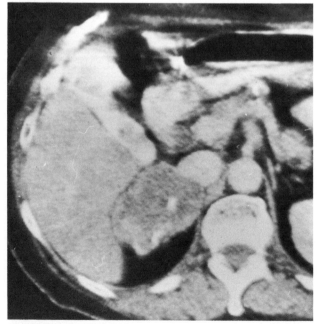

Figure 22–34. Myelolipoma, right adrenal, with calcification but no radiologically demonstrable fat. Computed tomogram, contrast material enhanced.

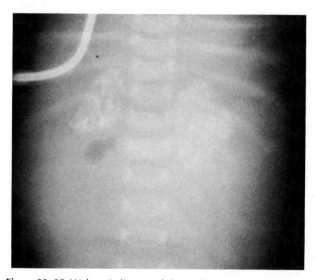

Figure 22–35. Wolman's disease. Abdominal radiograph. Both adrenal glands are enlarged and diffusely calcified.

Table 22–3. DIAGNOSTIC SET: SMALL (<5 cm) SOLID
MASS (See Fig. 22–6)

Hyperfunction
 Adenoma
 Hyperplasia
 Pheochromocytoma
 Neuroblastoma/Ganglioneuroblastoma
 Ganglioneuroma
Normal function
 Metastases
 Adenoma
 Myelolipoma
 Neuroblastoma/Ganglioneuroblastoma
 Ganglioneuroma

accumulation of triglyceride and cholesterol esters. Characteristically, affected patients are children with hepatosplenomegaly and enlarged adrenals with punctate calcifications in areas of tissue necrosis (Fig. 22–35).

DIAGNOSTIC SETS

When confronted with an adrenal mass, it is useful to categorize the lesion in one of the following diagnostic sets:

> **SMALL ADRENAL MASS (LESS THAN 5 CM DIAMETER)**
> **LARGE ADRENAL MASS (MORE THAN 5 CM DIAMETER)**
> **CYSTIC ADRENAL MASS**
> **MULTIPLE ADRENAL MASSES**
> **ADRENAL ENLARGEMENT**
> **ADRENAL CALCIFICATION**

Each of these diagnostic sets includes entities that can be further characterized as to whether the patient in question exhibits adrenal hyperfunction, normal function, or diminished function. Each diagnostic set is formulated in Tables 22–3 through 22–8. Other radiologic features that might enable a specific diagnosis should be sought. Usually, however, only a differential diagnosis is possible.

Table 22–4. DIAGNOSTIC SET: LARGE (>5 cm) SOLID
MASS (See Fig. 22–9)

Hyperfunction
 Carcinoma
 Pheochromocytoma
 Neuroblastoma/Ganglioneuroblastoma
 Ganglioneuroma
Normal function
 Carcinoma
 Metastases
 Myelolipoma
 Pheochromocytoma
 Neuroblastoma
 Granuloma (e.g., tuberculoma)
 Rare tumors (e.g., mesenchymal tumor)

Table 22–5. DIAGNOSTIC SET: CYSTIC ADRENAL
MASS (see Fig. 22–26)

Normal function
 Cyst
 Organizing hemorrhage
 Pheochromocytoma
 Neuroblastoma
Hyperfunction
 Pheochromocytoma
 Neuroblastoma

Table 22–6. DIAGNOSTIC SET: MULTIPLE ADRENAL
MASSES (see Fig. 22–17)

Normal function
 Metastases
 Pheochromocytoma
Hyperfunction
 Pheochromocytoma
 Multinodular hyperplasia

Table 22–7. DIAGNOSTIC SET: BILATERAL ADRENAL
ENLARGEMENT (see Fig. 22–2)

Hyperfunction
 Hyperplasia
 Pheochromocytoma
Normal or diminished function
 Granulomatous disease
 Metastases
 Hemorrhage
 Extramedullary hematopoiesis

Table 22–8. ADRENAL LESIONS THAT CALCIFY
(see Fig. 22–26)

Adenoma (14%)
Carcinoma (40%)
Neuroblastoma/ganglioneuroblastoma (85%)
Ganglioneuroma
Pheochromocytoma (10%)
Metastases (16%)
Mesenchymal tumors
Hemangioma (phleboliths)
Cyst (75%)
Hemorrhage (50%)
Myelolipoma
Granulomatous disease
Wolman's disease

Percentages refer to approximate frequency.

Bibliography

Atkinson, G. O., Jr., Zaatari, G. S., Lorenzo, R. L., Gay, B. B., Jr., and Garvin, A. J.: Cystic neuroblastoma in infants: Radiographic and pathologic features. AJR 146:113, 1986.

Baker, D. E., Glazer, G. M., and Francis, I. R.: Adrenal magnetic resonance imaging in Addison's disease. Urol. Radiol. 9:199, 1988.

Baker, M. E., Blinder, R., Spritzer, C., Leight, G. S., Herfkens, R. J., and Dunnick N. R.: MR evaluation of adrenal masses at 1.5T. AJR 153:307, 1989.

Berland, L. L., Koslin, D. B., Kenney, P. J., Stanley, R. J., and Lee, J. Y.: Differentiation between small benign and malignant adrenal masses with dynamic incremented CT. AJR 151:95, 1988.

Blevins, L. S., and Wand, G. S.: Primary aldosteronism: An endocrine perspective. Radiology 184:599, 1992.

Boechat, M. I., Ortega, J., Hoffman, A. D., Cleveland, R. H., Kangarloo, H., and Gilsanz, V.: Computed tomography in stage III neuroblastoma. AJR 145:1283, 1985.

Chezmar, J. D., Robbins, S. M., Nelson, R. C., Steinberg, H. V., Torres, W. E., and Bernardino, M. E.: Adrenal masses: Characterization with T1-weighted MR imaging. Radiology 166:357, 1988.

Chang, A., Glazer, H. S., Lee, J. K. T., Ling, D., and Heiken, J. P.: Adrenal gland: MR imaging. Radiology 163:123, 1987.

David, R., Lamki, N., Fan, S., Singleton, E. B., Eftekhart, F., Shirkhoda, A., Kumar, R., and Madewell, J. E.: The many faces of neuroblastoma. Radiographics 9:859, 1989.

Dietrich, R. B., Kangarloo, H., Lenarsky, C., and Feig, S. A.: Neuroblastoma: The role of MR imaging. AJR 148:937, 1987.

Doppman, J. L., Gill, J. R., Jr., Nienhuis, A. W., Earll, J. M., and Long, J. A., Jr.: CT findings in Addison's disease. J Comput. Assist. Tomogr. 6:757, 1982.

Doppman, J. L., Miller, D. L., Dwyer, A. J., Loughlin, T., Nieman, L., Cutler, G. B., Chrousos, G. P., Oldfield, E., and Loriaux, D. L.: Macronodular adrenal hyperplasia in Cushing disease. Radiology 166:347, 1988.

Doppman, J. L., Travis, W. D., Nieman, L., Miller, D. L., Chrousos, G. P., Gomez, M. T., Cutler, G. B., Loriaux, D. L., and Norton, J. A.: Cushing syndrome due to primary pigmented nodular adrenocortical disease: Findings at CT and MR imaging. Radiology 172:415, 1989.

Doppman, J. L., Gill, J. R., Jr., Miller, D. L., Change, R., Gupta, R., Friedman, T. C., Choyke, P. L., Feuerstein, I. M., Dwyer, A. J., Jicha, D. L., McClellan, M. W., Norton, J. A., and Linehan, W. M.: Distinction between hyperaldosteronism due to bilateral hypoerplasia and unilateral aldosteronoma: Reliability of CT. Radiology 184:677, 1992.

Dunnick, N. R.: Adrenal imaging: Current status. AJR 154:927, 1990.

Dunnick, N. R., Leight, G. S., Jr., Roubidoux, M. A., Leder, R. A., Paulson, E., and Kurylo, L.: CT in the diagnosis of primary aldosteronism: Sensitivity in 29 patients. AJR 160:321, 1993.

Francis, I. R., Gross, M. D., Shapiro, B., Korobkin, M., and Quint, L. E.: Integrated imaging of adrenal disease. Radiology 184:1, 1992.

Glazer, G. M., Francis, I. R., and Quint, L. E.: Imaging of adrenal glands. Invest Radiol 23:3, 1988.

Hamper, U. M., Fishman, E. K., Hartman, D. S., Roberts, J. L., and

Sanders, R. C.: Primary adrenocortical carcinoma: Sonographic evaluation with clinical and pathologic correlation in 26 patients. AJR 148:915, 1987.

Harrison, R. B., and Francke, P., Jr.: Radiographic findings in Wolman's disease. Radiology 124:188, 1977.

Ikeda, D. M., Francis, I. R., Glazer, G. M., Amendola, M. A., Gross, M. D., and Aisen, A. M.: The detection of adrenal tumors and hyperplasia in patients with primary aldosteronism: Comparison of scintigraphy, CT, and MR imaging. AJR 153:301, 1989.

Jafri, S. Z. H., Francis, I. R., Glazer, G. M., Bree, R. L., and Amendola, M. A.: CT detection of adrenal lymphoma. J. Comput. Assist. Tomogr. 7:254, 1983.

Kenney, P. J., Streeten, D. P., and Anderson, G. H.: Difficulties in the prospective diagnosis of functional adrenal disease by CT. Urol. Radiol. 8:184, 1986.

Kenney, P. J., and Stanley, R. J.: Calcified adrenal masses. Urol. Radiol. 9:9, 1987.

Korobkin, M.: Overview of adrenal imaging/adrenal CT. Urol. Radiol. 11:221, 1989.

Levine, E., deVries, P., and Wetzel, L. H.: MR imaging of inferior venal caval recurrence of extraadrenal pheochromocytoma. J. Comput. Assist. Tomogr. 11:717, 1987.

Mitchell, D. G., Crovello, M., Matteucci, T., Petersen, R. O., and Miettinen, M. M. Benign adrenocortical masses: Diagnosis with chemical shift MR imaging. Radiology 185:345, 1992.

Mitty, H. A.: Adrenal venous sampling and adrenal biopsy. Urol. Radiol. 11:227, 1989.

Murphy, B. J., Casillas, J., and Yrizarry, J. M.: Traumatic adrenal hemorrhage: Radiologic findings. Radiology 169:701, 1988.

Newhouse, J. H.: MRI of the adrenal gland. Urol. Radiol. 12:1, 1990.

Pagani, J. J.: Normal adrenal glands in small cell lung carcinoma: CT-guided biopsy. AJR 140:949, 1983.

Palmar, W. E., Gerard-McFarland, E. L., and Chew, F. S.: Adrenal myelolipoma. AJR 156:724, 1991.

Quint, L. E., Glazer, G. M., Francis, I. R., Shapiro, B., and Chenevert, T. L. Pheochromocytoma and paraganglioma: Comparison of MR imaging with CT and I-131 MIBG scintigraphy. Radiology 165:89, 1987.

Reinig, J. W.: MR imaging differentiation of adrenal masses: Has the time finally come? Radiology 185:339, 1992.

Remer, E. M., Weinfeld, R. M., Glazer, G. M., Quint, L. E., Francis, I. R., Gross, M. D., and Bookstein, F. L.: Hyperfunctioning and nonhyperfunctioning benign adrenal cortical lesions: Characterization and comparison with MR imaging. Radiology 171:681, 1989.

Sandler, M. P., and Delbeker, D.: Radionuclides in endocrine imaging. Radiol. Clin. North Am. 31:909, 1993

Sivit, C. J., Hung, W., Taylor, G. A., Catena, L. D., Brown-Jones, C., and Kushner, D. C.: Sonography in neonatal congenital adrenal hyperplasia. AJR 156:141, 1991.

Smith, S. M., Patel, S. K., Turner, D. A., and Matalon, A. S.: Magnetic resonance imaging of adrenal cortical carcinoma. Urol. Radiol. 11:1, 1989.

van Gils, A. P. G., Falke, T. H. M., van Erkel, A. R., Arndt, J. W., Sander, M. P., van der Mey, A. G. L., and Hoogma, R. P. L.: MR imaging and MIBG scintigraphy of pheochromocytomas and extraadrenal functioning paragangliomas. Radiographics 11:37, 1991.

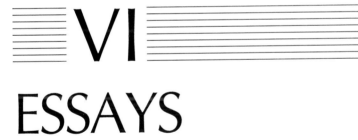

VI
ESSAYS

23

NEPHROGRAPHIC ANALYSIS

DEFINITIONS

Angiographic Nephrogram

Approximately 80 per cent of renal blood flows to the cortex; the remaining 20 per cent perfuses the medulla, pelvocalyceal system, and sinus fat. As a result, a bolus of contrast material flowing to the kidney renders the renal cortex radiodense relative to the medulla during that brief period—up to 30 seconds—in which distribution of contrast material is predominantly in the cortical microvasculature (Fig. 23–1). This phenomenon of selective cortical opacification is known as the *angiographic nephrogram.*

The density of the angiographic nephrogram depends on the amount of contrast material in the bolus and on the site of injection. Optimal visualization occurs with selective injection of contrast material (usual dose = 35 mg/kg of iodine) through a catheter in the renal artery and rapid sequence filming (Fig. 23–2).

The angiographic nephrogram can also be imaged during dynamic computed tomographic scanning for a period of approximately 30 seconds after intravenous injection of a bolus of approximately 200 mg/kg of iodine (Fig. 23–3). The angiographic nephrogram may sometimes be visualized during standard excretory urography when a film of optimal technical quality is exposed within 30 seconds of the rapid injection of a bolus of contrast material into a peripheral vein (usual dose = approximately 300 mg/kg of iodine).

The magnetic resonance equivalent of the angiographic nephrogram can be seen within 15 to 30 seconds of an intravenous bolus injection of 0.1 mmol/kg gadolinium-labeled DTPA. T1-weighted gradient-echo pulse sequences during suspended respiration depict the cortex as more hyperintense than the medulla owing to the T1-shortening effects of low dose Gd-DTPA (Fig. 23–4).

Urographic Nephrogram

The radiodensity of the medulla increases as the lumina of the proximal tubules fill with contrast material cleared from the plasma by glomerular filtration. There are two populations of nephrons with different proximal tubule length (Fig. 23–5). One population is composed of short proximal tubules whose extent is limited to the cortex and the juxtacortical medulla. The second population has long proximal tubules that extend from the corticomedullary region to the apex of the renal lobe at the level of the papilla. This anatomic arrangement ensures that the full thickness of the renal parenchyma is opacified by contrast material filtering into both sets of proximal tubules. Within approximately 1 minute after injection of contrast material into a peripheral vein, the radiodensity of the medullae of the renal lobes, when imaged by radiographic or computed tomographic techniques, equals that of the cortices. It is this homogeneous density of the entire renal parenchyma that is known as the *urographic nephrogram* (Fig. 23–6).

The radiodensity of the urographic nephrogram in a normal, unobstructed kidney is a function of the *filtered fraction,* which is the product of the plasma concentration of contrast material and the glomerular filtration rate. The plasma concentration, in turn, var-

Text continued on page 757

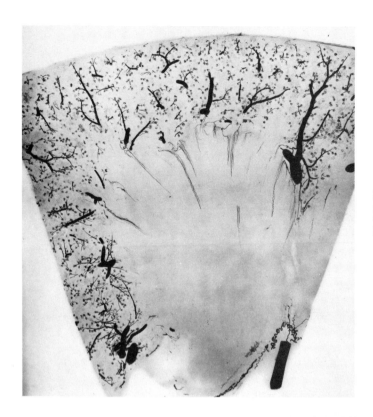

Figure 23–1. Microradiograph of a renal lobe from a human kidney that was injected post mortem with barium. The predominant vasculature is in the cortex. This distribution of blood vessels is the basis for the angiographic nephrogram.

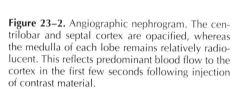

Figure 23–2. Angiographic nephrogram. The centrilobar and septal cortex are opacified, whereas the medulla of each lobe remains relatively radiolucent. This reflects predominant blood flow to the cortex in the first few seconds following injection of contrast material.

A, Selective renal arteriogram, late arterial phase.

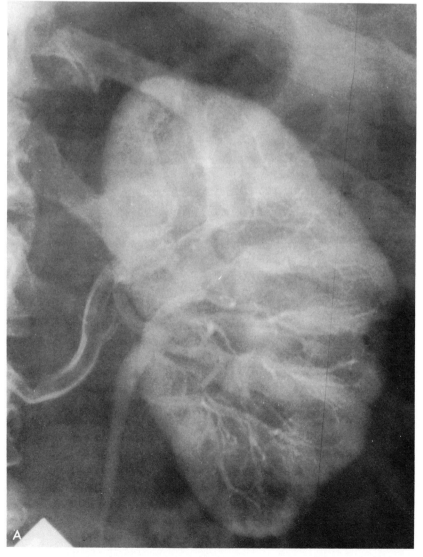

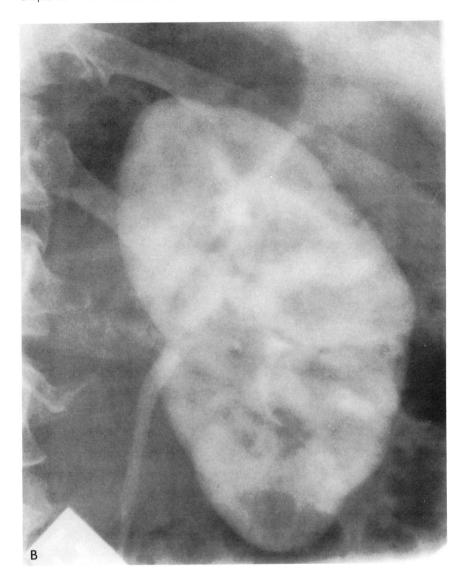

B

Figure 23–2 *Continued B,* Selective renal arteriogram, capillary or angiographic nephrogram phase.

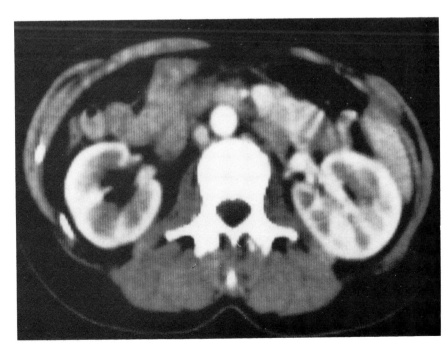

Figure 23–3. Angiographic nephrogram. There is opacification of centrilobar and septal cortex immediately after the intravenous injection of a bolus of contrast material. Note opacification of the aorta. Contrast material has not yet passed into the medulla. Dynamic computed tomogram. (Courtesy of Leon Love, M.D., Loyola University, Chicago, Illinois.)

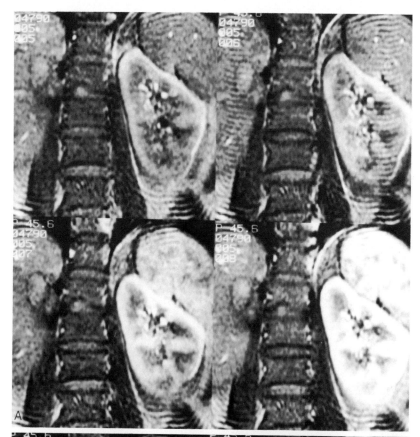

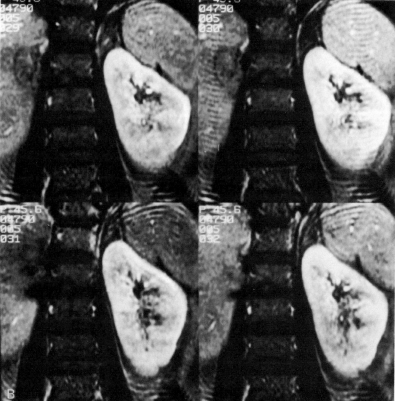

Figure 23–4. Angiographic and urographic nephrogram demonstrated by magnetic resonance imaging.

A, Early dynamic enhanced magnetic resonance images demonstrate cortical enhancement following a bolus injection of the paramagnetic contrast material gadolinium DTPA. Images were obtained with a spoiled gradient-echo technique during suspended respiration.

B, The urographic nephrogram develops as the cortical and medullary signal intensities equilibrate at 45 seconds after injection of contrast material.

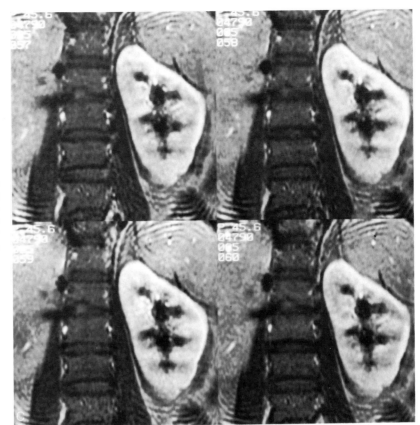

Figure 23–4 *Continued C,* Images obtained 5 minutes after injection of contrast material demonstrate low signal intensity within the renal pelvis and pyramids representing hyperconcentration of the paramagnetic contrast material and T2-shortening effects. (Kindly provided by Peter Choyke, M.D., National Institutes of Health, Bethesda, Maryland.)

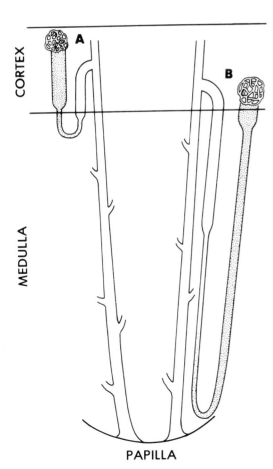

Figure 23–5. Distribution of nephrons and collecting ducts in the renal cortex and medulla. One population of nephrons (A) is limited to the cortex and adjacent parts of medulla. A second population (B) is composed of juxtamedullary glomeruli with tubules that extend deep into the medulla. Contrast material in the proximal tubules of both populations renders the full thickness of the renal parenchyma radiopaque and is the basis of the urographic nephrogram.

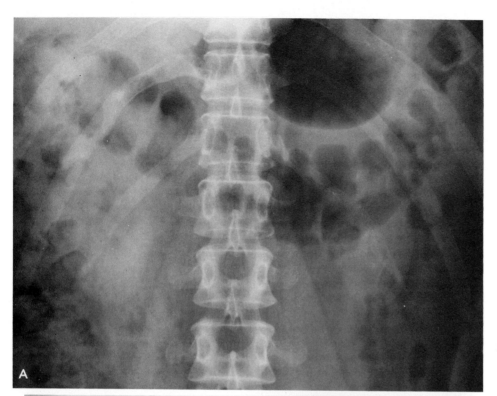

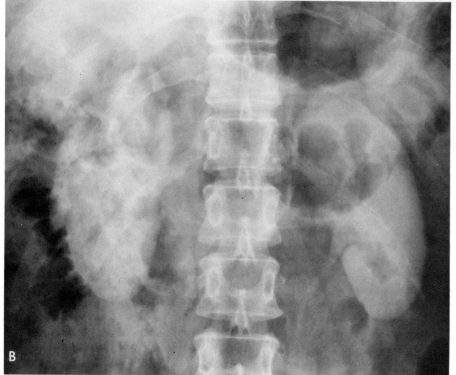

Figure 23–6. Urographic nephrogram. Sodium diatrizoate 50%, 1.0 ml/kg body weight.

A, Preliminary film. Bowel preparation is poor.

B, Excretory urogram, 1-minute film. There is intense radiodensity of the renal parenchyma, reflecting contrast material that is passing through the nephrons and the collecting ducts.

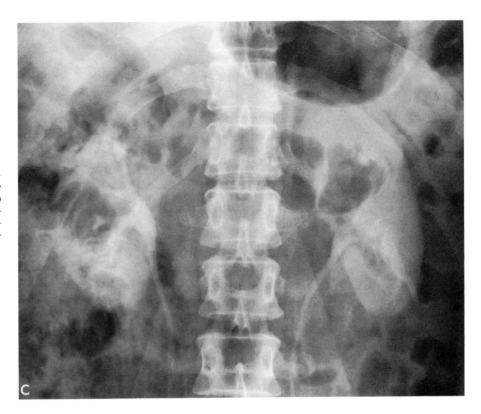

Figure 23–6 *Continued C,* Excretory urogram, 5-minute film. The intensity of the nephrogram has diminished owing to both the decrease in the plasma concentration of contrast material and the forward flow of opacified urine into the pelvocalyceal system.

ies with the amount of contrast material administered and the time elapsed after injection. The density of the urographic nephrogram is greatest approximately 1 minute after the bolus injection of contrast material (usual dose = 300 mg/kg of iodine) at which time the peak plasma level is reached. Beyond this point, the density of the nephrogram diminishes as the plasma level of the contrast material falls. Therefore, after each successive unit of time, fewer iodine-bearing molecules are cleared. Furthermore, the continued flow of contrast material from the nephrons and collecting ducts into the pelvocalyceal system contributes to the decrease in parenchymal (nephrographic) density beyond 1 minute.

Technical considerations also influence perceived nephrographic density. Film with low-contrast characteristics, high-kilovoltage x-ray beams, and a large amount of overlying tissue reduce apparent radiodensity. Liver overlying a portion of the right kidney and intestinal gas overlying the left kidney may cause differences in the baseline radiodensity of the kidneys as well as in the radiodensity of the subsequent urographic nephrograms. These variables undermine the value of comparing the nephrographic density of one kidney with that of another as an index of abnormality and also make the practice of using the intensity of the nephrogram as a measure of renal function unreliable.

The injection of a bolus of contrast material produces a higher plasma level than injection of an equal amount of iodine by drip infusion (Fig. 23–7). When contrast material is infused slowly, a greater amount than that used in a bolus injection must be given if equivalent diagnostic information is to be obtained.

Antidiuretic hormone does not influence water reabsorption in the proximal tubule. Therefore, the concentration of solutes, including contrast material, in the proximal tubule is uninfluenced by the state of a patient's water balance. In other words, dehydration does not influence the intensity of the urographic nephrogram.

The urographic nephrogram, therefore, is best visualized during excretory urography with a film obtained approximately 1 minute after the bolus injec-

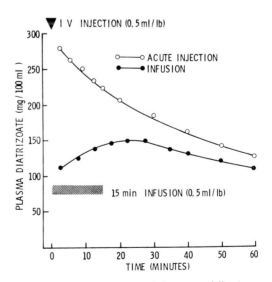

Figure 23–7. Plasma concentration of diatrizoate following a rapid bolus injection and a slow drip infusion. Drip infusion does not produce the same maximal level of contrast material as bolus injection. (From Cattell, W. R.: Invest. Radiol. *5:*473, 1970. With kind permission of the author and *Investigative Radiology.*)

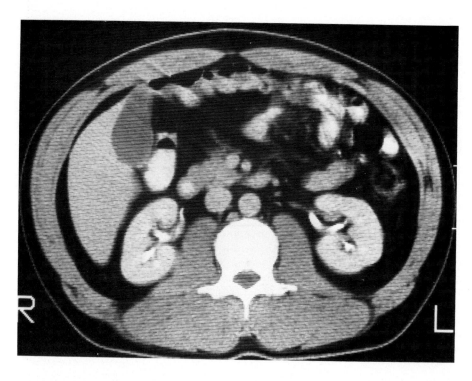

Figure 23–8. Urographic nephrogram. Contrast material in the nephrons and collecting ducts renders the cortex and medulla homogeneously radiodense. Computed tomogram.

tion of contrast material. Linear tomography; an increased dose of contrast material to compensate for impaired renal function, large body build, or obscuring intestinal contents; and a well-coned, low-kilovoltage x-ray beam enhance the quality of the image.

The urographic nephrogram is also seen during computed tomography once contrast material enters the tubules and obliterates the sharply defined corti-

comedullary junction that is a feature of the angiographic nephrogram (Fig. 23–8). Some computed tomography units with superior contrast resolution demonstrate persistently higher cortical density relative to the medulla throughout the entire period of renal opacification. This is presumably due to a summation of the angiographic and the urographic nephrograms (Fig. 23–9).

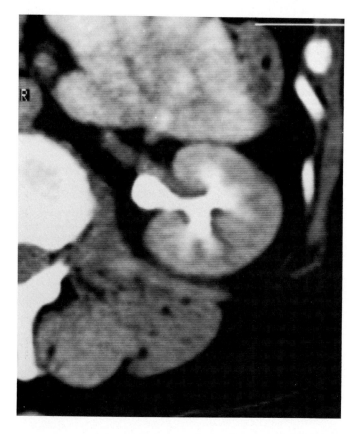

Figure 23–9. Combined urographic and angiographic nephrogram. With computed tomographic equipment capable of high-density resolution, the radiodensity of the cortex remains higher than that of the medulla, owing to the additive effect of contrast material in the microvasculature of the cortex. Computed tomogram.

With magnetic resonance imaging, the urographic nephrogram becomes apparent as the medulla equilibrates with the cortex following the intravenous injection of a bolus of 0.1 mmol/kg of Gd-DTPA (see Fig. 23–4). As the Gd-DTPA concentrates in the loop of Henle and collecting ducts, the medulla may become very hypointense owing to profound T2* (susceptibility weighted) shortening. If a highly T2-weighted gradient-echo sequence is employed, the cortex will be initially hypointense and become even darker as the intratubular concentration of Gd-DTPA increases.

Value of Nephrographic Analysis

The angiographic nephrogram, as a microvascular phenomenon, requires only an intact vascular system. Abnormality of the angiographic nephrogram, therefore, is a useful indicator of a disturbance in blood flow to the kidney.

The urographic nephrogram, in the simplest sense, permits accurate evaluation of the fundamentals of renal radiology: the kidney's size, position, and contour. A normal urographic nephrogram requires, in addition to normal blood flow, functional and structural integrity of the nephrons and an unobstructed flow of filtrate through the tubules. Therefore, information regarding these more complex aspects of the kidney can also be derived from nephrographic analysis.

The following sections of this chapter discuss the nephrogram in the context of renal perfusion, the dynamics of urine formation, and the structural integrity of the renal parenchyma. The appearance of the various nephrographic abnormalities and the principles that explain them apply regardless of whether the nephrogram is imaged by excretory urography, angiography, computed tomography, or magnetic resonance imaging.

ANALYSIS OF RENAL PERFUSION

Main Renal Artery Narrowing

In film radiography, there is frequently a difference in the baseline nephrographic density between the kidneys, caused by uneven distribution of overlying bowel gas and soft tissue. Because of this, a difference in radiodensity is not a reliable indicator of renal ischemia due to main renal artery stenosis unless the difference is of great magnitude (Fig. 23–10). With aortography, unequal nephrograms may result from incomplete mixing of the bolus of contrast material with the aortic blood before its flow to the kidneys. On the other hand, a reduced rate of nephrographic enhancement in one kidney compared with the other during computed tomography is presumptive evidence of decreased renal blood flow, assuming that unilateral renal parenchymal disease or obstructive uropathy is excluded.

Over time, the urographic nephrogram becomes increasingly dense in some patients with severe renal artery stenosis. This reflects an abnormality in the dynamics of urine formation, initiated by reduced renal perfusion pressure. This is discussed further in this chapter in the section "Increasingly Dense Nephrogram." Other aspects of ischemia due to focal main renal artery disease are discussed in Chapter 6.

Main Renal Artery Occlusion

The nephrogram in acute total occlusion of the main renal artery, as seen with an embolism, is either absent or extremely faint (Fig. 23–11). In complete acute occlusion without collateral flow, no nephrogram is seen and renal infarction ensues. Any opacification that does occur is the result of collateral blood flow. If the collateral flow bypasses the occluding lesion itself, contrast material passes into the distal part of the main renal artery. Thus, the entire population of nephrons is perfused, although at a level greatly reduced from normal, and a faint nephrogram develops.

There are circumstances in which the only collaterals that form in response to main renal artery occlusion are those of the perirenal capsular circulation. These collaterals are variably derived from the inferior adrenal, lumbar, gonadal, iliac, intercostal, or phrenic arteries. When this occurs, a 2- to 4-mm rim of outer cortex opacifies during contrast material–enhanced studies (Fig. 23–12). This opacification represents that portion of the subcapsular renal cortex that is perfused by capsular artery collateral circulation. The remainder of the kidney does not increase in density. In addition to acute, total main renal artery obstruction, a cortical rim nephrogram has been reported in renal vein thrombosis and acute tubular necrosis.

Segmental Renal Artery Occlusion

The considerations described for acute total occlusion of the main renal artery also apply to acute total occlusion of one or more of the major segmental branches of the renal artery (Figs. 23–13 and 23–14). Here, the nephrogram will be absent or markedly reduced only in the affected region. One pole or a set of ventral or dorsal lobes may be involved. A cortical rim nephrogram limited to the affected area may also be seen in acute segmental renal artery occlusion.

Interlobar or Arcuate Artery Occlusion

Occlusion of an interlobar or arcuate artery leads to infarction of a part or all of a renal lobe in a characteristic wedge-shaped pattern. During the period immediately following occlusion, the bulk of the infarcted tissue is preserved, although no blood flows to the area. This results in a triangle-shaped angiographic and urographic nephrogram defect without deformity of the renal contour (Fig. 23–15). Within 3 weeks, the affected area will be transformed into a deep, broad-based scar as the infarcted tissue is resorbed. This process is discussed in detail in Chapter 5.

Acute Cortical Necrosis

Acute cortical necrosis is a unique perfusion abnormality in which the cortical microvasculature is oblit-

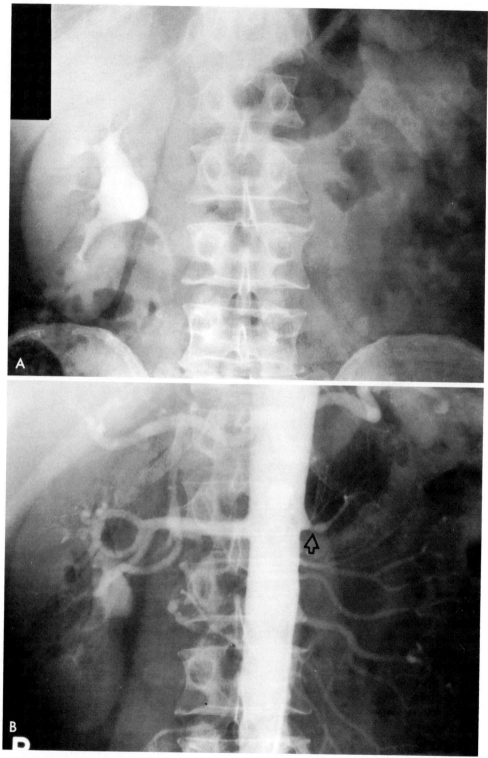

Figure 23–10. Diminished nephrographic density due to left main renal artery narrowing. The decreased radiodensity of the left urographic nephrogram relative to the right signals severe reduction in perfusion.

A, Excretory urogram, 4-minute film. In addition to the reduced radiodensity of the nephrogram, the left kidney is small and has delayed opacification of the pelvocalyceal system.

B, Aortogram. There is a high-grade stenosis of the left main renal artery *(arrow)* with post-stenotic dilatation.

(Courtesy of Department of Diagnostic Radiology, Hammersmith Hospital, Royal Postgraduate Medical School, London, England.)

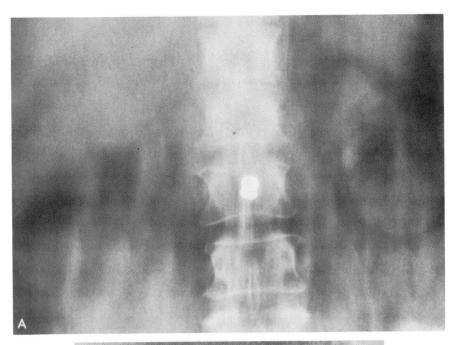

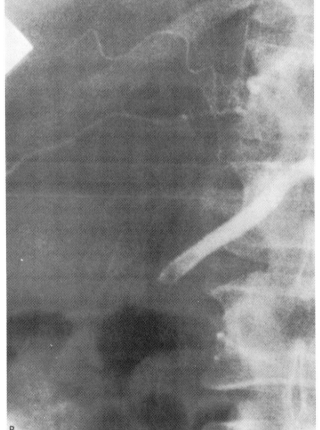

Figure 23–11. Acute embolus to the main right renal artery in a woman with rheumatic heart disease and atrial fibrillation.

A, Excretory urogram. Tomogram obtained at 30 minutes. The right kidney is enlarged (length = 14.5 cm) and has a faint nephrogram. The left kidney has evidence of old and recent lobar infarction.

B, Selective right renal arteriogram demonstrates complete occlusion of the main renal artery. (Same patient illustrated in Fig. 9–9.)

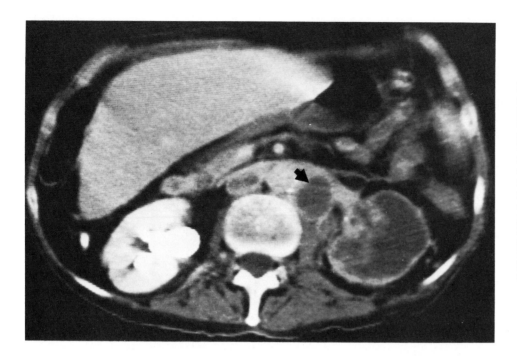

Figure 23–12. Occlusion of the left main renal artery by metastatic deposit from lung carcinoma. The low density metastasis *(arrow)* has occluded the left renal artery, causing smooth enlargement of the kidney and an absent nephrogram except where collateral circulation continues to perfuse the cortex. A rim nephrogram results. Lucency within the inferior vena cava is presumably due to a thrombus. Computed tomogram, contrast material enhanced. (Same patient illustrated in Fig. 9–8.) (Courtesy of Stuart London, M.D., Oakland, California.)

erated. In some instances, the process is incomplete, leading to a patchy angiographic nephrogram and a homogeneous urographic nephrogram. In most circumstances, however, there is complete necrosis of the cortex and the angiographic nephrogram does not develop at all (Fig. 23–16). However, even in this circumstance medullary enhancement may occur, presumably as a result of the continued function of viable juxtamedullary nephron units.

In other cases of acute cortical necrosis, the outer margin of the cortex receives blood from the perirenal capsular arterial system, which acts like a collateral pathway in acute main or segmental renal artery occlusion. When this happens, arterial blood perfuses the outer rim and the juxtamedullary portion of the cortex; however, the central zone between them infarcts. The result is a distinctive nephrogram characterized by a middle zone of nonenhanced cortex located between the opacified outer rim and the inner cortex and medulla. Chapter 8 includes an additional discussion of acute cortical necrosis.

ANALYSIS OF THE DYNAMICS OF URINE FORMATION

Normal Time–Density Curve

The density of the urographic nephrogram is greatest approximately 1 minute after a bolus of contrast material is injected into a peripheral vein. Thereafter, the nephrogram becomes progressively less dense. Fading of the nephrogram is due to the continuous flow of contrast material out of the nephrons and collecting ducts and into the pelvocalyceal system, while at the same time decreasing amounts of contrast material enter the tubules as plasma concentration falls. Thus, over time the decrease in nephrographic density or gadolinium-induced change in signal intensity parallels the plasma decay curve of contrast material con-

centration (see Fig. 23–7). There is a 50 per cent reduction in the plasma level concentration of iodinated contrast material approximately every 50 minutes. (This is discussed in Chapter 1.)

Abnormalities that affect the dynamics of urine formation may disturb the normal time–density pattern of nephrogram decay. Three abnormal time–density patterns are recognized: immediate, faint, and persistent; increasingly dense; and immediate, dense, and persistent.

Immediate, Faint, Persistent Nephrogram

With this nephrographic pattern, peak density is seen on the first film exposed at the completion of contrast material injection and is not commensurate with the amount of contrast material injected. The nephrogram, though faint, persists for several hours.

The immediate, faint, persistent nephrogram occurs when glomerular filtration is severely impaired by a reduction in the number of functioning nephrons. The faintness of the nephrogram reflects a low plasma clearance rate of contrast material. In fact, a high dose of contrast material is required if the nephrogram is to be seen at all during excretory urography.

The renal diseases associated with an immediate, faint, persistent nephrogram are often associated with a high urea load and impaired sodium reabsorption in the proximal tubules. These cause a diuresis that also contributes to the faintness of the nephrogram. Persistence of the nephrogram reflects a very slow rate of decay of plasma contrast material owing to impaired glomerular filtration.

An immediate, faint, persistent nephrogram is seen in patients with chronic glomerular disease and in those who have had a sudden loss of glomerular function as a result of widespread obliteration of the renal microvasculature, such as in atheroembolic renal disease (Fig. 23–17).

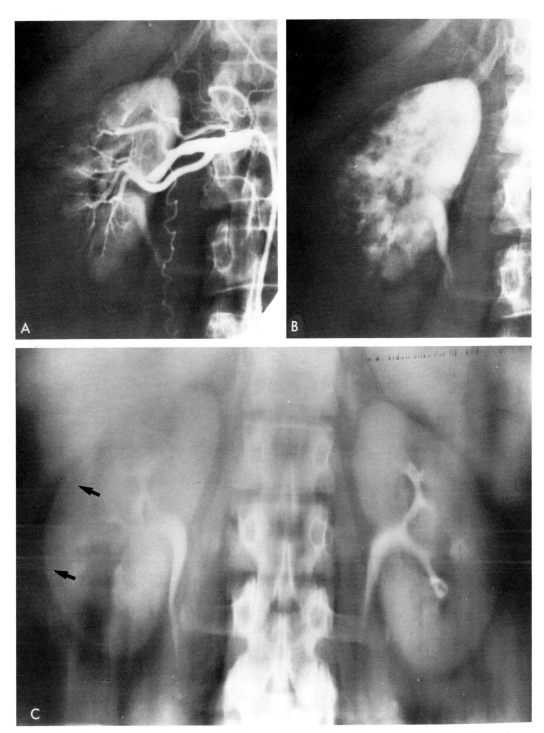

Figure 23–13. Segmental renal artery occlusion. Multiple emboli have occluded both interlobar and arcuate arteries. The nephrogram is absent in those portions of the kidney served by the occluded vessels. Collateral blood flow through capsular arteries causes a rim of nephrographic density in the cortex *(arrows).*

A, Selective right renal arteriogram, arterial phase. There are numerous points of occlusion.

B, Selective right renal arteriogram, nephrographic phase. The distribution of the perfusion abnormality is well visualized.

C, Excretory urogram. Tomogram. The nephrogram is absent in the lateral portion of the right kidney except in the rim of cortex.

(Same patient illustrated in Fig. 9–10.)

(Courtesy of Professor César Pedrosa and E. Ramirez, M.D., Hospital Clinico de San Carlos, Madrid, Spain.)

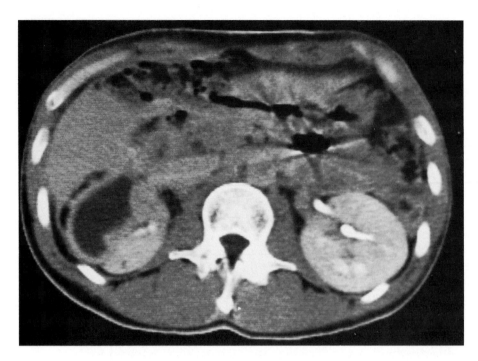

Figure 23–14. Acute occlusion of the segmental renal artery to the ventrolateral portion of the right kidney. The dorsomedial portion of the kidney continues to be perfused, while the affected part of the kidney has an absent nephrogram except for the rim of the cortex, which is perfused by capsular collaterals. Computed tomogram. (Courtesy of Stuart London, M.D., Oakland, California.)

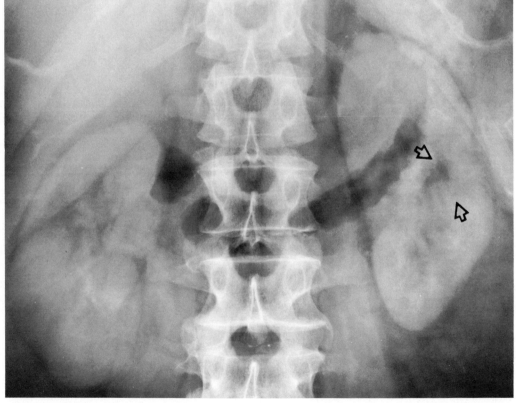

Figure 23–15. Acute lobar infarction in a 61-year-old man who experienced sudden left groin and flank pain with microscopic hematuria. Excretory urography was performed 3 days later. A triangular radiolucent nephrographic defect with its base on the renal margin is present in the interpolar region *(arrows).* Excretory urogram, early film. (Same patient illustrated in Figs. 5–17 through 5–19.) (Courtesy of Ira Kanter, M.D., Peralta Hospital, Oakland, California.)

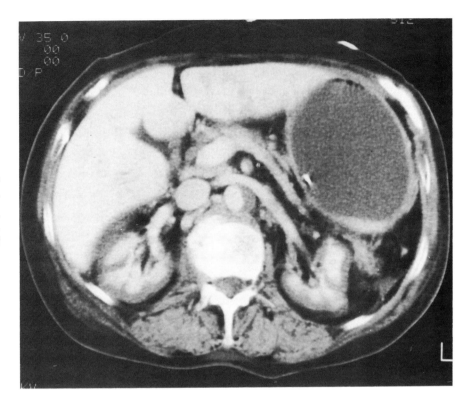

Figure 23–16. Acute cortical necrosis in a 74-year-old woman with recent surgery for thoracic and abdominal aortic dissection. Computed tomogram with contrast material enhancement demonstrates absence of enhancement of the cortex and selective enhancement of the medulla. (Same patient illustrated in Fig. 8–14.)

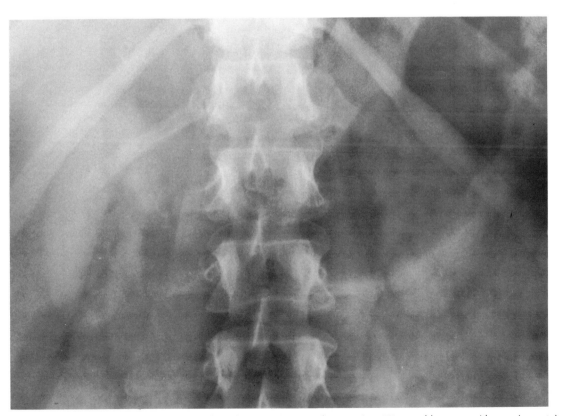

Figure 23–17. Chronic glomerulonephritis with an immediate, faint, persistent nephrogram in a 37-year-old woman with anemia, proteinuria, and creatinine clearance of 3 ml/min. Excretory urogram, 10-minute film. (Same patient illustrated in Fig. 7–12.)

Increasingly Dense Nephrogram

In this nephrographic pattern, the nephrogram is faint to begin with, but becomes increasingly dense over a period of hours to days. The mechanism for each of the many causes of an increasingly dense nephrogram is an increase in tubule transit time of filtrate combined with diminished clearance of contrast material from plasma. Leakage of contrast material into the renal interstitial space is an additional possible factor that may contribute to an increasingly dense nephrogram in certain etiologies.

Acute extrarenal obstruction, as occurs with ureteral calculus, is the most common cause of an increasingly dense nephrogram (Fig. 23–18). Pathophysiologically, a downstream ureteral obstruction leads to an increase in hydrostatic pressure that extends back to the nephron. The subsequent reduced glomerular filtration rate lowers the amount of contrast material entering the tubules during any given period, producing the reduced density of the nephrogram during the first few minutes of the excretory urogram or computed tomogram. However, continued reabsorption of water by the tubules compensates for the elevated hydrostatic pressure within the tubules, and thus glomerular filtration does not cease completely. There are other factors, less important and inconstant, that help to compensate for the increased hydrostatic pressure that follows acute extrarenal obstruction. These include distention of the collecting structures proximal to the obstructing lesion and leakage of urine into the renal sinus, interstices, lymphatics, or veins through rents in the fornices of the calyces. The net result is the continued formation of an iodine-bearing glomerular filtrate that moves sluggishly forward. Because of this, the nephrogram gradually increases over many hours, and calyceal opacification is delayed.

Diminished perfusion pressure of the kidney, as seen in systemic arterial hypotension or severe main renal artery stenosis, is another cause of an increasingly dense nephrogram. Here, a decrease in arterial perfusion pressure at the level of the glomerular capillary bed reduces the rate of contrast material clearance from the plasma into the proximal tubule lumina. Renal underperfusion also promotes increased reabsorption of salt and water by the tubules, causing the volume of tubule filtrate to diminish. The net effect of these alterations is a slow accumulation of contrast material molecules with an increasingly dense nephrogram.

In the case of systemic hypotension, the nephrograms of *both* kidneys become increasingly dense (Fig. 23–19). Only on restoration of normal blood pressure is there rapid pelvocalyceal opacification and the return of normal nephrographic density. This nephrographic pattern is most often seen in the clinical setting of an adverse reaction to contrast material. (See discussion in Chapter 7.) An increasingly dense nephrogram due to diminished perfusion pressure secondary to severe main renal artery stenosis, on the other hand, is usually *unilateral* and is accompanied by other radiologic signs of ischemia (Fig. 23–20), as discussed in Chapter 6.

Acute tubular necrosis is another cause of an increasingly dense nephrogram (Fig. 23–21), although more commonly this condition is associated with an immediate, dense, persistent nephrogram. The mechanism that leads to this pattern, which may evolve over a period of hours to days, has not been defined. The fact that this same pattern is seen with diminished perfusion is used by some clinicians as evidence that preglomerular ischemia is a factor in the genesis of acute tubular necrosis. This, too, is an unresolved issue.

Exposure of the kidney to contrast material is one uncommon cause of acute tubular necrosis. Contrast material nephrotoxicity is dose related and potentiated by pre-existing dehydration, low flow states, and chronic renal disease, especially diabetic nephropathy. The first manifestation of this complication may be an abnormal nephrogram and an absent pyelogram. This problem is discussed in fully in Chapter 1.

Intratubular obstruction by uric acid crystals, by casts of myeloma or Tamm-Horsfall protein, or by acute papillary necrosis is another circumstance in which an increasingly dense nephrogram is encountered (Fig. 23–22). Although the mechanism for this is not well understood, it is probably similar to the mechanism for extrarenal obstruction, except that the site of obstruction is within each tubule lumen or at swollen papillary tips rather than in the pelvocalyceal system or ureter. In some patients with intratubular obstruction there is opacification of a nondilated pelvocalyceal system during excretory urography. This suggests that some urine is formed by uninvolved nephrons and passes forward unimpaired.

Precipitation of Tamm-Horsfall protein is encountered in infants and children and may be a complication when contrast material is administered in severely dehydrated patients. Acute urate and myeloma nephropathy are discussed in detail in Chapter 8.

Acute glomerular disease and *acute renal vein thrombosis* are two additional circumstances in which an increasingly dense nephrogram has been reported on a few occasions. Speculation on the underlying mechanisms in acute glomerular disease centers on reduction of glomerular perfusion by obliterative changes in the renal microvasculature. In the case of renal vein thrombosis, possible explanations for an increasingly dense nephrogram include reduced arterial perfusion or obstruction of the tubules by interstitial edema and hemorrhage. Leakage of contrast material into interstitial spaces is another possible contributing factor.

Immediate, Dense, Persistent Nephrogram

In this pattern, the nephrogram is at least as dense as would be normally expected at 1 minute. Rather than fading, however, the level of density persists, and often slightly increases over a period of hours to days. When this pattern is associated with nonoliguric acute renal failure, the collecting system may opacify.

The mechanism for the production of an immediate, dense, persistent nephrogram has not been clarified.

Text continued on page 771

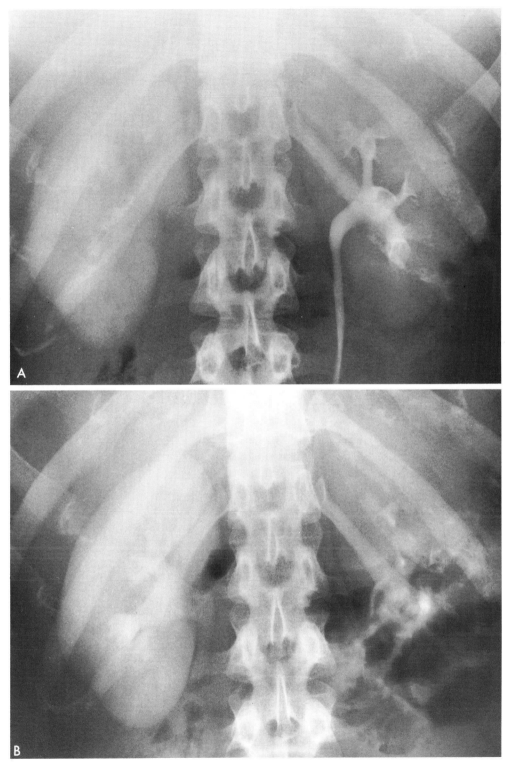

Figure 23–18. Acute extrarenal obstruction with an increasingly dense nephrogram. The patient was a young woman with right distal ureteral stone.

  A, Excretory urogram, 10-minute film. The right nephrogram is already more dense than the left.

  B, Excretory urogram, 4-hour film. The density of the nephrogram has increased. (Same patient illustrated in Figs. 9–11 and 9–22.)

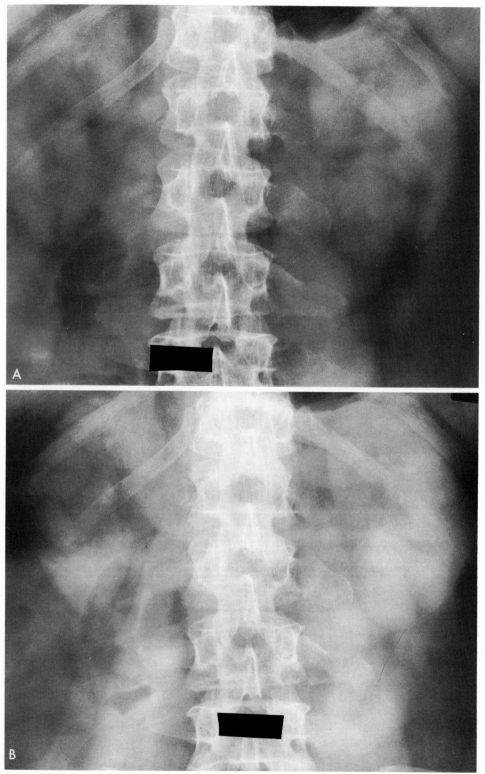

Figure 23–19. Arterial hypotension with increasingly dense nephrogram. The hypotension was associated with an adverse response to contrast material.

 A, Excretory urogram, 5-minute film. There is impaired nephrographic density and absent pelvocalyceal opacification.

 B, Excretory urogram, 10-minute film. The nephrographic density has increased, but the pelvocalyceal system remains unopacified. (Same patient illustrated in Fig. 7–31.)

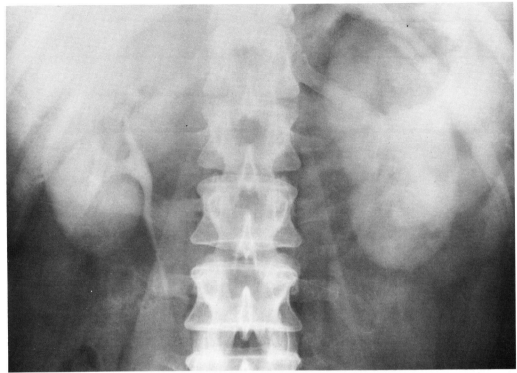

Figure 23–20. Renovascular ischemia of the left kidney associated with an increasingly dense urographic nephrogram. The nephrogram of the left kidney is more dense than the right, and the calyces are faintly opacified. Excretory urogram, delayed film.

Figure 23–21. Acute tubular necrosis associated with an increasingly dense nephrogram in a 60-year-old man with oliguric renal failure after severe trauma.
  A, Excretory urogram, 30-minute film.
  B, Excretory urogram, 18-hour film.
  (Same patient illustrated in Fig. 8–12.)
  (Courtesy of Professor Thomas Sherwood, M.B., University of Cambridge, Cambridge, England.)

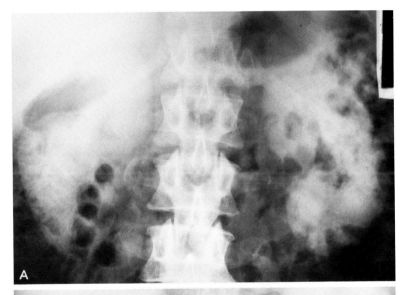

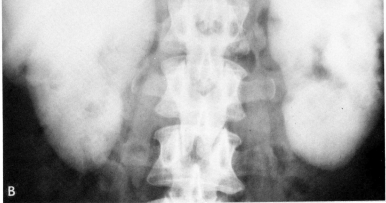

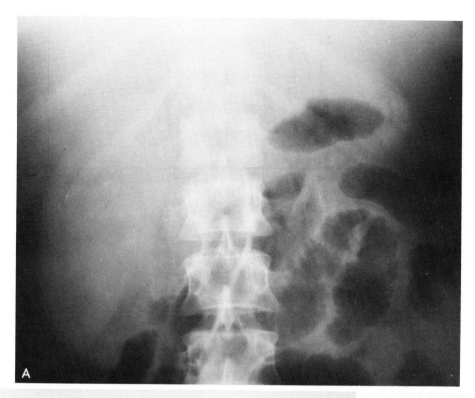

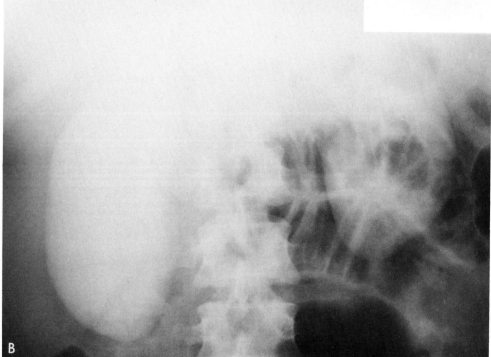

Figure 23–22. Acute urate nephropathy with increasingly dense nephrogram due to intratubular precipitation of urate crystals. The patient was a 31-year-old woman with extensive hepatic metastases from a poorly differentiated carcinoma and hyperuricemia.

A, Excretory urogram, 10-minute film.

B, Excretory urogram, 40-hour film.

(Same patient illustrated in Fig. 8–25.)

The early appearance of a dense nephrogram suggests unimpaired glomerular filtration. Since nephrographic density remains rather constant despite anuria or oliguria, there must be return of filtered contrast material to the circulation. This is believed to occur through diffusion of tubule fluid into the interstitial space and then into the systemic circulation through veins and/or lymphatics. Another mechanism that may contribute to an immediate, dense, persistent nephrogram is blockage of tubule lumina by casts and cellular debris shed from damaged tubule epithelium. This might add an obstructive component that could account for the slight increase in nephrographic density over time that is seen in some of these patients.

Acute tubular necrosis is most commonly associated with an immediate, dense, persistent nephrogram (Fig. 23–23). The evolution of this pattern following

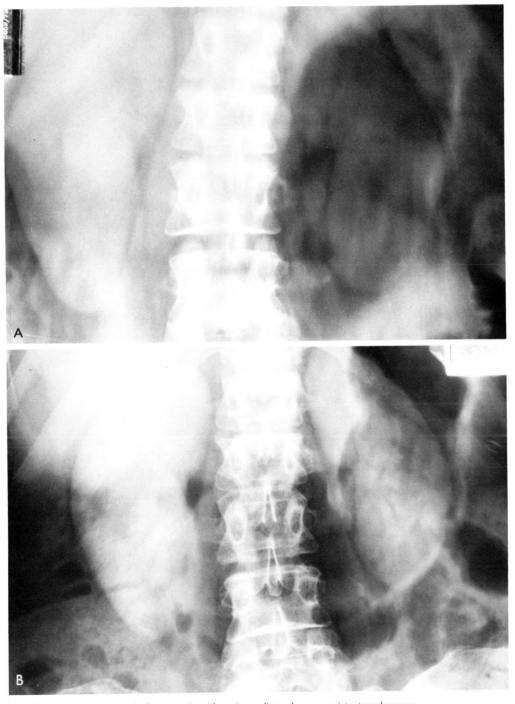

Figure 23–23. Acute tubular necrosis with an immediate, dense, persistent nephrogram.
A, Excretory urogram, 2-minute film. The nephrogram is denser than normally seen at 2 minutes.
B, Excretory urogram, 16-hour film. The nephrogram persists and becomes slightly denser over time.
(Same patient illustrated in Fig. 8–11.)
(Courtesy of Professor Thomas Sherwood, M.B., University of Cambridge, Cambridge, England.)

an initially normal excretory urogram suggests the development of contrast material–induced nephrotoxicity.

Acute bacterial nephritis is another condition in which an immediate, dense, persistent nephrogram with little or no collecting system opacification is sometimes observed. Here, the abnormality is almost always unilateral. Bilateral involvement is a rare, chance event. A striated urographic nephrogram is frequently encountered in patients with acute bacterial nephritis, especially with computed tomography. Additional discussion of this manifestation of acute pyelonephritis can be found in the following section of this chapter and in Chapter 9.

The reader is cautioned against using any of the various abnormal time–density nephrographic patterns described here as specific presentations of any given renal abnormality or as hard and fast rules in formulating a diagnosis. As always, careful integration of all radiologic, laboratory, and clinical data remains basic to accurate diagnosis.

Striated Urographic Nephrogram

Inhomogeneity of the urographic nephrogram, characterized by fine linear bands of alternating lucency and density uniformly oriented in a direction similar to that of tubules and collecting ducts, is encountered occasionally as a transitory phenomenon in acute ex-

trarenal obstruction (Fig. 23–24). A similar, sometimes extensive, pattern is consistently seen in acute bacterial nephritis, and in some cases of acute pyelonephritis (Fig. 23–25). A striated nephrogram is also seen in autosomal recessive (infantile) polycystic kidney disease, invariably in the neonatal form, and to a lesser degree, in the juvenile form (see Figs. 8–18 and 8–22). Isolated case reports of striated nephrograms have also been associated with systemic hypotension, intratubular obstruction due to Tamm-Horsfall proteinuria, renal vein thrombosis, and contusion of the kidney.

Stasis of urine in tubules underlies the development of nephrographic striations in acute extrarenal obstruction. During the course of excretory urography, the striated pattern emerges from a background of faint but homogeneous density, becomes progressively more apparent, reaches a plateau, and then fades.

The pathogenesis of the striated nephrogram in acute obstruction has been disputed. In one concept, the dense striae are believed to represent hyperconcentration of contrast material that has accumulated in dilated collecting ducts or in groups of ducts that form in the inner cortex and extend through the medulla to the tip of the papillae in bundles known as *medullary rays* (Bigongiari et al., 1975, 1977). The development of striae may require the presence of chronically dilated collecting ducts from prior epi-

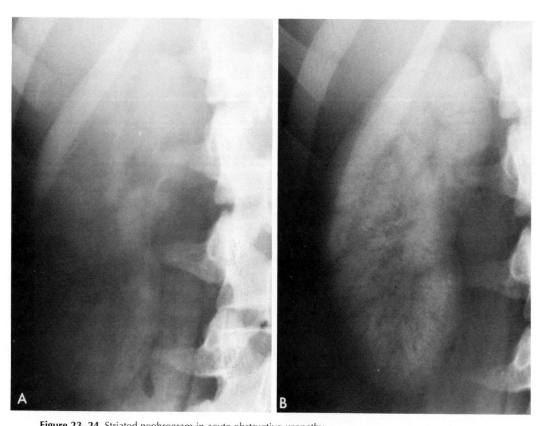

Figure 23–24. Striated nephrogram in acute obstructive uropathy.
A, Excretory urogram, 5-minute film. Delayed opacification.
B, Excretory urogram, 45-minute film. Striae are well illustrated. (Same patient illustrated in Fig. 9–16.)

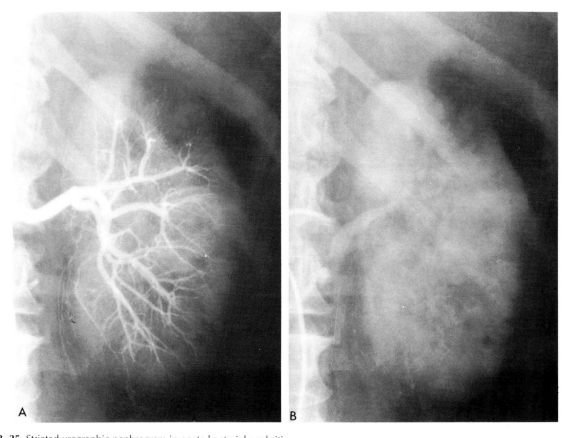

Figure 23–25. Striated urographic nephrogram in acute bacterial nephritis.
  A, Selective renal arteriogram. Arterial phase. There is stretching of arcuate arteries.
  B, Selective renal arteriogram. Nephrogram phase. A striated pattern is present. (Courtesy of Klaus Dehlinger, M.D., and Edward Drasin, M.D., Berkeley, California.)

sodes of obstruction, therefore explaining the low frequency of this finding in acute extrarenal obstruction.

Another concept that has been proposed to explain the striated nephrogram of acute extrarenal obstruction distinguishes the linear lucencies, rather than densities, as the abnormal components. This formulation proposes that the lucencies are the result of unopacified calyceal urine that has been forced retrograde into some of the collecting ducts dilated by obstruction (Bretland, 1974). It is suggested that the reflux occurs because the luminal hydrostatic pressure is known to be lower in collecting ducts draining long loops of Henle than in those draining nephrons with short loops of Henle. Collecting ducts with lower pressure would thereby contain nonopaque urine that is refluxed from the pelvocalyceal system, while ducts with higher pressure would contain opacified urine that is slowly progressing in a normal prograde direction.

The striated nephrogram in acute pyelonephritis and acute bacterial nephritis represents an acute tubulointerstitial nephritis in medullary or cortical rays served by incompetent papillary orifices, as described in Chapter 9. The acute inflammatory cell infiltrate increases interstitial pressure, which diminishes the perfusion and contrast enhancement of the affected portions of the kidney. This is seen as striated areas of relative radiolucency in the early stages of a contrast material–enhanced study. On delayed images, these linear radiolucent striations gradually become radiodense as iodine-containing urine slowly accumulates in collecting ducts that are partially obstructed by inflammatory exudate.

Ectasia of collecting ducts is the fundamental structural kidney abnormality in autosomal recessive (infantile) polycystic kidney disease, as discussed in Chapter 8. As contrast material initially passes through the nephrons, adjacent dilated collecting ducts in the cortical and medullary rays appear as striated nephrographic radiolucencies because they are filled with nonopacifed urine. Eventually. the collecting ducts opacify. However, the striated pattern may persist as the bundles of nephrons that are interposed with the cortical and medullary rays lose their radiopacity and become radiolucent relative to the collecting ducts.

The basis for a striated urographic nephrogram in hypotension, intratubular block, renal contusion, and renal vein thrombosis is entirely speculative. Suggestions for its existence have included prolonged tubule transit time and hyperconcentration due to decreased glomerular filtration (hypotension), increased intersti-

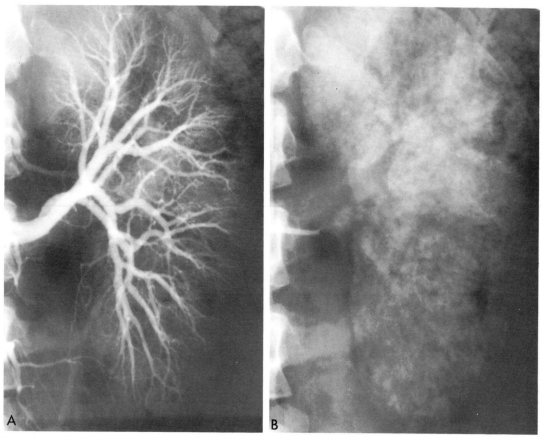

Figure 23–26. Patchy urographic nephrogram in acute lupus nephritis.
    A, Selective renal arteriogram. Arterial phase. The kidney is enlarged, and the intrarenal arteries are stretched.
    B, Selective renal arteriogram. Nephrogram phase. There is a patchy nephrogram indicative of diffuse, obliterative changes in the microvasculature.

tial pressure (renal vein thrombosis, renal contusion), intratubular block (Tamm-Horsfall proteinuria), and vasospasm (renal contusion).

Patchy Urographic Nephrogram

Inhomogeneous urographic nephrograms have been described in obliterative diseases of the renal microvasculature, such as polyarteritis nodosa, scleroderma, and necrotizing angiitis, and in catheter-induced vasospasm (Fig. 23–26). In these diseases, the nephrogram consists of patchy densities and does not have an orderly pattern of striations. This reflects random occlusive events in the microvasculature of the kidney.

ANALYSIS OF THE INTEGRITY OF RENAL STRUCTURE

The radiologist's ability to detect structural abnormalities of the kidney depends on identifying disruption of the homogeneity of the urographic nephrogram. Accomplishing this task with excretory urography requires an adequate dose of contrast material, low-kilovoltage radiographic technique, and linear tomography. Computed tomography is much more reliable than excretory urography in detecting structural de-

formities of the nephrogram and requires much less contrast material. The advantage of computed tomography over excretory urography is particularly noted when lesions are located on the anterior or posterior surface of the kidney, areas not seen in the standard profile views of excretory urography.

The urographic nephrogram is deformed by processes that cause loss of renal tissue (reflux nephropathy, lobar infarction), displacement of normal parenchyma (chronic obstructive uropathy, autosomal dominant (adult) and autosomal recessive (infantile) polycystic kidney disease, medullary cystic disease, simple cyst, focal hydronephrosis), or replacement of parenchyma (benign or malignant neoplasm and inflammatory mass). Each of these diseases is discussed in detail in other chapters.

Bibliography

Banner, M. P., and Pollack, H. M.: Evaluation of renal function by excretory urography. J. Urol. *124*:437, 1980.
Bigongiari, L. R., Patel, S. K., Appelman, H., and Thornbury, J. R.: Medullary rays: Visualization during excretory urography. AJR *125*:795, 1975.
Bigongiari, L. R., Davis, R. M., Novak, W. G., Wicks, J. D., Kass, E., and Thornbury, J. R.: Visualization of the medullary rays on excretory urography in experimental ureteric obstruction. AJR *129*:89, 1977.

Bowley, N. B.: Renal opacification during intravenous urography in acute cortical necrosis (the nephrogram in cortical necrosis). Br. J. Radiol. *54*:24, 1981.

Brennan, R. E., Curtis, J. A., Pollack, H. M., and Weinberg, I.: Sequential changes in the CT numbers of the normal canine kidney following intravenous contrast administration: I. The renal cortex. Invest. Radiol. *14*:141, 1979.

Brennan, R. E., Curtis, J. A., Pollack, H. M., and Weinberg, I.: Sequential changes in the CT numbers of the normal canine kidney following intravenous contrast administration: II. The renal medulla. Invest. Radiol. *14*:239, 1979.

Bretland, P. M.: Acute ureteric obstruction—clinical and radiological aspects. Proc. R. Soc. Med. *67*:1215, 1974.

Coel, M. N., and Talner, L. B.: Obstructive nephrogram due to renal vein thrombosis. Radiology *101*:573, 1971.

Frank, J. A., Choyke, P. L., Austin, H. A., and Girton, M. E.: Functional MR of the kidney. Magn. Reson. Med. *22*:319, 1991.

Frank, P. H., Nuttall, J., Brander, W. L., and Prosser, D.: The cortical rim sign of renal infarction. Br. J. Radiol. *47*:875, 1974.

Fry, I. K., and Cattell, W. R.: The nephrographic pattern during excretion urography. Br. Med. Bull. *28*:227, 1972.

Glazer, G. M., and London, S. S.: CT appearance of global renal infarction. J. Comput. Assist. Tomogr. *5*:847, 1981.

Goergen, T. G., Lindstrom, R. R., Tan, H., and Lilley, J. J.: CT appearance of acute renal cortical necrosis. AJR *137*:176, 1981.

Hann, L., and Pfister, R. C.: Renal subcapsular rim sign: New etiologies and pathogenesis. AJR *138*:51, 1982.

Heinz, E. R., Dubois, P. J., Drayer, B. P., and Hill, P.: A preliminary investigation of the role of dynamic computed tomography in renovascular hypertension. J. Comput. Assist. Tomogr. *4*:63, 1980.

Ishikawa, I., Onouchi, Z., Saito, Y. K., Kitada, H., Shinoda, A., Ushitani, K., Tabuchi, M., and Suzuki, M.: Renal cortex visualization and analysis of dynamic CT curves of the kidney. J. Comput. Assist. Tomogr. *5*:695, 1981.

Korobkin, M.: The nephrogram of hemorrhagic hypotension. AJR *114*:673, 1972.

Korobkin, M., Shanser, J. D., and Carlson, E. L.: The nephrogram of normovolemic renal artery hypotension. Invest. Radiol. *11*:71, 1976.

Lee, J. K. T., McClennan, B. L., Melson, G. L., and Stanley, R. J.: Acute focal bacterial nephritis: Emphasis on gray scale sonography and computed tomography. AJR *135*:87, 1980.

Martin, D. C., and Jaffe, N.: Prolonged nephrogram due to hyperuricaemia. Br. J. Radiol. *44*:806, 1971.

Newhouse, J. H., and Murphy, R. X., Jr.: Tissue distribution of soluble contrast: Effect of dose variation and changes with time. AJR *136*:463, 1981.

Newhouse, J. H., and Pfister, R. C.: The nephrogram. Radiol. Clin. North Am. *17*:213, 1979.

Paul, G. J., and Stephenson, T. F.: The cortical rim sign in renal infarction. Radiology *122*:338, 1977.

Rubin, B. E., and Schliftman, R.: The striated nephrogram in renal contusion. Urol. Radiol. *1*:119, 1979.

Sherwood, T., Doyle, F. H., Boulton-Jones, M., Joekes, A. M., Peters, D. K., and Sissons, P.: The intravenous urogram in acute renal failure. Br. J. Radiol. *47*:368, 1974.

Treugut, H., Andersson, I., Hildell, J., Nyman, U., and Weibull, H.: Diagnostik renaler Perfusionsstörungen durch Sequenz-CT. Fortshr. Röntgenstr. *135*:381, 1981.

White, E. A., Korobkin, M., and Brito, A. C.: Computed tomography of experimental acute renal ischemia. Invest. Radiol. *14*:421, 1979.

Wicks, J. D., Bigongiari, L. R., Foley, W. D., and Walter, J.: Parenchymal striations in renal vein thrombosis: Arteriographic demonstration. AJR *129*:95, 1977.

Young, S. W., Noon, M. A., and Marincek, B.: Dynamic computed time-density study of normal human tissue after intravenous contrast administration. AJR *129*:36, 1981.

Young, S. W., Noon, M. A., Nassi, M., and Castellino, R. A.: Dynamic computed tomography body scanning. J. Comput. Assist. Tomogr. *4*:168, 1980.

24

RADIOLOGIC TECHNIQUES IN THE DIAGNOSIS OF RENAL FAILURE

CLINICAL AND RADIOLOGIC BACKGROUND	THE USE OF CONTRAST MATERIAL IN THE AZOTEMIC PATIENT
Prerenal Failure	Selection of Patients
Postrenal Failure	Radiographic Techniques
Renal Failure	Contrast Material
	OTHER DIAGNOSTIC PROCEDURES

The physician who sees a patient with a first-time diagnosis of renal failure must ask certain practical questions that have diagnostic, therapeutic, and prognostic importance. The answers to some of these are frequently found in radiologic studies.

This chapter considers both the clinical aspects of renal failure relevant to the radiologist and the specific information that should be derived from the radiologic examination of patients. Administration of contrast material to the azotemic patient requires special techniques and precautions. These are discussed in Chapter 1 in the broader context of contrast material physiology and radiologic technique but are summarized here for the convenience of the reader and also to emphasize their importance. Specific pathologic, clinical, and radiologic features of the individual diseases that lead to renal failure can be found under the appropriate diagnostic set in other chapters.

CLINICAL AND RADIOLOGIC BACKGROUND

Renal failure occurs when kidney function is inadequate to maintain the volume and the composition of the internal environment. Invariably, this is associated with azotemia, the accumulation of nitrogenous wastes in the blood.

Distinction between acute and chronic renal failure can usually be made before radiologic examination. Acute renal failure develops rapidly in patients who previously were in good health. When acute renal failure occurs in the form of acute tubular necrosis, a precipitating event such as hypotension, severe dehydration, trauma, or exposure to a nephrotoxin can be

established. One of the acute glomerulonephritides is the other major form of acute renal failure, and this is occasionally preceded by an upper respiratory tract infection. Patients with acute renal failure have a normal hemoglobin value, and most are normotensive. The finding of bilaterally normal to large-sized kidneys supports the clinical diagnosis of acute renal failure except in autosomal dominant (adult) or autosomal recessive (infantile) polycystic kidney disease or bilateral hydronephrosis.

Chronic renal failure, on the other hand, is insidious in onset and is associated with pruritus, weight loss, anorexia, hypertension, and anemia. Hypocalcemia with secondary hyperparathyroidism and renal osteodystrophy occur. Chronic renal failure is identified by bilaterally small kidneys that are either smooth or scarred, depending on the initiating disease, except for autosomal dominant (adult) polycystic kidney disease in which the kidneys are large or acquired cystic kidney disease in which the kidneys vary from small to large.

Symptomatic disorders of the gastrointestinal, cardiovascular, and central nervous systems, collectively known as the *uremic syndrome*, develop in both acute and chronic renal failure.

The diseases and pathophysiologic states that cause either acute or chronic renal failure can be placed in one of three categories: *prerenal, postrenal,* or *renal.* Suspected prerenal failure can be excluded by clinical measures, whereas ultrasonography combined with an abdominal radiograph is the principal method for investigating possible postrenal and renal failures. Excretory urography should be used as the initial technique for evaluating the patient with renal failure only when ultrasonography or unenhanced computed tomography is not available.

Prerenal Failure

Prerenal failure results from hypoperfusion of the kidney due to causes other than primary disease of the kidney or urinary tract. These include hypovolemia (fluid loss from hemorrhage, burns, or gastrointestinal disorders), impaired cardiac function (heart failure, myocardial infarction, cardiac tamponade), and prolonged peripheral vasodilatation (bacteremia, antihypertensive medications). These usually produce acute renal failure *de novo*. However, hypoperfusion states can transform a case of pre-existing, but subclinical, renal failure into one of acute decompensation. The essence of prerenal failure, however, is that it is functional and reversible.

One of the first steps that the clinician must take in the evaluation of the patient with oliguric renal failure is to exclude a prerenal cause. This can be accomplished by an appropriate therapeutic trial, such as expansion of the intravascular fluid volume, administration of a diuretic drug, or correction of hypotension. If prerenal failure is present, these steps will correct the state of hypoperfusion and convert a small output of concentrated urine into a larger output of less concentrated urine. When this occurs, further diagnostic evaluation of possible diseases of the kidney or urinary tract is unnecessary.

The radiologist must depend on the clinician to eliminate prerenal failure as a cause of renal failure before the patient is referred for radiologic evaluation. This is particularly important if ultrasonography is not available and excretory urography must be used. In this circumstance, if renal hypoperfusion is present, it will increase the risk of contrast material–induced nephrotoxicity. Once prerenal factors are excluded, however, radiologic techniques are very useful in differentiating the remaining two categories of kidney failure.

Postrenal Failure

Processes that obstruct urine outflow from both kidneys will eventually result in renal failure. These are classified as postrenal. This condition is sometimes referred to as obstructive *nephro*pathy to indicate impairment of renal function, whereas obstructive *uro*pathy is more generally used to describe lesions that dilate the collecting structures proximal to a point of narrowing without necessarily affecting renal function. To cause impaired function, an obstruction must be bilateral or occur unilaterally in the presence of an absent or diseased contralateral kidney. Postrenal failure can be acute or chronic.

A large number of specific lesions cause mechanical outflow obstruction and postrenal failure. These include congenital and inflammatory processes, calculi, trauma, and tumors. Functional abnormalities such as megaureter, severe vesicoureteral reflux, and neuropathic bladder may also produce postrenal failure.

The exclusion of obstruction as a possible cause of renal failure is an important early step in the management of the patient with renal failure. Ultrasonography readily identifies the dilated, urine-filled upper collecting systems. This is the basis for the very high sensitivity of this technique in detecting urinary tract obstruction of sufficient duration to have caused dilatation of the upper tracts. False-negative results occur in four situations. First, if the obstruction leading to renal failure is acute, dilatation of the collecting system is often minimal to absent and the ultrasound examination of the kidney may be interpreted as normal. For this reason, a small amount of dilatation should be taken seriously in the presence of oliguric renal failure. Excretory urography, rather than ultrasonography, is a more sensitive test for the exclusion of acute obstruction as a cause of renal failure. Second, a staghorn calculus that forms in an obstructed system will generate dense echoes and an acoustic shadow, which may obscure the fact that the renal pelvis is dilated due to obstruction. Therefore, the ultrasonographic finding of staghorn calculus alone does not exclude the possibility of obstruction. Third, false-negative results sometimes occur when acute renal failure is superimposed on chronic obstruction. In this situation, urine production ceases and the previously dilated collecting system collapses. Finally, if an obstruction is caused by a retroperitoneal mass that surrounds the pelvocalyceal systems and proximal ureters, these structures will not be distensible despite the presence of obstruction. When these four sources of false-negative results are taken into account, the sensitivity of ultrasound examination for detecting urinary tract obstruction approaches 100 per cent.

It should be kept in mind, on the other hand, that all dilated pelvocalyceal systems and ureters are not obstructed. Nonobstructive causes of collecting system dilatation include vesicoureteral reflux, infection, high flow states, congenital megacalyces, postobstructive atrophy, pregnancy, prune-belly syndrome, and primary megaureter. These entities may lead to a false-positive ultrasound diagnosis of chronic obstruction and are the factors that underlie a specificity of only 75 per cent. This is discussed further in Chapter 17.

Ultrasonography is frequently employed in the evaluation of the patient with renal failure of recent onset because of its high sensitivity in the diagnosis of subacute and chronic obstruction. However, the positive yield for this investigation is exceedingly low unless the patient is screened using criteria that increase the probability of obstruction. These criteria include known pelvic malignancy, palpable abdominal or pelvic mass, suspected renal colic, known calculous disease, bladder outlet obstruction, recent pelvic surgery, and suspected urinary sepsis.

When imaging modalities that are not contrast material dependent (ultrasonography, unenhanced computed tomography) are not available, excretory urography is a suitable substitute in the assessment of postrenal failure. Delayed opacification of a dilated collecting system is the urographic hallmark of post-renal failure. Demonstration of this sometimes requires that films be taken up to 24 hours after the start of urography. This allows time for the depressed rate of contrast material clearance from the blood to accumulate enough atoms of iodine in the collecting structures for radiographic visualization. A less common but equally definitive urographic sign of obstruction is the radiolucent image of dilated calyces, which becomes apparent as contrast material accumulates in the compressed parenchyma surrounding the calyces (see Fig. 9–20). This finding is called the "negative pyelogram" and is associated with chronic postrenal failure (see Chapter 9). It is conceivable, but not very likely, that there are some cases in which the combination of renal failure and obstruction will produce no nephrogram and no pyelogram and cause the urographic diagnosis of obstruction to be missed by excretory urography.

Contrast material–enhanced computed tomographic findings in chronic obstruction are the same as those described for excretory urography. Similarly, this technique should be used only as an adjunct to ultrasonography, or when other, simpler methods are not available.

Renal Failure

Azotemia that occurs as a result of primary disease of the renal parenchyma is termed *renal failure* in the classification system used in this chapter. Patients are placed in this category after prerenal failure has been excluded by appropriate therapeutic trials and postrenal failure has been excluded by ultrasonography, or when necessary, by excretory urography.

Once the diagnosis of renal (i.e., primary parenchymal) failure has been established, uroradiologic studies can often suggest the nature of the process. Usually, large kidneys indicate acute renal failure, whereas small kidneys indicate chronic renal failure. Sometimes, a specific disease may be indicated either by the pattern on ultrasonography, as seen in autosomal dominant (adult) or autosomal recessive (infantile) polycystic kidney disease, or by contour scars, papillary abnormalities, or nephrographic features detected by excretory urography or computed tomography.

Renal parenchymal diseases that cause acute renal failure are usually associated with bilaterally enlarged, smooth kidneys (see Chapter 8). Most of these diseases are bilateral by nature. However, when some inherently unilateral diseases occur bilaterally by chance, they also cause renal failure (see Chapter 9). Virtually all of these diseases produce radiologic signs of global enlargement without specific abnormalities. The radiologic findings of large, smooth kidneys with nondilated calyces indicate that the azotemia is due to primary renal disease and that the process is acute and therefore potentially reversible. This information is important, since it directs the clinician to perform needle biopsy for a more specific diagnosis, while the patient is treated with appropriate measures, including short-term dialysis.

The finding of small kidneys indicates that renal failure is chronic. This information leads the clinician to consider the problems of long-term management, including hemodialysis and transplantation. Knowledge of the specific nature of the disease becomes less important, since the process is irreversible. Nevertheless, radiologic features often do provide a specific diagnosis, particularly in reflux nephropathy, lobar infarction, and renal papillary necrosis, and occasionally in medullary cystic disease. Renal disease that produces bilaterally small, smooth kidneys (see Chapter 7) usually cannot be specifically diagnosed by radiologic tests. The lack of discrimination of radiologic tests in this situation, however, is of little practical importance because the renal failure is irreversible.

THE USE OF CONTRAST MATERIAL IN THE AZOTEMIC PATIENT

Selection of Patients

Excretory urography should be performed in the patient with renal failure only when ultrasonography, unenhanced computed tomography, or magnetic resonance imaging is not available for the initial screening or when there is a need for information that cannot be provided by these other modalities. Certain precautions, discussed in detail in Chapter 1, must be taken whenever urographic contrast material is administered to any azotemic patient. The three major precautions are summarized below:

1. Dehydration must be avoided. The azotemic kidney does not concentrate urine normally because of a urea-induced osmotic diuresis as well as an increased rate of sodium loss in chronic disease. Fluid deprivation and cathartics used in standard patient preparation for urography can lead to a negative fluid balance and worsening of the patient's condition. Close cooperation between radiologist, clinician, and nurse is required to avoid this situation.
2. Dehydration must also be avoided in patients with hypergammaglobulinemia and/or hyperuricemia, to lessen the likelihood of intratubular blockage by precipitation of these substances. Urography should be delayed in patients with very high serum uric acid levels until they are lowered.
3. Prerenal azotemia should be excluded before excretory urography.

Radiographic Techniques

Tomograms of the kidney should be exposed before contrast material injection. These provide baseline data for the detection of accumulation of faint amounts of contrast material during urography.

Tomograms should be obtained within the first 20 minutes of the examination if standard films fail to reveal calyceal opacification. It is during this period that a faint amount of contrast material is likely to be identified in one or two nondilated calyces in the severely azotemic, nonobstructed patient. Kilovoltage in the 60- to 75-kV range is necessary for good quality tomograms.

If conclusive diagnostic information is not obtained within the first hour, periodic films with standardized technique should be obtained up to 24 hours. These films allow the detection of delayed opacification of dilated calyces and an analysis of the time–density characteristics of the nephrogram (see Chapters 8 and 23).

Contrast Material

For excretory urography in the azotemic patient, 600 mg of iodine per kilogram of body weight should be used. This level can be produced by a dose of 2 ml/kg of the commonly used contrast material listed in Table 1–1.

A reduction in the risk of further impairment of renal function by low osmolality contrast agents compared with high osmolality agents has been suggested but has not been conclusively established in patients with pre-existing renal failure. However, when high osmolality contrast agents are used in azotemic patients, N-methylglucamine salts should be chosen for those on sodium-restricted diets, while patients who are not on sodium-restricted diets should be given sodium salts of contrast material (see Table 1–1).

The radiologist should keep in mind that the glomerular filtration rate must fall below 25 per cent of normal before the blood urea nitrogen and serum creatinine levels begin to rise above normal limits. Thus, doses adjusted for renal failure may be necessary in some patients with normal blood urea nitrogen and serum creatinine levels.

OTHER DIAGNOSTIC PROCEDURES

A radiograph of the abdomen and renal ultrasonography are fundamental to the radiologic assessment of the azotemic patient. Other studies may yield information unique to an individual set of circumstances.

If obstruction is established as the cause of renal failure, antegrade pyelography is often useful in defining the site and etiology.

Radionuclide flow studies, described in Chapter 2, are often used to investigate suspected perfusion disorders of the kidney. Arteriography or venography may also be of value when occlusive disease of arteries or veins is considered as a cause of renal failure. Magnetic resonance angiography or color Doppler ultrasonography may serve a similar purpose. Other, less definitive indications for angiography are discussed in Chapter 26.

Computed tomography, like excretory urography, has adjunctive value in the assessment of the azotemic patient. Additionally, this technique is particularly well suited to the detection of nephrocalcinosis, urolithiasis, and obstructing lesions of the ureters as well as to the assessment of renal perfusion and the retroperitonial space.

Bibliography

Behan, M., Wixon, D., and Kazam, E.: Sonographic evaluation of the nonfunctioning kidney. J. Clin. Ultrasound 7:449, 1979.

Brown, C. B., Glancy, J. J., Fry, I. K., and Cattell, W. R.: High-dose excretion urography in oliguric renal failure. Lancet 2:952, 1970.

Brown, J. M.: The ultrasound approach to the urographically nonvisualizing kidney. Semin. Ultrasound 2:44, 1981.

Denton, T., Cochlin, D. L., and Evans, C.: The value of ultrasound in previously undiagnosed renal failure. Br. J. Radiol. 57:673, 1984.

Dhar, S. K., Chandrasekhar, H., and Smith, E. C.: Renosonogram in diagnosis of renal failure. Clin. Nephrol. 7:15, 1977.

Elkin, M.: Obstructive uropathy and uremia. Radiol. Clin. North Am. 10:447, 1972

Fry, I. K., and Cattell, W. R.: Radiology in the diagnosis of renal failure. Br. Med. Bull. 27:148, 1971.

Fry, I. K., and Cattell, W. R.: Excretion urography in advanced renal failure. Br. J. Radiol. 44:198, 1971.

Hennessy, W. T., Pollack, H. M., Banner, M. P., and Wein, A. J.: Radiologic evaluation of anuric patient: Systematized approach. Urology 18:435, 1981.

Mahaffy, R. G., Matheson, N. A., and Caridis, D. T.: Infusion pyelography in acute renal failure. Clin. Radiol. 20:320, 1969.

McClennan, B. L.: Current approaches to the azotemic patient. Radiol. Clin. North Am. 17:197, 1979.

Moccia, W. A., Kaude, J. V., Wright, P. G., and Gaffney, E. F.: Evaluation of chronic renal failure by digital gray scale ultrasound. Urol. Radiol. 2:1, 1980.

Papper, S.: Renal failure. Med. Clin. North Am. 55:335, 1971.

Platt, J. F., Rubin, J. M., and Ellis, J. H.: Distinction between obstructive and non-obstructive pyelocaliectasis with duplex Doppler sonography. AJR 153:997, 1989.

Platt, J. F., Rubin, J. M., and Ellis, J. H.: Acute renal failure: Possible role of duplex Doppler US in distinction between acute renal failure and acute tubular necrosis. Radiology 179:419, 1991.

Platt, J. F., Rubin, J. M., Bowerman, R. A., and Marn, C. S.: The inability to detect kidney disease on the basis of echogenicity. AJR 151:317, 1988.

Ritchie, W. W., Vick, C. W., Glocheski, S. K., and Cook, D. E.: Evaluation of azotemic patients: Diagnostic yield of initial US examination. Radiology 167:245, 1988.

Rosenfield, A. T.: Ultrasound evaluation of renal parenchymal disease and hydronephrosis. Urol. Radiol. 4:125, 1982.

Stage, P., Brix, E., Folke, K., and Karle, A.: Urography in renal failure. Acta Radiol. (Diagn.) 11:337, 1971.

Stuck, K. J., White, G. M., Granke, D. S., Ellis, J., and Weissfeld, J. L.: Urinary obstruction in azotemic patients: Detection by sonography. AJR 149:1191, 1987.

Talner, L. B.: Urographic contrast media in uremia: Physiology and pharmacology. Radiol. Clin. North Am. 10:421, 1972.

Talner, L. B., Scheible, W., Ellenbogen, P. H., Beck, C. H., Jr., and Gosink, B. B.: How accurate is ultrasonography in detecting hydronephrosis in azotemic patients? Urol. Radiol. 3:1, 1981.

Winston, M., Pritchard, J., and Paulin, P.: Ultrasonography in the management of unexplained renal failure. J. Clin. Ultrasound 6:1, 1978.

25

DIAGNOSTIC EVALUATION OF THE UNIFOCAL RENAL MASS

EVALUATION OF THE "PRESUMPTIVELY FLUID-FILLED" MASS

EVALUATION OF THE "PRESUMPTIVELY SOLID" MASS

EXTENUATING CIRCUMSTANCES AFFECTING THE MANAGEMENT OF A RENAL MASS

MISCELLANEOUS CONSIDERATIONS

The discovery of a kidney tumor results from either an investigation instigated by clinical findings suggestive of a urinary tract neoplasm or as an incidental finding. *Discovery* of a mass, however, is only the first step in its radiologic evaluation. Once a mass is found, the main challenge to the radiologist is to reliably predict its *nature* while giving recognition to the fact that a final tissue diagnosis is in the province of the pathologist, not the radiologist. Thus, a proper radiologic diagnosis should be viewed as a prediction that reflects a level of probability based on both the sensitivity of the imaging modality or modalities used and the inherent characteristics of the mass. In addition to its probable accuracy, the value of a radiologic diagnosis should also be measured by its influence on patient management. For example, a confident diagnosis of a simple cyst indicates no need for further investigation; a confident diagnosis of an angiomyolipoma supports renal-sparing conservative surgery; whereas a confident diagnosis of adenocarcinoma militates for radical nephrectomy. Information regarding local or distant spread and bilaterality or multiplicity of tumor sites within the kidneys also impacts management decisions. As a final consideration, the radiologist must strive to use means that are both precise and economic in the pursuit of these goals.

The approach taken in this chapter is to initially characterize a mass as either "presumptively fluid-filled" or "presumptively solid." Assigning a mass to one of these categories determines an imaging strategy that should be designed to impart the highest level of confidence to the final radiologic diagnosis. Each of the modalities that might be used contributes its own particular level of confidence to this process. The techniques most commonly employed are excretory urography, ultrasonography, and computed to-

mography. Needle aspiration, magnetic resonance imaging, radionuclide scan, angiography, inferior vena cavography, and percutaneous biopsy sometimes provide adjunctive information.

The specific entities that form unifocal masses in the kidney are discussed in Chapter 12. A summary of the concepts expressed in this chapter are presented in Figures 25–1 and 25–2 in the form of flow charts.

EVALUATION OF THE "PRESUMPTIVELY FLUID-FILLED" MASS

Excretory Urography

Presumptively fluid-filled masses are those that have an unenhanced nephrogram, a sharp interface between the mass and the renal parenchyma, a "beak" or "claw" sign, a thin, almost imperceptible wall, and, if present, smooth effacement or displacement of the adjacent collecting system. A very thin line of mural calcification may also be present. Based on prevalence considerations alone, most presumptively fluid-filled masses are simple cysts. Other causes of a presumptively fluid-filled mass include *focal hydronephrosis, multilocular cystic nephroma, mature liquefied abscess,* cavernous forms of *congenital arteriovenous malformation, renal artery aneurysm,* as well as the hypovascular or cystic forms of *renal adenocarcinoma* or *Wilms' tumor.*

Even with the advantage of excellent technique, excretory urography does not permit a confident diagnosis that a mass is, in fact, cystic (Figs. 25–3 and 25–4). When excretory urography alone is used, the overall accuracy for predicting the final pathologic diagnosis is about 50 per cent. Even with tomography, the accuracy only rises to slightly over 55 per cent. With the experienced eyes of a full-time uroradiologist, the

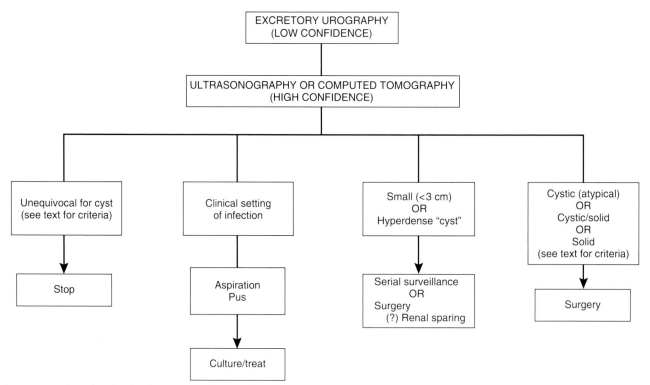

Figure 25–1. Flow chart for the diagnostic evaluation of a "presumptively fluid-filled" unifocal mass. This chart assumes initial evaluation is by excretory urography.

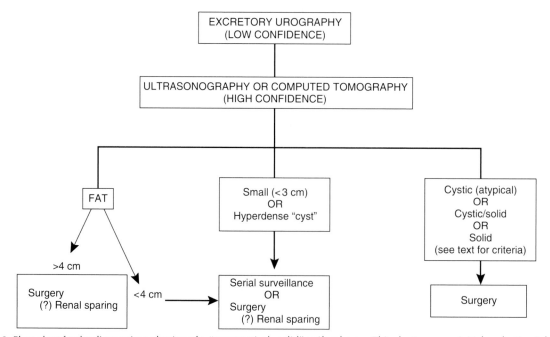

Figure 25–2. Flow chart for the diagnostic evaluation of a "presumptively solid" unifocal mass. This chart assumes initial evaluation is by excretory urography.

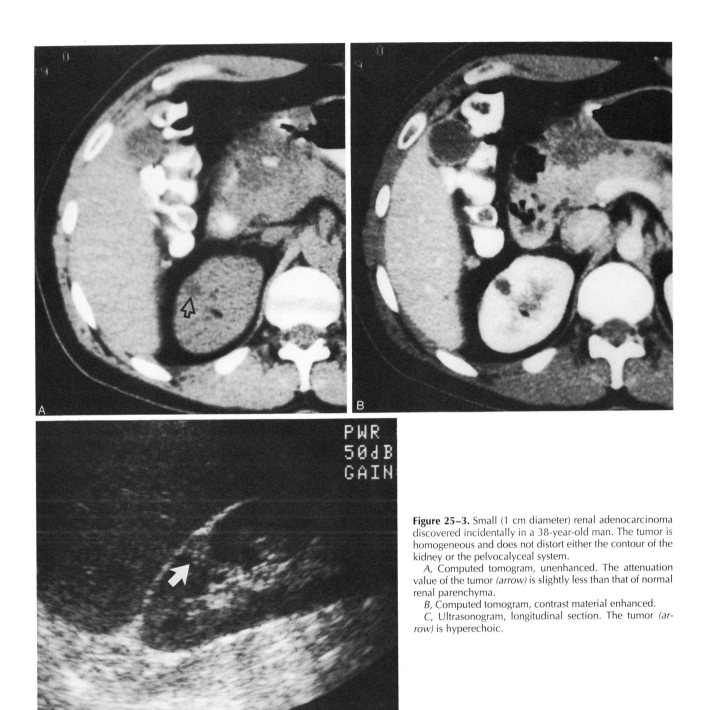

Figure 25–3. Small (1 cm diameter) renal adenocarcinoma discovered incidentally in a 38-year-old man. The tumor is homogeneous and does not distort either the contour of the kidney or the pelvocalyceal system.

A, Computed tomogram, unenhanced. The attenuation value of the tumor *(arrow)* is slightly less than that of normal renal parenchyma.

B, Computed tomogram, contrast material enhanced.

C, Ultrasonogram, longitudinal section. The tumor *(arrow)* is hyperechoic.

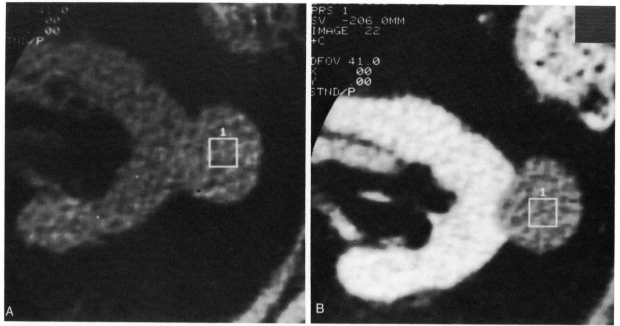

Figure 25–4. Small (2.5 cm in diameter) renal adenocarcinoma appearing as a hyperdense mass that does not enhance with contrast material. The tumor is round, smooth, and homogeneous, and most of its bulk extends outside the kidney. The findings illustrated correspond exactly to those that would be expected with a hyperdense simple cyst.

   A, Computed tomogram, unenhanced. The attenuation value is 44.5 Hounsfield units.

   B, Computed tomogram, contrast material enhanced. The attenuation value is essentially unchanged at 43.9 Hounsfield units.

   (From Hartman, D. S., et al.: Cystic renal cell carcinoma: CT findings simulating a benign hyperdense cyst. AJR *159*:1235, 1992. Reproduced with kind permission of the American Roentgen Ray Society.)

overall accuracy is still an unsatisfactory 70 per cent. Therefore, the low sensitivity of excretory urography requires further characterization of the mass to achieve a level of confidence secure enough for a decision regarding patient management.

In proceeding with the diagnostic workup, it is necessary to keep in mind that the challenge in the investigation of a fluid-filled mass is to not miss an adenocarcinoma and, because of the ubiquity of simple kidney cysts in older patients, to perform simple and inexpensive procedures. In this context, both ultrasonography and computed tomography provide a very high level of diagnostic confidence. The former is usually more readily available and less expensive to perform than the latter but is operator dependent and may be technically difficult, especially in patients with a mass in the left kidney or an unfavorable body habitus. Computed tomography, on the other hand, provides more standardized and comprehensive data including enhancement characteristics of the mass when studies are obtained both with and without the administration of contrast material.

Ultrasonography or Computed Tomography

Demonstration of an anechoic lesion with a sharply defined far wall and acoustic enhancement permits a diagnosis of simple cyst with an accuracy approaching 100 per cent. A similar level of confidence is achieved with the computed tomographic demonstration of a sharply defined, almost imperceptible thin-walled mass of homogeneous content that has a near-water attenuation value that does not vary by more than 15 Hounsfield units before and after contrast material enhancement. By using either modality, fine, curvilinear mural calcification or a few filamentous septa may be identified. With these findings, the mass can confidently be diagnosed as a simple cyst with the usual implication of clinical insignificance.

The radiologist must, however, take safeguards against certain pitfalls associated with some masses that mimic simple cyst on either ultrasonography or computed tomography. Some simple cysts have been complicated by infection or hemorrhage that cause deviation from the strict criteria described above for simple cyst. Other lesions that might simulate at least some characteristics of simple cyst are *multilocular cystic nephroma, focal hydronephrosis, liquefied abscess,* the cavernous form of *arteriovenous malformation, renal artery aneurysm, adenocarcinoma* or *Wilms' tumor* that is cystic, necrotic, or hypovascular, and *echinococcal disease.*

Diagnostic error as a result of these pitfalls can be minimized only by adhering rigidly to the strict ultrasonographic or computed tomographic criteria for simple cyst, as enumerated previously. Atypical findings include a calcified or uncalcified wall that is more than 1 mm thick, mural irregularity or nodule(s), thick septa, tissue or debris internal to the mass, or enhancement of internal contents, including septa, by more than 15 Hounsfield units after administration of contrast material. When any of these criteria are present, one of two strategies must be pursued. If the ultrasonographic or computed tomographic findings of an atypical fluid-filled mass are present *in the clinical setting of infection,* needle aspiration should be performed to exclude an infected simple cyst, a calyceal diverticulum, a hydrocalyx, or a mature abscess. If, on the other hand, the ultrasonographic or computed tomographic findings define features that are not unequivocally those of a simple cyst, then management decisions turn to obtaining either a tissue diagnosis or, if extenuating circumstances exist, continued observation. These alternatives are discussed later in this chapter.

Needle Aspiration

Needle aspiration should be performed only when there is a strong prior likelihood that the atypical fluid-filled mass is due to infection. The value of aspiration is in the potential for confirming the infectious nature of a mass by aspirating pus. This not only confirms the diagnosis but also allows for culture of the infecting organism. The aspiration of old blood, debris, or tissue militates for a strategy for the presumptively solid masses described below.

EVALUATION OF THE "PRESUMPTIVELY SOLID" MASS

The excretory urographic findings for a presumptively solid mass include an inhomogeneous nephrogram that enhances to a lesser degree than normal renal tissue, invasion and/or irregular displacement of the adjacent pelvocalyceal system, nonperipheral calcification, and an irregular interface with the renal parenchyma. With these findings the likelihood of the mass truly being solid is quite high, in contradistinction to the low level of confidence associated with the excretory urographic diagnosis of a presumptively fluid-filled mass. It is important to remember, however, that some or all of these urographic findings may represent diverse processes, including *anomalies* as well as all *malignant* and *benign tumors,* and evolving *inflammatory* or *hemorrhagic masses* (*bacterial nephritis, abscess, contusion, infarction,* or *hematoma*).

Although the urographic findings may be compelling enough to warrant surgery without further radiologic study, it is common practice to use computed tomography or, alternatively, ultrasonography to confirm the excretory urographic findings, to characterize the mass further as discussed later, and to evaluate important staging factors such as retroperitoneal or adjacent visceral invasion, contralateral kidney involvement, regional lymph node enlargement, or venous extension. Angiography, radionuclide scans, or magnetic resonance imaging may provide adjunctive information in selected cases. The radiologic findings in various unifocal solid masses are described in Chapter 12.

Whereas the goal for the imaging evaluation of a fluid-filled mass was to keep things simple and inexpensive while not missing a mass that required surgery, the goal for the evaluation of a presumptively solid mass is to identify characteristics of tumors (e.g., angiomyolipoma, adenoma/oncocytoma, multilocular cystic nephroma, or mesoblastic nephroma) that would support a conservative, renal-sparing surgical approach or to suggest a specific surgical approach such as nephroureterectomy for a transitional cell carcinoma invading the kidney. An additional objective is to detect those "tumors" that, in fact, are neither real (e.g., lobar dysmorphism) nor neoplastic (e.g., acute bacterial nephritis, infarction, or contusion).

Computed tomography or ultrasonography provide imaging data that satisfy the previously stated goals in most cases. Computed tomography is of particular value in identifying fat within a tumor and thereby establishing the basis for a confident diagnosis of angiomyolipoma. Similarly, a radionuclide scan is of particular value in investigating lobar dysmorphism as the basis for a "tumor." Angiography is of limited value in the contemporary evaluation of renal masses. The unique value of angiography is its ability to describe arterial anatomy as a guide for surgical approach. This is particularly so in the planning of renal-sparing, conservative surgery.

EXTENUATING CIRCUMSTANCES AFFECTING THE MANAGEMENT OF A RENAL MASS

The incidental discovery of a small (less than 3 cm diameter) solid mass in an asymptomatic patient or one that is "hyperdense" but otherwise has all the characteristics of a simple cyst are two conditions that were unrecognized before the era of modern imaging technology (see Figs. 25–3 and 25–4). Such events have provoked an interest in the biology and pathology of small renal tumors as a basis for developing appropriate management strategies (e.g., local excision, enucleation, or serial surveillance) other than radical nephrectomy.

Size alone cannot be used as a reliable determinant of the nature of a renal tumor. It is well established that there is a positive correlation between the size of a primary kidney adenocarcinoma and the probability of metastases. Most tumors less than 3 cm in diameter do not metastasize. There are, however, reports of small malignant tumors that have metastasized and caused death. Extenuating factors other than size that also must be considered in formulating the diagnostic and therapeutic approach to an incidentally discovered small renal tumor are patient age, general state of health, reliability for follow-up, and tolerance for living with the unknown on the part of the patient as well as the responsible physicians.

Similar reservations should be applied to the small renal mass that is hyperdense to renal parenchyma on unenhanced computed tomograms and does not increase in attenuation values after contrast material is given. Although it is probable that most lesions with these characteristics are simple cysts with altered fluid contents, probably due to prior hemorrhage, it is also established that adenocarcinoma can produce identical imaging results (Hartman et al., 1992). The relative frequency of both cysts and adenocarcinomas presenting as hyperdense masses is not known.

The concepts that an incidentally discovered very small, solid kidney tumor should not be removed until serial examinations demonstrate growth or that a hyperdense mass is a benign cyst and need not be removed are speculative and based on neither a broadly based, critically evaluated clinical experience nor specific insights into the biology of kidney tumors. A generally agreed on approach to these special circumstances must await greater understanding of the nature and malignant potential of small solid tumors and hyperdense masses. Both clinicians and the patient should recognize these uncertainties in formulating management strategies that do not include, at a minimum, excisional biopsy.

MISCELLANEOUS CONSIDERATIONS

The urinary tract signs or symptoms that originally brought a patient to a radiologic investigation should influence the diagnostic decision process at every step. Evaluation of a patient with hematuria should not stop with a negative excretory urogram and cystoscopy or a urogram that demonstrates only a simple renal cyst. This circumstance usually requires computed tomography for complete evaluation.

The identification of any amount of fat within a tumor that is clearly renal in origin permits a diagnosis of angiomyolipoma with nearly 100 per cent confidence (Fig. 25–5). Fat may be a component of adenocarcinoma, Wilms' tumor, or an intrarenal teratoma, but these are exceedingly rare occurrences. Another very rare potential source of error is an oncocytoma that entraps perirenal fat (Curry, 1990). On the other hand, the failure to detect fat in a kidney tumor, even with a technically thorough examination, does not exclude the diagnosis of angiomyolipoma, as discussed in Chapter 12. Small, exclusively fat-containing renal tumors are sometimes discovered as incidental findings during computed tomography or ultrasonography. These are presumed to be small angiomyolipomas of no clinical significance. It has been suggested that angiomyolipomas larger than 4 cm in diameter are more likely to be symptomatic than those of smaller size (Oesterling et al., 1986).

Confident differentiation of oncocytoma from adenocarcinoma or, more broadly speaking, benign from malignant solid tumors on the basis of imaging criteria is not possible. Homogeneous density and central "scar" occur with sufficient frequency in adenocarcinoma as to negate their value as predictors of oncocytoma regardless of the size of the tumor (Davidson et al., 1993). The same limitation applies to the angiographic demonstration of a "rim and spoke wheel" arterial pattern.

Needle biopsy of solid lesions is advocated by some radiologists, but the problem of sampling error is a

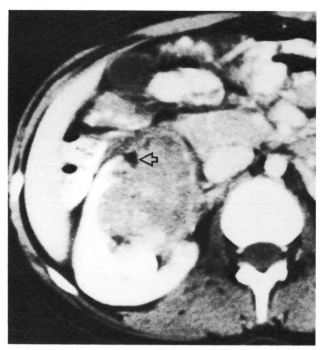

Figure 25–5. Angiomyolipoma containing a small amount of detectable fat in a 21-year-old woman. Computed tomogram, contrast material enhanced. Only a small portion of the tumor has the attenuation value of fat (arrow).

serious drawback. All the tissue within a carcinoma does not necessarily contain positive histologic or cytologic features of malignancy. Failure to identify malignancy in a percutaneous aspirate or biopsy specimen therefore cannot be taken as assurance that malignant change is not present in some portion of the mass. Adequate sampling requires access to the whole lesion, either at the time of surgical exploration or following surgical removal. Clearly, routine percutaneous needle biopsy of solid masses neither shortens the diagnostic process nor provides additional valuable information. Fear of spreading tumor cells along the needle track is sometimes used as an argument against needling any kind of unifocal mass, either fluid or solid. Extensive clinical experience indicates that this is not a valid argument in patients with adenocarcinoma, but it may be a risk in the biopsy of transitional cell carcinoma. Special circumstances in which biopsy may be of value in formulating a management strategy include patients with a single kidney, high surgical risk factors, a known primary malignancy, and bilateral, multiple tumors.

Bibliography

Ambrose, S. S., Lewis, E. L., O'Brien, D. P., III, Walton, K. N., and Ross, J. R.: Unsuspected renal tumors associated with renal cysts. J. Urol. 117:704, 1977.

Amendola, M. A., Bree, R. L., Pollack, H. M., Francis, I. R., Glazer, G. M., Jafri, S. Z. H., and Tomaszewski, J. E.: Small renal cell carcinomas: Resolving a diagnostic dilemma. Radiology 166:637, 1988.

Becker, J. A., and Schneider, M.: Simple cyst of the kidney. Semin. Roentgenol. 10:103, 1975.

Bell, E. T.: A classification of renal tumors with observation on the frequency of various types. J. Urol. 39:238, 1938.

Bennington, J. L., and Beckwith, J. B.: Tumors of the kidney, renal pelvis and ureter. In Atlas of Tumor Pathology, second series, fascicle 12. Washington, D. C., Armed Forces Institute of Pathology, 1975.

Birnbaum, B. A., Bosniak, M. A., Megibow, A. J., Lubat, E., and Gordon, R. B.: Observations on the growth of renal neoplasms. Radiology 176:695, 1990.

Bosniak, M. A.: The current radiological approach to renal cysts. Radiology 158:1, 1986.

Bosniak, M. A.: The small (≤ 3.0 cm) renal parenchymal tumor: Detection, diagnosis and controversies. Radiology 179:307, 1991.

Bush, W. H., Jr., Burnett, L. L., and Gibbons, R. P.: Needle tract seeding of renal cell carcinoma. AJR 129:725, 1977.

Cheng, W. S., Farrow, G. M., and Zincke, H.: The incidence of multicentricity in renal cell carcinoma. J. Urol. 146:1221, 1991.

Cohan, R., Dunnick, N., Degesys, G., Degesys, G., and Korobkin, M.: Computed tomography of renal oncocytoma. J. Comput. Assist. Tomogr. 8:284, 1984.

Cronan, J. J., Amis, E. S., Zeman, R. K., and Dorfman, G. S.: Obstruction of the upper-pole moiety in renal duplication in adults: CT evaluation. Radiology 161:17, 1986.

Curry, N. S., Reinig, J., Schabel, S. I., Ross, P., Vujic, I., and Gobien, R. P.: An evaluation of the effectiveness of CT vs other imaging modalities in the diagnosis of atypical renal masses. Invest. Radiol. 19:447, 1984.

Curry, N. S., Schabel, S. I., and Betsill, W. L.: Small renal neoplasms: Diagnostic imaging, pathologic features and clinical course. Radiology 158:113, 1986.

Curry, N. S., Schabel, S. I., Garvin, A. J., and Fish, G.: Intratumoral fat in a renal oncocytoma mimicking angiomyolipoma. AJR 154:307, 1990.

Davidson, A. J., and Davis, C. J., Jr.: Fat in renal adenocarcinoma: Never say never. Radiology 188:316, 1993.

Davidson, A. J., Hayes, W., S., Hartman, D. S., McCarthy, W. F., and Davis, C. J.: Renal oncocytoma and carcinoma: Failure of differentiation with CT. Radiology 186:693, 1993.

Davis, C. J., Sesterhenn, I. A., Mostofi, F. K., and Ho, C. K.: Renal oncocytoma: Clinicopathological study of 166 patients. J. Urogenital. Pathol. 1:41, 1992.

Delahunt, B., Gupta, R. K., and Nacey, J. N.: Diagnosis of renal oncocytoma. Urology 37:602, 1991.

Dunnick, N. R., Korobkin, M., and Clark, W. M.: CT demonstration of hyperdense renal carcinoma. J. Comput. Assist. Tomogr. 8:1023, 1984.

Dunnick, N. R.: Renal lesions: Great strides in imaging. Radiology 182:305, 1992.

Emmett, J. L., Levine, J. R., and Woolner, L. B.: Coexistence of renal cyst and tumor. Br. J. Urol. 35:403, 1963.

Endress, C., and Chita, M. A.: Renal cell carcinoma simulating oncocytoma (letter). AJR 158:920, 1992.

Forman, H. P., Middleton, W. D., Melson, G. L., and McClennan, B. L.: Hyperechoic renal cell carcinomas: Increase in detection at US. Radiology 188:431, 1993.

Fryback, D. G., and Thornbury, J. R.: Evaluation of a computerized Bayesian model for diagnosis of a renal cyst vs. tumor vs. normal variant from excretory urography information. Invest. Radiol. 11:102, 1976.

Goiney, R., Goldenberg, L., and Cooperberg, P. L.: Renal oncocytoma sonographic analysis of 14 cases. AJR 143:1001, 1984.

Goldman, S. M., and Hartman, D. S.: The simple cyst. In Hartman, D. S. (ed.): Renal Cystic Disease, fascicle I. In AFIP Atlas of Radiologic-Pathologic Correlation. Philadelphia, W. B. Saunders, 1989, pp. 6–37.

Hartman, D. S., Aronson, S., and Frazier, H.: Current status of imaging indeterminate renal masses. Radiol. Clin. North Am. 29:475, 1991.

Hartman, D. S., Weatherby, E., Laskin, W. B., Brody, J. M., Corse, W., and Baluch, J. D.: Cystic renal cell carcinoma: CT findings simulating a benign hyperdense cyst. AJR 159:1235, 1992.

Hélénon, O., Chrétien, Y., Paraf, F., Melki, P., et al.: Renal cell carci-

noma containing fat: Demonstration with CT. Radiology 188:429, 1993.

Hellsten, S., Berg, T., and Wehlin, L.: Unrecognized renal cell carcinoma: Clinical and pathological aspects. Scand. J. Urol. Nephrol. 15:273, 1981.

Jaschke, W., Kaick, G., Peter, S., and Palmtag, H.: Accuracy of computed tomography in staging of kidney tumors. Acta Radiol. (Diagn.) 23:593, 1982.

Kass, D. A., Hricak, H., and Davidson, A. J.: Renal malignancies with normal excretory urograms. AJR 141:731, 1983.

Lazzaro, B., Gonick, P., and Katz, S. M.: Renal cell carcinoma vs renal oncocytoma: Report of a case with overlap features and review of the literature. Urology 37:52, 1991.

Levine, E., Huntrakoon, M., and Wetzel, L. H.: Small renal neoplasms: Clinical, pathologic and imaging features. AJR 153:69, 1989.

Licht, M. R., and Novick, A. C.: Nephron-sparing surgery for renal cell carcinoma. J. Urol. 149:1, 1993.

Love, L., Churchill, R., Reynes, C., Schuster, G. A., Moncada, R., and Berkow, A.: Computed tomography staging of renal carcinoma. Urol. Radiol. 1:3, 1979.

Marshall, F. F., Taxy, J. B., Fishman, E. K., and Chang, R.: The feasibility of surgical enucleation for renal cell carcinoma. J. Urol. 135:231, 1986.

Marshall, F. F., Holdford, S. S., and Hamper, U. M.: Intraoperative sonography of renal tumors. J. Urol. 148:5, 1992.

Medeiros, L. J., Gelb, A. B., and Weiss, L. M.: Low grade renal cell carcinoma: A clinicopathologic study of 53 cases. Am. J. Surg. Pathol. 11:633, 1987.

Montie, J. E.: The incidental renal mass: Management alternatives. Urol. Clin. North Am. 18:427, 1991.

Oesterling, J. E., Fishman, E. K., Goldman, G. M., and Marshall, F. F.: The management of renal angiomyolipoma. J. Urol. 135:1121, 1986.

Plaine, L. I., and Hinman, F., Jr.: Malignancy in asymptomatic renal masses. J. Urol. 94:342, 1965.

Provet, J., Tessler, A., Brown, J., Golimbo, M., Bosniak, M., and Morales, P.: Partial nephrectomy for renal cell carcinoma: Indications, results, and implications. J. Urol. 145:472, 1991.

Smith, S. J., Bosniak, M. A., Megibow, A. J., Hulnick, D. H., Horii, S. C., and Ragharendra, B. N.: Renal cell carcinoma: Earlier discovery and increased detection. Radiology 170:699, 1989.

Steinbach, F., Stöckle, M., Müller, S. C., Thüroff, J. W., Melchior, S. W., Stein, R., and Hohenfellner, R.: Conservative surgery of renal cell tumors in 140 patients: 21 years of experience. J. Urol. 148:24, 1992.

Stephenson, T. F., Iyengar, S., and Rashid, H. A.: Comparison of computerized tomography and excretory urography in detection and evaluation of renal masses. J. Urol. 131:11, 1984.

Strotzer, M., Lehner, K. B., and Becker, K.: Detection of fat in a renal cell carcinoma mimicking angiomyolipoma. Radiology 188:427, 1993.

Talano, T. S., and Shonnard, J. W.: Small renal adenocarcinoma with metastases. J. Urol. 124:132, 1980.

Tikkakosi, T., Päiväsalo, M., Alanen, A., Nurmi, M., Taavitsainen, M., Farin, P., and Apaja-Sarkkinen, M.: Radiologic findings in renal oncocytoma. Acta Radiol. 32:363, 1991.

Tosuka, A., Ohya, K., Yamada, K., Ohashi, H., Kitahara, S., Sekine, H., Takehara, Y., and Oka, K.: Incidence and properties of renal masses and asymptomatic renal cell carcinoma detected by abdominal ultrasonography. J. Urol. 144:1097, 1990.

Wadsworth, D. E., McClennan, B. L., and Stanley, R. J.: CT of the renal mass. Urol. Radiol. 4:85, 1982.

Warshauer, D. M., McCarthy, S. M., Street, L., Bookbinder, M. J., Clicleman, M. G., Richter, J., Hammers, L., Taylor, C., and Rosenfield, A. T.: Detection of renal masses: Sensitivities and specificities of excretory urography/linear tomography, US and CT. Radiology 169:363, 1988.

Winters, W. D., Lebowitz, R. L.: Importance of prenatal detection of hydronephrosis of the upper pole. AJR 155:125, 1990.

Zagoria, R. J., Wolfman, N. T., Karstaedt, N., Hinn, G. C., Dyer, R. B., Chen, Y. M.: CT features of renal cell carcinoma with emphasis on relation to tumor size. Invest. Radiol. 25:261, 1990.

26

ANGIOGRAPHY IN DISEASES OF THE KIDNEY

The main renal artery and vein and their branches to the arcuate level are routinely visualized during arteriography or venography. Perfusion of the microvasculature of the kidney is represented by the angiographic nephrogram, the homogeneous radiodensity that appears during arteriography as contrast material flows through the cortex. Abnormalities that directly involve the vessels often create unique angiographic patterns that permit specific diagnosis. Diseases of the parenchyma, on the other hand, alter blood vessels indirectly. Here, angiographic abnormalities are nonspecific, and radiologic diagnosis is more limited.

This chapter first considers aspects of angiography of the large arteries and veins. Following that is a discussion of abnormalities of the microvasculature. Each section of the chapter describes normal anatomy, findings in primary diseases of blood vessels, and secondary effects caused by diseases of the renal parenchyma and interstitium. Congenital arteriovenous malformation and angiography of tumors are discussed in Chapter 12.

MAJOR ARTERIES AND VEINS

Normal Anatomy

The main renal artery bifurcates into anterior and posterior branches that divide several times in the renal hilus into segmental arteries. These arteries, also known as interlobar arteries, traverse the fat of the renal sinus and at the level of the calyx give rise to the arcuate arteries that penetrate the renal lobe between the cortex and the medulla (Fig. 26–1). The arcuate arteries continue along the corticomedullary junction, periodically giving off perpendicular branches (the interlobular arteries) that run to the cortex (Fig. 26–2). Most arcuate arteries are end-arteries, although a few may communicate with capsular arteries by way of an interlobular artery. Arcuate arteries are visualized in all normal angiograms, whereas interlobular arteries are only occasionally identifiable as discrete structures. A normal renal artery has a smooth wall and gentle curves and overlaps other vessels, tapers gradually, and has a multiplicity of branches. Blood vessels extend to the periphery of the normal kidney (Fig. 26–3).

The middle-sized and large veins of the kidney parallel arteries and are similarly named. Interlobular veins drain the cortex, become arcuate veins, and then interlobar and segmental veins. Unlike the renal arteries, the veins of the kidney freely anastomose. The arcuate veins form complete arches along the corticomedullary junction. Their opacification vividly depicts lobar architecture (Fig. 26–4).

Standard techniques for the study of the renal arteries and microvasculature are aortography and selective renal angiography with rapid-sequence filming or digitally subtracted images. Injection of epinephrine into the renal artery, balloon catheter occlusion, and performance of the Valsalva maneuver are useful adjuncts in renal venography.

Primary Diseases of the Renal Artery

Atherosclerosis. Atherosclerotic plaque is usually located in the proximal 2 cm of the main renal artery, but the distal artery or its branches may be involved, especially at points of bifurcation (see Fig. 23–10). The plaque is most often focal and eccentrically placed in the arterial lumen. Stenosis develops from direct growth of the plaque or from intermittent bleeding into the plaque wall. Complete obstruction, aneurysm formation, and dissection are occasional complica-

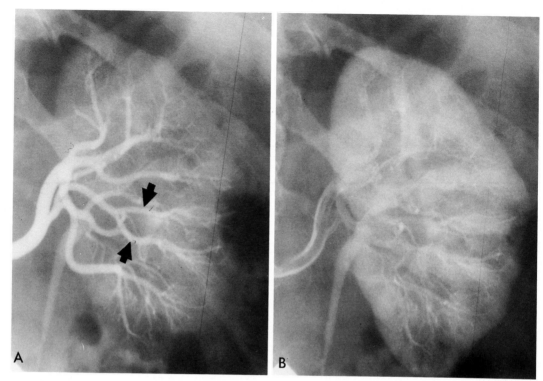

Figure 26–1. Normal renal arteries and angiographic nephrogram. Division of the main renal artery into anterior and posterior branches is followed by bifurcation into segmental, or interlobar, arteries. The arcuate arteries *(arrows)* form at the level of the calyx and run along the corticomedullary junction.

A, Selective renal arteriogram. Arterial phase.

B, Selective renal arteriogram. Late arterial and early nephrographic phase.

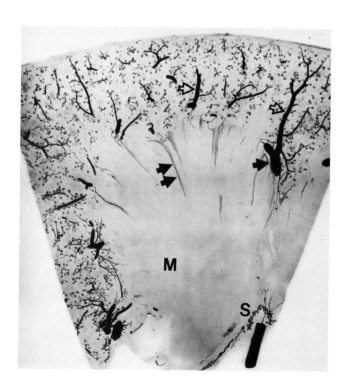

Figure 26–2. Microradiograph of a barium-injected normal human kidney. Arcuate artery *(single solid arrow)* runs between two fused lobes, periodically giving off interlobular arteries *(open arrow).* M, medulla; S, spiral artery to papilla; double solid arrows, vasa rectae.

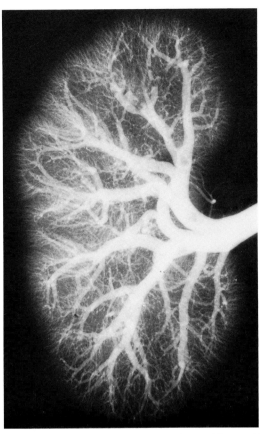

Figure 26–3. Radiograph of a barium-injected normal human kidney. Normal arteries are characterized by smooth walls, gentle curves, overlapping of vessels, gradual tapering, and a multiplicity of fine branches. Vessels extend to the periphery of the kidney.

tions of advanced atherosclerosis (see Fig. 6–2). With high-grade stenosis or complete obstruction, collateral vessels may develop (see Fig. 6–7). These vessels are derived variably from pre-existing lumbar, pelvic, ureteral, intercostal, adrenal, capsular, or other retroperitoneal arteries.

Renal angiography identifies the site and extent of an atherosclerotic lesion and is a part of the diagnostic and therapeutic approach to the patient with renovascular hypertension. Useful hemodynamic data can be derived from the thoroughly performed angiogram by observing factors such as the presence of collaterals, the dilution defects in opacified extrarenal vessels during pharmacologic manipulation of renal blood flow, and the spillover of contrast material into the aorta following selective injection at a constant, known rate (Bookstein and Ernst, 1973).

Atherosclerotic plaque is an inevitable part of the aging of the kidney. The impact of the aging process on the angiogram is discussed in the section on chronic renal disease.

Arterial Dysplasia. Dysplastic lesions result from a variable mixture of collagen deposition, hyperplasia of smooth muscle and fibroblasts, and disruption or thinning of the elastica interna. Some authors group all forms of dysplasia under the single heading of "fibromuscular hyperplasia." Others identify angio-

graphic-pathologic subtypes. These include "intimal fibroplasia," a symmetric, funnel-shaped band of narrowing (Fig. 26–5); "medial fibroplasia," multiple aneurysms larger in diameter than the renal artery itself (Fig. 26–6); "subadventitial fibroplasia," uneven stenosis that occurs singly or in a series, with bulges that do not exceed the diameter of the uninvolved parts of the artery; and "fibromuscular hyperplasia," an uncommon form with a variable angiographic picture. Subtypes may differ to some degree in clinical features relating to sexual predilection, age distribution, and propensity for bilaterality. Any of these lesions can cause renovascular hypertension.

Polyarteritis Nodosa and Drug Abuse. The angiographic abnormalities in these two conditions result from focal areas of mural necrosis in intermediate-sized (arcuate) arteries. In polyarteritis nodosa, the aneurysms that result are multiple, sharply defined, and 2- to 3-mm wide (Fig. 26–7). These occur only in the "classic" form and are not seen in the "microscopic" form in which the capillary bed, rather than larger vessels, is involved. The renal aneurysms of polyarteritis nodosa may heal with therapy. Thus, failure to demonstrate aneurysms does not exclude the diagnosis of polyarteritis nodosa. Unlike polyarteritis, angiitis associated with drug abuse has widespread irregularities of the arterial lumina. In addition, the aneurysms tend to be more irregular than those seen with polyarteritis (Fig. 26–8).

Trauma. Severe abdominal trauma can indirectly threaten the viability of the kidney by partial or complete avulsion of the renal pedicle or directly by infarction of the kidney parenchyma. Angiography provides useful information in these circumstances. Multiple aneurysms of middle-sized vessels, similar to those of polyarteritis nodosa or drug abuse angiitis, may appear following a blunt deceleration injury to the abdomen. Arteriovenous aneurysm (fistula) may follow either blunt or penetrating wounds to the kidney, including needle biopsy. If the volume of shunted blood is large enough, high-output heart failure or renal ischemia leading to hypertension may ensue. Small post-traumatic aneurysms usually heal spontaneously. Some may cause parenchymal hemorrhage to the degree that surgical or transcatheter embolic therapy is required. Chapter 27 discusses the comprehensive radiologic approach to the patient with possible renal trauma.

Secondary Effects of Parenchymal Disease on Large Vessels

Disease of the renal parenchyma or interstitium indirectly alters the appearance of medium- and large-sized blood vessels. Increased renal bulk from interstitial edema, cellular proliferation or infiltration, or protein deposition in the nephrons and the interstitial tissue causes the renal arteries and veins to attenuate, to taper acutely, and to separate from each other. Small branches disappear, and circulation time increases (Fig. 26–9). This occurs in widely diverse abnormalities, such as acute tubular necrosis, acute py-

Text continued on page 797

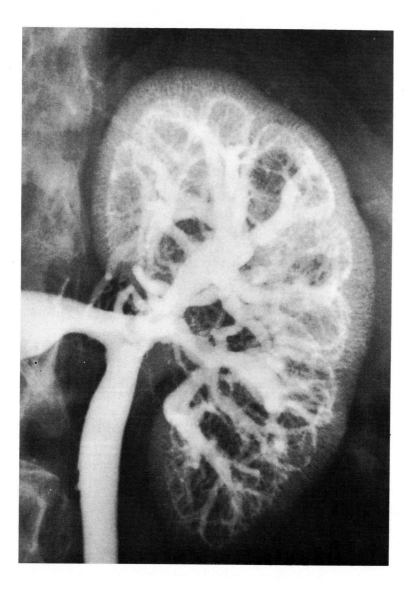

Figure 26–4. Normal renal venogram performed with a balloon-occluding technique. Veins parallel arteries but freely anastomose and form complete arches along the corticomedullary junction. Interlobular veins are opacified. (Courtesy of J. Rösch, M.D., University of Oregon, Portland.)

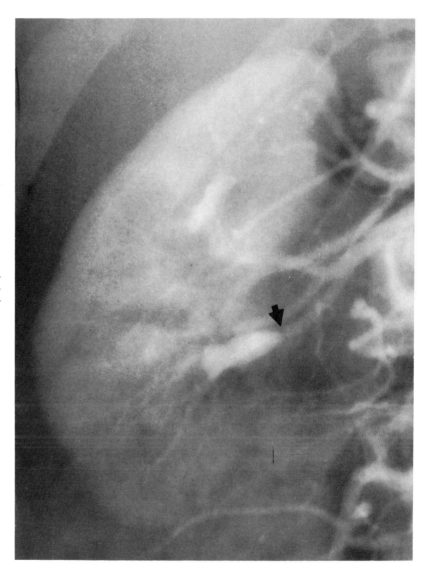

Figure 26–5. Renal artery dysplasia. Intimal fibroplasia subtype. There is post-stenotic dilatation immediately distal to a symmetric band of narrowing *(arrow)*. Aortogram.

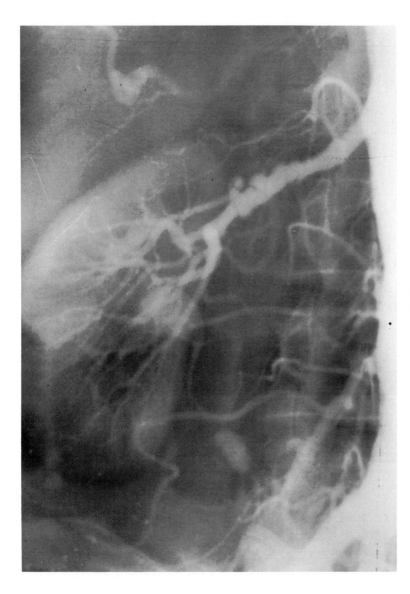

Figure 26–6. Renal artery dysplasia. Medial fibroplasia subtype. There are multiple aneurysms of the main renal artery, each larger than the renal artery itself. Aortogram. (Same patient illustrated in Fig. 16–19.)

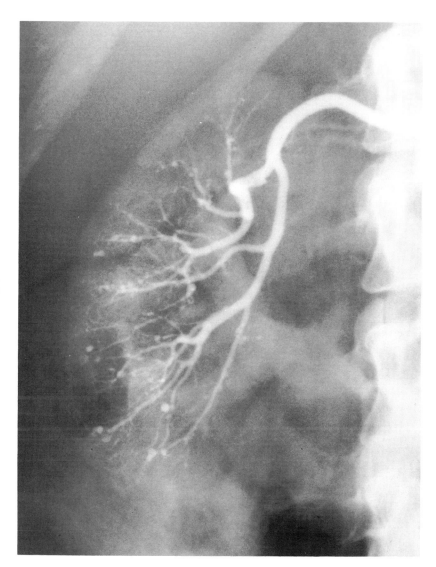

Figure 26–7. Polyarteritis nodosa, classic form. There are multiple, sharply defined aneurysms in the arcuate arteries. Selective renal arteriogram.

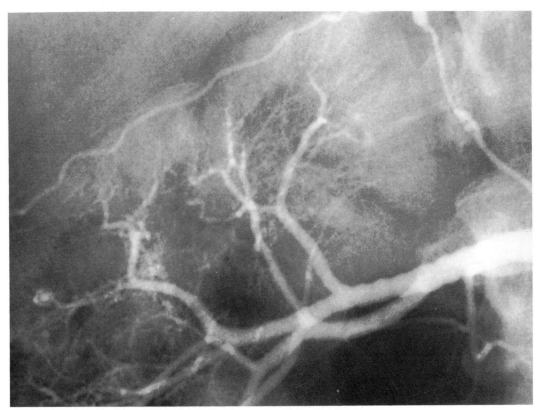

Figure 26–8. Drug abuse arteritis. View of the superior portion of the right kidney. There are widespread irregularities of the medium-sized arteries in addition to small aneurysms. Selective renal arteriogram. (Courtesy of Robert Clark, M.D., St. Francis Memorial Hospital, San Francisco, California.)

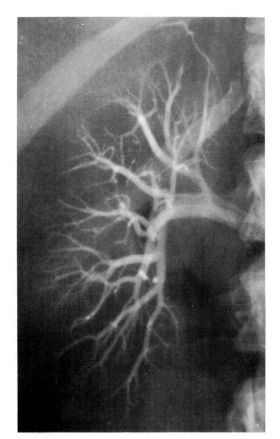

Figure 26–9. Secondary effects of acute glomerulonephritis on renal vasculature. The arteries are attenuated and separated from each other and have fewer branches than normal. Circulation time is prolonged. Selective renal arteriogram. (The film was exposed 1.75 seconds after the start of injection of contrast material.)

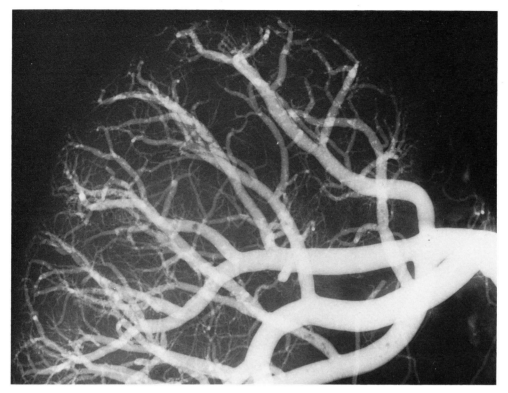

Figure 26–10. Radiograph of a barium-injected human kidney illustrating the effects of chronic parenchymal loss on the arterial tree. The interlobar arteries fail to taper normally and are tortuous distally. The arcuate arteries angle sharply and terminate abruptly. These changes follow a wide variety of chronic diseases but are also found in the aged although otherwise normal kidney, as in this illustration.

elonephritis, acute glomerulonephritis, and leukemic infiltration as well as in other forms of acute renal disease.

Chronic processes that lead to the generalized loss of nephrons and interstitial fibrosis cause loss of the normal, smooth tapering of arteries, increased tortuosity, and abrupt termination of the distal extent of arcuate arteries. Arteries crowd together as surrounding parenchyma is lost, and the number of arterial branches decreases. Irregularities of the arterial wall appear. The main renal artery may become smaller as total blood flow to the kidney diminishes. These changes follow a wide variety of chronic kidney diseases, such as pyelonephritis, glomerulonephritis, and nephrosclerosis. Similar changes occur in the nondiseased kidney as part of the aging process (Fig. 26–10).

Patients with chronic renal disease on long-term dialysis sometimes develop multiple aneurysms of medium-sized arteries as a component of acquired cystic kidney disease, which is described in Chapter 10. Acute retroperitoneal bleeding may result if these arteries rupture. Similarly, hemorrhage within and around the kidney may occasionally complicate polyarteritis nodosa and malignant nephrosclerosis.

Primary Abnormalities of the Main Renal Vein

Thrombosis is the principal abnormality of the renal vein, as discussed in Chapter 9. This may occur as an extension of clot previously formed in the inferior vena cava or as a primary event in the main renal vein or its intrarenal tributaries. Parenchymal disease of the kidney, especially amyloidosis and glomerulonephritis, as well as adenocarcinoma predisposes the renal vein to thrombosis. Occasionally, the renal vein is partially or completely occluded by tumors, cysts, hematomas, or fibrosis in the renal hilus. In any of these circumstances, the viability of the kidney depends on the suddenness and extent of compromise of the venous system and the degree to which collaterals provide effective drainage of the kidney. Varix of the left renal vein, usually associated with compression by the superior mesenteric artery, is an additional uncommon primary abnormality.

THE MICROVASCULATURE OF THE KIDNEY

Normal Anatomy

Approximately 80 per cent of the renal blood flow passes through the interlobar arteries and into the microvasculature of the cortical nephrons. From a radiologic viewpoint, this appears as a homogeneous density of the cortex that develops in the few seconds following injection of contrast material into the main renal artery (see Fig. 26–1). This density, the *angiographic nephrogram*, represents contrast material in afferent arterioles, glomerular capillaries, efferent arterioles, and the rich, freely anastomosing system of peritubular capillaries that surround the various parts

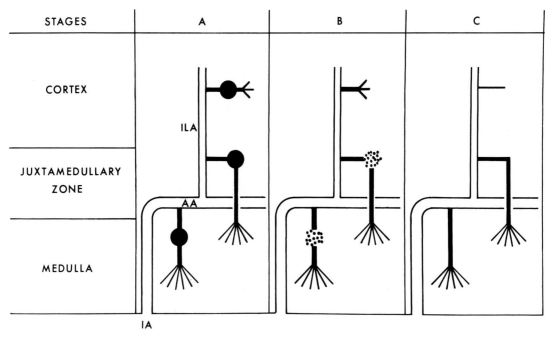

Figure 26–11. Schema of normal and abnormal microvasculature.

A, Normal adult pattern shows arteriolar-glomerular units in the cortex and vasa rectae spuriae in the juxtamedullary zone and medulla.

B, With both chronic parenchymal disease and advancing age, there is deterioration of glomeruli.

C, In advanced forms of aging and chronic parenchymal disease, many cortical arterioles are obliterated, and there is conversion of the vasa rectae spuriae into vasa rectae verae in the juxtamedullary and medullary zones.

IA, interlobar artery; AA, arcuate artery; ILA, interlobular artery.

(Adapted from Ljungqvist, A.: Acta Med. Scand. *174*[Suppl. 1401]:1, 1963.)

of the tubule in the cortex (Fig. 26–11; see Fig. 26–2). Blood flow continues into peritubular and interlobular veins and then into the arcuate veins. The possibility exists that contrast material in the extravascular space also contributes to the angiographic nephrogram.

A second system of microscopic blood vessels carries approximately 18 per cent of the renal blood flow to the medulla. This system is composed of the *vasa rectae* that originate directly from the arcuate arteries or the interlobular arteries in the juxtamedullary zone of the cortex (see Figs. 26–2 and 26–11). These are long, straight tubes that follow the descending limb of Henle's loop through the medulla and papilla, turn at the end of the loop, and return to the corticomedullary junction as venules draining into arcuate veins. Some vasa rectae include glomeruli near their origins; others do not. These vessels are not large enough to be visualized during angiography. During angiography in the normal state, the medulla remains radiolucent compared with its surrounding cortex because its blood supply is sparse compared with the supply flowing through the adjacent cortical microvasculature.

Rapid homogeneous opacification of the entire cortex and a sharply defined corticomedullary junction are the normal features of opacified blood flow through the renal microvasculature (see Fig. 26–1). The angiographic nephrogram appears within the first 2 seconds of selective injection of contrast material into the renal artery, then fades slightly as contrast

material leaves the microvasculature and moves into the venous drainage and the tubule lumen.

Primary Abnormalities

Acute cortical necrosis and *atheroembolic renal disease* are associated with obliteration of the arterial side of the renal microvasculature. The former is caused by afferent arteriolar and glomerular capillary thrombosis as well as interstitial edema and coagulation necrosis of tubule cells. In the latter, showers of microscopic cholesterol emboli, usually occurring after aortic surgery or catheter aortography, occlude the interlobular arteries and afferent arterioles. Under these circumstances, the angiographic nephrogram is absent; in the case of incomplete acute cortical necrosis, it is patchy (see Fig. 23–16). Circulation time is prolonged, and venous opacification is faint or absent. Changes due to interstitial edema are noted in addition to those reflecting loss of flow to the microvasculature.

Acute tubular necrosis is thought by some clinicians to be due to vasoconstriction of the afferent arteriole as a primary event. The angiographic abnormalities are similar to those of acute cortical necrosis and atheroembolic disease, but the nephrogram has a lesser degree of density impairment.

Acute lobar or *segmental infarction* can be diagnosed by careful analysis of the angiographic nephrogram as well as by identification of an occluded artery (see Figs. 5–17 through 5–19). A wedge-shaped radiolucency in the cortex reflects the blood flow defect in the area normally perfused by the obliterated artery.

Secondary Effects of Renal Parenchymal Disease

Alteration in cortical perfusion, seen as a diffusely decreased or patchy angiographic nephrogram, occurs in a wide variety of *acute diseases of the renal parenchyma*, including the acute glomerulonephritides, Wegener's granulomatosis, lupus nephritis, polyarteritis nodosa (microscopic form), and acute interstitial nephritis (see Fig. 23–26). Decreased cortical flow is due both to compression of the vascular bed that follows swelling of the kidney within its relatively nondistendable capsule and to obliteration of the small vessels by the direct pathologic process.

An abnormal pattern of linear striations in the angiographic nephrogram has been described in *acute bacterial nephritis* (see Fig. 23–25). These striations are probably due to obliteration of interlobular arteries by inflammatory infiltrate.

Characteristic changes in the microvasculature occur in *chronic diseases of the kidney parenchyma*, such as reflux nephropathy, glomerulonephritis, nephrosclerosis, and interstitial nephritis. As nephron loss progresses, *both* the glomeruli and their afferent and efferent arterioles are obliterated. At the same time, glomeruli in the juxtamedullary region degenerate but their afferent and efferent arterioles persist as dilated, directly communicating channels. These are the *vasa rectae verae* that carry a larger than normal amount of blood directly into the medulla at the expense of the cortex. These changes are schematized in

Figure 26–11. The redistribution of blood flow from the cortex to the medulla that results is reflected angiographically as a decrease in cortical opacification, an increase in medullary density, and a loss of the usually distinct corticomedullary junction (Fig. 26–12). The same process occurs in the normal aging kidney in the absence of hypertension, thus limiting the usefulness of angiography as a precise method in the diagnosis of chronic parenchymal diseases of the kidney.

PRACTICAL CONSIDERATIONS

Angiography traditionally has been used as a valuable method for eliminating arterial or venous occlusion as a cause of acute renal failure and for assessing the severely traumatized patient with shock and hematuria. Radionuclide studies, Doppler ultrasonographic techniques, magnetic resonance angiography, and computed tomography have largely supplanted angiography in these clinical situations. Angiography remains useful in evaluating selected hypertensive patients for arterial stenosis and for investigation of unexplained hematuria, especially when the source of blood has been lateralized at cystoscopy to one side. Demonstrating characteristic patterns in acute cortical necrosis, atheroembolic renal disease, polyarteritis nodosa, necrotizing angiitis of drug abuse, and arteriovenous malformations and aneurysms is another way in which angiography may aid diagnosis or clinical

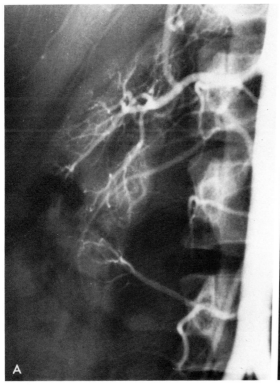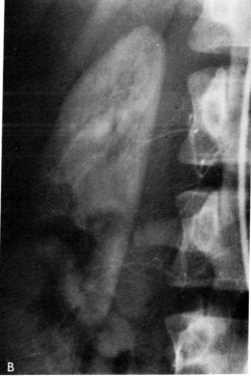

Figure 26–12. Chronic glomerulonephritis. There is loss of the usually distinct corticomedullary junction because of the redistribution of flow from the cortex to the medulla.

A, Aortogram. Arterial phase.

B, Aortogram. Nephrographic phase.

management. Angiography is no longer commonly used for preoperative diagnostic evaluation or embolization of tumors of the kidney.

For the diagnosis of chronic renal diseases, evaluation of clinical features, urine and blood analysis, and a properly performed ultrasonogram usually suffice. This is particularly true in light of the fact that the angiographic findings of most chronic diseases and of the normal aging process overlap.

Bibliography

Abrams, H. L., Obrez, I., Hollenberg, N. K., and Adams, D. F.: Pharmacoangiography of the renal vasculature. Curr. Probl. Diagn. Radiol. *1*:1, 1971.

Adams, D. F., Hollenberg, N. K., and Adams, H. L.: Angiography of renal failure. *In* Griffiths, H. J. (ed.): Radiology of Renal Failure. Philadelphia, W. B. Saunders Co., 1976, pp. 269–261.

Bennett, A. F., and Wiener, S. N.: Intrarenal arteriovenous fistula and aneurysm. AJR *95*:372, 1965.

Bookstein, J. J., and Ernst, C. B.: Vasodilatory and vasoconstrictive pharmacoangiographic manipulation of renal collateral flow. Radiology *108*:55, 1973.

Bookstein, J. J., and Mena, E.: Letter to Editor. Invest. Radiol. *8*:361, 1973.

Bookstein, J. J.: Angiography of the genitourinary tract: Techniques and applications. *In* Pollack, H. M. (ed.): Clinical Urography. Philadelphia, W. B. Saunders, 1990, pp. 456–496.

Castaneda-Zuniga, W., Zollikofer, C., Valdez-Davila, O., Nath, P. H., and Amplatz, K.: Giant aneurysms of the renal arteries: An unusual manifestation of fibromuscular dysplasia. Radiology *133*:327, 1979.

Citron, B. P., Halpern, M., McCarron, M., et al.: Necrotizing angiitis associated with drug abuse. N. Engl. J. Med. *283*:1003, 1970.

Cosgrove, M. D., Mendez, R., and Morrow, J. W.: Traumatic renal arteriovenous fistula: Report of 12 cases. J. Urol. *110*:627, 1973.

Davidson, A. J., Talner, L. B., and Downs, W. M., III.: A study of the angiographic appearance of the kidney in an aging normotensive population. Radiology *92*:975, 1969.

Davidson, A. J., and Talner, L. B.: Urographic and angiographic abnormalities in adult-onset acute bacterial nephritis. Radiology *106*:249, 1973.

Davidson, A. J., and Talner, L. B.: Lack of specificity of renal angiography in the diagnosis of parenchymal disease. Invest. Radiol. *8*:90, 1973.

Davidson, A. J., and Talner, L. B.: Letter to Editor. Invest. Radiol. *8*:361, 1973.

Deutsch, V., Frankl, O., and Drory, Y.: Bilateral renal cortical necrosis with survival through the acute phase with a note on the value of selective renal nephroangiography. Am. J. Med. *50*:828, 1971.

Easterbrook, J. S.: Renal and hepatic microaneurysms: Report of a new entity simulating polyarteritis nodosa. Radiology *137*:629, 1980.

Ekelund, L.: Renal vascular changes as reflected by angiography. Urol. Radiol. *1*:81, 1979.

Ekelund, L., Kaude, J., and Lindholm, T.: Angiography in glomerular disease of the kidney. AJR *119*:739, 1973.

Ekelund, L., and Lindholm, T.: Angiography in collagenous disease of the kidney. Acta Radiol. (Diagn.) *15*:413, 1974.

Engelbrecht, H. E., Keen, E. N., Fine, H., and VandenBulcke, C.: The radiological anatomy of the parenchymal distribution of the renal artery—a revised approach. S. Afr. Med. J. *43*:826, 1969.

Fine, H., and Keen, E. N.: The arteries of the human kidney. J. Anat. *100*:881, 1966.

Gill, W. M., Jr., and Pudvan, W. R.: The arteriographic diagnosis of renal parenchymal diseases. Radiology *96*:81, 1970.

Guyer, P. B.: Radiology of the loin pain—haematuria syndrome. Clin. Radiol. *29*:561, 1978.

Herschman, A., Blum, R., and Lee, Y. C.: Angiographic findings in polyarteritis nodosa. Radiology *94*:147, 1970.

Hessel, S. J., and Smith, E. H.: Renal trauma: A comprehensive review and radiologic assessment. CRC Crit. Rev. Diagn. Imaging *5*:251, 1974.

Hollenberg, N. K., Adams, D. F., and Oken, D. E.: Acute renal failure due to nephrotoxins: Renal hemodynamic and angiographic studies in man. N. Engl. J. Med. *282*:1329, 1970.

Hollenberg, N. K., Epstein, M., and Rosen, S. M.: Acute oliguric renal failure in man: Evidence for preferential renal cortical ischemia. Medicine (Balt.) *47*:455, 1968.

Hollenberg, N. K., Harrington, D. P., Garnic, J. D., Adams, D. F., and Abrams, H. L. Renal angiography in the oliguric state. *In* Abrams, H. L. (ed.): Angiography. 3rd ed. Boston, Little, Brown & Co., 1983, pp. 1299–1325.

Jander, H. P., Vilar, J. S., Kashlan, B. M., and Witten, D. M.: Selective angiography in renal and peri-renal inflammatory lesions: Correlation with histopathology. Br. J. Radiol. *52*:536, 1979.

Kassirer, J. P.: Atheroembolic renal disease. N. Engl. J. Med. *20*:812, 1969.

Lang, E. K., Trichel, B. E., and Turner, R. W.: Arteriographic assessment of injury resulting from renal trauma. An analysis of 74 patients. J. Urol. *106*:1, 1971.

Ljungqvist, A.: The intrarenal arterial pattern in the normal and diseased human kidney: A micro-angiographic and histologic study. Acta Med. Scand. (Suppl. 1401) *174*:1–38, 1963.

Mena, E., Bookstein, J. J., and Gikas, P. W.: Angiographic diagnosis of renal parenchymal disease. Radiology *108*:526, 1973.

Newhouse, J. H.: Fluid compartment distribution of intravenous iothalamate in the dog. Invest. Radiol. *12*:364, 1977.

Olin, T. B., and Reuter, S. R.: A pharmacoangiographic method for improving nephrophlebography. Radiology *85*:1036, 1965.

Palmer, J., Barry, B., Williams, R., and Briscoe, P.: Diagnosis of venous extension in renal cell carcinoma: The value of routine inferior vena-cavography. Australas. Radiol. *19*:265, 1975.

Poutasse, E. F., and Dustan, H. P.: Arteriosclerosis and renal hypertension: Indications for aortography in hypertensive patients and results of treatment of obstructive lesions of renal artery. JAMA *165*:1521, 1957.

Robins, J. M., and Bookstein, J. J.: Regressing aneurysms in periarteritis nodosa. Radiology *104*:215, 1972.

Scott, J. A., Rabe, F. E., Becker, G. J., Yum, M. N., Yune, H. Y., Holden, R. W., Richmond, B. D., Klatte, E. C., Grim, C. E., and Weinberger, M. H.: Angiographic assessment of renal artery pathology: How reliable? AJR *141*:1299, 1983.

Sidaway, M. E.: Small-vessel changes in renal disease. Br. Med. Bull. *28*:247, 1972.

Smailowitz, Z., Kaneti, J., and Sober, I.: Spontaneous perirenal hematoma: A complication of polyarteritis nodosa. J. Urol. *121*:82, 1979.

Stewart, B. H., Dustan, H. P., and Kiser, W. S.: Correlation of angiography and natural history in evaluation of patients with renovascular hypertension. J. Urol. *104*:261, 1970.

Takaro, T., Dow, J. A., and Kishev, S.: Selective occlusive renal phlebography in man. Radiology *94*:589, 1970.

Tsubogo, Y.: Angiography in chronic renal disease. Australas. Radiol. *17*:43, 1974.

Tuttle, R. J., and Minielly, J. A.: The angiographic diagnosis of acute hemorrhagic renal cortical necrosis. Radiology *126*:637, 1978.

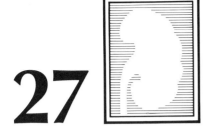

MICHAEL P. FEDERLE
R. BROOKE JEFFREY, JR.

27

RADIOLOGIC EVALUATION OF RENAL TRAUMA

ABDOMINAL RADIOGRAPHY	RADIONUCLIDE STUDIES
EXCRETORY UROGRAPHY	ULTRASONOGRAPHY
ANGIOGRAPHY	COMPUTED TOMOGRAPHY

Although the kidney is the most frequently injured organ in blunt abdominal trauma, most damage is minor and heals without specific therapy. Serious renal injury, however, is often associated with abnormalities in other organs. Multiorgan involvement occurs in 80 per cent of patients with penetrating trauma and in 20 per cent of those with blunt trauma.

The indications for radiologic evaluation of possible renal injury remain somewhat controversial. Twenty-five per cent of patients with gross hematuria after blunt abdominal trauma will have "significant" renal damage. On the other hand, microscopic hematuria is associated with important renal injury in less than 1 per cent of cases. Many experienced trauma surgeons and urologists now recommend imaging evaluation only for patients with gross hematuria or with microscopic hematuria and a compelling history or physical findings, such as a rapid deceleration injury or hemodynamic instability.

Renal injuries are classified into three categories, each of which has important implications for therapeutic management (Fig. 27–1). Category I lesions are minor and include contusion and small corticomedullary laceration. These constitute 75 to 85 per cent of cases in most series. Lesions in category II are more serious and account for about 10 per cent of cases.

Abnormalities in this group include parenchymal lacerations that communicate with the collecting system (complete laceration and renal fracture). Lesions in category III are catastrophic, constitute about 5 per cent of the total, and consist of shattered kidneys and injuries to the renal vascular pedicle. The relatively uncommon entities of ureteropelvic junction avulsion and laceration of the renal pelvis are assigned a separate status and may be designated as category IV lesions.

There is general agreement among surgeons that category I (minor) injuries are best managed nonoperatively, whereas category III (catastrophic) lesions require urgent surgery. Although opinion is divided over proper management of category II lesions, virtually all authors stress the need for prompt and accurate evaluation of the type and the extent of injury so that optimal therapy can be planned.

The goal of the radiologist in assessing the patient with possible renal trauma is to define the nature and the extent of renal injury so that the maximum amount of functioning renal tissue can be preserved with the fewest number of complications. This chapter reviews the various imaging modalities used to evaluate renal trauma, their advantages and limitations, and a reasonable approach to their use. Trauma to the

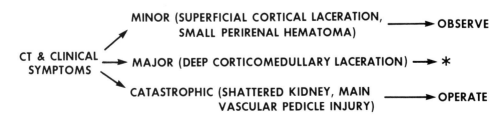

*Therapy depends on amount of nonviable tissue, extent of hemorrhage and extravasation of urine

Figure 27–1. Classification and management of renal injuries.

801

lower urinary tract is discussed in Chapter 19 (The Urinary Bladder) and in Chapter 20 (The Urethra).

ABDOMINAL RADIOGRAPHY

Standard radiographs of the abdomen should be obtained in all cases of abdominal trauma. Pneumoperitoneum or hemoperitoneum from associated nonrenal injuries may be detected and militate for urgent surgery. Perirenal hemorrhage may be evident as a mass displacing adjacent viscera such as the colon and the duodenum. Perirenal hematoma tends to obscure the upper one-third of the psoas shadow. Blood usually accumulates in the dorsal perirenal space, displacing the kidney anteriorly. Because of magnification, the displaced kidney appears enlarged on a supine abdominal radiograph. A streaked and mottled appearance of the perirenal fat due to irregular infiltration by blood is an additional sign of perirenal hemorrhage. Although radiographs may provide important clues, they are usually not sufficiently informative to direct management of renal trauma.

EXCRETORY UROGRAPHY

Technique

The most widely available and thoroughly investigated study for renal trauma is the excretory urogram. Refinements in technique have improved the accuracy of urography but are too often ignored in many practices. The recommended dose of iodinated contrast material for adults is 1.5 to 2.0 ml/kg of 50% sodium diatrizoate or 60% meglumine iothalamate. The dose for children is 2 to 3 ml/kg of the same materials. A film coned to the renal area is exposed immediately after the injection is completed, to image the maximally dense nephrogram. The appearance of intact renal contours during the nephrogram is one of the most important observations. The kidneys frequently are obscured by overlying gas and stool, making tomography an important adjunct to urographic evaluation. Oblique films and adequate views of the ureters and bladder are also essential. Ureteral compression should *not* be used. Optimal technique is sometimes not possible owing to other constraints, such as severe abdominal injury with hemodynamic instability. In such cases, the most important information an abbreviated excretory urogram can provide is whether two functioning kidneys are present, should emergency surgical exploration be required.

Findings

Excretory urography distinguishes various types of renal injuries with moderate success. A normal urogram usually excludes significant injury, although parenchymal lacerations of the anterior or posterior renal surface may not be detected. Renal contusion may result in diminished nephrographic density and less than normal pyelographic density. Uncommonly, a striated nephrogram occurs as a result of contusion.

A diminished nephrogram is a very nonspecific finding and may be due to parenchymal laceration or a shattered kidney, in addition to simple contusion. Unlike simple contusion, however, parenchymal laceration leads to perirenal hemorrhage, which cannot be measured precisely by urography. Moreover, perirenal hemorrhage may develop from nonrenal sites, such as a fractured pelvis, with normal kidneys.

Renal parenchymal laceration or intrarenal hematoma appears as a focal contour abnormality, nephrographic defect, or an intrarenal mass with splaying of calyces. Extravasation of opacified urine is indicative of a lacerated collecting system and usually implies serious injury (Fig. 27–2). When a small calyceal tear is associated with parenchymal laceration, the extravasation may be limited to the kidney. Laceration of the renal pelvis or the upper ureter even when the kidney is not injured is rare in blunt trauma; it occurs more frequently in penetrating trauma. More commonly, pelvocalyceal tear is associated with major parenchymal laceration and the extravasated urine accumulates in the perirenal space. Many urologists consider renal laceration with extravasation an indication for surgical repair. The term *renal fracture* should be reserved for deep lacerations of the collecting system, with separation of the two renal poles by hematoma.

Blunt or penetrating trauma can cause occlusion or avulsion of the renal artery or vein. Renal pedicle injuries commonly accompany multiple organ and skeletal trauma. Diagnosis of the renal injury may be delayed or missed owing to the priority of other injuries. In this situation, the mortality rate is approximately 40 per cent. Renal artery occlusion or avulsion is more common than injury to the renal vein and results in ischemia of that portion of the kidney supplied by the disrupted artery. Main renal artery occlusion causes an absent nephrogram.

Although an absent nephrogram suggests a renal pedicle injury or a shattered kidney, the same abnormality occurs following relatively minor injuries. The nephrogram may be difficult to define if the kidney is obscured by overlying bowel gas. It is also important to keep in mind that an absent nephrogram may be due to other conditions, such as congenitally absent or ectopic kidney or nonfunction due to pre-existing disease. Thus, an absent nephrogram is not a compelling criterion for immediate surgical intervention.

Chronic sequelae of renal trauma include parenchymal scars due to infarction and global wasting of the kidney, which are often asymptomatic. Persistent subcapsular or perirenal hemorrhage may form a fibrous capsule around the kidney, causing renal ischemia, the so-called Page kidney. The urographic findings in this situation often simulate those seen with renovascular ischemia due to main renal artery stenosis (Fig. 27–3). Computed tomography may demonstrate directly the perirenal fibrous capsule.

Advantages and Limitations

A normal excretory urogram is reliable evidence of insignificant renal trauma if the patient is clinically

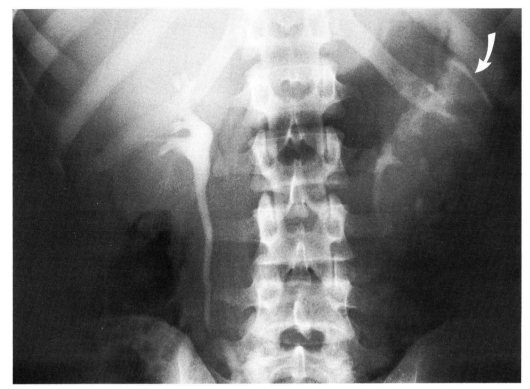

Figure 27–2. Decreased left nephrogram after blunt trauma. Perirenal extravasation of urine *(arrow)* indicates deep corticomedullary laceration that extends into the collecting system. Excretory urogram.

stable (decreasing hematuria and stable hematocrit and vital signs). An abnormal urogram is usually nonspecific, with a broad overlap between fundamentally different types and degrees of renal trauma. A decreased nephrogram may result from contusion, laceration, or even shattered kidney. Both false-negative and false-positive diagnoses of extravasation of urine may occur with urography owing to confusing overlying radiographic densities. Decreased renal function associated with severe parenchymal laceration may also result in failure to detect extravasated, poorly opacified urine.

The sensitivity and specificity of urography in trauma is difficult to assess owing to variations in radiographic technique, a prevalence of varying degrees of renal trauma, and an absence of a "gold standard" for comparison. Early reports suggested that in the acutely injured patient, the immediate excretory urogram was of diagnostic quality in only 50 per cent of cases; when of satisfactory quality, it correctly predicted the extent of renal damage in 50 to 80 per cent of cases. Optimal urographic technique, including tomography, probably indicates the true extent of injury in 75 to 85 per cent of cases. This still leaves a substantial number of patients, particularly those with major injuries, with a need for further evaluation.

ANGIOGRAPHY

Before the advent of high-resolution computed tomography, selective renal arteriography was a main-

stay in the evaluation of renal trauma. The use of angiography was advocated for almost all patients with urographic evidence of significant renal injury. When compared with surgical series, selective renal angiography is an accurate technique for detecting renovascular and parenchymal injuries and provides valuable information for guiding patient management and directing surgical intervention.

Technique

Percutaneous transfemoral angiography is performed using the Seldinger technique. An initial midstream aortogram is performed to evaluate the number and status of the renal arteries. Adequate evaluation of the kidneys may be achieved by using an aortogram, but optimal evaluation often requires selective renal artery injections. Digital subtraction imaging of intra-arterial or intravenous contrast material injections may be useful in some circumstances. Oblique projections are necessary to evaluate the renal contours completely. The filming sequence must be timed to include arterial, capillary, and venous phases.

Findings

Renal contusion and small laceration hematoma are frequently not detected on angiography or may present as subtle parenchymal swelling or slow flow during the arterial phase. A large laceration and hematoma result in separation and stretching of the arterial

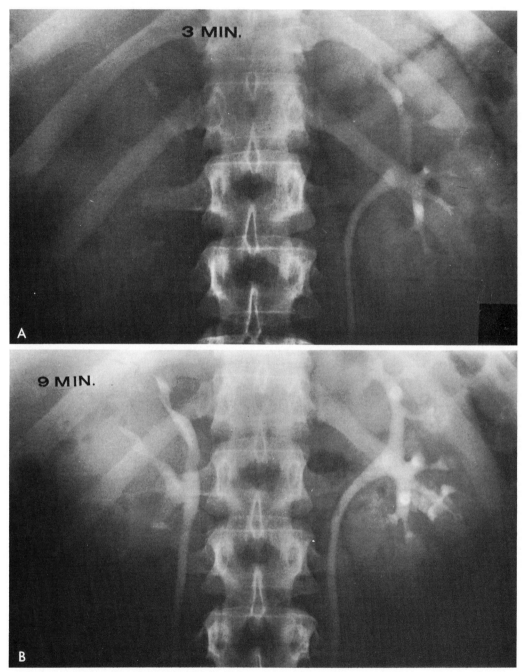

Figure 27–3. Organized perirenal hematoma as a late complication of renal trauma. This is a cause of renovascular hypertension ("Page" kidney).
   A, Excretory urogram, 3-minute film. There is delayed appearance of contrast material in the right kidney.
   B, Excretory urogram, 9-minute film. A mass effect from organized perirenal and subcapsular hematoma displaces the collecting system.
   (Courtesy of Ronald Castellino, M.D., Cornell University, New York, New York, and William Marshall, M.D., Stanford University, Stanford, California.)

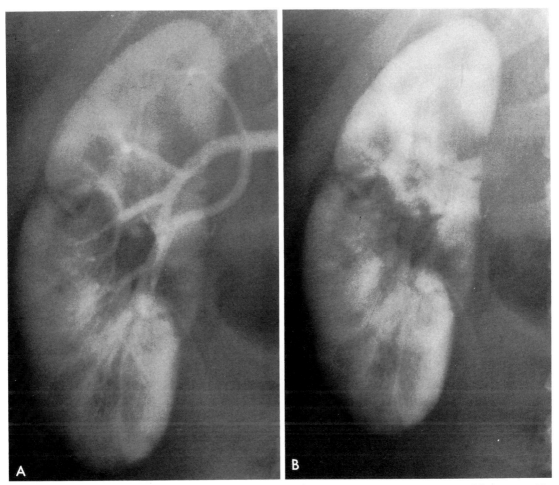

Figure 27–4. Renal fracture. There is a deep laceration extending through the renal parenchyma, with separation of the upper and lower poles.
A, Selective renal arteriogram, arterial phase.
B, Selective renal arteriogram, nephrographic phase.

branches. Sharply demarcated nephrographic defects related to devitalized tissue from traumatic thrombosis, vasospasm of small vessels, and the mass effect of intrarenal hematoma may be identified (Figs. 27–4 and 27–5). If active bleeding is present during angiography, extravasation of contrast material is seen during the arterial phase (Fig. 27–6).

Perirenal and subcapsular hematomas cause outward displacement or stretching of the capsular artery as it courses through the perirenal fat (see Fig. 27–13). Subcapsular collections flatten or indent the renal parenchyma, whereas perirenal hematoma may spread more diffusely through the perirenal space and cause less deformity of the renal contour.

Renal pedicle injury is detected as an abrupt termination of the renal artery just beyond its origin. The lesion is rarely a complete arterial avulsion. Occlusion, usually secondary to stretching and cracking of the arterial intima, is more common. Arteriovenous aneurysm (fistula) may result from blunt or penetrating trauma and is diagnosed by opacification of the draining vein during the arterial passage of contrast medium (Fig. 27–7). Angiography is unquestionably the most sensitive and specific method for detecting renal pedicle injuries or arteriovenous aneurysm (fistula).

Advantages and Limitations

The development of computed tomography and the realization that most renal injuries can be managed conservatively have greatly diminished the need for angiography in renal trauma. Compared with angiography, computed tomography has several distinct advantages as a noninvasive technique that can rapidly image the entire abdomen. Computed tomography with contrast material enhancement can accurately classify renal injuries, extrarenal hemorrhage, and associated abnormalities. Nevertheless, in selected patients, angiography may be both diagnostically and therapeutically valuable.

Patients with persistent hematuria following blunt or penetrating trauma are at risk for formation of an arteriovenous aneurysm (fistula). This may occlude vessels or resolve spontaneously. If persistent, however, hypertension or hematuria may follow. Angiography not only accurately defines this complication but can provide access for transcatheter embolization and thus obviate surgery.

Emergency angiography may be used for confirmation of suspected vascular pedicle injury. However, computed tomography has replaced angiography for this purpose in most situations. In some cases of renal

Text continued on page 811

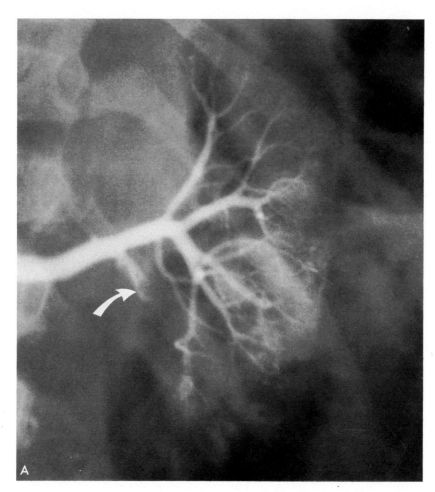

Figure 27–5. Nonopacification of the lower pole, probably related to devitalized tissue from traumatic arterial thrombosis *(arrow)*, vasospasm, and intrarenal hematoma.

A, Selective renal arteriogram, arterial phase.

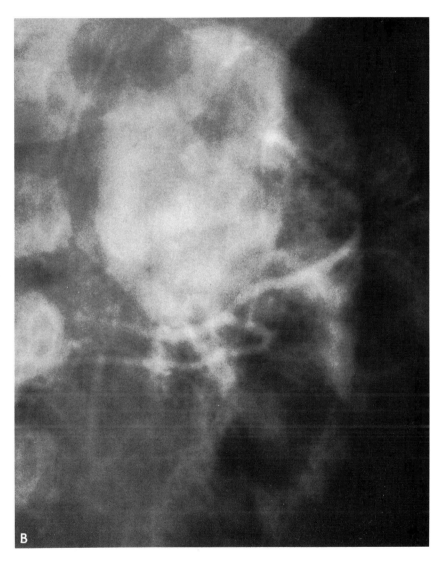

Figure 27-5. *Continued B*, Selective renal arteriogram, nephrographic phase.

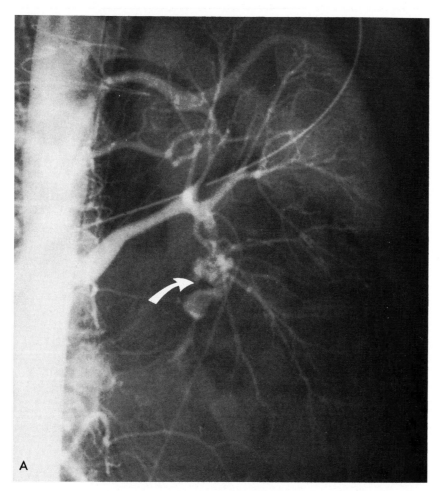

Figure 27–6. There is persistent collection of extravasated blood from a lacerated lower pole artery *(arrow)*. A defect in the nephrogram is noted that corresponds to the area supplied by the lacerated vessel.

A, Aortogram, arterial phase.

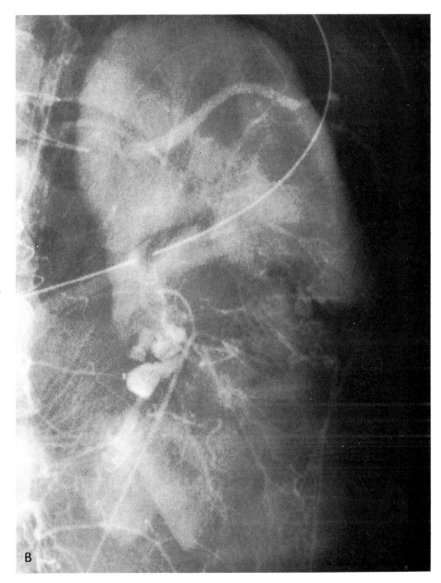

Figure 27–6. *Continued B,* Aortogram, nephrographic phase.

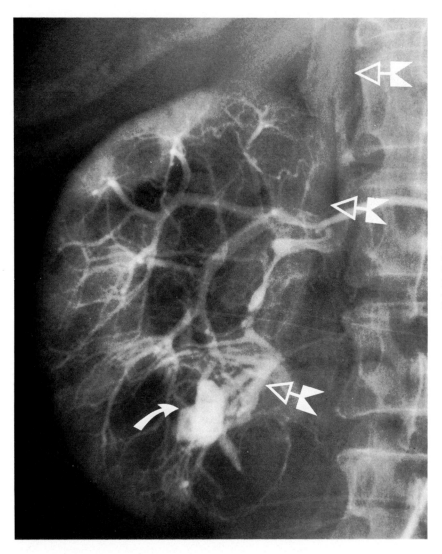

Figure 27–7. Traumatic arteriovenous aneurysm (fistula). There is an irregular collection of contrast material *(curved arrow)* within the lower pole, with early opacification of the renal vein and the inferior vena cava *(open arrows).* Selective renal arteriogram, arterial phase.

fracture or severe laceration, angiography may be useful for the definition of vascular anatomy before anticipated partial nephrectomy, although the primary diagnostic modality for this purpose is computed tomography.

RADIONUCLIDE STUDIES

Developments in radionuclide techniques have expanded their application to the evaluation of renal trauma (see also Chapter 2).

Technique

Both ^{99m}Tc-glucoheptonate and ^{99m}Tc-iron-ascorbate-DTPA have been used efficaciously for the study of trauma patients. The radionuclide scan has two components. The dynamic perfusion phase provides vascular flow information, and the static phase images tubular concentration and glomerular filtration. Both dynamic and static images are recorded on a gamma camera in posterior and both oblique projections.

Findings

Parenchymal lesions are visualized on static images as photopenic areas, with few features to distinguish between complete and incomplete lacerations, infarction, and arteriovenous aneurysm (fistula). Renal arterial occlusion is detected as nonperfusion of the kidney.

Advantages and Limitations

Radionuclide studies are noninvasive, relatively inexpensive, and generally available. These techniques may decrease the need for angiography in some cases in which excretory urography findings are nonspecific, such as the unilaterally decreased nephrogram. The abnormal radionuclide scan, however, is nonspecific, and perirenal hemorrhage and extravasation of opacified urine are not reliably diagnosed. Thus, even advocates of radionuclide scans have stressed the need for confirmatory studies such as angiography when the radionuclide scan is abnormal.

Radionuclide studies seem to have fallen victim to bad timing. Just as angiography captured the limelight in renal trauma imaging in the 1960s, computed tomography now similarly competes with radionuclide techniques. Computed tomography has the following advantages: it offers specific information about various types of renal trauma, is not limited to imaging a single organ, accurately quantitates perirenal hemorrhage, and rarely requires further confirmatory studies.

ULTRASONOGRAPHY

Published experience with evaluation of renal trauma by ultrasonography is limited, although the theoretical capability and limits are agreed on by most authors.

Technique

Technical limitations are a major factor hindering the utility of ultrasonography. Complete evaluation of the kidneys requires an uninterrupted ultrasound "window" from the skin surface to the kidneys. Since bowel gas limits the anterior approach, prone or decubitus scans are mandatory, particularly in studying the left kidney. Badly traumatized patients, however, frequently have difficulty in assuming such positions. Skin wounds and broken ribs may also restrict access.

Findings

Renal parenchymal laceration and hematoma may have a variety of appearances, depending on factors that include the frequency of the transducer and the elapsed time between bleeding and imaging. Renal hematoma appears as a sonolucent, hyperechoic, or mixed mass. A perirenal collection of urine or blood is usually detectable. Doppler ultrasonography may detect flow within suspected pseudoaneurysms or arteriovenous aneurysms (fistulas) (Fig. 27–8).

Advantages and Limitations

Ultrasonography provides morphologic detail about perirenal fluid collections and, to a lesser extent, the renal parenchyma. The absence of functional information provided by contrast material–dependent techniques limits the value of ultrasonography in the diagnosis of pedicle injuries, extravasation of urine, and parenchymal viability. Ultrasonography may be best used in follow-up studies of patients with previously defined injuries, particularly those with perirenal fluid collections.

COMPUTED TOMOGRAPHY

Broad experience has documented the accuracy of computed tomography in diagnosing the entire spectrum of abdominal trauma, including laceration and hematoma of the spleen, liver, pancreas, bowel, and kidney.

Technique

Because one of the major attributes of computed tomography is its capacity for multiorgan imaging, rarely is the study confined to the kidneys of patients with abdominal trauma. As previously noted, renal trauma is frequently accompanied by other visceral injuries. Scans are obtained at 10-mm intervals from the diaphragm to the bottom of the kidneys, then at 20-mm intervals through the pelvis. All scans are obtained after administration of diluted oral and intravenous contrast media. Urographic contrast material helps evaluate parenchymal function and extravasation of urine. Adult patients receive 100 to 150 ml of urographic contrast material. When computed tomography is performed soon after excretory urography, a "booster" dose of approximately 50 ml is recom-

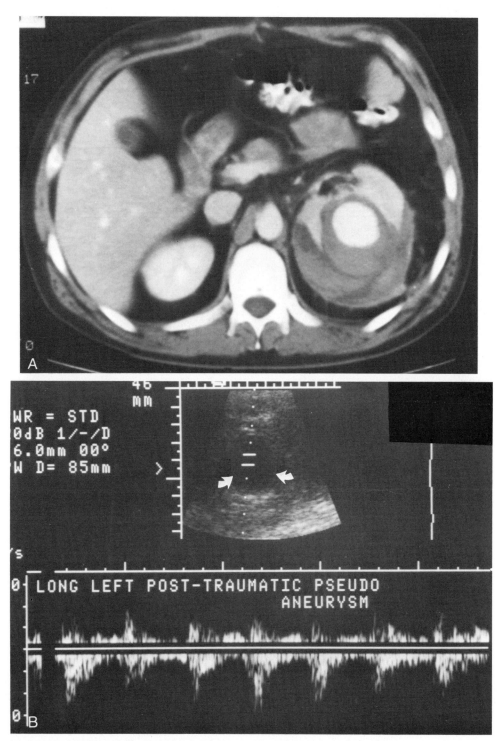

Figure 27–8. Pseudoaneurysm, left kidney, following stab wound.

   A, Computed tomogram with contrast material enhancement demonstrates intrarenal and perirenal hemorrhage as well as a well-circumscribed central lesion that enhances equally with the aorta.

   B, Ultrasonogram with Doppler interrogation. There is a "cystic" intrarenal lesion *(arrows)* with pulsatile disorganized flow.

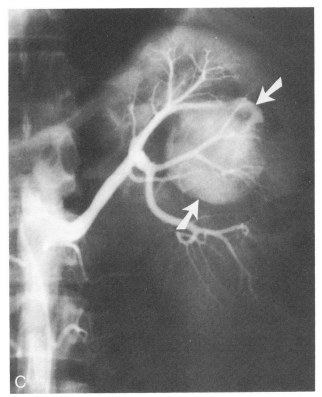

Figure 27–8. *Continued C,* Selective renal arteriogram directly demonstrates the pseudoaneurysm *(arrows).* Transcatheter embolization for control can be performed at this time.

(Courtesy of Philip Ralls, M.D., University of Southern California, Los Angeles, California.)

mended to reopacify blood vessels and optimally demonstrate parenchymal perfusion. Dynamic studies in which multiple sections through the kidneys are rapidly acquired following a bolus injection of contrast material have been advocated. The details of tim-

ing sequence and contrast material administration vary with the scanner used. Sagittal and coronal reformations of the axial slices are occasionally useful in understanding the three-dimensional nature of complex renal injuries.

Findings

The degree of anatomic resolution and functional information provided by computed tomography is unmatched by any other imaging modality. Minor, major, and catastrophic renal injuries can be precisely depicted and classified.

Minor injury, contusion, and small parenchymal laceration are often accompanied by a small subcapsular or perirenal hemorrhage (Fig. 27–9). Subcapsular collections appear as generally small and crescentic and flatten the underlying renal contour. Perirenal collections infiltrate or displace perirenal fat and may extend to the renal fascia. Contusion appears as diffuse or focal swelling, occasionally with prolonged and dense accumulation of contrast material, which is presumably in the renal interstitium. Scans obtained after intravenous infusion of contrast material show contusions or intrarenal lacerations as areas of decreased enhancement compared with normal renal parenchyma. A striated nephrogram that resolves without clinical sequelae has been noted on computed tomograms. This same feature has also been described on excretory urography and presumably results from stasis of urine in blood-filled tubules.

Major injuries, such as deep parenchymal lacerations, are almost always accompanied by perirenal hemorrhage. Extravasation of opacified urine, either into renal parenchyma or into the perirenal space, occurs when the laceration extends into the collecting system (Fig. 27–10; see also Fig. 27–13). Perirenal ex-

Figure 27–9. Minor laceration, left kidney. Computed tomogram, contrast material enhanced. A small ventral nephrographic defect and a small subcapsular hematoma *(arrow)* indicate a minor injury that will almost always heal spontaneously.

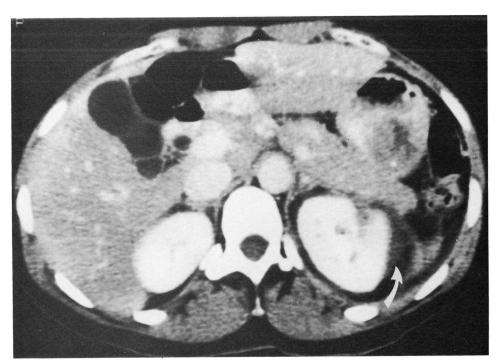

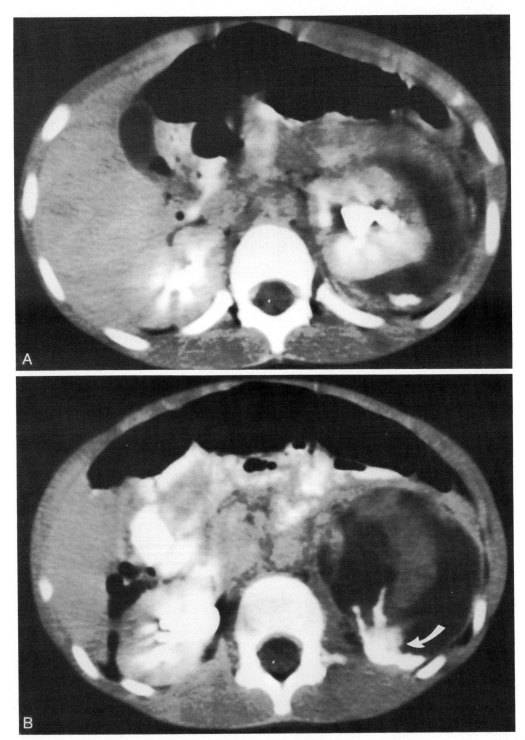

Figure 27–10. Fracture, left kidney, in a 7-year-old child after a bicycle accident. Computed tomogram, contrast material enhanced.
  A, Upper renal pole is intact and excretes urine.
  B, Urine in the perirenal space *(arrow)* indicates a tear of the collecting system.

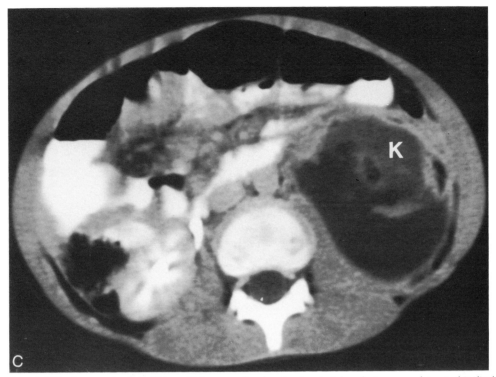

Figure 27–10. *Continued C,* The lower pole of the kidney (K) is nonperfused owing to arterial occlusion or avulsion and is displaced by perirenal urine and blood.

travasation is an important observation, one that many urologists consider a major criterion for surgical intervention. It can be detected by computed tomography when excretory urography is negative or equivocal. Extravasation accompanying severe renal laceration is less likely to be detected by excretory urography than is extravasation from focal lacerations caused by penetrating wounds.

Catastrophic injuries consist of a shattered kidney or a pedicle injury. A shattered or pulverized kidney is detected on computed tomography as multiple fracture planes separating functioning or devitalized renal fragments. A large perirenal hematoma is invariably present (Fig. 27–11).

Computed tomography can usually reliably diagnose a pedicle injury. Traumatic renal arterial occlusion is detected on computed tomography by a normal-sized, nonenhancing kidney, usually with little perirenal hemorrhage (Fig. 27–12). A rim of cortical tissue may be perfused by collateral vessels. This appears as an enhanced area that is quite different in appearance from renal laceration. Angiography is probably not necessary in this setting. Surgical repair, if it is to be attempted, should certainly not be delayed by more than a few hours by angiography.

Marked extravasation of opacified urine, especially if it is concentrated in the medial rather than the usual posterolateral part of the perinephric space, should suggest ureteral disruption. Failure of the ureter to opacify is further evidence of a ureteropelvic junction disruption, and this clinical and radiologic setting is virtually the only indication for retrograde pyelography in the trauma setting.

Penetrating renal trauma has been considered by many clinicians to be an indication for surgical exploration, regardless of urographic findings, which may correlate poorly with actual pathology. Some urologists now screen such patients with computed tomography and decide on management based on computed tomographic findings and clinical features. The criteria for choosing between nonoperative and surgical therapy for minor or major injury are the same as those previously described: amount of nonviable tissue, extravasation of urine, and extent of perirenal hemorrhage (Fig. 27–13). Prolonged hematuria or hypertension suggests arteriovenous aneurysm (fistula), which requires angiographic evaluation.

Kidneys that are abnormal by virtue of congenital anomaly, hypertrophy, ureteral obstruction, or underlying tumor are more prone to traumatic injury than normal kidneys. Findings on excretory urography may be difficult to interpret, or they may even be misleading. Underlying tumor may not be apparent. Often, bleeding is not proportional to the degree of trauma, and extravasation of urine may occur without parenchymal laceration. In such cases, computed tomography effectively distinguishes major from minor trauma, regardless of the size, position, or degree of hydronephrosis of the kidneys, and depicts underlying neoplasm or cyst (Fig. 27–14).

Advantages and Limitations

Because excretory urography is widely available, relatively inexpensive, and useful for diagnosis in cases of minor trauma, it remains the screening procedure of choice for suspected, isolated renal trauma. If urography findings are normal or indicative of only a small focal abnormality, and if the patient is clinically

Text continued on page 822

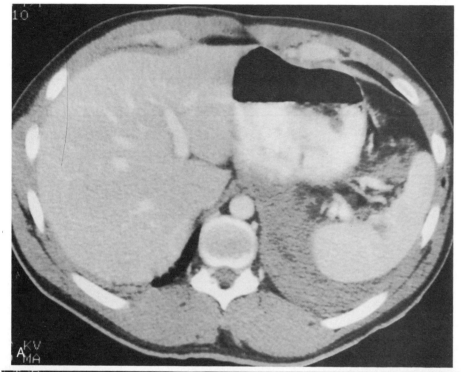

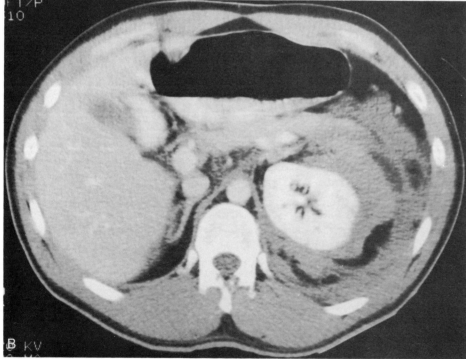

Figure 27–11. Lacerations, left kidney and spleen. Computed tomogram, contrast material enhanced.

  A, Splenic laceration with perisplenic and retroperitoneal hemorrhage.

  B, The upper pole of the left kidney is intact but surrounded by extensive perirenal hematoma.

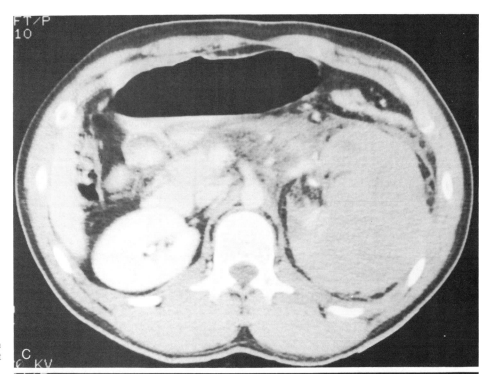

Figure 27–11. *Continued C,* There is a fracture completely through the left midkidney.

D, A small fragment of functioning lower pole renal parenchyma remains.

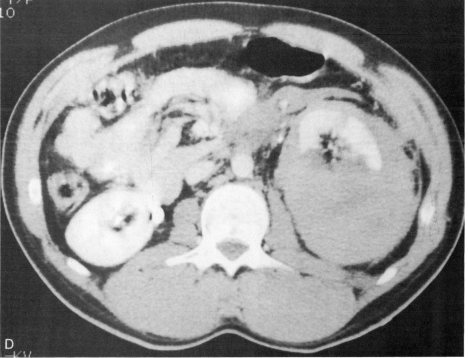

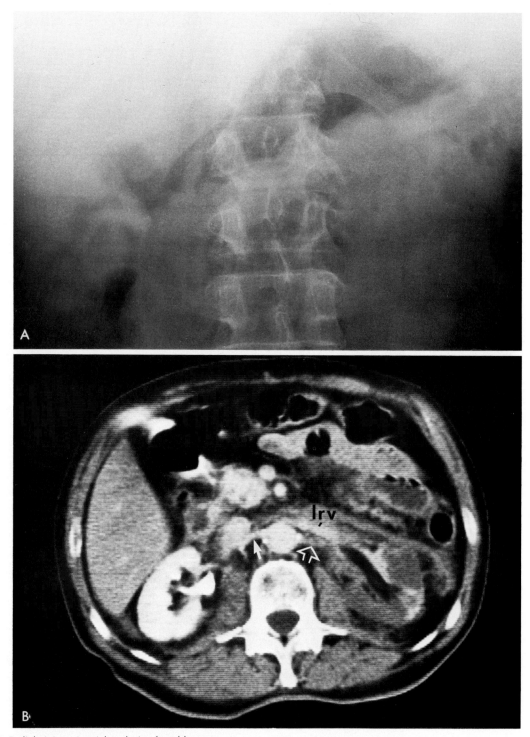

Figure 27–12. Pedicle injury. Arterial occlusion from blunt trauma.
    A, Excretory urogram shows decreased renal function on the right and no opacification of the left kidney.
    B, The computed tomogram shows a normal right kidney and a nonfunctioning left kidney. The left renal vein (lrv) and the right renal artery *(solid arrow)* are intact. The left renal artery *(open arrow)* does not opacify.

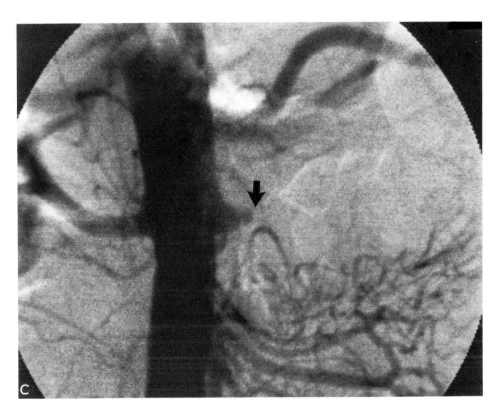

Figure 27–12. *Continued C,* Aortogram confirms occlusion of the left renal artery *(arrow).* (Angiography in this setting was unnecessary.)

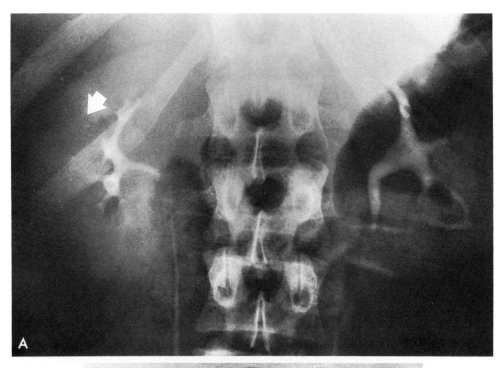

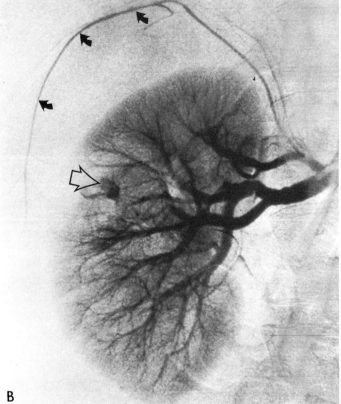

Figure 27–13. Stab wound in the right flank.
   A, Excretory urogram shows focal parenchymal defect *(arrow)* but no extravasation of urine.
   B, Arteriogram performed because of continuing hematuria and falling hematocrit shows parenchymal defect, subtle extravasation of urine *(open arrow)*, and displaced capsular artery *(solid arrows)*, indicating perirenal hemorrhage.

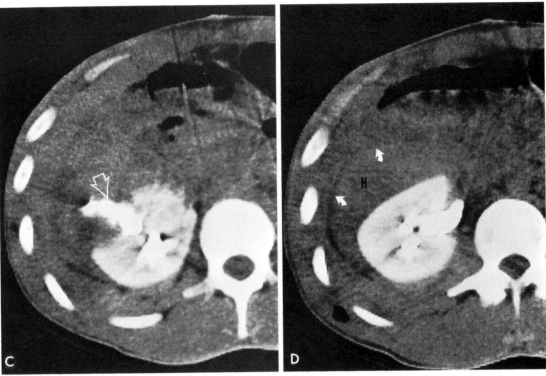

Figure 27–13 *Continued C* and *D,* Computed tomograms show extravasation of urine *(open arrow)* and large hematoma (H) distending the perirenal space and limited by renal fascia *(solid arrows).*

Figure 27–14. Relatively minor trauma with major consequence manifested by marked hematuria and falling hematocrit. Computed tomogram demonstrates a large perirenal hematoma with "hematocrit effect" due to settling of blood clot *(solid arrows).* A solid mass representing an adenocarcinoma of the kidney *(open arrows)* is evident but was not detected by excretory urography.

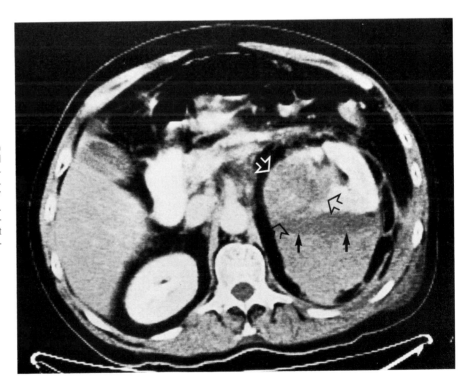

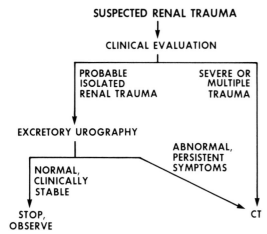

Figure 27–15. Suggested radiologic evaluation of renal trauma.

stable, no further studies are performed. However, if the patient has continued hematuria or falling hematocrit, or if the urogram suggests major injury, computed tomography is the next procedure to be performed. In severe or suspected multiple trauma, computed tomography is the initial diagnostic test used, since other organs must be evaluated. The combination of computed tomographic findings and clinical evaluation provides the basis for informed management decisions in all cases of major trauma. This approach is illustrated in Fig. 27–15.

Bibliography

Berg, B. C., Jr.: Nuclear medicine and complementary modalitities in renal trauma. Semin. Nucl. Med. 12:280, 1982.

Bretan, P. N., and McAninch, J. W.: Evaluation of renal trauma: Indications for computed tomography and other diagnostic techniques. In Lytton, B., Catalona, W. J., Lipshutz, L. I., McGuire, E. J. (eds.): Advances in Urology. Chicago, Year Book Medical Publishers, 1988, vol. 1, p 65.

Burbridge, B. E., Groot, G., Olenuik, F. F., et al.: Emergency excretory urography in blunt abdominal trauma. J. Can. Assoc. Radiol. 42:326, 1991.

Carroll, P. R., and McAninch, J. W.: Operative indications in penetrating renal trauma. J. Trauma 25:587, 1985.

Cass, A. S., and Luxenberg, M.: Conservative or immediate surgical management of blunt renal injuries. Radiology 130:11, 1983.

Cass, A. S., and Vieira, J.: Comparison of IVP and CT findings in patients with suspected severe renal injury. Urology 29:484, 1987.

Chopp, R. T., Hekmat-Ravan, H., and Mendez, R.: Technetium-99m glucoheptonate renal scan in diagnosis of acute renal injury. Urology 15:201, 1980.

Conrad, M. R., Freedman, M., Weiner, C., et al.: Sonography of the Page kidney. J. Urol. 116:293, 1976.

Evins, S. C., Thomason, W. B., and Rosenblum, R.: Nonoperative management of severe renal lacerations. J. Urol. 123:247, 1980.

Federle, M. P., Kaiser, J. A., McAninch, J. W., et al.: The role of computed tomography in renal trauma. Radiology 141:455, 1981.

Federle, M. P., Brown, T. R., and McAninch, J. W.: Penetrating renal trauma: CT evaluation. J. Comput. Assist. Tomogr. 11:1026, 1987.

Fisher, R. G., Ben-Menachem, Y., and Whigham, C.: Stab wounds of the renal artery branches: Angiographic diagnosis and treatment of embolization. AJR 152:1231, 1989.

Halpern, M.: Angiography in renal trauma. Surg. Clin. North Am. 48:1221, 1968.

Heyns, C. F., deKlerk, D. P., and deKock, M. L. S.: Nonoperative management of renal stab wounds. J. Urol. 134:239, 1985.

Jakse, G., Furtschegger, A., and Egender, G.: Ultrasound in patients with blunt renal trauma managed by surgery. J. Urol. 138:21, 1987.

Jakse, G., Putz, A., Gassner, I., and Zechman, W.: Early surgery in the management of pediatric blunt renal trauma. J. Urol. 131:920, 1984.

Karp, M. P., Jewett, T. C., Jr., Kuhn, J. P., et al.: The impact of computed tomography scanning on the child with renal trauma. J. Pediatr. Surg. 21:617, 1986.

Kay, C. J., Rosenfield, A. T., and Armm, M.: Gray-scale ultrasonography in the evaluation of renal trauma. Radiology 134:461, 1980.

Koehler, P. R., Talner, L. B., Friedenberg, M. J., and Kyaw, M. M.: Association of subcapsular hematomas with the nonfunctioning kidney. Radiology 106:537, 1973.

Kuhn, J. P., and Berger, P. E.: Computed tomography in the evaluation of blunt abdominal trauma in children. Radiol. Clin. North Am. 19:503, 1981.

Lang, E. K.: Arteriography in the assessment of renal trauma. J. Trauma 15:553, 1975.

Lang, E. K.: Assessment of renal trauma by dynamic computed tomography. Radiology 3:566, 1983.

Lang, E. K., Sullivan, J., and Fretz, G.: Renal trauma: Radiological studies: Comparison of urography, computed tomography, angiography and radionuclide studies. Radiology 154:1, 1985.

Mahoney, S. A., and Persky, L.: Intravenous drip nephrotomography as an adjunct in the evaluation of renal injury. J. Urol. 99:513, 1968.

McAninch, J. W., and Federle, M. P.: Evaluation of renal injuries with computerized tomography. J. Urol. 128:456, 1982.

McCort, J. J.: Perirenal fat infiltration by hemorrhage: Radiographic recognition and CT confirmation. Radiology 149:665, 1983.

Mee, S. L., McAninch, J. W., Robinson, A. L., Auerbach, P. S., and Carroll, P. R.: Radiographic assessment of renal trauma: 10-year prospective study of patient selection. J. Urol. 141:1095, 1989.

Mendez, R.: Renal trauma. J. Urol. 118:698, 1977.

Meyers, M. A.: Dynamic Radiology of the Abdomen. 3rd ed. New York, Springer Verlag, 1988.

Olsson, O., and Lunderquist, A.: Angiography in renal trauma. Acta Radiol. (Diagn.) 1:1, 1963.

Phillips, T., Sclafani, S. J. A., Goldstein, A., et al.: Use of the contrast-enhanced CT enema in the management of penetrating trauma to the flank and back. J. Trauma 26:593, 1986.

Pollack, H. M., and Popky, G. L.: Roentgenographic manifestations of spontaneous renal hemorrhage. Radiology 110:1, 1974.

Pollack, H. M., and Wein, A. J.: Imaging of renal trauma. Radiology 172:297, 1989.

Rhyner, P., Federle, M. P., and Jeffrey, R. B.: CT of trauma to the abnormal kidney. AJR 142:747, 1984.

Rous, S. N.: The value of serial selective renal angiography in the delayed management of renal trauma. J. Urol. 107:345, 1972.

Sandler, C. M., and Toombs, B. D.: Computed tomographic evaluation of blunt renal injuries. Radiology 141:461, 1981.

Schaner, E. G., Balow, J. E., and Doppman, J. L.: Computed tomography in the diagnosis of subcapsular and perirenal hematoma. AJR 129:83, 1977.

Stables, D. P.: Unilateral absence of excretion at urography after abdominal trauma. Radiology 121:609, 1976.

Steinberg, D. L., Jeffrey, R. B., Federle, M. P., and McAninch, J. W.: The CT appearance of renal pedicle injury. J. Urol. 132:1163, 1984.

Takahashi, M., Tamakawa, Y., Shibata, A., and Fukushima, Y.: Computed tomography of "Page" kidney. J. Comput. Assist. Tomogr. 1:344, 1977.

Thomas, S. D., Bogash, M., Popky, G., and Pollack, H.: Abnormal renal vasculature and renal trauma. J. Urol. 110:155, 1973.

Thompson, I. M., Latourette, H., Montie, J. E., and Ross, G., Jr.: Results of nonoperative management of blunt renal trauma. J. Urol. 118:522, 1977.

Yale-Loehr, A. J., Kramer, S. S., Quinlan, D. M., et al.: CT of severe renal trauma in children: Evaluation and course of healing with conservative therapy. AJR 152:109, 1989.

APPENDIX

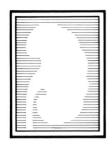

UROGRAPHIC CONTRAST MATERIAL: HISTORICAL DEVELOPMENT AND CHEMICAL CHARACTERISTICS

In 1897, Tuffier placed a rigid metal stylet through a ureteral catheter and thereby outlined the course of the ureter on a radiograph of the abdomen. In so doing, he began the history of the development of urographic contrast material. Reports of modifications of this method rapidly followed, first describing the use of flexible wires to outline the margins of the renal pelvis and later, replacement of metallic rods and wires with a diverse group of materials for retrograde instillation into the ureter. These materials included colloidal silver, bismuth, iodine-silver emulsions, thorium, potassium iodide, sodium iodide, sodium bromide, and strontium chloride. Even air, oxygen, and carbon dioxide were used as contrast agents. All of these techniques were abandoned after short periods of use, principally because of complications, usually of a common nature, such as infection and tissue trauma, but also because of exotic problems such as air embolism, silver deposits in the kidneys, and generalized argyry (silver poisoning).

The concept of radiographically visualizing the urinary tract by renal excretion rather than retrograde introduction of a radiopaque substance was discussed in a report of bladder opacification following oral or intravenous administration of 10% sodium iodide (Osborne et al., 1923). Osborne and Rowntree (Figs. A–1 and A–2), dermatologists at the Mayo Clinic, had been studying the therapeutic potential of iodine-containing compounds for the treatment of syphilis and other infections. It occurred to them that the known radiopacity and renal excretion of iodine might make this substance useful in rendering the urinary tract opaque to x-radiation. Charles G. Sutherland (Fig. A–3) was the only coauthor of this landmark article who was a radiologist. The value of the Mayo Clinic approach, which used sodium iodide, was soon confirmed by others. Other forms of iodine, bromide, and

sodium iodide–urea complexes were investigated during the 1920s. However, none of these agents consistently opacified the kidneys and ureters, large amounts of material were required for minimal density, and systemic reactions were common. Clearly, improvements were needed.

During this period of testing inorganic iodide radiopaque materials, two German chemists, Arthur Binz and C. Räth, were synthesizing pyridine compounds as potential therapeutic agents in the treatment of in-

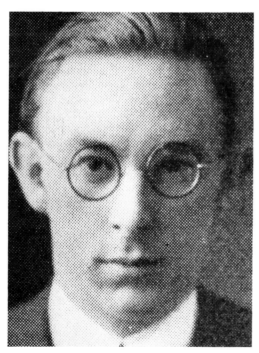

Figure A–1. Earl D. Osborne, M.D. (Courtesy of the late Glen W. Hartman, M.D., Mayo Clinic, Rochester, Minnesota.)

825

826

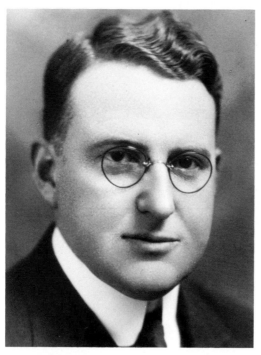

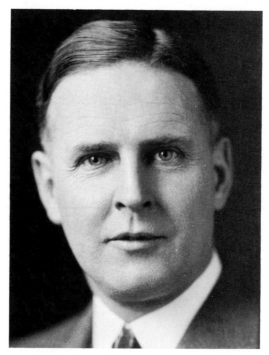

Figure A–2. Leonard G. Rowntree, M.D.

Figure A–3. Charles G. Sutherland, M.D.

(Courtesy of the late Glen W. Hartman, M.D., Mayo Clinic, Rochester, Minnesota.)

fections. One of these compounds, Selectan-neutral (Fig. A–4), was excreted by both the biliary system and the kidneys and therefore was used as treatment for infections of the gallbladder and urinary tract. Clinical trials were conducted in a hospital in Hamburg-Altona at which a young American urologist, Moses Swick (Fig. A–5), was working under the direction of Prof. Dr. Lichwitz. Swick, noting that Selectan-neutral was composed of 54 per cent iodine, realized the potential for urinary tract opacification and conducted simultaneous excretion, toxicity, and radiologic studies. Nausea, vomiting, headache, and diplopia limited the usefulness of Selectan-neutral. Paying particular attention to the diplopia, Swick reasoned that the toxicity might be diminished by modification of the N-methyl group at position 1. This change, along with other suggestions designed to increase solubility of the drug, was proposed to Binz, who synthesized sodium 5-iodo-2-pyridone-N-acetate, or Uroselectan, containing 42 per cent iodine (Fig. A–6). This

new material was tested by Swick, who by then had transferred to the service of Prof. von Lichtenberg at St. Hedwig's Krankenhaus in Berlin. It was found to offer improved water solubility over Selectan-neutral, was well tolerated, and provided a degree of opacification of the urinary tract that was never before achieved. Swick and von Lichtenberg reported their results to the German Urologic Congress, which met

Mol. Wt.: 238
Iodine Content: 54%
Trade Name: Selectan-neutral

N-methyl-5-iodo-2-pyridone

Figure A–4. Chemical characteristics of Selectan-neutral.

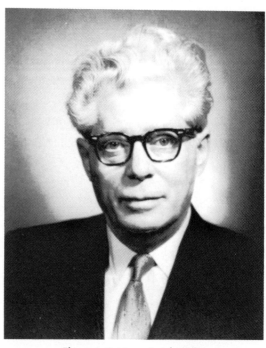

Figure A–5. Moses Swick, M.D.

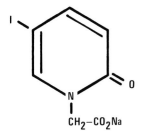

Mol. Wt.: 301
Iodine Content: 42%
Trade Names: Uroselectan
Iopax

Figure A–6. Chemical characteristics of Uroselectan (Iopax).

Sodium 5-iodo-2-pyridone-N-acetate

Figure A–7. Chemical characteristics of Uroselectan B (Neo-Iopax).

Mol. Wt.: 493
Iodine Content: 51.5%
Generic Name: sodium iodomethamate, U.S.P.
Iodoxyl, B.P.
Trade Names: Neo-Iopax, Uroselectan B

Disodium 1-methyl-3, 5 diiodo-
4-pyridone-2-6-dicarboxylate

in Munich in 1929. This report set the stage for the era of modern excretory urography. Uroselectan, marketed in the United States as Iopax, was modified by Binz into disodium 1-methyl-3, 5-diiodo-4-pyridone-2,6-dicarboxylate (Fig. A–7), which offered increased iodine content. The modified version was sold as Uroselectan B in Europe and as Neo-Iopax in the United States.

In 1930, Bronner, Hecht, and Schüller introduced sodium iodomethanesulfonate (Abrodil in Europe, Skiodan in the United States). At about the same time, Iopax was modified into 3,5-diiodo-4-pyridone-N-acetic acid diethanolamine salt, or Diodrast (Fig. A–8). Neo-Iopax and Diodrast were accepted rapidly as the contrast agents of choice for excretory urography; their predominance continued until the introduction of the benzoic acid derivative, acetrizoate, some 20 years later.

Whereas it was not until 1950 that acetrizoate was introduced into clinical radiology, the conceptual basis for the radiologic use of this compound was laid by Moses Swick in the early 1930s. Swick originated the idea of using an organic nucleus that was a normal product of metabolism—not a synthetic substance—as a carrier for a radiopaque element. He proposed the detoxification product of benzoic acid, sodium orthoiodohippurate, or Hippuran, as an iodine carrier that would be excreted by the kidneys. The Billings Gold Medal of the American Medical Association was awarded to Swick in 1933 for the introduction of this concept. Hippuran could be administered orally and did opacify the urinary tract. Unfortunately, its usefulness was impaired by adverse systemic effects related to the addition of iodine to the hippuric acid molecule. Additional factors that limited its use were obscuration of the urinary tract by the orally adminis-

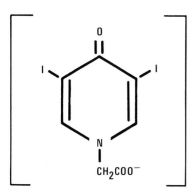

$H_2N^+(CH_2CH_2OH)_2$

Mol. Wt.: 510
Iodine Content: 49.8%
Generic Names: iodopyracet, U.S.P.
diodone, B.P.
Trade Names: Diodrast
Umbradil

Figure A–8. Chemical characteristics of Diodrast.

3, 5 diiodo-4-pyridone-N-acetic
acid, diethanoleamine salt

Figure A–9. Chemical characteristics of Urokon.

Mol. Wt.: **479**
Iodine Content: **65.8%**
Generic Name: **sodium acetrizoate, U.S.P.**
Trade Name: **Urokon**

Sodium 3-acetamido-2, 4, 6 triiodobenzoate

tered opaque material in the gut and the limitation of radiopacity imposed by one iodine atom on each molecule of Hippuran. Despite these drawbacks, the value of binding iodine to the 6-carbon benzoic acid ring rather than the 5-carbon pyridone-derived ring was established.

During the period of 1948–1950, V. H. Wallingford and his colleagues at the Research Laboratories of Mallinckrodt Chemical Works, St. Louis, studied a group of normal detoxication products obtained by acetylation of aminobenzoic acid. These workers reported on the synthesis and clinical usefulness of sodium 3-acetamido-2,4,6-triiodobenzoate, or acetrizoate (Fig. A–9). This was one of a group of iodinated acylaminobenzoic acids tested by Wallingford and associates that was selected as potentially useful for excretory urography because of its high iodine content (sodium salt, 65.8%) high water solubility, and urinary excretion. Initial biochemical, toxicologic, and clinical trials showed acetrizoate to be of low toxicity and efficacious for urinary tract opacification. Other studies indicated that this compound was excreted principally by glomerular filtration and that visualization of the urinary tract was more satisfactory than that possible with agents generally in use at that time. This achievement was due to acetrizoate's high iodine content and low toxicity relative to Diodrast. Acetrizoate was marketed as Urokon and began to replace Diodrast in clinical urography.

In the formulation of acetrizoate, the 5 position on the benzoic ring was unsubstituted. (See Figs. A–9

and A–13.) In 1955, J. O. Hoppe and his colleagues at the Sterling-Winthrop Research Institute reported their evaluation of a large number of di- and tri-iodinated benzoic acid derivatives in which the 5 position was substituted with a variety of radicals. Of the compounds studied, one stood out as fulfilling requirements for a urographic compound in humans, namely high radiopacity, high water solubility, low toxicity, and a minimum of pharmacodynamic activity. This substance, 3,5-diacetamido-2,4,6-triiodobenzoic acid, or diatrizoate, was registered by Winthrop Laboratories. The sodium salt was marketed as Hypaque (Fig. A–10). Development of sodium diatrizoate was reported independently by the Schering group in West Germany. As clinical experience and laboratory investigations into contrast material pharmacology accumulated, the relative safety of sodium diatrizoate compared with sodium acetrizoate and other previously used contrast agents (e.g., Diodrast and Neo-Iopax) became apparent. Every water-soluble urographic contrast agent in clinical use today is a modification or derivative of tri-iodinated, fully saturated benzoic acid.

The urographic contrast agents most commonly in use are monomers that ionize into a cation (sodium or N-methylglucamine) and a benzoate anion that bears three atoms of iodine. The formulas, chemical characteristics, and generic and trade names of these agents are illustrated in Figures A–10 through A–12. Table A–1 lists the sodium and iodine content of these preparations. All of these substances are fully substituted

Figure A–10. Chemical characteristics of Hypaque.

Mol. Wt.: **636**
Iodine Content: **59.8%**
Generic Name: **sodium diatrizoate, U.S.P.**
Trade Name: **Hypaque**

Sodium 3, 5, diacetamido-2, 4, 6 triiodobenzoate

COO⁻

I I

CH₃CONH NHCOCH₃

I

Na⁺ and CH₃NH₂⁺
|
CH₂
|
HCOH
|
HOCH
|
HCOH
|
HCOH
|
CH₂OH

Mol. Wt.: 810
Iodine Content: 47.6%
Generic Name: meglumine and sodium diatrizoate, U.S.P.
Trade Names: Renografin 60
Urografin

Figure A–11. Chemical characteristics of Renografin 60 (Urografin).

Sodium and N-methylglucamine 3, 5 diacetamido-2, 4, 6 triiodobenzoate

Figure A–12. Chemical characteristics of Conray.

COO⁻

I I

CH₃CONH CONHCH₃

I

CH₃NH₂⁺
|
CH₂
|
HCOH
|
HOCH
|
HCOH
|
HCOH
|
CH₂OH

Mol. Wt.: 810
Iodine Content: 62%
Generic Name: meglumine iothalamate, U.S.P.
Trade Name: Conray

N-methylglucamine-5-acetamido-2, 4, 6 triiodo-N-methylisophthalamate

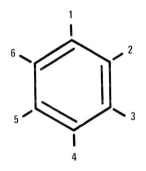

Position 1 – carboxyl group (–CO₂H) as sodium or N-methylglucamine salt
Positions 2, 4, 6 – iodine
Position 3 – acetamido
Position 5 – acetamido (diatrizoate)
    N-methyl carbamyl (iothalamate)
    N-methyl acetamido (metrizoate)

Figure A–13. Basic benzene ring common to all modern contrast agents. Variations at positions 3 and 5 distinguish the generic designation of various compounds. Variation at position 1 determines the form of the salt.

benzoic acid derivatives. The several agents are distinguished one from the other by the radical at position 3 or 5 and/or by the sodium or N-methylglucamine (meglumine) cation at position 1 (Fig. A–13).

A major factor in the toxicity of ionic monomers is their high osmolality (greater than 2000 mOsm/kg water in some products) relative to that of physiologic solutions (approximately 290 mOsm/kg water). Hyperosmolality of this magnitude is responsible for the injection site pain, heat, flushing, and nausea that are associated with contrast material injection. Serious adverse systemic reactions also are related in some

way to the osmolality of contrast agents. Other alterations that are considered due to hyperosmolality of ionic monomeric forms of contrast material include crenation of erythrocytes, increase in pulmonary artery pressure, injury to venous and capillary endothelium, disruption of the blood–brain barrier, and increase in circulating blood volume with associated alterations in heart rate. Depression of the kidney's ability to extract para-aminohippuric acid, changes in renal blood flow, decrease in glomerular filtration rate, abnormal urine enzyme output, and changes in urinary electrolyte excretion are a result of contrast

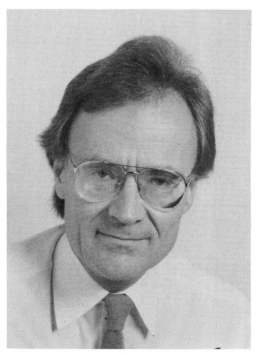

Figure A–14. Torsten Almén, M.D.

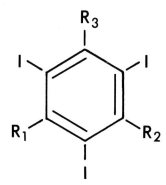

Figure A–15. Generic structure of radiopaque nonionic monomers. R_1, R_2, and R_3 are hydrophilic, nonionizing radicals.

material administration in both humans and laboratory animals. Hyperosmolality accounts for some, if not all, of these effects.

Although these toxic reactions to contrast material have not been of sufficient magnitude to prevent the widespread vascular use of monomeric ionic forms of contrast material in large doses, the need for agents of lower osmolality has been apparent for a long time. In 1969, the Swedish radiologist Torsten Almén (Fig. A–14) opened a new era in the history of water-soluble radiopaque compounds by theorizing that osmolality would be lower and radiopacity would be main-

tained with iodine-bearing compounds that were *nonionizing*. Metrizamide (Amipaque) was the first of the water-soluble nonionic monomeric compounds based on this concept to gain clinical use, principally for opacification of the subarachnoid space.

The development of low-osmolality water-soluble contrast agents for intravascular use that have followed Almén's concepts has been along two lines. The first has focused on a single benzene ring that is fully saturated with both iodine atoms (positions 2, 4, and 6) and hydrophilic radicals (positions 1, 3, and 5). The latter render the molecules water soluble without ionization. The architecture of nonionic monomers is illustrated in Figure A–15. These retain the same radiopacity as ionic monomers with three atoms of iodine on each molecule. The reduction of the number of particles in solution from two to one, however, substantially reduces the osmolality of these compounds. Characteristics of various nonionic monomers are listed in Table A–1 and illustrated in Figures A–16 through A–19.

The second line of development of low-osmolality contrast agents has been dimers of tri-iodinated ben-

Table A–1. COMMONLY USED CONTRAST MATERIAL FOR EXCRETORY UROGRAPHY AND COMPUTED TOMOGRAPHY

Generic Name	Trade Name	Sodium Content (mEq/ml)	Iodine Content (mg/ml)	Osmolality (mOsm/kg H_2O)
Ionic Monomers (Ratio 1.5)				
Sodium diatrizoate	Hypaque 50	0.8	300	1515
Meglumine and sodium diatrizoate	Renografin 60	0.16	292	1420
Sodium iothalamate	Conray 400	1.05	400	2300
Meglumine iothalamate	Conray		282	1400
Nonionic Monomers (Ratio 3)				
Iopamidol	Isovue 300		300	616
Iohexol	Omnipaque		300	709
Ioversol	Optiray		320	702
Iopromide	Ultravist		300	620
Ionic Dimer (Ratio 3)				
Meglumine and sodium ioxaglate	Hexabrix	0.15	320	600
Nonionic Dimers (Ratio 6)				
Iotrolan (under development)				
Iodixanol (under development)				

(S)-N,N'-bis[2-hydroxy-1-(hydroxymethyl)ethyl]-
2,4,6-triiodo-5-lactamidoisophthalamide

Mol. Wt.: 777
Iodine Content: 49%
Generic Name: iopamidol, U.S.P.
Trade Name: Isovue

Figure A–16. Chemical characteristics of Isovue.

N,N'-bis(2,3-dihydroxypropyl)-5-[N-(2,3-dihydroxypropyl)-
acetamidol]-2,4,6-triiodoisophthalamide

Mol. Wt.: 821
Iodine Content: 46%
Generic Name: iohexol, U.S.P.
Trade Name: Omnipaque

Figure A–17. Chemical characteristics of Omnipaque.

N,N'-bis(2,3-dihydroxypropyl)-5-[N-(2-hydroxyethyl)-
glycolamidol]-2,4,6-triiodoisophthalamide

Mol. Wt.: 807
Iodine Content: 47%
Generic Name: ioversol, U.S.P.
Trade Name: Optiray

Figure A–18. Chemical characteristics of Optiray.

5-Methoxyacetylamino-2,4,6-triiodoisophthalic acid
[(2,3-dihydroxy-N-methylpropyl)-(2,3-dihydroxypropyl)]diamide

Mol. Wt.: 791
Iodine Content: 48%
Generic Name: iopromide, U.S.P.
Trade Name: Ultravist

Figure A–19. Chemical characteristics of Ultravist.

831

Figure A–20. Generic structure of a mono-acid dimer contrast agent. R_1, R_2, and R_3 are hydrophilic, nonionizing radicals.

N-(2-hydroxyethyl)-2,4,6-triiodo-5-[2-[2,4,6-triiodo-3-(N-methylacetamido)-isophthalamic acid, compounded with 1-deoxy-1-(methylamino)-D-glucitol (1:1) and sodium N-(2-hydroxyethyl)-2,4,6-triiodo-5-[2-(2,4,6-triiodo-3-(N-methylacetamido)-5-(methylcarbamoyl)benzamido]acetamido]-isophthalamate.

Iodine Content: 32%
Generic Name: ioxaglate meglumine and sodium
Trade Name: Hexabrix

Figure A–21. Chemical characteristics of Hexabrix.

Figure A–22. Contrast material classification by ratio number.

zene rings, as illustrated in Figure A–20. The first product developed as a dimer, sodium-meglumine ioxaglate (Hexabrix), has one ionizing carboxyl group and is classified as an ionic, or monoacid, dimer (Fig. A–21). Under development are dimers that achieve water solubility by full substitution with hydrophilic radicals at all sites except for the six sites at which atoms of iodine are attached. These products are compounded with an osmolality essentially equivalent to that of plasma. The ionic dimeric contrast agent is characterized further in Table A–1 and is illustrated in Figure A–21. Nonionic dimers have not been introduced for general use.

The new classes of low-osmolality contrast agents are conveniently characterized by the ratio of the number of atoms of iodine to the number of particles in solution for each molecule. This expression relates, respectively, radiodensity to osmolality. Ionic monomers are *ratio 1.5* compounds by virtue of their three atoms of iodine for every two particles in solution. Nonionic monomers (three atoms of iodine to one particle in solution) and ionic dimers (six atoms of iodine to two particles in solution) are *ratio 3* compounds. Nonionic dimers (six atoms of iodine to one particle in solution) are *ratio 6* compounds. This nomenclature is summarized in Figure A–22.

Bibliography

Almén, T.: Contrast agent design. J. Theor. Biol. *24*:216, 1969.
Almén, T.: Experience from 10 years of development of water-soluble nonionic contrast media. Invest. Radiol. *15*:S283, 1980.
Almén, T.: Development of nonionic contrast media. Invest. Radiol. *20*(Suppl.):S2, 1985.
Bettmann, M. A.: Ionic versus nonionic contrast agents for intravenous use: Are all the answers in? Radiology *175*:616, 1990.
Bettmann, M. A.: Guidelines for use of low-osmolality contrast agents. Radiology *172*:901, 1989.
Bettmann, M.: Clinical summary with conclusions: Ionic versus nonionic contrast agents and their effects on blood components. Invest. Radiol. *23*(Suppl. 2):S378, 1988.
Brennan, R. E., Rapoport, S., Weinberg, I., Pollack, H. M., and Curtis, J. A.: CT determined canine kidney and urine, iodine concentrations following intravenous administration of sodium diatrizoate, metrizamide, iopamidol and sodium ioxaglute. Invest. Radiol. *17*:95, 1982.
Bruwer, A. J. (ed.): Classic Descriptions in Roentgenology. Springfield, Charles C Thomas, 1964, pp. 1606–1614.
Cochran, S. T., Ballard, J. W., Katzberg, R. W., Barbaric, A. L., Spataro, R., Iwamoto, K., and Lee, J. J.: Evaluation of iopamidol and diatrizoate in excretory urography: A double-blind study. AJR *151*:523, 1988.
Cohan, R. H., and Dunnick, N. R.: Intravascular contrast media: Adverse reactions. AJR *149*:665, 1987.
Danford, R. O., Talner, L. B., and Davidson, A. J.: Effect of graded osmolalities of saline solution and contrast media on renal extraction of PAH in the dog. Invest. Radiol. *4*:301, 1969.
Davidson, A. J.: Lysozymuric response to contrast agents. Invest. Radiol. *3*:65, 1968.
Davidson, A. J., Abrams, H. L., and Stamey, T. A.: Renal extraction of PAH in man following aortography. Radiology *85*:1043, 1965.
Dawson, P., Grainger, R. G., and Pitfield, J.: The new low-osmolar contrast media: A simple guide. Clin. Radiol. *34*:321, 1983.
Dawson, P., Heron, C., and Marshall, J.: Intravenous urography with low-osmolarity contrast agents: Theoretical considerations and clinical findings. Clin. Radiol. *35*:173, 1984.
Dawson, P.: Chemotoxicity of contrast media and clinical adverse effects: A review. Invest. Radiol. *20*(Suppl.):S84, 1985.
Evill, C. A., and Benness, G. T.: Solute excretion during intravenous urography: A comparison of sodium and methylglucamine iothalamates. Invest. Radiol. *10*:148, 1975.
Gale, M. E., Robbins, A. H., Hamburger, R. J., and Widrich, W. C.: Renal toxicity of contrast agents: Iopamidol, iothalamate and diatrizoate. AJR *142*:333, 1984.
Gavant, M. L., and Siegle, R. L.: Iodixanol in excretory urography: Initial clinical experience with a nonionic, dimeric (ratio 6:1) contrast medium. Radiology *183*:515, 1992.

Grainger, R. G.: The clinical and financial implications of the low-osmolar radiological contrast media. Correspondence. Clin. Radiol. 35:422, 1984.

Hoppe, J. O., Larsen, A. A., and Coulston, F.: Observations on the toxicity of a new urographic contrast medium, sodium 3,5-diacetamido-2,4,6-triiodobenzoate (Hypaque sodium) and related compounds. J. Pharmacol. Exp. Ther. 116:394, 1956.

Hryntschak, T.: Studien Zur röentgenologischen Darstellung von Nierenparenchym und Nierenbecken auf intravenösem Wege. Z. Urol. Nephrol. 23:893, 1929.

Katayama, H., Yamaguchis, K., Kozuka, T., Takashima, T., Seez, P., and Matsuura, K.: Adverse reactions to ionic and nonionic contrast media: A report from the Japanese committee on the safety of contrast media. Radiology 175:621, 1990.

Kaye, B., Howard, J., Foord, K. D., and Cumberland, D. C.: Comparison of the image quality of intravenous urograms using low-osmolar contrast media. Br. J. Radiol. 61:589, 1988.

Kennison, M. C., Powe, N. R., and Steinberg, E. P.: Results of randomized controlled trials of low- versus high-osmolality contrast media. Radiology 170:381, 1989.

Khoury, G. A., Hopper, J. C., Varghese, Z., Farrington, K., Dick, R., Irving, J. D., Sweny, P., Fernando, O. N., and Moorhead, J. F.: Nephrotoxicity of ionic and non-ionic contrast material in digital vascular imaging and selective renal arteriography. Br. J. Radiol. 56:631, 1983.

Kolbenstvedt, A., Andrew, E., Christophersen, B., Golman, K., Kvarstein, B., and Lien, H. H.: Metrizamide in high dose urography. Acta Radiol. (Diagn.) 10:39, 1979.

Lalli, A. F., Williams, B., and Maynard, E.: Iohexol in urography. Urol. Radiol. 5:95, 1983.

Langecker, H., Harward, A., and Junkman, K.: 3,5-Diacetylamino-2,4,6-trijodensoesäure als Röntgenkontrastmittel. Arch. Exper. Path. u. Pharmakol. 222:584, 1954.

Larsen, A. A., Moore, C., Sprague, J., Cloke, B., Moss, J., and Hoppe, J. O.: Iodinated 3,5-diaminobenzoic acid derivatives. J. Am. Chem. Soc. 78:3210, 1956.

Lasser, E. C., Walters, A., Reuter, S. R., and Lang, J.: Histamine release by contrast media. Radiology 100:683, 1971.

Lasser, E. R., and Berry, C. C.: Nonionic versus ionic contrast media: What do the data tell us? AJR 152:945, 1989.

Lasser, E. C.: Pretreatment with corticosteroids to prevent reactions to IV contrast material: Overview and implications. AJR 150:257, 1988.

Lenarduzzi, G., and Pecco, R.: Iniezioni endovenose di ioduro di sodio (richerche radiologiche sperimentali). Arch. Radiol. 3:1055, 1927.

Lichtenberg, A., and Swick, M.: Klinische Prüfung des Uroselectans. Klin. Wochenschr. 8:2089, 1929.

Longhran, C. F.: Clinical intravenous urography: Comparative trial of ioxoglate and iopamidol. Radiology 161:455, 1986.

Magill, H. L., Clarke, E. A., Fitch, S. J., Boulden, J. F., Ramirez, R., Siegle, R. L., and Somes, G. W.: Excretory urography with iohexal: Evaluation in children. Radiology 161:625, 1986.

McChesney, E. W., and Hoppe, J. O.: Studies of the tissue distribution and excretion of sodium diatrizoate in laboratory animals. AJR 78:137, 1957.

McClennan, B.: Ionic versus nonionic contrast media: Safety, tolerance and rationale for use. Urol. Radiol. 11:200, 1989.

McClennan, B. L.: Low-osmolality contrast media: Premises and promises. Radiology 162:1, 1987.

Miller, D. L., Chang, R., Wells, W. T., Dowjat, B. A., Malinovsky, R. M., and Doppman, J. L.: Intravascular contrast media: Effect of dose on renal function. Radiology 167:607, 1988.

Mindell, H. J., and Gibson, T. C.: ECG abnormalities during excretory urography: The effect of stress. AJR 150:1327, 1988.

Moore, T. D., and Mayer, R. F.: Hypaque: An improved medium for excretory urography: A preliminary report of 210 cases. South. Med. J. 48:135, 1955.

Moreau, J.-F., Droz, D., Sabto, J., Jungers, P., Kleinknecht, D., Hinglais, N., and Michel, J.-R.: Osmotic nephrosis induced by water-soluble triiodinated contrast media in man. Radiology 115:329, 1975.

Mudge, G. H.: Some questions on nephrotoxicity. Invest. Radiol. 5:407, 1970.

Narath, P. A.: Renal Pelvis and Ureter. New York, Grune & Stratton, 1951.

Neuhaus, D. R., Christman, A. A., and Lewis, H. B.: Biochemical studies on Urokon (sodium 2,4,6-triiodo-3-acetylaminobenzoate), a new pyelographic medium. J. Lab. Clin. Med. 35:43, 1950.

O'Reilly, P. H., Jones, D. A., and Farah, N. B.: Measurement of the plasma clearance of urographic contrast media for the determination of glomerular filtration rate. J. Urol. 139:9, 1988.

Osborne, E. D., Sutherland, C. G., Scholl, A. J., and Rowntree, L. G.: Roentgenography of urinary tract during excretion of sodium iodide. JAMA 80:368, 1923.

Palmer, F. J.: The RACR survey of intravenous contrast media reactions final report. Aust. Radiol. 32:426, 1988.

Porporis, A. A., Elliott, G. V., Fischer, G. L., and Mueller, C. B.: The mechanism of Urokon excretion. AJR 72:995, 1954.

Rapoport, S., Bookstein, J. J., Higgins, C. B., Carey, P. H., Sovak, M., and Lasser, E. C.: Experience with metrizamide in patients with severe anaphylactoid reactions to ionic contrast agents. Radiology 143:321, 1982.

Rockoff, S. D., Brasch, R., Kuhn, C., and Chraplyvy, M.: Contrast media as histamine liberators: I. Mast-cell histamine release in vitro by sodium salts of contrast media. Invest. Radiol. 5:503, 1970.

Rockoff, S. D., Kuhn, C., and Chraplyvy, M.: Contrast media as histamine liberators: IV. In vitro mast-cell histamine release by methylglucamine salts. Invest. Radiol. 6:186, 1971.

Rockoff, S. D., Kuhn, C., and Chraplyvy, M.: Contrast media as histamine liberators: V. Comparison of in vitro mast-cell histamine release by sodium and methylglucamine salts. Invest. Radiol. 7:177, 1972.

Rollins, M., Bonte, F. J., Rose, F. A., and Keating, D. R.: Clinical evaluation of a new compound for intravenous urography. AJR 73:771, 1955.

Root, J. C., and Strittmatter, W. C.: Hypaque, a new urographic contrast medium. AJR 73:768, 1955.

Roseno, A.: Die intravenöse Pyelographic: II. Mitteilung. Klin. Ergebnisse. Klin. Wochenschr. 8:1165, 1929.

Schrott, K. M., Behrends, B., Clauss, W., Kaufman, J., and Lehnert, J.: Iohexal in der Auscheidungsurographic: Ergelbnisse des drug-monitoring. Forshr. Med. 104:153, 1986.

Sherwood, T., and Lavender, J. P.: Does renal blood flow rise or fall in response to diatrizoate? Invest. Radiol. 4:327, 1969.

Spataro, R. F., Fischer, H. W., and Baylan, L.: Urography with low osmolality contrast media: Comparative urinary excretion of iopamidol, Hexabrix and diatrizoate. Invest. Radiol. 17:494, 1982.

Spataro, R. F., Katzberg, R. W., Fischer, H. W., and McMannis, M. J.: High-dose clinical urography with low-osmolality contrast agent Hexabrix: Comparison with conventional agent. Radiology 162:9, 1987.

Swick, M.: Darstellung der Niere und Harmwege im Röntgenbild durch intravenöse Einbringung eines neuen Kontrastoffes, des Uroselectans. Klin. Wochenschr. 8:2087, 1929.

Swick, M.: Intravenous urography by means of the sodium salt of 5-iodo-2-pyridon-n-acetic acid. JAMA 95:1403, 1930.

Swick, M.: Excretion urography by means of the intravenous and oral administration of sodium orthoiodohippurate: With some physiological considerations. Preliminary report. Surg. Gynecol. Obstet. 56:62, 1933.

Swick, M.: Excretion urography: With particular reference to a newly developed compound: Sodium ortho-iodohippurate. JAMA 101:1853, 1933.

Swick, M.: Intravenous urography in children. Radiology 26:539, 1936.

Swick, M.: The discovery of intravenous urography: Historical and developmental aspects of the urographic media and their role in other diagnostic and therapeutic areas. Bull. N.Y. Acad. Med. 42:128, 1966.

Swick, M.: Radiographic media in urology. Surg. Clin. North Am. 58:977, 1978.

Talner, L. B., and Davidson, A. J.: Renal hemodynamic effects of contrast media. Invest. Radiol. 3:310, 1968.

Talner, L. B., and Davidson, A. J.: Effect of contrast media on renal extraction of PAH. Invest. Radiol. 3:229, 1968.

Talner, L. B., Rushmer, H. N., and Coel, M. N.: The effect of renal artery injection of contrast material on urinary enzyme excretion. Invest. Radiol. 7:311, 1972.

Thompson, W. M., Foster, W. L., Jr., Halvorsen, R. A., Dunnick, N. R., Rommel, A. J., and Bates, M.: Iopamidol: New, nonionic contrast agent for excretory urography. AJR 142:329, 1984.

Törnquist, C., and Holtäs, S.: Renal angiography with iohexol and metrizoate. Radiology 150:331, 1984.

Volkmann, J.: Zur röntgenographischen Darstellung der Harnwege durch intravenöse Verabreiehung schattengebender Mittel. Dsch. Med. Wochenschr. 50:1413, 1924.

Wallingford, V. H., Decker, H. G., and Kruty, M.: X-ray contrast media: I. Iodinated acylaminobenzoic acids. J. Am. Chem. Soc. 74:4365, 1952.

Wallingford, V. H.: The development of organic iodine compounds as x-ray contrast media. J. Am. Pharm. Assoc. 42:721, 1953.

Webb, J. A. W.: The role of the distal nephron mechanisms in the distribution of contrast medium in the urine. Br. J. Radiol. 57:381, 1983.

Webb, J. A. W.: The effect of intravenous contrast medium on glomerular filtration rate. Br. J. Radiol. 57:387, 1983.

Wilcox, J., Evill, C. A., Sage, M. R., and Beness, G. T.: Urographic excretion studies with nonionic contrast agents: Iopamidol vs. iothalamate. Invest. Radiol. 18:297, 1983.

Winfield, A. C., Dray, R. J., Kirchner, F. K., Jr., Muhletater, C. A., and Price, R. R.: Iohexol for excretory urography: A comparative study. AJR 141:571, 1983.

Williams, T. C.: Detoxication Mechanisms. New York, John Wiley & Sons, 1947.

Wolf, G. L., Arenson, R. L., and Cross, A. P.: A prospective trial of ionic vs nonionic contrast agents in routine clinical practice. Comparison of adverse effects. AJR 152:939, 1989.

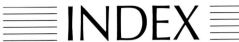

INDEX

Note: Page numbers in *italics* indicate illustrations; those followed by t refer to tables.

ISBN 0-7216-3552-0

90038